Klaus & Fanaroff's
Care of the High-Risk Neonate

6th Edition

Avroy A. Fanaroff, MD, FRCP, FRCPCH
Professor Emeritus
Department of Pediatrics and Neonatology in Reproductive Biology
Case Western Reserve University School of Medicine;
Eliza Henry Barnes Chair in Neonatology
Department of Pediatrics
Rainbow Babies and Children's Hospital
Cleveland, Ohio

Jonathan M. Fanaroff, MD, JD
Associate Professor
Department of Pediatrics
Case Western Reserve University School of Medicine;
Director, Rainbow Center for Pediatric Ethics
Co-Director, Neonatal Intensive Care Unit
Rainbow Babies and Children's Hospital/University
Hospitals Case Medical Center
Cleveland, Ohio

ELSEVIER
SAUNDERS

ELSEVIER
SAUNDERS

1600 JOHN F. KENNEDY BLVD.
STE 1800
PHILADELPHIA, PA 19103-2899

KLAUS & FANAROFF'S CARE OF THE HIGH-RISK NEONATE   ISBN: 978-1-4160-4001-9
Copyright © 2013, 2001, 1993, 1986, 1979, 1973 by Saunders, an imprint of Elsevier Inc.

Notices

Knowledge and best practice in this field are constantly changing. As new research and experience broaden our understanding, changes in research methods, professional practices, or medical treatment may become necessary.

Practitioners and researchers must always rely on their own experience and knowledge in evaluating and using any information, methods, compounds, or experiments described herein. In using such information or methods, they should be mindful of their own safety and the safety of others, including parties for whom they have a professional responsibility.

With respect to any drug or pharmaceutical products identified, readers are advised to check the most current information provided (i) on procedures featured or (ii) by the manufacturer of each product to be administered to verify the recommended dose or formula, the method and duration of administration, and contraindications. It is the responsibility of practitioners, relying on their own experience and knowledge of their patients, to make diagnoses, to determine dosages and the best treatment for each individual patient, and to take all appropriate safety precautions.

To the fullest extent of the law, neither the Publisher nor the authors, contributors, or editors assume any liability for any injury and/or damage to persons or property as a matter of products liability, negligence or otherwise, or from any use or operation of any methods, products, instructions, or ideas contained in the material herein.

Library of Congress Cataloging-in-Publication Data

Klaus & Fanaroff's care of the high-risk neonate / [edited by] Avroy A. Fanaroff,
Jonathan M. Fanaroff. — 6th ed.
     p. ; cm.
  Care of the high-risk neonate
  Rev. ed. of: Care of the high-risk neonate / [edited by] Marshall H. Klaus, Avroy A. Fanaroff.
5th ed. c2001.
  Includes index.
  ISBN 978-1-4160-4001-9 (hardcover : alk. paper)
  I. Fanaroff, Avroy A. II. Fanaroff, Jonathan M. III. Klaus, Marshall H., 1927- IV. Care of the
high-risk neonate. V. Title: Care of the high-risk neonate.
  [DNLM: 1. Infant, Newborn. 2. Infant Care. 3. Infant, Newborn, Diseases—therapy.
4. Intensive Care, Neonatal. WS 420]
  618.92'01—dc23   2012028210

Senior Content Strategist: Stefanie Jewell-Thomas
Content Development Specialist: Rachel Miller
Publishing Services Manager: Anne Altepeter
Senior Project Manager: Cheryl A. Abbott
Design Direction: Steven Stave
Cover image courtesy Bella Baby Photography

Printed in the United States

Last digit is the print number: 9 8 7 6 5 4 3 2 1

To all students of perinatology; our patients and their parents;
Roslyn and Kristy Fanaroff; Peter, Jodi, Austin, and Morgan Tucker;
and Amanda, Jason, Jackson, and Raya Lily Hirsh

Contributors

David H. Adamkin, MD
Professor of Pediatrics
Director of Neonatal Medicine
Director of Neonatal Research
Co-Director of Neonatal Fellowship
  Program
University of Louisville;
Attending Physician, Neonatal Intensive
  Care Unit
Kosair Children's Hospital;
Attending Physician, Neonatal Intensive
  Care Unit
University of Louisville Hospital
Louisville, Kentucky

Sanjay P. Ahuja, MD, MSc
Associate Professor
Department of Pediatrics
Case Western Reserve University School
  of Medicine
Director, Hemostasis and Thrombosis
  Center
Rainbow Babies and Children's Hospital
Cleveland, Ohio

Namasivayam Ambalavanan, MD
Professor
Department of Pediatrics
University of Alabama at Birmingham
Birmingham, Alabama

Jill E. Baley, MD
Professor
Department of Pediatrics
Case Western Reserve University School
  of Medicine;
Medical Director, Neonatal Transitional
  Care Unit
Department of Pediatrics
Rainbow Babies and Children's Hospital
Cleveland, Ohio

Sheila C. Berlin, MD
Assistant Professor of Radiology
Department of Radiology
Case Western Reserve University School
  of Medicine;
Pediatric Radiologist
Department of Diagnostic Radiology
Rainbow Babies and Children's Hospital
Cleveland, Ohio

Waldemar A. Carlo, MD
Edwin M. Dixon Professor of Pediatrics
Department of Pediatrics
Director, Division of Neonatology
University of Alabama at Birmingham
Birmingham, Alabama

Moira A. Crowley, MD
Assistant Professor
Department of Pediatrics
Case Western Reserve University School
  of Medicine;
Attending Physician
Division of Neonatology
Rainbow Babies and Children's Hospital
Cleveland, Ohio

Clifford L. Cua, MD
Associate Professor of Pediatrics, Heart
  Center
Department of Pediatrics
Nationwide Children's Hospital
The Ohio State University, College
  of Medicine
Columbus, Ohio

Arthur E. D'Harlingue, MD
Medical Director, Neonatal Intensive
  Care Unit
Division of Neonatology
Children's Hospital and Research Center,
  Oakland
Oakland, California

**Avroy A. Fanaroff, MD, FRCP,
FRCPCH**
Professor Emeritus
Department of Pediatrics and Neonatology
  in Reproductive Biology
Case Western Reserve University School
  of Medicine;
Eliza Henry Barnes Chair in Neonatology
Department of Pediatrics
Rainbow Babies and Children's Hospital
Cleveland, Ohio

Jonathan M. Fanaroff, MD, JD
Associate Professor
Department of Pediatrics
Case Western Reserve University School
  of Medicine;
Director, Rainbow Center for Pediatric Ethics
Co-Director, Neonatal Intensive Care Unit
Rainbow Babies and Children's Hospital/
  University Hospitals Case Medical Center
Cleveland, Ohio

Neil N. Finer, MD
Professor
Department of Pediatrics
University of California, San Diego School
  of Medicine;
Director, Division of Neonatology
Department of Pediatrics
University of California, San Diego
  Medical Center
San Diego, California

Kimberly S. Gecsi, MD
Assistant Professor
Department of Reproductive Biology
Case Western Reserve University School
  of Medicine;
Director, Obstetrics and Gynecology
  Clerkship
Department of Obstetrics and Gynecology
MacDonald Women's Hospital
University Hospitals Case Medical Center
Cleveland, Ohio

Maureen Hack, MBChB
Professor
Department of Pediatrics
Case Western Reserve University School
  of Medicine;
Co-Director, High-Risk Follow-Up Clinic
Department of Pediatrics
Rainbow Babies and Children's Hospital
Cleveland, Ohio

**Leta Houston Hickey, RN, MSN,
NNP-BC**
Neonatal Nurse Practitioner II
Division of Neonatology
Rainbow Babies and Children's Hospital/
  University Hospitals Case Medical Center
Cleveland, Ohio

Rosemary D. Higgins, MD
Program Scientist and Medical Officer
Pregnancy and Perinatology Branch
National Institute of Child Health
  and Human Development
National Institutes of Health
Bethesda, Maryland

David N. Kenagy, MD
Assistant Professor
Department of Pediatrics
Case Western Reserve University School
  of Medicine
Cleveland, Ohio

John H. Kennell, MD
Professor Emeritus
Department of Pediatrics
Case Western Reserve University School
  of Medicine
Cleveland, Ohio

Marshall H. Klaus, MD
Professor Emeritus
Department of Pediatrics
University of California, San Francisco
San Francisco, California

Robert M. Kliegman, MD
Professor and Chair
Department of Pediatrics
Medical College of Wisconsin;
Pediatrician-in-Chief
Pamela and Leslie Muma Chair in Pediatrics
Children's Hospital of Wisconsin
Milwaukee, Wisconsin

Justin R. Lappen, MD
Assistant Professor
Department of Reproductive Biology
  (Obstetrics and Gynecology)
Case Western Reserve University School
  of Medicine;
Assistant Director, Residency Program
Department of Obstetrics and Gynecology
Director, Fellowship in Advanced Obstetrics
Department of Family Medicine
University Hospitals Case Medical Center
Cleveland, Ohio

Linda Lefrak, RN, MS
Neonatal Clinical Nurse Specialist
Benioff Children's Hospital
University of California, San Francisco
San Francisco, California

Ethan G. Leonard, MD
Associate Professor
Department of Pediatrics
Case Western Reserve University School
  of Medicine;
Vice Chair for Quality
Department of Pediatric Infectious Disease
Rainbow Babies and Children's Hospital
Cleveland, Ohio

Tina A. Leone, MD
Associate Clinical Professor and Director,
 Neonatal-Perinatal Medicine Training
 Program
Department of Pediatrics, Division of
 Neonatology
University of California, San Diego School
 of Medicine;
Attending Physician
Department of Pediatrics, Division of
 Neonatology
University of California, San Diego
 Medical Center
San Diego, California

John Letterio, MD
Professor
Department of Pediatrics, Division of
 Pediatric Hematology/Oncology
Case Western Reserve University School
 of Medicine
Cleveland, Ohio

Jennifer Levy, MD
Attending Neonatologist
Division of Neonatology
Children's Hospital and Research Center,
 Oakland
Oakland, California

Salisa Lewis, MS, RD
Neonatal Nutritionist
Kosair Children's Hospital
Louisville, Kentucky

Tom Lissauer, MB BChir, FRCPCH
Honorary Consultant Pediatrician
Consultant Pediatric Program Director
 in Global Health
Imperial College London
London, United Kingdom

Carolyn Houska Lund, MS, RN, FAAN
Associate Clinical Professor
Department of Family Health Care
 Nursing
University of California, San Francisco
San Francisco, California;
Neonatal Clinical Nurse Specialist
Neonatal Intensive Care Unit
Children's Hospital and Research Center,
 Oakland
Oakland, California

M. Jeffrey Maisels, MB, BCh, DSc
Professor and Chair
Department of Pediatrics
Oakland University William Beaumont
 School of Medicine;
Physician in Chief
Beaumont Children's Hospital
Royal Oak, Michigan

Richard J. Martin, MD
Professor
Department of Pediatrics, Reproductive
 Biology, and Physiology & Biophysics
Case Western Reserve University School
 of Medicine;
Drusinsky/Fanaroff Professor
Department of Pediatrics
Rainbow Babies and Children's Hospital
Cleveland, Ohio

Jacquelyn McClary, PharmD, BCPS
Clinical Pharmacist Specialist
Neonatal Intensive Care Unit
Department of Pharmacy
Rainbow Babies and Children's Hospital
Cleveland, Ohio

Lawrence J. Nelson, PhD, JD
Associate Professor
Department of Philosophy
Santa Clara University
Santa Clara, California

Mary Elaine Patrinos, MD
Assistant Professor
Department of Pediatrics
Case Western Reserve University School
 of Medicine;
Attending Neonatologist
Department of Pediatrics
Rainbow Babies and Children's Hospital
Cleveland, Ohio

Agne Petrosiute, MD
Clinical Instructor
Department of Pediatrics
University Hospitals Case Medical Center
Rainbow Babies and Children's Hospital
Cleveland, Ohio

Christina M. Phelps, MD
Assistant Professor of Pediatrics, Heart
 Center
Department of Pediatrics
Nationwide Children's Hospital
Ohio State University, College of Medicine
Columbus, Ohio

Paula G. Radmacher, MSPH, PhD
Assistant Professor
Department of Pediatrics, Division
  of Neonatal Medicine
Neonatal Nutrition Research Laboratory
University of Louisville School of Medicine
Louisville, Kentucky

Roya L. Rezaee, MD, FACOG
Assistant Professor
Department of Reproductive Biology
Case Western Reserve University School
  of Medicine;
Medical Director, Women's Health Center
Co-Director, Division of Sexual and
  Vulvovaginal Health
Department of Obstetrics and Gynecology
MacDonald Women's Hospital
University Hospitals Case Medical Center
Cleveland, Ohio

Ricardo J. Rodriguez, MD
Associate Professor
Department of Pediatrics
Cleveland Clinic Lerner College
  of Medicine, Case Western Reserve
  University School of Medicine;
Chairman, Department of Neonatology
Pediatric Institute
Cleveland Clinic Children's Hospital
Cleveland, Ohio

Mark S. Scher, MD
Professor
Departments of Pediatrics and Neurology
Case Western Reserve University School
  of Medicine;
Division Chief, Pediatric Neurology
Director, Rainbow Neurological Center
Neurological Institute of University
  Hospitals;
Director, Pediatric Neurointensive Care
  Program/Fetal Neurology Program
Department of Pediatric Neurology
Rainbow Babies and Children's Hospital/
  University Hospitals Case Medical Center
Cleveland, Ohio

Phil Steer, Bsc, MD, FRCOG
Emeritus Professor of Obstetrics
  and Gynecology
Imperial College, London;
Consultant Obstetrician and Gynecologist
Chelsea and Westminster Hospital
London, United Kingdom

Philip T. Thrush, MD
Fellow, Heart Center
Department of Pediatrics
Nationwide Children's Hospital
The Ohio State University, College
  of Medicine
Columbus, Ohio

Michael R. Uhing, MD
Professor
Department of Pediatrics
Medical College of Wisconsin;
Medical Director
Neonatal Intensive Care Unit
Children's Hospital of Wisconsin
Milwaukee, Wisconsin

Beth A. Vogt, MD
Associate Professor
Department of Pediatrics
Case Western Reserve University School
  of Medicine;
Attending Pediatric Nephrologist
Department of Pediatric Nephrology
Rainbow Babies and Children's Hospital
Cleveland, Ohio

Michele C. Walsh, MD, MS Epi
Professor
Department of Pediatrics
Case Western Reserve University School
  of Medicine;
Chief, Division of Neonatology
William and Lois Briggs Chair
  in Neonatology
Rainbow Babies and Children's Hospital
Cleveland, Ohio

Jon F. Watchko, MD
Professor of Pediatrics, Obstetrics,
  Gynecology, and Reproductive Sciences
Division of Newborn Medicine
Department of Pediatrics
University of Pittsburgh School of Medicine;
Senior Scientist
Magee-Women's Research Institute
Pittsburgh, Pennsylvania

Deanne Wilson-Costello, MD
Professor
Department of Pediatrics
Case Western Reserve University School
  of Medicine;
Director, High Risk Follow-Up Program
Department of Pediatrics
Division of Neonatology
Rainbow Babies and Children's Hospital
Cleveland, Ohio

COMMENTERS

Michael Caplan, MD
Clinical Professor of Pediatrics
University of Chicago, Pritzker School
  of Medicine
Chicago, Illinois;
Chairman, Department of Pediatrics
NorthShore University HealthSystem
Evanston, Illinois

Waldemar A. Carlo, MD
Edwin M. Dixon Professor of Pediatrics
Department of Pediatrics
Director, Division of Neonatology
University of Alabama at Birmingham
Birmingham, Alabama

**Jonathan Hellmann, MBBCh,
FCP(SA), FRCP(C), MHSc**
Professor of Paediatrics
University of Toronto
The Hospital for Sick Children
Toronto, Ontario, Canada

John Kattwinkel, MD
Charles Fuller Professor of Neonatology
Department of Pediatrics
University of Virginia
Charlottesville, Virginia

Preface

It is with a great deal of humility, as well as satisfaction, that we present the sixth edition of *Klaus & Fanaroff's Care of the High-Risk Neonate*. There have been incredible advances in the field of neonatal-perinatal medicine in the 40 years since the book was first published. These include better understanding of the pathophysiology of neonatal disorders, as well as sophisticated technologic advances that permit monitoring, imaging, and support of even the tiniest, least mature infant. Over the same period, we have witnessed the development of therapeutic agents and strategies to enable maximal survival with the least morbidity for many complicated neonatal structural and metabolic disorders. Although these advances are gratifying, many challenges remain. Prematurity, birth defects, neonatal infections, birth asphyxia, and brain injury remain major causes of neonatal mortality and morbidity.

The dawning of the subspecialty in the late 1950s and the introduction of neonatal intensive care in the 1960s are often referred to as the era of anecdotal medicine, accompanied by many disasters. The first edition of *Klaus & Fanaroff's Care of the High-Risk Neonate*, published toward the end of this era in 1973, addressed the uncertainties in knowledge by offering multiple choices and approaches to management. Many of the gaps in knowledge have been filled, and there is now sufficient data to practice a more unified evidence-based neonatology. However, evidence-based medicine predicts what happens to the masses but not the individual. The next era, individualized medicine, will require the knowledge of the unique genetic makeup of the individual and the application of therapeutics based on predictable responses to pharmacologic agents.

The 10-year interval between the fifth and sixth editions of this book has been characterized by many changes in care practices and the accumulation of extensive data in randomized trials. To update this volume, each chapter has undergone comprehensive revision. To present fresh perspectives and ideas, once again one third of the chapters have been assigned to new authors. However, we have adhered to the basic format, utilizing text, case problems, and critical comments. To emphasize the importance of quality improvement and evidence-based medicine, we have inserted a new lead chapter on this topic, which includes the role and impact of the neonatal networks on modern neonatal intensive care.

Marshall H. Klaus, MD, has become an emeritus author of this book. However, his wisdom, philosophy, and yearning to provide quality, compassionate, and minimally invasive care with emphasis on human milk feeding, alleviation of pain, and psychosocial support for the family, strongly pervades the book. We thank him for his continuing support and inspiration. It has been a uniquely gratifying experience to have Jonathan M. Fanaroff, my son, assume the role of co-editor. We are all grateful that this book continues to serve as a companion and source of information for healthcare providers in many parts of the world. Bonnie Siner, RN, has once again served as in-house editor extraordinaire. Without her we could never have completed this edition, and we are most grateful to have had her skillful assistance. We thank, too, Rachel Miller and Judy Fletcher at Elsevier for their support and assistance. We thank the authors and commenters who gave of their time and knowledge. We also thank Bella Baby Photographers for use of the cover image.

Avroy A. Fanaroff, MD, FRCP, FRCPCH
Jonathan M. Fanaroff, MD, JD

Contents

Evidence-Based Medicine and the Role of Networks in Generating Evidence

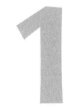

Michele C. Walsh and Rosemary D. Higgins

The explosion of clinical research has led to a conundrum in practice: Never before has so much evidence been generated to guide practice, but the sheer volume generated makes it difficult for practitioners to keep pace with the knowledge, and new knowledge rapidly eclipses existing practice. In 2009, it is estimated that more than 120 randomized clinical trials in neonatology were published.[1] This dilemma has made it imperative that every physician become skilled at evidence-based medicine (EBM), which, at its core as defined by Sackett in 1997 is "...a process of life-long, self-directed learning in which caring for our patients creates the need for clinically important information about diagnosis, prognosis, therapy, and other clinical and health issues...".[2] This chapter will review the components of EBM and the contribution of neonatal research networks to the generation of high-quality evidence.

THE EVOLUTION OF EVIDENCE-BASED MEDICINE

When first conceptualized in 1992 by Guyatt, the fundamental principle of EBM was real time application of the best available clinical evidence at the bedside. The chief barriers to such application in neonatology were the absence of high quality evidence and the tedious search for, and synthesis of, available evidence. The development of large research collaboratives has led to the generation of high-quality evidence. Advances in computer technology and information management have made evidence available on the desktop of every clinician. The Cochrane Collaboration in 1990 developed standard approaches to literature review and analyses that have placed the practice

of EBM within the reach of most practitioners.[3] Neonatologists are indeed fortunate that the Eunice Kennedy Shriver National Institute of Child Health and Human Development (NICHD) has funded online publication of the Neonatal Cochrane reviews for more than a decade. This has contributed to the rapid uptake of EBM among neonatal practitioners. The next innovation in EBM will incorporate rigorous assessments of quality improvement methods to aid us in determining which methods most rapidly lead to the incorporation of evidence-based treatments into practice. Many authors have documented that on average it takes more than 7 years for a new practice that has strong evidence of efficacy to achieve high penetration at the bedside.[4-6] Methods are needed to enhance the dissemination and uptake of these innovations. Physicians who are skilled in EBM are more likely to recognize and incorporate these advances.

A PRESCRIPTION FOR EVIDENCE-BASED MEDICINE FOCUSED PRACTICE

Sackett and colleagues synthesized the steps needed to ask and answer a relevant question using EBM (Box 1-1). To these steps we have added a first step using the phrase by Horbar, "developing the habit for using evidence and implementing change," which has been disseminated among neonatologists by the Vermont Oxford Collaborative.[7]

DEVELOPING THE HABIT FOR EVIDENCE USE

Medical students and residents who are educated in a culture that values, teaches, and models the use of EBM are more likely to apply the method themselves in later

1

Box 1-1.	**Steps in the Practice of Evidence-Based Medicine**

1. Develop the habit for the use of evidence.
2. Frame the question in a manner that can be answered.
3. Search for evidence with maximum efficiency from the most reliable sources.
4. Critically appraise the evidence for its validity (closeness to the truth) and usefulness (clinical application).
5. Apply the results of this appraisal in practice.
6. Evaluate the performance of the treatment.

Adapted from Strauss SE, Richardson WS, Glasziou P, et al: Evidence-based medicine: how to practice and teach EBM, ed 4, Churchill Livingstone, 2011.

---

practice.[8] Nevertheless, all physicians can learn and practice the steps needed. Research has shown that physicians who use EBM are more likely to be current in practice 15 years out of training than those who are not practicing EBM.[9] Today, the American Board of Medical Specialties has mandated continuous maintenance of certification, rather than permanent or intermittent recertification, as the best practice for documenting physician competency.[10] EBM will facilitate self-directed lifelong learning and support maintenance of certification.

FRAMING THE QUESTION

To be easily answered, the exact question must be carefully framed. Strauss and colleagues have summarized the four elements of a good question as "PICO": Patient population, Intervention, Comparison, Outcome.[2]

Patient Population

Describe precisely the patient population under consideration; for example, "infants born at <28 weeks' gestation," OR "inborn infants <28 weeks' gestation," OR "very low-birth-weight (VLBW) neonates who remain intubated and mechanically ventilated at 14 days of age." The more precisely the population is defined, the more targeted the search for evidence will be.

Intervention

Describe the main intervention in which you are interested. For example: "Is clindamycin superior to ampicillin in the treatment of necrotizing enterocolitis?" Other questions that may be explored may relate to prognostic factors or to risk factors.

Comparison

What is the main alternative to compare with the intervention (e.g., when compared with supportive therapy alone).

Outcome

State the outcome of interest in as specific terms as possible including a time horizon. For example: "Will adding clindamycin to ampicillin in a VLBW infant with stage 2 necrotizing enterocolitis reduce mortality prior to hospital discharge?"

A busy clinician will generate more questions than they have time to address. To avoid frustration, the questions may be prioritized by how critical the patient is, or which question is of most interest to the clinician. Other questions can be added to a list, which can be used when off-service time can be directed to self-education. Through this process the clinician will be actively practicing lifelong learning.

SEARCHING FOR EVIDENCE

Searching for evidence to answer clinically relevant questions is the most time consuming aspect of practicing evidence-based medicine. Strauss and others have suggested that this is the major barrier to effective implementation.[11,12] Nordenstrom has recommended that clinicians search for evidence using online sources that contain critically reviewed data directed at clinical questions.[13] By prioritizing sources, the clinicians' time is used most efficiently. Nordenstrom recommends that the first source should be the Cochrane Collaboration, followed by meta search engines including Google Scholar. The next step is to search secondary sources focused on clinical questions such as the United Kingdom's National Institute for Health and Clinical Excellence (www.nice.org.uk), the United States Agency for Healthcare Research and Quality Effective Health Care Program (http://effectivehealthcare.ahrq.gov) or Up To Date (www.uptodate.com), a commercial online source generated by content experts. Perhaps surprisingly, Nordenstrom recommends that PubMed be searched last, because 75% of the PubMed content deals with basic science research topics versus clinically relevant questions. Thus, for a

Table 1-1.	The GRADE System	
Study Design	**Quality of Evidence**	**Lower/Higher Level of Quality if:**
Randomized trial	• High (further research is very unlikely to change our confidence in the estimate of effect) • Moderate (further research is likely to have an important impact on our confidence in the estimate of effect and may change the estimate)	• Risk of bias (serious [−1]; very serious [−2]) • Inconsistency (serious [−1]; very serious [−2]) • Indirectness (serious [−1]; very serious [−2]) • Imprecision (serious [−1]; very serious [−2]) • Publication bias (likely [−1]; very likely [−2]) • Large effect (large [+1]; very large [+2]) • Evidence of a dose-response gradient (+1)
Observational trial	• Low (further research is very likely to have an important impact on our confidence in the estimate of effect and is likely to change the estimate) • Very low (any estimate of effect is very uncertain)	• All plausible confounding: would reduce a demonstrated effect (+1); would suggest a spurious effect when results show no effect (+1)

Adapted from Scott IA, Guyatt GH: Clinical practice guidelines: the need for greater transparency in formulating recommendations, *Med J Aust* 195(1):29, 2011.

busy clinician other sources are likely to yield a better answer faster.

CRITICALLY APPRAISE THE EVIDENCE FOR VALIDITY, APPLICABILITY AND IMPORTANCE

In this discussion, we will focus on the appraisal of evidence regarding treatments. The highest hierarchy of evidence for these are results from a randomized controlled trial. The following critical questions to ask when assessing the validity of a trial are:

1. Were patients randomly assigned to the treatment?
2. Were all patients who were randomized accounted for in the analysis? Were they analyzed in the group to which they were assigned (intent-to-treat analysis)?
3. Were patients, the clinicians caring for them, and those assessing the outcome kept masked to the treatment assignment?
4. Were the groups similar at the beginning of the trial?

Randomized trials provide the most non-biased assessment of the effect of a treatment. If the trial is not randomized, it may be best to stop reading and search for other sources. If the only evidence available is from a nonrandomized study, one must view the stated effects with some skepticism because the odds ratios from randomized trials are generally smaller than those from nonrandomized studies.

There are a number of different systems proposed for grading the quality of evidence. The proliferation of systems has made it difficult to adopt and understand any one method. Recently, a group of clinical epidemiologists have proposed a system that combines many of the elements of other systems and termed this the GRADE (Grading of Recommendations Assessment, Development, and Evaluation) system.[14] The *British Journal of Medicine* has required a GRADE assessment of recommendations since 2006, and now more than 25 groups who generate systematic reviews, including the World Health Organization, the American College of Physicians, the American Thoracic Society, UpToDate (www.uptodate.com), and the Cochrane Collaboration have adopted the GRADE standard (Table 1-1). The Grade system synthesizes the evidence into a recommendation based first on the quality of the evidence and second on the magnitude of effects, thereby yielding a recommendation which is either "strong" or "weak." The GRADE system classifies quality of evidence into four levels: high, moderate, low, or very low. Evidence from randomized controlled trials (RCTs) begins as high quality, but may be rated down if trials demonstrate one of five categories of limitations. Observational studies begin as low-quality evidence, but may be rated up if associated with one of three categories of special strengths.

The GRADE system suggests that when the desirable effects of a treatment clearly outweigh the undesirable effects, or the contrary, that guideline offers strong recommendations. When the data are less clear, such as when the quality of existing evidence is low or when undesirable effects outweigh desireable effects, the recommendations should be rated as weak, or equivocal. Such a standardized approach to rating the evidence would clearly benefit clinicians.

Applying the Evidence in Daily Practice

The Institute of Medicine (IOM) focuses on the promise of evidence-based medicine to improve the quality and effectiveness of health care, and has also highlighted barriers in the current system. The IOM cites "an irony of the information-rich environment is that information important to clinical decision making is often not available, or is provided in forms that are not relevant to the broad spectrum of patients—with differing levels of health, socioeconomic circumstances, and preferences—and the issues encountered in clinical practice."[15] In the IOM view, these limitations are driven by a paucity of clinical effectiveness research, poor dissemination of the evidence that is available, and too few incentives and decision supports for evidence-based care. Glenton and colleagues described several factors hindering the effective use of systematic reviews for clinical decision making.[15] They found that reviews often lacked details about interventions and did not provide adequate information on the risks of adverse events, the availability of interventions, and the context in which the interventions may or may not work.

Evaluate the Performance of the Treatment

The final step in EBM is to assess the outcome of the treatment. Did the patient (or their parents) judge their condition to be improved? Was the treatment cost-effective? Did the treatment fit within the context of the unique circumstances and biology of the family? If a similar scenario was encountered again, what would the clinician do differently? This habit for critical self-appraisal and unremitting learning is at the heart of EBM. Only by widespread implementation of the principals of EBM is healthcare quality and value likely to improve.[16,17]

CRITICAL PROGRESS IN GENERATING THE EVIDENCE: THE ROLE OF NEONATAL RESEARCH NETWORKS

Neonatal-perinatal medicine was recognized as a subspecialty by the American Board of Pediatrics in 1975.[18] In the past 2 to 3 decades, it has become increasingly apparent that neonatal research requires observational studies and interventional trials to provide the basis for evidence-based care for newborns. Several groups, including the NICHD the Neonatal Research Network, the Canadian Neonatal Network, the Vermont Oxford Network, as well as international networks, have been established and maintained to investigate evidence-based strategies, including observational studies, interventional clinical trials, and quality improvement initiatives. These networks have made significant contributions to patient care and quality improvement. This chapter will discuss advantages, opportunities, and challenges for research networks as well as selected highlights from the various networks.

Clinical networks can offer large numbers of patients for study. For uncommon or rare conditions, networks can provide the numbers of patients needed to study diseases in an observational or interventional study. Generally, networks are set up to look at specific disease categories. The neonatal networks and collaborations concentrate on diseases of the newborn, particularly those affecting preterm infants and critically ill, late preterm and term infants. Many of the neonatal networks have access to high-risk obstetrics or maternal-fetal medicine consultants at their institutions. In addition, most have level III newborn intensive care units (NICUs) for care of patients and recruitment of patients for clinical studies. Well-developed and established networks have provisions for follow-up of the infants and children after hospital discharge.

The NICHD Neonatal Research Network (NRN) was established in 1986 to form a set of academic centers to conduct common protocols for observational and interventional studies of newborns.[19,20] The goal of the NRN is to provide the research evidence to facilitate advancement of neonatal care by providing infrastructure for a network of academic centers to study required numbers of patients to provide data more rapidly than individual center studies. The perceived advantages of a network of centers included large patient numbers to provide evidence more rapidly than individual study sites, availability of patients with rare or rarer diseases (such as hypoxic-ischemic encephalopathy), and available infrastructure for clinical studies (Table 1-2). Further, specialized needs including high-risk pregnancy study subjects, preterm infants, capability of short-term outcome ascertainment, and longer term follow-up can be mandated in a request for application (RFA).

Table 1-2. Impact of Interventional Randomized Trials of the Eunice Kennedy Shriver NICHD Neonatal Research Network*

Study	Patient Enrollment	Outcome	Impact
A Controlled Trial of Intravenous Immune Globulin to Reduce Nosocomial Infections in Very Low Birth Weight Infants *N Engl J Med* 330:1107, 1994	2416 infants 501-1500 grams randomized by 72 hours of life to IVIG or placebo (phase I)/no infusion (phase II).	IVIG failed to significantly reduce nosocomial infections (17% IVIG vs 19% control). Increased NEC in infused groups.	Routine use of IVIG not recommended for prevention of infection in VLBW infants.
The Effect of Antenatal Phenobarbital Therapy on Neonatal Intracranial Hemorrhage in Preterm Infants *N Engl J Med* 337:466, 1997	610 women with gestation ≥24 and <33 weeks anticipated to deliver within 24 hours randomized to receive phenobarbital or placebo daily until delivery or 34 weeks.	Antenatal administration of phenobarbital did not reduce the incidence of intracranial hemorrhage or early death (24% vs 23%) in infants born <34 weeks.	Prophylactic use of antenatal phenobarbital to prevent intracranial hemorrhage in preterm infants not recommended.
Vitamin A Supplementation for Extremely Low Birth Weight Infants *N Engl J Med* 340:1962, 1999	807 infants ≤1000 grams randomized to receive IM injection of vitamin A or control (sham injection) 3 times per week for 4 weeks.	Vitamin A supplementation significantly reduced risk of CLD or death (55% vs 62%).	Routine use of vitamin A supplementation recommended for infants ≤1000 grams in the first month of life.
Effects of Early Erythropoietin Therapy on the Transfusion Requirements of Preterm Infants Below 1250 Grams Birth Weight: A Multicenter, Randomized Controlled Trial *Pediatrics* 108(4):934, 2001	290 infants 401-1250 grams birth weight randomized to erythropoietin or placebo until 35 weeks' post menstrual age.	Combination of erythropoietin and iron-stimulated erythropoiesis but did not affect transfusion requirements (4.3 vs 5.2 transfusions) in treated vs. control preterm infants ≤1250 grams.	Early use of erythropoietin and iron to reduce transfusion number and exposure of infants to the risks of multiple transfusions not warranted.
Parenteral Glutamine Supplementation Does Not Reduce the Risk of Mortality or Late-Onset Sepsis in Extremely Low Weight Infants *Pediatrics* 113(5):1209, 2004	1433 infants 401-1000 grams randomized to parenteral nutrition with glutamine supplementation or control (standard parenteral nutrition).	Parenteral glutamine supplementation did not decrease rate of mortality or late-onset sepsis (51% vs. 48%) in infants ≤1000 grams.	Routine use of parenteral glutamine supplementation to reduce the risk of death or late-onset sepsis in ELBW infants not recommended. Importance of early protein administration recognized, changing practice.
Randomized Clinical Trial of Dexamethasone Therapy in Very Low Birth Weight (VLBW) Infants at Risk for Chronic Lung Disease (CLD) *N Engl J Med* 338:1112, 1998	371 infants 501-1500 grams treated DOL 14-42 with dexamethasone/placebo or placebo/dexamethasone.	No clear pulmonary benefit starting dexamethasone at 2 weeks vs. 4 weeks of age (39% vs. 42%). Dexamethasone increased GI perforation, hypertension, and hyperglycemia.	Awareness of harmful effects of dexamethasone therapy for ventilator-dependent premature infants. Decreased use of postnatal steroids.
Inhaled Nitric Oxide for Premature Infants with Severe Respiratory Failure *N Engl J Med* 353:13, 2005	420 infants <34 weeks' gestation with BW 401-1500 grams with severe respiratory failure randomized to receive inhaled nitric oxide or placebo.	No difference in incidence of BPD or death in the inhaled nitric oxide and placebo groups (80% vs. 82%).	No benefit to the early use of inhaled nitric oxide in premature infants with severe respiratory failure.
Whole-Body Hypothermia for Neonates with Hypoxic-Ischemic Encephalopathy *N Engl J Med* 353:1571, 2005	208 term infants with moderate or severe HIE randomized by 6 hours of age to whole-body cooling for 72 hours or usual care (normothermia).	Whole-body cooling safe and effective in reducing the risk of death or moderate or severe disability (44% vs. 62%) among infants with HIE.	Whole-body cooling instituted as standard of care for term infants with moderate or severe hypoxic-ischemic encephalopathy.

Continued

Table 1-2. Impact of Interventional Randomized Trials of the Eunice Kennedy Shriver NICHD Neonatal Research Network*—cont'd			
Study	**Patient Enrollment**	**Outcome**	**Impact**
Aggressive vs Conservative Phototherapy for Infants with Extremely Low Birth Weight *N Engl J Med* 359:1885, 2008	1974 infants with BW 501-1000 grams randomized to aggressive or conservative phototherapy by 12-36 hours of age.	No significant effect of aggressive vs conservative phototherapy on death or NDI. Aggressive phototherapy significantly reduced overall rate of NDI, but showed trend toward increased mortality in infants 501-750 grams.	Treatment still not standardized.
Target Ranges of Oxygen Saturation in Extremely Preterm Infants *N Engl J Med* 362:1959, 2010	1316 infants 24^0 to 27^6 weeks' gestation randomized at birth to targeted oxygen saturation ranges of low (85%-89%) vs. high (91%-95%) until 36 weeks' postmenstrual age or no longer receiving oxygen or respiratory support.	No significant difference in the combined primary outcome of severe ROP or death between the low and high saturation groups (28% vs. 32%) but with increased risk of in-hospital death and reduced risk of severe ROP (9% vs. 18%) in the low saturation ranges.	Caution for the use of low saturation ranges due to the increased risk of mortality among preterm infants. Current practice to keep saturation ranges of 90%-94%.
Early CPAP versus Surfactant in Extremely Preterm Infants *N Engl J Med* 362:1970, 2010	1316 infants 24^0 to 27^6 weeks randomized at birth to begin treatment with CPAP and limited ventilation or intubation and early surfactant followed by conventional ventilation.	No significant difference in combined outcome of death or bronchopulmonary dysplasia when defining BPD by the physiological definition (48% vs. 51%) or the need for supplemental oxygen at 36 weeks (49% vs. 54%).	Consideration for the use of CPAP as an alternative to intubation and surfactant administration in preterm infants.

Table prepared by N. Newman BA, RN, from data at neonatal.rti.org/studies.cfm.
BPD, Bronchopulmonary dysplasia; *BW*, birth weight; *CLD*, chronic lung disease; *CPAP*, continuous positive airway pressure; *DOL*, day of life; *ELBW*, extremely low birth weight; *GI*, gastrointestinal; *HIE*, hypoxic-ischemic encephalopathy; *IM*, intramuscular; *IVIG*, intravenous immunoglobulin; *IVH*, intraventricular hemorrhage; *NDI*, neurodevelopmental impairment; *NEC*, necrotizing enterocolitis; *PVL*, periventricular leukomalacia; *ROP*, retinopathy of prematurity; *VLBW*, very low birth weight.

The network is subject to open competition on 5-year cycles and undergoes peer review and a second level of review by the NICHD advisory council. The collective knowledge of the principal investigators, follow-up investigators, and coinvestigators at the individual study sites, are a clear advantage in determining appropriate studies, feasibility, and experimental design. Policies and procedures that are explicitly formulated are allowed to change over time, depending on NICHD programmatic needs and input from the Steering Committee.

The NICHD also has issued RFAs on 5-year cycles for a data coordinating center (DCC). The DCC provides critical assistance with study development and implementation. Statistical expertise, as well as staff for data collection, programming, study logistics and training, data analysis, and manuscript writing is required. The DCC also assumes responsibility for study monitoring, including activities required for data safety and monitoring committee functions. The DCC tracks patient enrollment and assists the clinical sites with day-to-day activities necessary for the conduct of studies.

The NICHD NRN has been successful with respect to recruiting and retaining patients. Figure 1-1 shows a graphic representation of NRN studies over time. Further, follow-up rates at 18 to 22 months' corrected age generally exceed 90% for clinical studies. The clinical sites have various measures in place to achieve optimum compliance, including early identification of infants for follow-up, maintaining contact with families, scheduling and procedures for rescheduling missed visits, and home visits for follow-up in specific cases.

The NICHD NRN has challenges in conducting multicenter research. Center differences are a large challenge: populations may be different, practice styles vary, and equipment varies. Many units have written policies or guidelines for specific management such as nutrition, respiratory care, monitors, and so forth. Developing a clinical study oftentimes requires compromise as opposed to consensus. Simple definitions can be a challenge if there is variation across sites. Determination of primary and secondary outcomes can be an area of lively debate. Further, determination of equipoise at any site may be a challenge, particularly if there are passionate views on management strategies or entrenched systems of belief in patient care. Agreement from the staff in the intensive care nursery, including physicians, nurses, therapists, and consultants to participate in the studies can be challenging. Education and in-service training are performed on a routine basis. Time to study start can be highly variable depending on staff, institutional review board lead time for submission, review and approval, and appropriate training at individual sites and centers. Studies or trials that require recruitment in a short time window or at the time of delivery can pose significant challenges with research staff coverage on nights, weekends, and holidays. Many successful clinical research sites participate in multiple projects at any one time, so the issue of conflicting trials must be addressed for each study.

The Canadian NICU Network was established in 1995 and funded by the Medical Research Council of Canada. The primary objectives of the network were to establish a standardized database of practices and outcomes, to examine variations in outcomes, and for improving efficiency and efficacy of treatment in the NICU.[21] Currently, there are members from 30 hospitals and 17 universities in Canada. The network maintains a standardized neonatal intensive care unit (NICU) database and conducts collaborative projects with the goal to improve neonatal health. The Canadian NICU Network has provided multiple publications in the areas of practice variation and neonatal outcomes, including mortality as well as morbidity.

The Vermont Oxford Network (VON) consists of more than 800 institutions and has worldwide representation.[22] The VON is invested in quality and safety of medical care for the newborn.[23] The Network provides an infrastructure for research, education, and quality improvement. The VON database is the largest data collection of infants weighing less than 1500 grams accruing over 56,000 births annually. It includes information on baseline characteristics, interventions in the NICU serial, and acute hospital outcome information. The network provides a confidential Nightingale Internet Reporting System for centers to compare their data with data from other VON hospitals. The VON also established a neonatal encephalopathy registry (NER) in 2006 with the advent of cooling therapy for hypoxic-ischemic encephalopathy (HIE) with the primary objective of characterizing infants with neonatal encephalopathy.[24]

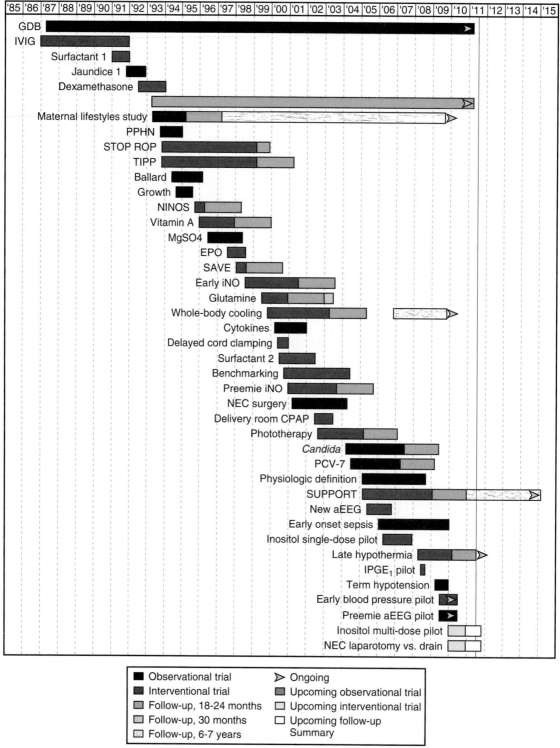

Figure 1-1. Neonatal Research Network Trial Timeline, 1987 to present. *aEEG*, Amplitude integrated electroencephalogram; *CPAP*, continuous positive airway pressure; *EPO*, erythropoietin; *GDB*, generic database; *iNO*, inhaled nitric oxide; *IPGE₁*, inhaled prostaglandin E_1; *IVIG*, intravenous immune globulin; *NEC*, necrotizing enterocolitis; *NINOS*, neonatal inhaled nitric oxide study; *PPHN*, persistent pulmonary hypertension; *ROP*, retinopathy of prematurity; *SAVE*, steroids and ventilation; *STOP ROP*, supplemental therapeutic oxygen for prethreshold ROP; *TIPP*, Trial of indomethacin prophylaxis.

Monitoring the introduction and dissemination of hypothermic therapy was a secondary objective for the NER. The VON provides various tools and resources with emphasis on high quality and safe care for newborns and their families.

The Australian and New Zealand Neonatal Network (ANZNN) was established in 1994 following a recommendation from the National Health and Medical Research Council's (NHMRC) Expert Panel on Perinatal Medicine. The goal is to improve the care of high-risk newborn infants and their families through collaborative audits and research.[25] The network's achievements are in areas including follow-up outcome, mortality, retinopathy of prematurity, and chronic lung disease.

Various other networks and individual study groups have been organized in neonatology. The international perspective, as well as an international perspective devoted to sepsis in very low-birth-weight infants, has recently been reviewed.[26,27] Region-specific networks including China and the Middle East have been developed to investigate neonatal-perinatal medicine and genetics.[28,29]

Regional initiatives are rapidly growing in the United States. The California Perinatal Quality Care Collaborative (CPQCC) was established as a regional collaboration to improve perinatal care.[30] This entity is largely focused on quality improvement, and has research and collaboration as vital components. There are now additional statewide neonatal improvement collaborative centers active in Ohio, New York, North Carolina, and Tennessee.

Various neonatal networks have been established over the past 25 years with common goals, including improvement of patient care and outcome, as well as quality improvement. Well-designed observational studies and interventional trials have provided evidence for practice recommendations from the various networks. Care and management of high-risk newborns continues to be advanced by existence of these networks to provide the evidence to guide optimum medical treatment.

REFERENCES

The reference list for this chapter can be found online at www.expertconsult.com.

Antenatal and Intrapartum Care of the High-Risk Infant

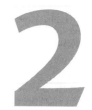

Roya L. Rezaee, Justin R. Lappen, and Kimberly S. Gecsi

Everything ought to be done to ensure that an infant be born at term, well developed, and in a healthy condition. But in spite of every care, infants are born prematurely.

Pierre Budin, The Nursling

IDENTIFICATION OF THE PREGNANCY AT RISK

The goal of prenatal care is to ensure optimal outcomes for both baby and mother. Prenatal care involves a series of assessments over time as well as education and counseling that help guide the interventions that may be offered. A significant part of the process involves identifying a pregnancy as high risk. Early and accurate establishment of gestational age, identification of the patient at risk for complications, anticipation of complications, and the timely implementation of screening, diagnosis, and treatment help to achieve these goals. The distinction between a high-risk versus a low-risk pregnancy and/or mother gives the provider the opportunity to potentially intervene prior to the advent of adverse outcomes. This chapter will discuss the identification of the high-risk pregnancy focusing on some of the more commonly encountered fetal and maternal conditions.

Many of the principal determinants of perinatal morbidity and mortality have been delineated. Included among these are maternal age, race, socioeconomic status, nutritional status, past obstetric history, family history, associated medical illness, and current pregnancy problems. Ideally, the process of risk identification is established prior to conception because it is the time when counseling for and against certain behaviors, foods and nutritional supplements, medications, work and environmental risks is likely to have the most beneficial outcome.[1]

Preparations can be made for certain medical and obstetrical conditions long before untoward effects have occurred. Therefore, any such assessment should include a detailed history that involves elements of personal and demographic information, personal and family medical, psychiatric and genetic histories, past obstetrical, gynecological, menstrual and surgical histories, current pregnancy history, domestic violence history, and drug and tobacco use history. The care provider should also assess for any barriers to care and whether the patient has any social concerns that would be better evaluated and managed by someone with social services expertise.[2]

Accurate estimation of date of delivery (EDD) is crucial to the timing of interventions, monitoring fetal growth and timing of delivery, as well as for overall management. This is usually calculated from the date of a known last menstrual period (LMP) and can be confirmed by ultrasound if dating is uncertain due to irregular menses or if conception occurred on hormonal contraception. A standard panel of tests is ordered for all pregnant women at their first prenatal visit. This work-up is modified based on the woman's risk profile. What constitutes optimal prenatal care and performed by whom and how often may still be up for debate.[3] Screening and treatment of asymptomatic bacteriuria, group B beta-hemolytic *Streptococcus* (GBS), and sexually transmitted diseases for at-risk women to prevent the consequences of horizontal and vertical transmission is indicated. Screening should also be offered for fetal structural and chromosomal abnormalities and women who are Rh (D)-negative should receive anti (D)-immune globulin to prevent alloimmunization and reduce the risk of hemolytic disease of the newborn. Screening for malpresentation of the fetus, as well as development of preeclampsia in the mother, is also likely to have a great impact on pregnancy outcomes.

In the United States, about 12% to 13% of all live births are premature and about 2% are born at less than 32 weeks.[4] Approximately 50% of these births are the result of spontaneous preterm labor, 30% from preterm rupture of membranes, and 20% from induced delivery secondary to maternal or fetal indications. Prematurity remains a significant perinatal problem, because prematurity along with the associated low birth weight is the most significant contributor to infant mortality. Mortality increases with both decreasing gestational age and birth weight. Additional causes of mortality include congenital anomalies, as well as delivering in a hospital with a lower level of resources and experience in providing such complex neonatal care. Improvements in obstetric and neonatal care, including surfactant, antenatal steroids, and maternal transport to an appropriate delivery facility capable of caring for high-risk neonates have decreased the mortality rates except in those at the limit of viability.

The goal remains to identify at-risk women as soon as possible. Careful analysis indicates that determinants of morbidity and mortality are composed of historical factors existing before pregnancy as well as factors and events associated directly with pregnancy. Historically, an attempt was made to put these together into some type of assessment technique capable of distinguishing most of the high-risk patients from the low-risk patients before delivery (Table 2-1). Unfortunately, when these scoring systems have been applied to a large population base, they have not resulted in significant changes in the prematurity rates. Still, the grouping of risk factors may be of some use to the obstetrical provider because it allows for the identification of the woman who might need additional surveillance, counseling, referral, and resources.

BIRTH DEFECTS AND CONGENITAL DISORDERS

Birth defects affect approximately 2% to 4% of liveborn infants. Contributing factors include genetic and environmental influences such as maternal age, illness, industrial agents, intrauterine environment, infection, and drug exposure. The frequency of the various etiologies of birth defects can be broken down as follows: unknown and multifactorial origin, about 65% to 75%; genetic origin, about 25%; and environmental exposures, about 10% (Table 2-2).

The terminology used to describe these anomalies is based on their underlying cause: malformation, deformation, disruption, and dysplasia. Dysmorphology is the study of individuals with abnormal features, and increased scholarship in this area has led to specialists who study birth defects

Table 2-1.	Scoring System* for Risk of Preterm Delivery		
	Socioeconomic Status	**Past History**	**Daily Habits**
1	Two children at home Low socioeconomic status	One abortion <1 year since last birth	Works outside home
2	<20 years >40 years Single parent	Two abortions	>10 cigarettes/day
3	Very low socioeconomic status Height <150 cm Weight <45 kg	Three abortions	Heavy work Long, tiring trip
4	<18 years	Pyelonephritis	
5		Uterine anomaly Second-trimester abortion Diethylstilbestrol exposure	
10		Premature delivery Repeated second-trimester abortion	

Adapted from Creasy R, Gummer B, Liggins G: System for predicting spontaneous preterm birth, *Obstet Gynecol* 55:692, 1980.
*Score is computed by addition of number of points given any item. 0-5 = Low risk; 6-9 = medium risk; ≥10 = high risk.

and establish patterns. The result has been a better understanding of many conditions, which has improved the quality of counseling for families including possible recurrence rates in future pregnancies.

Malformations are considered major if they have medical or social implications and many times they require surgical repair. Defects are considered to be minor if they have only cosmetic relevance. They can arise from genetic or environmental factors.

Deformations are defects in the position of body parts arising from some intrauterine mechanical force that interferes with the normal formation of the organ or structure. Such uterine forces could include oligohydramnios, uterine malformations or tumors, and fetal crowding from multiple gestations. Disruptions refer to defects that result from the destruction of or interference with normal development. These are typically single events that may involve infection, vascular compromise, or mechanical factors. Amniotic band syndrome is the most common example of a disruption and the timing occurs from 28 days' postconception to 18 weeks' gestation. Dysplasias are defects that result from the abnormal organization of cells into tissues. There are recognizable patterns in many congenital defects. The terminology to describe these patterns includes syndrome, sequence, association, and developmental field defect.

The study of congenital malformations caused by environmental or drug exposure is called teratology. An agent that causes an abnormality in the function or structure of a fetus is called a teratogen (Table 2-3). About 4% to 6% of birth defects are caused by teratogens and include maternal illnesses, infectious agents, physical agents and drugs, and chemical agents. Timing of exposure to the agent plays a great role in the resulting malformation. Exposure during the first 10 to 14 days postconception can result in cell death and spontaneous miscarriage. The all-or-none theory refers to the possibility that if only a few cells are damaged, then the other cells may compensate for their loss

Table 2-2.	Leading Categories of Birth Defects
Birth Defect	**Estimated Incidence (births)**
STRUCTURAL/METABOLIC	
Heart and circulation	1 in 115
Muscles and skeleton	1 in 130
Genital and urinary tract	1 in 135
Nervous system and eye	1 in 235
Chromosomal syndromes	1 in 600
Club foot	1 in 735
Down syndrome (trisomy 21)	1 in 900
Respiratory tract	1 in 900
Cleft lip/palate	1 in 930
Spina bifida	1 in 2000
Metabolic disorders	1 in 3500
Anencephaly	1 in 8000
Phenylketonuria (PKU)	1 in 12,000
CONGENITAL INFECTIONS	
Congenital syphilis	1 in 2000
Congenital HIV infection	1 in 2700
Congenital rubella syndrome	1 in 100,000
OTHER	
Rh disease	1 in 1400
Fetal alcohol syndrome	1 in 1000

Table 2-3.	Common Teratogens	
Type of Teratogen	**Agent**	**Defect**
Chemical	Retinoic Acid	Hydrocephalus, CNS migrations
	Thalidomide	Limb reduction
	Valproic acid	Neural tube defects
	Phenytoin	Heart defects, nail hypoplasia, dysmorphic features
	Lithium	Ebstein anomaly
	ACE inhibitors	Renal and skull defects
	Misoprostol	Fetal death, vascular disruptions
	DES (diethylstilbestrol)	Cervical cancer in daughters, genital anomalies in males and females
Physical	Ionizing radiation	Fetal death, growth restriction, leukemia
	Hyperthermia	Microcephaly, mental retardation, seizures
Biological	Cytomegalovirus	Microcephaly, mental retardation, deafness
	Toxoplasmosis	Hydrocephalus, mental retardation, chorioretinitis
Maternal	Diabetes	Congenital heart anomalies, neural tube defects, sacral anomalies
	Phenylketonuria (PKU)	Microcephaly, mental retardation

Adapted from Reece EA, Hobbins JC: Developmental toxicology, drugs and fetal teratogenesis. In Reece EA, Hobbins JC, editors: *Clinical obstetrics: the fetus and mother,* ed 3, Malden, Mass., 2008, Blackwell, p 215.

and result in no abnormality. Most effects are seen after fertilization, but exposure prior to conception can cause genetic mutations. Mechanisms of teratogenesis are varied and include cell death, altered cell growth, proliferation, migration, and interaction. The embryo is most vulnerable during the period of organogenesis and this occurs up to the eighth week postconception, but certain organ systems including the eye, central nervous system (CNS), genitalia, and hematopoietic systems continue to develop through the fetal stage and remain susceptible.

Maternal illness that can present a teratogenic risk involves conditions in which a metabolite or antibody travels across the placenta and affects the fetus. Maternal illness can include pregestational diabetes, phenylketonuria, androgen-producing tumors, maternal obesity, and systemic lupus erythematosus. The mother may be infected but asymptomatic. Ultrasonic findings suggestive of fetal infection include microcephaly, cerebral and/or hepatic calcifications, intrauterine growth restriction, hepatosplenomegaly, cardiac malformations, limb hypoplasia, hydrocephalus, and hydrops. Maternal fever or hyperthermia has also been associated with teratogenesis when it occurs in the first trimester and may be associated with miscarriage and/or neural tube defects (Table 2-4).[5]

Maternal ingestion of certain drugs can cause birth defects or adverse fetal outcomes. It is important that nonpregnant women are counseled about the need for contraception when using a medication that is classified as category X by the U.S. Food and Drug Administration. Maternal exposure to numerous physical and environmental agents has also been implicated as a cause of birth defects. High plasma levels of lead, mercury, and other heavy metals have been associated with central nervous system damage and negative neurobehavioral effects in infants and children.[6] More controversial are the recent concerns over maternal exposure to so-called endocrine disruptors, bisphenol A (BPA), and phthalates, and airborne polycyclic aromatic hydrocarbons. These entities are chemicals that mimic the action of naturally occurring hormones such as estrogen. These chemicals can be found in pesticides, leaching from plastics found in water and infant bottles, medical devices, personal care products, tobacco smoke, and other materials. Exposure to them is widespread, and a large portion of the population has measurable levels.[7] The chemicals have been associated with adverse changes in behavior, the brain, male and female reproductive systems, and mammary glands.

Our knowledge of the effects of ionizing radiation on the fetus has been based on case reports and extrapolation of data from survivors of atomic bombs and nuclear reactor accidents. Radiation exposure during pregnancy is a clinical issue when diagnostic imaging in a pregnant woman is required. Possible hazards of radiation exposure include: pregnancy loss, congenital malformation, disturbances of growth and/or development, and carcinogenic effects.[8] The U.S. Nuclear Regulatory Commission recommends that occupational radiation exposure of pregnant women not exceed 5 mGy

Table 2-4.	Viral-Induced Teratogenesis and Selected Fetal Infections	
Agent	**Observed Effects**	**Exposure Risk**
Cytomegalovirus (CMV)	Birth defects, low birth weight, developmental disorders	Health care workers, childcare workers
Hepatitis B virus	Low birth weight	Health care workers, household members, sexual activity
Human immunodeficiency virus (HIV)	Low birth weight, childhood cancers, lifelong disease	Health care workers, sexual partners
Human parvovirus B19	Miscarriage, fetal heart failure	Health care workers, childcare workers
Rubella (German measles)	Birth defects, low birth weight	Health care workers, childcare workers
Toxoplasmosis	Miscarriage, birth defects, developmental disorders	Animal care workers, veterinarians
Varicella-zoster virus (chicken pox)	Birth defects, low birth weight	Health care workers, childcare workers
Herpes simplex virus	Late transmission, skin lesions, convulsions, systemic disease	Sexual activity

Adapted from Reese EA, Hobbins JC, editors: Teratogenic infections. In Reece EA, Hobbins JC, editors: *Clinical obstetrics: the fetus and mother,* ed 3, Malden, Mass., 2008, Blackwell, p 248.

(500 mrad) to the fetus during the entire pregnancy. Diagnostic procedures typically expose the fetus to less than 0.05 Gy (5 rad) and there is no evidence of an increased risk of fetal anomalies or adverse neurologic outcome.

Diagnostic x-rays of the head, neck, chest, and limbs do not result in any measurable exposure to the embryo/fetus, but it is advised that the pregnant woman wear a shield for such studies. Fetal exposure from nonabdominal pelvic computed tomography (CT) scans is minimal, but again, the pregnant woman should have her abdomen shielded. Ultrasound (US) imaging has demonstrated no untoward biologic effects on the fetus or mother because the acoustic output does not generate harmful levels of heat. US has been used extensively over the last 3 decades. Magnetic resonance imaging (MRI) also has not demonstrated any negative effects.

Genetic Origins

Chromosomal abnormalities affect about 1 of 140 live births. In addition, approximately 50% of spontaneous abortions have an abnormal chromosomal pattern. More than 90% of fetuses with chromosomal abnormalities do not survive to term. In fetuses with congenital anomalies, the prevalence of chromosomal abnormalities ranges from 2% to 35%.[9] A comprehensive, three-generation family history and ethnic origin assessment should be taken, whether evaluating preconceptionally or after birth. Congenital anomalies of a genetic origin can be sporadic or heritable and have a number of etiologies. They can involve nondisjunction, nonallelic homologous recombination, inversions, deletions and duplications, and translocations. Infants are also at a risk for having birth defects if their parents are carriers of genetic mutations. This single gene transmission pattern in humans follows three typical patterns: autosomal dominant, autosomal recessive, and x-linked conditions. These typically follow traditional mendelian genetics. Nonmendelian patterns of transmission include unstable DNA and fragile X syndrome, imprinting, mitochondrial inheritance, germline or gonadal mosaicism, and multifactorial inheritance. The most common genetic disorders for which prenatal screening may be offered are trisomy 21, trisomy 18, hemoglobinopathies (such as hemoglobin C disease, hemoglobin S-C disease, sickle cell anemia, thalassemia), cystic fibrosis, fragile X syndrome, and a variety of disorders seen most commonly in the Ashkenazi Jewish population.

Prenatal Genetic Testing for Trisomy 21

Caring for a special needs child or adult has a significant impact on a couple and family. Down syndrome is the most common chromosomal abnormality causing mental disability in the United States. In addition to cognitive deficits, these children are also at risk for congenital heart disease, duodenal atresia, urinary tract malformations, epilepsy, and leukemia. Prenatal testing for chromosomal abnormalities is a matter of weighing the risks of the genetic condition in question with the ultimate risks of the tests available to identify that abnormality. This should include the risks of a false-negative result in an affected pregnancy and the false-positive result in the unaffected pregnancy and the possible riskier diagnostic tests that may follow. Over the last 2 to 3 decades, the ability to more effectively and safely diagnose Down syndrome has improved.

Prenatal testing for Down syndrome has moved away from the traditional invasive diagnostic testing based on age alone. Presently, a combination of maternal blood tests and ultrasound screening provide women with choices beyond routine chorionic villus sampling or amniocentesis. Optimally, this prenatal screening should minimize the number of women identified as screen-positive while maximizing the overall detection rate. These screening tests, therefore, require a high sensitivity and a low false-positive rate. The improvements in testing have achieved this and ultimately reduced the number of invasive tests performed and, in turn, decreased the rate of procedure-related losses. Historically, the first screening tests used maternal age as a cut-off for risk assessment because the prevalence of trisomy 21 rises with age. Women age 35 and above were eligible for screening based on a cost-benefit analysis and an attempt to match the risk of an affected fetus with a procedure-related loss. Screening based on this parameter of advanced maternal age alone had a detection rate of about 30% with a false-positive rate of 5% when implemented in the 1970s.

From 1974 to 2002, the mean age of women giving birth in the United States has increased from 24.4 to 27.4 years, and the percentage of women aged 35 years and older at birth increased from 4.7% to 13.8%. Using advanced maternal age (AMA) as the main parameter became less efficacious.[10] In 1984, the association between aneuploidy and low levels of maternal serum alpha-fetoprotein (MS-AFP) was reported. In 1987, the association between high maternal serum human chorionic gonadotropin (hCG) value and a low conjugated estriol level in Down syndrome pregnancies was reported. In 1988, this information was first integrated and called the "Triple Screen Test." Combining MS-AFP, hCG, and unconjugated estriol values with maternal age risk and performing it between 15 and 22 weeks, doubled the age-related detection rate to 60% and maintained the false-positive rate at 5%. The test is considered positive when the result, stated as an estimate of risk, is above the set cut-off range. This is usually about 1:270 and based on the second trimester age-related risk of a 35-year-old woman. In 1996, the "Quad Screen" was created when the level of inhibin-A was added to the Triple Screen. This test has a detection rate of 76% and a false-positive rate that remains at 5%.

Over the last 3 decades, the addition of ultrasonography to the practice of obstetrics has allowed for the detection of significant fetal abnormalities prior to delivery (Fig. 2-1). About 20% to 27% of second trimester fetuses with Down syndrome have a major anatomic abnormality.[11] Over time, sonographic markers were identified that, when present, increase the likelihood that a chromosomal abnormality may exist. The risk increases as the number of markers increases. Sonographic markers are seen in 50% to 80% of fetuses with Down syndrome. The most common markers are cardiac defects, increased nuchal-fold thickness, hyperechoic bowel, shortened extremities, and renal pyelectasis. When a second trimester ultrasound is performed to search for these markers, it is called a "genetic sonogram." The overall sensitivity of this ultrasound is 70% to 85%.

Nuchal translucency is a standard ultrasound technique and is most accurately measured in skilled hands between 10 to 14 weeks (Figs. 2-2 and 2-3). There is a direct correlation between an increased measurement and a risk for Down syndrome, other aneuploidy,

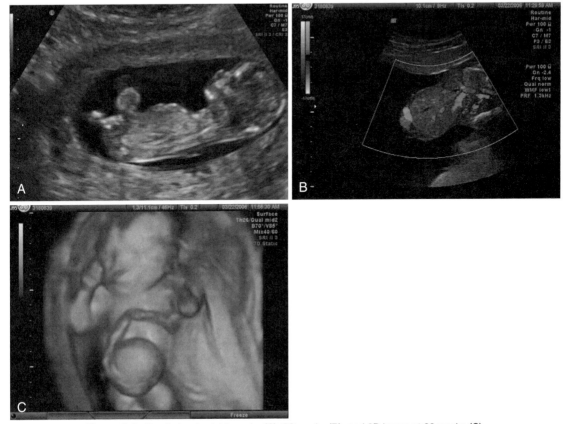

Figure 2-1. Omphalocele at 12 weeks **(A)**, 26 weeks **(B)**, and 3D image at 22 weeks **(C)**.

and major structural malformations.[12] In fact, a very large nuchal translucency suggests a very high risk for aneuploidy. Down syndrome, trisomy 18, and Turner syndrome are the most likely chromosomal abnormalities and cardiac defects are the most likely malformations.

Serum genetic screening and genetic sonography evolved into a combined testing approach. With this method, the sensitivity of Down syndrome screening increased whereas the false-positive rate decreased. The rationale involves modifying the a priori maternal age risk up or down. If the pattern seen is similar to the pattern in a Down syndrome pregnancy, then the risk is increased; if it is the opposite, then it is decreased. The magnitude of this difference is expressed in multiples of the median and it determines how much the risk is modified. For sonographic markers, the magnitude of these differences is measured by a likelihood ratio (LR = sensitivity/false-positive rate) that is then multiplied by the a priori risk.

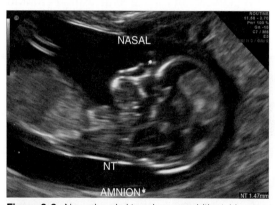

Figure 2-2. Normal nuchal translucency width at 11 weeks, 6 days.

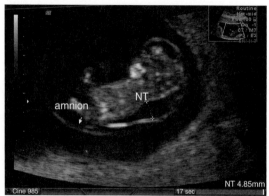

Figure 2-3. Abnormally thickened nuchal translucency at 10 weeks, 5 days.

This next phase of screening became the "first-trimester screening" protocol. The ultrasound component involves the sonographic measurement of the nuchal translucency. If this measurement is increased for the gestational age, it can indicate an affected fetus. This is an operator-dependent measurement, but has demonstrated a 62% to 92% detection rate. The serum markers that are measured are maternal serum beta-hCG and maternal serum pregnancy-associated plasma protein A (PAPP-A). In the first trimester, pregnancies in which the fetus has Down syndrome have higher levels of hCG and lower levels of PAPP-A than do unaffected pregnancies. This combination of maternal age, nuchal translucency, hCG, and PAPP-A is now the standard first trimester screening and is called the "first trimester combined test." It has a detection rate of 85% and a false-positive rate of 5%. This is better than the quadruple screen detection rate of 80% and a false-positive rate of 5% and, therefore, it became the recommended screen for women who presented early in pregnancy.

It makes sense to offer Down syndrome screening as early in pregnancy as possible. Performed between 11 and 13 weeks, the first trimester screening combined test provides for as early an evaluation and diagnosis as possible for fetal abnormalities. It also provides for maximum decision making time and adjustment, privacy, and safer termination options if desired. One of the issues with such sophisticated screening protocols is the timing and availability of such methods. The American College of Obstetricians and Gynecologists (ACOG) recommends that all women be offered screening before 20 weeks and all women should have an option of invasive testing regardless of age.[13] They also recommend that prenatal fetal karyotyping should be offered to women of any age with a history of another pregnancy with trisomy 21 or other aneuploidy, at least one major or two minor anomalies in the present pregnancy, or a personal or partner history of translocation, inversion, or aneuploidy.

The impact of prenatal screening is significant. During this age of first trimester screening, the number of amniocentesis and chorionic villus sampling procedures performed has dropped. In areas where Down syndrome screening tests have been implemented, there has been an increase in the detection of affected fetuses and a drop in the number of live births with Down syndrome.

Trisomy 18

Trisomy 18 is also called *Edwards syndrome* and is the second most common autosomal trisomy, occurring in 1 in 8000 births. Many fetuses with trisomy 18 die in utero and so the prevalence of this abnormality is three to five times higher in the first and second trimesters than at birth. Prenatal screening for trisomy 18 is included with screening for Down syndrome. The analyte pattern of the first trimester test is a very low beta-hCG and a very low PAPP-A with an increased nuchal translucency.[14] Advanced maternal age increases the risk of having a pregnancy affected with trisomy 18. These fetuses have an extensive clinical spectrum disorder and many organ systems can be affected. Fifty percent of these infants die within the first week of life and only 5% to 10% survive the first year of life. The combined and integrated tests are especially effective at detecting these affected pregnancies. The earliest detection provides for the most comprehensive counseling and earliest intervention, if desired.

Prenatal Screening for Neural Tube Defects

The incidence of neural tube defects (NTDs) in the United States is considered to be highly variable because it depends on geographic factors and ethnic background. Typically seen in 1 in 1000 pregnancies, they are considered to be the second most prevalent congenital anomaly in the United States, with only cardiac anomalies being seen more often. It has been recommended by ACOG that screening for NTDs should be offered to all pregnant women. The American College of Medical Genetics also recommends screening using the MS-AFP and/or ultrasonography between 15 and 20 weeks.[15]

The majority of NTDs are isolated malformations caused by multiple factors such as folic acid deficiency, drug exposure, excessive vitamin A intake, maternal diabetes mellitus, maternal hyperthermia, and obesity. A genetic origin is also suggested by the fact that a high concordance rate is found in monozygotic twins. NTDs are also more common in first-degree relatives and are more often seen in females versus males. Family history also supports a genetic mode of transmission. The recurrence risk for NTDs is about 2% to 4% when there is one affected sibling and as high as 10% when

there are two affected siblings.[16] There is also some evidence that NTDs are associated with the genetic variance seen in the homocysteine pathways (*MTHFR* gene) and the *VANGL1* gene.[17] There is also a high prevalence of other karyotypic abnormalities and trisomy 18 is typically the most common aneuploidy found.

In the 1970s through the 1980s, maternal serum screening programs were instituted and combined with preconception supplementation with folic acid. In the 1990s, folic acid food fortification was implemented. During this time, screening protocols were also instituted and initially they involved just the MS-AFP and amniocentesis for abnormal results and then went on to include sonography. Where these methods were employed, a decrease in the prevalence of NTDs was seen—largely due to the prevention of folic acid-deficient women preconceptually.[18]

Screening for open NTDs typically involves the MS-AFP, which is most optimally drawn between 16 and 18 weeks' gestation. It is made by the fetal yolk sac, gastrointestinal tract, and liver and is a specific fetal-specific globulin. It is similar to albumin and can be found in the maternal serum, amniotic fluid (from fetal urine), and fetal plasma. It is found in much lower concentrations in the maternal serum than in the amniotic fluid or fetal plasma. The primary intent is to detect open spina bifida and anencephaly, but when concentrations are abnormal, it can also suggest the presence of other nonneural abnormalities such as ventral wall defects.

For each gestational week, these results are expressed as multiples of the median (MoM). A value above 2.0 to 2.5 MoM is considered abnormal. Some characteristics can significantly affect the interpretation of the results. A screen performed before 15 weeks and after 20 weeks will falsely raise or lower the MoM. Maternal weight affects the results because the AFP is diluted in the larger blood volume of obese women.[19] Women with diabetes mellitus have an increased risk of NTDs and so their threshold value has to be adjusted to have a more accurate sensitivity. The presence of other fetal anomalies increases the level of the MS-AFP. The MoM level also has to be adjusted in pregnancies with multiple gestations because the MS-AFP level is proportional to the number of fetuses. Race can affect the results of the MS-AFP because African-American women have a baseline level that is 10% higher than that of non–African-American women. Finally, MS-AFP cannot be interpreted in the face of fetal death; therefore, it cannot be used as a screening method when there is a nonviable fetus present in a multiple gestation.

Ultrasound can potentially detect more NTDs than MS-AFP.[20] Detection rates depend on the type of anomaly and the trimester during which it is used. Anencephaly and encephalocele have detection rates between 80% and 90% in the first trimester, whereas detection rates of >90% for spina bifida are not seen until the second trimester.[21] Although the vast majority of NTDs can be seen on ultrasound and the sensitivity of the ultrasound evaluation is high, the ultimate diagnosis depends on the position of the fetus, the size and location of the defect, the maternal body habitus, and the skill of the ultrasonographer.

Women who have a screen-positive pregnancy will be counseled to undergo an ultrasound to document accurate gestational age, fetal viability, and possible presence of multiple gestation. A detailed anatomic survey of the fetus will also be performed. The use of amniocentesis may also be employed if there is some discrepancy found on ultrasound that does not explain the abnormal MS-AFP. Elevations in both amniotic fluid AFP and amniotic fluid acetylcholinesterase (AChE) suggests an open NTD with almost 96% accuracy. There is some conflict today regarding the use of amniocentesis, and some experts believe that ultrasound alone should be used given its high detection rate, absent procedure loss rate, and cost savings advantage. After reviewing the data, ACOG still recommends that the most sensitive approach to prenatal diagnosis of NTDs is the MS-AFP screening followed by ultrasound examination when elevated, and then amniocentesis if there are discrepant findings or the patient desires more information to help formulate a management decision. Magnetic resonance imaging (MRI) of the fetus can also be used when there is some factor that is interfering with ultrasound diagnosis of the defect.[22] This additional modality can be of great significance when planning for potential fetal or neonatal surgery, route of delivery, and overall counseling of the parents.

Fetal surgery for myelomeningocele was recently compared in a randomized trial comparing outcomes of in utero repair to standard postnatal repair.[23] The trial was stopped early because of the improvements seen with prenatal surgery. A composite outcome of fetal or neonatal death or the need for placement of cerebrospinal fluid shunt by the age of 12 months was seen in 98% of the postnatal-surgery group versus 68% of the infants in the prenatal surgery group. Prenatal surgery, however, was associated with more preterm delivery as well as uterine dehiscence at delivery.

MULTIPLE GESTATION

Multiple gestation has been increasing in the United States. In the most recent data for 2008, the twin birth rate rose 1% to 32.6 per 1000 births.[24] This rate has now remained essentially stable between 2004 and 2008 after rising almost 80% between 1980 and 2004. The natural occurring rate of twins and triplets in the Unites States is 1 in 80 and 1 in 8000, respectively. The likely reason for the increasing numbers of multiple births has to do with the increasing maternal age at childbirth and the use of assisted reproductive technology (ART). Maternal age, ART, parity, race, geographic origin, family history, maternal weight and height have all been associated with an increased risk of twins.

Zygosity is an important concept for multiple gestation. Twins are most commonly referred to as either di- or monozygotic. Dizygotic twins result from ovulation and fertilization of two separate oocytes. Monozygotic twins result from the ovulation and fertilization of one oocyte then followed by division of the zygote. The timing of the egg division determines placentation. Diamniotic, dichorionic (DA/DC) placentation occurs with division prior to the morula stage. Diamniotic, monochorionic (DA/MC) placentation occurs with division between days 4 and 8 postfertilization. Monoamniotic, monochorionic (MA/MC) placentation occurs with division between days 8 and 12 postfertilization. Division after day 12 results in conjoined twins. Placentation is typically dichorionic for dizygotic twins and can be mono- or dichorionic for monozygotic twins. Sixty-nine percent of naturally occurring twins are dizygotic, whereas 31% are monozygotic. Dizygotic twins are also more common with ART pregnancies and account for 95% of all twins conceived with ART.

Chorionicity is also an important concept because the presence of monochorionicity places those monzygotic twins at an increased risk for complications:

twin-to-twin transfusion syndrome (TTTS), twin anemia-polycythemia sequence (TAPS), twin reversed arterial perfusion sequence (TRAP), and selective intrauterine growth restriction.[25] The risk of neurologic morbidity and perinatal mortality in these twins is higher than that of dichorionic twins.

Early ultrasound assessment is a reliable way to not only diagnose multiple gestation, but to also establish amnionicity and chorionicity. It provides accurate assessment of gestational age, which can be of vital importance given the risk of preterm birth and intrauterine growth abnormalities in multiple gestation. The optimal time for this ultrasound would be in the first and early second trimester. Offering early ultrasound can also include screening for Down syndrome because each fetus is at the same risk for having a chromosomal abnormality based on maternal age and family history and all women should be offered options for risk assessment. Maternal serum analyte interpretation can be difficult in multiple gestation because all fetuses, living or not, contribute to the concentration. Measurement of the nuchal translucency can improve the detection rate by helping to identify the affected fetus. The first trimester combined test can be offered to the woman carrying multiples when chorionic villus sampling is available.

Although twins are not predisposed to any one type of congenital anomaly, monozygotic twins are two to three times more likely to have structural defects than singletons and dizygotic twins. Anencephaly, holoprosencephaly, bladder exstrophy, VATER association (*v*ertebral defects, imperforate *a*nus, *t*racheo*e*sophageal fistula, *r*adial and *r*enal dysplasia), sacrococcygeal teratoma, and sirenomelia are the anomalies seen with increasing frequency. Most often the co-twin is structurally normal. The diagnosis of an anomalous twin is especially problematic if management might require early delivery or therapy that ultimately affects both twins. In the setting of conjoined twins, this process is even more complicated. The incidence ranges from 1 in 50,000 to 1 in 100,000 live births.[26] Additional causes for concern in monozygotic twins are monochorionic placentas that have vascular connections. The connections occur frequently and can lead to artery-to-artery shunts and, ultimately, the TRAP sequence with reversed arterial perfusion. This results in the fetal malformation,

acardiac twins. Acardia is lethal in the affected twin, but also can result in a mortality rate of 50% to 75% in the donor twin. This condition occurs in about 1% of monozygotic twins.

Growth restriction and premature birth are major causes of the higher morbidity and mortality in twins compared to singletons. The growth curve of twins deviates from that of singletons after 32 weeks' gestation and, 15% to 30% of twin gestations may have growth abnormalities. This is more likely to be seen in monochorionic twins, but discordant growth can be seen in dichorionic twins depending on the placental surface area available to each. Twin growth should be monitored with serial ultrasound, and if there is evidence of discordance, then additional evaluation is needed. Starting in the second trimester, monochorionic pregnancies are followed every 2 to 3 weeks, whereas dichorionic pregnancies are followed every 4 to 6 weeks. There is no consensus on the optimal definition of discordance because a difference of 15% to 40% has been found to be predictive of a poor outcome.[27] Presently, an estimated fetal weight below the tenth percentile using singleton growth curves or a 20% discordance in estimated fetal weight between the twins is the working definition of abnormal growth. Doppler velocimetry of the umbilical artery can be added to the ultrasound evaluation and may improve the detection rate of growth restriction.

The risk of preterm birth is higher for multiple gestations than for singletons and represents the most serious risk to these pregnancies. When compared to singletons, the risk of preterm birth for twins and triplets was five and nine times higher. As the number of fetuses increases, the gestational age at the time of birth decreases. In 2008, the average gestational ages were 35.3, 32, 30.7, and 28.5 weeks for twins, triplets, quadruplets, quintuplets, and higher order multiples, respectively. The rate of preterm birth for twins in the United States in 2008 was 59% before 37 weeks and 12% before 32 weeks. Additionally, 57% of these twins were of low birth weight (<2500 g) and 10% were of very low birth weight (<1500 g). Interestingly, the outcomes after delivery are similar between twins and singletons born prematurely.[28] Preterm premature rupture of membranes is also a cause of preterm birth in multiple gestations and most often occurs in the presenting sac, but can occur in the nonpresenting twin. It seems that multiple gestations have a shorter period of latency before delivery when compared to singleton gestations.

Triplet Gestation

The incidence of natural spontaneous triplet births is about 1 in 8000. Triplet pregnancy has a higher risk of maternal, fetal, and neonatal morbidity than does twin pregnancy. As the number of fetuses increases to that of the higher order multiples, these risks increase even more significantly. Some consequences found more often in these pregnancies include growth restriction, fetal death, preterm labor, premature preterm rupture of membranes, preterm birth, neonatal neurologic impairment, pregnancy-related hypertension, eclampsia, abruption, placenta previa, and cesarean delivery.[29]

Diagnosis of a triplet or higher order multiple gestation is done by ultrasound and most instances are found in the first trimester because the vast majority of these pregnancies are conceived via ART. As with twin pregnancy, chorionicity identification is important. Monozygotic gestations can occur even though most of these pregnancies originate from three or more separate oocytes, especially in those that are spontaneously conceived. Spontaneous loss is common and it occurs in 53% of triplet pregnancies. Given the inherent increased maternal and fetal risks involved with these pregnancies, historically, fetal reduction has been offered in hopes that fewer fetuses would translate into a reduced risk. For triplet gestation, this presumption may be changing.

The risk of premature delivery or fetal death in utero of one fetus is specific to multiple gestation. The surviving fetus(es) is affected by the chorionicity and the number of fetuses. There is an ethical dilemma not seen in singleton pregnancies because one must weigh the benefits for the affected fetus against the risks of the potential interventions to the remaining fetus(es). Typically, delivery before 26 weeks is not considered because the risk of mortality is significant for all fetuses. After 32 weeks, it is appropriate to move to deliver all if one is at risk because the morbidity is considered low. Between 26 and 32 weeks is a more difficult period and remains a time when parental preference is taken into great consideration after counseling has occurred. Chorionicity helps to guide delivery when fetal death occurs because

optimal management is unclear. As with twins, the risk is associated with monochorionicity and mortality is worse when this fetal demise occurs later in pregnancy.

A majority of triplets are born prematurely and 95% of them weigh less than 2500 g (low birth weight) and 35% are less than 1500 g (very low birth weight). The primary cause of these preterm births is premature labor. Multiple protocols have been tried to reduce the risk of preterm birth including decreased activity, bed rest hospitalization, home uterine activity monitoring, and tocolysis. Unfortunately, elective cerclage, progesterone supplementation, and sonographic cervical assessment also do not seem to have reduced the spontaneous preterm birth rate.

Although great strides have been made in the management of the neonate, the goal remains to reduce the risk and numbers of preterm birth or at least uncover a reliable method to predict women at the highest risk of developing preterm labor or premature rupture of membranes. This will be discussed in more detail in a separate section.

ANTEPARTUM ASSESSMENT OF THE FETAL CONDITION

Improved physiologic understanding and multiple technologic advancements provide the obstetrician with tools for objective evaluation of the fetus. In particular, specific information can be sought and obtained relative to maternal health and risk, fetal anatomy, growth, well-being, and functional maturity, and these data are used to provide a rational approach to clinical management of the high-risk infant before birth. It is important to emphasize that no procedure or laboratory result can supplant the data obtained from a careful history and physical examination and these have to be interpreted in light of the true or presumed gestational age of the fetus. The initial prenatal examination and subsequent physical examinations are approached with these facts in mind to ascertain whether the uterine size and growth are consistent with the supposed length of gestation. In the era prior to routine ultrasound dating, the milestones of quickening (16 to 18 weeks) and fetal heart tone auscultation by Doppler ultrasound (12 to 14 weeks) were important and needed to be systematically recorded. Although most of this information is gathered early in pregnancy, the significance may not be appreciated until later in gestation when decisions regarding the appropriateness of fetal size and the timing of delivery are contemplated.

Ultrasonography

A clear role for antenatal ultrasound has been established in dating pregnancies, diagnosing multiple gestations, monitoring intrauterine growth, and detecting congenital malformations. It is also integral to locating the placental site and documenting any pelvic organ abnormalities. Ultrasound is valuable when performing chorionic villus sampling or amniocentesis. Ultrasound may be used during labor to detect problems related to vaginal bleeding, size or date discrepancies, suspected abnormal presentation, amniotic fluid levels, loss of fetal heart tones, delivery of a twin, attempted version of a breech presentation, and diagnosis of fetal anomalies.

Ultrasound is a technique by which short pulses (2 μsec) of high-frequency (approximately 2.5 MHz), low-intensity sound waves are transmitted from a piezoelectric crystal (transducer) through the maternal abdomen to the uterus and the fetus. The echo signals reflected back from tissue interfaces provide a two-dimensional picture of the uterine wall, placenta, amniotic fluid, and fetus. Some indications for ultrasound are contained in Box 2-1. In certain instances, ultrasound is performed to comply with the mother's request only.

As noted earlier, gestational age is most accurately determined the earlier it is performed during pregnancy. In the first trimester, the gestational age of the fetus is assessed by a crown-to-rump measurement and this is the most accurate means for ultrasound dating.[30] After the thirteenth week of gestation, measurement of the fetal biparietal diameter (BPD) or cephalometry is the most commonly used technique. Before 20 weeks' gestation, this measurement provides a good estimation of gestational age within a range of plus or minus 10 days. After 20 weeks' gestation, the predictability of the measurement is less reliable, so an initial examination should be obtained before this time whenever possible. Such early examination also assists in interpretation of prenatal genetic screening as well as in detection of major malformations. Follow-up examinations can then be done to ascertain whether fetal growth in utero is proceeding at a normal rate.

> **EDITORIAL COMMENT:** In countries with great access to prenatal care, the problem of attending a delivery with uncertain gestational age occurs much less frequently.[3]

When fetal growth is restricted, however, brain sparing may result in an abnormal ratio of growth between the head and the rest of the body. Because the BPD may then be within normal limits, other measurements are needed to detect the true restriction of growth. The measurement of the ratio between the circumferences of head and abdomen is particularly valuable under these circumstances.[31]

Femur length (FL), which may be less affected by alterations in growth than the head or abdomen, is used to aid in determining gestational age and to identify the fetus with abnormal growth. Serial assessment of growth and deviations from normal, including both macrosomia and growth restriction, helps to identify the fetus at risk during the perinatal period. Calculation of estimated fetal weight (EFW) based on various fetal biometric parameters (BPD, head circumference [HC], abdominal circumference [AC], and FL) plotted against gestational age using various sonographic nomograms is an extremely useful method for serial assessment of fetal growth. Sophisticated computer software to serially plot

---

Box 2-1.   Uses of Ultrasound

Confirmation of pregnancy
Determination of
Gestational age
Fetal number, chorionicity, presentation
Placental location, placentation
Fetal anatomy (previous malformations)

Assessment of
Size/date discrepancy
Fetal well-being (biophysical profile, Doppler measurements of umbilical vessels, middle cerebral artery)
Volume of amniotic fluid (suspected oligohydramnios or polyhydramnios)
Fetal arrhythmias
Fetal anatomy (abnormal alpha-fetoprotein)

Assist with procedures
CVS, amniocentesis, PUBS, intrauterine transfusion, external version

Amniocentesis
Intrauterine transfusion

CVS, chorionic villus sampling; PUBS, percutaneous umbilical blood sampling.

EFW and provide percentile ranking of a given fetus is commonly used.

Three-dimensional and four-dimensional ultrasonography have added technological advancement to the imaging possibilities. Using these modalities, the volume of the targeted anatomic area can be acquired and displayed. When the vectors have been formatted, the anatomy can be demonstrated topographically. This has been a promising technique for delineating malformations of the fetal face, neural tube, and skeletal systems, but proof of clinical advantage over two-dimensional sonography is still lacking.

Antepartum Surveillance

Early identification of any risk for neurologic injury or fetal death is the primary goal of any fetal assessment technique. The process of antenatal assessment was introduced to help pursue this underlying risk of fetal jeopardy and thereby prevent adverse outcomes. It is based on the rationale that fetal hypoxia and acidosis create the final common pathway to fetal injury and death and that prior to their development, there is a sequence of events that can be identified.

There is a general pattern of fetal response to an intrauterine challenge or chronic stress. The most widely used tests to evaluate the function and reserve of the fetoplacental unit and the well-being of the fetus before labor are maternal monitoring of fetal activity, contraction stress test (CST) and nonstress test (NST) monitoring of the fetal heart rate (FHR), fetal biophysical profile (BPP), and Doppler velocimetry.

Formal Maternal Monitoring of Fetal Activity

Fetal movement perception is routinely taught in obstetrical practice as an expression of fetal well-being in utero and its counting is purported to be a simple method of fetal oxygenation monitoring. With a goal of decreasing the stillbirth rate near term, there has been an increased tendency to use fetal movements as an indicator of fetal well-being. It is monitored by maternal recording of perceived activity or using pressure-sensitive electromechanical devices and real-time ultrasound. A diagnosis of decreased fetal movement is a qualitative maternal perception of reduced normally perceived fetal movement. There is no consensus regarding a perfect definition nor is there consensus regarding the most accurate method for counting. Whereas evidence of an active or vigorous fetus is reassuring,

an inactive fetus is not necessarily an ominous finding and may merely reflect fetal state (fetal activity is reduced during quiet sleep, by certain drugs including alcohol and barbiturates, and by cigarette smoking). Three commonly used methods for fetal kick counts include perception of at least 10 fetal movements during 12 hours of normal maternal activity, perception of at least 10 fetal movements over 2 hours when the mother is at rest and concentrating on counting and perception of at least 4 fetal movements in 1 hour when the mother is at rest and focused on counting. Fetal movement does decrease with hypoxemia, but there are conflicting data regarding its use to prevent stillbirth.[32] Nonetheless, maternal perceived fetal inactivity requires prompt reassessment including real-time ultrasound or electronic FHR monitoring.

> **EDITORIAL COMMENT:** Just as pediatricians are taught to "listen to the parents," prudent obstetricians pay attention when a pregnant woman thinks something is different about the pregnancy.

Antepartum Fetal Heart Rate Monitoring

Antepartum electronic monitoring of the FHR has provided a useful approach to fetal evaluation (Table 2-5). It essentially involves the identification of two fetal heart rate patterns: nonreassuring (associated with adverse outcomes) and reassuring (associated with fetal well-being). These patterns are interpreted in the context of gestational age, maternal conditions, and fetal conditions, and compared to any prior evaluations. Electronic fetal monitors use a small Doppler ultrasound device that is placed on the maternal abdomen. It focuses a small beam on the fetal heart and the monitor interprets these signals of the heart beat wave and reflects its peak in a continuously recording graphic form. This pattern is then evaluated for the presence and absence of certain components that help to identify fetal well-being.

Antepartum testing is performed to observe pregnancies with an increased risk of fetal death or neurologic consequences (Box 2-2). The nonstress test (NST) is the most commonly used method. It is performed at daily or weekly intervals, but there are no high-quality data regarding the optimal interval of testing. Frequency is based on clinical judgment and the presence of a reassuring test only indicates that there is no fetal hypoxia at that time. It is commonly

Table 2-5.	Criteria for Interpreting Nonstress Test and Acoustic Stimulation Test
Reactivity Terms	**Criteria**
Reactive NST	Two fetal heart rate (FHR) accelerations of at least 15 beats per minute (bpm), lasting a total of 15 sec, in 10-min period
Nonreactive NST	No 10-min window containing two acceptable (as defined by reactive NST) accelerations for maximum of 40 min
Reactive AST	Two FHR accelerations of at least 15 bpm, lasting a total of 15 sec, within 5 min after application of acoustic stimulus or one acceleration of at least 15 bpm above baseline lasting 120 sec
Nonreactive AST	After three applications of acoustic stimulation at 5-min intervals, no acceptable accelerations (as defined by reactive AST) for 5 min after third stimulus

AST, Acoustic stimulation test; *NST,* nonstress test.

Box 2-2.	Indications for Antepartum Fetal Surveillance

Maternal antiphospholipid syndrome
Poorly controlled hyperthyroidism
Hemoglobinopathies
Cyanotic heart diseases
Systemic lupus erythematosus
Chronic renal disease
Type 1 diabetes mellitus
Hypertensive disorders
Pregnancy complications
Preeclampsia
Decreased fetal movement
Oligohydramnios
Polyhydramnios
Intrauterine growth restriction
Postterm pregnancy
Isoimmunization
Previous unexplained fetal demise
Multiple gestation

Adapted from the American College of Obstetricians and Gynecologists: Antepartum fetal surveillance. Practice Bulletin No. 9, October 1999.

---

understood that a reactive NST assures fetal well being for 7 days, but this is not proven. The management of a nonreactive NST depends on the gestational age and clinical context. The false-positive rate of an NST may be as high as 50% to 60%, so additional testing such as vibroacoustic stimulation, BPP, and possibly CST are useful adjuncts.

The oxytocin challenge test or contraction stress test (CST) records the responsiveness of the FHR to the stress of induced uterine contractions and thereby attempts to assess the functional reserve of the placenta. A negative CST (no FHR decelerations in response to adequate uterine contractions) gives reassurance that the fetus is not in immediate jeopardy. The CST evaluates uteroplacental function and was traditionally performed by initiating uterine contractions with oxytocin (Pitocin). Because continuous supervision and an electronic pump is required for regulated oxytocin infusion, and because of the invasiveness of intravenous infusion, attempts have been made to induce uterine contractions with nipple stimulation either by automanipulation or with warm compresses. Nipple stimulation has a variable success rate and, because of inability to regulate the contractions, as well as concerns raised by the observation of uterine hyperstimulation accompanied by FHR decelerations, it has not gained wide acceptance. Nonetheless, breast stimulation provides an alternative, cheap technique for initiating uterine contractions and evaluating placental reserve. Similar information may be obtained by evaluating the response of the FHR to spontaneous uterine contractions and perhaps also from the resting heart rate patterns without contractions. Because the CST requires the presence of contractions and has the major drawback of a high false-positive rate, its use has diminished with the better understanding of the NST and the use of the BPP and Doppler velocimetry.

As understanding of the NST evolved, it was noted that the absence of accelerations on the fetal heart rate tracing was associated with poor fetal outcomes and the presence of two or more accelerations on a CST was associated with a negative CST. Although the false-negative and false-positive rates are higher for an NST than a CST, it is more easily used and, therefore, the initial method of choice for first line antenatal testing.

The modified NST has become the initial testing scheme of choice. The modified NST comprises vibroacoustic stimulation, initiated if no acceleration is noted within 5 minutes

Table 2-6.	Technique of Biophysical Profile Scoring	
Biophysical Variable	**Normal (score = 2)**	**Abnormal (score = 0)**
Fetal breathing movements	At least one episode of at least 30 sec in 30-min observation	Absent or no episode of ≥30 sec in 30 min
Gross body movement	At least three discrete body/limb movements in 30 min (episodes of active continuous movement considered as single movement)	Two or fewer episodes of body/limb movements in 30 min
Fetal tone	At least one episode of active extension with return to flexion of fetal limb(s) or trunk; opening and closing of hand considered normal tone	Either slow extension with return to partial flexion or movement of limb in full extension or absent fetal movement
Reactive fetal heart rate	At least two episodes of acceleration of ≥15 beats per minute (bpm) and at least 15 sec associated with fetal movement in 30 min	Less than two accelerations or accelerations <15 bpm in 30 min
Qualitative amniotic fluid volume	At least one pocket of amniotic fluid that measures at least 1 cm in two perpendicular planes	Either no amniotic fluid pockets or a pocket <1 cm in two perpendicular planes

From Manning F, Morrison I, Lange I, et al: Antepartum determination of fetal health: composite biophysical profile scoring, *Clin Perinatol* 9:285, 1982.

during the standard NST. Because reactivity is defined by two accelerations within 10 minutes, the sound is repeated if 9 minutes have elapsed since the first acceleration. Vibroacoustic stimulation, using devices emitting sound levels of approximately 80 dB at a frequency of 80 Hz, results in FHR acceleration and reduces the rate of falsely worrisome NSTs. Thus, the specificity of the NST may be improved by adding sound stimulation.

Amniotic Fluid Volume

The amniotic fluid volume (AFV) is measured via ultrasound using the value of the amniotic fluid index (AFI). This is the sum of the measured vertical amniotic fluid pockets in each quadrant of the uterus that does not contain umbilical cord. The value can be associated with a number of potential complications depending on whether it is too high (polyhydramnios) or too low (oligohydramnios), although set recommendations for monitoring are not established.[33] When found, alterations in amniotic fluid volume can suggest the presence of premature rupture of membranes, fetal congenital and chromosomal anomalies, fetal growth restriction, and the potential for adverse perinatal outcomes such as intrauterine fetal demise. Pregnancies that are at risk for AFV abnormalities where surveillance may be indicated include those with such conditions as preterm premature rupture of membranes, hypertension, certain fetal congenital abnormalities, maternal infection conditions, diabetes, intrauterine growth restriction, and postterm pregnancies.

Fetal Biophysical Profile

Five components—the NST, fetal movements of flexion and extension, fetal breathing movements, fetal tone, and amniotic fluid volume—constitute the fetal biophysical profile (Table 2-6). It is performed over a 30-minute period and the presence of each component is assigned a score of 2 points for a maximum of 10 of 10. A normal score is considered to be 8 of 10 with a nonreactive NST or 8 of 8 without the NST. Equivocal is 6 of 10 and abnormal is ≤4 of 10. This test assesses the presence of acute hypoxia (changes in the NST, fetal breathing, body movements) and chronic hypoxia (decreased AFV). A modified biophysical profile refers to an NST and an AFI. The risk of developing fetal asphyxia within the next 7 days is about 1 in 1000 with a score of 8 to 10 of 10 (when the amniotic fluid index is normal). The false-negative rate is 0.4 to 0.6 per 1000. A normal fetal biophysical profile appears to indicate intact central nervous system (CNS) mechanisms, whereas factors depressing the fetal CNS reduce or abolish fetal activities. Thus, hypoxemia decreases fetal breathing and, with acidemia, reduces body movements. The biophysical profile offers a broader approach to fetal well-being than does the NST, but still allows for a noninvasive, easily learned and performed method for predicting fetal jeopardy. Guidelines for implementation parallel that for other antenatal fetal assessment techniques and so the BPP is usually initiated at 32 to 34 weeks' gestation for most pregnancies at risk for stillbirth.

Doppler Velocimetry
Doppler velocimetry has been used to assess the fetoplacental circulation since 1978, but still has a limited role in fetal evaluation. Because the placental bed is characterized by low resistance and high flow, the umbilical artery maintains flow throughout diastole. Diastolic flow steadily increases from 16 weeks' gestation to term. A decrease in diastolic flow, indicated by an elevated systolic-to-diastolic ratio, reflects an increase in downstream placental resistance. A normal waveform is considered reassuring and presumes normal fetal oxygenation. Elevated systolic-to-diastolic ratios are best interpreted in conjunction with NSTs and the fetal biophysical profile. The information gathered from the study of Doppler waveform patterns depends on the vessel being studied. Measurement of these velocities in the maternal and fetal vessels suggests information about blood flow through the placenta and the fetal response to any negative changes, and so, any challenge to the fetoplacental circulation can ultimately result over time in a compromise of the vascular tree. These indices in the umbilical artery will rise when 60% to 70% of the vascular tree has been altered. The ultimate development of absent or reversed diastolic flow (defined as the absence or reversal of end-diastolic frequencies before the next systolic upstroke) in the umbilical artery is regarded as an ominous finding and is associated with fetal hypoxia and fetal acidosis with subsequent adverse perinatal outcome.[34] Umbilical artery Doppler evaluation is most useful in monitoring the pregnancy that is associated with maternal disease (hypertension or diabetes), uteroplacental insufficiency, and fetal intrauterine growth restriction, and it is not supported in the routine surveillance in other settings.

When a fetus is compromised, the systemic blood flow is redistributed to the brain.[35] Doppler assessment of the fetal middle cerebral artery is presently the best tool for evaluating for the presence of fetal anemia in the at-risk pregnancy. It has all but replaced the use of percutaneous fetal umbilical blood sampling (cordocentesis or PUBS) in the evaluation of pregnancies involving Rh isoimmunization and other causes of severe fetal anemia such as parvovirus-induced hydrops fetalis or hemolytic anemia.

Fetal Blood Sampling
In the past, fetal blood sampling was indicated for rapid karyotyping and diagnosis of the heritable disorders of the fetus, diagnosis of fetal infection, and determination and treatment of fetal Rh(D) disease and severe anemia. Historically, PUBS, or cordocentesis, provided direct access to the fetal circulation for both diagnostic and therapeutic purposes. Presently, the procedures of chorionic villus sampling and amniocentesis allow for the acquisition of the same information at an earlier time and with lower risk to the fetus. Fetal diagnostic tests for karyotype can be performed on the amniocytes or chorionic villi. Fetal involvement in maternal infections, such as parvovirus B19, can also be determined through identification of infection in amniotic fluid, fetal ascites or pleural fluid, and Doppler of the middle cerebral artery is used to evaluate and follow subsequent fetal anemia. Inherited coagulopathies, hemoglobinopathies, and platelet disorders can also be identified through chorionic villus sampling and amniocentesis, but the immunologic platelet disorders such as idiopathic thrombocytopenia purpura (ITP) and alloimmune thrombocytopenia may benefit from fetal blood sampling with antepartum PUBS and during labor through fetal scalp sampling. Preparations for and ability to transfuse must be available. Suspected fetal thyroid dysfunction remains an area where fetal blood sampling by PUBS may be necessary and plays a critical role in the diagnosis and management of the disease.[36]

Chorionic Villus Sampling and Amniocentesis
Chorionic villus sampling (CVS) is a method of prenatal diagnosis of genetic abnormalities that can be used during the first trimester of pregnancy. Small samples of placenta are obtained for genetic analysis. It can be performed either transcervically or transabdominally. The major indication for chorionic villus sampling is an increased risk for fetal aneuploidies owing to advanced maternal age, family history, and abnormal first trimester screening for Down syndrome. It can also be used to detect hemoglobinopathies. Amniocentesis is a transabdominal technique by which amniotic fluid is withdrawn so it may be assessed. The most common indications include prenatal genetic analysis and assessment for intrauterine infection and fetal lung maturity. It may also be used to evaluate for other fetal conditions associated with hemoglobinopathies, blood and platelet disorders, neural

tube defects, twin-to-twin transfusion, and polyhydramnios. It is usually performed under ultrasound guidance and has a low rate of direct fetal injury from placement of the needle.

Procedure-related loss rates for CVS have been identified as 0.7% and 1.3% within 14 and 30 days, respectively, after a transabdominal procedure. It has been found that the loss rate may be higher with a transcervical approach. The pregnancy loss rate associated with amniocentesis has been reported to be 1 in 300 to 1 in 500. Although the safety and efficacy of both procedures has been established, CVS is considered to be the method of choice for first trimester evaluation because it has a lower risk of pregnancy-related loss than does amniocentesis before 15 weeks. Second trimester amniocentesis is associated with the lowest risk of pregnancy loss.

Assessing Fetal Maturity
Because respiratory distress syndrome (RDS) is a frequent consequence of premature birth, both spontaneous and iatrogenic, and is also a major component of neonatal morbidity and mortality in many high-risk situations, it is critical that an antenatal assessment of pulmonary status be performed when indicated. The main value of fetal lung maturity testing is predicting the absence of RDS. It is not typically performed prior to 32 weeks because physiologically the fetus is likely to have not yet matured. Fetal pulmonary maturity should be confirmed in pregnancies scheduled for delivery before 39 weeks unless the following criteria can be satisfied: ultrasound measurement at less than 20 weeks of gestation that supports gestational age of 39 weeks or greater; fetal heart tones (FHT) by Doppler ultrasonography have been present for 30 weeks; or it has been 36 weeks since a positive serum or urine pregnancy test. If any of these confirm a gestational age of 39 weeks, amniocentesis can be waived for delivery. Lung maturity does not need to be performed when delivery is mandated for fetal or maternal indications.

Historically, the introduction of amniocentesis for study of amniotic fluid and Rh-immunized women paved the way for development of the battery of tests currently available to assess fetal maturity. The initial methods developed were based on amniotic fluid levels of creatinine, bilirubin, and fetal fat cells, and these provided a good correlation with fetal size and gestational age. They were, however, inadequate predictors of fetal pulmonary maturity.

Amniocentesis to assess fetal pulmonary maturity is the currently accepted technique. Fetal lung secretions can be found in amniotic fluid. Evaluation of the amniotic fluid either tests for the components of the fetal pulmonary surfactant (biochemical tests) or the surface-active effects of these phospholipids (biophysical tests). The lecithin to sphingomyelin ratio, and the presence of phosphatidylglycerol are biochemical tests, whereas the fluorescence polarization or the surfactant to albumin ratio (TDx-FLM II) is a biophysical test. Lamellar body counts can also be used. No test has been shown to be more superior to the other at predicting RDS and each has its own defined level of risk. The predictive values of RDS vary with gestational age and with the population.[37]

The risk of respiratory distress syndrome is least when the ratio of lecithin to sphingomyelin (L:S) is greater than 2.0. However, this does not preclude the development of RDS in certain circumstances (e.g., infant of a diabetic mother or erythroblastosis). Given the physiology of fetal lung maturity, the presence of phosphatidylglycerol is a good indication of advanced maturity and, therefore, a correlated lessened risk of RDS with fewer false-negative results. Phosphatidylglycerol can be measured by rapid tests and is not influenced by blood or vaginal secretion, and can be sampled from a vaginal pool of fluid. The surfactant to albumin ratio is a true direct measurement of surfactant concentration. Levels greater than 55 mg of surfactant per gram of albumin correlate well with maturity, whereas those less than 40 mg are considered immature. Lamellar body count, with a size similar to platelets, is a direct measurement of surfactant production by type I pneumocytes. Given their size, a standard hematology counter can be used for their measurement; values of greater than 50,000/μL indicate maturity.[38] The negative predictive value of these tests is high so that when one result is positive, the development of RDS is unlikely.

INTRAPARTUM FETAL SURVEILLANCE
The ultimate goal of fetal heart rate (FHR) monitoring is to identify the fetus that may suffer neurologic injury or death, and to intervene prior to the development of these events. The rationale behind this goal

is that FHR patterns reflect states of hypox-emia and subsequent acidosis. It is the relationship between the condition of the mother, fetus, placenta, and labor course that can result in a poor neonatal outcome. Although one can identify risk factors such as maternal hypertension and diabetes, fetal growth restriction, and preterm birth, these conditions account for only a small number of the neonates with asphyxia at birth.[39]

The two most common approaches are intermittent auscultation and continuous electronic FHR monitoring. There are no studies comparing the efficacy of electronic fetal monitoring (EFM) to no fetal moni-toring to decrease complications such as neonatal seizures, cerebral palsy, or intra-partum fetal death.[40] A recent metaanaly-sis compared intermittent auscultation to continuous EFM found as follows: the use of EFM increased the risk of both operative vaginal delivery and cesarean delivery, did not reduce cerebral palsy or perinatal mor-tality, and did not change Apgar scores or neonatal unit admission rates, although it did reduce the risk of neonatal seizures. The reason for this is unknown, although it is suspected that 70% of cases of cerebral palsy occur before the onset of labor.[41] Also, the use of EFM instead of intermittent aus-cultation has not resulted in a decrease of the overall risk of perinatal death. Given these findings, the American College of Obstetricians and Gynecologists stated that high-risk pregnancies should be monitored continuously during labor and that either EFM or intermittent auscultation is accept-able in uncomplicated patients.

At present, continuous EFM is the pre-ferred method of identifying the FHR pat-tern. This is typically performed externally through a Doppler ultrasound device belted to the maternal abdomen. The device plots the continuous FHR while another pressure transducer attached to the maternal abdo-men simultaneously plots the frequency and duration of uterine contractions. These patterns can also be obtained from internal measurement of the FHR and uterine tone by a fetal scalp electrode and intrauterine pressure catheter. The scalp electrode yields a fetal electrocardiogram (ECG) and calcu-lates the FHR based on the interval between the R waves. External monitoring is usually as reliable as internal and is the preferred method as long as it remains interpretable. A fetal scalp pH can be measured when the FHR record is difficult to interpret or in the presence of decelerations.[42] Complications of fetal scalp blood sampling and fetal scalp electrode monitoring may include significant fetal blood loss and infections in the new-born, although these occur rarely. Fetal scalp pH sampling has largely been abandoned due to its problematic collection and poor sensitivity and positive predictive value. An alternative to fetal scalp pH determination is digital stimulation of the fetal scalp in the absence of uterine contractions and when the FHR is at the baseline. A positive test (i.e., an acceleration [15 bpm for 15 seconds] response to such stimulation) is considered fairly reliable evidence of the absence of fetal acidosis and a pH of 7.2 or greater, and clini-cal investigation supports its use.

Principles Related to FHR Monitoring

Despite the frequency of its use, the EFM has poor inter- and intraobserver reproducibil-ity and a high false-positive rate.[43] Almost 99% of nonreassuring FHR abnormalities are not associated with the development of cerebral palsy. For this reason, in 2008, the National Institutes of Child Health and Human Development convened a workshop with experts from the American College of Obstetricians and Gynecologists and the Society for Maternal-Fetal Medicine to try to reach a consensus on the definitions of FHR patterns. This is a standard that has been adopted and endorsed by ACOG (Table 2-7). Two major assumptions that have been made is that these definitions are primarily for visual interpretation of FHR patterns, and that they should be applied to intrapar-tum patterns, but are applicable to antepar-tum testing as well.

Terminology used to describe uterine activity has been revised to include[44] the following:

Normal: five contractions or less in 10 min-utes averaged over a 30-minute period.

Tachysystole: more than five contractions in 10 minutes, averaged over a 20-minute window.

The terms hyperstimulation and hypercon-tractility are not defined and should be abandoned.

Tachysystole should always be qualified as to the presence or absence of associated FHR decelerations. The term tachysystole applies to both spontaneous and stimu-lated labor.

The FHR pattern is usually identified as either reassuring or nonreassuring in order to guide clinical management.

Table 2-7.	**2008 Electronic Fetal Monitoring Definitions**
Pattern	**Definition**
Baseline	Bradycardia = below 100 beats per minute (bpm) Normal = 110 to 160 bpm Tachycardia = over 160 bpm The baseline must be for a minimum of 2 min in any 10 min period or the baseline for that time is indeterminate. May refer to prior 10 minute segment to exclude periodic changes, areas of marked variability.
Variability	Fluctuations in the baseline that are irregular in amplitude and frequency Absent = amplitude undetectable Minimal = amplitude is 0-5 bpm Moderate = amplitude is 6-25 bpm Marked = amplitude greater than 25 bpm Measured in a 10 min window, peak to trough. There is no longer a distinction between short- and long-term variability.
Acceleration	A visually abrupt increase in the fetal heart rate (FHR) (onset to peak is less than 20 sec) Before 32 wk, 10 beats above the baseline for 10 sec After 32 wk, 15 beats above the baseline for 15 sec A prolonged acceleration lasts 2 min or more, but less than 10 min If it lasts longer than 10 min, then it is a baseline change.
Early Deceleration	A gradual, usually symmetrical decrease from the baseline of the FHR with a contraction The nadir occurs at the same time as the peak of the contraction.
Late Deceleration	A gradual, usually symmetrical decrease from the baseline of the FHR with a uterine contraction. The deceleration is delayed in timing, with the nadir occurring after the peak of the contraction.
Variable Deceleration	An abrupt decrease in the FHR below the baseline The decrease is ≥15 bpm, lasting ≥15 sec and <2 min from the onset to return to baseline. The onset, depth, and duration of the variable commonly vary with successive contractions.
Prolonged Deceleration	A decrease in FHR below the baseline of more than 15 bpm lasting at least 2 min but <10 min from the onset to return to baseline A prolonged deceleration of 10 min or more is considered a change in baseline.

Adapted from Macones GA, Hankins GD, Spong CY, et al: The 2008 National Institute of Child Health and Human Development workshop report on electronic fetal monitoring: update on definitions, interpretation, and research guidelines, *Obstet Gynecol* 112:661, 2008.

The presence of a reassuring tracing suggests that there is no fetal acidemia at that point in time. To be considered reassuring, a tracing must have the following components: a baseline fetal heart rate of 110 to 160 beats per minute (bpm), absence of late or variable FHR decelerations, moderate FHR variability, and age-appropriate FHR accelerations (2 accelerations in 20 minutes of 15 beats above the baseline for 15 seconds for 32 weeks' gestation and above, and 2 of 10 beats above the baseline for 10 seconds for less than 32 weeks' gestation).

Nonreassuring tracings are associated with an altered fetal acid-base status and require immediate attention and intervention. In addition to the new definitions, a three-tiered interpretation system was established to help facilitate management (Box 2-3).

A category I tracing represents a normal FHR pattern, category II represents an indeterminate tracing, and category III represents an abnormal tracing.

Serial evaluation of the tracing is necessary because the FHR pattern represents only a risk of acidosis at that point in time and does not predict future status because the pattern can change in response to labor and maternal and fetal predisposing conditions. Transient tachycardia with heart rates of more than 160 beats per minute (Fig. 2-4, *A*) may be an isolated finding. It frequently precedes a variable deceleration pattern as a brief episode (see Fig. 2-4, *B* and *C*), which may reflect umbilical cord venous compression.

A late deceleration pattern (Fig. 2-5) is commonly associated with uteroplacental insufficiency. Either of these patterns may be compatible with fetal stress (Box 2-4).

Some additional principles include[39,44] the following:

- The presence of FHR accelerations with moderate variability almost always indicates a fetus that is not acidotic.
- In the presence of normal FHR variability, a fetus without accelerations is unlikely to

Box 2-3.	**Three-Tiered Fetal Heart Rate Interpretation System**

Category I

All of the following criteria must be present and, when present, are predictive of normal acid-base status at that time:

- Baseline rate: 110-160 beats per minute (bpm)
- Moderate variability
- Absent late or variable decelerations
- Present or absent early decelerations
- Present or absent accelerations

Category II

Includes all fetal heart rates (FHRs) that are neither Category I nor Category III. They are considered indeterminate.

Category III

These tracings are predictive of abnormal fetal acid-base status at the time of observation and need to be promptly evaluated.

FHR tracings include either:

- Absent baseline FHR variability *and* any of the following:

      Recurrent late decelerations

      Recurrent variable decelerations

      Bradycardia

      Sinusoidal pattern

Adapted from Macones GA, Hankins GD, Spong CY, et al: The 2008 National Institute of Child Health and Human Development workshop report on electronic fetal monitoring: update of definitions, interpretation, and research guidelines, Obstet Gynecol 112:661, 2008.

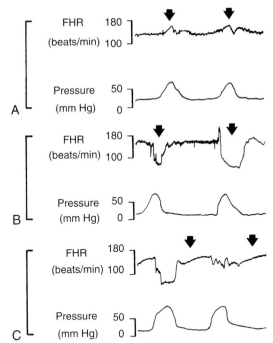

Figure 2-4. Changes in fetal heart rate (FHR) during uterine contractions as reflection of fetal distress. *Arrows* indicated transient tachycardia (**A**), variable deceleration (**B**), and variable deceleration with slow recovery after uterine relaxation (**C**). Pressure is uterine pressure. (See text for explanation.)

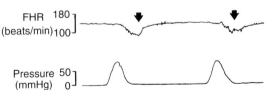

Figure 2-5. Changes in fetal heart rate (FHR) during uterine relaxation as reflection of fetal distress. *Arrows* indicate late deceleration pattern with slow recovery after uterine relaxation. Pressure is uterine pressure. (See text for explanation.)

be acidotic because moderate variability is strongly associated with an umbilical cord pH of greater than 7.15. An attempt can be made via vibroacoustic stimulation or scalp stimulation to elicit an acceleration.

- Neither baseline bradycardia (FHR <120 bpm) nor tachycardia (FHR >160 bpm) alone is predictive of acidosis.
- Baseline tachycardia may be due to early asphyxia but is more frequently the result of maternal fever, fetal infection, maternal drugs, or prematurity.
- Persistent fetal bradycardia with good variability is generally not associated with acidosis. It is more likely to be the result of drugs (medications) or fetal arrhythmias. Persistent bradycardia below 100, even with variability present, is nonreassuring because this level of FHR may not be able to perfuse tissue adequately.
- Variability is a measure of fetal reserve. Absent or minimal variability is suggestive

of fetal acidosis, especially when combined with recurrent late decelerations. Normal baseline variability and accelerations occurring spontaneously or after stimulation indicate intact fetal reserves.

- Recurrent variable decelerations may be relieved with intrauterine amnioinfusion of saline to relieve cord compression.
- A sinusoidal pattern is no longer considered a preterminal condition in all cases and may not be due to acidosis. An attempt should be made to identify the cause. Fetal scalp stimulation may provide some reassurance.
- With any FHR tracing, if there is an increase in FHR at the time of digital

Box 2-4.	Fetal Heart Rate Patterns and Underlying Mechanisms

Reflecting fetal reserve

Normal baseline heart rate and fetal heart rate (FHR)

Tachycardia (>160 beats per minute [bpm])

Diminished variability (<6 bpm variation)

Bradycardia (<120 bpm)

Sinusoidal pattern

Reflecting acute environmental change

Early deceleration

Variable deceleration

Late deceleration

Acceleration

Head compression

Cord compression, acute hemorrhage

Contraction-induced hypoxia

Intact autonomic response to intrinsic or extrinsic stimuli

Underlying mechanisms

Intact autonomic cardiovascular reflexes

Prematurity, maternal fever, acidosis

"Sleep cycle," drug effects, acidosis, congenital anomaly

Normal variant, congenital heart block, cardiac anomaly, maternal hypothermia

Anemia, hypoxia, drug effect

Modified from Clark SL, Miller FC: Scalp blood sampling—fetal heart rate patterns tell you when to do it, Contemp Obstet Gynecol 21:47, 1984.

stimulation of the fetal scalp, then the pH is likely to be greater than 7.15.

- Transient episodes of hypoxemia due to contraction or temporary cord occlusion are generally well tolerated, but prolonged or repeated episodes, especially if severe and/or associated with decreased variability, can lead to acidosis.

Treatment of the Category II and III Tracings

Most category II and III tracings require expeditious intervention. Administration of a high concentration of oxygen to the mother of a fetus under stress is one of the few methods of treating acute fetal hypoxemia. Maternal position changes are made to displace the gravid uterus or an occult cord. Treatment of maternal hypotension with intravenous crystalloid fluid bolus or ephedrine is given if hypotension is related to neuraxial anesthesia. Medications such as pitocin are discontinued if tachysystole is present. Beta-adrenergics such as terbutaline

can be used for tachysystole that is unrelenting; these agents contribute to intrauterine resuscitation. These are just a few of the measures that can be taken to correct the nonreassuring FHR pattern changes. If the FHR tracing continues to indicate fetal compromise and it remains unresolved by interventions, a prompt delivery may be indicated. The method of delivery, operative vaginal or cesarean section, will depend on cervical dilation, station, position of the fetal head, maternal obstetrical history, and urgency of the situation.

Adequate preparation is desirable for prompt effective resuscitation of the newborn. The pediatrician should be alerted when a decision is being made to intervene operatively for a fetus in distress (Box 2-5; also see Chapter 3). A nonreassuring FHR tracing may or may not be associated with birth asphyxia because only 30% to 40% of newborns who have low Apgar scores at birth (depressed) are actually acidotic as well. Historically, low 1- and 5-minute Apgar scores were used to define birth asphyxia. In our modern understanding of the development of cerebral palsy and neurologic impairment, this is considered a misuse of the Apgar score. In general, because measurement of the process that leads to birth asphyxia is almost impossible in the fetus, asphyxia is described as the presence of hypoxia and metabolic acidosis that is severe enough to result in hypoxic encephalopathy.[45]

Neonatal encephalopathy is the present preferred terminology to describe central nervous system abnormalities during the newborn period of a neonate who was born after 36 weeks' gestation.[46] Birth asphyxia, now called hypoxic-ischemic (anoxic) encephalopathy (HIE), is a subset of neonatal encephalopathy. The underlying cause of brain injury in the neonate is oftentimes poorly understood, so the criteria for diagnosing HIE have not been completely established. The task force that was convened by ACOG and the AAP determined that four criteria must be met in order to define an intrapartum event as the cause of neonatal encephalopathy that would lead to cerebral palsy[47]: profound metabolic acidosis (pH <7.0 and base deficit >12 mmol/L) on umbilical cord arterial sample; early onset of severe or moderate neonatal encephalopathy in infants past 34 weeks' gestation; cerebral palsy of the spastic quadriplegic or dyskinetic type; and exclusion of other identifiable etiologies. Additional supportive

---

Box 2-5.	**Planning Care of the High-Risk Infant**

Fetal disorders (suspected or confirmed)
Size for date discrepancy
Abnormal karyotype
Polyhydramnios or oligohydramnios
Hydrops fetalis
Fetal anomalies
Abnormal alpha-fetoprotein determination
Abnormal stress or nonstress contraction test
Reduced biophysical profile score
Reduced fetal movement
Immature L:S ratio
Cardiac dysrhythmias

Maternal problems
Pregnancy-associated hypertension
Diabetes
Previous stillbirth or neonatal death
Maternal age <18 or >34 years
Anemia or abnormal hemoglobin
Rh sensitization
Maternal infection
Prematurity or postmaturity
Malnutrition or poor weight gain
Premature rupture of membranes
Antepartum hemorrhage
Collagen vascular disorders
Drug therapy
Maternal drug or alcohol abuse
Multiple gestation

Intrapartum factors associated with Maternal/fetal compromise
Extreme prematurity or postmaturity
Placenta previa or abruptio placentae
Abnormal presentation
Prolapsed cord
Prolonged rupture of membranes >24 h
Maternal fever or chorioamnionitis
Abnormal labor pattern
Prolonged labor >24 h
Prolonged second stage of labor >2 h
Persistent fetal tachycardia
Persistent abnormal fetal heart rate (FHR)
    pattern
Loss of beat-to-beat variability in FHR
Meconium-stained amniotic fluid
Fetal acidosis
General anesthesia
Narcotic administered to mother within 4 h of
    delivery
Cesarean delivery
Difficult delivery

findings of an intrapartum origin that are discussed also include a sentinel hypoxic event in labor, electronic FHR abnormalities, Apgar score of 0 to 5 after 5 minutes, onset of multiorgan involvement within 72 hours, and early neuroimaging studies that show evidence of an acute nonfocal abnormality.

There are a number of antenatal risk factors that are associated with neonatal encephalopathy and cerebral palsy and it is not surprising that they include maternal medical conditions, placental abnormalities, postterm gestation, preeclampsia, prematurity, maternal fever and infection, and intrauterine growth restriction. Further discussion of the etiologies, diagnostic options, and management strategies of this condition will be discussed in subsequent chapters.

FETAL TREATMENT

A combination of medical and surgical therapies is available for the prevention and treatment of fetal disorders. As noted in (Box 2-6), these range from simple dietary supplements (which prevent birth defects) to complex surgical procedures, usually mandated by severe fetal compromise with hydrops fetalis or gross disturbances in the volume of amniotic fluid. The development of invasive fetal therapy can be attributed to advances in prenatal ultrasonography. Ultrasonography has been critical in following the natural history of many of the birth defects and disorders. It has also permitted early identification of structural anomalies and served as a guide for the minimally invasive prenatal therapy as well as intraoperative monitoring during open fetal surgery. MRI can now be used when ultrasound is limited or its evaluation is incomplete.

Direct or indirect treatment of the fetus continues to evolve slowly. These treatments include short-term oxygen therapy for IUGR, blood transfusions for fetal anemia, antibiotics and antiretrovirals for toxoplasmosis and HIV, steroid replacement for congenital adrenal hyperplasia, stem cell therapy for immune deficiency disorders, therapy for fetal arrhythmias, and thyroxine instillation for severe hypothyroidism.

The field of fetal surgery has continued to grow and even diaphragmatic hernias, cystadenomatous malformations of the lung, neural tube defects, hydrocephalus, and hydronephrosis, are conditions that may be managed with in utero interventions and surgery.

Box 2-6. An Overview of Fetal Therapy

Prevention of birth defects
Folic acid
Periconceptual glucose control in diabetes

Hormonal therapy
Thyroid hormone
Antenatal corticosteroids for acceleration of
    pulmonary maturation
Corticosteroids for congenital adrenal
    hyperplasia

**Prevention and treatment of anemia/
jaundice**
Anti-D globulin (Rhogam) at 28 weeks to
    prevent erythroblastosis
Direct transfusions for severe anemia/hydrops

Treatment and prevention of infection
Spiramycin for toxoplasmosis
Zidovudine or other agents for human immu-
    nodeficiency virus
Antibiotics for premature rupture of membranes
Intrapartum penicillin for group B streptococ-
    cal disease

Treatment of cardiac arrhythmias
Agents administered to mother, injected into
    amniotic fluid or directly into the fetus

Fetal surgery: highly selected cases
Usually with hydrops fetalis or gross altera-
    tions in amniotic fluid volume
Congenital diaphragmatic hernia
Congenital cystic adenomatoid malformation
Fetal hydrothorax
Sacrococcygeal teratoma
Obstructive uropathy
Fetal airway obstruction due to giant neck
    masses
Neural tube defects

Box 2-7. Criteria for the Diagnosis of Severe Preeclampsia

Blood pressure of 160 mm Hg systolic or
    higher or 110 mm Hg diastolic or higher on
    two occasions at least 6 hours apart while
    the patient is on bed rest
Proteinuria of 5 g or higher in a 24-hour urine
    specimen or 3+ or greater on two random
    urine samples collected at least 4 hours
    apart
Oliguria of less than 500 mL in 24 hours
Cerebral or visual disturbances
Pulmonary edema or cyanosis
Epigastric or right upper quadrant pain
Impaired liver function
Thrombocytopenia
Fetal growth restriction

SELECTED DISORDERS OF THE MATERNAL-FETAL INTERFACE
PREGNANCY-RELATED HYPERTENSION

Hypertensive disorders in pregnancy can be grouped into four main classes: chronic hypertension, preeclampsia and eclampsia, preeclampsia superimposed on chronic hypertension, and gestational hypertension. This system was prepared by the National Institutes of Health (NIH) Working Group on Hypertension in Pregnancy.[48] Chronic hypertension is defined as persistent blood pressure greater than 140/90 mm Hg observed prior to pregnancy or in the first 20 weeks of gestation. Hypertension that is diagnosed after the 20th week of gestation and accompanied by proteinuria (>300 mg in 24-hour specimen) is defined as preeclampsia. Preeclampsia can be further divided into mild and severe categories based on the presence of at least one of the criteria in Box 2-7. When seizure activity is present, the diagnosis of eclampsia is made. Preeclampsia superimposed on chronic hypertension can have a worse prognosis for mother and fetus than either condition alone. The diagnosis of superimposed preeclampsia can be difficult, and should be suspected when worsening hypertension and new onset or worsening proteinuria is noted. A woman who is noted to have new onset hypertension without proteinuria after 20 weeks' gestation can be classified as having gestational hypertension. Many of these women will go on to develop preeclampsia or be diagnosed post pregnancy with chronic hypertension.

Preeclampsia occurs in about 4% of pregnancies and two thirds of cases occur in nulliparous women.[49] Other risk factors include advanced maternal age, chronic hypertension, chronic renal insufficiency, obesity, diabetes, systemic lupus erythematosus, and multiple gestation. Numerous tests have been proposed for the prediction or early detection of preeclampsia. At present, there is no single screening test that is considered reliable and cost-effective for predicting preeclampsia.[50] Concurrently, numerous trials have described the use of various methods to reduce the rate or severity of preeclampsia. Magnesium, zinc, vitamin C, vitamin E, fish oil, calcium, and low-dose aspirin have all been proposed. Many of these studies show minimal to no benefit or conflicting results and at present none are recommended.

Maternal and neonatal outcomes in preeclampsia depend on the severity of the disease and the gestational age affected, as well as presence of other comorbidities. In a study that examined 10,614,679 singleton pregnancies in the United States from 1995 to 1997 after 24 weeks' gestation, the relative risk for fetal death was 1.4 for any hypertensive disorder and 2.7 for those born to women with chronic hypertensive disorders compared to low-risk controls.[51] Causes of perinatal death in preeclampsia include abruption, placental insufficiency, and prematurity. The perinatal mortality rate is greatest for women with preeclampsia superimposed on preexisting vascular disease. Maternal morbidity and mortality is also increased with preeclampsia. Seizures, pulmonary edema, acute renal or liver failure, liver hemorrhage, disseminated intravascular coagulopathy, and stroke can be seen in severe preeclampsia and are more common in women who develop the disease before 32 weeks' gestation or in those with preexisting medical conditions.[52] The currently used combination of magnesium sulfate and antihypertensive drugs, followed by timely delivery, has reduced the maternal mortality rate to almost zero.

Given the progressive deteriorating course of severe preeclampsia and the increased risk of maternal and neonatal morbidity and mortality, prompt delivery after 34 weeks' gestation is recommended. However, in women with severe persistent symptoms, eclampsia, multiorgan dysfunction, severe fetal growth restriction, abruptio placentae, or nonreassuring fetal testing, the recommendation is to undergo prompt delivery regardless of gestational age.[53] There is disagreement about the treatment of severe preeclampsia before 34 weeks' gestation in which the maternal condition is stable and fetal status is reassuring. Although delivery is always appropriate for the mother, it may not be optimal for the premature fetus. Several studies have shown that with close monitoring, pregnancies with severe preeclampsia can be expectantly managed with good maternal and neonatal outcomes. Continuing a pregnancy long enough to administer corticosteroids has been shown to be beneficial for infants born before 34 weeks' gestation in the setting of severe preeclampsia to reduce the rate of respiratory distress syndrome, neonatal intraventricular hemorrhage, neonatal infection, and neonatal death.

Mild preeclampsia can be expectantly managed until 37 weeks' gestation, when delivery is recommended. At gestational ages less than 37 weeks, inpatient or outpatient management is acceptable depending on patient compliance with home blood pressure and symptom monitoring, resources available to return to the hospital if needed, and ability to maintain modified bed rest. These women need to have twice weekly testing including NST and ultrasound evaluation. Women with gestational hypertension at term with a favorable cervix should be considered for induction of labor.[54]

Intrapartum management of preeclampsia centers on prevention of seizures, detection of fetal heart rate abnormalities, and detection and treatment of worsening maternal disease. Magnesium sulfate is the drug of choice to prevent seizures in women with preeclampsia. The efficacy of magnesium for seizure prevention in severe disease is well established; however, the benefit for women with mild disease remains unclear.[55] Most U.S. investigators recommend prophylactic anticonvulsant therapy for all women with the diagnosis of preeclampsia, regardless of severity. Control of severe hypertension is imperative to prevent cardiovascular and cerebrovascular complications. Recommended agents include hydralazine, labetalol and nifedipine. The mode of delivery is based on obstetric considerations, and a vaginal delivery should be attempted in most women. Continuous fetal heart rate monitoring and evaluation for vaginal bleeding is essential during the labor process. Monitoring for signs of worsening disease with laboratory evaluation is also recommended for some patients. Women with HELLP syndrome—intravascular *h*emolysis, *e*levated *l*iver function test results, and *l*ow *p*latelets (thrombocytopenia)—require more intense monitoring and evaluation.

OBESITY IN PREGNANCY

Obesity is an epidemic in the United States and worldwide. The NIH and the World Health Organization define normal weight and obesity according to body mass index (BMI) as shown in Table 2-8. The Centers for Disease Control and Prevention (CDC) reports that in women of reproductive age in the United States, the prevalence of obesity was 30.2% and the prevalence of overweight was 56.7%. Obesity is a risk factor

Table 2-8.	Normal Weight and Obesity According to Body Mass Index
Weight	**BMI**
Normal	18.5-24.9
Overweight	25-29.9
Obesity class I	30-34.9
Obesity class II	35-39.9
Obesity class III	>40

Adapted from World Health Organization: Obesity: preventing and managing a global epidemic, *World Health Organ Tech Rep Ser* 894:1, 2000.
BMI, Body mass index.

for a number of pregnancy complications. Therefore, as recommended by ACOG in Committee Opinion No. 315, obese women should be encouraged to decrease weight before considering pregnancy.[56] Given the high number of unplanned pregnancies, this goal is often not achieved. In 2009, the Institute of Medicine revised the recommendations for weight gain in pregnancy to account for the increasing prevalence of obesity and the resultant complications.[57]

Miscarriage and recurrent miscarriage are increased in obese women compared to normal weight controls. Fetal malformations, specifically neural tube defects, heart defects, and omphalocele are increased in obesity. Obese gravidas have an increased incidence of gestational diabetes above that in the general obstetrical population (6% to 12% vs. 2% to 4%), and the magnitude of this risk is positively correlated with increases in maternal weight. An association between obesity and hypertensive disorders during pregnancy also exists. A review of 13 cohort studies comprising nearly 1.4 million women found that the risk of preeclampsia doubled with each 5 to 7 kg/m^2 increase in prepregnancy BMI. Because of the underlying medical issues and pregnancy complications present in morbidly obese women, an increased risk of preterm delivery (OR, 1.5; 95% CI, 1.1 to 2.1) is observed compared to normal weight controls.[58]

Obesity is also associated with an increased risk of unexplained stillbirth. Data from the Danish National Birth Cohort noted an increased hazard rate of stillbirth in obese women from 37 to 39 weeks of 3.5 (95% CI, 1.9 to 6.4) and at 40 weeks of 4.6 (95% CI, 1.6 to 13.4).[59] Furthermore, a Canadian study revealed that the factor most strongly associated with unexplained fetal death was increased prepregnancy weight. Fetal

macrosomia, defined as weight greater than 4000 g, is increased in the obese population from 8.3% in nonobese women to 13.3% in the obese, and 14.6% in the morbidly obese. Although the risk of macrosomia is greater in women with gestational diabetes (OR 4.4 versus 1.6), the high prevalence of obesity correlates to a fourfold higher number of large-for-gestational age and macrosomic infants than is seen as a result of diabetes. Being born macrosomic or large for gestational age correlates with an increased risk of obesity in the adolescent and adult years.[60] Macrosomia also contributes to the increased risk for cesarean section in obese gravidas and decreased success when attempting vaginal birth after cesarean section. Increased difficulties with regional and general anesthesia are also concerns and should prompt consideration for antepartum anesthesia consultation.

DIABETIC PREGNANCY

Major advances in the knowledge of carbohydrate metabolism provide the opportunity for improved screening and identification of the gestational diabetic woman.[61] Physiologic studies currently offer a better rationale for management of the chemical and the overt diabetic pregnant woman and her fetus. The increased risks for stillbirth, prematurity, and neonatal morbidity associated with diabetes pose a direct challenge to the efficacy of antenatal surveillance and neonatal intensive care.

Pregnancy increases the risks of adverse outcomes for mother and infant in women with type 1 diabetes. Reducing the risk of adverse outcomes in diabetic pregnancies to the level of risk in nondiabetic pregnancies is a major goal in diabetes care. Tight glycemic control before and during pregnancy is crucial. Preconception care is effective with an approximately threefold reduction in the risk of malformations. Supplementation with folic acid may also reduce the risk of malformations.[62,63] Rapid-acting insulin analogs are regarded as safe to use in pregnancy, and studies on long-acting insulin analogs are in the pipeline. It is imperative to minimize episodes of severe hypoglycemia during pregnancy to optimize outcomes. Screening for diabetic retinopathy, diabetic nephropathy, and thyroid dysfunction is important, and indications for antihypertensive treatment and treatment of thyroid dysfunction need to be in focus before and during pregnancy. Pregnancy in women with pregestational diabetes is associated with high perinatal morbidity and mortality. Stillbirth accounts for the majority of cases of perinatal death. Maternal smoking, hypertension (preeclampsia), and substandard utilization of antenatal care are significantly associated with stillbirths in diabetic women. Intrauterine growth restriction, fetal hypoxia, and congenital malformations may be additional contributing factors, but more than 50% of stillbirths remain unexplained. The majority of stillbirths are characterized by suboptimal glycemic control during pregnancy. Better glycemic control together with regularly scheduled antenatal surveillance tests, including ultrasound examinations of the fetal growth rate, kick counting, and nonstress testing of fetal cardiac function are necessary but do not ensure a favorable outcome. In summary, all known diabetic women should plan their pregnancies and optimize glycemic control preconceptually and throughout pregnancy to reduce the frequency of congenital abnormalities, obstetric complications, and perinatal mortality.

Because of the increasing incidence of type 1 diabetes, the recent emergence of type 2 diabetes as a condition that can begin during childhood, and the increasing prevalence of gestational diabetes mellitus, the number of women who have some form of diabetes during their pregnancies is increasing. Together diabetes and obesity are the most common and important metabolic disorders. These women and their babies are at increased risk of morbidity, not just during pregnancy and birth but for the long term as well. Between 1989 and 2004, the prevalence of gestational diabetes mellitus (GDM) in the United States increased by 122%. Glycosylated hemoglobin, as measured by hemoglobin A1C (A1C), can potentially identify pregnant women at high risk for adverse outcomes associated with GDM, including macrosomia and postpartum glucose intolerance. An elevated hemoglobin A1C at GDM diagnosis was positively associated with postpartum abnormal glucose tolerance. A 1% increase in A1C at GDM diagnosis was associated with 2.36 times higher odds of postpartum abnormal glucose 6 weeks after delivery.[64] Women with pregnancies complicated by preeclampsia or GDM had an increased risk of later diabetes, especially those having GDM.

Leary and associates wrote "The impact of gestational diabetes on maternal and fetal health has been increasingly recognized."[65]

However, universal consensus on the diagnostic methods and thresholds has long been lacking. Published guidelines from major societies differ considerably from one another, ranging in recommendations from aggressive screening to no routine screening at all. As a result, real-world practice is equally varied. The recently published Hyperglycemia and Adverse Pregnancy Outcomes (HAPO) Study,[66] and two randomized controlled trials evaluating treatment of mild maternal hyperglycemia, have confirmed the findings of smaller, nonrandomized studies solidifying the link between maternal hyperglycemia and adverse perinatal outcomes. In response to these studies, the International Association of Diabetes and Pregnancy Study Groups (IADPSG) have formulated new guidelines for screening and diagnosis of diabetes in pregnancy. Key components of the IADPSG guidelines include the recommendation to screen high-risk women at the first encounter for pregestational diabetes, to screen universally at 24 to 28 weeks' gestation, and to screen with the 75-g oral glucose tolerance test interpreting abnormal fasting, 1-hour, and 2-hour plasma glucose concentrations as individually sufficient for the diagnosis of gestational diabetes. The diagnosis of gestational diabetes is made when any of the following three 75-g, 2-hour oral glucose tolerance test thresholds are met or exceeded:

- *Fasting*—92 mg/dL
- *1 hour*—180 mg/dL
- *2 hours*—153 mg/dL

Increases in each of the three values on the 75-g, 2-hour oral glucose tolerance test are associated with graded increases in the likelihood of pregnancy outcomes such as large for gestational age, cesarean section, fetal insulin levels, and neonatal fat content. Furthermore, to translate the continuous association between maternal glucose and adverse outcomes demonstrated in the HAPO cohort, they recommend thresholds for positive screening tests at which the odds of elevated birth weight, cord C-peptide, and fetal body fat percent are 1.75 relative to odds of those outcomes at mean glucose values.[65]

Despite insulin therapy, the perinatal mortality rate among offspring of diabetic mothers remains higher than the general population. Note that the infant survival rate at the Joslin Clinic from 1922 to 1938 was only 54%. From 1938 to 1958, the survival rate improved to 86%, and from 1958 to 1974, a 90% survival was achieved. Thus, the combined toll from stillbirth and neonatal death may persist at five times the rate of nondiabetic women, even at major medical centers. Where care is less intensive, perinatal mortality rate for diabetics of 20% to 30% still exists. Congenital malformations are responsible for 30% to 50% of perinatal deaths in diabetics compared with 20% to 30% in nondiabetics.

Based on the increased risk of stillbirth during the last month of pregnancy, preterm delivery at 36 to 37 weeks' gestation was the generally accepted recommendation for many years. Möller was one of the first to strive for an avoidance of premature deliveries.[67] In 1970, she reported from Sweden a series of diabetic women carried closer to term when blood sugar regulation comparable to the nondiabetic pregnancy had been achieved and when evidence of fetal jeopardy or pregnancy complications such as toxemia did not appear. The perinatal mortality rate in her series of 47 patients was 2.1% as compared with a 21% mortality rate in a prior series from the same obstetric unit.

Similar favorable results have been reported from other institutions in Europe and in the United States.[68-70] Gyves and coworkers described a reduction in perinatal mortality rate from 13.5% to 4.1% in a group of 96 diabetic patients in whom the modern technology was applied and preterm delivery was not routinely employed.[68] These statistics continue to improve.

> **EDITORIAL COMMENT:** On the basis of a literature review, Syed and colleagues concluded that optimal control of serum blood glucose versus suboptimal control was associated with a significant reduction in the risk of perinatal mortality but not stillbirths.[71] Preconception care of diabetes (information about need for optimization of glycemic control before pregnancy, assessment of diabetes complications, review of dietary habits, intensification of capillary blood glucose self-monitoring, and optimization of insulin therapy) versus none was associated with a reduction in perinatal mortality. They estimate that the stillbirth rate can be reduced by 10%.

For many years, good control of maternal blood sugar concentration has been considered important for the well-being of the fetus of the diabetic mother. However, wide differences of opinion exist as to what constitutes good control. The fasting plasma glucose concentration in pregnancy, in normal and diabetic mothers, has been shown to be lower than in women in the nongravid state. The continuous siphoning of glucose by the fetus profoundly affects maternal carbohydrate metabolism and, as a result, fasting glucose levels are 15 to 20 mg/dL lower during pregnancy than postpartum. Physiologic studies describing diurnal profiles for blood glucose concentrations in normal pregnancies have shown a remarkable constancy of these concentrations throughout the day. The fetus is thus, under normal circumstances, provided with a constant glucose environment.

These physiologic principles have provided a rational basis for the care of pregnant diabetic women, and the importance of rigid blood glucose control has been illustrated by several clinical studies. The marked improvement in perinatal mortality rates and morbidity obtained by Möller and Gyves and colleagues was with a mean preprandial blood glucose concentration kept close to 100 mg/dL, particularly during the third trimester.[67,68] The latter series also described a significant reduction in macrosomia among the infants of such well-controlled diabetic mothers. Karlsson and Kjellmer reported that their perinatal mortality rate could be directly correlated with maternal mean blood glucose concentrations.[72] When mean concentrations were greater than 150 mg/dL, the mortality rate was 23.6%. At concentrations between 100 and 150 mg/dL, the rate declined to 15.3%, and at less than 100 mg/dL, mortality of 3.8% was achieved. The King's College group in London reported on deliveries of 100 diabetic pregnant women in whom the mean preprandial blood glucose concentrations were maintained at approximately 100 mg/dL. There was no perinatal loss in this series.

Because improvements in obstetric and neonatal management have evolved over the same time span as these studies of intensive blood sugar control, it is difficult to attribute marked improvements in outcome to only one variable. Nevertheless, it seems prudent that the therapeutic objective in pregnant diabetic patients be an effort at normalization of plasma glucose throughout the day. This approach should apply to the woman with gestational diabetes as well as to the woman who was diabetic before pregnancy.[73]

Principles of Management of Diabetes in Pregnancy

1. Metabolic derangements are the major abnormality affecting individuals with diabetes mellitus.

Table 2-9.	Clinical Status of Diabetes: Timing of Assessments		
Assessment	**Noninsulin-Dependent**	**Insulin-Dependent, No Vasculopathy**	**Insulin-Dependent, with Vasculopathy**
MATERNAL			
History/physical examination	Preconceptual/initial visit	Preconceptual/initial visit	Preconceptual/initial visit
Ophthalmologic evaluation*			
No known abnormality	Preconceptual/initial visit	Preconceptual/early first trimester	Preconceptual/early first trimester
Known abnormality	Each trimester	Each trimester	Each trimester as indicated
Electrocardiogram[†]	NI	Preconceptual/initial visit[‡]	Preconceptual/initial visit[†]
Prenatal screen panel and bacteriuria screen	Preconceptual/initial visit	Preconceptual/initial visit	Preconceptual/initial visit
Glycosylated proteins[‡]	NI	Initial visit/delivery[‡]	Initial visit/delivery[‡]
Thyroid panel screen	NI	Preconceptual/initial visit (repeat monthly until normal)	Preconceptual/initial visit (repeat monthly until normal)
Creatinine clearance	NI	Preconceptual/initial visit (if abnormal, each trimester)	Preconceptual/initial visit (if abnormal, each trimester)
Urine protein			
Dipstick	Serially	Serially	Serially
24 h	NI	≥1 + by dipstick	≥1 + by dipstick
Lipid profile	NI	Preconceptual/initial visit	Preconceptual/initial visit
FETAL		**Weeks' Gestation**	
Alpha-fetoprotein (maternal serum)	16-18	16-18	16-18
Ultrasonography			
Dating/anomaly screen	18-22	18-23	18-22
Echocardiography	NI	20-24	20-24
Fetal growth/development	37-39[§]	30-32; 37-39	30-32; 37-39
Fetal movement[§]	36 to intervention[§]	34 to intervention[§]	30 to intervention[§]
CST/NST (biophysical profile: backup)[§]	NI	32-34 to intervention[§]	32-34 to intervention[§]
Lung maturity documentation	If intervention <38 wk	If intervention <39 wk	If intervention <39 wk

From *Guidelines for care: California diabetes and pregnancy program,* Maternal and Child Health Branch, Department of Health Services, 1986.
NI, Not routinely indicated.
*Implies pupillary dilation.
[†]Advised with diabetes >10 yr duration or known cardiovascular disease or abnormal lipid profile.
[‡]More frequently if used as compliance evaluator.
[§]Earlier or more frequent assessment dependent on clinical status (e.g., evidence of intrauterine growth restriction or multiple gestation).

2. Pregnant women with diabetes should be managed by suitably trained individuals and teams who comprehensively monitor mother and fetus throughout pregnancy (Table 2-9).
3. Optimal care of women with diabetes must begin before conception because it has been demonstrated that careful preconception control of diabetes reduces the incidence of major anomalies.
4. All pregnancies should be screened so that women with gestational diabetes can be identified and appropriately managed.

Management of Diabetic Women Before Conception

The rationale of the preconception program for diabetic women is to optimize the pregnancy outcome for the woman and her offspring. Optimal care of gravidas with prepregnancy diabetes must begin before conception. A well-disciplined, well-coordinated, and well-organized multidisciplinary team and a compliant patient are the prime ingredients for a successful pregnancy outcome. The team comprises internists, perinatologists, and selected other medical subspecialists; a nutritionist, a social worker, and other perinatal nurse specialists who coordinate the dietary needs; and specialists in ongoing education, exercise, and blood glucose regulation. The goal is to achieve a mean fasting glucose of less than 92 mg/dL and a 2-hour postprandial level around 120 mg/dL. Glycosylated hemoglobin should be maintained within the normal range. The objective is to achieve glycemic control before conception and throughout embryogenesis and then continue throughout gestation. In this way, major abnormalities may be averted. In addition, prophylactic folate supplementation is advocated during the periconceptual period to reduce the risk of neural tube defects. Strict glucose control may also diminish other perinatal complications including intrauterine demise, macrosomia, and neonatal disorders such as hypoglycemia and polycythemia in addition to a cardiomyopathy. Ongoing surveillance, continued education, and careful monitoring throughout the pregnancy are necessary to achieve optimal maternal and perinatal outcome.

Outpatient management of the diabetic pregnancy has replaced the obligatory period of hospitalization. However, in the face of deteriorating glycemic control, maternal complications including hypertensive disorders, infection, preterm labor, or evidence of fetal compromise, hospitalization is mandated. A comprehensive program devised by the California Maternal and Child Health Division is outlined in Table 2-9.

A critical determinant of the outcome of diabetic pregnancy is the timing of delivery. The risk of intrauterine death increases as term approaches. Alternatively, the infant delivered preterm is exposed to the risks of prematurity, particularly that of respiratory distress, which may result in neonatal loss. The risk of RDS is higher in diabetic pregnancies compared with nondiabetic pregnancies. Over the past 35 years, the feasibility of extending the gestational period and of individualizing delivery timing for the diabetic mother has been enhanced by the availability of objective tests for fetal surveillance.

Because the major consequence of premature birth is respiratory distress, fetal pulmonary functional maturity is the most critical objective of current care. Biochemical estimations of this maturity can be obtained from the amniotic fluid with either the L:S ratio or the foam stability test.[74,75] These determinations provide an important dimension in the management of the pregnant diabetic woman, particularly when maternal blood sugar control has been good and a normal physiologic milieu has been approximated.

> **EDITORIAL COMMENT:** Despite technological advances in the field, testing for fetal lung maturity at a more advanced gestational age (>36 weeks) is neither reliable nor cost effective. Data mandate reconsideration of our current recommendation of amniocentesis to confirm fetal lung maturity prior to elective delivery at 36 to 39 weeks' gestation in well-dated pregnancies.

Congenital malformations have assumed a major role in diabetic pregnancies. In a prospective study, Simpson et al[76] documented a 6.6% incidence of major anomalies among offspring of diabetic mothers as compared with a 2.4% incidence in control mothers. (Other centers report even higher rates.) Because the anomaly rate in those patients whose diabetes was aggressively managed was similar to that observed by others in patients whose diabetes was less vigorously managed, the researchers hypothesized that abnormal development had occurred before the patients entered the study. There is a major emphasis on carefully managing diabetes before conception and even in the first trimester to reduce the high anomaly rate associated with diabetic pregnancies.

Patients with high hemoglobin (Hb) A_{1C} (variably defined as greater than 7.99 or greater than 9.0) have extremely high (22.5% to 40%) risk of congenital malformation compared with women whose HbA_{1C} is less than that level (5%). This is supported by data generated by Ylinen et al,[77] who measured maternal HbA_{1C} as an indication of maternal hyperglycemia during pregnancy to determine its relationship to fetal malformations. Maternal HbA_{1C} was measured at least once before the end of the fifteenth week of gestation in 139 insulin-dependent patients who delivered after 24 weeks' gestation. The mean initial HbA_{1C} was 9.5% of the total hemoglobin concentration in the 17 pregnancies complicated by malformations, which was significantly higher than in pregnancies without malformations (8.0%). Fetal anomalies occurred in 6 of 17 cases (35%) with values initially of 8% to 9.9%, and only 3 of 63 (5%) anomalies occurred in babies of patients who had an initial level less than 8%. These data support the notion that there is an increased risk of malformation associated with poor glucose control. Unplanned pregnancies should be avoided in diabetic women, and determination of HbA_{1C} before conception may assist in planning the optimal time for conception.

The application of current technology provides the clinical team with the means of minimizing both fetal death in utero and preventable neonatal morbidity and mortality from the hazards of prematurity. Together with intensive control of maternal blood glucose, the technology of fetal surveillance offers the possibility of normalizing perinatal outcomes in large numbers of diabetic pregnancies.

The definition of macrosomia may be a birth weight more than 4000 or 4500 or 5000 g or, if you are a stickler for taking gender and gestational age into consideration, a birth weight above the 90th percentile for gestation, or, if you are a statistical purist, above the 97.75th percentile of a reference population corrected for gestational age and sex have been proposed. Whatever you select, these are large babies with considerable risk for morbidity before, during, and after birth. Because the number of adverse outcomes increases substantially above 4500 g, this is widely accepted. Macrosomia

is associated with a higher risk of emergency cesarean section, longer maternal hospital stay of >3 days, and a four times higher risk of shoulder dystocia, together with a greater need for neonatal resuscitation and intensive care admission of the babies.

PRETERM LABOR AND PRETERM DELIVERY

Preterm birth, defined as birth before 37 weeks' gestation, remains an unsolved problem of paramount importance in perinatal medicine. The rate of preterm delivery in the United States has increased over 33% in the past 25 years from 9.4% in 1981 to approximately 12.8% in 2006 (one in eight births).[79] Although advances in neonatal intensive care have improved outcomes for preterm infants, the complications of prematurity remain the most common underlying cause of perinatal and infant morbidity and mortality. Approximately 75% of preterm births occur between 34 and 36 weeks' gestation, and although these infants experience morbidity, the majority of perinatal mortality and serious morbidity occurs among the 15% of preterm infants who are born before 32 weeks' gestation.

Preterm birth may fall into two broad categories: spontaneous preterm birth or indicated preterm birth. Spontaneous preterm birth includes preterm labor with intact membranes, preterm premature rupture of membranes (PPROM) prior to the onset of labor, and cervical insufficiency. Indicated preterm births are those that occur secondary to an underlying fetal or maternal medical conditions or compromise. Seventy-five percent of all preterm births are spontaneous, whereas the remaining 25% are indicated. Although a distinction between indicated and spontaneous preterm birth may not always be clear or clinically evident, the distinction provides a conceptual framework for evaluating etiologies and trends of preterm birth. Notably, the overall rise in preterm birth rate in the United States is largely attributed to indicated preterm birth. This rise in preterm birth has been accompanied by an overall decline in fetal mortality, which suggests that this rise may reflect improved perinatal care (Fig. 2-6).

Spontaneous preterm birth represents a multifactorial disorder in which multiple modifiable and nonmodifiable risk factors interact, predispose, and cause disease. Maternal characteristics and behavior,

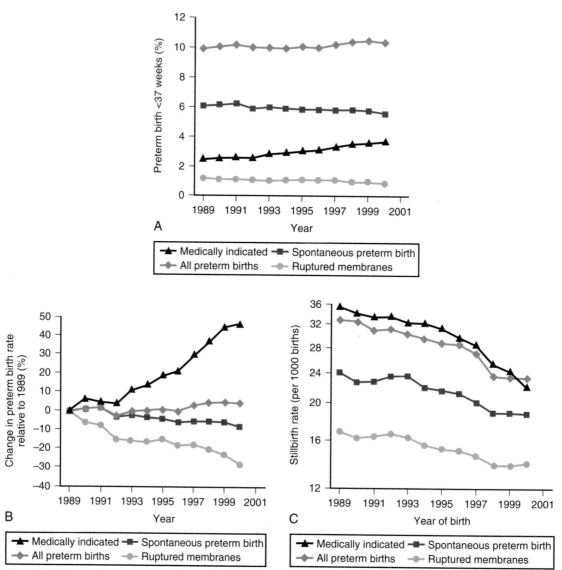

Figure 2-6. Temporal change in singleton preterm births < 37 weeks: overall, medically indicated, from spontaneous preterm labor, from ruptured membranes, and from stillbirth. **A,** Rates in each group by year. **B,** Change (%) in rates relative to 1989. **C,** Trend of stillbirth by year. *(Adapted from Ananth CVP, Joseph KSM, Oyelese YM, et al: Trends in preterm birth and perinatal mortality among singletons: United States, 1989 through 2000,* Obstet Gynecol *105:1084, 2005.)*

maternal reproductive history, and characteristics of the index pregnancy all affect the risk of preterm delivery (Box 2-8). Although risk factors may identify patients at risk for preterm birth, many preterm deliveries occur in women without risk factors.

The diagnosis and treatment of preterm labor remains a challenging, inexact process for a multitude of reasons: the signs and symptoms of early preterm labor are often noted in normal pregnancy (menstrual-like cramping, low back or abdominal pain, nausea), the progression from subclinical to overt preterm labor may be gradual and

unpredictable, and no threshold of contraction frequency has been shown to correlate with the risk of preterm delivery. Traditional diagnostic criteria—persistent uterine contractions accompanied by dilation and/or effacement of the cervix—demonstrate reasonable accuracy if contraction frequency is greater than 6 per hour and cervical dilation is greater than or equal to 3 cm and effacement is 80% or greater. However, many symptomatic women present with lower thresholds of cervical dilation or progression, and therefore, over-diagnosis remains prevalent. Initial evaluation includes a detailed

Box 2-8.	Risk Factors that Increase Risk of Spontaneous Preterm Delivery

Nonmodifiable

Familial Risk

Low socioeconomic status

Low education status

Low or high maternal age (<18 or >40 years)

African-American race

Uterine anomalies

Prior spontaneous PTD

Multiple gestation

ART (singleton or multiple gestation)

Uterine volume

Cervical length ("short cervix")

Modifiable

Maternal smoking

Substance abuse

Nutritional status (low BMI)

Genital tract infection/colonization

Prior pelvic surgery

?Antenatal stress or depression

ART, Assisted reproductive technology; PTD, preterm delivery.

obstetric and medical history, physical examination, establishment of gestational age, evaluation of fetal status (monitoring or ultrasound), and a consideration of other etiologies (PPROM, cervical insufficiency, abruption), and an evaluation for underlying infection. Transvaginal ultrasound and/or fetal fibronectin (fFN) testing in cervicovaginal fluid may improve diagnostic accuracy and decrease false-positive diagnoses. Women with a cervical length of 30 mm by transvaginal ultrasound are at a very low risk for preterm delivery.[80] These women may be discharged home after a period of observation with confirmation of fetal well being, lack of cervical change, and exclusion of a precipitating event. Fetal fibronectin, a glycoprotein thought to promote cellular adhesion at the fetal-maternal interface, is released into cervicovaginal secretions when the chorionic/decidual interface is disrupted. Although this is a likely candidate to predict preterm labor and preterm delivery if present, numerous studies have demonstrated that the principal utility of fFN testing rests in the very high negative predictive value (>99% for prediction of preterm labor and preterm delivery in the next 14 days). The positive predictive value (less than 30% in most populations) limits the utility of a positive test.[81] Therefore, negative tests remain highly useful in the initial triage of patients presenting with symptoms of preterm labor because patients with negative tests may reliably be discharged home.

After diagnosis of acute preterm labor and prior to the initiation of treatment, contraindications must be excluded and gestational age must be established. Contraindications to tocolysis include placental abruption, chorioamnionitis, fetal demise, and acute fetal or maternal compromise, among others. Regarding gestational age, the lower limit at which therapy should be offered is controversial and no definitive data from randomized trials exist to support a recommendation. However, greater consensus regarding an upper gestational age limit exists. At 34 weeks' gestation, the perinatal morbidity and mortality are too low to justify the potential maternal and fetal complications or cost associated with inhibition of labor. Treatment of preterm labor consists of administration of GBS prophylaxis, magnesium sulfate for neuroprotection if appropriate (see later discussion), and the administration of tocolytic therapy to inhibit uterine contractions and antenatal corticosteroids.

The goal of tocolysis is to reduce neonatal morbidity and mortality long enough to allow for the administration of antenatal corticosteroids and maternal transport to an appropriately equipped hospital. Metaanalyses have demonstrated the utility of tocolytic therapy for preterm labor in that all agents were more effective than no therapy or placebo at delaying delivery for 48 hours to 7 days. However, this prolongation was not associated with a statistically significant decrease in respiratory distress or neonatal death.[82] Tocolytic therapy includes many classes of drugs: calcium channel blockers, cyclooxygenase inhibitors, magnesium sulfate, oxytocin antagonists, nitric oxide donors, and beta-mimetics. However, no tocolytic drug is currently FDA-approved for the indication of arresting labor. Selection of appropriate tocolytic therapy requires consideration of the maternal and fetal risk, efficacy, and side effects. A detailed discussion of the numerous trials comparing tocolytic agents is beyond the scope of this discussion. However, recent evidence shows the following:[83]

- Nifedipine and indomethacin are suggested first-line agents, with some authorities suggesting indomethacin as the first-line agent in patients less than 32 weeks who are also receiving magnesium sulfate for

Table 2-10.	Impact of 17-OHP on Spontaneous Preterm Delivery			
	N*	<37 wk (%)	<35 wk (%)	<32 wk (%)
Placebo	153	54.9	30.7	19.6
17OHP	306	36.3	20.6	11.4

Adapted from Meis PJ, Klebanoff M, Thom E, et al: Prevention of recurrent preterm delivery by 17α-hydroxyprogesterone caproate, *N Engl J Med* 348:2379, 2003.
17-OHP, 17α-hydroxyprogesterone.

neuroprotection (potential for increased maternal adverse events with simultaneous use of magnesium sulfate and a calcium channel blocker).

- Magnesium sulfate should be used with caution as a primary tocolytic, given that data support less efficacy and increased side effects or adverse events.
- The use of multiple tocolytic agents ("double tocolysis") should be performed with caution because the propensity for adverse events increases and no evidence supports increased efficacy.
- Data from poorly designed studies do not support maintenance or repeat tocolysis after initial inhibition of preterm labor.

Although the identification and inhibition of acute preterm labor remains an important strategy aimed at reducing neonatal morbidity and mortality, primary prevention strategies have remained slow to develop owing to the multifactorial, complex pathophysiology of preterm labor and delivery. However, over the past 10 years, secondary prevention has made a marked impact on recurrent preterm delivery. Meis et al published a landmark trial in 2003 demonstrating a decrease in recurrent,[84] spontaneous preterm delivery for women receiving weekly intramuscular (IM) injections of 17α-hydroxyprogesterone caproate (17-OHP) from 16 to 36 weeks (Table 2-10). Notably, the risk reduction increased with earlier gestational age of the index preterm delivery. Subsequent studies confirmed that supplementation in multiple gestation does not provide any benefit. With primary preventive strategies still in development, secondary prevention with 17-OHP has been estimated to save in excess of $2 billion annually in the United States alone.[85]

PRETERM PREMATURE RUPTURE OF THE MEMBRANES

Preterm premature rupture of the membranes (PPROM), defined as spontaneous membrane rupture before labor *and* before 37 weeks' gestational age, occurs in

Box 2-9.	Factors and Etiologies of PPROM

Amniocentesis
Cerclage
Cervical insufficiency
Cigarette smoking
Collagen defect or degradation
Low socioeconomic status
History of cervical conization
History of preterm delivery
History of PPROM
Sexually transmitted infection
Other choriodecidual infection or inflammation
Uterine overdistention (polyhydramnios, multifetal gestation)
Vaginal bleeding in pregnancy (subchorionic hemorrhage, abruption, abnormal placentation)

PPROM, Prolonged premature rupture of membranes.

approximately 3% of pregnancies and affects more than 120,000 pregnancies annually in the United States. PPROM is responsible for more than one third of all preterm births and remains an important cause of maternal, fetal, and neonatal morbidity and mortality. The etiology of PPROM is multifactorial, and many patients will have multiple risk and etiologic factors (Box 2-9). Many of these factors are involved with pathways that result in accelerated membrane weakening such as increased stretch or degradation from local inflammation or ascending infection. A history of early preterm birth (23 to 27 weeks) after PPROM is the strongest risk factor for PPROM, which carries a three-fold increase in risk of recurrence. In the majority of cases, an exact etiology of PPROM remains unknown after diagnosis.

The frequency and severity of neonatal complications after PPROM vary with gestational age at which membrane rupture and delivery occur. Additional factors that increase perinatal morbidity and mortality are perinatal infection, placental abruption, and umbilical cord compression. The most notable morbidities include respiratory distress syndrome, necrotizing enterocolitis, intraventricular hemorrhage, and sepsis, which are common with early preterm birth. However, the risk of sepsis is twofold higher in the context of PPROM relative to preterm labor without PPROM. With conservative management after PPROM, the risk of intrauterine fetal demise is approximately 1% to 2%. Additionally, with expectant or conservative management of PPROM in the early midtrimester, the risk of pulmonary hypoplasia increases with estimated risks of 0% to 26% of births after PPROM at 16 to 26 weeks' gestation and approximately 50% when PPROM occurs before 20 weeks.

In the majority of cases, PPROM can be diagnosed clinically by a combination of clinical suspicion, patient history, and physical examination. Notably, patient history has 90% accuracy for diagnosis of PPROM. Physical examination should include a sterile speculum investigation with collection of fluid from the posterior vaginal fornix to evaluate by the nitrazine and ferning tests. Both of these tests are highly sensitive and specific for the diagnosis of PPROM, with nitrazine being more susceptible to contamination. In rare cases where history and examination remain equivocal, a dye test by amniocentesis (intrauterine injection of indigo carmine followed by observation for passage of blue fluid onto a perineal pad) may be performed to confirm PPROM. Notably, digital cervical examination should be avoided because multiple trials have demonstrated decreased latency periods with one to two cervical examinations in patients with PPROM.

Given that gestational age at membrane rupture and delivery substantially affects the risk of perinatal morbidity and mortality, a gestational-age based model guides management in the context of PPROM. This model balances the risks of fetal and neonatal complications with immediate delivery compared with the potential risks and benefits of conservative management to prolong pregnancy. Although practice variation exists, a few general principles and trials deserve attention:
- Gestational age must be established based on clinical history and ultrasound evaluation.
- Ultrasound should be performed to evaluate fetal growth, position, amniotic fluid volume, and anatomy.
- Women with PPROM must undergo clinical evaluation for preterm labor, chorioamnionitis, placental abruption, or fetal distress, which are indications for delivery independent of gestational age.
- A patient must be admitted to a facility that is appropriately equipped to provide emergent obstetric services as well as neonatal intensive care, and therefore transfer may be appropriate.

A large National Institute of Child Health and Human Development Maternal-Fetal Medicine Units Network (NICHD-MFMU) study demonstrated the safety and efficacy of intravenous erythromycin and ampicillin followed by oral therapy to complete a 1-week course. In this trial, antibiotics improved neonatal outcomes by reducing the risk of death, RDS, early neonatal sepsis, severe intraventricular hemorrhage, severe necrotizing enterocolitis, patent ductus arteriosus, and bronchopulmonary dysplasia (from 53% to 44%; $p < .05$). A decrease in amnionitis and increase in latency of at least 1 week was also demonstrated.[86]

Several studies have evaluated other antibiotic regimens. The use of oral amoxicillin-clavulanic acid has been associated with an increased risk of necrotizing enterocolitis and should be avoided. The algorithm in Figure 2-7 outlines the management of PPROM by gestational age.

CERVICAL INSUFFICIENCY

Cervical insufficiency describes a presumed physical or structural weakness that causes or contributes to the loss of an otherwise healthy pregnancy. Classically, cervical insufficiency manifests in the midtrimester with painless cervical dilation. Although anatomic, biochemical, and clinical evidence supports structural weakness as an underlying cause of midtrimester birth, cervical integrity or competence represents only one variable of a multifactorial problem. Other factors such as uterine overdistention, hemorrhage, decidual infection, or inflammation may trigger the parturition process leading to changes that ripen, shorten, or weaken the cervix. When this occurs, the clinical presentation may be indistinguishable from so-called "weakness"-mediated cervical insufficiency. Therefore, in the absence of definitive tests to discriminate between underlying etiologies or mechanisms, cervical insufficiency may be defined when other variables (labor, intrauterine infection, hemorrhage, etc.) that may precipitate midtrimester loss are not clinically evident.

Many patients who present with cervical insufficiency do not have underlying

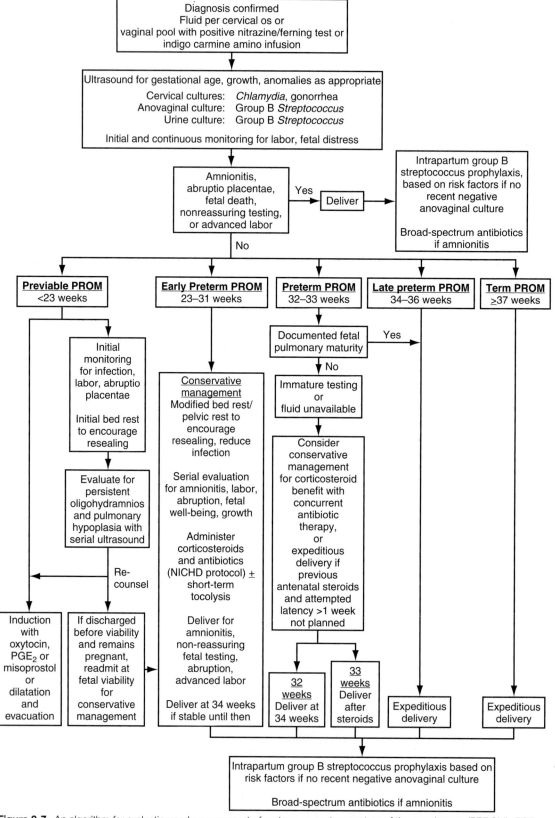

Figure 2-7. An algorithm for evaluation and management of preterm premature rupture of the membranes (PPROM). *PGE₂;* Prostaglandin E₂; *NICHD,* National Institute of Child Health and Human Development (Maternal-Fetal Medicine Units Network). *(From Mercer BM: Treatment of preterm premature rupture of the membranes,* Obstet Gynecol *101(1):178, 2003.)*

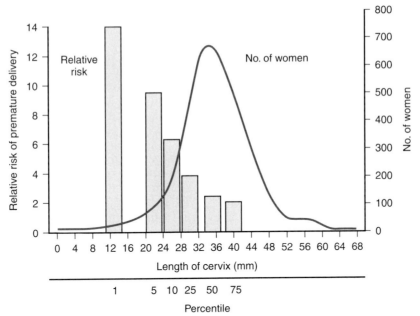

Figure 2-8. Distribution of subjects among percentiles for cervical length measured by transvaginal ultrasonography at 24 weeks of gestation (*solid line*) and relative risk of spontaneous preterm delivery before 35 weeks of gestation according to percentiles for cervical length (*bars*). *(From Creasy RK, Resnik R: Preterm labor and delivery. In Creasy RK, Resnik R, editors:* Maternal-fetal medicine, *ed 4, Philadelphia, 1999, WB Saunders.)*

risk factors. However, some patients may have congenital or acquired forms of cervical insufficiency that include those with a history of collagen disorders (e.g., Ehlers-Danlos syndrome), uterine anomalies, diethylstilbestrol (DES) exposure, prior cervical trauma, or surgery. Notably, the cervix is a dynamic organ and it undergoes various biological changes during normal pregnancy, parturition, and postpartum, which include softening, ripening, dilation, and repair.[87] In normal pregnancies, the cervix begins to efface at 32 to 34 weeks' gestation in preparation for term birth. Over the past 15 years, cervical length (measured by transvaginal ultrasound) has emerged as a notable risk factor for preterm delivery. A landmark study by Iams and coworkers, published in 1996, demonstrated a few important principles: (1) cervical length is normally distributed in the population (Fig. 2-8); (2) the risk of spontaneous preterm birth before 35 weeks' gestation increases as cervical length shortens, particularly for those in the lowest quartile of the distribution. Although ultrasound may identify women at risk for preterm delivery due to a "short" cervix, ultrasound cannot distinguish the diagnosis of cervical insufficiency compared to other causes of premature cervical effacement. Attempts to characterize the cervix with percentile cervical length alone

or in combination with other sonographic characteristics to predict cervical insufficiency have been unsuccessful.

Therefore, cervical insufficiency remains a clinical diagnosis informed by history, physical examination, and ultrasound evaluation. Notable historical factors include the following: history of cervical trauma; repeat midtrimester pregnancy loss; absence of painful contractions, bleeding or infection; advanced cervical dilation or effacement on presentation; and ultrasound findings of a cervical length less than the tenth percentile before 24 weeks' gestation. Notable elements of a physical exam include a speculum evaluation for prolapsing or "hourglassing" membranes, which are always abnormal, and a sterile vaginal exam to evaluate for advanced dilation or effacement. A comprehensive physical evaluation for symptoms of intrauterine infection (tachycardia, uterine tenderness) should also be completed. Laboratory evaluation includes a white blood count to exclude leukocytosis. Some authorities recommend amniocentesis to exclude intrauterine infection (glucose >20 mg/dL) prior to offering treatment with an emergent cerclage. The treatment of cervical insufficiency may vary based on gestational age at presentation and on the history and clinical scenario.

Presentation with Unanticipated Advanced Cervical Dilation or Effacement

Management of cervical insufficiency in the emergent setting (when advanced dilation or effacement is discovered <24 weeks' gestation in the absence of infection, hemorrhage, or labor) remains controversial. Very limited data exist to guide management; however, data from one small randomized trial and a larger observational trial suggest that increased gestational time can be gained by placement of an emergent cerclage compared with expectant management.[88] The benefits of this increased latency remain unclear because many patients deliver children at the threshold of viability who suffer from the complications and sequelae of extreme prematurity. A retrospective study of 116 patients with emergent cerclage placement concluded that nulliparity, the presence of prolapsing membranes beyond the external cervical os, and gestational age less than 22 weeks at the time of cerclage placement are associated with a decreased likelihood of delivery at or after 28 weeks' gestation.[89] Additionally, the risks of cerclage placement, particularly membrane rupture, increase with the degree of cervical dilation and effacement as well as the gestational age at the time of placement. These factors should inform counseling regarding emergent cerclage and the decision should be individualized to the clinical scenario at hand.

Documented History of Cervical Insufficiency

Patients with a history of cervical insufficiency in a previous pregnancy may be followed by either serial ultrasound surveillance of cervical length or with prophylactic cerclage, which is generally placed between 12 to 15 weeks' gestation. Recommendations may include history-indicated prophylactic cerclage over ultrasound surveillance when history is confirmed. Prophylactic cerclage is an accepted treatment in this subset of patients with success rates reported to be as high as 75% to 90%.

Incidental Observation of Short Cervix by Ultrasound

This increasingly common scenario has no evidence-based recommendation for management. Many of these women are asymptomatic and short cervix is discovered incidentally by a midtrimester ultrasound to assess fetal anatomy. Women with singleton pregnancies with cervical shortening and normal obstetric histories do not benefit from cerclage.[90] Preliminary evidence for treatment with vaginal progesterone to decrease the risk of preterm delivery in asymptomatic women with an incidentally discovered short cervix exists, and an ongoing multicenter randomized control trial of 17-OHP in nulliparous women with incidentally discovered short cervix is ongoing.[91]

Women with a History of Spontaneous Preterm Delivery

Data from a recent randomized controlled trial supports a role for cerclage placement for women with a history of preterm birth (defined between 16 and 34 weeks). As a part of this trial, 301 women with a history of preterm birth were screened with serial cervical length assessment beginning at 16 weeks, and those with a cervical length below 25 mm were randomly assigned to cerclage or no cerclage. Cerclage did not result in a significant reduction in the primary outcome of preterm birth before 35 weeks for the study cohort (OR 0.67, 95% CI 0.42 to 1.07) except in the women with cervical length less than 15 mm (OR 0.23, 95% CI 0.08 to 0.66). Additionally, the cerclage group was noted to have improvement in the following secondary outcomes: perinatal death (8.8% vs. 16%), birth before 24 weeks (6.1% vs. 14%), and birth before 37 weeks (45% vs. 60%).[92] This benefit was also reaffirmed by an individual, patient-level metaanalysis that demonstrated a reduction in composite perinatal morbidity and mortality as well as preterm birth at <24, 28, 32, and 37 weeks' gestation.[93]

INTRAUTERINE GROWTH RESTRICTION (IUGR)

Identifying a fetus at risk for or with growth restriction remains a major focus of prenatal care. The classification of newborns by birth weight percentile cannot be understated because there is an inverse relationship between birth weight and adverse perinatal outcomes: newborns in the lowest percentiles are at increased risk of immediate perinatal morbidity and mortality (Fig. 2-9) as well as subsequent adult cardiovascular disease (hypertension, hyperlipidemia, coronary artery disease, diabetes mellitus) as described in the Barker hypothesis. In the 1960s, Lubchenco and colleagues published a series of classic papers with detailed graphs depicting birth weight as a function of gestational age and adverse outcomes. Since

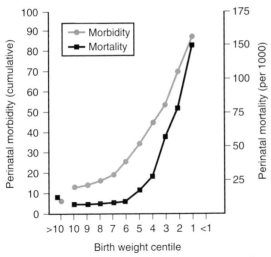

Figure 2-9. Relationship between birth weight percentiles and adverse perinatal outcomes in infants with intrauterine growth restriction. *(From Creasy RK, Resnik R: Intrauterine growth restriction. In Creasy RK, Resnik R, editors: Maternal-fetal medicine, ed 4, Philadelphia, 1999, WB Saunders.)*

Box 2-10.	**Factors and Disorders Associated with Intrauterine Growth Rate**

Maternal factors
Hypertensive disease, chronic or preeclampsia
Renal disease
Diabetes mellitus
Antiphospholipid syndrome
Hemoglobinopathy
Collagen vascular disease
Severe nutrition deficiency (inflammatory bowel disease, poor weight gain, low pregnancy BMI)
Smoking and substance abuse
Maternal hypoxia (cyanotic heart disease, lung disease, high altitude)
Medications

Fetal factors
Multiple gestation
Placental abnormalities
Infection (viral, protozoal)
Congenital anomalies
Chromosomal abnormalities

BMI, Body mass index.

that time, various classification schemes and terminology have been adapted to describe infants that fail to reach their growth potential, such as "premature," "low birth weight," "small for gestational age," "small for dates," or "growth restricted." The evolution of these differing terms highlights the complexity of this problem as well as the difficulty of establishing uniform diagnostic criteria. The most common definition for IUGR today is an estimated fetal weight less than the 10% for gestational age by ultrasound evaluation. However, this criteriun remains controversial given that it relies on a population-based reference standard and does not provide a means to distinguish fetuses that are constitutionally small, growth restricted and small, and growth restricted but not small. Studies evaluating customized, individual fetal growth curves have been published in Spain, France, and New Zealand and demonstrate improved accuracy in detecting fetuses at risk for adverse outcome but are not currently employed in the United States.[94-97]

Numerous maternal and fetal factors have been associated with IUGR and these etiologies are listed in Box 2-10. Often, the underlying etiology is clinically apparent and in such cases a diagnosis and management plan can be established. In other cases, the underlying cause may be more elusive. Importantly, an attempt should be made to determine the cause antenatally to provide appropriate counseling and management plans. Additionally, the underlying etiology may have implications for future pregnancies. Therefore, when IUGR is identified, additional testing such as a detailed anatomic ultrasound evaluation, karyotype, or evaluation for viral infections may be warranted—depending on the clinical scenario.

Typically, the fundal height measurement in centimeters should approximate the weeks of gestational age. Therefore, a fundal height measurement significantly less than the estimated gestational age may suggest an IUGR fetus. However, clinical diagnosis of IUGR is inaccurate. In fact, studies demonstrate that with the use of physical exam alone, IUGR remains undetected or is incorrectly diagnosed in about 50% of cases. Currently, ultrasound is the preferred modality for the diagnosis of IUGR. Therefore, one essential principle of the antenatal recognition of IUGR is identification of the maternal and fetal risk factors that may prompt ultrasound surveillance.

Ultrasound measurements of the biparietal diameter, head circumference, abdominal circumference, and femur length are four standard measurements used to estimate fetal weight and allow for the determination of the pattern of growth aberration.

Symmetrical IUGR, which accounts for approximately 20% to 30% of cases, occurs after an insult early in pregnancy (infection, drug or environmental exposure, chromosomal abnormality) affects fetal growth equally at all morphologic parameters. Conversely, asymmetrical IUGR occurs more frequently and results from placental insufficiency later in pregnancy. In asymmetrical IUGR, the femur length and head circumference are preserved but the abdominal circumference is decreased secondary to the redistribution of blood flow to vital organs (heart, brain, placenta) at the expense of less vital organs (lungs, abdominal viscera, skin). Notably, the finding of a normal abdominal circumference reliably excludes IUGR with a false-negative rate of less than 10%.

An optimal or standard management of pregnancies complicated by IUGR has not been established. The cornerstones of management for a fetus with IUGR include antenatal testing with serial NSTs or BPPs; serial ultrasound surveillance of fetal growth, amniotic fluid volume, and umbilical artery Doppler velocimetry; and the administration of antenatal corticosteroids if preterm delivery is anticipated. Notably, the weekly monitoring of umbilical artery Doppler velocimetry is the recommended primary surveillance tool for the fetus with IUGR. Numerous studies and metaanalyses have demonstrated a reduction in perinatal mortality and iatrogenic prematurity (premature or unnecessary induction of labor) for a preterm infant with IUGR when umbilical artery Doppler is utilized in decisions regarding timing of delivery. Normal or decreased umbilical artery flow is rarely associated with significant morbidity whereas absence or reversal of end-diastolic flow suggests poor fetal condition.

The optimal timing of delivery for the IUGR fetus remains controversial and without consensus. However, although opinions vary, experts generally agree that the growth-restricted infants should be delivered close to term, assuming that growth continues and antenatal testing remains reassuring. The Growth Restriction Intervention Trial highlighted the difficulty in selecting the appropriate timing of delivery. This trial randomized 548 preterm IUGR pregnancies for which both fetal compromise and uncertainty regarding delivery were identified to immediate or delayed delivery. In the delayed group delivery occurred when the primary obstetrician felt certainty regarding delivery timing (median delay 4.9 days). The primary finding was that delayed delivery results in more stillbirths than immediate delivery; however, the number of stillbirths was equal to the increase in neonatal deaths observed in the immediate delivery arm. The long-term outcomes failed to demonstrate any neurodevelopmental differences in either group among survivors.[98]

Therefore, timing of delivery should be individualized and based on gestational age and fetal condition. The following principles may guide management of pregnancies complicated by IUGR:

- Remote from term, conservative management to prolong pregnancy may be performed safely with serial antepartum surveillance as described earlier to achieve further fetal maturity.
- The term or late preterm (>34 weeks) IUGR fetus should be delivered when there is evidence of maternal hypertension, poor interval growth (over 2- to 4-week intervals), nonreassuring antenatal testing (NST, BPP), and/or umbilical artery Doppler testing to demonstrate absence or reversal of flow.
- When growth restriction is mild, no complicating maternal or fetal factors are present, and the umbilical artery Doppler and fetal testing are reassuring, delivery can be delayed until at least 37 weeks to minimize the risks of prematurity.
- Each specific clinical scenario requires close consideration and an individualization of management plans.

MAGNESIUM FOR NEUROPROTECTION

Cerebral palsy (CP) comprises a heterogeneous group of chronic, nonprogressive disabilities of the central nervous system, primarily of movement and/or posture. CP represents the most common cause of childhood motor disability and the prevalence has remained stable over time at approximately 1 to 2 per 1000 live births. Prematurity is one of the most powerful risk factors for CP, and in one study the prevalence of CP rose from 0.1% in term infants to 0.7% at 32 to 36 weeks, 6% at 28 to 31 weeks, and to 14% at 22 to 27 weeks.[99] Observational studies, primarily secondary analyses of trials involving very low-birth-weight infants whose mothers received magnesium sulfate either for tocolysis or eclampsia prophylaxis, emerged in the 1980s-1990s, describing an association between magnesium sulfate exposure and neurologic outcomes. Many of these studies noted that exposure conferred a protective effect against the development of CP. Importantly, animal models have supported the biological plausibility for a neuroprotective effect, which may involve the inhibition of N-methyl-D-aspartate (NMDA) excitotoxic neuronal damage, promotion of cerebral vasodilation, scavenging of free radicals, or reduction of inflammatory cytokines.

Subsequently, multiple randomized controlled trials were conducted to evaluate the efficacy of magnesium sulfate specifically for neuroprotection in women at risk for preterm delivery.[100-102] Notably, all trials demonstrated a decrease in the risk of moderate or severe CP in the magnesium-exposed trial arms. In the largest trial, the Benefits of Antenatal Magnesium (BEAM) by Rouse and associates,[102] magnesium reduced the risk of moderate to severe CP from 7.3% to 4.2% (P<.004). Although there was no statistically significant difference noted in the primary composite outcome (death or cerebral palsy) in the larger two trials, the published analysis included data demonstrating that there was no impact of magnesium on the risk of death, thereby eliminating the possibility that the lower rate of CP in the treatment arm was caused by increased death with magnesium. No increase in serious maternal adverse events was reported in any trial. Additionally, multiple metaanalyses have been performed that confirm the findings of the individual trials (reduction in moderate to severe CP, no impact on death alone) and also demonstrate a statistically significant reduction in the primary outcome of death or CP (summary RR 0.85, 95% CI 0.74 to 0.98.[103])

Therefore, the weight of the available evidence supports the use of magnesium for neuroprotection, and ACOG published a Committee Opinion in March 2010 supporting its use.[104] Notably, the number of women who must be treated to prevent one case of CP decreases with decreasing gestational age: at less than 32 weeks' gestation 63 women must receive magnesium to prevent one case of moderate-to-severe cerebral palsy; at less than 28 weeks, 29 women must be treated. If magnesium sulfate were administered uniformly to women at risk of preterm delivery before 32 weeks in the United States more than 1000 cases of handicapping CP would be prevented yearly. Institutions adopting the use of magnesium sulfate for neuroprotection should develop specific treatment protocols, guidelines, and inclusion criteria in accordance with trials that have demonstrated benefit.

ANTENATAL CORTICOSTEROIDS

In a landmark paper published in 1972, Liggins and Howie demonstrated a decrease in respiratory distress syndrome and neonatal mortality in the offspring of women treated with antenatal corticosteroids. Subsequently, the efficacy of antenatal glucocorticoid therapy has been confirmed by more than 12 randomized controlled trials and multiple metaanalyses. In 1994, the NIH held a consensus conference to address antenatal corticosteroids use, which resulted in the recommendation for the administration of a single course of corticosteroids to all pregnant women between 24 and 34 weeks' gestation at risk for preterm delivery within 7 days, including patients with PPROM prior to 32 weeks' gestational age. A recent committee opinion notes that although data remain inconclusive, steroid administration for women with PPROM between 32 0/7 and 33 6/7 may be beneficial, particularly if pulmonary immaturity is documented.[105] See Figure 2-7 recommendations for steroids in the context of PPROM.

Corticosteroid therapy is thought to improve neonatal lung function through multiple mechanisms: accelerating the morphologic development and maturation of both type I and type II alveolar pneumocytes, stimulating surfactant production from type II pneumocytes, and increasing the synthesis of surfactant-binding proteins and lung antioxidant enzymes. The cumulative effect is a maturation of the lung architecture and the biochemical pathways that improve the mechanical function of the lungs and gas exchange. Regarding clinical respiratory morbidity and mortality outcomes, a Cochrane systematic review concluded that treatment with antenatal corticosteroids was associated with an overall reduction in RDS as well as severe RDS (relative risk reduction of approximately 40% to 50%), thereby decreasing requirements for respiratory support. Importantly, numerous studies and systematic reviews have demonstrated that antenatal corticosteroid administration decreases the risk of other severe morbidities related to prematurity. The aforementioned Cochrane review also concluded that corticosteroid treatment decreases the risk of intraventricular hemorrhage (RR 0.54, 95% CI 0.43 to 0.69), necrotizing enterocolitis (RR 0.46, 95% CI

0.29 to 0.74), neonatal mortality (RR 0.69, 95% CI 0.58 to 0.81), and systemic infection within the first 48 hours of life (RR 0.56, 0.38 to 0.85).

Betamethasone and dexamethasone are the preferred corticosteroids for antenatal treatment and have been the most widely studied agents. Both drugs cross the placenta in their active form and have similar biological activity. Although comparative trials between betamethasone and dexamethasone exist, results have been inconsistent and conflicting, and there is insufficient evidence to recommend one steroid over the other. The most commonly used regimens that constitute a single course include the following:

- *Betamethasone*—12 mg intramuscularly every 24 hours for two doses
- *Dexamethasone*—6 mg intramuscularly every 12 hours for four doses

There is no evidence to support the efficacy or safety of increasing the quantity of the dose or accelerating a dosing regimen should prompt delivery be expected.

The initial data of Liggins and Howie suggested that the benefits of antenatal corticosteroid administration decreased beyond 7 days after administration, which was also evident in the aforementioned Cochrane analysis. However, other retrospective studies have challenged this view and, subsequently, various trials have examined the role for repeat courses of corticosteroids.[105,106] In 2000, the NIH reconvened another consensus panel to update the 1994 recommendations with regard to repeat courses of antenatal corticosteroids. The panel concluded that although existing evidence suggested a possible benefit in respiratory outcomes, animal and human studies demonstrated evidence of adverse fetal effects on fetal growth (head circumference), lung growth and organization, retinal development, insulin resistance, renal glomerular number, and maturation and myelination of the central nervous system. Two studies with long-term follow-up of children exposed to multiple courses of steroids to 2 years of age did not demonstrate any significant difference in neurocognitive outcomes.[100,107] However, a large randomized controlled trial demonstrated a trend, albeit statistically insignificant, toward an increased incidence of cerebral palsy with repeat courses of corticosteroids.[107] Both the NIH and ACOG do not recommend repeat courses of corticosteroids.[105]

However, a single rescue course of antenatal corticosteroids may significantly improve short-term neonatal respiratory morbidity. A recent multicenter randomized control trial of a single rescue course was conducted in 437 patients without PPROM who had completed a course of antenatal corticosteroids before 30 weeks of gestation. Other inclusion criteria included completion of a course of corticosteroids more than 14 days before randomization and a recurring threat of preterm delivery before 33 weeks' gestation. The study demonstrated a significant reduction in respiratory distress syndrome, surfactant use, and composite morbidity in those delivering before 34 weeks' gestation and for the overall cohort without any increase in other fetal, neonatal, or maternal outcomes.[108] Long-term data have not yet been published. Since publication of this trial, ACOG has released a committee opinion stating that in the appropriate candidates a single rescue course of steroids "may be considered."[105]

Little evidence supports the use of antenatal corticosteroids for the previable fetus. Administration prior to 24 weeks' gestation will unlikely have a significant impact on the improvement of lung function, given that lungs are still in the canalicular phase of development with few primitive alveoli available on which steroids can exert an effect. Few studies regarding neonatal outcomes after steroid administration prior to 24 weeks have been conducted, and the available data are limited to case series and observational studies. The largest study conducted to date evaluated 181 neonates born between 23 0/7 and 23 6/7 weeks' gestation and noted that neonates exposed to a complete course of corticosteroids had a decreased mortality risk (OR 0.18, 95% CI 0.06 to 0.54). However, exposure to corticosteroids had no impact on the risk of severe intraventricular hemorrhage or necrotizing enterocolitis.[109] Although a detailed discussion of the management of the periviable fetus is beyond the scope of this chapter, the authors believe that the administration of antenatal corticosteroids prior to 24 weeks may be considered in select circumstances. This decision should be individualized after a careful consideration of the clinical scenario, prognostic factors (weight, fetal gender, presence of intraamniotic infection, etc.), and parental wishes regarding neonatal resuscitation.

NORMAL AND ABNORMAL LABOR

Labor and delivery is dependent on the complex interaction of three variables: the powers, the passenger, and the passage. The powers refer to the forces generated by the uterus. Uterine activity is characterized by the intensity, frequency, and duration of contractions. The passenger is the fetus: the absolute size, lie, position, presentation, attitude, and number. The passage refers to the pelvis and its ability to allow for delivery of the fetus. The bony limits of the pelvis can be assessed using clinical pelvimetry or, rarely, radiography and CT.

Labor occurs in three distinct stages. First stage is the interval between the onset of labor and full cervical dilation. This stage has been further subdivided into three phases: latent, active, and deceleration. The second stage is the interval between full cervical dilation and delivery of the infant. The mother assists in this stage with active pushing, although this is not a requirement. The third stage is the interval between delivery of the infant and delivery of the placenta and fetal membranes. Each of these stages has an expected length, although recent research has questioned this older data.[110] Abnormalities of the labor process can occur at any of these stages.

Intrapartum management depends on assessment of risk and evaluation for current or pending complications. Complications can arise rapidly during labor. Approximately 20% to 25% of all perinatal morbidity and mortality occurs in pregnancies with no underlying risk factors.[111] The presence of medical comorbidities such as diabetes, hypertension, asthma, HIV, and obesity, will affect management. Labor will also be affected by complications of pregnancy; preeclampsia, macrosomia, chorioamnionitis, preterm premature rupture of membranes preterm labor, and fetal anomalies. When possible, the assessment and management of these complications and comorbidities antenatally is essential for the proper care of the patient during her labor course.

During labor, all pregnant women require surveillance of vital signs and fetal heart rate. The value of routine continuous electronic fetal monitoring during labor is controversial. The United States Preventive Services Task Force states that: "routine electronic fetal monitoring for low-risk women in labor is not mandatory and there is insufficient evidence to recommend for or against intrapartum electronic fetal monitoring for high-risk pregnant women." Regardless, some form of FHR monitoring has become a standard of care for all women in the United States, either by continuous electronic or manual auscultation.

Assessment of contractions and cervical change are also done at regular intervals to follow the progress of labor and guide the need for intervention. There is no standard interval for cervical assessment and many practitioners weigh the risk of chorioamnionitis with frequent cervical exams versus the prolongation of labor due to lack of progress. Contraction frequency and duration can be monitored using simple observation and palpation of the fundus or with internal or external tocodynamometry. However, only internal tocodynamometry with an intrauterine pressure catheter (IUPC) can measure the strength of contractions. Contractions or cervical change that is not deemed adequate for labor, a lack of powers, can be augmented using oxytocin. The use of oxytocin in most institutions is given under a standard protocol to ensure safe administration and low incidence of hyperstimulation that can lead to fetal heart rate abnormalities and acidemia.

Abnormalities in labor progression that lead to arrest or protraction disorders can occur in the first or second stages. Typically first stage arrest that is not amenable to oxytocin administration is treated with cesarean delivery. Second stage arrest can also be treated by cesarean delivery if an operative vaginal delivery cannot be safely completed. In the United States, 4.5% of births are completed by operative vaginal delivery and the success rate is high.[112] Choice of instrument is determined by level of training with either forceps or vacuum. Other considerations include the degree of maternal anesthesia, gestational age of the fetus, and anticipated difficulty of the procedure. Maternal and fetal complications rates depend on a number of factors and may be more related to abnormal labor than to the devices themselves. A metaanalysis of 10 trials comparing vacuum with forceps delivery found vacuum deliveries were associated with less maternal soft tissue trauma and required less anesthesia, but were less likely to result in successful vaginal delivery. Neonates delivered by vacuum extraction had more cephalohematoma and retinal hemorrhages than those delivered by forceps. Sequential attempts at operative vaginal delivery using different instruments should be avoided due to an increased risk of fetal injury.

Reducing infectious complications in the mother and the neonate are important in the management of labor. In the United States, a universal screening program for Group B *Streptococcus* (GBS) has been implemented. This screening program combined with the chemoprophylaxis of screen-positive patients has dramatically reduced the incidence of early onset GBS infections in neonates.[113] The diagnosis of chorioamnionitis can contribute to significant morbidity for the mother and infant. Risk factors for intrauterine infection include nulliparity, spontaneous labor, prolonged rupture of membranes (>18 hours), multiple digital vaginal examinations, meconium-stained fluid, internal fetal or uterine monitoring, and the presence of genital tract pathogens. Maternal fever and two of the following symptoms contribute to the diagnosis: maternal or fetal tachycardia, uterine fundal tenderness, foul-smelling amniotic fluid, or elevated maternal white blood cell count. Prompt treatment with broad spectrum intravenous antibiotics is recommended to improve maternal and neonatal outcomes. Typically ampicillin, gentamycin, and clindamycin or metronidazole is used. Alternative regimens include ampicillin-sulbactam or cefoxitin.

Labor is a painful process and women use different methods to relieve this discomfort. While some prefer nonpharmacologic methods, ACOG supports the concept that maternal request alone is a sufficient medical indication for labor analgesia. Pharmacologic approaches can be classified as systemic, regional, or local. Systemic methods involve intravenous or intramuscular administration of typically opioid agents or opioid agonist-antagonists. These agents provide only minimal relief unless high dosages are used. When used in higher dosages, opioid analgesics can cause respiratory depression and an increased risk of aspiration in the mother as well as neonatal respiratory depression. Regional techniques include epidurals, spinals, and combined spinal-epidurals. The methods typically use a mixture of a local anesthetic and opioid agent. Neuraxial anesthesia is very widely used in the United States with approximately 70% of patients receiving this type of labor pain relief.[114] Maternal risks of neuraxial anesthesia are rare, including systemic toxicity, high spinal, hypotension resulting in fetal bradycardia, postdural puncture headache, infection, hematoma, and urinary retention. The effects on the neonate have been studied and show either no difference or improvement in neonatal neurobehavior after epidural compared to systemic opioid analgesia or no medication. The effect of neuraxial analgesia in labor on breast feeding is controversial and studies to date are inconclusive. ACOG concluded that breast feeding is not affected by choice of anesthetic; thus anesthetic choice should be based on other considerations. Local injections of anesthesia in the area of the pudendal nerve (pudendal block) can be used in the second or third stage of labor without any effect on the neonate.

HUMAN IMMUNODEFICIENCY VIRUS

Pregnant women with HIV require comprehensive medical care to achieve good maternal outcomes and low rates of perinatal HIV transmission. Antiretroviral therapy is recommended to reduce perinatal transmission. Transmission can occur during pregnancy, labor and delivery, or the breast-feeding period. The risk has been reduced to less than 2% in the United States with the administration of antiretroviral prophylaxis and viral suppression.[115] The first study in 1994 showed the benefit of administering a single agent, zidovudine, intrapartum and to the infant after delivery. It was effective in significantly decreasing transmission from 25% to 8%. Since that time, other studies have shown benefit of multiple agents and administration earlier in pregnancy.[116] The current recommendation is to start antiretroviral therapy immediately if the patient requires it for her own health, or otherwise after the first trimester. Delaying treatment until after 28 weeks may result in an increased risk of transmission. Treatment regimens for pregnant patients with HIV are the topic of guidelines produced and regularly updated by the U.S. Department of Health and Human Services.[117]

In addition to standard screening, pregnant women with HIV should be screened for other infectious diseases including hepatitis B and C, toxoplasmosis, tuberculosis, and cytomegalovirus. For women with CD4 counts <200 cells/mm^3, pneumocystis pneumonia prophylaxis is recommended. Counseling on sexually transmitted disease prevention and reduction of other risk factors should be performed. Women should be informed that in resource-rich areas, such as the United States, breast feeding is not recommended because of the increased risk of transmission to the infant.

True or False

Insulin is the first line of treatment for gestational diabetics with elevated glucose levels.

When pharmacologic therapy is required, oral antidiabetic agents have been almost universally endorsed as first-line drugs in the treatment of gestational diabetes mellitus (GDM). This recommendation is based on well-designed studies that have found these agents are as efficacious as insulin for all severities of gestational diabetes. Also there is no association between these agents and congenital malformations.[118] Therefore, the answer is false.

REFERENCES

The reference list for this chapter can be found online at www.expertconsult.com.

Resuscitation at Birth

Tina A. Leone and Neil N. Finer

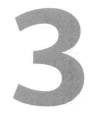

The transition from fetal to neonatal life is a dramatic and complex process involving extensive physiologic changes that are most obvious at the time of birth. Individuals who care for newly born infants during these first few minutes of neonatal life must monitor the progress of the transition and be prepared to intervene when necessary. In the majority of births, this transition occurs without a requirement for any significant assistance. However, when the need for intervention arises, the presence of providers who are skilled in neonatal resuscitation can be life saving. Each year approximately 4 million children are born in the United States and more than 30 times as many are born worldwide.[1,2] It is estimated that approximately 5% to 10% of all births will require some form of resuscitation beyond basic care, thereby making neonatal resuscitation the most frequently practiced form of resuscitation in medical care. Throughout the world, approximately 1 million newborn deaths are associated with birth asphyxia. Although it cannot be expected that neonatal resuscitation will eliminate all early neonatal mortality, it has the potential for helping save many lives and for significantly reducing associated morbidities.

Attempts at reviving nonbreathing infants immediately after birth have occurred throughout recorded time with references in literature, religion, and early medicine. Although the organization and sophistication has changed, the basic principle and goal of initiating breathing has remained constant throughout time. It has just been over the last 20 years that the process of neonatal resuscitation has been more officially regimented. Resuscitation programs in other areas of medicine were initiated in the 1970s in an effort to improve knowledge about effective resuscitation and provide an action plan for early responders. The first of such programs was focused on adult cardiopulmonary resuscitation.[3] These programs then began increasing in complexity and becoming more specific to different types of resuscitation needs. With the collaboration of the American Heart Association and the American Academy of Pediatrics, the Neonatal Resuscitation Program (NRP) was initiated in 1987 and was designed to address the specific needs of the newly born infant. Since the origination of the NRP, on-going evaluation of the program has resulted in changes when new evidence becomes available. The most recent edition of the NRP textbook published in 2011 made several revisions including specific recommendations for the preterm infant.[4] Various groups throughout the world also provide resuscitation recommendations that may be more specific to the practices in certain regions. An international group of scientists, the International Liaison Committee on Resuscitation (ILCOR), meets on a regular basis to review available resuscitation evidence for all the different areas of resuscitation and puts forth a summary of its review.[5]

The overall goal of the NRP is similar to other resuscitation programs in that it intends to teach large groups of individuals of varying backgrounds the principles of resuscitation and to provide an action plan for providers. Similarly, a satisfactory end-result of resuscitation would be common to all forms of resuscitation, namely to provide adequate tissue oxygenation to prevent tissue injury and restore spontaneous cardiopulmonary function. When comparing neonatal resuscitation with other forms of resuscitation, several distinctions can be noted. First, the birth of an infant is a more predictable occurrence than most events that require resuscitation in an adult, such as an arrhythmia or a myocardial infarction. Although not every birth will require "resuscitation," it is more reasonable to expect that skilled individuals can be present when the need for neonatal resuscitation arises. It is possible to anticipate with some accuracy which neonates will more likely require resuscitation based on perinatal factors and thus allow time for preparation. The second distinction of neonatal resuscitation compared with other forms of resuscitation involves the unique physiology involved in the normal fetal transition to neonatal life.

The fetus exists in the protected environment of the uterus where temperature is closely controlled, continuous fetal breathing is not essential to provide gas exchange, the lungs are filled with fluid, and the gas exchange organ is the placenta. The transition that occurs at birth requires the neonate to increase heat production, initiate continuous breathing, replace the lung fluid with air/oxygen, and significantly increase pulmonary blood flow so that gas exchange can occur in the lungs. The expectations for this transitional process and knowledge of how to effectively assist the process help guide the current practice of neonatal resuscitation.

FETAL TRANSITION TO EXTRAUTERINE LIFE

The key elements necessary for a successful transition to extrauterine life involve changes in thermoregulation, respiration, and circulation. In utero, the fetal core temperature is approximately 0.5° C greater than the mother's temperature.[6] Heat is produced by metabolic processes and is lost over this small temperature gradient through the placenta and skin.[7] After birth, the temperature gradient between the infant and the environment becomes much greater and heat is lost through the skin by radiation, convection, conduction, and evaporation. The newly born infant must begin producing heat through other mechanisms such as lipolysis of brown adipose tissue.[8] If heat is lost at a pace greater than it is produced, the infant will become hypothermic. Preterm infants are at particular risk because of increased heat loss through immature skin, a greater surface area to body weight ratio, and decreased brown adipose tissue stores. Preterm hypothermic infants who are admitted to the nursery have decreased chances of survival.[9] Routine measures during neonatal resuscitation, such as the use of radiant warmers and drying the infant are aimed at preventing heat loss. For the preterm infant, special measures for temperature management, such as the use of plastic wrap as a barrier to evaporative heat loss, are necessary to ensure adequate thermoregulation.

The fetus lives in a fluid-filled environment and as lung development occurs, the developing alveolar spaces are filled with lung fluid. Lung fluid production decreases in the days prior to delivery and the remainder of lung fluid is resorbed into the pulmonary interstitial spaces after delivery.[10,11] As the infant takes the first breaths after birth, a negative intrathoracic pressure of approximately 50 cm H_2O is generated.[12,13] The alveoli become filled with air, and with the help of pulmonary surfactant, the lungs retain a small amount of air at the end of exhalation known as the functional residual capacity (FRC). Although the fetus makes breathing movements in utero, these efforts are intermittent and are not required for gas exchange. Continuous spontaneous breathing is maintained after birth by several mechanisms including the activation of chemoreceptors, the decrease in placental hormones, which inhibit respirations, and the presence of natural environmental stimulation. Spontaneous breathing can be suppressed at birth for several reasons, most critical of which is the presence of acidosis secondary to compromised fetal circulation. The natural history of the physiologic responses to acidosis has been described by researchers creating such conditions in animal models. Dawes described the breathing response to acidosis in different animal species.[14] He noted that when pH was decreased, animals typically have a relatively short period of apnea followed by gasping. The gasping pattern then increases in rate until breathing ceases again for a second period of apnea. Dawes also noted that the first period of apnea or primary apnea could be reversed with stimulation, whereas the second period of apnea, secondary or terminal apnea, required assisted ventilation to establish spontaneous breathing. In the clinical situation, the exact timing of onset of acidosis is generally unknown and, therefore, any observed apnea may be either primary or secondary. This is the basis of the resuscitation recommendation that stimulation may be attempted in the presence of apnea, but if not quickly successful, assisted ventilation should be initiated promptly. Without the presence of acidosis, a newborn may also develop apnea because of recent exposure to respiratory-suppressing medications such as narcotics, anesthetics, and magnesium. These medications, when given to the mother, cross the placenta, and depending on the time of administration and dose, may act on the newborn.

Fetal circulation is unique because gas exchange takes place in the placenta. In the fetal heart, oxygenated blood returning via the umbilical vein is mixed with deoxygenated blood from the superior and inferior vena cava and is differentially distributed throughout the body. The most oxygenated blood is directed toward the brain, while the most deoxygenated blood is directed toward the placenta. Thus, blood returning from the placenta to the right atrium is preferentially streamed via the foramen ovale to the left atrium and ventricle, and then to the ascending aorta, providing the brain with the most oxygenated blood. Fetal channels, including the ductus arteriosus and foramen ovale, allow blood flow to mostly bypass the lungs with their intrinsically high vascular resistance, which will receive only approximately 8% of the total cardiac output. Thus, the fetal circulation is unique in that the pulmonary and systemic circulations are not equal as occurs after these channels close. In the mature postnatal circulation, the lungs must receive 100% of the cardiac output. When the low resistance placental circulation is removed after birth, the infant's systemic vascular resistance increases while the pulmonary vascular resistance begins to fall as a result of pulmonary expansion, increased arterial oxygen tension, and local vasodilators. These changes result in a dramatic increase in pulmonary blood flow. The average fetal oxyhemoglobin saturation as measured in fetal lambs is approximately 50%,[15] but ranges in different sites within the fetal circulation between values of 20% to 80%.[16] The oxyhemoglobin saturation rises gradually over the first 5 to 15 minutes of life to 90% or greater as the air spaces are cleared of fluid. In the face of poor transition secondary to asphyxia, meconium aspiration, pneumonia, or extreme prematurity, the lungs may not be able to develop efficient gas exchange, and the oxygen saturation may not increase as expected. In addition, in some situations the normal reduction in pulmonary vascular resistance may not fully occur, resulting in persisting pulmonary hypertension and decreased effective pulmonary blood flow with continued right to left shunting through the aforementioned fetal channels. Although the complete transition from fetal to extrauterine life is complex and much more intricate than can be discussed in these few short paragraphs, a basic knowledge of these processes will contribute to the understanding of the rationale for resuscitation practices.

ENVIRONMENTAL PREPARATION

The environment in which the infant is born should facilitate the transition to neonatal life as much as possible and should readily accommodate the needs of a resuscitation team when necessary. Hospitals may vary in the approach to the details of how to prepare for resuscitation. For example, some hospitals may have a separate room designated for resuscitation where the infant will be taken after birth, others bring all the necessary equipment into the delivery room when resuscitation is expected, and some have every delivery room already equipped for any resuscitation. Wherever the resuscitation will take place, a few key elements should be ensured. The room should be warm enough to prevent excessive newborn heat loss, bright enough to assess the infant's clinical status, and large enough to accommodate the necessary personnel and equipment to care for the baby.

When no added risks to the newborn are identified, the term birth frequently may occur without the attendance of a specific neonatal resuscitation team. However, it is frequently recommended that one individual be present who is only responsible for the infant and can quickly alert a neonatal resuscitation team if necessary. Even the best neonatal resuscitation triage systems will not anticipate the need for resuscitation in all cases. Using a retrospective risk assessment scoring system, Smith and colleagues found that 6% of newborns requiring resuscitation would not be identified based on risk factors.[17] Antenatal determination of neonatal risk allows the neonatal resuscitation team to be present for the delivery and to be more thoroughly prepared for the situation. Preterm infants require resuscitation more frequently than term infants and, therefore, require the presence of a prepared neonatal resuscitation team at the delivery. Any situation in which the infant's respirations may be suppressed or the fetus is showing signs of distress should signal the need for a neonatal resuscitation team. A list of factors that may be associated with an increased risk of need for resuscitation can be found in Box 3-1. Hospitals may vary to some extent about which conditions require presence of the neonatal resuscitation team at delivery.

The composition of the neonatal resuscitation team will also vary tremendously among institutions. Probably the most important factor in how well a team functions is how well the group has prepared for the delivery. When there is a high index of suspicion that the newborn infant will be born in a compromised state, the minimally effective team should have at least three members, including one member with significant previous experience leading neonatal resuscitations. Preparation involves both

Box 3-1.	**Risk Factors Related to Resuscitation at Birth**

Maternal factors	**Fetal factors**	**Placental factors**
Diabetes mellitus	Preterm birth	Placenta previa
Preeclampsia	Known fetal anomalies	Placenta accreta
Chronic illness	Multiple gestation	Vasa previa
Poor prenatal care	Hydrops fetalis	Placental abruption
Substance abuse	Oligohydramnios	Premature rupture of membranes
Uterine rupture	Polyhydramnios	
General anesthesia	Intrauterine growth restriction	
Chorioamnionitis	Signs of fetal distress	
	Decreased fetal movement	

the immediate tasks of readying equipment and personnel, as well as the more broad institutional preparation of training team members and providing appropriate space and equipment. Teams that regularly work together and divide tasks in a routine manner will have a better chance of functioning smoothly during a critical situation. Although much attention has been raised in the literature regarding teamwork and team and leadership training, minimal evidence is available to recommend a specific team composition or training approach.

ASSESSMENT

Immediately after birth, the infant's condition is evaluated by general observation as well as measurement of specific parameters. Typically after birth, a healthy newborn will cry vigorously and maintain adequate respirations. The color will transition from blue to pink over the first 2 to 5 minutes, the heart rate will remain in the 140s to 160s, and the infant will demonstrate adequate muscle tone with some flexion of the extremities. The overall assessment of an infant who is having difficulty with the transition to extrauterine life will often reveal apnea, bradycardia, cyanosis, and hypotonia. Resuscitation interventions are based mainly on the evaluation of respiratory effort and heart rate. These parameters need to be continually assessed throughout the resuscitation. Heart rate can be monitored by auscultation or by palpation of the cord pulsations with auscultation being a more reliable method. In many situations, the use of a device for more extensive monitoring such as a pulse oximeter can be helpful during resuscitation. A pulse oximeter can provide the resuscitation team with a continuous audible and visual indication of the newborn's heart rate throughout the various steps of resuscitation while allowing

all team members to perform other tasks. In addition, the pulse oximeter can be used as a more accurate measure of oxygenation than the evaluation of color alone. It has been well established that color alone is an unreliable measure to accurately assess the infant's oxygen saturation, especially where the room lighting is suboptimal. Whenever interventions beyond brief mask positive pressure ventilation are required, a pulse oximeter should be considered for additional monitoring of the infant.

The overall assessment of a newborn was quantified by Virginia Apgar in the 1950s with the Apgar score.[18] The score describes the infant's condition at the time it is assigned and consists of a 10-point scale with a maximum of 2 points assigned for each of the following categories: respirations, heart rate, color, tone, and reflex irritability. The score was initially intended to provide a uniform, objective assessment of the infant's condition and was used as a tool to compare different practices, especially obstetrical anesthetic practices. Despite the intent of objectivity, there is often disagreement in score assignment among various practitioners.[19,20] Low scores have been consistently associated with increased risk of neonatal mortality,[21,22] but have not been predictive of neurodevelopmental outcome.[23] Interpreting the score when interventions are being provided may be difficult and current recommendations suggest that clinicians should document the utilized interventions at the time the score is assigned.[24]

INITIAL STEPS: TEMPERATURE MANAGEMENT AND MAINTAINING THE AIRWAY

In the first few seconds after birth, all infants are evaluated for signs of life and a determination of the need for further assistance is made. This is done both formally, as described in the NRP, and informally as the initial care providers observe the infant in the first few moments of life. When the determination that further assistance and formal resuscitation is necessary, the infant is then placed on a radiant warmer and positioned appropriately for resuscitation to proceed. Appropriate positioning includes placing the infant supine on the warmer in such a way that care providers have easy access, traditionally with the baby's head toward the open end of the warmer. In addition, the head should be in a neutral or "sniffing" position to facilitate maintenance of an open airway. Frequently, the oropharynx contains large amounts of fluid which can be removed by suctioning with a standard bulb syringe.

An infant born through meconium-stained amniotic fluid is at risk for aspirating meconium and developing significant pulmonary disease known as *meconium aspiration syndrome,* which may also be accompanied by persistent pulmonary hypertension. For many years, routine management of all infants with meconium-stained amniotic fluid included endotracheal intubation and tracheal suctioning in an attempt to remove any meconium from the trachea and prevent the development of meconium aspiration syndrome. Recognizing that intubation may not be necessary for all infants, while the procedure may be associated with complications, a more selective approach was proposed and evaluated.[25,26] A metaanalysis of studies that have evaluated this question supported the notion that universal endotracheal suctioning does not result in a lower incidence of meconium aspiration syndrome when compared with selective endotracheal suctioning.[27] The likelihood that an infant with meconium-stained amniotic fluid will develop meconium aspiration syndrome is increased in the presence of fetal distress. The selective approach to endotracheal suctioning requires a quick evaluation of the infant after delivery. If the infant is vigorous with good respiratory effort, normal heart rate and tone, the steps of resuscitation should proceed as usual. However, if the infant is not vigorous, has poor respiratory effort, a heart rate less than 100 beats per minute (bpm) and/or decreased tone, endotracheal intubation and tracheal suctioning are performed as quickly as possible.

The provision of warmth is particularly important for the extremely preterm infant. Preterm infants are commonly admitted to the neonatal intensive care unit (NICU) with core temperatures well below 37° C, and in a population-based analysis of all infants less than 26 weeks' gestation, greater than one third of these preterm infants had admission temperatures less than 35° C. More disturbing is the fact that infants with such admission temperatures survived less often than those with admission temperatures greater than 35° C.[10] Vohra and colleagues have shown that admission temperatures may be improved in infants less than 28 weeks' gestation by immediately covering the infant's body with polyethylene wrap prior to drying the infant.[28,29] With this approach, the infant's head is left out of the wrap and is dried, but the body is not dried prior to wrap application. Other measures for maintaining infant temperatures include performing resuscitation in a room that is kept at an ambient temperature of approximately 25° C to 26° C (77° F to 79° F), using modern radiant warmers with servo controlled temperature probes placed on the infant within minutes of delivery, and the use of accessory prewarmed mattress/heating pads for the tiniest of such infants. It is important to note that as a required safety feature, radiant warmers will substantially decrease their power output after 15 minutes of continuous operation in full power mode. If this decrease in power is unrecognized, the infant will be exposed to a much cooler radiant temperature. By applying the temperature probe and using the warmer in servo mode, the temperature output will adjust as needed and the power will not automatically decrease.

ASSISTING VENTILATION

As the newborn infant begins breathing and replaces the lung fluid with air, the lung becomes inflated and a functional residual capacity is developed and maintained. With inadequate development of FRC, the infant will not adequately oxygenate, and if prolonged, the infant will develop bradycardia. The steps involved in performing resuscitation include providing assisted positive pressure ventilation when the infant shows signs of inadequate lung inflation. The indications for provision of positive pressure ventilation include apnea or inadequate respiratory effort, poor color, and heart rate less than 100 bpm. Positive pressure ventilation can be delivered noninvasively with a pressure delivery device and a face mask or invasively with the same pressure delivery device and an endotracheal tube.

Pressure delivery devices can include self-inflating bags, flow-inflating or anesthesia bags, and T-piece resuscitators, each with its own advantages and disadvantages. A self-inflating bag requires a reservoir to provide nearly 100% oxygen, may deliver very high pressure if not used carefully, but is easy to use for inexperienced personnel and will work in the absence of a gas source. These devices have pressure blow-off valves, but these valves do not always open at the target blow-off pressures.[30] An anesthesia bag or flow-inflating bag requires a gas source for use, allows the operator to "instinctively" vary delivery pressures, but requires significant practice to develop expertise with use. A T-piece resuscitator is easy to use, requires a gas source for use, delivers the most consistent levels of pressure, but requires intentional effort to vary pressure levels.[31] The flow-inflating bag and T-piece resuscitator allow the operator to deliver continuous positive airway pressure (CPAP) or positive end expiratory pressure (PEEP) relatively easily.[32,33]

A level of experience is required to perform assisted ventilation using a face mask and resuscitation device, especially for an extremely low-birth-weight infant. It is important to maintain a patent airway for the air to reach the lungs. The procedure of obtaining and maintaining a patent airway includes, at minimum, clearing of fluid with a suction device, holding the head in a neutral position, and sometimes lifting the jaw slightly anteriorly. The face mask must make an adequate seal with the face for air to pass to the lungs effectively. No device will adequately inflate the lungs if there is a large leak between the mask and the face. Until recently, there were no masks that were small enough to provide an adequate seal over the mouth and nose for the tiniest infants. Such masks are now readily available and facilitate bag and mask resuscitation of very small infants. Signs that the airway is patent and air is being delivered to the lungs include visual inspection of chest rise with each breath and improvement in the clinical condition, including heart rate and color. The use of a colorimetric carbon dioxide detector during bagging will allow confirmation that gas exchange is occurring by the observed color change of the device or alerting the operator of an obstructed airway with lack of such color change.[34] It is important to remember that these devices will not change color in the absence of

pulmonary blood flow, as occurs with inadequate cardiac output. At times, multiple maneuvers are required to achieve a patent airway, such as readjusting the head and mask positions, choosing a mask of more appropriate size, and further suctioning of the pharynx. Alternate methods of providing a patent airway include the use of a nasopharyngeal tube,[35] a laryngeal mask airway device,[36] or an endotracheal tube.

The amount of pressure provided with each breath during assisted ventilation is critical to the establishment of lung inflation and therefore adequate oxygenation. Although it is important to provide adequate pressure for ventilation, excessive pressure can contribute to lung injury. Achieving the correct balance of these goals is not simple and is an area of resuscitation that requires more study. A specific level of inspiratory pressure will never be appropriate for every baby. Initial inflation pressures of 25 to 30 mm Hg are probably adequate for most term babies. The current NRP textbook recommends initial pressures of 20 to 25 mm Hg for preterm infants.[5] The first few breaths may require increased pressure if lung fluid has not been cleared, as occurs when the infant does not initiate spontaneous breathing, and infants with specific pulmonary disorders, such as pneumonia or pulmonary hypoplasia, also frequently require increased inspiratory pressure. It has been shown that using enough pressure to produce visible chest rise may be associated with hypocarbia on blood gas evaluation and excessive pressure may decrease the effectiveness of surfactant therapy.[37,38] It may be possible to establish FRC without increasing peak inspiratory pressures by providing a few prolonged inflations (3 to 5 seconds inspiration)[37], although the use of prolonged inflations has not been associated with better outcomes than has conventional breaths during resuscitation.[39] Choosing the actual initial inspiratory pressure is less important than continuously assessing the progress of the intervention.

EDITORIAL COMMENT: Current neonatal resuscitation guidelines recommend using visual assessment of chest wall movements to guide the choice of inflating pressure during positive pressure ventilation (PPV) in the delivery room. The accuracy of this assessment has not been tested. Poulton et al compared the assessment of chest rise made by observers standing at the infant's head and at the infant's side with measurements of tidal volume. Airway pressures and expiratory tidal volume (V[Te]) were measured during neonatal resuscitation using a respiratory function monitor. After 60 seconds of PPV, resuscitators standing at the infant's head (head view) and at the side of the infant (side view) were asked to assess chest rise and estimate V(Te). These estimates were compared with V(Te) measurements taken during the previous 30 seconds. Agreement between clinical assessment and measured V(Te) was generally poor. During mask ventilation, resuscitators were unable to accurately assess chest wall movement visually from either head or side view.

Poulton DA, Schmölzer GM, Morley CJ, et al: Assessment of chest rise during mask ventilation of preterm infants in the delivery room, Resuscitation 82:175, 2011.

A manometer in the circuit during assisted ventilation provides the clinician with an indication of the actual administered pressure, although if the airway is blocked, this pressure is not delivered to the lungs. The most critical component of continued assessment is evaluation of the infant's response to the intervention. If after initiating ventilation, the condition of the infant does not improve (specifically improved heart rate, breathing, and color), then the ventilation is most likely inadequate. Two most common reasons for inadequate ventilation are a blocked airway or insufficient inspiratory pressure. The blocked airway frequently can be corrected with changes in position or suctioning, whereas inadequate pressure is corrected by adjusting the ventilating device.

In addition to consideration of inspiratory pressure, use of continuous pressure throughout the breathing cycle seems to be beneficial for the establishment of FRC and improvement in surfactant function.[40,41] This is accomplished during assisted ventilation with the use of PEEP or CPAP when additional inspiratory pressure is not needed. In the absence of PEEP, a lung that has been inflated with assisted inspiratory pressure will lose on expiration most of the volume that had been delivered on inspiration. This pattern of repeated inflation and deflation is frequently thought to be associated with lung injury. In preterm infants, a general approach of using CPAP as a primary mode of respiratory support in neonatal intensive care units has been associated with a low incidence of chronic lung disease.[42] The recently published SUPPORT trial found no significant difference

in death or bronchopulmonary dysplasia between infants randomly assigned CPAP beginning in the delivery room versus those who received intubation and early surfactant.[43]

If assisted ventilation is necessary for a prolonged period of time or if other resuscitative measures have been unsuccessful, ventilation should be provided via an endotracheal tube. If it has been difficult to maintain a patent airway by ventilating with a face mask, the appropriately placed endotracheal tube will provide a stable airway. This will allow more consistent delivery of gas to the lungs and, therefore, provide for the ability to establish and maintain FRC. At this time, intubation is required for administering surfactant and may be used to administer other medications necessary for resuscitation. Finally, for depressed infants born through meconium-stained amniotic fluid, intubation is performed for suctioning of the airway.

EDITORIAL COMMENT: Videotaping resuscitations to review in detail, techniques, timing, and so on are extremely helpful. The debriefing is a valuable lesson for all involved, and it helps prepare the team for all emergencies. Furthermore, simulation provides a unique opportunity to test the team, establish team leadership, and test the techniques. For example, Schilleman et al established that mask ventilation during simulated neonatal resuscitation was often hampered by large leaks at the face mask. Moderate airway obstruction occurred frequently when effort was taken to minimize the leaks. Training in mask ventilation reduced mask leaks, but should also focus on preventing airway obstruction. In the delivery room, it is neither possible for the observers to accurately determine tidal volume nor to determine degree of leak (Schmölzer et al).

Schilleman K, Witlox RS, Lopriore E, et al: Leak and obstruction with mask ventilation during simulated neonatal resuscitation, Arch Dis Child Fetal Neonatal Ed 95:F398, 2010.
Schmölzer GM, Kamlin OC, O'Donnell CP, et al: Assessment of tidal volume and gas leak during mask ventilation of preterm infants in the delivery room. Arch Dis Child Fetal Neonatal Ed 95:F393, 2010.

The intubation procedure, although potentially critical for successful resuscitation, requires a significant amount of skill and experience to perform reliably and may be associated with serious complications. The procedure entails using a laryngoscope to visualize the vocal cords and passing the endotracheal tube between the vocal cords. The placement of the laryngoscope in the pharynx often produces vagal nerve stimulation, which leads to bradycardia. Assisted ventilation must be paused for the procedure, which if prolonged, will lead to hypoxia and bradycardia. Intubation has been shown to increase blood pressure and intracranial pressure.[44] Trauma to the mouth, pharynx, vocal cords, and trachea are all possible complications of intubation. Performing the intubation procedure when the infant already has bradycardia and is hypoxic can lead to further decline in heart rate and oxygenation.[45] Therefore, it seems most appropriate to make an attempt to stabilize the infant with noninvasive ventilation prior to performing the procedure, limit each attempt to 30 seconds or less, and stabilize the infant between attempts. If misplacement of the endotracheal tube into the esophagus goes unrecognized, the infant may experience further clinical deterioration. Clinical signs that the endotracheal tube has been correctly placed in the trachea include the following: auscultation of breath sounds over the anterolateral aspects of the lungs (near the axilla); mist visible on the endotracheal tube; chest rise; and clinical improvement in heart rate and color or oxygen saturation. The use of a colorimetric carbon dioxide detector to confirm intubation decreases the amount of time necessary to determine correct placement of the endotracheal tube,[46] and is now recommended by the NRP as one of the primary methods of determining endotracheal tube placement.

Oxygen Use

The use of pure oxygen for ventilation became routine practice in resuscitation because it seemed logical that oxygen would be beneficial. However, the recognition that oxygen could also be toxic led many investigators to question this previously well-accepted practice. Several worldwide trials have compared the use of pure (100%) oxygen with room air (21% oxygen) for newborn resuscitation. These trials found that room air was as successful as oxygen in achieving resuscitation, and infants resuscitated with room air had a shorter time to initiate spontaneous breathing and less evidence of oxidative stress.[47-50] Metaanalyses of several of the trials indicated that infants resuscitated with room air had less risk of mortality than those resuscitated with pure

oxygen.[51-53] The latest NRP guidelines advocate starting resuscitation of term babies with room air (21% oxygen).

The preterm infant may be more susceptible to any harmful effects of excessive oxygen delivery because of decreased antioxidant enzyme capacity. Some of the infants in the previous oxygen trials were preterm, but few were less than 1000 grams. Neonatal intensive care units generally attempt to reduce oxygen toxicity by limiting the amount of oxygen delivered to neonates using an upper limit for oxygen saturation and adjusting delivered oxygen levels to maintain oxygen saturation levels within that limit. The unlimited use of oxygen during resuscitation will expose the preterm infant to higher oxygen saturation levels than would routinely be accepted in the neonatal intensive care unit. When initiating resuscitation of very preterm infants with room air, desired oxygen saturation targets may be achieved without providing supplemental oxygen.[54] The most recent NRP guidelines recommend resuscitating preterm babies using a pulse oximeter and an oxygen blender so that the amount of oxygen can be adjusted based on the needs of the infant. The use of oxygen concentrations between 21% and 100% requires compressed air and a blender. When choosing oxygen saturation targets, it is important to remember that the neonate transitioning from fetal life begins with an oxygen saturation of approximately 50% and gradually increases to 90% over the first 5 to 10 minutes of life. The most recent NRP guidelines recommend that supplemental oxygen be delivered via a blender and that an oximeter probe be placed on the newborn, with the amount of oxygen titrated to maintain SpO_2 within the ranges shown in Table 3-1. Clearly, targeted oxygen delivery requires the early use of pulse oximeters and blended oxygen in the resuscitation area.

Table 3-1.	Target Oxygen Saturation According to Time after Birth
Time After Birth (min)	**Target SpO_2 (%)**
1	60-65
2	65-70
3	70-75
4	75-80
5	80-85
10	85-95

Assisting Circulation

In newly born infants, the need for resuscitative measures beyond assisted ventilation is extremely rare. Additional circulatory assistance can include chest compressions, administration of epinephrine, and volume infusion. In a large urban delivery center with a resuscitation registry, 0.12% of all infants delivered received chest compressions and/or epinephrine from 1991 to 1993 and 0.06% of all infants delivered received epinephrine from 1999 to 2004.[55,56]

The importance of chest compressions in resuscitation is currently being emphasized in adult resuscitation programs.[57] Although neonatal resuscitation is clearly distinct from adult resuscitation as previously discussed, any situation in which circulation has been sufficiently compromised will require support with chest compressions until spontaneous circulation is initiated. Ventilation remains the most critical priority in neonatal resuscitation. However, if an airway is established (either with a face mask and good positioning or an endotracheal tube), adequate ventilation is provided for 30 seconds, and bradycardia of <60 bpm persists, chest compressions are initiated. Further attention to ventilation with the use of increased pressures and/or intubation may be required. Chest compressions may be provided with either two fingers of one hand or two thumbs. The preferred method according to current guidelines is the two-thumb method which involves encircling the chest with both hands and placing the thumbs on the sternum. During placement of an umbilical catheter, the two-finger technique may be necessary to allow access to the umbilical cord. With either method, the chest is then compressed in a 3:1 ratio coordinated with ventilation breaths to provide 90 compressions to 30 breaths per minute.

Further circulatory support may be necessary if adequate chest compressions do not result in an increase in heart rate after 30 seconds. Epinephrine is then indicated as a vasoactive substance, which increases blood pressure by alpha-receptor agonist effects, improves coronary perfusion pressure, and increases heart rate by beta-receptor agonist effects. The strongly recommended method of epinephrine administration is intravenous in a dose of 0.01 to 0.03 mg/kg (0.1 to 0.3 mL/kg of a 1:10,000 solution). Therefore, early placement of an umbilical venous catheter during a difficult resuscitation is important for both volume and epinephrine administration. If there is any prenatal indication that substantial resuscitation will be required, the necessary equipment for umbilical venous catheter placement should be prepared before delivery as completely as possible. It is probably advisable to initiate the process of umbilical venous catheter placement when the need for chest compressions arises. Epinephrine may be given by endotracheal tube but the delivery is not as certain and, therefore, an increased dose of 0.05 to 0.1 mL/kg of a 1:10,000 solution is currently recommended. Epinephrine doses may be repeated every 3 minutes if heart rate does not increase. Excessive epinephrine administration may result in hypertension, which in preterm infants may be a factor in the development of intraventricular hemorrhage. However, the risks are balanced by the benefit of successful resuscitation in an infant who might not otherwise survive.

If the infant has not responded to all of the prior measures, a trial of increasing intravascular volume should be considered by the administration of crystalloid or blood. Situations associated with fetal blood loss are also frequently associated with the need for resuscitation. These include placental abruption, cord prolapse, and fetal maternal transfusion. Some of these clinical circumstances will have an obvious history associated with blood loss, whereas others may not be readily evident at the time of birth. Signs of hypovolemia in the newly born infant are nonspecific but include pallor and weak pulses. Volume replacement requires intravenous access for which emergent placement of an umbilical venous catheter is essential. Any infant who has signs of hypovolemia and has not responded to other resuscitative measures should have an umbilical venous line placed and a volume infusion administered. The most common volume replacement (and currently recommended fluid) is isotonic saline. A trial volume of 10 mL/kg is given initially and repeated if necessary. If a substantial blood loss has occurred, the infant may require infusion of red blood cells to provide adequate oxygen-carrying capacity. This can be accomplished emergently with uncrossmatched O-negative blood, with blood collected from the placenta, or with blood drawn from the mother who will usually have a compatible antibody profile with her infant at the time of birth. Because not all blood loss is obvious, and resuscitation algorithms usually discuss volume replacement as a last resort of a difficult resuscitation, the clinician needs to keep an index of suspicion for significant hypovolemia so that action may be taken to correct the problem as promptly as possible. Therefore, in situations where the possibility for hypovolemia is known prior to birth, it would be wise to prepare an umbilical catheter, an initial syringe of isotonic saline, and discuss with the blood bank the possibility that uncrossmatched blood may be required.

Specific Problems Encountered During Resuscitation

Neonatal Response to Maternal Anesthesia/Analgesia

Medications administered to the mother during labor can affect the fetus by transfer across the placenta and acting on the fetus or by adversely affecting the mother's condition, thereby altering uteroplacental circulation and placental oxygen delivery. The most commonly discussed complication of intrapartum medication exposure is perinatal respiratory depression after maternal opiate administration. Because opiates can cross the placenta, the fetus may develop respiratory depression from the direct effect of the drug. Naloxone has been used during neonatal resuscitation as an opiate receptor antagonist to reverse the effects of fetal opiate exposure. Despite a lack of evidence of beneficial effect, naloxone hydrochloride in a dose of 0.1 mg/kg (intravenous route preferred, intramuscular route acceptable, endotracheal administration NOT recommended) may be given if the newborn does not develop spontaneous respirations after adequate resuscitation and the mother has received an opiate analgesic during labor. Do not give this medication to a newborn when the mother has either been on methadone maintenance or is suspected of being addicted to narcotics, because seizures may occur. It is also critical that assisted ventilation be provided as long as spontaneous respirations are inadequate. It should be noted that the administration of a narcotic antagonist is never an acutely required intervention during neonatal resuscitation because such infants can be adequately ventilated with a bag and mask.

Conditions Complicating Resuscitation

When resuscitation has proceeded through the described steps without improvement in the infant's clinical condition, other problems should be considered. Some of these problems may be modifiable with interventions that could improve the course of the resuscitation. For example, an unrecognized pneumothorax could prevent adequate pulmonary inflation, and if under tension, could impair cardiac function. If the pneumothorax is recognized and drained, both gas exchange and circulation can be improved. Some congenital anomalies that were not diagnosed antenatally make resuscitation more difficult. Congenital diaphragmatic hernia is one such anomaly that is difficult to recognize on initial inspection of the infant but can cause significant problems with resuscitation. The abdominal organs are displaced into one hemithorax and the lungs are unable to develop normally, causing ventilation to be quite difficult. If the intestines are displaced into the thorax and mask ventilation is provided, the intestines will become inflated making ventilation even more difficult. If the congenital diaphragmatic hernia is known before delivery or a presumptive diagnosis is made in the delivery room, the baby should be intubated early to prevent intestinal inflation. A large (10 F) orogastric suction tube should also be placed to decompress the inflated intestines. Many other congenital anomalies that can lead to a difficult resuscitation will be more visibly obvious when the baby is born. For example, hydrops fetalis occurring for any reason can be associated with very difficult resuscitation. Although most cases are diagnosed on fetal ultrasound before delivery, severe hydrops would be visible on examination with skin edema and abdominal distention. Frequently, peritoneal and/or pleural fluid will need to be drained to achieve adequate ventilation.

A situation which may create a particularly difficult resuscitation is an airway obstruction, especially if not diagnosed prior to delivery. If a significant airway obstruction is diagnosed antenatally, an EXIT procedure (EX-utero Intrapartum Treatment) can be planned. This allows for establishment of a stable airway prior to clamping of the umbilical cord, which maintains placental function until the airway is secure. The therapy will vary depending on the cause of obstruction. An alternate airway (oral or nasopharyngeal) can be helpful if endotracheal intubation is not possible as can occur with micrognathia. Tracheal suctioning can be attempted if a tracheal plug is suspected. In extreme situations of airway obstruction, an emergency cricothyroidotomy may be attempted.

After Resuscitation

In infants born without a heart rate or any respiratory effort, if resuscitation is performed to the full extent without any response, discontinuation may be appropriate after 10 minutes. This recommendation is based on the high incidence of mortality and morbidity among infants born without any signs of life and poor response to resuscitation.[58,59] The new NRP guidelines do recognize that the decision of when to discontinue resuscitation is complicated and influenced by a number of factors.

Infants who do survive a significant resuscitation may require special attention in the hours to days that follow. Frequent complications immediately following resuscitation include hypoglycemia, hypotension, and persistent metabolic acidosis. In addition, infants with evidence of hypoxic-ischemic encephalopathy may benefit from mild therapeutic hypothermia.[60] This therapy is most beneficial when initiated as quickly as possible after an insult and is not available at every center. Institutions that do not provide this therapy should coordinate in advance with centers that do to ensure that treatment is started in a timely manner.

CASE 1

A woman presents to labor and delivery in active labor after having had no prenatal care. She precipitously delivers the baby and you are called urgently to the room. Who will go with you to the delivery room?

Each institution must decide the composition of their delivery resuscitation team. The individuals intended to participate on any given day should be identified prior to the start of the day. A team that has worked well together consistently would be expected to work well together in difficult situations.

The baby is handed to you; you place the baby on a radiant warmer and begin to evaluate the baby. You suction the mouth and remove the wet linens. The baby is making intermittent respiratory effort and the heart rate is over 100 bpm.

As you are drying the baby, you are stimulating him and his breathing becomes more regular by one minute of life. His heart rate always remains greater than 100 bpm, his color transitions from blue to pink centrally by 2 minutes of life. You note that his extremities are flexed and he cries when you examine him.

What Apgar score do you assign him at 5 minutes of life?

By 5 minutes of life, the baby has a heart rate greater than 100 bpm (2 points), adequate regular spontaneous respirations (2 points), good tone (2 points), good reflex irritability (2 points), and is centrally pink (1 point). Therefore, the Apgar score at 5 minutes of life is 9.

Once the initial stabilization has been completed, what do you look for in this infant whose mother had no prenatal care?

Among the most important observations to make is an approximation of gestational age. In addition to evaluating the size of the baby, a quick physical examination with attention to physical maturity findings will indicate an approximate gestational age which will be important in determining the further care necessary for this newborn. A brief physical examination will also be important as a preliminary screen for congenital anomalies. Further evaluation and observation will be necessary because of the lack of prenatal screening. Some of these routine prenatal screens may be completed by testing the mother at the time of admission. The pediatrician needs to be aware of these screens to treat the baby properly. Urgent considerations for the baby include rapid HIV testing, hepatitis B screening, syphilis screening, blood type assessment, and a sepsis risk assessment as group B *Streptococcus* carrier status is unknown. An urgent or early therapy for each of these conditions can be life altering. Further evaluation may also be indicated but is not necessarily as urgent.

CASE 2

A woman with a twin gestation at 25 weeks is admitted to labor and delivery with preterm labor. Fetal monitoring is initiated, a dose of betamethasone is administered, and a course of antibiotics is begun. You have a chance to talk with the parents; in addition to discussing general issues of prematurity at 25 weeks, what do you tell them to expect in the delivery room?

To begin the discussion, it would be helpful to inform the parents who will be caring for the babies at the delivery and where they will be cared for immediately after delivery. When multiples are delivered, it is best to have a separate resuscitation team planned for each infant. This may take extra preparation to ensure that enough resources are available at the time of delivery. It would be appropriate to inform the parents that preterm babies at 25 weeks have a higher chance of requiring resuscitation, including the need for intubation, but that currently survival for such infants is 70% or greater in most institutions.

Later that evening her labor is progressing and late decelerations develop on fetal heart rate monitoring. Your team is called to the delivery and a cesarean section is performed. The first baby is handed to you and does not have any apparent respiratory effort. Describe what you expect to occur in the first 1 minute of life.

The infant will be brought to a radiant warmer and wet linens will be removed. On the warmer there will be a plastic wrap/bag waiting which will cover the infant's body as soon as the wet linens are removed. While one team member assesses the heart rate by auscultation and providing a visual display for the entire team, a second team member will bulb suction the infant's mouth, position the baby on the bed in a straight fashion with the neck neutral. After suctioning the mouth, the second team member will place a face mask and initiate assisted ventilation. The third person will place a pulse oximeter and adjust the delivered oxygen concentration to meet the saturation targets recommended by NRP, which is 60% to 65% at 1 minute of life, and 65% to 70% at 2 minutes of life.

You begin positive pressure ventilation because the baby's spontaneous respiratory effort was inadequate. The nurse auscultates the heart rate and finds it to be approximately 80 bpm and not yet increasing. How do you proceed?

Because you are already giving positive pressure ventilation, you need to assess whether the breaths are being delivered adequately—in other words, whether the airway is open. The first step would be to readjust the head position ensuring that there is a good seal with the face mask and the neck is neutral. It can be helpful to gently hold upward pressure on the corners of the mandible while stabilizing the face mask. Observe the chest for movement with breaths, although this is sometimes difficult to see in very small babies. An additional indication of an open airway is detection of carbon dioxide on a disposable device placed in line with the face mask and breathing device. If the heart rate does not improve with these initial measures, the positive inspiratory pressure of the delivered breaths should be increased (done differently depending on the device used) or the inspiratory time of each breath should be increased. A prolonged breath with an inspiratory time of approximately 5 seconds may be attempted for one or two breaths as well. These measures may be attempted and frequently lead to improvement but should not be prolonged and delay more definitive therapy.

At this point (it is now approximately 1.5 minutes of life), the baby has a functioning pulse oximeter on the right hand which displays a heart rate of 85 bpm and an oxygen saturation of 30%. The baby has made some attempts at breathing but does not have sustained spontaneous respirations. Why do you think the baby is not making further improvements and what is your next step?

The most likely cause of the continued bradycardia is lack of development of an adequate functional residual capacity. Because attempts to stabilize the baby with noninvasive ventilation have failed, it is necessary to intubate the baby to provide a more direct and secure method of providing positive pressure. One may try a further increase in the inspiratory pressure because inadequate ventilation is the most frequent cause for continuing bradycardia and desaturation, and add 5 cm H_2O end-expiratory pressure to assist in establishing and maintaining FRC. It would also be appropriate at this time to increase the delivered oxygen concentration if an amount <100% is being administered.

The equipment necessary for intubation had been prepared and inspected prior to delivery and is waiting at the bedside. An appropriately sized endotracheal tube is available. The designated operator performs the procedure with the assistance of a second team member. Because the pulse oximeter is functioning, the baby will be monitored throughout the procedure. An additional team member will track the time and notify the operator if 30 seconds has elapsed prior to passing the endotracheal tube. If the attempt is unsuccessful, the laryngoscope will be removed from the baby's mouth and the positive pressure ventilation will be reinstituted to allow the baby to recover prior to another attempt. Once the endotracheal tube is positioned, a carbon dioxide detector will be used to ensure placement in the trachea. Breath sounds will be auscultated and the depth of the tube will be adjusted as necessary.

When the endotracheal tube is inserted and positive pressure is restarted, the heart rate increases to 150 bpm and the baby becomes pink with an oxygen saturation that increases to 95%. How would you care for the baby until you are able to arrive in the neonatal intensive care unit?

Attention will be paid to the infant's temperature, breathing, and heart rate throughout the entire time in the delivery room and through transport to the NICU. A temperature probe will be placed and the radiant warmer switched to servo mode. The pulse oximeter will be kept in place throughout the time in the delivery room and transport to the NICU. The delivered oxygen concentration will be adjusted to maintain the oxygen saturation appropriate for the time of life. Continued positive pressure ventilation with end expiratory pressure will be provided with delivered pressures adjusted as needed for the infant. In this case, the pressure was increased prior to intubation. If a T-piece resuscitator is being used for ventilation, the pressure will need to be manually adjusted to obtain desired levels and should be decreased once the intubation is performed and the heart rate and oxygen saturation have improved. The most consistent methods of providing continued ventilation with consistent levels of pressure would be either with a T-piece resuscitator or a ventilator. The use of either the self-inflating bag or flow-inflating bag for prolonged periods of time will likely lead to inconsistent pressure delivery with the potential for delivery of excess peak inspiratory pressure or inadequate positive end expiratory pressure levels, both of which may contribute to lung injury. Some institutions determine the level of pressure provided by measuring the tidal volume delivered, targeting an exhaled volume of 5 to 6 mL/kg. Additional care for an infant of this gestational age who has required intubation would be administration of exogenous surfactant. Although the provision of surfactant early, particularly within the first 15 minutes of life, is a proven intervention that will reduce the severity and mortality from respiratory distress syndrome, later administration up to 2 hours of age is also beneficial. Administration of surfactant may vary in preferred location (delivery room versus NICU) and timing.

CASE 3

A 27-year-old gravida 2 para 0 woman presents to labor and delivery at 30 weeks' gestation with rupture of membranes. She is admitted to the hospital, betamethasone is administered, and fetal monitoring is initiated. After she has been hospitalized for 4 days, the fetal heart rate is noted to increase to the 170s. On examination, it is noted that the umbilical cord is palpable in the vagina. The mother is rushed to the operating room and an emergency cesarean section is performed. The pediatric team is called to the delivery room and is handed the baby who is limp, pale, and has no respiratory effort. How do you proceed?

The baby is positioned on a radiant warmer, quickly dried, wet linens are removed, and the mouth is bulb suctioned. If these simple measures, which also act to stimulate the baby, do not cause the infant to begin breathing spontaneously, then assisted ventilation must be initiated without delay. The face mask and ventilating device are then immediately applied and positive pressure ventilation is initiated. At the same time, a second team member is evaluating the heart rate.

The heart rate is not appreciable by auscultation or palpation. What is your next step?

The effectiveness of ventilation is evaluated looking for evidence of a patent airway. The head position is adjusted and the level of positive pressure delivered is increased. If these actions have made no difference in heart rate, chest compressions are initiated. At this point, a third team member is placing a pulse oximeter, while the team member who had been evaluating the heart rate begins chest compressions. Chest compressions and breaths are coordinated in a three compressions to one breath rhythm with the team member performing chest compressions counting the actions out loud. The pace will be such that in 1 minute there will be approximately 90 compressions and 30 breaths.

The heart rate is reevaluated after 30 seconds of assisted ventilation and chest compressions and continues to be undetectable. What do you do now?

At this point, endotracheal intubation is necessary. This is performed by the team member who was providing positive pressure ventilation previously, with assistance from the team member who had placed the pulse oximeter. Chest compressions are paused during the intubation. If the intubation attempt is unsuccessful within 30 seconds, chest compressions and mask ventilation are reinitiated for at least 10 seconds before another intubation attempt is made. Depending on the number of individuals present at the resuscitation, more help should be called at this point, if necessary. Because the baby is being intubated with a low (absent) heart rate, it will most likely be necessary to give epinephrine. Therefore, an additional (fourth) individual could be preparing the epinephrine dose, and if a fifth skilled individual is available, an umbilical line should be prepared for placement. When the intubation is complete, if the heart rate is still low, the dose of epinephrine could be given in the endotracheal tube. Ensure that this dose is adequately flushed through the ETT so that it reaches the lung. At the same time that this is being done, the umbilical venous catheter is being placed so that a dose of epinephrine can be given intravenously.

Can you do anything else to help the baby at this point?

A dose of intravenous epinephrine should be given as soon as the umbilical venous catheter is placed because the effectiveness of intravenous epinephrine is more consistent than endotracheal epinephrine.

Because the baby appeared pale from the start and there was a history of cord prolapse, it may be helpful to provide intravenous fluid volume. A bolus of 10 mL/kg of normal saline can be given initially and repeated if necessary. If suspicion of blood loss is high, a transfusion of emergency blood may be provided. In addition, repeat doses of epinephrine can be administered every 3 minutes. An evaluation for other causes of cardiopulmonary insufficiency should be done. A pneumothorax may cause circulatory compromise and may be evaluated by auscultation of breath sounds and transillumination of the chest. A brief survey for congenital anomalies might disclose a cause for difficulty with resuscitation.

After you have given one dose of intravenous epinephrine and one bolus of normal saline, the baby's heart rate becomes detectable and steadily increases to greater than 100 bpm. How long would you have continued resuscitation if there had been no improvement?

In a situation where there are no signs of life (no heart rate or respiratory effort), and full resuscitative efforts are continued for 10 minutes with no effect, it is considered appropriate to stop the resuscitation. Each team may vary the time frame based on when resuscitative efforts were felt to be truly adequate, and whether there is any clinical evidence of signs of life.

CASE 4

You are called to the delivery room emergently because a woman at 40 weeks' gestation is delivering an infant vaginally. She has just ruptured her membranes and thick meconium is noted. You arrive at the delivery room as the baby's head is being delivered. How do you quickly prepare your equipment?

A glance at the power display on the radiant warmer will determine whether the device is in the full power mode. If not, this can be done quickly. A laryngoscope with blade is prepared and the function of light bulb is tested. The blade is then left in place in the off position and the laryngoscope is placed on the bed. An endotracheal tube with meconium aspirator is opened and placed on the bed in the packaging. Confirmation that a source of suction is available and functioning properly is made. The flow of air and oxygen to a ventilating device is initiated and function of the ventilating device is tested. If additional time is available, extra warm blankets can be prepared and any other usual preparations can be made. Information about the prenatal history can also be solicited at this time.

The baby is delivered and is limp and apneic. After he is handed to you, you place him on the radiant warmer with his head to you. What do you do next?

This infant's tone and respiratory effort are poor. He is, therefore, not vigorous and immediate intervention is indicated. Before any other action is taken, a direct laryngoscopy is performed. The pharynx is suctioned to clear any fluid that is obstructing the view of the larynx, and you then pass the endotracheal tube through the glottis. As you continue to hold the endotracheal tube in place, another team member connects the suction tubing directly to the endotracheal tube by the meconium aspirator and applies suction as you remove the endotracheal tube. As you are doing this, a third team member is continuously assessing the heart rate.

As you were suctioning, you saw a small amount of meconium in the tubing before the endotracheal tube was pulled back to the pharynx. At this point, the baby has made weak respiratory effort, the heart rate is approximately 100 bpm and the tone is still poor. What is your next step?

If meconium is suctioned from the trachea and the baby's heart rate is not decreasing, another endotracheal intubation and suctioning could be performed. Frequently at this time, the infant has either begun crying or has a decreasing heart rate because there has been inadequate breathing. In this case, there may be benefit to attempting a second suctioning since there is an indication that the baby did aspirate and he seemed to tolerate the first procedure well.

As you place the laryngoscope into the pharynx, the heart rate begins to drop which you note by the indication of slower tapping from your fellow team member. How do you proceed?

At this point, you abandon the second effort to suction the trachea, remove the laryngoscope, and begin positive pressure ventilation. As you initiate positive pressure ventilation, you note the heart rate being tapped out begins increasing. You continue providing assisted breaths and the baby develops a stronger regular respiratory effort. You stop providing assisted breaths when the respiratory effort is adequate and the heart rate is about 140 bpm. You do, however, continue to provide supplemental oxygen and place a pulse oximeter.

The baby is now vigorous and crying with good muscle tone. You note, however, that he has developed severe intercostal retractions and grunting. The oxygen

saturation level on the right hand is 95% while blow-by oxygen is being delivered. What is your plan for the baby at this point?

You know that the baby is at risk for developing a severe respiratory illness and persistent pulmonary hypertension of the newborn. You want to monitor the baby closely and begin any necessary therapy in a timely manner. You decide to transport the baby to the NICU while providing oxygen. When in the NICU, you will place an intravenous catheter, obtain a blood gas level, a glucose level, and a chest x-ray. You will place pre- and postductal oxygen saturation monitors, and start intravenous fluids and antibiotics. It is likely that you will need to intubate the baby to assist ventilation and place umbilical venous and arterial lines for medication delivery and closer monitoring. One might choose to perform intubation in the delivery room based on the description of the infant that was given. However, the choice to return to the NICU allows you to obtain intravenous access and provide medications for intubation which may be particularly beneficial in an infant who is now vigorous and will likely fight the procedure.

CASE 5

A 30-year-old gravida 2 para 1 woman presents to labor and delivery at 35 weeks' gestation with spontaneous rupture of membranes and early labor. She develops a fever and is started on antibiotics for presumed chorioamnionitis. Labor is progressing slowly but ultimately a cesarean section is performed. You are called to the cesarean section and your team of three individuals attends the delivery. The baby is handed to you and you place her on the radiant warmer. She is dried and the wet blankets are removed. You suction her mouth and note that she is not breathing. How do you proceed?

The drying and suctioning that you previously performed would be adequate to stimulate breathing if breathing could have been stimulated. It is, therefore, necessary to initiate positive pressure ventilation. You do this while a second team member auscultates the heart rate and taps out the beats. You ensure that the assisted breaths that you are providing are being adequately delivered to the lungs by looking for chest rise and continuously monitoring the heart rate to determine the occurrence and direction of change. Throughout these initial steps, the third team member is placing a pulse oximeter.

The heart rate prior to starting ventilation was 70 bpm and it has increased slightly to 90 bpm when ventilation was initiated. You note that there appears to be chest rise and you have used a carbon dioxide detector between the mask and ventilating device which is changing color indicating that you have an open airway. The baby continues to be apneic and the heart rate remains at approximately 90 bpm. What would you do next?

Ventilation was somewhat effective, but did not improve the heart rate to normal and spontaneous respirations have not yet begun. An increase in the amount of positive pressure may help to develop the functional residual capacity and improve the heart rate. After increasing the pressure for several breaths, if there is no further improvement, the next step would be to intubate the baby.

You now have a functioning pulse oximeter which indicates that the heart rate is 95 bpm and the oxygen saturation on the right hand is 35%. The baby is now 2 minutes old and you proceed with the intubation. Describe the procedure.

The baby is positioned on the bed with the body straight, neck in the neutral position, and back flat against the bed. You obtain the correctly-sized endotracheal tube (a 3.5 mm for this infant of 35 weeks' gestational age) and you insert a stylet to the appropriate depth above the side hole if so desired. You ensure that the pharynx is suctioned and you quickly test the function of the light bulb before inserting the laryngoscope into the mouth. Because the pulse oximeter is functioning, you are comfortable that the baby is being monitored while you are performing the procedure and you ask another team member to watch the time while you are performing the procedure. You move the laryngoscope blade to the locked and functioning position. You open the baby's mouth with your right hand, insert the laryngoscope blade into the mouth with your left hand and advance it toward the base of the tongue. The laryngoscope handle should be along the baby's midline making an approximate 45 degree angle with the baby's chin. You then lift the tongue with the laryngoscope blade using a straight upward motion, but maintaining the same angle of the laryngoscope handle with the chin. The tendency when lifting the tongue is to make a rocking motion with the laryngoscope handle which will increase the angle that the laryngoscope handle makes with the chin and will obscure the view of the larynx. After you have inserted the blade and have lifted the tongue, you identify the normal airway landmarks including the epiglottis and vocal cords. When you see the vocal cords, a second team member places the endotracheal tube in your right hand and you pass it through the glottis.

You then remove the laryngoscope while holding the endotracheal tube with your right hand and a second team member helps remove the stylet and attach a carbon dioxide detector and ventilating device. You look for cyclical color change on the carbon dioxide detector and mist on the tube. You listen for breath sounds bilaterally. You can also palpate the tip of the tube in the suprasternal notch to ensure that the tube is not placed too far distally, which could potentially result in a right main stem bronchus intubation. When you have confirmed tube placement, you tape the tube in place.

After you successfully intubate the baby, the heart rate increases to approximately 100 to 110 bpm, the baby begins to make gasping respirations and the oxygen saturation is 40%. Despite continued assisted ventilation, the heart rate and oxygen saturation do not increase beyond these levels. How do you proceed at this point?

This baby has not followed the usual pattern of improvement after provision of what seems to be adequate ventilation. It is, therefore, necessary to evaluate for other problems that might be hindering resuscitation. You have a second team member providing ventilation and the third team member is ensuring adequate temperature control. You do a quick survey of the baby for any obvious anomalies. You note that the face appears normally formed; there is no evidence of compression deformations which would be associated with longstanding oligohydramnios and could lead to pulmonary hypoplasia. There is no obvious edema to suggest hydrops fetalis or ascites, which could lead to compression of the thoracic cavity and respiratory compromise. You auscultate the chest on both sides and hear breath sounds louder on the right, and note that the abdomen appears scaphoid. Transillumination of the chest is unremarkable. You, therefore, suspect a congenital diaphragmatic hernia on the left and insert an orogastric tube. You aspirate the syringe and obtain 10 mL of air. The heart rate slowly increases and the oxygen saturation has increased slowly to 55%. You now consider administering surfactant and move the infant to the NICU for further management.

QUESTIONS

The International Liaison Committee on Resuscitation recommends starting positive pressure ventilation (PPV) in the delivery room when the heart rate (HR) is less than 100 beats per min (bpm) and giving cardiac compressions when the HR is less than 60 bpm. How soon does the heart rate rise with positive pressure ventilation in babies born at less than 32 weeks' gestation?

It takes more than a minute for newly born infants less than 30 weeks' gestation with a HR less than 100 bpm to achieve a HR above 100 bpm. In these infants, HR does not stabilize until it reaches 120 bpm (Yam et al). Also, there was no significant difference in arterial oxygen saturation (SpO_2) at 5 minutes after birth in infants less than 29 weeks' gestation given PPV with a T-piece or a self-inflating bag (Dawson et al).

Yam CH, Dawson JA, Schmölzer GM, et al: Heart rate changes during resuscitation of newly born infants <30 weeks' gestation: an observational study. Arch Dis Child Fetal Neonatal Ed 96:F102, 2011.

Dawson JA, Schmölzer GM, Kamlin CO, et al: Oxygenation with T-piece versus self-inflating bag for ventilation of extremely preterm infants at birth: a randomized controlled trial, J Pediatr 158:912, 2011.

True or False

The majority of extremely preterm infants are apneic at birth?

O'Donnell et al reviewed the videos of 61 extremely preterm infants taken immediately after birth. The majority cried (69%) and breathed (80%) without intervention. Most preterm infants are not apneic at birth. Therefore, the answer is false.

O'Donnell CP, Kamlin CO, Davis PG, et al: Crying and breathing by extremely preterm infants immediately after birth, J Pediatr 156:846, 2010.

True or False

Some neonatologists state that at the delivery of extremely premature infants they rely on "how the baby looks" when deciding whether to initiate resuscitation. This is a reliable and precise method to determine whether to initiate resuscitation.

Previous studies have reported poor correlation between early clinical signs and prognosis. To determine if neonatologists can accurately predict survival to discharge of extremely premature infants on the basis of observations in the first minutes after birth, Manley et al showed videos of the resuscitation of 10 extremely premature infants (<26 weeks' gestation) to 17 attending neonatologists and 17 fellows from the three major perinatal centers in Melbourne, Australia. Antenatal information was available to the observers. A monitor visible in each video displayed the heart rate and oxygen saturation of the infant. Observers were asked to estimate the likelihood of survival to discharge for each infant at three time points: 20 seconds, 2 minutes, and 5 minutes after birth. Observers' ability to predict survival was poor and not influenced by their level of experience.

CONCLUSION: Neonatologists' reliance on initial appearance and early response to resuscitation in predicting survival for extremely premature infants is misplaced. Therefore, the answer is false.

Manley BJ, Dawson JA, Kamlin CO, et al: Clinical assessment of extremely premature infants in the delivery room is a poor predictor of survival, Pediatrics 125:e559, 2010.

REFERENCES

The reference list for this chapter can be found online at www.expertconsult.com.

Recognition, Stabilization, and Transport of the High-Risk Newborn

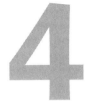

Jennifer Levy and Arthur E. D'Harlingue

At delivery, the newborn infant makes a complicated transition from intrauterine to extrauterine life. Although most newborns adapt without difficulty, the first few hours of life can be a precarious time for the high-risk infant. Health care professionals who provide care to newborns must anticipate potential problems for the high-risk infant before delivery. Early recognition of high-risk factors in the maternal history and of significant findings in the newborn allows for timely and appropriate monitoring and treatment. The goal of this approach of active anticipation and intervention is to prevent the development or progression of more serious illness and to minimize the risk of morbidity and mortality in the high-risk newborn. A newborn infant should receive a level of care specific to his or her unique needs. If an infant is critically ill, it is essential to intervene rapidly and effectively to stabilize the infant. In contrast, some infants with perinatal risk factors may do quite well postnatally. After an initial assessment and careful observation, such an infant might be advanced to well newborn care. This chapter outlines an approach to the preparation for, and management of, the high-risk infant in the first hours of life, including initial stabilization and transport.

MATERNAL HISTORY

During fetal growth the infant is somewhat protected in the intrauterine environment. However, in the course of a pregnancy the health of the mother affects the well-being of the fetus.[1] Both acute and chronic maternal illnesses can adversely affect embryogenesis and fetal growth and maturation. Maternal nutrition, medications, smoking, and drug use all affect the growth and development of the fetus. Such prenatal maternal factors may continue to have effects on the postnatal course of the newborn. Intrapartum factors, including obstetric complications, maternal therapy, and mode of delivery may also affect the condition of the newborn infant.

It is essential to obtain a complete maternal history to anticipate and prepare for a high-risk newborn. The physician should obtain this information before the delivery of the infant whenever possible. The maternal record should be reviewed, including the current hospital chart and, as available, the prenatal care record. Particular attention should be paid to the results of maternal prenatal laboratory studies, peripartum cultures, underlying maternal illnesses, and peripartum complications (Box 4-1). Maternal illnesses and medical problems have an important impact on the well-being of the fetus and the newborn (Table 4-1). Discussions with the obstetrician and nursing staff are essential to clarify the status of the mother and infant. When high-risk factors are identified, the physician and nursery staff are then prepared to deal with the anticipated problems of the newborn during delivery and subsequent hospital course.

MATERNAL DISEASES

Maternal diabetes mellitus affects the fetus before conception and throughout the entire pregnancy. Uncontrolled diabetes during the periconceptional period and during early embryogenesis increases the risk for fetal malformations, including congenital heart disease, limb abnormalities, and central nervous system anomalies.[2] Small left colon syndrome, femoral hypoplasia–unusual facies syndrome, and caudal regression syndrome are particularly associated with maternal diabetes. Poor diabetic

---

Box 4-1. Review of Obstetric and Perinatal History

Routine prenatal care
Last menstrual period
Estimated date of conception (by dates and ultrasound)
Onset of prenatal care

Previous pregnancies
Number
Outcome of each
Previous prenatal, intrapartum, neonatal complications

Maternal laboratory studies
Blood type and Rh
Antibody screen
Rapid plasma regain (syphilis)
Hepatitis B surface antigen
Rubella immunity
Human immunodeficiency virus antibody
Alpha-fetoprotein and other prenatal markers
Results of cultures or antibody titers

Maternal illnesses and infections
Diabetes
Hypertension
Thyroid disease
Seizure disorder
Infections (gonorrhea, syphilis, chlamydia, herpes simplex, HIV)

Pregnancy-related and perinatal conditions
Pregnancy-induced hypertension, eclampsia
Chorioamnionitis, maternal fever
Premature labor (use of tocolytics)

Maternal medications and drug use
Steroids
Tocolytics
Antibiotics
Psychotropics
Analgesics
Anesthetics
Tobacco
Alcohol

Marijuana
Cocaine
Amphetamines
Heroin or methadone
Phencyclidine (PCP)

Fetal laboratory studies
Amniotic fluid lung maturity studies
Fetal karyotype and other genetic tests
Amniotic fluid delta 450 to assess fetal bilirubin
Cordocentesis labs (complete blood count, platelet count)
Scalp pH

Fetal status
Singleton, twins, higher multiples
Ultrasound findings (weight, gestational age, anomalies, intrauterine growth restriction)
Amniotic fluid (polyhydramnios, oligohydramnios, meconium staining)
Time of rupture of membranes
Cord injuries or prolapse
Results of fetal heart rate monitoring
Maternal bleeding; placenta previa, abruptio placentae

Delivery
Method of delivery: vaginal or cesarean section (indication)
Instrumentation at delivery: forceps, vacuum
Presentation and position
Prolonged second stage
Shoulder dystocia
Cord complications: nuchal cord, true knot, laceration, avulsion

Social factors
Maternal support system
History of family violence, neglect, or abuse
Previous childen in foster care
Stable living situation, homelessness
History of depression, psychosis

---

control with resulting chronic hyperglycemia during the third trimester leads to fetal macrosomia, which increases the risk for birth trauma and the need for cesarean delivery. Fetal lung maturation is also delayed by maternal diabetes, increasing the risk for respiratory distress syndrome even in near-term infants. The infant of the diabetic mother is at risk for hypoglycemia, hypocalcemia, hypomagnesemia, polycythemia, and hyperbilirubinemia.

Maternal thyroid disease can have a wide variety of effects on the newborn, depending on the combined effects of maternal transplacental antithyroid antibodies and thyroid medications. The neonate born to a mother with Graves disease can be hypothyroid, euthyroid, or hyperthyroid at birth. When the mother's Graves disease is well controlled with medications (e.g., propylthiouracil) during the pregnancy, then the infant is usually euthyroid at birth. However, as the effects of maternal antithyroid medication wear off, persistent maternal antithyroid antibodies may stimulate the neonatal thyroid gland and cause thyrotoxicosis.

Table 4-1.	Maternal Medical Conditions and the Newborn
Maternal Condition	**Potential Effects on the Fetus or Newborn**
ENDOCRINE, METABOLIC	
Diabetes mellitus	Hypoglycemia, macrosomia, hyperbilirubinemia, polycythemia, increased risk for birth defects, birth trauma, small left colon syndrome, cardiomyopathy, and respiratory distress syndrome
Hypoparathyroidism	Fetal hypocalcemia, neonatal hyperparathyroidism
Hyperparathyroidism	Neonatal hypocalcemia and hypoparathyroidism
Graves' disease	Fetal and neonatal hyperthyroidism, intrauterine growth restriction, prematurity
Obesity	Macrosomia, birth trauma, hypoglycemia
Phenylketonuria (poorly controlled)	Mental restriction, microcephaly, congenital heart disease
Vitamin D deficiency	Neonatal hypocalcemia, rickets
CARDIOPULMONARY	
Asthma	Increased rates of prematurity, toxemia, and perinatal loss
Congenital heart disease	Effects of cardiovascular drugs; risk of maternal mortality
Pregnancy-induced hypertension	Premature delivery due to uncontrolled hypertension or eclampsia. Uteroplacental insufficiency, abruptio placentae, fetal loss, growth restriction, thrombocytopenia, neutropenia
HEMATOLOGIC	
Severe anemia (hemoglobin <6 mg/dL)	Impaired oxygen delivery, fetal loss
Iron deficiency anemia	Reduced iron stores, lower mental and developmental scores in follow-up
Idiopathic thrombocytopenic purpura	Thrombocytopenia, central nervous system (CNS) hemorrhage
Fetal platelet antigen sensitization	Thrombocytopenia, CNS hemorrhage
Rh or ABO sensitization	Jaundice, anemia, hydrops fetalis
Sickle cell anemia	Increased prematurity and intrauterine growth restriction
INFECTIOUS	
Chorioamnionitis	Increased risk for neonatal sepsis, prematurity
Gonorrhea	Ophthalmia neonatorum
Hepatitis A	Perinatal transmission
Hepatitis B and C	Perinatal transmission, chronic hepatitis, hepatic carcinoma
Herpes simplex	Encephalitis, disseminated herpes (risk of neonatal disease is much higher with primary versus recurrent maternal infection)
Human immunodeficiency virus	Risk of transmission to the fetus or newborn
Syphilis	Congenital syphilis, intrauterine growth restriction
Tuberculosis	Perinatal and postnatal transmission
INFLAMMATORY, IMMUNOLOGIC	
Systemic lupus erythematosus	Fetal death, spontaneous abortions, heart block, neonatal lupus, thrombocytopenia, neutropenia, hemolytic anemia
Inflammatory bowel disease	Increase in prematurity, fetal loss, and growth restriction
RENAL, UROLOGIC	
Urinary tract infection	Prematurity, intrauterine growth restriction
Chronic renal failure	Prematurity, intrauterine growth restriction
Transplant recipients	Prematurity, intrauterine growth restriction, possible effects of maternal immunosuppressive therapy and mineral disorders

Maternal preeclampsia has a number of adverse effects on the fetus and the newborn. When preeclampsia occurs early in the pregnancy, it may have severe effects on fetal growth. Fetal distress caused by preeclampsia may necessitate premature delivery of the infant before maturation of the lungs. Preeclampsia also causes neonatal neutropenia and thrombocytopenia.

Particular attention must be paid to infectious illnesses during the pregnancy and in the perinatal period. The results of the prenatal RPR (rapid plasma reagin), as well as any maternal treatment for syphilis, should be recorded in the neonatal record. In communities with a high prevalence of syphilis or in high-risk patients, repeat testing (despite negative prenatal results) of the mother for syphilis at the time of delivery should be considered. All women should be tested for hepatitis B surface antigen during pregnancy, and all neonates born to positive mothers should receive both hepatitis B immunoglobulin and hepatitis B vaccine. Maternal testing for antibody to the human immunodeficiency virus (HIV) should be recommended for all women prenatally. Treatment of the HIV-positive mother during the pregnancy and through the intrapartum course, combined with postnatal treatment of the infant, greatly reduces the risk of transmission of HIV to the infant. Any infant born to a mother who tests positive for HIV antibody or other evidence of HIV infection should be referred, when possible, to an infectious disease specialist for appropriate evaluation and possible treatment.

Active maternal genital infection with herpes simplex virus (HSV) in a woman with ruptured membranes or who delivers vaginally puts the infant at risk for neonatal herpes disease. The risk for vertical transmission of HSV is particularly high when the mother has active primary infection at the time of delivery or the infant is born prematurely. In contrast, with recurrent maternal herpes, the risk for vertical transmission of HSV is about 2%.[3]

Maternal chorioamnionitis increases the risk for bacterial sepsis in the newborn, particularly in the premature infant. It is strongly encouraged to follow the recommendations of the Centers for Disease Control and Prevention (CDC) regarding the use of intrapartum prophylactic antibiotics for mothers at risk to transmit group B STREPTOCOCCUS to their infants.[4] When clinical chorioamnionitis is diagnosed in a mother, the risk for sepsis in the newborn is greatly increased. Such infants should have a sepsis screen—a blood culture obtained and the infant started on broad spectrum antibiotics (e.g., ampicillin and gentamicin) pending culture results.

MATERNAL MEDICATIONS

Medications given to the mother may have adverse effects on the fetus (Table 4-2).[5,6] One area of great concern has been the risk for fetal malformations caused by maternal drug use. Because organogenesis occurs primarily in the first 12 weeks of gestation, the fetus can easily be exposed to a variety of potentially teratogenic toxins and drugs before a woman knows that she is pregnant or before the first prenatal visit. Appropriate counseling about the dangers of maternal drug use on the fetus is further complicated if prenatal care is delayed or lacking. Hence, the issue of medications and drugs during pregnancy is truly a public health issue. Women of childbearing age need to be educated about the potential risks associated with use of medications (both prescribed and over the counter) and illicit drugs before conception and embryogenesis. Besides their teratogenic potential, medication used by the mother can have a variety of other effects on the fetus and newborn. Fetal growth can be impaired by antineoplastic agents, heroin, cocaine, irradiation, and some anticonvulsants. Drugs used for tocolysis of labor can cause symptoms in the neonate. Beta-sympathomimetics are associated with neonatal hypoglycemia resulting from the mobilization of glycogen from the fetal liver. Magnesium sulfate, which is used for treatment of preterm labor and preeclampsia, depresses respiratory effort and can lead to respiratory failure in the newborn. In contrast, prenatal steroids for fetal lung maturation are generally safe and without adverse effects on the newborn.

Psychotropic drugs used during pregnancy have the potential for effects on the fetus and newborn. Fluoxetine, a selective serotonin reuptake inhibitor (SSRI), has been reported to increase the risk for neonatal problems and may have some neurobehavioral effects.[7] SSRIs in general may put the neonate at risk for pulmonary artery hypertension.[8] Benzodiazepines may increase the risk for oral clefts. Lithium is associated with a small increased risk for Ebstein anomaly.

Illicit and recreational drug use among pregnant women remains a major problem that affects both the fetus and the newborn. Maternal heroin and methadone use cause neonatal abstinence syndrome, which is characterized by irritability, hypertonia, jitteriness, seizures, sneezing, tachycardia, diarrhea, and difficulties with feedings.[9,10] Withdrawal symptoms can be prolonged, particularly with methadone exposure. Intrauterine opiate exposure is also associated with intrauterine growth restriction, poor postnatal growth, and abnormal neurodevelopmental outcome. Maternal cocaine exposure has also been reported to be associated with neurobehavioral disturbances in the newborn, although true withdrawal symptoms are less pronounced than with heroin or methadone.[11] In utero cocaine exposure affects fetal growth, and such infants tend to have a lower birth weight and smaller head circumference. Cocaine use in pregnancy is associated with neonatal cerebral hemorrhage, premature delivery, abruptio placentae, and stillbirth. There are conflicting data about the role of prenatal cocaine exposure and the risk for congenital

Table 4-2.	Maternal Medications and Toxins: Possible Effects on the Fetus and Newborn
Medication	**Effect on Fetus and Newborn**
ANALGESICS AND ANTI-INFLAMMATORIES	
Acetaminophen	Generally safe except with maternal overdose
Aspirin	Hemorrhage, premature closure of ductus arteriosus, pulmonary artery hypertension (effects not seen at ≤100 mg/day)
Opiates	Neonatal abstinence syndrome with chronic use
Ibuprofen	Reduced amniotic fluid volume when used in tocolysis; risk for premature ductus arteriosus closure and pulmonary hypertension
Indomethacin	Closure of fetal ductus arteriosus and pulmonary artery hypertension
Meperidine	Respiratory depression peaks 2 to 3 hours after maternal dose
ANESTHETICS	
General anesthesia	Respiratory depression of infant at delivery with prolonged anesthesia just before delivery
Lidocaine	High serum levels cause central nervous system (CNS) depression; accidental direct injection into the fetal head causes seizures
ANTIBIOTICS	
Aminoglycosides	Ototoxicity reported after use of kanamycin and streptomycin
Cephalosporins	Some drugs in this group displace bilirubin from albumin
Isoniazid	Risk for folate deficiency
Metronidazole	Potential teratogen and carcinogen, but not proven in humans
Penicillins	Generally no adverse effect
Tetracyclines	Yellow-brown staining of infant's teeth (when given at ≥5 months' gestation); stillbirth and prematurity due to maternal hepatotoxicity
Sulfonamides	Some drugs in this group displace bilirubin from albumin; can cause kernicterus
Trimethoprim	Folate antagonism
Vancomycin	Potential for ototoxicity
ANTICONVULSANTS	
Carbamazepine	Neural tube defects; midfacial hypoplasia
Phenobarbital	Withdrawal symptoms, hemorrhagic disease; midfacial hypoplasia
Phenytoin	Hemorrhagic disease; fetal hydantoin syndrome: growth and mental deficiency, midfacial hypoplasia, hypoplasia of distal phalanges
Trimethadione	Fetal trimethadione syndrome: growth and mental deficiency, abnormal facies (including synophrys with upslanting eyebrows), cleft lip and palate, cardiac and genital anomalies
Valproic acid	Neural tube defects, midfacial hypoplasia
ANTICOAGULANTS	
Warfarin (Coumadin)	Warfarin embryopathy: stippled epiphyses, growth and mental deficiencies, seizures, hypoplastic nose, eye defects, CNS anomalies including Dandy-Walker syndrome
Heparin	No direct adverse effects on the fetus
ANTINEOPLASTICS	
Aminopterin	Cleft palate, hydrocephalus, meningomyelocele, intrauterine growth restriction
Cyclophosphamide	Intrauterine growth restriction, cardiovascular and digital anomalies
Methotrexate	Absent digits, CNS malformation
ANTITHYROID DRUGS	
Iodide-containing drugs	Hypothyroidism
Methimazole	Hypothyroidism, cutis aplasia
Potassium iodide	Hypothyroidism and goiter, especially with chronic use
Propylthiouracil	Hypothyroidism
Iodine 131	Hypothyroidism, partial to complete ablation of thyroid gland
ANTIVIRALS	
Acyclovir	No definite adverse effects
Ribavirin	Teratogenic and embryolethal in animals
Zidovudine	Potential for fetal bone marrow suppression; combined maternal and neonatal treatment reduces perinatal transmission of human immunodeficiency virus
CARDIOVASCULAR DRUGS AND ANTIHYPERTENSIVES	
Angiotensin-converting enzyme inhibitors	Fetal hypocalvaria, oligohydramnios and fetal compression, oliguria, renal failure
β-Blockers (propranolol)	Neonatal bradycardia, hypoglycemia
Calcium channel blockers	If maternal hypotension occurs, this could affect placental blood flow
Diazoxide	Hyperglycemia; decreased placental perfusion with maternal hypotension

Continued

Table 4-2.	**Maternal Medications and Toxins: Possible Effects on the Fetus and Newborn—cont'd**
Medication	**Effect on Fetus and Newborn**
Digoxin	Fetal toxicity with maternal overdose
Hydralazine	If maternal hypotension occurs, this could affect placental blood flow
Methyldopa	Mild, clinically insignificant decrease in neonatal blood pressure
DIURETICS	
Furosemide	Increases fetal urinary sodium and potassium levels
Thiazides	Thrombocytopenia, hypoglycemia, hyponatremia, hypokalemia
HORMONES AND RELATED DRUGS	
Androgenics (danazol)	Masculinization of female fetuses
Corticosteroids	Cleft lip/palate
Diethylstilbestrol (DES)	DES daughters: vaginal adenosis, genital tract anomalies, increased incidence of clear cell adenocarcinoma, increased rate of premature delivery in future pregnancy DES sons: possible increase in genitourinary anomalies
Estrogens, progestins	Risk for virilization of female fetuses reported with progestins; small, if any, risk for other anomalies
Insulin	No apparent direct adverse effects, uncertain risk related to maternal hypoglycemia
Tamoxifen	Animal studies suggest potential for DES-like effect
SEDATIVES, TRANQUILIZERS, AND PSYCHIATRIC DRUGS	
Barbiturates	Risk for hemorrhage and drug withdrawal
Benzodiazepines	Drug withdrawal; possible increase in cleft lip/palate
Selective serotonin reuptake inhibitors (SSRIs)	Pulmonary artery hypertension, jitteriness, irritability
Lithium	Ebstein anomaly, diabetes insipidus, thyroid depression, cardiovascular dysfunction
Thalidomide	Limb deficiency, cardiac defects, ear malformations
Tricyclic antidepressants	Jitteriness, irritability
SOCIAL AND ILLICIT DRUGS	
Alcohol	Fetal alcohol syndrome, renal and cardiac anomalies
Amphetamines	Withdrawal, prematurity, decreased birth weight and head circumference, cerebral injury
Cocaine	Decreased birth weight, microcephaly, prematurity, abruptio placentae, stillbirth, cerebral hemorrhage; possible teratogen: genitourinary, cardiac, facial, limb, intestinal atresia/infarction
Heroin	Increased incidence of low birth weight and small for gestational age, drug withdrawal, postnatal growth and behavioral disturbances; decreased incidence of respiratory distress syndrome
Marijuana	Elevated blood carboxyhemoglobin; possible cause of shorter gestation, dysfunctional labor, intrauterine growth restriction, and anomalies
Methadone	Increased birth weight as compared to heroin, drug withdrawal (worse than with heroin alone)
Phencyclidine (PCP)	Irritability, jitteriness, hypertonia, poor feeding
Tobacco smoking	Elevated blood carboxyhemoglobin; decreased birth weight, increased prematurity rate, increased premature rupture of membranes, placental abruption and previa, increased fetal death, possible oral clefts
TOCOLYTICS	
Magnesium sulfate	Respiratory depression, hypotonia, bone demineralization with prolonged (weeks) use for tocolysis
Ritodrine	Neonatal hypoglycemia
Terbutaline	Neonatal hypoglycemia
VITAMINS AND RELATED DRUGS	
A (preformed, not carotene)	Excessive doses ($\geq$50,000 IU/day) may be teratogenic
Acitretin	Activated form of etretinate (see later)
D	Megadoses may cause hypercalcemia, craniosynostosis
Etretinate	Limb deficiency, neural tube defect; ear, cardiac, and CNS anomalies
Folate deficiency	Neural tube defects
Isotretinoin (13-*cis*-retinoic acid)	Ear, cardiac, CNS, and thymic anomalies
Menadione (vitamin K_3)	Hyperbilirubinemia and kernicterus
Phytonadione (vitamin K_1)	No adverse effect

Table 4-2.	Maternal Medications and Toxins: Possible Effects on the Fetus and Newborn—cont'd
Medication	**Effect on Fetus and Newborn**
MISCELLANEOUS	
Anticholinergics	Neonatal meconium ileus
Antiemetics	Doxylamine succinate and/or dicyclomine HCl with pyridoxine reported to be teratogens, but bulk of evidence is clearly negative
Aspartame	Contains phenylalanine; potential risk to fetus of a mother with phenylketonuria
Chorionic villus sampling (CVS)	Limb deficiency with early CVS
Irradiation	Adverse effects primarily associated with therapeutic, not diagnostic doses, and is dose dependent: fetal death, microcephaly, intrauterine growth restriction
Lead	Decreased IQ (dose related)
Methylene blue	Hemolytic anemia, hyperbilirubinemia, methemoglobinemia; intraamniotic injection in early pregnancy associated with intestinal atresia
Methylmercury	CNS injury, neurodevelopmental abnormalities, microcephaly
Misoprostol	Möebius sequence
Oral hypoglycemics	Neonatal hypoglycemia
Polychlorinated biphenyls	Cola skin coloration, minor skeletal anomalies, neurodevelopmental deficits

malformations (including intestinal atresia, urogenital anomalies, and limb reduction anomalies), and necrotizing enterocolitis.[12] Prenatal opiate and cocaine exposure is associated with an increased incidence of sudden infant death syndrome.[13] Persistent illicit drug activity in the mother or other family members can continue to affect the care of the high-risk infant throughout hospitalization and at the time of discharge, especially if the infant requires any type of special treatment at home. The management of the dysfunctional drug-exposed family can complicate the care of the sick newborn.

Prenatal alcohol use has serious adverse effects on the fetus that can manifest as problems in the neonatal period and beyond. The greatest risk to the fetus seems to be associated with heavy chronic drinking during the pregnancy (four to six drinks per day). However, with even more modest alcohol consumption (e.g., two drinks per day), effects have been noted in some studies. The most extreme result of maternal alcohol use is fetal alcohol syndrome.[14,15] Signs of this syndrome at birth may include symmetrical intrauterine growth restriction, central nervous system problems (microcephaly, irritability, tremulousness), facial dysmorphic features, congenital heart disease, and ear, eye, and limb (joint contractures, nail hypoplasia) anomalies. The facial dysmorphic features include short palpebral fissures, thin upper lip, smooth philtrum, maxillary hypoplasia, and a short nose. Later in life, these infants may have continued poor growth, neurobehavioral problems, and low IQ scores. Many infants exposed to alcohol in utero do not have sufficient physical features or anomalies required to make the diagnosis of fetal alcohol syndrome. However, these same infants may still demonstrate neurobehavioral and motor problems, which have been referred to as *fetal alcohol effects*.

Maternal smoking increases blood levels of carboxyhemoglobin and impairs oxygen delivery to the fetus. Smoking is associated with a decrease in birth weight of 175 to 250 grams. Several studies have suggested that nonsmoking mothers who are exposed to environmental tobacco smoke are more likely to have low-birth-weight infants than mothers with minimal tobacco exposure. Maternal smoking has also been implicated in placental abruption, preterm delivery, and postnatal respiratory illnesses. Whether prenatal exposure to tobacco causes an increased incidence of congenital malformations is unclear.[16,17]

PREPARATIONS FOR DELIVERY

After the maternal record has been reviewed, the physician should meet with the parents before the delivery of a high-risk infant. Important information regarding the prenatal course is not always reflected in the hospital obstetric record, particularly if prenatal care was lacking or fragmented, and this information may be available from the mother. This is particularly relevant regarding familial and genetic disorders. If the delivery of a premature infant is expected, it is appropriate to explain the role of the pediatrician, neonatal nurse practitioner, neonatologist, or other health care professionals in the delivery room, as well as resuscitation and subsequent management procedures (Box 4-2). Aspects of the anticipated hospital course for a sick premature infant should be discussed. Preparing parents for the prolonged hospitalization of a premature infant begins to build the foundations of trust and communication that will be needed between the family and the medical team. If time is limited because of the imminent delivery of the infant, the physician should, at the least, introduce himself or herself to the parents and briefly explain how the infant will initially be managed.

Depending on the type and severity of anticipated problems, specific equipment or extra personnel may be needed in the delivery room. For example, if an infant is known to have hydrops with pleural effusions and ascites, then the resuscitation team should have equipment fully prepared before the delivery for needle thoracentesis, chest tube drainage, intubation, ventilation, and umbilical catheterization. For such a high-risk delivery, the presence of two physicians to care for the infant may be indicated. Neonatal nursing personnel should be kept informed regarding the admission of high-risk mothers and possible pending deliveries. The pediatric surgeon should be notified of the anticipated delivery of any infants with abdominal wall defects, possible gastrointestinal anomalies or obstruction, diaphragmatic hernia, or tracheoesophageal fistula. The cardiology team, including cardiothoracic surgery, should be informed of impending deliveries of infants with known cardiac defects.

The pediatrician can also play an important role in the appropriate prepartum management of a high-risk mother. Aggressive tocolysis and use of prenatal steroids to induce fetal lung maturity should be strongly encouraged for the mother in preterm labor. Despite the multiple postnatal benefits for premature infants who were given prenatal steroids (Box 4-3)[18], maternal steroids are sometimes withheld in the presence of ruptured membranes, extreme prematurity, or an anticipated interval of less than 24 hours before delivery. Assessing the gestational age of the fetus can be very important in extremely premature infants. The discussion with the parents regarding outcomes will be markedly different for a 23-week as opposed to a 26-week fetus or newborn. Unless there are clear contraindications to steroid treatment or proven fetal lung maturity, in the setting of anticipated premature delivery, the mother should be given steroids.[19] The pediatrician should also advocate for delivery of high-risk mothers in the most appropriate setting. The needs of the mother, the fetus, and the newborn infant must all be recognized, and the personnel, equipment, and expertise must be available to meet these needs. Certain high-risk mothers, if stable for transport, should be transferred to a perinatal center. In particular, if premature delivery is anticipated before 32 weeks' gestation or if there are known major fetal congenital anomalies

---

Box 4-2. Subjects to Discuss with Parents Before Delivery of a Premature Newborn

Anticipated birth weight and gestational age
Approximate risk of death and major morbidities
Anticipated length of hospitalization
Respiratory distress syndrome, oxygen, ventilation, surfactant
Procedures: intubation, intravenous catheters, umbilical catheterization, lumbar puncture
Blood transfusion: risks, benefits, alternatives, use of designated donor
Potential problems: patent ductus arteriosus, intraventricular hemorrhage, jaundice
Possible need for transport (if not delivered in a tertiary center)
Role of the parents in the intensive care nursery
Importance of providing breast milk

Box 4-3. Effects of Prenatal Steroids on the Premature Newborn

Increased tissue and alveolar surfactant
Maturational effects on the lung: structural and biochemical
Possible maturational effects on brain, gastrointestinal tract, and other organs
Decreased mortality rate
Decreased incidence and severity of respiratory distress syndrome
Decreased incidence of necrotizing enterocolitis
Decreased incidence of intraventricular hemorrhage
Decreased incidence of significant patent ductus arteriosus
Decreased length of stay and costs of hospitalization

that would affect the stabilization of the newborn, then maternal transfer to a perinatal center with an intensive care nursery is most appropriate.[20]

LABOR AND DELIVERY

Appropriate supplies and a well-trained staff are essential in the delivery room. Whether the birth occurs in a birthing room or in the operating room, the equipment and procedures need to be the same—an infant warming table with working lights, Apgar timer, air and oxygen supply, and an oxygen blender. A person needs to be delegated to ensure that the infant table is adequately prepared. There needs to be mechanical suction and a device to deliver positive pressure ventilation. Endotracheal tubes of different sizes, meconium aspirators, and a laryngoscope must be readily available. If a multiple delivery is anticipated, there must be a stocked infant table for each infant. An emergency crash cart designated specifically for neonates must be close by and well stocked in case of emergency.

The value of a staff that is well trained and prepared cannot be overstated. Health care workers who attend deliveries should have appropriate training in NRP (neonatal resuscitation program). Additionally, emergency procedures for alerting more subspecialized health care professionals (e.g., neonatologists or pediatricians) must be in place in the event of an acutely ill infant.

There are additional special considerations in the delivery room when anticipating the delivery of a preterm infant. Preterm infants are especially prone to cold stress and hypothermia. Infants less than 29 weeks should be placed in a polyurethane bag up to the neck to minimize heat loss.[21] Most premature infants should have a pulse oximeter applied shortly after birth in the delivery room. A proportion of infants born at 32 weeks or less will develop respiratory distress syndrome from surfactant deficiency. Preparations to support such an infant should include the potential to provide nasal continuous positive airway pressure (CPAP), intubation, and surfactant administration as needed. If available, a neonatal respiratory therapist should be present to facilitate the stabilization of these infants. There has been increasing evidence that infants resuscitated in the delivery room with room air, rather than 100% oxygen, have lower levels of oxygen-free radicals, which may affect the incidence of retinopathy of prematurity. In addition, oxygen may have an adverse affect on cerebral circulation and breathing physiology.[22] Most extremely low-birth-weight (ELBW) infants will need some supplemental oxygen in the delivery room, and it is suggested to begin with about 30% O_2 in such infants who require resuscitation and then adjust Fio_2 as needed, guided by pulse oximetry.

TRANSITION

Transition is a term used to describe a series of events that are centered around birth itself, beginning in utero and continuing into the postnatal period. The fetus is well adapted to the intrauterine environment. However, during this intricate symbiotic relationship with the mother, the fetus must also prepare for transition to extrauterine life. This transition requires striking adaptive changes in multiple organ systems of the newborn. Some of these dynamic changes are largely completed in the first minutes to hours after birth. Others are initiated at birth, but continue to evolve over the first weeks of life. The ability of the newborn to make this transition safely and expeditiously affects the health and survival of the infant. Recognition of the factors that may adversely affect the transitional period allows the health professional to act promptly and judiciously for the benefit of the infant.

The most dramatic changes during transition involve the cardiovascular and respiratory systems. During fetal life, gas exchange is accomplished by the placenta, whereas the fetal lungs are gasless and filled with fluid. In the several days before delivery, fetal lung water begins to decrease and is accelerated by labor. Various hormones, including epinephrine and vasopressin, decrease fluid secretion into the pulmonary intraluminal space. Plasma protein levels increase with labor, and this augmented oncotic pressure likely increases pulmonary intraluminal water reabsorption. Intraluminal fluid is transported to the interstitium and is removed primarily by augmented postnatal pulmonary blood flow as pulmonary artery pressure decreases. Some intraluminal fluid is transported by the lymphatics through the mediastinal tissues or across the pleural space. Previously, it has been suggested that thoracic compression during vaginal birth played a prominent role in the expulsion of lung fluid through the oropharynx, but such a mechanism does not seem to have a major role in the reduction of lung water in the newborn.

Fetal breathing is episodic and occurs primarily during periods of low-voltage electrocortical activity. It likely plays a role in the conditioning of respiratory muscles and may have other effects on chest wall, lung, and muscle growth. A variety of phenomena contribute to the onset of continuous breathing, which occurs shortly after birth in relatively healthy nonasphyxiated infants. Aspects of the physical environment may play a role, such as light, sound, cutaneous stimulation, and heat loss. Cord occlusion and an increase in blood oxygen appear to be potent stimulants of continuous breathing by the newborn. The fetus prepares for air breathing by the synthesis and release of surfactant into the alveolar space. The process can be accelerated by premature rupture of fetal membranes, β-mimetic tocolysis, and the administration of steroids to the mother. Delivery of a term infant by elective cesarean section without labor may prevent maturation of this late process of surfactant production and release, resulting in an infant with respiratory distress syndrome. If an infant is scheduled to be delivered via elective cesarean section before 39 weeks, fetal lung maturity should be checked to avoid the sequelae of surfactant deficiency.[23]

The transitional changes in the cardiovascular system are primarily an adaptation to the elimination of the placental circulation and an adaptation to pulmonary gas exchange. As the lungs expand at birth, pulmonary artery pressure declines, and there is a dramatic increase in pulmonary blood flow. Systemic arterial resistance increases with cord occlusion and elimination of the low resistance placental circulation. These factors combine to favor an increase in pulmonary blood flow rather than the passage of blood via the ductus arteriosus into the distal aorta. Because of the increase in pulmonary blood flow, left atrial pressure increases and functionally closes the foramen ovale, thereby eliminating this source of previous right-to-left shunting. The right and left ventricles now function primarily in series versus pumping in parallel as in the fetal state. The ductus arteriosus remains open for a variable period, but it begins to close in response to exposure to highly oxygenated blood. It generally functionally closes by 1 to 2 days in a term infant, but frequently remains open in the premature or the seriously ill term newborn with pulmonary artery hypertension. The ductus venosus closes within 1 to 2 days (contributing to the technical difficulty of passing an umbilical venous catheter to the right atrium beyond the first day of life). Pulmonary artery pressure continues to decline through the first weeks of life. During these dramatic changes in the cardiovascular system, the sick newborn may demonstrate difficulties in making these transitions. Because of the parallel pumping systems of the fetal cardiovascular system, most infants with complex congenital heart disease are well adapted to the in utero state. However, these infants often do poorly in the transition to extrauterine life. In infants with ductal dependent cyanotic congenital heart disease, progressive cyanosis develops as the ductus arteriosus closes. In those infants with left-sided obstructive lesions (e.g., hypoplastic left heart), acidosis and shock develop as the ductus arteriosus closes and distal aortic blood flow is lost. Infants with pulmonary artery hypertension shunt right to left at the foramen ovale or patent ductus arteriosus. Recognition of infants at risk for pulmonary artery hypertension (e.g., meconium aspiration) may lead the physician to earlier interventions (e.g., endotracheal suctioning, oxygen, ventilation) to reverse or prevent this problem.

The uterine environment is relatively quiet, very dark, and rather unchanging until labor and passage through the birth canal. At birth, the newborn is bombarded with stimuli, including exposure to light, different sounds, and tactile stimuli. In addition, the newborn must begin to defend its core temperature against heat loss, despite being born both wet and into a much cooler environment. These multiple stresses result in a surge of sympathetic nervous system activity. Catecholamines increase dramatically at birth. Brown fat (nonshivering) thermogenesis causes the hydrolysis of stored triglycerides and the release of fatty acids. Box 4-4 summarizes these and other events during transition.

Specific physical and behavioral changes, which occur in the healthy newborn in the hours after birth, have been described (Fig. 4-1). The healthy newborn may have some initial bradycardia or tachycardia, and cutaneous perfusion may be mottled or pale. Respirations may be initially somewhat irregular but should improve steadily and become regular and vigorous. There may be some mild transient grunting and flaring, but true respiratory distress with retractions should not

---

Box 4-4.	**Summary of Transitional Events in the Newborn**

Pulmonary
Reabsorption of intraluminal fluid
Onset of continuous breathing
Expansion of pulmonary air spaces
Pulmonary gas exchange replaces placental
   circulation
Surfactant synthesis and release

Cardiovascular
Removal of the placental circulation
Decline in pulmonary artery pressure and
   increase in pulmonary blood flow
Closure of ductus arteriosus, foramen ovale,
   and ductus venosus

Glucose homeostasis
Loss of transplacental glucose transport with
   decline in serum glucose
Increase in glucagon and decrease in insulin
   levels

Thermogenesis
Sympathetic nervous system activation caused
   by cold stress
Nonshivering thermogenesis (brown fat)

Hormonal and metabolic
Shift from primarily glucose metabolism (RQ =
   1) to glucose and fat (RQ = 0.8-0.85)
Increase in oxygen consumption
Increase in levels of epinephrine and norepi-
   nephrine
Acute increase in TSH with subsequent decline
Peak increase in T_4, free T_4, and T_3 at 48 hours
Decrease in reverse T_3

Decline in serum calcium with nadir at 24 hours
   and subsequent elevation
Increase in parathyroid hormone, 1,25 OH
   vitamin D, and calcitonin
Increase in glycerol and free fatty acids

Nervous system
Adaptive interaction with parents and environ-
   ment
Movement between states
Increase in motor activity

Renal
Increase in renin production
Increase in sodium reabsorption
Onset of long-term maturational changes with
   improving glomerular filtration rate
Reduction of extracellular fluid compartment
   (diuresis)

Hematologic
Marked reduction in erythropoietin and erythro-
   genesis
Postnatal increase in blood leukocyte and neutrophil count
Improved vitamin K-dependent carboxylation of
   coagulation factors

Gastrointestinal
Evacuation of meconium
Induction of intestinal enzymes with feeding
Establishment of effective coordinated suck,
   swallow, breathing

---

be present. If the infant has made a stable transition, these parameters stabilize within the first hour of life. After birth, the healthy newborn often undergoes a quiet alert phase, which has been referred to as the *first phase of reactivity*. When placed skin-to-skin on the mother's chest shortly after birth, the infant often becomes quiet or exploring.[24] Rhythmic, pushing movements of the lower extremities have been described as the infant searches for the mother's breast. If left undisturbed, the infant crawls and searches for the areola in an attempt to attach and suckle (Fig. 4-2). Suckling causes release of oxytocin in the mother, stimulating milk production and uterine contractions. Sucking movements in the infant stimulate the release of multiple gastrointestinal hormones, which prepare the infant to digest enteral nutrients.[25] The warmth provided by the mother's chest maintains a stable temperature in the infant, as long as a blanket is also placed over the infant and the room is not too cold.[26] Early contact with the mother has been shown to increase the success of breast feeding, and it is an important first step in the bonding process. Most hospital staff in birthing centers recognize the importance of this early contact between the mother and infant. Sometimes mothers are encouraged to promptly attempt to nurse their infant immediately after birth. It may be more appropriate to quickly dry the infant and to rapidly determine that the infant is healthy and requires no immediate interventions. Then the infant can be placed on the mother's chest, skin to skin, and allowed to have a private quiet time with the parents.

PHYSICAL EXAMINATION OF THE NEWBORN

The first 24 hours of life are particularly precarious as the infant makes the transition from intrauterine to extrauterine life.

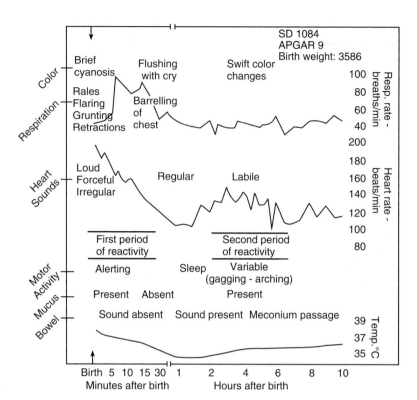

Figure 4-1. A summary of the physical findings in normal transition (the first 10 hours of extrauterine life in a representative high-Apgar-score infant delivered under spinal anesthesia without premedication). *(From Desmond M, Rudolph A, Phitaksphraiwan P: The transitional care nursery.* Pediatr Clin North Am *13:651, 1966.)*

During this critical period, a thorough physical examination is essential to identify problems and institute early intervention. Physicians should continually strive to improve their observational skills and the quality of their newborn examinations. Nothing can replace years of clinical experience with the many normal variations and abnormal findings with which a newborn may present.[27,28]

After initial resuscitation and stabilization in the delivery room, the newborn should receive an initial examination to identify any significant problems or anomalies. The infant's respiratory effort and air exchange should be observed closely. An infant with persistently shallow and irregular respirations needs further resuscitation and appropriate monitoring. Symptoms of respiratory distress such as grunting, flaring, retractions, and cyanosis should be identified promptly. Particular attention should be paid to the adequacy of the infant's heart rate and clinical indicators of cardiovascular function. Pallor and poor perfusion need immediate further evaluation and possible intervention. It should be established that the infant is appropriately responsive and has good muscle tone. The extremities, facies, genitalia, abdomen, and back should be quickly inspected for any anomalies.

Such a quick examination of an apparently healthy infant in the delivery room can usually be performed in 1 to 2 minutes. Any major abnormalities should be discussed with the parents as soon as feasible.

In a stable, healthy, term or near-term newborn, a more detailed examination by the physician may be deferred. However, admitting nursing personnel should perform a thorough assessment of the infant within 2 hours of birth. This allows the infant to be with the parents and to start breast feeding. The nursing personnel should evaluate the infant for high-risk factors, review the pertinent maternal history (usually included on the labor and delivery record), and examine the infant. The physician should be notified of any high-risk factors in the history or significant findings on examination. This nursing assessment should be recorded in a standardized format. It should include measurement of weight, length, head circumference, estimate of gestational age, and vital signs. The physician should perform a complete physical examination no later than 24 hours after birth, but preferably within 12 hours of birth. The normal newborn should also be examined by the physician within the 24 hours before discharge. High-risk infants, including those with respiratory distress, poor cardiac output, gestational age

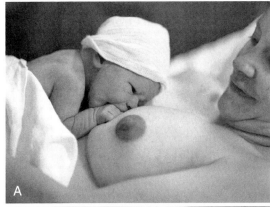

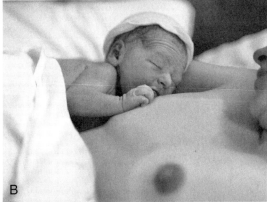

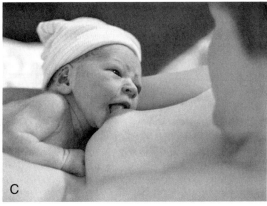

Figure 4-2. A, Infant about 15 minutes after birth, sucking on the unwashed hand and possibly looking at mother's left nipple. **B,** An arm push-up, which helps the infant to move to mother's right side. **C,** At 45 minutes of age, the infant moved to the right breast without assistance and began sucking on the areola of the breast. The infant has been looking at the mother's face for 5 to 8 minutes. *(Photographed by Elaine Siegel. From Klaus PH: Your amazing newborn, Cambridge, Mass., 1998, Perseus, pp 13, 16, and 17.)*

of less than 35 weeks, congenital anomalies, infants of a diabetic mother, or clinical signs of asphyxia or sepsis should be assessed immediately by the nursing staff and examined by the physician.

VITAL SIGNS, BODY MEASUREMENTS, AND GESTATIONAL AGE ASSESSMENT

The admitting nursing personnel should measure the temperature, respiratory rate, and heart rate of all newborn infants within the first hour of life. In the past, the initial measurement of temperature was commonly performed rectally to additionally determine patency of the anus. This practice of an initial rectal temperature has been largely abandoned by birth centers because of the small but real risk of bowel perforation with rectal measurement. The nurse should not only record the respiratory rate, but also should observe for any signs of respiratory distress, irregularities in respiratory pattern (e.g., apnea), and the degree of work of breathing. In the first day of life most newborns have a respiratory rate of 40 to 60 breaths per minute. However, in transition, some newborns have a respiratory rate as high as 80 to 100 breaths per minute with little or no signs of distress. Heart rate should be checked by auscultation and any irregularities in rhythm should be noted. Healthy term newborns do not require routine blood pressure determination on admission. Any sick newborn and any premature infant (less than 35 weeks' gestational age) should have at least an initial blood pressure measurement, which is easily performed by an oscillometric technique.

Every newborn should have assessment of gestational age performed.[29] In some nurseries, the gestational age examination is performed by the nursing staff on admission of all newborns. We encourage physicians to continue to perform a gestational age assessment as part of their evaluation of a premature infant. The results of this examination should then be compared with the maternal estimated date of confinement (by ultrasound and last menstrual period). The nursing staff should record the weight (in kilograms), and the length and head circumference (in centimeters) of the infant on admission. These measurements should be plotted on the appropriate intrauterine growth curves. This facilitates the identification of infants who are small or large for gestational age, or who are microcephalic or macrocephalic.

GENERAL EXAMINATION

It is useful to observe the overall condition of the infant, including major anomalies, respiratory effort, color, perfusion, activity, and responsiveness. In infants with respiratory distress, it is important to note the presence of grunting, flaring, and retractions and to assess the work of breathing. The quality and the strength of the infant's cry and overall motor activity are especially useful indicators of the infant's general condition. Such general observations are useful to quickly categorize an infant and to focus one's attention on a critically ill newborn. A vigorous, screaming, pink infant clearly does not demand the same immediate intervention required by the infant who is pale and hypotonic with labored or irregular breathing.

Edema is readily noted in any initial examination. The presenting part at birth may be edematous, bruised, and covered with petechiae. Edema of the dorsum of the feet may be seen as a focal finding in Turner syndrome, or it may be part of a more generalized picture of edema. Infants with hydrops, whether immune or nonimmune, often have generalized edema, which can include the trunk, extremities, scalp, and face. In critically ill infants who require fluid volume resuscitation, generalized edema may develop over the course of their illness. Such edema often localizes to the face and trunk, and especially the flanks.

The initial examination should also include a quick survey for dysmorphic features, whether malformations or deformations. The presence of a major congenital anomaly or multiple minor anomalies may indicate the need for an aggressive investigation of other major organ defects.

SKIN

In the extremely premature infant (23 to 28 weeks' gestation) the skin can be translucent with little subcutaneous fat and superficial veins that are easily visualized. Because the stratum corneum is quite thin, the skin of the extremely premature infant is easily injured by seemingly innocuous procedures or manipulation that results in denudation of the stratum corneum and a raw weeping surface. With advancing gestational age, the fetal skin matures as the stratum corneum thickens, subcutaneous fat increases, and the skin loses its translucent appearance. By term, the fetal skin is relatively opaque with considerable subcutaneous fat.

By 35 to 36 weeks' gestational age, the infant is covered with vernix. The vernix thins by term and is usually absent in the postterm infant. Meconium staining of the skin, nails, and cord is evident when meconium has been present in the amniotic fluid for a number of hours. The postmature infant has parchment-like skin with deep cracks on the trunk and extremities. Fingernails may be elongated, and peeling of the distal extremities is often evident in the postmature infant.

Erythema toxicum neonatorum is a benign rash seen generally in term infants beginning on the second or third day of life. It is characterized by 1- to 2-mm white papules, which may become vesicular, on an erythematous base. Wright or Giemsa stain of the lesions demonstrates large numbers of eosinophils. Milia, which are 1- to 2-mm whitish papules, are frequently found on the face of newborns. Transient neonatal pustular melanosis, which is seen predominantly in black infants, is a benign generalized eruption with a mixture of superficial pustules that progress to hyperpigmented macules. Congenital dermal melanocytosis (Mongolian spot) is a gray-blue nonraised area of hyperpigmentation seen predominantly over the buttocks or trunk and is seen most commonly in black, Asian, and Hispanic infants.

The newborn infant can have a variety of color changes in the first day of life, some of which are due to cardiovascular lability during transition. The harlequin sign is a benign transient finding in which the infant is pale on one side and flushed on the contralateral side with a distinct border in the midline. Mottling of the skin is common in the first days to weeks of life in some infants. The color and perfusion of the skin can provide information regarding cardiac output and oxygenation. Acrocyanosis is a common finding in the first 6 to 24 hours of life, but is usually of little significance by itself. Central cyanosis persisting beyond the first few minutes of life may indicate inadequate oxygen delivery and demands further evaluation. Infants can have cyanosis over just the lower half of the body in the presence of right-to-left shunting across a patent ductus arteriosus. Capillary refill time can be sluggish in the first hours of life as the infant adapts to extrauterine life. Persistent pallor and poor perfusion may reflect inadequate cardiac output as a result of perinatal hypoxia and ischemia, congenital heart disease, or sepsis. Infants with anemia may have pallor, but this is an inconsistent finding even in the presence of severe anemia. Marked plethora may occur with polycythemia, but this finding is also inconsistent. Hence, the physician must have a high index of suspicion for those infants at risk for either anemia or polycythemia. Jaundice at birth is abnormal and requires immediate investigation. Physiologic jaundice is generally not seen before 24 hours of age. Petechiae and bruising are very common on the presenting fetal parts. However, in the presence of thrombocytopenia or platelet dysfunction, petechiae are more likely to be generalized.

A careful examination of the newborn's skin should be made to identify congenital nevi, hemangiomas, areas of abnormal pigmentation, tags, and pits. A port wine stain of the face should alert the physician to the possibility of Sturge-Weber syndrome. Congenital strawberry hemangiomas should be identified and their progression monitored. Large hemangiomas of the face and neck can potentially cause airway obstruction. Massive hemangiomas of the extremities or trunk can result in large systemic shunts and high-output cardiac failure. Congenital defects in the skin are important in the identification of underlying structural problems or systemic disorders. Localized scalp defects are associated with trisomy 13. Midline posterior defects of the skin are particularly important to identify. Sacral dimples should be carefully examined to ensure that the base is clearly visualized and the possibility of a sinus tract to the spinal cord is excluded. Such dermal sinuses can communicate with the cerebrospinal fluid and result in meningitis.

HEAD AND SCALP

The occipital-frontal head circumference should be measured and recorded for all newborns. Ideally, three careful measurements should be taken at various positions over the occipital-frontal area, and the largest measurement is then recorded. The head should be palpated carefully and visually inspected to detect any unusual distortions, hematomas, or caput. Because the fetal skull is molded by the delivery process, abnormal skull shapes may need to be reevaluated in 1 to 2 days. Caput succedaneum is a common and expected finding after vaginal vertex delivery. Bruising and edema caused by caput is usually soft, crosses suture lines, and does not significantly expand in size postnatally. Subperiosteal hematomas, which are common, are easily identified by their distinct margins which stop at the suture lines. Subperiosteal hematomas are generally soft

and fluctuant on palpation and can give a sensation of absence of the bony skull beneath the hematoma. In contrast, subgaleal hematomas are not limited by suture margins and usually cross the midline. A rapidly expanding subgaleal hematoma can be life threatening because of the blood loss into the hematoma. Such patients require close monitoring and aggressive volume replacement.

The skull sutures should be checked to note whether they are widened or overriding. A widely open full anterior fontanelle with split sutures suggests increased intracranial pressure, which may be caused by intracranial hemorrhage, cerebral edema, or hydrocephalus. Unusual scalp hair patterns can be an indication of underlying brain dysmorphogenesis, particularly if the infant has other dysmorphic features. A midline mass protruding from the skull may be an encephalocele and requires thorough evaluation.

EYES, EARS, MOUTH, AND FACIAL FEATURES

The overall configuration of the face should be inspected including the profile, which helps in the detection of micrognathia. Such overview reveals areas of maxillary or mandibular hypoplasia, any distortion, or hemifacial hypoplasia. The eyes should be inspected for abnormalities in the size of the globes or orbits, and for any malposition (e.g., proptosis as in neonatal hyperthyroidism). Abnormalities of the eyebrows may be a clue to specific syndromes, such as synophrosis in Cornelia de Lange syndrome. The eyelids of the newborn may be edematous or may display ecchymosis from the delivery process. Nevus flammeus is commonly noted on the upper eyelids. After vaginal delivery, the conjunctivae are often injected and scleral hemorrhages may be present. The parents may need reassurance regarding these generally benign features.

Abnormal slanting of the palpebral fissures is associated with a number of syndromes. Notably, an upward slant is seen in trisomy 21, whereas down-slanting eyes are a feature of Treacher Collins, Apert, and DiGeorge syndromes. Short palpebral fissures with a smooth philtrum and thin upper lip suggest fetal alcohol syndrome. Hypertelorism or inner epicanthal folds are associated with a large number of syndromes (most notably trisomy 21). Marked hypotelorism is associated with holoprosencephaly and trisomy 13. The eyes should be examined with an ophthalmoscope to check for the red reflex and the presence of cataracts. Leukocoria, or a white pupil, mandates a thorough ophthalmologic examination. Cloudiness of the cornea may be seen at birth, especially in the premature infant. The pupils should be round and equal in size. Pupillary reactivity to light is minimal beginning at 30 to 32 weeks' gestation and increases with gestational age. The lenticular pattern can be useful in gestational age assessment.

The oral cavity should be inspected using a tongue blade and a light source. Important findings to note include the presence of neonatal teeth, the arch of the palate, the integrity of both the hard and soft palate, the shape and movement of the tongue, and the presence of any oropharyngeal masses or mucosal lesions. Although cleft lip and palate are frequently isolated anomalies, the infant with these anomalies should be carefully examined for any other associated anomalies. Abnormal masses (e.g., tumors, hemangiomas) in the area of the mouth and pharynx demand prompt attention in view of their potential to cause airway obstruction. Neonatal teeth are generally a benign finding, but may be associated with several syndromes (Ellis-van Creveld, Hallermann-Streiff, and Sotos syndromes). Protrusion of the tongue from the mouth is seen in trisomy 21, or it may be due to macroglossia, which may be associated with storage diseases, Beckwith-Wiedemann syndrome, or hypothyroidism.

The position, rotation, and shape of the ears should be noted. In very premature infants, the pinna is soft, flat, and easily folded back on itself. In term infants, the outer helix of the pinna should be well formed with a definite curvature. Infants of diabetic mothers may have unusually hairy ears. The presence of abnormally shaped or malformed (e.g., microtia) ears should prompt a careful examination of the infant for other potential dysmorphic features. In particular, low set and posteriorly rotated ears are associated with a number of syndromes. The ears are carefully inspected to ensure patency of the external auditory canal. Otoscopy is not routinely needed in the newborn infant with normal external ear anatomy. Amniotic fluid debris and secretions often prevent easy viewing of the tympanic membrane in the first days of life.

NECK AND THORAX

The neck should be supple and easily turned from side to side, and the trachea should be in the midline. Gentle extension of the neck is performed looking for any mass, cystic hygroma, or goiter. Large masses in the neck require urgent evaluation because of their potential for airway obstruction. A webbed neck or redundant skin is associated with trisomy 21, Turner, Noonan, or Zellweger syndromes. The clavicles should be palpated to check for deformities. A clavicular fracture often results in crepitance and swelling, and an asymmetrical Moro reflex.

The thorax may appear to be small or malformed in a number of neuromuscular disorders, or in lung hypoplasia. With congenital disorders of generalized muscle weakness, the thorax assumes a bell-shaped appearance. In term infants, the areolae of the nipples are raised and there is an underlying breast bud with a diameter of 0.5 to 1 cm. The nipples may be enlarged secondary to the effects of maternal hormones, and a milky discharge (so-called "witch's milk") is not uncommon in both male and female infants. Mastitis, which is usually unilateral, causes swelling, erythema, warmth, and tenderness. In extremely premature infants, the areola may be quite small, flat, and difficult to identify. Abnormal displacement of the nipple or supernumerary nipples should be noted. The nipples are widely spaced in Turner syndrome, Noonan syndrome, and trisomy 18.

RESPIRATORY SYSTEM

When breathing at rest, the healthy newborn should move air easily and comfortably at a rate of 40 to 60 breaths per minute. Because most air exchange in newborns is accomplished by the effects of diaphragmatic excursion, there is considerable abdominal wall motion with breathing. Respiratory distress, whether because of lung disease or airway obstruction, is evident by the presence of subcostal or sternal retractions. Suprasternal retractions may be evident in the presence of severe respiratory distress. Audible grunting occurs as the infant expires against a partially closed glottis and is an extremely reliable indicator of any process causing alveolar collapse or atelectasis. Asymmetrical movement of the chest wall with respirations occurs with a variety of unilateral lesions of the diaphragms or pleural space (e.g., pneumothorax, diaphragmatic hernia, diaphragmatic paralysis, pleural effusion). The quality of the infant's cry should be noted. A high-pitched shrill cry may suggest a central nervous system disorder. A weak cry may occur in the presence of respiratory distress or a depressed central nervous system. A hoarse or muffled cry may occur with vocal cord swelling, intratracheal narrowing, or a mass.

The lungs should be auscultated anteriorly, posteriorly, and at the sides of the chest. Comparison should be made between the two sides. The breath sounds should be checked for the amount of air exchange (whether with spontaneous or with assisted ventilation). Asymmetrical breath sounds may be caused by pneumothorax (Box 4-5), an improperly placed endotracheal tube, diaphragmatic hernia, or any other space-occupying lesion in the hemithorax. Crepitant breath sounds or crackles are often heard in the initial transitional period. These sounds generally clear as the newborn expands the lungs and clears fluid from the pulmonary airspaces. However, crackles may be heard with respiratory distress syndrome, pneumonia, and various types of aspiration syndromes. Stridor occurs with a variety of causes of airway obstruction, but may be absent or difficult to appreciate in the infant who is moving little air. An audible leak during the inspiratory phase of a ventilator may be heard around the endotracheal tube of intubated infants and may obscure the quality of the breath sounds. The sounds caused by air leak are often transmitted through the mouth and are audible by the unassisted ear. These sounds, when auscultated by a stethoscope, are sometimes mistakenly attributed to wheezing caused by bronchoconstriction. Coarse breath sounds or rhonchi may suggest the need for suctioning to clear secretions in the upper airway or in an endotracheal tube.

For ventilated infants, auscultation of the lungs is routinely used to confirm appropriate position of the endotracheal tube. The breath sounds should be symmetrical and there should be adequate chest excursion

with good air entry during the inspiratory phase of positive-pressure ventilation. Diminished breath sounds on the left may indicate that the endotracheal tube has passed into the right mainstem bronchus. In such a situation, the tube should be gradually withdrawn until the breath sounds are equal. The depth of the endotracheal tube (in centimeters from the tip) is an important part of the physical examination of an intubated infant. Small movements of the endotracheal tube in a newborn can result in inadvertent right mainstem placement or accidental extubation. However, auscultation of breath sounds alone for confirmation of intubation is not always adequate. The small size of the neonatal chest allows for wide transmission of breath sounds. The sounds created by ventilation through an endotracheal tube inadvertently misplaced into the esophagus can transmit through the newborn's chest. Even with a properly placed endotracheal tube, chest movement and air entry may be inconsistent with positive pressure breaths if the infant is fighting the ventilator. If lung compliance is very poor, chest movement may also be diminished except with high pressures. Devices that detect exhaled CO_2 are widely used to confirm intubation, and their routine use is highly recommended.

During high-frequency ventilation, whether by oscillation or jet, the lungs are not capable of being auscultated. The amplitude of the "chest wiggle" in such infants (by visual inspection or palpation) can be a useful guide to the effectiveness of the high-frequency pulsations. Such infants should routinely be removed from high-frequency ventilation for a brief time in order to auscultate the chest while the infant is given positive-pressure tidal breathing by bagging.

CARDIOVASCULAR SYSTEM

The apical cardiac impulse can be appreciated by visual inspection and palpation. A hyperdynamic precordium may occur with a large left-to-right shunt or with marked cardiomegaly. The cardiac impulse in a normally positioned heart is most prominent at the lower left sternal border. Prominence of the apical cardiac impulse at the lower right sternal border suggests dextrorotation or dextroposition of the heart. A shift of the apical impulse is a useful sign to detect tension pneumothorax.

Auscultation of the heart should include right and left second intercostal space, right

---

Box 4-5.	Signs of Tension Pneumothorax

Shift of cardiac apical impulse
Decreased breath sounds on the affected side
Asymmetrical subcostal retractions and chest wall movement
Ballooning of the chest on the affected side
Increased halo of light with transillumination

and left fourth intercostal space, the cardiac apex, and the axillae. Both the diaphragm and bell (with a good seal) of the stethoscope should be used. The infant should be as quiet as possible. It is sometimes necessary to briefly disconnect the ventilator for intubated infants who can tolerate this procedure. The quality of the heart tones (S_1 and S_2) and any clicks, murmurs, or additional heart tones (S_3, S_4) should be noted. The heart rate in the first day of life is generally between 120 and 160 beats per minute while the infant is at rest. During quiet sleep, some term infants have a resting heart rate as low as 90 to 100 beats per minute. Normal sinus arrhythmia with breathing can be more difficult to discern because of the relatively rapid neonatal heart rate. S_1 is relatively loud in the newborn and is best heard at the apex. S_2 is loudest at the left upper sternal border. Because of the relatively fast heart rate of the newborn, it may be difficult to appreciate the splitting of S_2. With the normal postnatal decline in pulmonary artery pressure, splitting of S_2 may be easier to appreciate. A loud S_2 that is narrowly split may suggest pulmonary artery hypertension. Absence of a split S_2 may occur with various anomalies of the great vessels: aortic atresia, pulmonary atresia, transposition, and truncus arteriosus. Any murmurs should be noted with regard to timing, intensity, and location. A soft systolic murmur in a term infant during the first day of life may be due to a closing ductus arteriosus or to flow across the pulmonary valve as pulmonary resistance declines. Harsh or loud murmurs, particularly in the presence of other cardiovascular symptoms or respiratory distress, require further evaluation. The absence of a cardiac murmur does not exclude the possibility of congenital heart disease. Infants with persistent cyanosis or hypoxemia despite oxygen administration may have cyanotic congenital heart disease, primary lung disease, or pulmonary artery hypertension. Intubation and positive-pressure ventilation can sometimes distinguish an infant with pulmonary artery hypertension and lung disease from an infant with cyanotic congenital heart disease. Echocardiography should be promptly obtained in any critically ill infant with hypoxemia despite oxygen administration and ventilation. Peripheral pulmonary stenosis, which is common in premature infants during the first weeks of life, usually manifests as a high-pitched soft systolic murmur. This murmur

is best heard at the cardiac base and radiates widely to the axillae and the back. Hemodynamically significant patent ductus arteriosus (PDA) in a premature infant usually has a systolic murmur best heard along the left sternal border. It is rarely a continuous murmur in the neonatal period and it may be silent. PDA with a large left-to-right shunt may further be associated with a hyperdynamic precordium, bounding pulses, low diastolic pressure, and wide pulse pressure.

The femoral and brachial pulses should be palpated and compared. Pulses may be diminished as a result of hypovolemia, depressed myocardial contractility, sepsis, or left-sided obstructive heart lesions. In left-sided obstructive heart lesions (e.g., coarctation of the aorta and hypoplastic left heart syndrome), the femoral pulses are usually diminished, but may be readily palpable if distal flow is maintained by right-to-left shunting at the ductus arteriosus. While the normal newborn does not routinely require blood pressure measurement, blood pressure should be checked by palpation or by an automated technique (e.g., oscillometric) in any unstable infant, including those infants with respiratory distress, poor perfusion, presence of a cardiac murmur, or depressed neurologic status. All premature infants admitted to an intensive care nursery should also have blood pressure monitored. The blood pressure of critically ill infants is optimally monitored continuously by a transducer connected to an indwelling umbilical or peripheral arterial catheter. Reference can be made to normal values of blood pressure by both birth weight and postnatal age (see Appendix C). However, a normal blood pressure does not ensure adequate cardiac output. The quality of the pulses, skin perfusion, capillary refill time, and color are further indirect measures of cardiac output. The presence or absence of acidosis, measurement of mixed venous saturation, and the monitoring of urine output can be further useful indices of tissue perfusion.

Infants with congestive heart failure may have left-to-right shunting from congenital heart disease. Symptoms may include tachycardia, tachypnea, respiratory distress, poor feeding, and hepatomegaly. The cause of such symptoms may be obvious from echocardiography. However, more subtle etiologies of congestive heart failure may escape easy detection. The skull and abdomen (especially over the liver) should be auscultated for bruits resulting from an arteriovenous malformation. Large hemangiomas or sacrococcygeal teratomas can also cause high output failure. An enlarged thyroid gland suggests hyperthyroidism, but specific laboratory studies are needed to confirm this diagnosis.

ABDOMEN

The abdominal shape, size, and color should be noted. Abdominal wall defects (e.g., gastroschisis, omphalocele) are readily apparent at birth and demand immediate attention. Most newborns have a slightly protuberant abdomen, which becomes more evident as air is swallowed after birth. Bowel obstruction caused by distal atresias, stenosis, meconium plug, and Hirschsprung disease usually manifests within the first 1 to 2 days of life with distention, visible loops of bowel, and emesis. In duodenal atresia, there may be only mild distention in the epigastric area resulting from an enlarged stomach. Distention is usually apparent at birth when there is massive ascites, meconium ileus, and peritonitis, or intrauterine midgut volvulus. Intestinal perforation usually gives the abdomen a bluish-gray tint, but frank abdominal wall erythema develops with the onset of peritonitis. Diaphragmatic hernia may result in a scaphoid abdomen resulting from the herniation of abdominal contents into the thorax. Visible loops of bowel suggest intestinal obstruction, particularly in the presence of bilious emesis or gastric aspirates. Bilious emesis should always be considered abnormal and requires further evaluation. In extremely premature infants, some loops of bowel may be seen through a thin abdominal wall without clinical signs of overt obstruction. In prune belly (Eagle-Barrett) syndrome, the abdominal musculature is lax and the abdominal wall is quite thin, resulting in visible loops of bowel.

Abdominal palpation should be performed with warm hands, patience, and a quiet infant. Under such conditions, the infant's abdominal muscles generally relax after some initial resistance, thus permitting a careful palpation of the internal organs. However, if the abdomen is tense and distended, palpation may only reveal the absence or presence of tenderness. Abdominal tenderness may be obscured if the infant is obtunded, sedated with medications, or extremely premature. The size and position of the liver can be determined by a combination of percussion and palpation, but palpation is primarily used in the newborn. The liver may normally extend 1 to 2 cm below the right costal margin. A midline or left-sided liver should initiate a careful search for other anomalies and appropriate imaging studies. Hepatomegaly may be due to heart failure, congenital infection, congenital anemia, hydrops, intrahepatic tumors, hemangiomas, or hematomas. Pulmonary hyperinflation causes the liver to extend deeper into the abdomen and can give a false impression of hepatomegaly. The spleen is generally not palpable in the healthy newborn, but may be appreciated at the costal margin. Splenomegaly may occur with congenital infection, immune hemolytic disorders, and portal venous hypertension. The kidneys should be carefully palpated bilaterally with the infant relaxed. Bimanual examination can be helpful to evaluate kidney size and shape. Common causes of an enlarged kidney in the newborn include hydronephrosis, renal vein thrombosis, and multicystic renal dysplasia. Enlargement of the adrenal gland is difficult to discern from a renal mass by palpation. Causes of adrenal masses include hemorrhage and tumors (e.g., neuroblastoma). The urinary bladder is palpable only if it is distended with urine. The sick newborn can have transient urinary retention and bladder distention in the presence of a critical illness and the use of sedative drugs, particularly morphine. Reduction of an enlarged bladder by Credé's method (manual pressure) is discouraged, because it may cause ureteral reflux or bladder perforation. Infants with pathologic urinary bladder retention should undergo sterile bladder catheterization as initial management. Palpable intraabdominal masses should be described by their location, size, shape, mobility, and consistency. It should be noted whether the mass adheres to or is contiguous with other internal organs.

UMBILICUS, CORD, AND PLACENTA

The number of arteries and veins in the cord should be noted. The presence of a single umbilical artery is associated with an increased incidence of renal anomalies. The base of the cord and umbilicus should be inspected for any herniation of intestinal contents. A short umbilical cord has been associated with an increased risk for psychomotor abnormalities,[30] cord injuries, and abruptio placentae. About 1% of singleton and about 5% of multiple pregancies (twins, triplets, or more) have an umbilical cord that contains a single umbilical artery. The cause is unknown, but it is associated with an increased risk of birth defects, including heart, central nervous system, and renal structures, in addition to chromosomal abnormalities. The consensus is that it is unnecessary to do a renal ultrasound in all babies with single umbilical artery because the yield is very low. A moist cord raises the spectrum of a persistent urachus which connects from the cord to the dome of the bladder. Persistent omphalo mesenteric cysts are another set of anomalies. There may also be massive cord cysts or even herniation of bowel into the cord. Major anomalies are gastroschisis, which always occurs to the right of the cord and omphaloceles, which may be small or very large containing liver and bowel.

Placental pathology, which may readily explain an infant's problems, is often overlooked. Abruption and infarcts of the placenta can lead to inadequate blood and oxygen delivery to the fetus. Vasa previa may lead to acute fetal blood loss. Histopathologic examination of the placenta should be performed after any complicated delivery, including multiple gestation pregnancies, premature delivery, cases of abruption or other acute blood loss, and stillbirth.

GENITALIA AND INGUINAL AREA

The physician should become familiar with the normal variations of newborn genitalia and be able to recognize those abnormalities that require evaluation. The genitalia may be abnormal as a result of primary errors in morphogenesis, but other abnormalities may result from secondary hormonal effects. Clues to underlying systemic hormonal disorders or dysmorphic syndromes may be obtained by careful examination of the genitalia. Gender assignment should never be made for the infant with ambiguous genitalia until a full assessment has been performed. The parents should be reassured that gender assignment will be made as soon as feasible.

To fully examine the female genitalia, the infant should be examined with the hips abducted while lying supine. The labia majora, labia minora, and clitoris should be inspected for size and surface characteristics. The labia majora may have some mild wrinkling, but should not have frank rugae. In the term female infant, the labia majora are more prominent than the labia minora and generally cover the latter. The female urethra may be difficult to visualize, but is found just anterior to the vaginal opening. Outpouching of the vaginal mucosa (vaginal tags) is common because of the effect of maternal hormones on the fetus. In contrast, the premature female infant may have more prominent labia minora and relative protrusion of the clitoris beyond the labial folds. Such findings are part of the normal morphogenesis of the growing fetus, but parents often need reassurance that the anatomy is normal. The groin and labia majora should be palpated for masses (gonads or herniae). Female infants often have a whitish mucous vaginal discharge. As the effects of maternal hormones subside in the first week, female infants may have a small amount of vaginal bleeding. Clitoromegaly, increased pigmentation, genital hair, and labioscrotal fusion are signs of virilization. Causes include congenital adrenal hyperplasia, virilizing tumors, and maternal androgenic medications. In females, obstructive lesions of the genital tract, such as imperforate hymen and vaginal atresia, cause retention of secretions or blood in the uterine cavity. This condition manifests as an abdominal mass or with symptoms of urinary tract obstruction.

The male infant's genitalia are also first evaluated by visual inspection. The size, color, and surface texture of the scrotum should be noted. In the term male infant, the scrotum is thin-skinned, rugated, and pendulous. In the premature infant, the scrotum is thicker, smoother, and less pendulous. Superficial abrasions, ecchymosis, and swelling of the scrotum may occur after breech birth. The length and girth of the phallus are noted visually. Sometimes the phallus may appear to be small, but its true size is merely hidden by the depth of the surrounding tissues. If there is a question of micropenis, then the phallus should be palpated and stretched, so its length can be measured. Micropenis may be associated with hypothalamic dysfunction and hypopituitarism. The phallus should be observed for any unusual angulation, ventral chordee, or web, and the completeness of the foreskin. If the foreskin is complete, then there is no need to retract it in order to identify the urethral opening. The urethra should be slitlike and open on the glans penis. An incomplete ventral foreskin should alert the examiner for the possibility of hypospadias.

If there is hypospadias, the site of the urethral orifice(s) should be determined by inspection and, if possible, by observation of the urinary stream. Infants with hypospadias should not be circumcised because the foreskin is often used in the repair. Hypospadias may also be associated with bifid scrotum.

The scrotal sacs should be palpated to determine the presence of a testis on each side. The size of the testes should be noted. If the testes are undescended, then the inguinal area should be carefully palpated for incomplete descent of the testis. In the neonatal period, the testes may be very mobile between the inguinal canal and the scrotum. Torsion of a testis results in a swollen hard scrotal mass and bluish discoloration of the scrotum. Viability of the testis is established by ultrasound detection of blood flow. The groin should be checked for the presence of an inguinal hernia. In male infants, it is useful to hold the testes in the scrotum while palpating the ipsilateral inguinal area in order to avoid confusing an undescended testis with a hernia. Hydrocele, a common cause of scrotal swelling, is nontender, often obscures the testis, and causes the scrotum to brightly transilluminate. If no gonads are palpable in an apparent male, then it is particularly important to examine the genitalia for other abnormalities and to exclude the possibility that the infant is a masculinized female. Observation of the urinary stream can be useful. Infants with neurogenic bladders typically "dribble" urine in small volumes with some frequency. Males with posterior urethral valves typically have a poor stream during spontaneous micturition.

Exstrophy of the bladder is evident in the suprapubic region. It is associated with a widening of the pubic symphysis, and there is epispadias or a rudimentary penis. There are often associated gastrointestinal anomalies (imperforate anus and intestinal atresia).

ANUS

Determination of patency of the anus by inspection alone is usually sufficient. If there is a question of anal patency, then a small catheter should be carefully passed through the orifice. The position of the anal orifice in relation to the genitalia and the presence of fistulas or rectal prolapse should be noted. Infants with imperforate anus may pass meconium through a fistula to the genitourinary tract. Sacrococcygeal teratomas may distort the perianal anatomy, displace the anal orifice, and cause intestinal obstruction. These lesions, which can be very large and highly vascular, may rapidly enlarge after birth as a result of internal hemorrhage, causing anemia and shock. In infants with meningomyelocele or other disorders that may affect anal function, the anus should be checked for sphincter tone. An anal wink can be elicited by gently stroking the perianal area.

BACK AND EXTREMITIES

The back should be inspected for symmetry or any abnormal postures. The vertebral column should be palpated along its length with the fingertips. This combination is usually sufficient to detect any moderate to severe scoliosis. Vertebral anomalies may be difficult to appreciate by palpation on a routine examination. If there are clinical reasons to suspect vertebral anomalies (e.g., VATER [vertebral defects, imperforate anus, tracheoesophageal fistula, radial and renal dysplasia] syndrome), then radiographs should be obtained. If a meningomyelocele is noted, it should be carefully inspected and minimally manipulated. The size and location of a meningomyelocele should be noted, and then it should be covered with an appropriate saline-soaked sterile dressing. When an infant is identified to have a meningomyelocele, the child should be kept in a prone or decubitus position to keep pressure off the defect. This creates a significant challenge to thoroughly perform the remainder of the physical examination. The midline of the back and sacrum should be carefully inspected for any unusual tufts of hair, dimples, or pits. Any midline palpable masses, however small, need further evaluation. Ultrasound of the spine can be very helpful in the evaluation of any vertebral or spinal cord anomaly.

Careful inspection alone usually determines whether the extremities are well formed. If there are any deformities, then careful palpation, measurements of length, and testing for range of motion may provide further information. For example, limb shortening may be visually evident in an infant with osteogenesis imperfecta. However, the bony swelling and tenderness of multiple fractures may only be evident by palpation. Fractures of long bones of the extremities are associated with swelling, distortion of shape, tenderness, and discoloration. There is often decreased spontaneous movement of the affected extremity owing to pain. Humerus fractures may occur with birth trauma. Fractures of the femur and humerus occur spontaneously in infants with severe osteopenia of prematurity. Direct comparisons between any aspect of the right and left extremities can be very helpful to discern any abnormalities in size, shape, or function. The hands and feet of every newborn should be carefully inspected. Abnormalities of the digits, including reduction, tapering, syndactyly, polydactyly, duplication, and nail hypoplasia, can be important clues to dysmorphic syndromes. Postaxial polydactyly, which can be inherited as an autosomal dominant trait, is relatively common and is often an isolated finding. In contrast, preaxial polydactyly is more commonly associated with other anomalies. Transverse amputations or limb reductions may be a clue to amniotic band syndrome.

Circumferential girth of the extremities can be an initial clue to muscle mass, and this can be further assessed by palpation. However, marked edema (as in a hydropic infant) or increased adipose tissue (as in an infant of a diabetic mother) can make muscle palpation more difficult. Extremely premature infants have relatively little muscle mass. Observation of motor activity and muscle tone is often sufficient in a healthy term newborn. Neuromuscular disorders may be associated with a decrease in muscle mass and contractures caused by the lack of fetal movement. Infants with a high myelomeningocele can have marked muscle wasting of the lower extremities with flexion contractions of the hips and knees and clubfoot bilaterally.

The hips should be examined for range of motion, and they should be fully abducted to check for hip clicks or dislocation. Useful techniques for dislocated hip are the Barlow maneuver (hip is flexed and abducted; the femoral head is pushed downward; if dislocatable, the femoral head will be pushed posteriorly out of the acetabulum) and Ortolani test (hip is abducted with upward leverage of femur; a dislocated hip will return with a palpable clunk into the acetabulum). Additional useful findings are discrepancies in length and asymmetrical creases of the lower extremities. Maternal hormones and abnormal fetal positions (e.g., breech) can cause laxity in the newborn's hips. If findings are uncertain, then repeated examinations should

be performed until the findings are clarified. If there is frank dislocation or suspicious findings, then hip ultrasound should be obtained. If there is any evidence of hip dysplasia, then orthopedic consultation should be obtained in a timely manner. Specific testing for range of motion for joints other than the hips is generally not indicated unless there are contractures or gross anomalies noted. Many aspects of joint function and range of motion are indirectly tested during the neurologic examination by passive range of motion.

NEUROLOGIC EXAMINATION

The neurologic examination of a healthy newborn is based on a combination of observations of behavior and specific testing on examination. The normal newborn certainly does not require a lengthy complete neurologic examination; however, certain aspects of neurologic function should be assessed. A more detailed neurologic examination should be performed in any infant with known neurologic disorders (seizures, intracranial hemorrhage, encephalopathy) or who is at high risk for neurologic injury.

A number of behaviors provide information about global brain function. Observations of an infant's overall responsiveness, quality of the cry, interaction with the mother, and general motor activity provide a broad useful perspective on cortical function. Although newborns sleep a great deal (18 to 20 hours per day), they do have periods of awake activity. The newborn infant goes through several states of alertness throughout each day. The neurologic examination of the newborn is significantly affected by the state of the infant. Tone and motor activity are decreased during active or rapid eye movement (REM) sleep. Examination of an infant in this state alone may give an incomplete impression of the infant's neurologic status. Important observations can be made as to whether an infant responds to comforting or withdraws from noxious stimuli.

Tone should be assessed by observation of posture and by passive movement of the extremities. Term infants have primarily a flexion posture at the knees and elbows with the fingers generally closed. However, the term newborn spontaneously opens the hands and periodically extends the arms and legs. A term infant with tight persistent flexion of the extremities, tightly clenched fists with adducted thumbs, and hypertonia suggests that there has been a previous cortical injury. Premature infants, in contrast, have relatively more extension, especially with decreasing gestational age. At 23 to 24 weeks' gestation, the premature infant likely has fully extended extremities, relatively decreased tone, and irregular, twitchy, spontaneous motor activity as normal findings. Head control and neck tone may be tested by gently lifting the infant by the arms slightly off the bed and assessing for head lag. Head control is generally poor in the premature infant, but some neck muscle tone is present in healthy term infants.

Motor activity of the infant should be observed to detect any asymmetry or abnormality in movement. Motor strength is assessed by the degree of resistance to passive range of motion, spontaneous movement, and active effort against restraint by the examiner. Jitteriness is very common in the newborn. In otherwise apparently healthy term infants, such jitteriness is generally benign unless the movements are particularly coarse or of a large amplitude. Occasionally, such jitteriness can be due to hypoglycemia or hypocalcemia. In an irritable, hypertonic infant, jitteriness may be due to drug withdrawal or neurologic injury.

For most infants, testing of deep tendon reflexes can be limited to the biceps and knee jerk. The ability to elicit deep tendon reflexes is dependent on the infant's activity and state, the patience of the examiner, and the effects of medications. There are a large number of elicitable reflexes in the newborn, but the physician rarely needs to test more than a few of these responses in most routine examinations. The Moro reflex is particularly useful to detect Erb palsy. The palmar reflex and asymmetrical tonic neck response may reveal asymmetries in motor function or strength. Sucking can be evoked even in extremely premature infants as early as 28 weeks. Rooting is easily demonstrated in term infants by stroking the side of the mouth.

Cranial nerve function should be thoroughly and specifically evaluated in the comatose infant or as part of an assessment for brain death. However, a less formal assessment of the cranial nerves suffices in most infants. The term newborn is capable of following an object from 30 to 60 degrees. Shining a bright light into the eyes should cause the term infant to close the eyes. Pupillary response to light may be absent in the premature infant because of immaturity and cloudiness of the cornea. However, the pupils of the term or near-term infant should constrict in response to light. Eye movements should be observed for any abnormal deviation or sustained nystagmus. Conjugate gaze is often inconsistent in the newborn. Facial nerve palsy may be apparent by the observation of asymmetry during crying. The gag reflex can be checked at the same time the mouth and tongue are being evaluated as part of the general physical examination. Ineffective sucking, swallowing, and handling of oral secretions may be an indicator of cranial nerve dysfunction or central nervous system depression. Hearing may be crudely assessed by the response to the mother's voice or sudden sounds. Universal hearing testing of all newborns is recommended prior to discharge to home.

ROUTINE EVALUATION DURING TRANSITION

The first hours of life are a period during which the newborn should be carefully monitored and evaluated. It is during this transition period that many of the problems of the high-risk infant manifest themselves. Because this is also an important period for the mother and family to bond with the infant, most of the monitoring and evaluating can be done by skilled obstetric and nursery nurses. Fortunately, most infants are healthy and require little intervention other than observation.

Where the infant is observed during the first few hours depends on the parents, the infant, and the hospital. Reasonable alternatives range from close observation of the mother and infant together in the mother's room to temporary admission to a transitional or intermediate nursery. Regardless of the setting for this transitional period, the emphasis must always be on careful observation with the ability to intervene in time to prevent significant problems.

For the high-risk infant, a number of problems may manifest themselves within the first hour. A systematic approach to these infants is important so that problems can be identified and responded to in a timely fashion, without overtreatment of infants. The most important evaluation of the infant within the first several hours is repeated physical examinations. These "mini-exams" require little intervention with the infant, but they can identify evolving problems.

RESPIRATORY

Is there any evidence of increasing respiratory distress? Many newborns have some mild grunting during the first few minutes of life. This grunting, often audible only with a stethoscope, decreases over the first 30 minutes in a healthy infant. The infant with increasing grunting at 15 to 30 minutes of age, particularly if it is associated with other signs of respiratory distress, should be considered abnormal. In the preterm infant, respiratory distress syndrome is, by far, the most common cause of respiratory distress that increases during the first hour of life—although other processes, such as pneumonia or pneumothorax, may present a similar picture. In the term infant, continued grunting is most often associated with pneumonia, aspiration syndrome, or retained lung fluid.

Is there tachypnea without grunting? This is most often either a benign finding or it represents transient tachypnea of the newborn. The differentiation between these two entities depends on whether the infant requires supplemental oxygen.

Is the infant pink and well saturated? All infants with any signs of respiratory distress should be placed on a pulse oximeter to more accurately assess oxygen saturation. Immediately after delivery, even without any need for resuscitation, oxygen saturation values for preterm infants increase more slowly than those for term infants. It takes about 4 minutes for term infants and nearly 8 minutes in preterm infants to reach a median saturation of greater than 90%.[31]

CARDIOVASCULAR

Is the infant well perfused? Hypoperfusion often accompanies sepsis or significant asphyxia. Does the infant have a murmur? Cardiac murmurs are detected on routine examination in 1% to 2% of normal infants. Many are transient flow murmurs related to circulatory changes following birth, including tricuspid flow as pulmonary hypertension resolves. Pulmonary artery branch stenosis is a common cause of a cardiac murmur as is congenital heart disease. Four extremity blood pressures should be measured in newborns with murmurs, and the definitive diagnosis is made with ultrasound. Although murmurs are present in a large percentage of healthy newborns during the first day of life secondary to the closing ductus arteriosus, a murmur in the presence of cyanosis, poor perfusion, or poor pulses is often associated with cardiac disease.

NEUROLOGIC

Is the infant lethargic and hypotonic, or, conversely, is the infant jittery? The former can be due to sepsis, hypoxic-ischemic insult, metabolic disorders, or neuromuscular disorders. The latter may indicate early drug withdrawal or hypoglycemia. Coarse high-amplitude jitteriness is sometimes seen in infants with hypoxic-ischemic encephalopathy.

TEMPERATURE

Temperature must be followed closely in the preterm infant who, because of a larger surface-to-volume ratio, is more likely to quickly become hypothermic. See Chapter 6 for a more detailed discussion of temperature regulation.

LABORATORY EVALUATION

The two laboratory tests most commonly performed during the transition period are an assessment of blood glucose and hematocrit (or hemoglobin). Some nurseries routinely check blood glucose on all newborns. Although healthy newborns without any risk factors probably do not need routine blood glucose monitoring, infants with risk factors do require glucose monitoring. Any sick newborn, in particular those with respiratory distress or cardiovascular problems, need glucose monitoring. Other at-risk groups for hypoglycemia include premature infants, small or large for gestational age infants, infants of diabetic mothers, and those who had hypoxic-ischemic perinatal insults. Signs of hypoglycemia include jitteriness, lethargy, or seizures (newborns rarely sweat with hypoglycemia). However, many hypoglycemic infants are asymptomatic. The frequency and duration of glucose monitoring depends on whether an infant has hypo- or hyperglycemia and the rate at which it resolves.

Either hematocrit or hemoglobin (or CBC) should be checked in newborns who fall into a high-risk group. In particular, such testing should be done in the setting of discordant twins, an infant of a diabetic mother, signs of plethora or hyperviscosity, hypovolemia or hypotension, history of maternal bleeding (abruption, previa), fetal or neonatal blood loss, suspected sepsis, or pathologic jaundice.

In addition to these tests, routine newborn screening is widely performed. The scope of testing ranges regionally. Typically, the newborn screen includes tests for hypothyroidism, phenylketonuria (PKU), galactosemia, congenital adrenal hyperplasia, hemoglobinopathies, and a variety of tests for genetic metabolic disorders is also available. These tests are run in batches at reference laboratories and are usually not available for at least several days or weeks. Newborn screening tests should be obtained before discharge from the hospital; however, the PKU test may not be valid if it is performed before 12 hours of age. In most states, the hypothyroidism screen is designed to detect only primary hypothyroidism by measuring thyroid-stimulating hormone (TSH). Hypothyroidism, which is caused by hypopituitarism, is not detected by TSH screening alone. Infants with suspected secondary hypothyroidism need specific testing of free thyroxine (T_4) to evaluate thyroid status. Prior transfusion invalidates the results of hemoglobinopathy and galactosemia screening tests. The hormone 17-hydroxy progesterone is measured to test for congenital adrenal hyperplasia. Establishing normal refernce values for premature infants, however, is under investigation. This leads to frequent false-positive values in premature infants. Many areas have begun testing for cystic fibrosis by measuring immunoreactive trypsinogen (IRT). If an infant has a positive IRT, then further mutation analyses are done on the sample.

ROUTINE TREATMENT

All newborns should receive vitamin K and ophthalmic treatment to prevent ophthalmia neonatorum resulting from gonococcal infection. We recommend the use of erythromycin, rather than silver nitrate treatment, because of the efficacy of erythromycin in treating chlamydial conjunctivitis.

Vitamin K is given as a single intramuscular dose, 1.0 mg to infants who weigh more than 2.5 kg and 0.5 mg to infants who weigh less than 2.5 kg. Whereas some studies have evaluated routine use of oral vitamin K,[32] this is not recommended for routine use at this time. Failure to provide vitamin K places the newborn (especially if breast fed) at risk for the development of hemorrhage in the first weeks of life because of vitamin K deficiency.

In most healthy infants, these routine treatments, like the routine monitoring of blood glucose and hematocrit, can be deferred until the infant is at least 1 hour old and the mother has been able to spend some private time with her infant.

MANAGEMENT OF THE HIGH-RISK INFANT DURING TRANSITION

The areas that most often need to be addressed in the high-risk infant are monitoring, vascular access, oxygen and ventilatory support, and evaluation of suspected sepsis. As with most other areas of newborn care, anticipation of potential problems leads to a practical and successful plan for the care of these infants.

MONITORING

Sick infants should be placed on a cardiorespiratory monitor. Blood pressure should be evaluated in all infants who are not having a normal transition after birth. Blood pressure is easily measured with automated cuff devices, which are noninvasive and simple to use. In any infant with an arterial catheter in place, arterial pressure should be continuously monitored, and the arterial waveform displayed on the cardiorespiratory monitor. Not only does this provide important information about the infant's cardiovascular status, but it provides important alarms in case the arterial catheter becomes disconnected. An arterial catheter that is not connected to a pressure transducer and that is not displayed with appropriate alarms could potentially cause massive undetected hemorrhage.

VASCULAR ACCESS

The first question about vascular access is whether the infant will need ongoing blood gas monitoring. Because of the less than ideal nature of capillary blood gas and arterial puncture blood gas monitoring, we recommend the placement of an umbilical or peripheral arterial catheter in any newborn requiring frequent blood gas monitoring.

The next question that needs to be answered is whether the infant will need vascular access for fluid support. In general, infants with a birth weight less than 1.8 kg do not tolerate immediate institution of entirely enteral nutrition and should be given intravenous fluids. Hypoglycemia, which is relatively common in premature and stressed infants, often requires ongoing intravenous glucose infusion until feedings can be established. Infants of diabetic mothers, who have either severe or recurrent hypoglycemia, need intravenous dextrose. Any infant with significant respiratory distress, gastrointestinal anomaly or obstruction, or suspected serious congenital heart disease needs intravenous access.

SUPPLEMENTAL OXYGEN, NASAL CPAP, AND VENTILATORY SUPPORT

Decisions about the correct amount of supplemental oxygen to deliver are usually straightforward. Patients should receive an Fio_2 that is adequate to prevent hypoxia and hyperoxia. Usually, maintaining arterial saturation by pulse oximetry (SpO_2) between 88% and 95% is a safe range. A lower range of SpO_2 (85% to 89%) in VLBW infants reduces retinopathy, but increases mortality.[33]

Infants with respiratory distress (oxygen need, retractions, tachypnea, grunting) in the delivery room or soon thereafter, often benefit from a trial of nasal continuous positive airway pressure (NCPAP). Even the smallest and most immature infants may benefit from NCPAP rather than immediate intubation and ventilation.[34,35] Decisions about institution of mechanical ventilation are more complex. The assessment of approaching respiratory failure depends on the infant's gestational age, postnatal age, pulmonary disease, physical examination, and blood gas measurements. General rules for instituting ventilation are as follows:

1. Inability to achieve adequate oxygenation, despite a trial of NCPAP, requires positive pressure. In most cases, the premature infant on NCPAP who requires an Fio_2 above 0.50 to 0.60 should be intubated and ventilated. Some premature infants may benefit from a trial of nasal ventilation. Term infants who require an Fio_2 above 0.70 to 0.80 often need to be intubated and ventilated.
2. Inability to spontaneously provide adequate CO_2 exchange requires ventilation. In most cases, infants with a $Paco_2$ between 50 and 65 mm Hg should be followed up closely for potential need for ventilation. Most newborns with a $Paco_2$ that remains above 60 to 70 mm Hg during the first hours of life need mechanical ventilation.
3. Respiratory fatigue, usually manifested by poor air exchange, a markedly abnormal respiratory pattern or apnea, should be considered an indication for mechanical ventilation.

EVALUATION AND TREATMENT OF SUSPECTED SEPSIS

Because of the potentially lethal nature of neonatal sepsis, and because it may be difficult to detect early in its course, one should always err in the direction of overevaluating and overtreating potential sepsis. Pneumonia in the neonate has a wide range of clinical and radiographic appearances, often mimicking either hyaline membrane disease (respiratory distress syndrome) or aspiration syndrome. For this reason, all infants with any significant degree of respiratory distress, whether from surfactant deficiency, aspiration syndrome, or an idiopathic cause, should be considered potentially septic.

No single screening test for sepsis is both sufficiently sensitive and specific. Leukocytosis and a high immature-to-mature white blood cell count may indicate sepsis, but these elements are often seen in normal newborns. Leukopenia is more specific for sepsis than is leukocytosis, but it is also often seen in newborns without sepsis, especially after maternal pregnancy-induced hypertension. Thrombocytopenia is a late finding that may be seen in infants with overwhelming sepsis and disseminated intravascular coagulopathy, but it should not be seen as a screening tool for sepsis. C-reactive protein may be increased (≥ 1 mg/dL) in cases of proven bacterial sepsis at the time of initial evaluation. However, there is a significant false-negative rate at the time of presentation. C-reactive protein may be more useful to determine whether to discontinue antibiotic therapy at 48 to 72 hours after the start of treatment. It has been shown that bacterial infection is very unlikely if two sequential (24 hours apart) C-reactive protein levels are less than 1 mg/dL in the 8 to 48 hours after presentation.[36]

The minimum evaluation for sepsis includes a complete blood count with differential, platelet count, and blood culture. C-reactive protein may also be a useful test to determine the length of treatment, but its utility in the decision whether to start antibiotics remains unclear. The infant who is at more than minimal risk of sepsis should also have a lumbar puncture for cell count, glucose, protein, Gram stain, and culture. However, there is considerable controversy regarding selective use of lumbar puncture in the evaluation of neonatal sepsis.[37-40]

Because early onset sepsis rarely manifests with urinary tract infection, a urinalysis or urine culture is not part of the routine evaluation of early onset sepsis. A number of factors are associated with an increased risk of neonatal infection including preterm delivery, rupture of membranes after 18 or more hours, maternal fever or chorioamnionitis, and positive maternal cultures for Group B *Streptococcus.*

Useful algorithms have also been proposed for the newborn at risk for group B streptococcal infection.[4] An infant with symptoms strongly suggestive of sepsis should be cultured and started on antibiotics, usually ampicillin and gentamicin, even in the absence of risk factors. If the infant's blood and cerebrospinal fluid cultures are negative and if the patient is clinically well, antibiotics can be stopped at 48 hours. For further discussion of antibiotics and their dosage, see Chapter 14 and Appendix A.

BREAST FEEDING: EFFECT OF MATERNAL ILLNESS AND DRUGS

Mothers should be encouraged and supported in their efforts to establish breast feeding. Human milk is the preferred source of nutrition for healthy newborn infants.[41,42] Breast feeding not only provides nourishment to the infant, but it also promotes the process of bonding. Human milk contains factors that support intestinal cell proliferation and bowel mucosal mass. A number of factors, including secretory IgA, lysozyme, lactoferrin, C3, C4, and maternal leukocytes, influence neonatal bacterial flora and the incidence of gastrointestinal infections. However, maternal illnesses or drugs can have adverse effects on lactation, which may preclude the use of maternal milk or may require special precautions in its use.

Viral agents can be transmitted into human milk and result in infection in the infant. HIV is secreted into human milk and transmission to the breast-fed infant has been reported.[43] The American Academy of Pediatrics (AAP) and the CDC recommend that infants born to mothers with human immunodeficiency virus (HIV) infection should be fed infant formula and not be breast fed.[44] However, in underdeveloped countries where a safe water supply and sufficient resources for infant formula are lacking, as per the World Health Organization recommendation, mothers with HIV should continue to breast feed. Herpes simplex virus has also been reported to be transmitted via maternal milk, suggesting that breast feeding should be withheld in young infants during an episode of acute primary maternal herpes infection or if there are herpes lesions on the breasts. Mothers with recurrent cervical or oral herpes are generally allowed to breast feed, provided good hygiene is used to prevent transmission, and the infant is not directly exposed to lesions. If there are lesions on the mother's breast, the mother should not feed the infant from the affected breast until lesions are resolved. Although hepatitis B virus is transmitted via human milk in mothers who are positive for hepatitis B surface antigen, these mothers are usually allowed to breast feed. Their infants should be protected if they are given hepatitis B vaccine and hepatitis B immunoglobulin at birth, and the infant then completes the hepatitis B vaccine series thereafter. Mothers who are seropositive for cytomegalovirus (CMV) also secrete virus into human milk, but this does not appear to pose any risk to the healthy term infant. Many infants born to seropositive mothers begin to excrete CMV postnatally, whether or not they are breast fed. For the premature infant, postnatal acquisition of CMV (via blood transfusion) has been associated with respiratory morbidity. Pasteurization, a process used at breast milk banks, has had good success with eliminating CMV transmission. However, the efficacy of freezing breast milk to eliminate CMV is still under debate. Human T-lymphotropic virus (HTLV) type 1 is likely transmitted from mother to infant through breast feeding. The AAP's *Redbook* recommends that women in the United States who are HTLV-1 seropositive should be advised not to breast feed.[43]

Almost all maternal medications are secreted to some extent into human milk.[5,42,45] Factors that affect the degree of secretion are the pKa of the drug, its lipid solubility, molecular size, and protein binding. Drugs that are small in molecular size or that are lipid soluble pass more readily into the breast milk. Drugs with a more alkaline pKa are in the nonionized form in the plasma, permitting easier passage across membranes and into the milk. Drugs that are poorly bound to plasma proteins are more readily secreted into human milk than drugs that are tightly bound. The time of collection or feeding of human milk affects the level of the drug in the milk. Less drug is delivered to the infant if breast feeding is performed just before the mother's dose of drug. Although the concentration of a drug in human milk provides an estimate of how much maternal drug to which an infant is exposed, the bioavailability of the drug may be limited by intestinal absorption. For example, although phenytoin is excreted into human milk, its intestinal absorption is quite poor in the newborn.

In counseling a mother regarding breast feeding, it should be emphasized that virtually all drugs are excreted into human milk and that caution should be taken with regard to any drug. The lactating woman should always make her physician aware that she is breast feeding when medications are prescribed for her. Although with most maternal medications, breast feeding can be maintained, the data regarding adverse effects of drugs in infants are incomplete. Most reports about breast feeding and maternal medications involve small numbers of infants; hence, adverse effects that occur infrequently are not easily recognized. The physician is often forced to make a judgment regarding the use of a drug in a lactating woman based on incomplete data. The mother should be informed of these uncertainties when appropriate. Medications for use in a lactating woman should be chosen in such a way as to minimize any risk to the infant and yet provide a therapeutic effect for the mother. Very few maternal medications are an absolute contraindication to breast feeding.[45] Because lactose is the predominant carbohydrate in breast milk, infants with galactosemia should not breast feed.

Maternal cocaine use during breast feeding may cause hypertension, seizures, and other toxic effects in the infant. Maternal heroin use or other illicit intravenous drug use puts both the mother and infant at risk for HIV infection. Although breast feeding by mothers on methadone has been reported to facilitate the control of neonatal abstinence syndrome, this may not be a sufficient reason to continue to expose the infant to such a long-acting opiate and infectious risks (e.g., HIV infection).

TRANSPORT

One of the major developments in modern neonatal care was the concept of regionalization of perinatal care. Central to this concept is transport, both of high-risk mothers and of high-risk infants, to centers that specialize in the care of these high-risk patients. Although the ideal situation is to transfer the prepartum mother to a center that can provide both high-risk perinatal care to the mother and intensive care to the newborn, this is often not possible. Because of the unpredictable nature of preterm labor and of the often unexpected pathology of an infant following a normal pregnancy, high-risk infants are often born at centers that are not equipped to provide total support and therapy for them. In these situations, it is necessary to transfer the infant to a higher level center.

Nurseries are commonly classified as level I, level II, and level III.[46] Level I nurseries are those that provide routine well newborn care and should be able to stabilize high-risk infants before transfer to a higher level center. Level II nurseries provide all of the services of a level I nursery, plus some support for smaller and sicker infants. Typically, healthy growing preterm infants, infants needing intravenous support, or infants needing hood oxygen but not prolonged mechanical ventilation, can be cared for in level II nurseries. Level III nurseries provide complete neonatal intensive care, including access to pediatric surgical support, multiple pediatric subspecialists, and all of the support services that are required to care for the smallest and sickest newborns.

A subgroup of level III nurseries, sometimes referred to as level IIID nurseries, provide therapies that are new or so specialized that they are not needed at all level III nurseries. Previously, therapies such as extracorporeal membrane oxygenation (ECMO), high-frequency ventilation, and nitric oxide were available only at a level IIID or regional intensive care nursery. Although ECMO will likely continue to be limited to a small number of centers, high-frequency ventilation is becoming increasingly available at most level III nurseries. Surgical repair of serious congenital heart anomalies is also reserved for level IIID nurseries. Inhaled nitric oxide (iNO), which was approved by the U.S. Food and Drug Administration in 1999, is now widely available in the United States. However, wide availability of iNO does not necessarily correlate with expertise in its use.

Infants are transported from lower level to higher level nurseries if conditions that cannot be treated at the lower level nursery develop or if the infant is at risk for development of such conditions. The exact indications for transferring an infant often depend on multiple factors other than the degree of pathology in the infant. The skill and comfort of the physicians caring for the infant, the skill and comfort of the nursing staff, the availability of adequate numbers of skilled nurses, and the availability of ancillary services all must be considered when deciding whether to continue treating an infant at a level I or II nursery. Only if all members of the nursery team are comfortable with their ability to provide optimal care for the infant should a high-risk infant remain at a lower level center. Because the high-risk infant is often a rapidly changing patient, decisions about transferring or not transferring a given infant must be flexible. These decisions should be made in conjunction with neonatologists at the regional level III center who remain in close telephone contact with the team treating the infant.

All level III nurseries and some level II nurseries have neonatal transport teams. Whereas the composition of these teams varies widely, they should all have similar skills for stabilizing and transporting a sick newborn. The goal of a transport team is to provide total support of the newborn from the time the team arrives at the referring hospital to the time the infant is delivered to the accepting hospital. The transport team should be an extension of the intensive care nursery, minimizing the risks of transport as much as possible.

Transport teams should have the ability to rapidly and accurately assess the infant and to immediately institute appropriate therapy. This includes the ability to intubate and ventilate, gain venous and arterial access, treat pneumothoraces, treat shock, institute pharmacologic therapy for cyanotic congenital heart disease, and support the infant with congenital or surgical anomalies. In addition, the team must be able to lucidly explain the infant's condition, prognosis, and treatment plans to the parents.

Indications for instituting therapies before transport are only slightly different than the indications for instituting those therapies in an intensive care nursery. In general, because of the difficulty of instituting therapies when an infant is in an ambulance, the transport team should provide early, rather than late, intervention. For the infant who is at high risk for needing ventilation, consideration should be given whether to intubate the infant prior to transport, rather than risking the need to intubate and begin ventilation during the transport. Similarly, one should decide whether to place a chest tube to evacuate a pneumothorax, which is not yet large or under tension, prior to leaving the referral hospital.

The entire transport process should involve the referring physician and nursing staff, the neonatal staff at the accepting institution, the staff of the transport team, and the parents. Clearly, communication before, during, and after the transport are of paramount importance.

RECOMMENDATIONS FOR CARE

Although the care of the newborn should be individualized to the needs of each infant, the perinatal service of each hospital must establish and maintain policies that ensure high quality of care for all newborns within each institution. However, current practices in perinatal and neonatal care are being driven by a variety of forces. Parents, as consumers, are demanding a more comfortable, almost homelike, environment for labor and delivery of their infant. Payors are carefully scrutinizing costs and will continue to pressure hospitals to reduce both costs and patient length of stay. Health care professionals must respond to these forces of change in a careful manner so that the medical needs of the mother and infant are thoroughly met. The following general recommendations are made:

1. Every delivery of a newborn, whether anticipated to be routine or high risk, should be attended by a person skilled in neonatal resuscitation. This person, whether a nurse, nurse anesthetist, neonatal nurse practitioner, or physician, should be skilled in bag-and-mask ventilation, endotracheal intubation, and neonatal cardiopulmonary resuscitation (CPR). This person cannot be available just on call or standby, but should be there to immediately attend to the infant after delivery. The principles of neonatal delivery room resuscitation as outlined by the American Academy of Pediatrics and the American Heart Association's Neonatal Resuscitation Program (NRP) should be followed. Health care professionals who are responsible for delivery room resuscitation should be trained in these principles. However, completion of NRP training alone is inadequate by itself. There is no substitute for practical experience to achieve expertise in newborn resuscitation.

2. For higher-risk deliveries, a physician, a neonatal nurse practitioner, or a neonatologist may need to be present in order to immediately evaluate and, if needed, to resuscitate the newborn. Each perinatal-neonatal service should establish its own criteria for when a physician, or more specifically a

neonatologist, should be called to attend a high-risk delivery. Physicians who attend high-risk deliveries and care for seriously ill newborns must be skilled in neonatal resuscitation and certain technical procedures, including endotracheal intubation, umbilical catheterization, needle thoracentesis, and chest tube placement.

3. After delivery, a sick or premature infant should be placed on a warming table, dried, evaluated, and resuscitated as appropriate. Apgar scores are assigned at 1 and 5 minutes of age. If the 5-minute Apgar score is less than 7, then Apgar scores should continue to be assigned every 5 minutes up to 20 minutes. There should be the capability, if needed, to perform intubation, provide positive pressure ventilation via the endotracheal tube, needle thoracentesis, and umbilical catheterization within the delivery room. If an infant is critically ill and further personnel are needed, assistance should be called for promptly. The sick newborn is moved from the delivery room to the intensive care nursery when the infant is initially stabilized with a patent airway, adequate ventilation, and stable heart rate.

4. The apparently stable healthy newborn can be readily evaluated in several minutes in the delivery room with careful attention to respiratory effort, heart rate, color, perfusion, and tone. The infant should then be dried and a quick physical examination should be performed to ensure that there are no significant anomalies or cardiopulmonary compromise before being allowed to return to the mother. The infant can be placed skin to skin on the mother's chest. This time shortly after birth is especially important to allow the parents to be close to their infant. Such a time for private bonding between the parents and the infant should not preclude close observation of the infant. Administration of eye prophylaxis and vitamin K to the healthy newborn can generally be delayed until 1 to 2 hours of age.

5. Within the first 1 to 2 hours of life, the healthy newborn should have a full assessment performed by the nursing staff. This should include measurement of temperature, heart rate, respiratory rate, and a full physical examination. The nursing staff should pay particular attention to adequacy of the respiratory effort and observe for any signs of respiratory distress. Infants with persistent poor perfusion, poor capillary refill, cyanosis, or respiratory distress should have measurement of blood pressure. Gestational age is assessed using standard techniques such as the Dubowitz or Ballard examination. Weight, length, and occipital frontal head circumference are measured and plotted on an appropriate growth chart. The physician should be promptly notified of any significant findings or abnormalities. For stable healthy newborns, the physician should examine the infant by 12 to 18 hours of age. Infants with significant respiratory distress, major anomalies, signs of sepsis, or prematurity should be examined and evaluated promptly by the physician. The initial assessment of the apparently healthy newborn infant need not occur in the "transitional nursery" or "well newborn" nursery. When possible, the healthy infant should be evaluated in the mother's room, rather than separating her from her infant. This is particularly appropriate as labor and delivery services move to combine the care of the mother and well newborn infant, the so-called model of a "mother-infant" dyad. It is essential, however, that the nursing staff caring for such mother-infant dyads continue to have the training and resources they need to fully evaluate the newborn infant and to be able to expeditiously provide for the infant's needs. The newborn infant should be regularly observed with frequent measurement of the heart rate, respirations, and temperature in the first 6 hours of life to ensure that the infant has made a stable transition to extrauterine life.

6. For the sick newborn, a full assessment should be performed immediately. If an infant has respiratory distress, poor perfusion or hypotension, signs of asphyxia, or other significant problems that require close monitoring or intervention, the child should be moved to the intensive care nursery. Infants who require intubation and ventilation for more than several hours should be transferred to an intensive care nursery that regularly ventilates newborns. Every effort should be made before transport to stabilize the infant to ensure a safe and expeditious transfer. A physician, neonatal nurse practitioner, or other individual with the training and ability to manage an intubated and ventilated newborn should remain in attendance during

the stabilization, transport, and ongoing care of ventilated infants. Complex neonatal intensive care should remain regionalized at tertiary centers that maintain a well-organized program of services to provide the specialized care needed by critically ill newborns. Health care professionals should advocate for the best care of the newborn and not allow themselves to be forced to provide a lower quality of care in response to economic and social pressures.

7. Mothers should be encouraged and supported in their efforts to breast feed. Nurses and physicians should be knowledgeable regarding issues of lactation support. Lactation counseling needs to be available for all breast-feeding mothers as needed.

8. Newborn infants and their mothers should be allowed to stay in the hospital for at least 48 hours after birth to ensure a stable transition of the infant and a safe postpartum course for the mother.[47] A 48-hour stay also provides a more ample opportunity to support the mother's efforts at breast feeding, to ensure adequate oral intake by the infant, and to evaluate the infant for significant jaundice before discharge. Outpatient follow-up plans for the infant and mother should be clearly defined before discharge.

CASE 1

At 41 weeks' gestation, a mother is about to deliver vaginally through thick meconium-stained amniotic fluid. There have been late fetal heart rate decelerations. In the past 2 minutes, the heart rate decreased to 80 bpm. Vacuum extraction is being performed to facilitate delivery.

What considerations should be taken in preparing for the delivery of the infant? What general principles should guide the delivery room resuscitation? Are there any special risk factors for vacuum extraction?

Those meconium stained infants, who are delivered through *thin* meconium, who have *uncomplicated* deliveries and are *vigorous* at birth, do not require intubation and tracheal suctioning. Intubation and suctioning for meconium should be performed in this case, however, because of two factors: thick meconium and a complicated delivery. As for the method of tracheal suctioning, the use of a meconium aspirator attached to the endotracheal tube (ETT) and wall suction is preferred. The ETT is withdrawn as the suction is applied. The direct insertion of a suction catheter alone into the trachea is not recommended. The patient should be repeatedly reintubated and suctioned as needed to remove thick or particulate meconium. However, in an infant with respiratory depression and a low heart rate, apnea, or poor respiratory effort, it may be necessary to proceed with resuscitation after the first suctioning of the ETT for meconium. With respect to vacuum extraction, if not applied properly, this procedure may increase the risk for intracranial and subgaleal hemorrhage.

This particular infant is critically ill with meconium aspiration syndrome, and is intubated and ventilated. The first blood gas has a pH of 7.15, Pco_2 of 40 mm Hg, Pao_2 of 40 mm Hg in 100% O_2, and mean airway pressure of 16. Blood pressure is 40/20; heart rate is 190. UAC and UVC have been placed. Chest radiograph shows the catheters and ETT in good position, and the lungs have fluffy dense infiltrates bilaterally.

The patient is in a community level I nursery. What measures might be taken immediately to help stabilize the patient for transport?

Give volume expander 10 mL/kg (normal saline or lactated Ringer's solution) in repeated boluses as needed to correct hypovolemia and hypotension. After volume repletion, consider starting dopamine at 5 μg/kg/min. Previously, for such patients, most practitioners would have given $NaHCO_3$ to correct metabolic acidosis, especially if it persists after a volume expander has been given. However, the use of $NaHCO_3$ to correct metabolic acidosis is now controversial.[48] In patients with hypoxic respiratory failure and pulmonary hypertension, past treatments have included intentional hyperventilation, hyperoxia, and $NaHCO_3$ infusions to cause intentional metabolic alkalosis in an attempt to reverse pulmonary hypertension. These therapies are no longer considered effective. Moderate ventilation is advised to maintain a normal Pco_2 and to avoid prolonged hyperoxia.

To what type of intensive care nursery should such a patient be ideally transferred?

This patient likely has pulmonary artery hypertension and myocardial dysfunction in addition to meconium aspiration syndrome. The patient may need high-frequency ventilation, surfactant administration, inhaled nitric oxide (iNO), and possibly ECMO. The patient will need an echocardiogram and cranial ultrasound before the initiation of ECMO. The patient should go to a level III nursery, preferably an ECMO center, that is capable of applying these treatments and evaluations expeditiously. Critically ill infants who are near or at ECMO criteria can be managed with high-frequency ventilation and iNO in an attempt to avoid ECMO. However, application of such therapies in a non-ECMO center must allow sufficient time to transfer the patient to an ECMO center in case the patient's clinical course deteriorates.

CASE 2

A mother presents to labor and delivery emergently with profuse vaginal bleeding of 2 hours' duration. She is 38 weeks pregnant and has had a benign pregnancy before this. She is 41 years old and this is her third child. When placed on an external fetal monitor, a sinusoidal heart tracing is appreciated and she is taken to the operating room immediately for a cesarean section.

What arrangements need to be made for preparation for this delivery? Which staff needs to be present for the resuscitation of this infant?

With the history of vaginal bleeding and the abnormal heart tracing, an acute hemorrhage is high on the differential diagnosis list. Staff well versed in neonatal resuscitation need to be present. At minimum, three caregivers need to be ready because this infant may need intubation, CPR, and blood or volume administration. A neonatologist needs to be notified of the delivery as soon as possible. Equipment must be available, including a crash cart stocked with medications necessary for resuscitation. The blood bank should be notified immediately and O negative blood should be sent to the operating room emergently.

The infant is delivered pale, blue, and apneic. The obstetrician notes a complete placental abruption. A cord arterial blood gas revealed a pH 6.96, Pco_2 of 45, Po_2 38, and base excess (BE)-20. What are the next necessary steps in resuscitation of this infant?

The infant should be warmed, dried, and assessed. Each person of the neonatal resuscitation team should be assigned a job (i.e., one for the airway, one for the heart rate, etc.) The neonatal resuscitation guidelines should be followed with assessment of airway, breathing, and circulation. This infant likely has severe birth depression secondary to a profound hemorrhage. If the infant continues to be apneic, intubation is necessary. The heart rate needs to be evaluated and CPR begun if the heart rate is 60 per minute or lower. The infant will need venous access. The most efficient method is via the umbilical vein, so umbilical catheters need to be

prepared for emergent placement. O negative blood or crystalloid volume bolus can be given when access is established. Apgar scores need to be recorded. If the infant has an Apgar score of 0 at 10 minutes of life, despite adequate resuscitation, cessation of further resuscitative efforts should be considered.

The infant is stabilized in the operating room and has Apgar scores of 1 at 1 minute, 4 at 5 minutes, and 5 at 10 minutes. He is comatose, without spontaneous respirations, and is seizing. What steps should be done next in treatment and evaluation of this infant?

The infant has a hypoxic injury as a result of the abruption. This has resulted in decreased oxygen delivery to all major organ systems. The rules of airway, breathing, and circulation still apply here. Establishing venous and arterial access is paramount. A blood gas and glucose should also be checked quickly. There is increasing evidence that moderately encephalopathic infants have an improved neurodevelopmental outcome if given cerebral or whole body cooling. The cooling must begin within the first 6 hours of life. Identifying a NICU that is equipped to transport, evaluate, and treat these infants is vital.

What is the definition of hypoxic-ischemic encephalopathy (HIE)?

Profound acidemia with a pH of less than 7, an Apgar score of less than 6 for 5 minutes, neurologic sequelae (seizures, hypotonia, coma), and multiple organ dysfunction.

What is the pathophysiology of HIE?

An acute asphyxia event elicits a diving reflex. This results in preferred blood flow to the brain, heart, and adrenal glands with vasoconstriction to other organs. Initially, there is an increase in cerebral blood flow and glucose influx to the brain. There is also an increase in glycogenolysis, glycolysis, lactate and hydrogen ions. Soon after, there is a decrease in oxidative phosphorylation, a decrease in brain glucose, and a decrease in adenosine triphosphate (ATP). These changes seem to be more pronounced in the white matter.

What is the best way to manage the infant's seizures?

It's imperative to correct metabolic abnormalities, especially hypoglycemia. Phenobarbital continues to be the first-line drug to manage seizures. Fosphenytoin and lorazepam should also be considered.

CASE 3

You are called to attend a delivery of a 27-year-old gravida 2, para 1 female with good prenatal care. She is scheduled to have a repeat cesarean section. Her first child was breech. She had an uncomplicated pregnancy aside from a low alpha-fetoprotein (aFP) at 16 weeks' gestation. She refused an amniocentesis. Her 20-week anatomy scan was reported as normal. The infant is delivered with clear amniotic fluid. The infant cries spontaneously and is assigned Apgars of 9 at 1 minute and 9 at 5 minutes. She is taken to the warmer and you note facial features consistent with trisomy 21.

What is your next step?

The infant requires a complete physical examination in the operating room. Whenever a caregiver has a high suspicion of an anomaly, the parents should be notified as soon as possible. In this situation, it is fair to wait until the mother is awake and stable in the recovery room. It should be emphasized that the diagnosis is suspected, and not confirmed. Establishing a trustful and honest relationship with the parents immediately is important.

The karyotype comes back 47, XX, trisomy 21. The parents are in shock. What do you say to them?

Although the risk of having an infant with Down syndrome is increased in women older than 35 years, the majority of children born with trisomy 21 have mothers younger than 35 years. This is due to the higher reproductive rate of this age group. It is important to emphasize to the mother that she did not do something in her pregnancy to cause this. The parents must understand the spectrum of medical problems associated with the diagnosis (i.e., cardiac, neurologic, endocrine, etc.). A social work referral should be made to inform the family of the support services available to them.

MATCHING

Match the maternal medications on the left that might cause the listed neonatal problems on the right.

Maternal Medication or Drug
1. Beta-blockers
2. Diethylstilbestrol (DES)
3. Carbamazepine
4. Cyclophosphamide
5. Oral hypoglycemics
6. Isotretinoin
7. Tobacco/smoking
8. Cocaine
9. Phenytoin
10. Methadone

Neonatal Condition or Disorder
a. CNS, ear, cardiac and thymus anomalies
b. Neural tube defect, midfacial hypoplasia
c. Neonatal abstinence syndrome
d. Prematurity, lower birth weight
e. Hypoglycemia
f. Bradycardia, hypoglycemia
g. Vaginal adenosis, genital tract anomalies
h. Growth restriction, cardiovascular and digital anomalies
i. Hypoplastic nails, midfacial hypoplasia, hemorrhagic disease
j. Abruptio placentae, preterm labor

Answers: 1 (f); 2 (g); 3 (b); 4 (h); 5 (e); 6 (a); 7 (d); 8 (j); 9 (i); 10 (c)

Match the birth trauma on the left with the symptom on the right.

Birth Trauma
1. Erb-Duchenne palsy
2. Spinal cord injury
3. Facial nerve palsy
4. Clavicular fracture
5. Pneumothorax
6. Cephalohematoma
7. Subgaleal hemorrhage
8. Fetal scalp electrode placement

Symptom
a. Asymmetrical cry
b. Tachypnea and decreased respirations on one side
c. Swelling on one side of the head, not crossing suture lines
d. Paralyzed abdominal muscles with rounded, distended appearance
e. Tachycardia, pallor, and bluish discoloration along the neck and behind the ears
f. Abrasion on crown of the head with minimal bleeding
g. No Moro reflex on left side
h. Arm adducted and internally rotated, extension of elbow, pronation of forearm

Answers: 1 (h); 2 (d); 3 (a); 4 (g); 5 (b); 6 (c); 7 (e); 8 (f)

Match the genetic abnormality with the common clinical finding.

Genetic Abnormality
1. Cystic fibrosis
2. DiGeorge syndrome
3. Williams syndrome
4. Down syndrome
5. Hemophilia A
6. Osteogenesis imperfecta
7. Galactosemia
8. Fanconi pancytopenia syndrome
9. Pierre Robin sequence
10. Turner syndrome

Common Clinical Finding
a. Meconium ileus
b. Macroglossia
c. *E.coli* infection
d. Aplastic thymus
e. Micrognathia
f. Supravalvular aortic stenosis
g. Excessive bleeding after a circumcision
h. Congenital lymphedema
i. Blue sclera
j. Radial hypoplasia

Answers: 1 (a); 2 (d); 3 (f); 4 (b); 5 (g); 6 (i); 7 (c); 8 (j); 9 (e); 10 (h)

REFERENCES

The reference list for this chapter can be found online at www.expertconsult.com.

Size and Physical Examination of the Newborn Infant

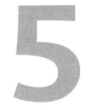

5

Tom Lissauer and Phil Steer

There are tiny, puny infants with great vitality. Their movements are untiring and their crying lusty, for their organs are quite capable of performing their allotted functions. These infants will live, for although their weight is inferior ... their sojourn in the womb was longer.

Pierre Budin, *The Nursling*

As indicated in the above quotation, a newborn infant's problems and prognosis are determined by birth weight and gestational age. The designation *low birth weight* (LBW) is applied to all infants weighing less than 2500 g at birth, regardless of the duration of gestation. Subsequently, the terms *very low birth weight* (VLBW) and *extremely low birth weight* (ELBW) have been used to categorize those infants with birth weights less than 1500 g and 1000 g, respectively. The classification of infants as *preterm* is reserved for those having completed less than 37 weeks of pregnancy, whereas *term* gestation refers to those infants delivered between 37 and 41 completed weeks of pregnancy, and *postterm* indicates birth after or equal to 42 completed weeks of pregnancy. The proportion of LBW infants who are preterm versus those with abnormal intrauterine growth varies around the world. In developed countries, the majority of LBW babies are premature, whereas in developing countries, the major contributor to the LBW rate is growth-restricted term infants. As the standard of living improves in developing countries, there is a shift toward the pattern of developed nations with regard to LBW infants.

Infants are classified as small for gestational age (SGA) if their birth weight is below the 10th percentile and large for gestational age (LGA) if their birth weight is above the 90th percentile (Fig. 5-1)[1]. Intrauterine growth restriction (IUGR) describes failure of a fetus to reach its genetic growth potential. The limitations and complexity of these concepts are considered further in this chapter.

DETERMINANTS OF FETAL GROWTH

Normal fetal growth requires contributions from the mother, the placenta, and the fetus. Numerous maternal metabolic adjustments are made during pregnancy, the unifying goal of which appears to be provision of an uninterrupted supply of nutrients to the developing fetus. Foremost among these are adjustments in carbohydrate metabolism. Mild fasting hypoglycemia and postprandial hyperglycemia associated with an increased basal insulin level and relative insulin resistance characterize the normal pregnancy. Maternal glucose use is attenuated, with ketones and free fatty acids increasingly serving as fuels for maternal tissues. The mechanisms for these alterations are not entirely clear. However, the effect is the provision of a continuous supply of glucose, the primary source of fetal oxidative metabolism, to the fetus, particularly during periods of maternal fasting. During relatively extended periods of fasting, the fetus uses ketones to serve his or her energy and synthetic needs as well. Maternal serum levels of lipids increase during gestation. In midpregnancy, fat is stored for fetal use during late pregnancy when demands increase. These, and a variety of other adjustments, are so effective in supplying the fetus with required nutrients that only with severe maternal malnutrition (e.g., wartime famine), and only then if starvation

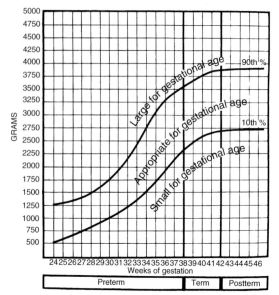

Figure 5-1. Birth weights of liveborn singleton white infants at gestational ages from 24 to 42 weeks. *(From Battaglia F, Lubchenco L: A practical classification of newborn infants by weight and gestational age, J Pediatr 7:159, 1967.)*

occurs during the third trimester, is birth-weight reduced. If starvation occurs in the first trimester, the placenta grows larger to compensate for the reduced energy supply to the fetus, and if nutrition is restored in the second and third trimester, birth weight is actually increased. The human placenta, in addition to its role of transmitting nutrients from mother to fetus, functions as an incredibly active endocrine organ, producing an array of hormones unsurpassed in the animal kingdom. Among those products with direct growth-promoting action are growth factors and human placental lactogen (HPL), also known as chorionic somato-mammotropin. HPL is produced by the syncytiotrophoblast cells of the placenta. Its growth-promoting effects are mediated by the stimulation of fetal insulin-like growth factor (IGF) production and increasing nutrient availability. The previously mentioned elevation of maternal serum lipids plays a role here as well. The expression of the HPL gene is regulated, in part, by apo-protein A1, the major protein component of high-density lipoprotein. The fetus plays a role in his own growth by producing a variety of polypeptide IGF molecules and modulating binding proteins. These substances are produced by a spectrum of fetal tissues, with site, timing, and control of expression varying with each IGF. The biologic and

clinical significance of serum levels of the various growth factors and binding proteins in the fetus and newborn is an area of active research.

THE CONCEPT OF INTRAUTERINE GROWTH RESTRICTION

The growth trajectory of any individual fetus results from the combined effects of its genetic programming and the growth support it receives from its mother. Clearly, the genetic growth potential of a fetus is determined by the contribution of the mother and the father and how they interact. This does not happen on the basis of equality of parental contribution. For example, approximately 30 genes are known to be active only if they are acquired from the mother, or from the father. This phenomenon is known as "genomic imprinting." Paternal imprinting tends to encourage fetal growth, whereas maternal imprinting tends to restrict fetal growth. Although maternal and paternal genes have an approximately equal contribution to adult height and weight, the height and weight of the mother contribute more than 90% of the influence on birth weight compared with the father. This was dramatically illustrated in the 1930s by Walton and Hammond who crossed very large Shire horses with very small Shet-land ponies,[2] and demonstrated that birth weight was appropriate to the mother's size, whereas adult size was intermediate (although foals born to the small mothers never quite reached the same size as those born to large mothers, showing that severe intrauterine growth restriction can result in reduced adult size). A similar phenomenon has been demonstrated in humans, such that the birth weight of babies born from ovum donation is appropriate to the size of the birth mother rather than that of the genetic mother.[3] Although a convenient definition of intrauterine growth restriction is failure of the fetus to reach its genetic growth potential, in practice this simple definition is not comprehensive because the genetic potential is not invariable, but is modifiable according to nutrient supply. In addition, some babies' genetic growth potential is abnormal in the first place, for example, a high proportion of babies with Down syndrome exhibit many of the characteristics of intrauterine growth restriction.

So how should we decide whether a fetus is growth restricted? Ideally, we should base our classification on functional measures,[4] the most obvious of which is the risk of stillbirth or neonatal death. Other typical indicators of inadequate growth status include an inability to cope with the hypoxia of labor, resulting in fetal acidosis and neonatal depression, the passage of meconium during labor, and neonatal dysfunction such as hypoglycemia and hypothermia. In the longer term, catch up growth may be incomplete, resulting in reduced adult size. Alternatively, catch-up growth can be excessive, leading to adult obesity, hypertension, and insulin resistance with an increased risk of diabetes. The concept of intrauterine growth restriction leading to long-term sequelae has led to the "fetal origins of adult disease" hypothesis proposed by Barker and his colleagues.[5,6]

Intrauterine growth restriction does not relate directly to percentile birth weight. Although babies that are small for gestational age are at increased risk of the dysfunction typical of intrauterine growth restriction, many of them will be normal small babies. There is no clear threshold of percentile birth weight below which the risk of dysfunction increases; instead the risk rises steadily as the percentile birth weight falls.[7] One approach that can improve the correlation of percentile birth weight with function is that of using "customized birthweight percentiles," in which the percentile birth weight of a particular baby is adjusted to take into account the mother's height, weight, racial origin, and other relevant factors.[8] However, these variations can be pathologic as well as physiologic. For example, severely underweight or overweight mothers are more likely to have babies that are born preterm or become macrosomic (with all its attendant problems), and it would be inappropriate to correct percentiles to this extent.[9] Mothers from some racial groups are more likely to have small babies that are twice as likely to be stillborn,[10] and again, correction for this would clearly be inappropriate. It has also been argued that using percentile charts based on estimated fetal weights of fetuses growing normally instead of percentiles based on actual birth weights may give a better indication of the incidence and role of fetal growth restriction on neonatal disease.[11] However, this approach is limited by the difficulty to obtain accurate measurements to establish growth charts based on estimated fetal weights.[12]

Perhaps the most appropriate way of defining intrauterine growth restriction is using serial ultrasound measurements of fetal size. Scans from 22 weeks' gestation onward can be used to establish the "normal" growth velocity for an individual fetus, and a subsequent decline in this growth trajectory clearly fulfills the requirements for the definition of growth restriction. Prospective studies have shown that such measurements are at least as good a predictor of intrapartum dysfunction as percentile birth weight (and the latter cannot be known accurately before birth anyway).[13] Some babies initially growing on the 90th percentile show slowing of growth typical of growth restriction, and sustain perinatal problems despite having a birth weight within the "normal" range. This phenomenon is sometimes called *normal weight growth restriction*.

PATTERN OF FETAL GROWTH

With the use of anthropometric measurements, including fetal weight, length, and head circumference, fetal growth standards have been determined for different reference populations from various locations.[14-16] From these data, it is apparent that there are variations in "normal" weight at any given gestational age from one locale to another. This variation is related to a number of factors including sex, race, socioeconomic class, and even altitude. Of course, the key issue here is what is meant by "normal." For example, babies born at high altitude are, on average, smaller than those born at sea level. Thus, when percentile birth weights for babies born at altitude are constructed, the 10th percentile (commonly used as the boundary between "normal" and "abnormal") will be at a lower birth weight than that for babies born at sea level. For example, babies that are on the 11th percentile for altitude might be on the 8th percentile for sea level and would be categorized as "normal weight" for altitude but as "below normal weight" for sea level. However, we also know that babies born at altitude have a higher stillbirth rate. Should we also regard it as "normal" for more babies to be stillborn? It is vital to remember that, ideally, the purpose of customized percentiles is to correct for variations in birth weight due to physiologic variations in the mother and her environment that are associated with variations in birth weight but not associated with a worse outcome.

For example, the Colorado data, presented by Lubchenco et al. in the 1960s,[15] summarized standards of intrauterine growth for white (55%), black (15%), and Hispanic (30%) newborns born between 1948 and 1961 in the vicinity of Denver. The graphic display of this relationship provides a useful and simple method for determining the appropriateness of growth with respect to gestational age and with respect to the local population. What such standards cannot do, however, is indicate whether the population as a whole (e.g., Hispanics compared with whites) is disadvantaged. This can only be determined by looking at perinatal mortality and morbidity rates. Ideally, to be most useful, equivalent measures of weight for gestational age between two different populations should be based on equivalent risk of poor outcome, rather than simply the population distribution of birth weight.

Ten years after the Colorado data were published, Brenner et al. presented fetal weight curves based on more than 30,000 pregnancies, including terminations of pregnancy and miscarriages as well as spontaneous births,[17] with correction factors for parity, race, and sex. Although these and other such curves differ in details, all demonstrate nearly linear growth between 20 and 38 weeks of gestation, with slowing thereafter. Using such nomograms, one can plot fetal growth and detect a decline in growth velocity, indicating growth restriction. Although the use of customized reference ranges for normal fetal growth can highlight intrauterine growth restriction by making a decline in growth more obvious, it must be emphasized that failing growth indicates increased risk to the fetus—irrespective of the percentile birth weight that the baby is currently on. So, for example, a fall in relative intrauterine size from the 80th percentile to the 40th percentile can be as significant as a fall from the 10th percentile to the 5th percentile. Thus, many workers consider that the best descriptor of intrauterine growth restriction is "a fall in growth velocity," rather than being on, or falling below, a particular percentile.

ANTENATAL ASSESSMENT OF INTRAUTERINE GROWTH

CLINICAL ASSESSMENT OF GESTATIONAL AGE

Optimal management of the pregnant woman and her fetus is highly dependent on an accurate knowledge of the gestational age of the fetus. Knowledge of the gestational age is important for interpretation of common tests (e.g., nuchal translucency screening for Down syndrome), scheduling invasive procedures (e.g., amniocentesis), planning the delivery of high-risk fetuses (e.g., assessing the risk of respiratory distress syndrome [RDS]), and assessing fetal size for gestational age. Determination of the expected date of delivery (due date) can be made with varying degrees of certainty by history of menstrual cycles, physical examination of the pregnant woman, and a variety of clinical obstetrical milestones. Regular ultrasound examination of the developing fetus is the most accurate (unless of course the date of conception is precisely known, as with in vitro fertilization and associated techniques).

The average duration of pregnancy is 280 days from the first day of the last menstrual period in white mothers. Because conception occurs on average on day 14 of the menstrual cycle, the true duration of pregnancy is 266 days. There is now good evidence that gestational age varies in different racial groups, being 5 to 7 days shorter, for example, in South Asians and black Africans.[18] Between 22 and 34 weeks' gestation, there is a reasonable correlation between the age of the normally growing, single fetus in weeks and the height of the uterine fundus in centimeters when measured as the distance over the abdominal wall from the upper border of the symphysis pubis to the top of the fundus. This can be used for screening, but it is very unreliable in the 30% or more of western populations who are obese. For this reason, the efficiency of screening for growth restriction is particularly poor in obese women (obesity also makes ultrasound measurements more difficult and therefore less reliable). The size of the uterus changes more slowly in late pregnancy because as the fetus grows, the relative proportion of amniotic fluid decreases. Although physical examination estimates of gestational age have a standard deviation of plus or minus 2 weeks in the first trimester, this extends to 4 weeks in the second trimester, and 6 weeks in the third trimester.

ASSESSMENT OF GESTATIONAL AGE

Forty percent of pregnant women have an uncertain last menstrual period (20% have no idea of the date), making accurate estimation of gestational age by history difficult at best. Since the 1970s, antenatal determination of gestational age using serial ultrasound studies of the fetus has become universal in developed countries. The type of ultrasound, the parameters measured, and the accuracy of the study vary with the progression of pregnancy. In the first trimester, although it is possible to visualize the early gestational sac as early as 5 weeks, the optimal time for scanning is between 7 and 9 weeks, with measurement of the crown-rump length using a high-resolution vaginal probe. Routine ultrasound screens for dating, however, are usually carried out during the second trimester, typically between 11 and 14 weeks' gestation, which is when the nuchal translucency assessment of Down syndrome risk is most accurate. It is also usual to perform a further scan at 20 to 22 weeks' gestational age, for comprehensive fetal anomaly screening. Measurements at this stage of pregnancy are less reliable for assessing gestational age, because to estimate gestational age from the size of the fetus, one has to assume that the fetus is of average size. Some babies will be small and some will be large for any particular gestational age. When the baby is growing rapidly in the first trimester, the change in size from 1 week to the next is substantial; therefore, the standard deviation of likely gestational age is small. Typically, 2 standard deviations are only 3 to 4 days different from the mean. It can be assumed that the fetus is likely to be of the average gestational age for a particular size, plus or minus 3 to 4 days. Fetuses smaller than 2 standard deviations below the average size for gestational age are likely to be heading for demise. However, the normal range of size increases as gestation advances, and accuracy of dating in the second trimester is generally no better than plus or minus 7 days. Ultrasound measures size and not gestational age. A very small baby on ultrasound examination may be just that, rather than having an incorrect gestational age assignment and, similarly, a very large baby may be macrosomic. The most commonly used parameters for determining estimated gestational age during the second trimester are head circumference, biparietal diameter, abdominal circumference, and femur length. Each of these measurements has its own advantages and disadvantages, but all have in common a decreasing level of accuracy with increasing gestational age, particularly after 20 weeks, because of increasing normal biological variation with advancing gestation. To enhance the accuracy of the assessment, a composite fetal size based on the average of these four measurements is used and incorporated into the software of the ultrasound machine for instantaneous calculations. Estimates of fetal weight and growth patterns are most accurately assessed by measuring the fetal abdominal circumference.

INTRAUTERINE GROWTH

Substandard growth rates, *intrauterine growth restriction (IUGR)*, can result from a multitude of pathologic and nonpathologic processes (see later discussion). The original term "intrauterine growth retardation" is no longer used, because the use of the word "retardation" often alarmed parents who took it to mean that their baby would be "retarded" or mentally deficient.

At times, the existence of two terms that describe less-than-desired growth (IUGR) and small for gestational age (SGA) can cause confusion. Perhaps the easiest way to think about these terms is that IUGR is a term used to describe a pattern of fetal growth over a period, whereas SGA is the term used by pediatricians to describe a baby's weight compared with its contemporaries born at the same gestational age. The significance of the label "small for gestational age" depends on the cut-off percentile used to define small. It is common to use the 10th percentile in population studies, because this gives a substantial number of babies to study while including probably 70% of babies that are genuinely growth restricted. However, most babies less than the 10th percentile will be "small normal," and will therefore function normally. If a 3rd or 2nd percentile cut-off is used (approximately 2 standard deviations below the mean), a much higher proportion of babies will actually show dysfunction secondary to growth restriction. The term *small for gestational age*, despite its lack of specificity in relation to growth restriction, is still widely used, and is useful because it can be defined for all babies, whereas the growth trajectories of most babies remains unknown.

EPIDEMIOLOGY AND ETIOLOGY OF FETAL GROWTH RESTRICTION

As previously discussed, normal fetal growth is dependent on the contributions of the mother, the placenta, and the fetus. The corollary to this is that aberrant fetal growth may result from disturbances in any of these same areas.

RACE

Almost without exception, studies in the United States have demonstrated a significantly higher rate of LBW and its subcomponents, IUGR, and preterm birth, in African Americans when compared with their white contemporaries. However, the differences between the patterns of birth weight and mortality in the different races are not simple. First, studies in Europe have shown that black African mothers have an average gestational length that is about five days shorter than that of white mothers.[18] This is compensated for by accelerated maturity in black Africans.[19] An important study was carried out in South Carolina over a 20-year period, which showed that between 1975 and 1979,[20] African-American babies younger than 37 weeks consistently had a lower perinatal mortality for gestational age than did white babies. However, this relationship reversed at term, a particular problem for African American babies being obstructed labor and meconium aspiration. Analysis of data between 1990 and 1994 showed that although gestation-specific perinatal mortality had reduced in both groups, the same pattern of lower mortality before 37 weeks, and higher mortality after 37 weeks in the black babies, persisted. A more recent study on 22 million births in the United States of mortality from 1989 to 1991, and then from 1999 to 2001, gave a similar result.[21] In contrast to the findings with African Americans in the United States, European studies have shown that babies of South Asian origin have a raised perinatal mortality at all gestations compared with white babies.[10] This is likely to be due to the fact that South Asian babies have a lower birth weight across the gestational age range. Babies born in India are on average approximately 600 g lighter than those born in Europe. However, studies of babies of South Asian racial origin born in developed countries shows that the deficit reduces to 300 g, but it persists. This highlights one of the potential pitfalls in correcting for racial origin in relation to birth weight by using "customized birth-weight percentile." The reason there should be a systematically lower birth weight in South Asian babies remains conjectural, but it seems likely that it is an adaptation to the average smaller maternal size, thus minimizing deaths from obstructed labor.[22] However, the long-term sequelae in this population include a very high incidence of diabetes and cardiovascular disease.[23-25]

PRIOR OBSTETRIC AND FAMILY HISTORY

Women who are younger than 15 years of age, older than 45 years of age, have a history of miscarriages or unexplained stillbirths after 20 weeks' gestation, or have prior preterm deliveries, are at increased risk for delivering a growth-restricted baby.[26] Familial factors also appear to play a role in the birth weight of babies. Mothers of LBW infants were frequently LBW infants themselves and are more likely to have subsequent LBW babies than other mothers, as are their siblings.[27,28] However, the pathological implications of being small depend on the context. Being small in an otherwise large family cohort is likely to be pathologic, whereas being small in a family that is usually small is likely to be less of a problem.

ALTITUDE

When comparing growth curves, most authors note that Lubchenco's data were generated in Denver, the "mile-high city," and that the 10th percentile thus generated is lower than the 10th percentile of data collected from centers closer to sea level. Yip was able to demonstrate a "dose-dependent" effect of altitude on the LBW rate,[29] with a two- to threefold greater rate of LBW seen at altitudes greater than 2000 meters than at sea level.

MATERNAL FACTORS CONTRIBUTING TO INTRAUTERINE GROWTH RESTRICTION

In developed countries, a handful of maternal characteristics and behaviors have consistently been associated with an increased risk of growth restriction. In addition to race and prior obstetric history, the list includes maternal nutritional status (prepregnancy weight and weight gain during pregnancy), short stature, smoking, preeclampsia/hypertension, multiple gestation, and female sex of the infant. In developing nations, malaria is a significant factor.

Maternal Nutritional Status

Prepregnancy weight and weight gain during pregnancy, although indicators of maternal nutritional status, are independent variables. There is some evidence of the potential benefits of nutritional intervention in the mother who is poorly nourished before pregnancy but this remains controversial.[30] Nutritional supplements provided to well-nourished women do not provide additional benefit. An obese mother is unlikely to deliver a growth-restricted baby, even if her pregnancy weight gain is low.

Smoking

Cigarette smoking, a habit practiced by 20% of pregnant Americans, has consistently been identified as a dose-dependent contributor to abruptio placentae, late fetal death, LBW, and IUGR. In developed nations, it is by far the single most important contributor to LBW. Rates of IUGR in smokers are 3 to 4.5 times that of nonsmokers, with average birth weights decreasing by 70 to 400 g. These adverse effects are particularly pronounced in babies born to older mothers. Elimination of smoking would diminish SGA rates by 20% to 30%. Multiple mechanisms may contribute to the detrimental effect of smoking during pregnancy. Nicotine and subsequent catecholamine release along with reduced synthesis of prostacycline result in placental vasoconstriction and elevated vascular resistance, decreasing delivery of nutrients and oxygen across the placenta. Levels of fetal carboxyhemoglobin are increased, further interfering with delivery of oxygen to the developing fetal tissues. Indirect effects by way of suboptimal nutritional status both before and during pregnancy have been suggested and are likely due to an increased rate of maternal metabolism rather than decreased maternal caloric intake. Smoking mothers consume more calories than their nonsmoking counterparts, and supplementing the diet of smoking mothers is ineffective in offsetting the detrimental effects on the fetus. If smoking mothers can be convinced to stop smoking before the third trimester, their infant's birth weight will be indistinguishable from those babies whose mothers did not smoke at all.

A variety of other recreational drugs, including alcohol, marijuana, cocaine, and amphetamines, have likewise been associated with adverse fetal effects. With the exception of the fetal alcohol syndrome, the effect of these agents is not as well established or as pervasive as is tobacco. Certain prescription drugs, particularly the anticonvulsants, can result in fetal growth restriction and specific malformation syndromes.

Preeclampsia/Hypertension

Maternal chronic hypertension is an independent risk factor for SGA infants. Infants born to older mothers are at increased risk of being SGA (Table 5-1). The worst perinatal

| Table 5-1. | Effect of Chronic Hypertension on the Risk of Small for Gestational Age by Maternal Age |

	SGA Births (%)	
Maternal Age	Normotensive	Chronic Hypertension
<26 years	10	6
26-30 years	7	14
>30 years	5	18

SGA, Small for gestational age.

outcome in hypertensive pregnancies is seen in those complicated by the superimposition of preeclampsia. Preeclampsia is not only a contributor to fetal growth restriction, but it also carries the most unfavorable prognosis in terms of severity of growth deficit. Both of these vascular-based problems are likely to produce their effects through a common placental disorder.

MULTIPLE GESTATIONS

The presence of more than one fetus in the uterus often results in SGA offspring. The onset of the growth restriction is determined by the number of fetuses: the more fetuses, the earlier growth restriction is likely to be observed.

OTHER

Finally, a variety of other maternally related factors have been proposed to play a role in the development of an SGA infant. Chronic medical conditions that interfere with maternal nutrition (inflammatory bowel disease, short gut syndrome), fetal oxygenation caused by decreased amounts of saturated hemoglobin (sickle cell disease, cyanotic heart disease), or oxygen and nutrient delivery caused by vasculopathies (advanced diabetes mellitus, chronic renal failure) can result in IUGR. The role of psychosocial stressors in IUGR is unclear.[31,32] A summary of the relative contributions of the various factors with direct causal impact is provided in Figure 5-2.

PLACENTAL CONTRIBUTIONS

Placental tissue is fetal tissue. It follows that if circumstances exist that ultimately result in abnormal fetal growth, then the placenta will likewise be similarly affected. This has certainly been observed, with a significant correlation between birth weight and both placental weight and villus surface area.

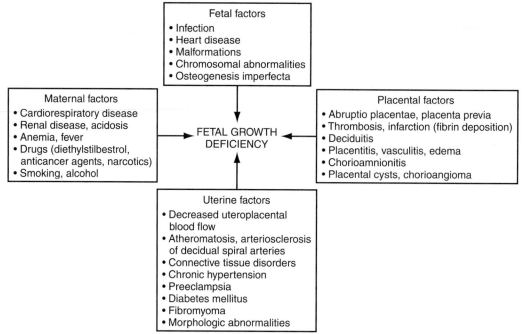

Figure 5-2. Causes of growth restriction by compartment. *(From James D, Steer P, Weiner C, Gonik B, editors:* High risk pregnancy, *ed 4, Philadelphia, 2010, Saunders.)*

Likewise, there are placental pathologic correlates of known causes of IUGR (intrauterine infections, chromosomal anomalies, hypertensive disorders, twins) and gross placental and cord abnormalities (chronic abruptio placentae, choriohemangioma, extensive infarction, and abnormal cord insertions), which are likely to result in restricted fetal growth. On the other hand, the majority of cases of IUGR are idiopathic, with the epidemiologic risk factors discussed earlier (e.g., previous fetal losses, extremes of maternal age, previous preterm or SGA infant, substance abuse) as the only clue. The cause of growth failure in these infants is presumed to be the result of the ill-defined *uteroplacental insufficiency*. Human and animal in vivo studies, Doppler ultrasound investigations, and pathologic evaluations have identified an array of placental abnormalities that may well shed a unifying light on these apparently disparate groups of mother-infant dyads[26,33] (Box 5-1). As a result of these investigations, the central role of the placenta in the development of the growth-restricted baby is coming to the forefront.

DIMINISHED POTENTIAL: FETAL CONTRIBUTIONS

As described earlier, the genetic potential for growth is inherited from both parents and is the major determinant of early fetal growth,

Box 5-1.	Findings in the Placenta in Fetal Growth Restriction

Uteroplacental blood flow
Diminished blood flow
Increased vascular resistance
Absent spiral artery remodeling
Atherosis of vessels of parietal decidua

Fetoplacental blood flow
Increased irregularity of luminal size
Abnormal umbilical Doppler flow studies
Decreased number of placental arterial vessels
Decreased size of placental vessels
Decreased artery to villus ratio

Interface of maternal and fetal circulations
Cytotrophoblastic hyperplasia
Thickened basement membrane
Chronic villitis

which is subsequently modulated by environmental factors. IUGR can also result from a variety of conditions (e.g., congenital infections) in which an otherwise normal fetus is prohibited from growing normally or if there is a genetic aberration that precludes the fetus from growing normally.

CONGENITAL INFECTIONS

During the rubella pandemic of 1962 to 1964, IUGR was found to be the most consistent characteristic of congenitally infected infants. In this episode, 60% of the affected infants were less than the 10th percentile for weight at birth and 90% were less than the 50th percentile.[34] Cytomegalovirus (CMV) is the infective organism most commonly associated with IUGR, although 90% of infants congenitally infected with CMV are asymptomatic. Hepatosplenomegaly and microcephaly with paraventricular calcifications are common findings in the symptomatic infant. Diagnosis is made most reliably with viral cultures of the urine obtained after birth. Human immunodeficiency virus has *not* been consistently associated with IUGR because other confounding variables have been difficult to separate. Although numerous other bacterial, protozoal, and viral pathogens are known to invade the developing fetus, most of these infants develop appropriately.

GENETIC FACTORS

About 8% of all SGA infants have a major congenital anomaly.[35] Conversely, the incidence of growth restriction in infants with significant congenital anomalies is 22%, nearly three times that of the general population, and a correlation exists between the number of malformations and frequency of IUGR.[36] A wide array of chromosomal aberrations (aneuploidy, deletions, translocations) are associated with IUGR. The likelihood of finding a chromosomal disorder in an SGA infant with a congenital anomaly is approximately 6%.[37] Chromosomal disorder, uniparental disomy, wherein a pair of homologous chromosomes are inherited from the same parent, has been associated with IUGR. Single-gene disorders and inborn errors of metabolism (maternal and fetal phenylketonuria) are likewise represented in this population. In addition there are well over 100 nonchromosomal syndromes associated with IUGR.

IDENTIFICATION AND MANAGEMENT OF GROWTH RESTRICTION

A major problem is knowing which babies are at risk of growth restriction and should, therefore, have their growth monitored. Using classic risk factors, and even including regular fundal height measurements of the uterus, at best two thirds of babies with growth restriction can be detected antenatally, and in routine clinical practice the proportion is often much lower, typically about 30%. Attempts have been made to detect intrauterine growth restriction in low-risk populations using a single assessment at 32 to 34 weeks' gestation; however, these have proved to be inefficient because a single measurement cannot indicate growth trajectory as opposed to size. Indeed, a Cochrane review showed that the harm from false-positive ultrasound diagnoses exceeds the benefit when screening is done in this way.[38] Regular growth velocity profiling for every baby would be prohibitively expensive.

Currently, usual policy is to measure the fetuses thought to be at risk of growth restriction from maternal (e.g., hypertension) and epidemiologic factors (e.g., a previous growth-restricted baby) every 2 weeks. Measurements at more frequent intervals are not reliable indicators of poor growth because the change in fetal size is within the error of the measurement. If growth slows, then the next step is to measure umbilical artery blood flow velocity waveforms.[39] A raised pulsatility index (ratio of systolic velocity to diastolic velocity), or even worse, absent or reversed end-diastolic flow, indicates increased resistance to perfusion of the placenta, putting the baby at risk of hypoxia. This investigation is well established as valuable and is part of routine surveillance in most tertiary centers; it can be carried out reliably by trained ultrasonographers. More expert fetal medicine specialists can move on to assessing fetal vascular redistribution as a response to early hypoxia. This redistribution can be detected by Doppler studies of key fetal organs, including the brain (by study of the middle cerebral artery), to detect the maintenance of the oxygen supply to them, thereby protecting their vital functions. At the same time, flow to less vital organs is reduced. Impaired cardiac function in the fetus can be demonstrated using venous Doppler examination of the precordial veins (ductus venosus, inferior vena cava, or superior vena cava), hepatic veins, and head and neck veins. Combining the umbilical artery, middle cerebral artery, and venous Doppler examinations provides information about the degree of placental disease, the level of redistribution, and the degree of cardiac compromise respectively. Changes in the venous Doppler usually precede abnormalities of the fetal heart rate pattern.[40] However, at present, the use of venous Doppler remains largely a research tool, and data from prospective trials of its utility in preventing unexpected intrauterine demise are required before it is widely adopted.

There is no currently known effective treatment to improve the growth pattern of a fetus. If it is likely, because of failing growth, that delivery will be necessary at <34 weeks' gestation, antenatal steroids should be given to improve pulmonary maturity before elective delivery. Prenatal management is aimed at determining the best time and mode of delivery. Gestational age is a critical factor in this decision. Deciding on the appropriate time of delivery is particularly difficult before 30 weeks' gestation, when the risks to the neonate are substantial. Early delivery of growth-restricted fetuses with an abnormal umbilical artery waveform results in a high liveborn rate but at the cost of a high neonatal mortality and morbidity. Alternatively, delaying delivery until the fetal heart rate pattern is abnormal has been reported to result in a nearly five-fold increase in stillbirths; neonatal deaths before discharge fall by more than one third; overall, the total mortality is unchanged; and there is some evidence that long-term outcome may be improved.[41] Therefore, if a fetus with growth restriction has an abnormal umbilical artery waveform, twice daily monitoring of the fetal heart rate pattern is recommended, and delivery should be undertaken as soon as the heart rate pattern becomes abnormal.

SMALL FOR GESTATIONAL AGE INFANTS

Lubchenco et al. defined SGA as being birth weight less than the 10th percentile. By definition then, 10% of all newborns in a given population are too small. Others have proposed or have indeed used other cut-off values (e.g., the 25th, 15th, 5th, or 3rd percentile) or 2 standard deviations from the mean, which would correspond to approximately 2.5% of the population. No matter what cutoff is used, there may be multiple factors that result in a large discrepancy in absolute weights seen at the lowest "normal" percentile. Goldenberg reviewed several reports wherein the 10th percentile was used as the definition of IUGR.[42] More than a 500-g difference was noted across these studies. This observation, however, may have been a reflection of the disparate methodologic approaches among the studies. Goldenberg's plea for a concerted effort by a variety of national professional academies and federal agencies to endorse a national standard has, so far, gone unheeded. The approach of using *any* percentile as an absolute criteria

has been thoughtfully challenged by Chard et al., who point out that not only is there no statistical evidence of a subpopulation of growth-restricted babies at term,[43] but also, by using the 10th percentile, many cases of IUGR (defined as a failure to achieve growth potential) will be missed. Although these may be seen as interesting, if somewhat arcane academic issues, the practical importance becomes apparent when one is responsible for making decisions regarding expensive and painful laboratory evaluations; when there is the need to monitor the infant in a more costly special care nursery; and when there are future referrals for formal developmental evaluations.

Excluding SGA infants who have significant congenital anomalies and infections, there is a group of SGA infants with a relatively characteristic physical appearance. Their heads are often disproportionately large for their trunks, and their extremities typically appear wasted. The nails are long. The facial appearance has been likened to that of a "wizened old man." The anterior fontanelle is often larger than expected, and the cranial sutures may be widened or overlapping. The umbilical cord is typically thin with little Wharton's jelly and may be meconium stained; the abdomen is scaphoid, which may mislead the examiner into considering a congenital diaphragmatic hernia. Subcutaneous fat and tissue are diminished, resulting in loose skin on the arms, legs, back, abdomen, and buttocks. Like the umbilical cord, the skin may be stained from meconium passed in utero and be unusually dry and flaky with little protective vernix caseosa present.

It is often suggested that measuring the weight, length, and head circumference allows further classification of the SGA infant as either symmetrically growth restricted (those infants with decreased length and head circumference) or asymmetrically growth restricted (relatively normal length with relative "head sparing"). Such a distinction has been proposed as both a diagnostic tool and prognostic marker. The symmetrically growth-restricted newborn, historically representing 20% of all SGA infants, is thought to result from an injury or process (congenital infection, genetic disorders) that occurred or began in the early stages of the pregnancy, during the phase of growth primarily characterized by cellular hyperplasia. The prognosis for eventual growth and development of these infants is somewhat guarded, in large part because of the underlying etiology. The asymmetrical ("wasted") SGA baby, on the other hand, has been proposed to result from a third trimester insult interfering with delivery of oxygen and nutrients (the effect of maternal hypertensive disorders, maternal starvation, advanced diabetes) during the cellular hypertrophy phase of fetal growth. This latter group has been projected to expect a much brighter future than their symmetrical brethren. Various indices such as the Ponderal Index (PI = Birth weight × 100/Length[44]) have been used to further describe or quantify the relationship between length and weight and identify these subgroups.

Whereas such an outline may appeal to one's sense of logic, recent data have necessitated a reevaluation of this approach. Chard et al. demonstrated that there is a continuous relationship between the PI and weight throughout the entire range of normal birth weight.[45] Infants in the lower half of the population have a lower PI than those in the upper half. In other words, smaller infants tend to be thinner, and larger infants tend to be fatter. Kramer et al.[46] when excluding infants with evidence of major malformations and congenital infections, likewise found a direct relationship between severity of growth restriction and a decreasing PI, arguing against distinct subgroups of proportional and disproportional infants. Similarly, a normal frequency distribution of head-to-abdominal circumference ratio is seen in antenatal ultrasound assessments of growth-restricted fetuses, with increased severity of growth restriction being associated with increased asymmetry.[47] Even the relative frequency of the two groups has come under question; in some populations, symmetrical SGA infants are found more frequently than asymmetrical infants.[48] The concept of asymmetry serving as a diagnostic tool has been further challenged by Salafia,[33] who found that IUGR preterm infants born to mothers suffering from preeclampsia were far more likely to be symmetrical than asymmetrical, and David,[47] who found an equal distribution of a small number of chromosomal abnormalities between the symmetrical and asymmetrical populations. In summary, although it may be premature to completely discard the framework of symmetry and asymmetry in intrauterine growth restriction, one should feel uncomfortable with a dogmatic approach to its use in the SGA infant.

CLINICAL PROBLEMS

PERINATAL AND NEONATAL MORBIDITY AND MORTALITY

The growth-restricted fetus and newborn have a higher perinatal mortality at each gestation compared with those of appropriate weight for gestation infants, whether preterm, term, or postterm (Fig. 5-3). They also have a variety of other adverse outcomes, reflecting the underlying plethora of diagnoses and chronic and acute deprivations of oxygen and nutrients. Overall, the perinatal mortality among growth-restricted infants is eight to ten times greater than for infants who have grown normally. The risk of perinatal morbidity and mortality increases markedly with the degree of growth restriction[49] (Fig. 5-4).

ACUTE NEONATAL PROBLEMS

Asphyxia
Perinatal asphyxia is the most significant risk for the growth-restricted fetus and newborn, who is often marginally oxygenated and who has limited carbohydrate reserves. With the stresses associated with labor and delivery, fetal death or hypoxic-ischemic encephalopathy may ensue.

Respiratory Difficulties
In association with the relative intolerance of the stresses of labor and delivery, passage of meconium and subsequent in utero or postpartum aspiration of this material poses

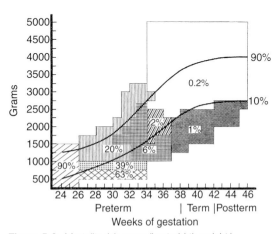

Figure 5-3. Mortality risk according to birth weight/ gestational age relationship. Based on 14,413 live births at University of Colorado Health Sciences Center (1974 to 1980). *IUGR*, Intrauterine growth restriction. *(From Koops B, Morgan LJ, Battaglia FC: Neonatal mortality risk in relation to birth weight and gestational age: update, J Pediatr 101:969, 1982.)*

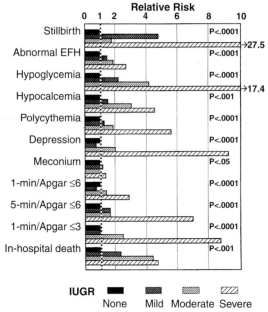

Figure 5-4. Morbidity and mortality varies with degree of growth restriction. EFH, Electronic fetal heart pattern. *(From Kramer MS, Olivier M, McLean FH, et al: Impact of intrauterine growth retardation and body proportionality on fetal and neonatal outcome, Pediatrics 86:707, 1990.)*

a risk to the term or near-term growth-restricted infant. Because of concerns regarding risk of in utero fetal demise, SGA infants are more likely to be electively delivered prematurely, with the attendant risks of prematurity, including RDS.

Hypoglycemia and Hypocalcemia
The SGA infant is at risk of hypoglycemia during the first 48 to 72 hours of life. Hypoglycemia can result from inadequate glycogen stores, diminished gluconeogenesis, a reduction in alternative energy substrates (e.g., free fatty acids, hyperinsulinemia and/or increased sensitivity to insulin and, in some, asphyxia, polycythemia/hyperviscosity, or hypothermia). Severe hypoglycemia can result in adverse long-term neurologic morbidity and, therefore, must be consistently sought and appropriately managed. Hypocalcemia is seen less frequently, but must be considered as a possible complication in these babies (see Chapter 12).

Thermoregulation
SGA babies often have difficulty with maintaining body temperature in the normal range. This may stem from a diminished supply of glucose, diminished insulating fat, and impaired lipid metabolism. The brown

adipose tissue is not consistently depleted in these infants, but, in some, this may diminish the infant's ability to respond to hypothermia. The range of thermoneutral environmental temperatures for SGA infants is narrowed when contrasted with appropriate for gestational age (AGA) infants of the same gestational age.

Hematologic Issues
Spun, central venous hematocrit values greater than 65% occur in as many as 40% of term or near-term SGA babies. Poor placental function with resultant relative fetal hypoxia and subsequently elevated levels of erythropoietin is thought to be the cause. Elevated levels of fetal hemoglobin and nucleated red blood cells have both been observed in SGA newborns. Polycythemia has been associated with a myriad of cardiopulmonary, metabolic, and neurologic effects. The need to reduce the level of red cell mass, the benefits derived, and at what level of hematocrit to intervene have been a matter of debate. The following elements are certain: (1) the value should be checked before any corrective action is taken (some nurseries routinely perform a heel stick to determine the hematocrit; if this is high, a free-flowing venous sample must be obtained and a spun hematocrit must be determined); (2) if a partial exchange transfusion is to be carried out, saline is the diluent of choice; it is as effective and less hazardous and less expensive than any blood-derived products; (3) immunologic function of the growth-restricted infant may be compromised; (4) serum IgG concentrations are depressed in term SGA infants when compared with their AGA peers; (5) deficiencies in lymphocyte function have been observed; (6) neutropenia and thrombocytopenia are seen in some SGA infants. Infants with congenital infections and those infants delivered to mothers with systemic hypertension/preeclampsia are particularly at risk for these latter problems.

THE PRETERM GROWTH-RESTRICTED INFANT
Animal data, as well as clinical research and experience, have led many to conclude that the growth-restricted preterm infant has a more favorable respiratory prognosis than the equally premature AGA infant because of in utero stress-induced acceleration of lung maturation. Several investigations make a cogent argument against this

Table 5-2.	Incidence of Respiratory Distress in Small for Gestational Age and Appropriate for Gestational Age Infants According to Gestational Age	
	Infants with RDS (%)	
Gestation (wk)	**SGA**	**AGA**
27-28	50	37
29-30	43	23
31-32	39	13
33-34	16	2.5
35-36	6	0
37-38	1.5	0.1

AGA, Appropriate for gestational age; *RDS,* respiratory distress syndrome; *SGA,* small for gestational age; *wk,* weeks.

hypothesis. Age-matched preterm growth-restricted neonates, in fact, appear to be at a significant disadvantage when compared with other premature infants (Table 5-2). Another study and analysis of a very large number of VLBW infants without major birth defects and between 25 to 30 weeks' gestation showed that SGA infants were at increased risk of neonatal death (odds ratio 2.77), necrotizing enterocolitis (odds ratio 1.27), and RDS (odds ratio 1.19).[50]

GROWTH AND LONG-TERM OUTCOME

GROWTH

Most small for gestation infants show some catch-up growth in the first year of life. In general, they remain somewhat shorter and lighter and have a smaller head circumference than those with birth weights appropriate for gestational age. As many as 44% of preterm and 29% of term SGA infants remain below the 5th percentile.[51] Some do not have catch-up growth; about one half of them remain short as adults. Infants with poor prenatal and postnatal head growth are at most risk of growth problems and poor developmental outcomes. The presence or absence of symmetry does not reliably predict poor or good growth in early childhood.[51]

NEURODEVELOPMENTAL OUTCOME

In light of the varied causes of growth impairment, it is not surprising that the literature regarding long-term neurodevelopmental outcome is contradictory. Overall,

fetal growth restriction in infants >32 weeks' gestation appears to be associated with an increased incidence of cerebral palsy, cognitive deficits, and behavior problems.[52,53] Poor prenatal head growth is associated with worse cognitive outcome, but impaired cognitive development is also seen in those with appropriate head growth. However, a comparison of health-related quality of life indices in 50-year-old adults who were born at term did not find an adverse effect of being born SGA.[54] In infants <32 weeks' gestation, the problems associated with prematurity overwhelm those of growth restriction.[55]

LARGE FOR GESTATIONAL AGE

Like SGA infants, babies whose birth weight exceeds the 90th percentile for gestational age (LGA) represent a heterogeneous group. Maternal risk factors associated with fetal macrosomia include multiparity, weight of 70 kg or more at the end of pregnancy, a prolonged or postterm pregnancy, abnormal glucose tolerance, and previous history of a macrosomic infant. In one study, the overall prevalence of macrosomic infants subsequent to a previous macrosomic birth was 22%, a proportion that did not vary notably with parity or when paternity changed between successive births.[56]

One of the more commonly recognized clinical associations with LGA infants is their increased likelihood of being delivered to diabetic mothers. Even in expert centers, the rates of fetal macrosomia are between 20% and 40% for offspring of women with insulin-dependent diabetes, noninsulin-dependent diabetes, and gestational diabetes.[57]

Because the delivery of an excessively large baby is potentially associated with significant perinatal morbidity and increased mortality rate, efforts are made to predict and confirm the presence of fetal macrosomia in an affected pregnancy before labor to facilitate appropriate management of the mother and infant. The neonatal morbidity anticipated among LGA infants includes birth trauma, hypoglycemia, polycythemia, and, more infrequently, congenital heart disease (in particular, transposition of the great vessels), and Beckwith-Wiedemann syndrome, all of which, when anticipated, are more likely to be detected and treated quickly. However, although antenatal prediction of fetal macrosomia is associated with a marked increase in cesarean deliveries, there has been no significant reduction documented in the incidence of shoulder dystocia or fetal injury secondary to the surgical delivery of macrosomic infants, challenging its cost effectiveness.[58-60]

PHYSICAL EXAMINATION OF THE NEWBORN INFANT

PREPARATION

Before embarking on the physical examination of the infant, the clinician must review the mother's medical and pregnancy history to help focus the examination and to ensure that no pertinent findings are overlooked. For example, a history of maternal insulin-dependent diabetes should alert the examiner to the risk of a variety of congenital anomalies as well as aberrant growth. A history of polyhydramnios raises the suspicion of a proximal gastrointestinal obstruction or underlying neurologic problem. A history of oligohydramnios may raise the question of structural renal anomalies. Knowing that a fetus presented in breech position should lead the examiner to focus on examination of the hips. As noted in the previous sections of this chapter, the presence of IUGR should alert the examiner to search for the stigmata of intrauterine infections and various syndromes.

Transfer of pathogenic microbes from the examiner to the baby must be prevented by thorough hand hygiene, and the stethoscope to be used should be cleaned with alcohol. For all newborns, but in particular the premature or sick neonate, the thermal environment must be appropriate. Attention must also be given to the lighting and noise in the examination area. Lighting needs to be adequate but must avoid very bright light because it interferes with the processes of stabilization and transition. Finally, a thorough examination of the newborn should take no more than 5 to 10 minutes.

VARYING PURPOSE OF THE EXAMINATION

The extent and focus of the examination varies with circumstances. There are typically three distinct periods during which the infant is examined: (1) a brief examination immediately after birth; (2) a complete examination in the newborn nursery or mother's room within 24 hours after birth; and (3) a focused examination within 24 hours before discharge, which may be accomplished with a single examination for shortened hospital stay.

The initial examination may be carried out by the labor and delivery nurse, the newborn nursery nurse assigned to the delivery area, or the physician or nurse practitioner attending the infant, depending on the circumstances surrounding the birth. The purpose of this initial examination is twofold: (1) to ensure that there is no evidence of significant cardiopulmonary instability that requires intervention; and (2) to identify significant congenital anomalies. For the high-risk neonate, it may be advantageous to use this setting to perform as complete an examination as possible to forgo a subsequent examination and thereby avoid an unnecessary disturbance of the baby in the intensive care nursery.

The assessment of cardiopulmonary adaptation begins as soon as the infant is delivered, and this initial evaluation is, in part, quantified by the Apgar score. Assessment of the presence, regularity, and effectiveness of respiratory effort is the first step in evaluating any newborn. The presence of apnea or signs of respiratory distress must be noted to determine the need for intervention. It is not unusual for a healthy newborn to require a few minutes to establish a regular respiratory pattern, and unlabored respiratory rates of 60 to 80 breaths per minute may be seen for the first 1 to 2 hours in some normal infants.

Cardiovascular adaptation is simultaneously assessed with the pulmonary adjustment to extrauterine life. The normal heart rate of a baby in the delivery area is greater than 100 beats per minute and may exceed 160 beats per minute for brief periods. Sustained tachycardia is not a normal finding and may indicate hypovolemia, inadequate oxygen delivery to the tissues, or, rarely, an arrhythmia. Autonomic instability may cause an asymptomatic irregular heart beat in the first few hours of life, which is not uncommon.

It is important to assess color of the infant centrally (gums and inner lips); acrocyanosis (blue discoloration of the hands and feet and perioral area) is often present in the normal infant during the first 24 hours of life. Pallor and poor perfusion require further evaluation.

As soon as the initial cardiopulmonary assessment is complete, evaluation of responsiveness and muscle tone is carried out as a further indicator of the success of transition and well-being of the infant. Normal tone varies considerably with gestational age, but the finding of flaccidity, hypertonicity, or asymmetry of tone is always abnormal.

When these initial steps are taken, an efficient survey of the face, mouth, abdomen, back, extremities, genitalia, and perineum is carried out. Major congenital anomalies must be sought while the infant is in the delivery area, and their presence and significance, and preliminary plans for their evaluation are discussed with the family. Even relatively minor anomalies can precipitate strong reactions from anxious parents.

After this initial assessment, assuming the condition of the baby and mother permits, baby and parents should be provided with some private time. The baby is usually in a state of quiet alertness, facilitating parent-infant bonding. This state of quiet alertness will allow the mother to suckle her infant, which increases the likelihood of breast-feeding success. The infant should be briefly assessed at least once every 30 minutes until there has been continued stability for 2 hours.[44]

TRANSITION PERIOD

During the initial 15 to 30 minutes of life, the *first period of reactivity*, the observed changes reflect a state of sympathetic discharge. In addition to the irregular respiratory efforts and relative tachycardia, the normal infant is alert and responsive, and exhibits spontaneous startle reactions, tremors, bursts of crying, side-to-side movements of the head, smacking of the lips, and tremors of the extremities. Bowel sounds, passage of meconium, and saliva production become evident as a reflection of parasympathetic discharge. Normal premature and term infants who are ill or were abnormally stressed by labor and delivery have a prolonged period of initial reactivity. During the first hour of life, the infant spends up to 40 minutes in a quiet alert state. This is often the longest period of quiet alert behavior during the first 4 days of life. After this burst of activity, the baby passes into a 1- to 2-hour period of decreased activity and sleep. A *second period of reactivity* subsequently emerges between 2 and 6 hours of age with many of the same motor and autonomic manifestations previously described for the first period of reactivity. Gagging and vomiting are often observed during this time. The duration of this phase is variable, lasting from 10 minutes to several hours. For more information on the transition period, see Chapter 4.

POSTNATAL ASSESSMENT OF GESTATIONAL AGE

A variety of methods for assessing the gestational age of the newborn infant have been developed. However, even in the most experienced hands, one can expect up to a 2-week variance in the postnatal assessment from well-established antenatal dating.

Currently, the most widely used system for the postnatal assessment of gestational age in the United States is the New Ballard Score (NBS) (Box 5-2 and Fig. 5-5).[61] This system, like many others, including the Dubowitz Score from which the Ballard system is derived, includes both physical and neurologic characteristics.[62] The advantages of the NBS are the relative ease with which it can be carried out, even in the newborn requiring ventilatory assistance, and the improved accuracy (within 1 week) for the extremely premature infant.

THE COMPLETE EXAMINATION

The complete examination of the healthy newborn can be carried out in the nursery or in the mother's room. In the latter location, the family is more able to express any concerns about the baby's physical features and the physician is better able to observe parent-infant interactions.

The purpose of the complete examination is to
- Detect any physical abnormalities—A significant congenital anomaly is present at birth in 10 to 20 per 1000 live births.
- Confirm and/or consider the further management of any abnormalities detected antenatally.
- Consider potential problems related to maternal pregnancy history or familial disorders.
- Allow the parents to ask any questions and raise any concerns about their baby.
- Determine whether there is concern by caregivers about the adequacy of parental care of the baby following discharge.
- Provide advice about preventive care.
- Ensure that appropriate follow-up arrangements are in place.

The clinician needs to find a method that will enable him or her to perform a comprehensive examination while minimizing the disturbance of the baby. General observation (hands and stethoscope off) is combined with a head-to-toe review. In practice, these examinations are done simultaneously, and an opportunistic approach is adopted, for example checking

---

Box 5-2.   Technique for New Ballard Score

Neuromuscular maturity

There is a general replacement of extensor tone by flexor tone in a cephalocaudal progression with advancing gestational age.

Posture: Observe the unrestrained infant in the supine position.

Square window: Flex the wrist and measure the minimal angle between the *ventral* surface of the forearm and the palm.

Arm recoil: With the infant supine and the head midline, hold the forearm against the arm for 5 seconds, then fully extend and release the arm. Note the time it takes the infant to resume a flexed posture.

Popliteal angle: Flex the hips with the thighs on the abdomen. Then, without lifting the hips from the bed surface, extend the knee as far as possible until resistance is met. (One may overestimate the extent of exten-sion if one attempts to continue extending the knee beyond the point where resistance is first met.)

Scarf sign: Keeping the head in the midline, pull the hand across the chest to encircle the neck as a scarf and note the position of the elbow relative to the midline.

Heel to ear: With the infant supine and the pelvis kept on the examining surface, the feet are brought back as far as possible toward the head, allowing the knees to be positioned alongside the abdomen.

Physical maturity

Skin: With maturation, the skin becomes thicker, less translucent and, eventually, dry and peeling.

Lanugo: This fine, nonpigmented hair is evenly distributed over the body and is most promi-nent at 27 to 28 weeks' gestation, then it gradually disappears, usually first from the lower back. Although present over the entire body, the lanugo over the back is used for gestational age assessment.

Plantar surface: As with the hands, the presence of creases in the foot is a reflection of intrauterine activity as well as maturation. The absence of creases may indicate an underlying neurologic problem as well as immaturity. Accelerated crease development is observed when oligohydramnios was present. An addition in the New Ballard Score (NBS) is the requirement for measuring the plantar surface.

Breast: The areola development is not dependent on adequacy of intrauterine nutrition. There is no difference in male or female infants.

Ear cartilage: With maturation, the ear cartilage becomes increasingly stiff and the auricle thickens. Fold the top of the ear and assess the recoil.

Eyelid opening: Used (incorrectly) by some as a sign of nonviability. Dr. Ballard included the degree of fusion of the lids as a new assessment tool. She defined *tightly fused* as both lids being inseparable by gentle traction, and *loosely fused* as either lid being able to be partly separated by gentle traction. Tightly fused lids were observed in 20% of infants born at 26 weeks' gesta-tion, and only 5% of babies delivered at 27 weeks. The presence of fused eyelids alone should never be used as a sign of nonviability.

External genitalia, male: Palpate for level of testicular descent and observe the degree of rugation.

External genitalia, female: The labia minora and clitoris are prominent in the immature newborn, at times leading the inexperienced examiner to suspect clitoromegaly. With maturation, the labia majora becomes fat-filled and therefore prominent. The under-nourished fetus may have relatively thin labia majora.

---

for red reflexes when the infant's eyes are open, but making sure that all aspects of the examination are covered.

BODY MEASUREMENTS AND GESTATIONAL AGE ASSESSMENT

Note the birth weight and gestational age and plot them on a growth chart. The ges-tational age is usually based on the maternal estimated date of delivery from ultrasound and last menstrual period. Gestational age can also be assessed by physical examination of the infant, using the New Ballard system, as already described. Familiarity with the scoring system is helpful to be able to recog-nize discrepancy between the infant matu-rity and maternal date of confinement or when maternal date is uncertain. During the

Neuromuscular maturity

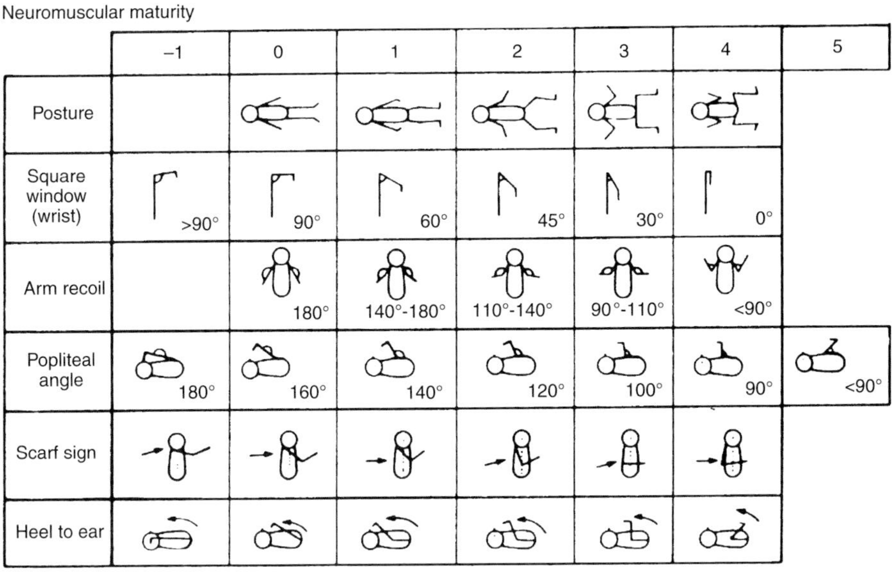

	−1	0	1	2	3	4	5
Posture							
Square window (wrist)	>90°	90°	60°	45°	30°	0°	
Arm recoil		180°	140°-180°	110°-140°	90°-110°	<90°	
Popliteal angle	180°	160°	140°	120°	100°	90°	<90°
Scarf sign							
Heel to ear							

Physical maturity

Skin	Sticky, friable, transparent	Gelatinous, red, translucent	Smooth, pink, visible veins	Superficial peeling &/or rash, few veins	Cracking pale areas, rare veins	Parchment, deep cracking, no vessels	Leathery, cracked, wrinkled
Lanugo	None	Sparse	Abundant	Thinning	Bald areas	Mostly bald	
Plantar surface	Heel-toe 40-50 mm: −1 <40 mm: −2	>50 mm no crease	Faint red marks	Anterior transverse crease only	Creases anterior 2/3	Creases over entire sole	
Breast	Imperceptible	Barely perceptible	Flat areola, no bud	Stippled areola 1-2 mm bud	Raised areola 3-4 mm bud	Full areola 5-10 mm bud	
Eye/ear	Lids fused Loosely:−1 Tightly:−2	Lids open, pinna flat, stays folded	slightly curved pinna; soft; slow recoil	Well-curved pinna; soft but ready recoil	Formed & firm, instant recoil	Thick cartilage, ear stiff	
Genitals, male	Scrotum flat, smooth	Scrotum empty, faint rugae	Testes in upper canal, rare rugae	Testes descending, few rugae	Testes down, good rugae	Testes pendulous, deep rugae	
Genitals, female	Clitoris prominent, labia flat	Prominent clitoris, small labia minora	Prominent clitoris, enlarging minora	Majora & minora equally prominent	Majora large, minora small	Majora covers clitoris & minora	

Maturity Rating

Score	Weeks
−10	20
−5	22
0	24
5	26
10	28
15	30
20	32
25	34
30	36
35	38
40	40
45	42
50	44

Figure 5-5. New Ballard Score. *(From Ballard J, Wednig K, Wang L, et al: New Ballard Score, expanded to include extremely premature infants,* J Pediatr *119:417, 1991.)*

examination, the head circumference and the length are also measured and plotted on a growth chart. This will assist identification of infants who have microcephaly or macrocephaly or who are abnormally short.

Vital Signs

The respiratory rate and heart rate of the normal newborn vary considerably in the first few hours of life. During the remainder of the first day of life, most newborns have a respiratory rate of 40 to 60 breaths per minute and a heart rate of 120 to 160 beats per minute. The temperature of the newborn will have been assessed using an axillary measurement. A temperature between 35.5° C and 37.5° C is normal. An elevated temperature may represent a fever, but more commonly it is the result of external factors such as overbundling or ambient heat source.

OBSERVATION

Initially, the examiner uses only his or her eyes and unaided ears to evaluate the baby (hands and stethoscope off). This is usually best done in stages, observing the exposed part of the baby in turn while undressing the baby.

Respiratory Effort

The respiratory effort of the newborn varies with the sleep state of the infant. During deep sleep, the infant usually has a regular breathing pattern, whereas during awake states, bursts of more rapid breathing are often observed. Because of the newborn's compliant chest wall and almost exclusive diaphragmatic breathing, it is not unusual to observe mild subcostal and intercostal retractions, as well as paradoxical movement during inspiration, with the thorax being drawn inward accompanied by outward abdominal excursion. Even though this "see-saw" pattern is often seen in neonates with respiratory distress, in the absence of further evidence of respiratory difficulties, this movement should not cause alarm. However, suprasternal and supraclavicular retractions are not normal findings. Likewise, asymmetrical chest wall movement is abnormal and may indicate unilateral lesions of the diaphragm (diaphragmatic hernia or diaphragmatic paralysis associated with a difficult delivery) or pleural space (effusion or pneumothorax). The normal newborn thorax is configured as an oval, with a relatively narrow anteroposterior diameter. A barrel chest appearance suggests cardiomegaly or air trapping, as may be seen with transient tachypnea of the newborn, meconium aspiration, or a pneumothorax. Audible grunting results from the infant expiring against a partially closed glottis in an effort to maintain a functional residual capacity in the face of atelectasis. This finding should be assumed to indicate a potentially significant cardiopulmonary disorder until proven otherwise.

Color and Perfusion

The normal newborn is pink. The finding of other colors such as blue, purple, yellow, or green; pallor; or mottling requires closer examination. Acrocyanosis (blue discoloration of the hands, feet, and perioral area) is common in the first day of life. Central cyanosis (involving the tongue and mucous membranes of the mouth) persisting beyond the first few minutes of life is always abnormal and may indicate significant cardiopulmonary disease. Occasionally, infants with polycythemia appear cyanotic despite adequate oxygenation because they have a relatively high concentration of reduced hemoglobin. As noted previously, polycythemia is more likely to present in postdate, LGA, and IUGR infants, and in infants of mothers with diabetes. The presenting fetal parts may be bruised during the process of birth, resulting in a localized bluish discoloration. This can be particularly striking in a face presentation or when a transient venous obstruction developed intrapartum (perhaps as the result of a nuchal cord), resulting in a purple-headed baby. To differentiate between cyanosis and bruising, apply pressure to the area. A bruise remains blue, whereas an area of cyanosis blanches. In addition, petechiae often accompany the ecchymosis. Finally, the vigorous infant may turn nearly purple when performing a Valsalva maneuver in preparation for crying. Occasionally, the harlequin color change is observed, wherein there is a striking division into pale and red halves in an infant (typically positioned on the side), with a line of demarcation along the midline from head to foot. This finding is of no consequence outside of initial consternation in the nursery.

Although jaundice develops in many, if not most, newborns, this finding in the first 24 hours of life is abnormal and requires investigation. Jaundice is best assessed in natural light, by applying gentle pressure and assessing the color of the underlying skin and subcutaneous tissue. The cephalopedal progression of jaundice with increasing bilirubin levels has been observed for more than a century, and the distribution of jaundice can assist in estimating serum bilirubin levels. However, Jaundice is suspected within the first 24 hours of life, transcutaneous or serum measurement should be performed because clinical estimation is unreliable. Rarely, direct hyperbilirubinemia is seen in the first hours of life, providing a green cast to the infant's skin. More commonly, greenish discoloration of the skin is the result of in utero staining by meconium. Mottling may be observed in the well preterm or chilled newborn, or can be a sign of significant systemic illness. Pallor, in contrast, is never normal, and may result from poor cardiac output, subcutaneous edema, asphyxia, or anemia. Finally, a grayish hue may be associated with significant metabolic acidosis.

Position and Movement

Observation of an infant's position at rest (an indicator of underlying tone) and spontaneous movement provides a great deal of information about his or her neurologic status. Gestational age, illness, maternal medications, and sleep state influence tone and spontaneous movements and must be considered during the evaluation. As is evident in the New Ballard examination, muscle tone generally progresses in a caudocephalad direction with advancing gestational age. In the infant of 28 weeks' gestation, there is little tone in either upper or lower extremities, and the infant generally remains in the position in which the care provider places him or her. By 32 weeks, the infant should have developed tone of the legs, resulting in flexion at the hips and knees. One month later, strong flexor tone is present in the lower extremities, and the arms begin to display some flexion. The normal, supine term infant in the quiet awake state holds all four extremities in moderate flexion. The hands intermittently open, but most often, they are fisted with the thumb adducted and folded (cortical thumbs). Finally, when in the prone position, the term infant should be able to briefly lift his or her head above the plane of the body, and often elevates the pelvis above the flexed hips and knees.

The character of normal spontaneous movements varies with gestational age. Before 32 weeks, infants demonstrate random, slow writhing movements with interspersed myoclonic activity of the extremities. This writhing quality often persists through 44 weeks' gestational age. By 32 weeks, flexor movements of the lower extremities begin to predominate and typically occur in unison. A month later, these movements alternate, a pattern seen more frequently in the term infant. This progression of findings is entirely dependent on gestational, not postnatal, age.

Normal babies of all gestational ages have symmetrical tone and movements. Finding more than mild asymmetry in position and range of spontaneous movement may indicate the presence of local birth trauma (brachial plexus injury or fractures of the clavicle, humerus, or femur), or, rarely, a central nervous system insult, lesion, or anomaly. Asymmetry of position may also reflect in utero positioning, which should improve with time. The finding of extremes of flexion or extension requires a more in-depth neurologic evaluation.

Face and Crying

The examiner must not become frustrated if the baby begins to cry. There is much to be gained by observing the face of both the quiet and crying baby, and then by listening to the cry. Symmetry of the mouth and eyes is the normal finding. An asymmetric mouth (the abnormal side does not "droop" with crying) with an ipsilateral eye that does not close and a forehead that does not wrinkle usually indicates an injury to the peripheral facial nerve (cranial nerve VII). This situation must be differentiated from a congenital degeneration or maldevelopment of the cranial nerve VI and VII nuclei (Möbius sequence), which is typically manifested by bilateral palsy. A palsy confined to the lower portion of the face (central facial palsy) may indicate an intracranial hemorrhage or infarct. This latter finding should be distinguished from congenital absence of the depressor anguli oris muscle (asymmetrical crying facies), a generally benign condition, but one that may be associated with congenital cardiac anomalies.

Most reassuring to a pediatrician is the lusty cry of a newborn baby. An abnormal cry, on the other hand, often heralds underlying problems. A weak or whining cry may indicate illness, developing respiratory distress, depression from maternal narcotics, or central nervous system disturbance. Central nervous system problems may also result in persistent high-pitched crying. Hoarseness can be caused by laryngeal edema resulting from airway manipulation in the delivery room, hypocalcemia, or airway anomalies. Conditions resulting in either internal obstruction or external compression of the airway often cause stridor, which is exacerbated by crying; therefore, stridor in the newborn infant must always be considered a potentially serious finding.

Congenital Anomalies

Finally, a quick survey for dysmorphic features, whether malformations or deformations, must be undertaken. All nurseries should have immediate access to detailed descriptions and illustrations of common neonatal malformation and deformation syndromes, either in a reference book or electronically.

HEAD-TO-TOE REVIEW

Skin

In the extremely premature infant (23 to 28 weeks' gestation), the skin can be translucent with little subcutaneous fat and easily visualized superficial veins. Because the stratum corneum is thin, the skin of the extremely premature infant is easily injured by seemingly innocuous procedures or manipulation that results in denudation of the stratum corneum and a raw weeping surface. Insensible losses of water through this immature integument can be considerable, resulting in marked fluid and electrolyte imbalances if measures such as high humidity in the incubator are not taken to reduce these losses. The stratum corneum of even the extremely premature infant quickly matures so that by 1 to 2 weeks of age the insensible water losses are reduced to levels seen in the mature infant. By term, skin is relatively opaque with considerable subcutaneous fat.

By 35 to 36 weeks' gestational age, at birth the infant is covered with greasy vernix caseosa. The vernix thins by term and is usually absent in the postterm infant. The postmature infant has parchment-like skin with deep cracks on the trunk and extremities. Fingernails may be elongated, and peeling of the distal extremities is often evident in the postmature infant.

A variety of transient skin conditions are found in the newborn. Erythema toxicum neonatorum is a benign rash seen generally in term infants beginning on the second or third day of life. It is characterized by 1- to 2-mm white papules (that may become vesicular) on an erythematous base of varying diameter. The lesions appear and disappear on different parts of the body, are never found on the palms or soles, and are relatively infrequent on the face. They contain eosinophils. Milia, which are 1- to 2-mm whitish papules, are frequently found on the face of newborns. Miliaria is a result of eccrine sweat duct obstruction, and it manifests as glistening vesiculopapular lesions over the forehead and on the scalp and skinfolds. Miliaria appears during the first day and disappears within the first week after birth. Transient neonatal pustular melanosis, which is seen predominantly in African-American infants, is a benign generalized eruption of superficial pustules overlying hyperpigmented macules. The pustules, which can be found on any body surface, including the palms and soles, may be removed when vernix is being wiped off or during the first bath, so that the physician may see only macules surrounded by a fine, scaly collarette. White infants may

not exhibit the hyperpigmentation, making the diagnosis more difficult. The lesions contain an occasional polymorphonuclear leukocyte and cellular debris. Mongolian spots are macular areas of slate-blue hyperpigmentation seen predominantly over the buttocks or trunk; they are seen most commonly in African-American, Native American, and Asian infants.

A large number of skin, nail, and hair abnormalities may be found in the newborn. Some of these are important clues in the identification of an underlying syndrome or generalized disease process. Examination of the newborn's skin should be made to identify any congenital nevi, hemangiomas, areas of abnormal pigmentation, tags, pits, unusual scaling, blistering, abnormal laxity, or dysplasia. The color, distribution, and texture of the body and head hair are noted. Nail hypoplasia, dysplasia, aplasia, or hypertrophy should be further investigated. A large hemangioma on the face or neck can potentially cause airway obstruction. Port wine stains (capillary malformations), are usually on the face, but can be anywhere on the body. They are pink macular lesions which become purple with time. Satisfactory cosmetic treatment may be achieved with laser therapy, starting in infancy. When the port wine stain involves the distribution of the trigeminal nerve, it may be associated with a vascular malformation of the meninges and cerebral cortex and cause seizures and developmental delay (Sturge-Weber syndrome). If the port wine stain involves the distribution of the first and second divisions of the trigeminal nerve, congenital glaucoma may occur.

Head

The scalp and size and shape of the head are next considered. Small lacerations or puncture wounds may result from the placement of a fetal scalp electrode. Use of forceps can result in superficial marks, edema, or bruising of the skin on the sides of the skull and face, whereas the vacuum extractor can leave a circumferential area of edema, bruising, and occasionally blisters. Use of either forceps or vacuum extractor is associated with an increased likelihood of injuries to the extracranial structures. Caput succedaneum is a boggy area of edema located at the presenting part of the often molded head; it is present at birth, crosses suture lines, and disappears within a few days. Cephalohematomas, present in 1% to 2% of all newborns, are subperiosteal collections of blood that do not cross suture lines. They are often bilateral, and they usually increase in size after birth. Depending on the amount of blood present, cephalohematomas may be fluctuant or tense. Cephalohematomas rarely cause problems, but they may take weeks to months to resolve. The subgaleal hemorrhage is the least common of the extracranial injuries, but it is also the most dangerous. Newborns can lose tremendous amounts of blood from this injury, and they must be monitored carefully for shock once the diagnosis is suspected. Like the caput, this swelling can cross suture lines, but, as in the cephalohematoma, the lesion grows after birth, at times covering the entire scalp and extending into the neck.

Unusual configuration of the scalp hair, such as double or anterior whorls or prominent cowlicks, may be associated with abnormalities of the skull or brain, particularly if there are associated unusual facies. Especially unruly hair is associated with both trisomy 21 and Cornelia de Lange syndrome. A low-set posterior hairline may indicate a short or webbed neck as in Turner syndrome. Ectodermal defects, wherein a 2- to 5-cm diameter portion of the scalp appears to be totally absent, may be an isolated problem, but it is also a common finding in trisomy 13.

Accurate measurement of the head circumference is an important aspect of the physical examination. Abnormally large or small heads may indicate significant underlying neuropathology. The final configuration and even the circumference of the skull may be difficult to ascertain immediately after birth because of the molding that occurs during the birth process, and some time may be required before one can be sure of the presence or absence of an abnormality.

Babies delivered by cesarean section without a trial of labor typically have little to no molding, whereas vaginal delivery usually results in an enhanced occipitomental dimension with a relatively narrow biparietal diameter. Those infants who were in breech presentation characteristically have an accentuation of the occipitofrontal measurement with a resultant occipital shelf and apparent frontal bossing. The effects of intrauterine positioning and birth are transient, and should recede within days. If not, underlying abnormalities should be considered. A head with a short occipitofrontal dimension (brachycephaly) is characteristic

of trisomy 21. Palpation of the skull should reveal bones with mobile edges along the sagittal, coronal, and lambdoidal suture lines. Initial overlapping of the sutures is normal. A palpable ridge along suture lines should always be considered abnormal, possibly indicating premature closure of the sutures (craniosynostosis). The impact of craniosynostosis on the final configuration of the skull depends on the suture involved. The most commonly involved is the sagittal suture, with resultant dolichocephaly ("keel head"). Even though most instances of craniosynostosis are isolated events, some syndromes (Apert, Crouzon) are characterized, in part, by this finding. The normal width of the various sutures of the skull is quite variable. African-American infants tend to have wider metopic and sagittal sutures. Wide lambdoidal and squamosal sutures in term infants may be a sign of raised intracranial pressure. Craniotabes, soft pliable parietal bone along the sagittal suture, is a common finding in preterm infants as well as in the term infant whose head had been resting on the pelvic brim for the last few weeks of pregnancy. As its name implies, craniotabes can be seen in congenital syphilis, but this is clearly the exception.

Palpation of the anterior and posterior fontanelles should take place when the infant is relatively quiet. The normal anterior fontanelle has slight pulsations accompanying the heart beat and is flat to slightly sunken. There is a wide range of normal for fontanelle size, and racial differences have been noted. African-American babies have statistically larger fontanelles than do whites. Routine measurement of fontanelles is not particularly useful and not recommended. Finally, in infants with unexplained heart failure, auscultation of the head for bruits over the anterior fontanelle and temporal arteries may identify an arteriovenous malformation.

Eyes

Salmon patches on the eyelids, mid-forehead, and nape of the neck are common. Those on the face fade at 1 year, those on the nape are more persistent and may be present in adults but covered by hair. Dysmorphism of the eye and ocular region are the most frequently cited findings in malformation syndromes. Abnormal eyes may also indicate inborn errors of metabolism, central nervous system defects, or congenital infections. Although careful evaluation of the eyes is clearly important, it is potentially one of the most difficult aspects of the examination. Most infants will open their eyes during the course of the examination. The eyes of a crying baby cannot be examined. Gently holding the infant upright and rocking backward and forward often prompts the baby to open his or her eyes.

The size, orientation, and position of the eyes should be noted. The diameter of the cornea and eye at term is approximately 10 mm and 17 mm, respectively. Microphthalmia is seen in a number of malformation syndromes, including trisomy 13, whereas an enlarged cornea should suggest congenital glaucoma. The eye that is positioned with the palpebral fissures slanting upward from the inner canthus is typically seen in trisomy 21, whereas Treacher Collins, Apert, and DiGeorge syndromes are characterized in part by downward slanting palpebral fissures. A large number of syndromes are associated with hypertelorism (a wide interpupillary distance) (e.g., Apert syndrome and trisomy 13), whereas hypotelorism is less commonly seen (holoprosencephaly and, again, trisomy 13).

Newborns often demonstrate random and, at times, disconjugate movements of the eyes. Persistent strabismus should be further evaluated. Subconjunctival hemorrhage is, at times, frightening in appearance, but it resolves spontaneously. The iris is blue in nearly all newborns, although some more heavily pigmented infants have dark irises at birth. Reaction of the pupil to light begins to appear by 30 weeks' gestation, but reaction may not be consistently seen for another 2 to 5 weeks. Detailed visualization of the retina is unnecessary in most infants. The goal of routine funduscopic examinations is to ensure the absence of intraocular pathology and opacities of the cornea and lens by establishing the presence of a normal light reflex (red reflex). Whereas the normal light reflex is red in white infants, more darkly pigmented infants have a pearly gray reflex. The finding of a white pupillary reflex (leukocoria) can suggest the presence of a variety of ocular pathologies (cataracts, trauma, persistent hyperplastic primary vitreous, tumor, retinopathy of prematurity) and requires urgent evaluation by an ophthalmologist.

Ears

Recognition of the wide variation of normal for the external ear configuration develops with experience. Many syndromes include malformed auricles as part of their spectrum, but the findings are not pathognomonic. The "low-set ears" so often mentioned in physical examinations is usually incorrect, the result of having the head positioned at the incorrect angle or an unusual skull shape. The patency of the external ear canals should be ensured. If a preauricular skin tag is present, consult a plastic surgeon. Check that the ear and hearing are normal. If there is an ear anomaly, some centers perform ultrasound evaluation of the kidneys because there is a slight increase in risk of renal abnormalities.

Nose

The nose may appear misshapen because of in utero deformation, and it usually self-corrects in a few days. Conversely, nasal asymmetry may be the result of septal displacement, which requires evaluation by an otolaryngologist. Several syndromes and teratogens have nasal manifestations including small (fetal alcohol syndrome) to large (trisomy 13) noses, and low (achondroplasia) to prominent (Seckel syndrome) nasal bridges. Nasal obstruction may be caused by mucus or it may represent true anatomic obstruction caused by tumors, encephalocele, or choanal atresia. Choanal atresia may be unilateral or bilateral, and may require the use of an oral airway or endotracheal intubation to maintain a patent airway. Choanal atresia is often part of the CHARGE association (*c*oloboma, *h*eart disease, *a*tresia choanae, *r*estricted growth and development and/or CNS anomalies, *g*enital anomalies and/or hypogonadism, and *e*ar anomalies and/or deafness).

Mouth

Micrognathia is a component of many malformation syndromes, with the Pierre-Robin sequence perhaps being the most obvious example. The interior of the mouth should be evaluated with a light and tongue blade (if necessary) as well as a gloved finger. The frenulum labialis superior is a band of tissue that connects the central portion of the upper lip to the alveolar ridge of the maxilla. It may be prominent and be associated with a notch in the maxillary ridge where it originates. Likewise, the frenulum linguae is a band of tissue that connects the floor of the mouth to the tongue. This may extend to the tip of the tongue (tongue-tie) but does not usually interfere with suckling or later speech. Natal (present at birth) and neonatal (present in the first month of life) teeth are usually found in the mandibular central incisor region, and are bilateral approximately half of the time. They are removed if loose, to avoid the risk of aspiration. White epithelial cysts on the palate known as Epstein pearls are present in most babies, and similar lesions may be seen along the gums. Clefts of the palate may be obvious to the eye, or only found by palpation (submucous cleft). This latter abnormality may be accompanied by a bifid uvula.

Face

One should be careful during the examination not to focus too much on specific problems, but to consider the overall picture. Take a moment, step back, and just observe the baby to ensure that, as the saying goes, you don't "miss the forest for the tress." Is there anything that just looks unusual?

Neck, Lymph Nodes, and Clavicles

The neck of the newborn is relatively short; coincidentally, it has a relatively short list of possible abnormal findings. Redundant skin along the posterolateral line (webbing) is seen in approximately one half of girls with Turner syndrome (XO), whereas the neck of the infant with trisomy 21 is notable for excess skin concentrated at the base of the neck posteriorly. A variety of branchial cleft remnants are manifested by pits, tags, and cysts. The most common neck mass is a lymphangioma (cystic hygroma), which is a multiloculated cyst composed of dilated lymphatics. Occasionally containing a hemangiomatous component, these are usually posterior to the sternocleidomastoid muscle with potential extension into the scapulae and thoracic and axillary compartments. The anterior neck should be evaluated for a midline trachea, thyromegaly, and thyroglossal duct cysts. Lymph nodes are sometimes palpable in the inguinal or cervical areas in healthy newborns; congenital infections can also result in lymphadenopathy. Supraclavicular nodes are never normal. The clavicles are palpated for their presence or absence (cleidocranial dysostosis) and the presence of fractures, which typically manifest as asymmetrical arm movements, tenderness, and crepitus.

Respiratory System and Chest

As stated previously, the most important part of the respiratory system examination is performed while simply watching the infant breathe. If the infant has respiratory distress, the stethoscope is used to assess the quantity, quality, and equality of breath sounds. Alveolar pathology (atelectasis, pneumonia) may be suggested by the presence of inspiratory crackles, whereas crepitant sounds heard both in inspiration and expiration are usually the result of airway secretions.

The chest is evaluated for size, symmetry, bony structure, musculature, and position of the nipples. The thorax may be malformed or small in a variety of neuromuscular disorders, osteochondrodysplasias, and processes associated with pulmonary hypoplasia. The presence of pectus excavatum (funnel chest) and carinatum (pigeon breast) can be of considerable concern to the family, and both can be associated with Marfan, Noonan, and other syndromes. Palpable pectoralis major muscle tissue in the axillae assures the presence of the muscle, the absence of which is suggestive of Poland syndrome. Supernumerary nipples, found inferomedial to the true breasts, are seen in approximately 1% of the general population, with a higher incidence in African Americans. Breast hypertrophy, at times asymmetrical, can be seen in both male and female infants in response to maternal hormones, and may be accompanied by the secretion of "witch's milk," a thin milky fluid, for a few days to weeks. Erythema and tenderness of the breasts do not accompany this normal variant.

Cardiac System

The goal of the cardiac examination generally falls into one of two categories: (1) to ensure the absence of heart disease during the routine examination and (2) to determine whether the heart is the source of the problem in the sick neonate.

The normal resting heart rate of the term newborn is between 100 and 160 beats per minute, although occasional brief fluctuations well above and below these values are expected. The premature infant's baseline heart rate tends to be slightly higher. Persistent bradycardia or tachycardia can be an indication of primary cardiac or, more commonly, other systemic processes.

Examination of the cardiovascular system begins with an assessment of general appearance, color, perfusion, and respiratory status. The presence of congenital anomalies increases the likelihood of associated congenital heart defects. Central cyanosis accompanied by a comfortable respiratory effort is suggestive of a structural heart defect with diminished pulmonary blood flow (pulmonary atresia). Because of the relative hypertrophy of the right ventricle, the point of maximal impulse (PMI) of the newborn is found just to the left of the lower sternum. In the term newborn, the precordial impulse is visible during the first few hours of life, but generally disappears by 6 hours of age. Because of the lack of subcutaneous tissue in the preterm and growth-restricted newborn, the point of maximal impulse may be visible for a somewhat longer time. Abnormal persistence of the visible or easily palpated point of maximal impulse is seen in transposition of the great vessels and structural defects characterized by right-sided volume overload. Palpation of the femoral pulses should be carried out. The femoral pulses are diminished in coarctation of the aorta, but may initially be palpable if blood flow is maintained by right-to-left shunting across the ductus arteriosus.

Auscultation should begin with a warmed stethoscope. Identifying abnormal heart sounds is made difficult by the fast heart rate in the neonatal period. The first heart sound is typically single and is accentuated at birth and in conditions in which there is increased flow across an atrioventricular valve. The second heart sound is best heard at the upper left sternal border. In most infants, the second heart sound (S_2) is split, although this can be difficult to appreciate because of the high heart rate. The presence of a normally split S_2 is an important physical finding. The absence of a split S_2 can indicate the presence of a single ventricular valve (aortic atresia, pulmonary atresia, and truncus arteriosus) or transposition of the great vessels (as a result of the orientation of the valves). Widely split S_2 is seldom indicative of increased pulmonary blood flow (atrial septal defect) in neonates, but it can be heard in total anomalous venous return and lesions characterized by an abnormal pulmonary valve. A narrowly split, accentuated S_2 is characteristic of persistent pulmonary hypertension of the newborn.

The absence of a heart murmur does not eliminate the possibility of important structural heart defects, and classic murmurs ascribed to specific lesions in older children may not be present in the neonate. Even though some infants may have a heart murmur noted during their first week of life, most of these murmurs are related to ongoing circulatory adaptation to an extrauterine environment and they are transient and inconsequential. Innocent murmurs are soft, systolic, at the left sternal edge or pulmonary area. The infant is well and examination is otherwise normal. The murmur of pulmonary artery branch stenosis is best heard in the pulmonary area, is a systolic flow murmur best heard in the pulmonary area, and radiates to the axilla and back. It resolves in a few weeks. Although uncommon, the most concerning murmurs are those from congenital heart disease, especially ductal-dependent lesions that may result in circulatory failure or cyanosis when the ductus arteriosus closes. Harsh grade 2 or 3 murmurs in the first hours of life (ventricular outflow tract obstruction), pansystolic (atrioventricular valve insufficiency), and to-and-fro, systolic-diastolic (absent pulmonary valve, valvular regurgitation) murmurs require more extensive evaluation with echocardiography. Finally, the disappearance of a previously noted murmur in a baby who is clinically deteriorating should make one suspect the closure of the ductus arteriosus with a ductal-dependent lesion (coarctation of the aorta, tricuspid atresia, or pulmonary atresia).

If a murmur is heard, the cardiac system is carefully evaluated. The definitive diagnosis is by echocardiography. A chest x-ray and ECG are of limited value in establishing a diagnosis. Pulse oximetry will establish if the arterial oxygen saturation is normal (>95%). If there are features of an innocent flow murmur, reassess the infant within a few days to check that the murmur has disappeared. The parents need to be informed that they should seek medical assistance should the infant develop symptoms suggestive of heart failure (slow feeding, breathlessness, and sweating). If the murmur persists or has pathologic features, or if the infant becomes unwell, referral to a pediatric cardiologist and echocardiography are indicated.

Blood pressure is not measured routinely but it is performed in infants who are unwell or preterm and require admission to a neonatal unit. If the femoral pulses are diminished and coarctation of the aorta is suspected, blood pressure is measured in the arms and legs. Blood pressure in the legs is normally the same or slightly higher than that found in the arms, but is markedly reduced if coarctation of the aorta is present. Normal systemic blood pressure varies with postnatal and gestational age.

Abdomen

Patience and warm hands are the keys to a successful abdominal examination. In most infants, inspection reveals a rounded abdomen. A flat or scaphoid abdomen may be observed in the presence of a diaphragmatic hernia. A full upper abdomen in the presence of a flattened lower abdomen suggests a proximal bowel obstruction. Distention is usually apparent at birth when there is massive ascites, meconium ileus and peritonitis, or intrauterine midgut volvulus. Clearly visible intestinal loops are not normal in the term infant, but the thin abdominal wall of the extremely premature baby may result in easily observed loops and peristalsis. Abdominal wall defects (omphaloceles and gastroschisis) are usually readily apparent; these require urgent surgical intervention. Bowel sounds are nearly always heard if auscultation is performed, and their absence is a concerning finding.

Palpation of the abdomen is facilitated by having the infant's legs in a flexed position. Palpation should begin in the lower abdomen, with the hand allowed to rest there until the infant relaxes. The kidneys are normally palpable bilaterally. Enlargement of the kidneys caused by hydronephrosis or cystic kidney disease is the most common abdominal mass found in the newborn. The liver is usually palpable 1 to 3 cm below the right costal margin, and the left lobe extends across the midline. The liver should be smooth and its edge should be soft and thin. It may be enlarged from cardiac failure, congenital infections, extramedullary hematopoiesis, tumors, and a variety of inborn errors of metabolism. The spleen is less frequently palpable than the liver and should be considered abnormally large if palpable more than 1 cm below the left costal margin.

The umbilical cord normally has two umbilical arteries and one umbilical vein. A "two-vessel cord" (single umbilical artery) is a soft marker for chromosomal abnormalities; in an otherwise normal newborn there is an increased risk of renal malformation.[63] Infants with limited fetal activity as a result of congenital neuromuscular disorders, including Down syndrome, often have relatively short umbilical cords, which the obstetrician may note at the delivery.

The Genitalia

The appearance of the genitalia is certainly one of the first, if not *the* first, areas of interest to the parents. If there is a disorder of sexual differentiation, assignment of the infant's gender should never be made until a detailed assessment has been performed.

Male

The penile size, position of the meatus, appearance of the scrotum, and position of the testes must all be assessed. A penis of the term infant stretched along its length until resistance is met should be at least 2.5 cm long. It is not necessary, and potentially painful and damaging, to retract the foreskin over the glans penis to determine the placement of the meatus. A meatal opening on the ventral surface of the penis (hypospadias) is relatively common and is readily apparent on inspection. Far less common is an epispadias, in which the meatus is present on the dorsal surface of the penis. This is usually not an isolated defect, more often being associated with exstrophy of the bladder. At the tip of the foreskin may be found a 1-mm diameter pearly white sebaceous cyst. This is of no concern. The testes should be palpable in the scrotum of the term infant. In approximately 2% to 4% of term infants, either one or both testes have not descended, but in three fourths of these infants the testes have descended at 3 months of age. Premature infants are far more likely to have an undescended testis at birth than the term infant. A hydrocele can usually be distinguished from a hernia by a combination of palpation and transillumination.

Female

The appearance of the female genitalia undergoes a maturational metamorphosis. The premature infant has a prominent clitoris and labia minora, whereas in the term infant, the labia majora completely covers these structures. The prominence of the clitoris in the premature infant is a result of this structure being fully developed by 27 weeks' gestation combined with a lack of fat in the labia majora. In the term female, outpouching of the vaginal mucosa (vaginal skin tags) is often seen at the posterior fourchette. Vaginal skin tags are inconsequential and regress within a few weeks. A mucous vaginal discharge, which is at times bloody, is often seen and may be of concern to parents. The passage of large amounts of blood, or clots, is not normal. The hymen has some opening in the majority of females. A completely imperforate hymen may result in the development of hydrometrocolpos. This is usually heralded by the bulging hymen which is particularly prominent with crying. Virilization of the female infant consists of varying degrees of clitoral hypertrophy and labioscrotal fusion. A mass in the labia or groin may be a hernia, but consideration must be given to the possibility of an ectopic gonad, which may be either an ovary or a testis.

Anus

The presence, patency, and location of the anus should be noted. An absent (imperforate) anus will require surgery, but should also bring to mind the possibility of other associated anomalies, in particular, esophageal atresia (VATER association—vertebral defects, anal defects, tracheoesophageal atresia, renal defects or VACTERL association—vertebral defects, anal defects, cardiac defects, tracheoesophageal atresia, renal defects, limbs defects).

Hips

Examination of the hips of the neonate is performed on all infants to detect developmental dysplasia of the hip (DDH). This disorder is more common in females, if there is a family history, infants with underlying neurologic abnormalities, and those presenting in the breech position. The infant must be relaxed because crying or kicking results in tightening of the muscles around the hip. There may be asymmetry of skinfolds around the hip and shortening of the affected leg. It should be possible to abduct both hips; full abduction may not be possible if the hip is dislocated. The Barlow maneuver is performed to check if the hip is dislocatable posteriorly by adducting a flexed hip with gentle posterior force to push the femoral head posteriorly out of the acetabulum. The Ortolani maneuver checks if a dislocated hip can be relocated into the acetabulum by abducting a flexed hip with gentle anterior leverage of the femur. If the examination is abnormal, a hip ultrasound and orthopedic consultation should be arranged. The American Academy of Pediatrics does not recommend routine ultrasound screening of all infants but only for female infants born in the breech position and optional hip ultrasound for boys born in the breech position

or girls with a positive family history.[64] Although screening leads to earlier identification, 60% to 80% of the hips identified as abnormal by physical examination and more than 90% of those identified by ultrasound resolve spontaneously. Avascular necrosis of the hip is reported in up to 60% of treated children and no screening method has been shown to reduce the need for operation for the disorder.[65]

The Extremities

Careful inspection of the extremities alone usually determines whether the extremities are well formed. Joint contractures, asymmetries, or dislocations should be noted. Erb palsy is manifested by an arm that is extended alongside the body with internal rotation and demonstrates limited movement. The humerus and femur are the second and third most commonly fractured bones at delivery. Abnormalities of the digits (shortening, tapering, syndactyly, polydactyly), single palmar creases, and nail hypoplasia can be important clues to dysmorphic syndromes. Variations caused by intrauterine positioning are seen and need to be differentiated from true equinovarus deformities. Positional deformities of the foot can usually be distinguished by the presence of a normal range of motion and ability to establish a normal position and appearance of the foot with gentle pressure.

The Back

The back is examined for the presence of abnormal curvatures and evidence of an abnormality overlying the spine. The presence of a tuft of hair, a subcutaneous lipoma, sinus, hemangioma, dimples separate from the gluteal crease, aplasia cutis, or skin tag should raise suspicion regarding the possibility of an underlying occult dysraphic state. If these abnormalities are found, an ultrasound examination of the involved area of the spine should be undertaken. Finding of a structural aberration requires intervention in the neonatal period or at least in very early infancy to prevent the development of neurologic deficits.

CONCLUDING THE PHYSICAL EXAMINATION

After completion of the examination, the infant's parents can usually be reassured that the examination was normal, and can be congratulated on their baby's birth. Any abnormalities or potential problems should be explained to them. Parents should be provided with the opportunity to inquire about any concerns they have about their baby. It also provides an opportunity to check on feeding and preventive care including immunization, universal neonatal biochemical screening, hearing screening, and advice about prevention of sudden infant death syndrome (SIDS). It also provides the opportunity to check that appropriate follow-up arrangements are in place.

CASE 1

Baby Boy K is born at 40 weeks' gestation with a birth weight of 2200 g, a length of 46 cm, and a head circumference of 32 cm. The physical examination is remarkable for short palpebral fissures, a small jaw, a smooth filtrum, and thin upper lip.

What is this combination of features most consistent with?

A. Trisomy 21
B. Fetal alcohol syndrome
C. Congenital cytomegalovirus infection
D. Beckwith-Wiedemann syndrome

This constellation of findings is most suggestive of (B), fetal alcohol syndrome (FAS). All but (D) can be associated with growth restriction, often "symmetrical." Beckwith-Wiedemann syndrome is typically associated with macrosomia. Other physical findings suggestive of FAS include eyelid ptosis, short nose, small distal phalanges, and small fifth fingernails. Long-term prognosis for these children is somewhat guarded, with the majority being developmentally delayed, often to a severe degree.

CASE 2

You are called to attend the delivery of Baby Boy G at uncertain gestation, who is to be delivered by emergency cesarean section after fetal distress is manifested by late fetal heart rate decelerations with uterine contractions. The fetal membranes are intact. The estimated fetal weight (determined by ultrasound during labor) is 2 kg. The mother is a 15-year-old nulliparous female who had a prenatal course notable for smoking, a weight gain of 12 pounds, and infrequent visits to the clinic. She was admitted in active labor and was found to have a blood pressure of 160/110 and proteinuria. She was subsequently given magnesium sulfate for preeclampsia for several hours before the delivery.

What types of problems can you anticipate that you will need to address in the delivery room, and what measures will you take to be prepared?

This is a complicated, but not uncommon, scenario. With a lack of regular obstetrical care, the gestational age of the baby is uncertain. The baby may be preterm or term. In either case, the infant care center must be warm, and towels for drying the baby must be available. If the infant is at term, he appears to be growth restricted and has shown evidence of not tolerating the stress of labor. The necessary supplies for airway management and suctioning must be present in the area. If the infant is preterm, meconium aspiration is less likely, but respiratory distress is still a distinct possibility.

At delivery, there was no meconium, and the baby needed only towel drying, clearing of the airway, and a brief period of supplemental oxygen for resuscitation. In the delivery room, the following are noted: bilaterally descended testes, stiff ear cartilage, scant vernix caseosa, well-developed areolae but poor breast tissue development, and decreased muscle tone. The baby's weight is 1800 g, length is 48 cm, and head circumference is 32 cm. There are no obvious anomalies on the initial examination, and the examination of the abdomen, heart, and lungs is normal.

What is your assessment of his gestational age and his classification?

This baby is likely a term, SGA infant. The findings of the descended testes, stiff ear cartilage, lack of vernix, and well-developed areolae support this contention. The decreased muscle tone may be related to exposure to magnesium. A complete Ballard examination needs to be carried out during the first 24 hours to confirm the gestational age.

What problems will you anticipate for this infant in the next 24 to 48 hours?

As an apparently term SGA infant, he is at risk for thermoregulation difficulties, hypoglycemia, polycythemia, and possibly hypocalcemia.

Why is this baby so small?

Several features place this baby at risk for poor growth: teenage mother, poor maternal weight gain during pregnancy, smoking, and apparent pregnancy-associated hypertension. How far to pursue further evaluation for other etiologies (chromosomal abnormalities, congenital infections) will vary among clinicians, but in the absence of other clinical abnormalities, the yield from further investigations is very low.

REFERENCES

The reference list for this chapter can be found online at www.expertconsult.com.

The Physical Environment  6

Avroy A. Fanaroff and Marshall H. Klaus

The foetus was no larger than the palm of his hand, but the father...put his son in an oven, suitably arranged...making him take on the necessary increase of growth, by the uniformity of the external heat, measured accurately in the degrees of the thermometer.

Laurence Sterne

An understanding of the thermal requirements of the high-risk infant was slow to develop. Pierre Budin,[1] historically the first neonatologist, had perhaps the earliest insight into the clinical importance of the thermal environment. In 1907 in his book, *The Nursling*, he emphasized the need for temperature control after noting a markedly increased survival rate when the infant's rectal temperature was maintained (Table 6-1). He recommended an air temperature of 30° C (86° F) for the small (1 kg), fully clothed infant. Sadly, his observations were neither fully understood nor appreciated in the first 50 years of the 20th century. In addition, during this period, the clinical value of two variables (temperature and humidity) was confused.

The modern era of neonatology was heralded by Silverman et al. in three sequential analyses,[2-4] whereby they resolved the importance and relationships between the incubator temperature and relative humidity. In the first study, the researchers compared high and low humidity in two groups of infants. Infants in the high humidity group had a lower mortality rate but higher rectal temperatures. In the second study, to end the confusion caused by two variables, they controlled the humidity and examined the effect of varying only environmental temperature. They noted a striking difference in survival rates. With only a 4° F increase in incubator temperature (from 85° F to 89° F), they observed a 15% increase in survival rate at the higher temperature (68.1% versus 83.5%), with the biggest difference affecting the smallest infants. In a further study, controlling environmental temperatures but varying humidity caused no difference in survival.

Hill, in part, clarified the profound effects of environmental temperature on survival observed by Silverman et al.[4-6] working with kittens and guinea pigs; she found that in 20% oxygen, oxygen consumption and rectal temperatures varied with the environmental temperature (Fig. 6-1). She noted a set of thermal conditions at which heat production (measured as oxygen consumption) is minimal, yet core temperature is within the normal range (neutral thermal environment). When the animals were cooled while breathing room air, their oxygen consumption markedly increased and body temperature was maintained. However, when they were given 12% oxygen and cooled, oxygen consumption did not increase, and the animals' body temperatures decreased. This, as well as the work of Bruck and others,[7] has emphasized that the human infant is a homeotherm and not a poikilotherm, as is a turtle. If a nonhypoxic infant is cooled, the infant maintains body temperature by increasing the consumption of calories and oxygen to produce additional heat. Homeotherms possess mechanisms that enable them to maintain body temperature at a constant level, more or less accurately, despite changes in the environmental temperature. In contrast, the body temperature of a turtle decreases if it is placed in a cool environment.

The increased survival rate in the warmer environment observed by Budin and Silverman presumably resulted from the decreased oxygen consumption and carbon dioxide production as environmental conditions approximated the neutral thermal environment. An

Table 6-1.	Infants' Temperatures and Survival Rate	
Temperature	**Survival Rate**	
32.5° C to 33.5° C	10%	
36.0° C to 37.0° C	77%	

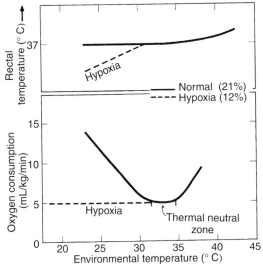

Figure 6-1. Effect of environmental temperature on oxygen consumption, breathing air, or a hypoxic mixture.

immature infant with a minimal ability to transfer oxygen and excrete carbon dioxide across his or her lungs has the least chance of becoming hypoxic or developing a respiratory acidosis—increased $Paco_2$—if maintained in an environment that minimizes oxygen consumption or metabolic rate.

Maintaining the neutral thermal environment became the first and foremost foundation of the modern era of neonatal intensive care. Recently, controlled cooling has been introduced to reduce the metabolic requirements of the brain and so to reduce injury in full-term infants with moderate to severe hypoxic-ischemic encephalopathy.

This chapter will summarize key elements of thermal regulation in addition to other important factors in the physical environment as they relate to the sick newborn.

PHYSIOLOGIC CONSIDERATIONS

HEAT PRODUCTION

The heat production within the body is a byproduct of metabolic processes and must equal the heat that flows from the surface of

the infant's body and the warm air from the lungs over a given period if the mean body temperature is to remain constant. A characteristic of the homeothermic infant is the ability to produce extra heat in a cool environment. In the adult, additional heat production can come from (1) voluntary muscle activity, (2) involuntary tonic or rhythmic muscle activity (at high intensities, characterized by a visible tremor known as "shivering"), and (3) nonshivering thermogenesis. The latter is a cold-induced increase in oxygen consumption and heat production, which is not blocked by curare, a drug that prevents muscle movements and shivering. In the adult, shivering is quantitatively the most significant involuntary mechanism of regulating heat production, whereas in the infant, nonshivering thermogenesis is probably most important. From animal and human studies, it can be inferred that, in the human infant, the thermogenic effector organ—brown fat—contributes the largest percentage of nonshivering thermogenesis.

BROWN FAT

More abundant in the newborn than in the adult, brown fat accounts for about 2% to 6% of total body weight in the human infant. Sheets of brown fat may be found at the nape of the neck, between the scapulae, in the mediastinum, and surrounding the kidneys and adrenals.[8] Brown fat differs from the more abundant white fat. The cells are rich in mitochondria and contain numerous fat vacuoles (as compared with the single vacuoles in white fat). Brown fat contains a dense capillary network and is richly innervated with sympathetic nerve endings on each fat cell. The special property of brown fat is the uncoupling protein, which results in the oxidation of food to heat rather than energy-rich phosphate bonds. Its metabolism is stimulated by norepinephrine released through sympathetic innervation, resulting in triglyceride hydrolysis to free fatty acids (FFAs) and glycerol.

The initiation of nonshivering thermogenesis at birth depends on cutaneous cooling, separation from the placenta, and the euthyroid state. The acute surge in thyroid hormones at birth appears to be of limited importance with regard to the immediate control of thermogenesis, whereas the intracellular conversion of T_4 to T_3 and the effects of norepinephrine appear to be of greater significance.[9] Stimulation of the sympathetic nervous system by cold exposure markedly increases local norepinephrine turnover within brown adipose tissue, which may not be reflected by an increase in circulating catecholamines.[10] This results in a marked increase in oxygen consumption without any appreciable increase in physical activity.

Interesting observations made in sheep noted that cooling of the fetus results in very small increases in FFAs and a significant decrease in body temperature. Ventilation of the fetus with increasing P_{O_2} resulted in a slight increase in FFAs, whereas clamping the cord resulted in a sharp increase in FFAs and glycerol. These and other observations suggest that before birth there is an inhibitor to thermogenesis, probably produced by the placenta.[11] Possible candidates for the inhibitor are adenosine or prostaglandin E_2. The nonshivering thermogenesis occurring in the brown fat during cooling can be turned off with hypoxia (see Fig. 6-1), and the sensory receptors for this are most probably the carotid body afferents.

EDITORIAL COMMENT: There also appears to be a relationship between feeding and brown adipose tissue (BAT) activity in rats. Initiation of feeding is mediated by a transient dip in blood glucose concentration caused by stimulated glucose utilization in BAT. Feeding continues while BAT and core temperature continue to rise. Termination is induced by the high level of core temperature brought about by the episode of stimulated BAT thermogenesis. The time between initiation and termination determines the size of the meal and depends on the balance between BAT thermogenesis and heat loss, and thus on ambient temperature. The underlying cause of the episodic stimulation of sympathetic nervous system activity is a decline in core temperature to a level recognized by the hypothalamus as needing a burst of increased heat production. Thus, BAT thermogenesis is important in control of meal size, relating it to thermoregulatory needs. The phenomenon is termed *thermoregulatory feeding*, to distinguish it from feeding initiated by other stimuli.[12]

The physiologic control mechanisms of the infant may alter the internal gradient (i.e., vasomotor) to change skin blood flow. The external gradient is of a purely physical nature. The large surface-to-volume ratio of the infant (especially those weighing less than 2 kg) in relation to the adult and the thin layer of subcutaneous fat increase the heat transfer in the internal gradient.

The heat transfers from the surface of the body to the environment of water. This heat transfer is complex, and the contribution of each component involves four means of loss: (1) by radiation; (2) by conduction; (3) by convection; and (4) by evaporation—influenced by the temperature of the surroundings (air and walls), air speed, and water vapor pressure, Of special clinical importance to the pediatrician is the considerable increase in radiant heat loss from the infant's skin to the cold walls of incubators.

Radiant heat loss is related to the temperature of the surrounding surfaces, not air temperature. When incubators are in cool surroundings (e.g., during transfer) the inner surface temperature of the single-walled incubator declines well below that of the air temperature in the incubator. In caring for the infant, this problem is easily solved by wrapping him or her in a light covering (transparent if necessary). The surrounding radiant temperature is then close to body temperature and more under the influence of the incubator air temperature.[13]

EDITORIAL COMMENT: Because heat may be transferred by four different routes, the physical characteristics of the newer incubators and radiant heaters should be familiar to the caretakers. Devices used to maintain thermal stability in preterm infants have advanced over time so that the latest, most advanced, user friendly, and developmentally supportive microenvironment is possible for even the smallest, least mature infants. Engineers continue to design the most efficient and effective means of assisting clinicians to achieve the neutral thermal environment, and at the same time offering the clinicians clear observation and access to the infant. The current generation of combined incubator-radiant warmers improves their chances of survival (Giraffe ®, Omnibed ®, Versulet). Furthermore, as noted, meticulous attention to keeping babies warm in the delivery room has become the standard of care.

In very small infants (<1500 g), evaporative heat loss is increased in the first days of life, the result of very thin skin that is unusually permeable to water (Fig. 6-2). For further discussion, see Chapter 9.

The effect of environmental temperature on heat production (oxygen consumption) is considered in Figure 6-3. As the environmental temperature is decreased below point A (critical temperature), oxygen consumption increases. Body temperature, however, is maintained if heat production is adequate.

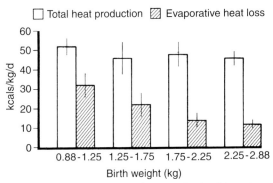

Figure 6-2. Relative role of evaporative heat loss at different birth weights.

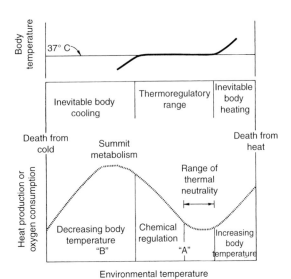

Figure 6-3. Effect of environmental temperature on oxygen consumption and body temperature. *(Adapted from Merenstein G, Blackmon L:* Care of the high-risk newborn, *San Francisco Children's Hospital, 1971.)*

If cooling is severe and body temperature drops below point B, with cold paralysis of the temperature regulation center, oxygen consumption also drops—two-to three-fold for every 10° decrease in body temperature. Homeothermy can also be abolished by sedative drugs and brain injury. Not all babies are homeotherms all the time.

Figure 6-3 shows that oxygen consumption is minimal in two areas: the neutral thermal environment and severe hypothermia. For many years, cardiac surgeons have taken advantage of the minimal metabolic rate with body cooling (temperatures below point B). More recently, cooling has been added to neuro-intensive care for term infants with hypoxic-ischemic encephalopathy. Under normal circumstances in the neonatal intensive care unit, caregivers strive to maintain the infant in a warm environment (the neutral thermal environment, or the so-called "zone of thermal comfort"). It is important clinically to note that the infant may not be in a neutral thermal environment and yet the rectal temperature may be in the normal range. As emphasized by Hey and Katz,[14] "body temperature alone fails to indicate whether a baby is subjected to thermal stress: it can only alert us to situations in which the thermal stress has been so severe that the baby's normal thermoregulatory mechanisms have been at least partially overpowered." Rectal temperature drops only when the baby's maximum effort to preserve and produce heat fails. The first mechanism to preserve heat is vasoconstriction, and this phenomenon can easily be detected by measuring skin temperature at a peripheral part of the body. A sensitive method to detect vasoconstriction is to measure both rectal and sole of the foot temperatures.[15]

EDITORIAL COMMENT: Claiming that the optimal thermal environment for sick preterm infants is unknown, Genzel-Boroviczény et al.[16] in a random manner, compared the effect of setting the incubator temperature to an abdominal wall temperature of 36.5° C (neutral temperature [NT]) or to a minimal temperature difference (<2° C) between abdominal wall and extremities (comfort temperature [CT]). They correctly speculated that this could affect the microcirculation perfusion, which they assessed with near-infrared photo-plethysmography (NIRP) at these two target temperatures between days 1 and 4 of life in preterm infants with normal or impaired (RED group) microcirculation as determined by a clinical score. They concluded that increasing the incubator temperature to CT changes thermoregulatory flow to the extremities in preterm infants with impaired microvascular perfusion and **might** improve tissue flow. So the issue of how to best set the neutral thermal zone without measuring energy expenditure remains unresolved. The old-fashioned increase in toe-tummy temperature differential is still a valuable indicator of ill health and potential sepsis.

Hypothermia and hyperthermia develop more rapidly in the neonate than in the adult. The infant has a lower capacity for heat storage because of the higher temperature of the body shell in relation to the environment and the larger surface-to-volume ratio. Thus, the thermoregulatory system of the homeothermic infant adjusts and balances heat production, skin blood flow, sweating, and respiration in such a way that the body temperature remains constant within a control range of environmental temperatures. The control range refers to the range of environmental temperatures at which body temperature can be kept constant by means of regulation. The control range of the infant is more limited than that of the adult because of less insulation. For the nude human adult, the lower limit of the control range is 0° C (32° F), whereas for the full-term infant it is 20° C to 23° C (68° F to 73.4° F).

The insufficient stability of body temperature in the small premature infant does not indicate an immaturity of temperature regulation because the system is intact. As pointed out by Bruck,[7] the insufficient stability "seems to be due to the discrepancy between efficiency of the effector systems and body size." The newborn infant has a well-developed temperature regulation but a narrower control range than the adult.

> **EDITORIAL COMMENT:** As emphasized by the late Albert Okken, the body surface-to-mass ratio of very immature and very low birth rate infants is about five times higher than in adults. The disadvantage of this relatively very large surface area of the premature infant observed at both ends of the thermal spectrum. There is rapid heat loss in a cool environment and rapid overheating in a heat-gaining environment.

IN UTERO

While the fetus is in utero, the heat produced is dissipated through the placenta to the mother. If complete placental separation occurs in utero, the temperature of the fetus increases rapidly. Normally the temperature of the fetus is 0.6° C above the mother's temperature. When the mother's temperature increases secondary to infection or move commonly with the use of an epidural analgesia for labor, the fetal temperature increases to about 0.6° C higher than the mother's. Approximately 30% to 40% of women receiving an epidural anesthetic in early labor are noted to have a fever in late labor, the cause of which is unknown.[17] The thermoregulatory system works well for the fetus except during periods when the mother has an increasing body temperature.

Schouten et al. studied the temperatures of women during labor and observed that the mean temperature increased from 37.1° C at the beginning of labor to 37.4° C after 22 hours.[18] Circadian temperature patterns were not observed during labor. Epidural

analgesia is associated with maternal fever due to inability of the mother to dissipate heat. Nulliparity and dysfunctional labor are also significant cofactors in the fever attributed to epidural analgesia. Lieberman noted intrapartum fever higher than 100.4° F in 14.5% of women receiving an epidural,[19] but in only 1.0% of women not receiving an epidural (adjusted odds ratio [OR] = 14.5, 95% CI = 6.3, 33.2). Neonates whose mothers received epidurals were more often evaluated for sepsis and treated with antibiotics. Although 63% of women received epidurals, 96.2% of intrapartum fevers, 85.6% of neonatal sepsis evaluations, and 87.5% of neonatal antibiotic treatment occurred in the epidural group. Compared with continuous infusion, intermittent epidural injections appear to protect against intrapartum fever in the first 4 hours of labor analgesia. This may be due to intermittent partial recovery of heat loss mechanisms between injections.[20]

> **EDITORIAL COMMENT:** As noted above, the association between the use of epidural analgesia for pain relief in labor and intrapartum maternal fever has been established in both observational and randomized trials. There has been a suggestion, too, of an increase in adverse neonatal outcomes with intrapartum maternal fever. Greenwell et al.* confirm that maternal temperature above 100.4° F developed during labor in 19.2% (535/2784) of women receiving epidural compared with 2.4% (10/425) not receiving epidural. Furthermore, maternal temperature above 99.5° F was associated with adverse neonatal outcomes. The rate of adverse outcomes (hypotonia, assisted ventilation, 1-and 5-min Apgar scores below 7, and early-onset seizures) increased two- to six-fold with maternal temperature above 101° F. Without temperature elevation, epidural use was not associated with adverse neonatal outcomes.
>
> ─────────────────────────────
> *Greenwell E et al: Intrapartum temperature elevation, epidural use, and adverse outcomes in term infants, Pediatrics 129:e447, 2012.

AFTER BIRTH

Hypothermia is a major cause of morbidity and mortality in infants; therefore, maintaining normal body temperatures in the delivery room is crucial. An understanding of how infants produce heat and what can be done to maintain normal body temperatures in full-term and preterm infants is essential for the preservation of thermal stability in this population.

At birth, the infant's core temperature decreases rapidly, owing mainly to evaporation from his or her moist body. The infant's small amount of subcutaneous tissue and large surface area-to-mass ratio compared with the adult, together with the cold air and walls of the delivery room, also result in large radiant and convective heat losses. Oxygen should always be warmed. Thus, under the usual delivery room conditions, deep body temperature of human newborns can decrease 2° C to 3° C unless special precautions are taken.

Although moderate to severe cooling may result in metabolic acidosis, a lower arterial oxygen level, and hypoglycemia in the newborn infant, very slight cooling of the infant may be beneficial in his or her adaptation to extrauterine life. Cooling of the skin receptors may play a significant role in initiating respiration and stimulating thyroid function. The vasoconstriction and peripheral resistance observed with mild cooling also alters systemic vascular resistance, thereby reducing the right-to-left shunting of blood through the ductus arteriosus. With severe cooling, a vicious circle can result in severe hypoxia and even death (Fig. 6-4). The neonatologist chooses to keep the infant warm following delivery to prevent metabolic acidosis and possibly dangerous reflex responses to cooling.

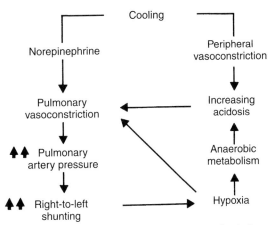

Figure 6-4. The vicious circle resulting from cooling in the neonate.

Keeping vulnerable preterm infants warm is problematic even when recommended routine thermal care guidelines are followed in the delivery suite. McCall et al. performed a Cochrane review to assess efficacy and safety of interventions designed for prevention of hypothermia in preterm and/or low-birth-weight infants applied within 10 minutes after birth in the delivery suite compared with routine thermal care.[23] Barriers to heat loss such as plastic wraps or bags were effective in reducing heat losses in infants less than 28 weeks' gestation but not in infants 28 to 31 weeks' gestation. Plastic caps were effective in reducing heat losses in infants less than 29 weeks' gestation. There was insufficient evidence to suggest that either plastic wraps or plastic caps reduce the risk of death during the hospital stay. There was no evidence of significant differences in other clinical outcomes for either the plastic wrap/bag or the plastic cap comparisons. Stockinet caps were not effective in reducing heat losses.

External heat sources, including transwarmer mattresses and SSC, were shown to be effective in reducing the risk of hypothermia when compared to conventional incubator care. The authors concluded that plastic wraps or bags, plastic caps, skin-to-skin care (SSC), and transwarmer mattresses all keep preterm infants warmer, leading to higher temperatures on admission to neonatal units and less hypothermia. However, the small numbers of infants and studies and the absence of long-term follow-up mean that firm recommendations for clinical practice cannot be given.

Simon et al. compared thermal mattresses (sodium acetate) with a plastic wrap for extremely low gestational age newborns (ELGANs) between 24 and 28 weeks' gestation with a birth weight less than 1250 grams.[24] Although the mattress was superior to the plastic wrap and both improved the thermal status of ELGANs, they concluded that all current interventions fall short of fully protecting all these vulnerable infants from thermal stress.

Trevisanuto et al. conducted a randomized trial and concluded that for very preterm infants,[25] polyethylene caps are comparable with polyethylene occlusive skin wrapping to prevent heat loss after delivery. Both these methods are more effective than conventional treatment; however, many babies are still admitted with low temperatures.

TEMPERATURE CONTROL IN THE VERY LOW-BIRTH-WEIGHT INFANT

Even though infants with a birth weight less than 1250 g make up less than 1% of the total babies born annually in the United States, they frequently constitute a significant percentage of the babies in the intensive care nursery. Very low-birth-weight (VLBW) infants' limited ability to produce heat, their increased evaporative water loss at birth secondary to extremely thin skin, as well as their small heat capacity (the result of their large surface-to-volume ratio) make them unusually susceptible to cold stress.[10,26]

Because one of the first responses to thermal stress in these infants is a change in peripheral vasomotor tone with vasodilation when overheated and vasoconstriction with cooling, a continuous assessment of central and peripheral temperatures and their difference is clinically helpful in promptly interpreting the effect of the thermal environment on the infant.[15]

In a study of the first 5 days of life in 79 infants weighing less than 1000 g and 71 infants weighing 1000 to 1500 g, central temperature (Tc) was measured with an abdominal skin probe over the liver and peripheral temperature (Tp) on the sole of the foot to calculate the central-peripheral temperature difference (Td). The nursing care attempted to keep the abdominal skin temperature between 36.8° C and 37.2° C to maintain a Td of less than 1° C. The infants were nursed in a double-walled incubator with 80% humidity, and the nurses altered the air temperature.[27] In the heavier babies, the Tc had a constant median value of 36.7° C and increased to 36.9° C for the next 4 days.

During the first day, the Tc was lower than the sole of the foot nearly 20% of the time, suggesting a slow vasomotor response to cold stress in these very immature infants. To prevent cold stress in this group, Tc was greater than 37.5° C 12% of the time. The normal pattern of Tc greater than Tp was seen more commonly after the first day. In infants weighing less than 1000 g, a Td greater than 2° C can be caused by poor perfusion resulting from hypovolemic shock. In these infants, there was other evidence of hypovolemia 11% of the time (such as increasing heart rate or decreasing blood pressure). With hyperthermia (Td less than 1° C) heart rate increased. If the Tc was greater than 38° C with Td greater than 1° C, the infant was investigated to rule out hypovolemia and sepsis.

For appropriate for gestational age infants weighing less than 1500 g, it is recommended that the infants be nursed in double-walled incubators, with low air velocity and additional humidity for the first week of life. Td should be maintained at less than 1° C. Modern incubators provide such an environment.

NUTRITION AND TEMPERATURE

Because of the relationship between metabolic rate and body temperature, both fluid and nutritional requirements for growth are intimately linked with temperature regulation. This is especially important to the small premature infant maintained in a slightly cool environment. Caloric intake is limited by the small capacity of his or her stomach. Fewer calories would be required for maintenance of body temperature if the infant was in a warmer environment; thus, in the neutral thermal environment, caloric intake can be more effectively used for growth.

The insensible loss of water parallels the metabolic rate, with 25% of total heat produced being dissipated in this manner. Thus, an elevated metabolic rate results in elevated fluid losses and, hence, increased fluid requirements. The neutral thermal temperature allows for small feedings and reduced caloric requirements for growth.

Glass et al. were able to quantitate the effect of temperature control on growth,[28] comparing 12 matched, healthy, small infants aged 1 week -who weighed between 1 and 2 kg. These infants were divided into a "warm" group (abdominal skin temperature maintained at 36.5° C [97.7° F]) and a "standard" group (abdominal skin temperature maintained at 35° C [95° F]). Both groups received 120 kcal/kg/d. Those in the warm group showed a significantly more rapid increase in body weight and length; however, their cold resistance (ability to prevent a decrease in deep body temperature in a cool environment) was diminished. Identical growth rates could be obtained by increasing caloric input intake the standard group.

It is, therefore, difficult to decide whether the premature infant, after the early neonatal period, should be maintained in the neutral thermal environment for optimal growth or be prepared for some of the rigors of a cold apartment or house.

EDITORIAL COMMENT: Longitudinal data on resting energy expenditure (REE) in extremely immature infants and full-term neonates are scarce, but are necessary to understand the energy requirements in neonatal nutrition during the first weeks of life. REE values increased in all gestational age groups from the first week to 5 to 6 weeks of postnatal age, with the most pronounced increase in the smallest infants (+140%) and the smallest increase in the full-term neonates (+47%).[29] Knowledge of the energy requirements is critical to meet the goals and ensure growth. Furthermore, the ability to modify energy expenditure (EE) is extremely helpful when energy intake is limited, which is why careful attention to the thermal environment is so important for very immature babies. Music such as Mozart may help, too. Lubetsky et al. present evidence that music generally may help premature infants by lowering stress hormone levels, leading to enhanced weight gain and growth.[30]

PRACTICAL APPLICATIONS

DELIVERY ROOM

The temperature of the delivery room is frequently set for the comfort of the medical staff rather than for the comfort of the newborn. Careful and immediate drying of the infant's entire body remains critical in minimizing evaporative heat loss. Many pieces of equipment are available to warm the infant—in particular, incubators and radiant warmers. However, the warm body of the mother is well-suited to meet this need. Christensson compared body temperatures over the first 90 minutes of life in healthy full-term neonates cared for with skin-to-skin with their mothers.[31] Infants

were thoroughly dried immediately after birth and placed either on their mother's chest and abdomen and covered with a light blanket or wrapped in cotton blankets and placed in a cot. The infants placed skin-to-skin warmed significantly faster than those in the cot. Oxygen consumption measurement while skin-to-skin revealed that they were in a neutral thermal environment.[32] Thus, for the normal full-term infant, skin-to-skin on the mother's chest is an ideal location for the first 2 hours of life. Also, this would allow the infant to crawl to the mother's breast and begin to suckle on his or her own.

Skin-to-skin care has been practiced in primitive and high technology cultures for body temperature preservation in neonates. Karlsson measured regional skin temperature and heat flow in moderately hypothermic term neonates (mean rectal temperature of 36.3° C) and observed that the mean rectal temperature increased by 0.7° C when placed skin-to-skin on their mothers' chests.[33] Caution must be exercised when attempting this in very immature infants. Bauer noted no significant changes in temperature or oxygen consumption in the first postnatal week for infants between 28 and 30 weeks' gestation[34]; however, infants of 25 to 27 weeks of gestational age lost heat during skin-to-skin contact. They recommended postponing skin-to-skin care for these infants until week 2 of life, when their body temperature remains stable and they are calmer during skin-to-skin contact than in the incubator.

INCUBATORS

In the United States, most intensive care units have double-walled incubators in which the temperature of the inner wall of the incubator is not affected by a cooler room temperature. However, because single-walled incubators are still found in the United States and many countries throughout the world and the temperature of the single walls cannot be controlled, it should be emphasized that the radiant heat loss of the infant to the wall of these incubators varies. Figure 6-5 indicates how the temperature of the inner wall of the incubator decreases with cooler room temperatures—a major disadvantage when nursing a sick infant. If the nursery is cool (23.8° C to 15.6° C [75° F to 60° F]) or if the incubator is placed near a cool window or wall, it is difficult—usually impossible—to locate and

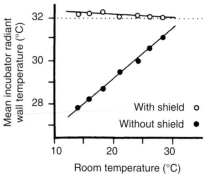

Figure 6-5. Effect of using heat shield (see Fig. 6-6) on mean incubator wall radiant temperature at varying room temperatures.

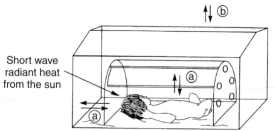

Figure 6-6. Inner heat shield provides warm inner walls to minimize radiant heat loss in cool nursery (a). Long wave radiant exchange between baby and heat shield and between inner wall of incubator and heat shield. Long wave radiant exchange between incubator walls and surroundings (b).

maintain the neutral thermal environment. The infant loses heat to the cold incubator wall and needlessly increases oxygen and caloric consumption in his or her efforts to stay warm. The magnitude of this loss can be predicted if room temperature is known. Hey and Katz found that operative temperature (true environmental temperature, taking into account radiation and convection) decreased 1° C below incubator temperature for every 7° C that incubator air exceeded room temperature.[14] Unless the incubator, room air, and radiant surfaces have similar temperatures, innumerable thermal conditions can exist.

Different types of adaptations prevent radiant heat loss and allow a precise and controlled thermal environment. One method is to warm the nude infant with warm air and heated incubator walls (using either a layer of warm water or electrically conductive plastic paneling).

These expensive procedures have been obviated by Hey, who has developed a small clear plastic heat shield to be used within the traditional single-walled incubator (Fig. 6-6). The warm incubator air heats the plastic wall of the shield to the same temperature as the air within the incubator. The infant radiates heat only to the warm inner plastic shield because radiant waves from the infant (2 to 9 μm) do not penetrate the plastic wall.

When the thermal conditions can be described and controlled, the neutral thermal environment for any nude infant can easily be located by using the studies of Scopes and Ahmed.[35] Generally, the thinner, smaller, and younger the infant, the higher the environmental temperature required to achieve the neutral thermal environment.[36]

Table 6-2 and Figure 6-7 are general guides for roughly locating the neutral temperature if the walls of the incubator are warm and within 1° C of the incubator air temperature. When estimating neutral temperatures in single-walled incubators, add 1° C to all the temperatures in the table for every 7° C that incubator air temperatures exceed room temperatures. The abdominal skin temperatures in very low-birth-weight infants during the first 5 days of life are depicted in Figure 6-9, *B*.

If an incubator is placed in the sunlight, the short wavelength radiant emission goes through the plastic wall and can overheat the infant because long wave re-radiation through the plastic wall is prevented (the "greenhouse effect") (see Fig. 6-6).

RADIANT HEATERS

When radiant heat panels are placed above the infant without a complete enclosure, there is a large increase in insensible water loss. A minimal oxygen consumption can be achieved by servo-controlling the heat panel according to the abdominal skin temperature and maintaining skin temperature between 36.2° C and 36.5° C (97° F and 98° F). Darnall et al.[37] comparing radiant warmers with an incubator, found no difference in minimal oxygen consumption, whereas LeBlanc found a significant increase in metabolic rate.[38] Under a radiant warmer, radiant losses were markedly reduced, or there was a net gain, whereas convective and evaporative losses were increased. Increasing the skin temperature above a set point of 36.5° C resulted in significant hyperthermia in a minority of infants studied. Baumgart concluded that a moderate abdominal skin temperature

Table 6-2. Neutral Thermal Environmental Temperatures

Age and Weight	Range of Temperature (° C)	Age and Weight	Range of Temperature (° C)
0-6 hr		**72-96 hr**	
<1200 g	34.0-35.4	<1200 g	34.0-35.0
1200-1500 g	33.9-34.4	1200-1500 g	33.0-34.0
1501-2500 g	32.8-33.8	1501-2500 g	31.1-33.2
>2500 g (and >36 wk)	32.0-33.8	>2500 g (and >36 wks)	29.8-32.8
6-12 hr		**4-12 days**	
<1200 g	34.0-35.4	<1500 g	33.0-34.0
1200-1500 g	33.5-34.4	1501-2500 g	31.0-33.2
1501-2500 g	32.2-33.8	>2500 g (and >36 wks)	
>2500 g (and >36 wk)	31.4-33.8	4-5 days	29.5-32.6
12-24 hr		5-6 days	29.4-32.3
<1200 g	34.0-35.4	6-8 days	29.0-32.2
1200-1500 g	33.3-34.3	8-10 days	29.0-31.8
1501-2500 g	31.8-33.8	10-12 days	29.0-31.4
>2500 g (and >36 wk)	31.0-33.7	**12-14 days**	
24-36 hr		<1500 g	32.0-34.0
<1200 g	34.0-35.0	1501-2500 g	31.0-33.2
1200-1500 g	33.1-34.2	>2500 g (and >36 wk)	29.0-30.8
1501-2500 g	31.6-33.6	**2-3 wk**	
>2500 g (and >36 wk)	30.7-33.5	<1500 g	32.2-34.0
36-48 hr		1501-2500 g	30.5-33.0
<1200 g	34.0-35.0	**3-4 wk**	
1200-1500 g	33.0-34.1	<1500 g	31.6-33.6
1501-2500 g	31.4-33.5	1501-2500 g	30.0-32.7
>2500 g (and >36 wk)	30.5-33.3	**4-5 wk**	
48-72 hr		<1500 g	31.2-33.0
<1200 g	34.0-35.0	1501-2500 g	29.5-32.2
1200-1500 g	33.0-34.0	**5-6 wk**	
1501-2500 g	31.2-33.4	<1500 g	30.6-32.3
>2500 g (and >36 wk)	30.1-33.2	1501-2500 g	29.0-31.8

Adapted from Scopes J, Ahmed I: Range of critical temperatures in sick and newborn babies, *Arch Dis Child* 41:417, 1966.
For their table, Scopes and Ahmed had the walls of the incubator 1° C to 2° C warmer than the ambient air temperatures. Generally speaking, the smaller infants in each weight group require a temperature in the higher portion of the temperature range. Within each time range, the younger the infant, the higher the temperature that is required.

between 36.5° C and 37° C would probably best correspond to a thermal neutral zone for a naked infant supine on an open bed platform.[39] He noted that there is a risk of hyperthermia much above this level.[40] A semipermeable polyurethane membrane (Saran) used as an artificial skin resulted in significantly less radiant heat needed for infants to remain in a neutral thermal environment and also reduced evaporative water loss by 30%.[41,42] Another concern is the effect of the infrared spectrum emanating from the radiant warmer on immature skin and eyes. To date, relatively small

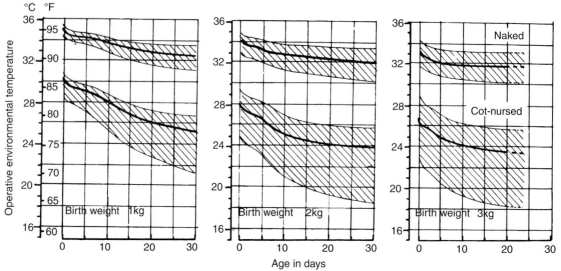

Figure 6-7. Range of temperatures to provide neutral environmental conditions for baby lying either dressed in cot or naked on warm mattress in draft-free surroundings of moderate humidity (50% saturation) when mean radiant temperature is same as air temperature. Hatched area shows neutral temperature range for healthy babies weighing 1, 2, or 3 kg at birth. Approximately 1° C should be added to these operative temperatures to derive appropriate neutral air temperature for single-walled incubators when room temperature is less than 27° C (80° F) and more if room temperature is much less than this.

studies reveal no cataracts, corneal opacities, or ulcerations.[43]

COT NURSING

An alternative approach that has been revived and studied in detail by Hey and O'Connell is to care for the infant dressed (cot nursed) rather than naked.[44] In a nude infant, the resistance to heat loss is 1.07 clo units, which is increased by 1.25 units when the infant is dressed in a shirt, diaper, and gown; additional resistance of 0.61 unit is added when a flannelette sheet and two layers of cotton blankets are added.

As emphasized by Hey, the major advantage of cot nursing is the larger latitude of safe environmental temperatures. If the incubator temperature decreases 2° C, the naked infant must increase heat production by 35% to prevent a decrease in deep body temperature, whereas a 2° C increase results in the infant becoming febrile. Similar changes in room temperature would have a negligible effect on the cot-nursed infant. Hey calculated that for the same effects in the cot-nursed infant, the room temperature must decrease to 19° C (66.2° F) or increase to 31° C (87.8° F). Lightly dressing the infant minimizes the effects of fluctuation in environmental temperature. Cot nursing is inexpensive and is clinically useful when close, continuous observation is

not required. The development in full-term infants of a nighttime temperature rhythm (with a temperature decrease with sleep) first begins to be noted between 6 and 12 weeks of age.[45]

HEATED WATER-FILLED MATTRESS

The 8-L polyvinylchloride heated water-filled mattress (HWM) is an effective low-cost device that has been evaluated using a thermal mannequin and trials with premature infants.[46] The mattress is heated by a thermocontrolled heating plate, and the temperature display records the actual water temperature. The low electric power (50 W) makes the heating slow (4.4° C/hour) so that the mattress must be warm even when not in use. The large heat storage capacity of the water, however, results in slow cooling (several hours) in case the electric current is interrupted.

A disadvantage in the use of the HWM is that the quality of the thermocontrol of the mattress must be exact because the safe temperature range is narrow, from 35° C to only 38° C. Below this range, there is cooling, with the infant losing heat by conduction to the mattress; above this range, there is the possibility of overheating and burns. In several clinical studies in which preterm infants were either in a cot with an HWM or in an air-heated single-walled incubator, the metabolic rate was lower during cot nursing with an HWM.

HATS

The relatively larger brain of the newborn is a major heat source. (The brain of the infant is 12% of body weight compared with 2% in the adult.) Studies by Stothers reveal that heat loss from the head is clinically important and can be significantly reduced with a three-layered hat made of wool and gauze.[47,48] Figure 6-8 illustrates how the neutral thermal range is extended 1° C and oxygen consumption is reduced in a cool environment when a three-layered hat is worn by a nude 1200-g infant. A tube gauze hat had no effect. The use of double-layered hats is recommended for all infants in the home and hospital who would benefit by a controlled thermal environment.

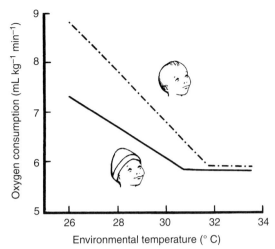

Figure 6-8. Extension of neutral thermal range and reduction of oxygen consumption in cool environment with wearing of a three-layered hat by nude 1200-g infant.

SERVO-CONTROL

A completely different approach to caring for an infant in the neutral thermal environment is to servo-control the heating device (whether it is a heat panel or incubator) to the infant's abdominal skin temperature. If the infant's skin temperature decreases, the warming device increases its heat output. The temperature of the skin at which the incubator is servo-controlled is critical. Maintaining the abdominal skin temperature at 36.5° C (97.7° F) minimizes oxygen consumption; at an abdominal skin temperature of 35.9° C (96.6° F), oxygen consumption increases 10%.[49,50]

Servo-control has been further refined by Perlstein et al. who developed a computerized system to control the heat input into the incubator.[51] Their system was designed to maintain the infant in a thermoneutral zone, avoid wide temperature fluctuations that might induce apneic episodes, and recognize the point at which an infant can be weaned from the incubator. The use of this system led to fewer deaths, although the impact of other portions of the computer information on the infant's survival could not be separated from the effect of incubator control.

Two disadvantages of servo-controlled equipment are the increased expense and required reorientation of nurses and physicians when evaluating the infant's condition—both the infant and the incubator temperatures must be compared together, so the infant's true condition is not masked. When an infant who is under servo-control starts to become febrile, the incubator temperature drops, but there is no change in body temperature. In the other direction, when an infant who is being servo-controlled dies, his or her body temperature is maintained because the incubator temperature elevates.

DISORDERS OF TEMPERATURE REGULATION

HYPOTHERMIA

Hypothermia should be anticipated in low-birth-weight infants, and the routine use of low-reading thermometers (from 29.4° C [85° F]) is advocated in their care, because temperatures less than 34.4° C (94° F) are frequently not immediately detected with the routine clinical thermometers. Hypothermia is seen particularly following resuscitation of asphyxiated premature infants. It may be an early sign of sepsis or evidence of an intracranial pathologic condition, such as meningitis, cerebral hemorrhage, or severe central nervous system (CNS) anomalies. CNS disease can also result in hyperthermia.

NEONATAL COLD INJURY

Neonatal cold injury following extreme hypothermia occurs under both warm and cool climatic conditions, particularly with domiciliary maternity services. Low-birth-weight infants are almost exclusively affected, except for full-term infants with problems such as intracerebral hemorrhage and major malformations of the CNS.

Clinical Features

A slight decrease in temperature may produce profound metabolic change; however, a significant decrease must occur before clinical features are evident.

The infants feed poorly, are lethargic, and feel cold to the touch. Mann and Elliott describe an "aura" of coldness about the body and skin over the trunk[52]; the periphery feels intensely cold and "corpselike." Core temperatures are depressed, often below 32.2° C (90° F).

The most striking feature is the bright red color of the infant. This red color (which may lead the physician astray because the infant "looks so well") is due to the failure of dissociation of oxyhemoglobin at low temperatures. Central cyanosis or pallor may be present. Respiration is slow, very shallow, irregular, and often associated with an expiratory grunt. Bradycardia occurs proportionate to the degree of temperature decrease.

Activity is lessened. Shivering is rarely observed. The CNS depression is constant, and reflexes and responses are diminished or absent. Painful stimuli (e.g., injections) produce minimal reaction, and the cry is feeble. Abdominal distention and vomiting are common.

Edema of the extremities and face is common, and sclerema is seen, especially on the cheeks and limbs. Sclerema is hardening of the skin; it is associated with reddening and edema. It is observed particularly with cold injury and infection and near the time of death.[53,54]

Metabolic derangements include metabolic acidosis, hypoglycemia, hyperkalemia, elevated blood urea nitrogen, and oliguria.[52] Pulmonary hemorrhage in association with a generalized bleeding diathesis is a common finding at autopsy.

Treatment

The infant should be warmed as mortality is reduced significantly. The use of a saline push (10 mL/kg) early in the rewarming period also may reduce mortality rate.

In addition to the rewarming, oxygen is administered, blood sugar is monitored closely, and metabolic acidosis is monitored and corrected. The infant should be fed only by intravenous (IV) infusion or gavage of dextrose solution until the temperature is 35° C (95° F). Hypothermic infants should not be permitted to feed by nipple. Antibiotics are administered only when infection is suspected or documented.

INDUCED HYPOTHERMIA

There is strong experimental evidence that prolonged cerebral hypothermia initiated after a severe hypoxic-ischemic insult can reduce subsequent neuronal loss in neonatal and adult animals.[55,56]

Acute brain injury results from the combined effects of cellular energy failure, acidosis, glutamate release, intracellular calcium accumulation, lipid peroxidation, and nitric oxide neurotoxicity that disrupt essential components of the cell, resulting in cell death. Many factors, including the duration or severity of the insult, influence the progression of cellular injury after hypoxia-ischemia. A secondary cerebral energy failure occurs from 6 to 48 hours after the primary event and may involve mitochondrial dysfunction secondary to extended reactions from primary insults (e.g., calcium influx, excitatory neurotoxicity, oxygen-free radicals, or nitric oxide formation). Some evidence suggests that circulatory and endogenous inflammatory cells or mediators also contribute to ongoing brain injury.

The goals of management of a newborn infant at risk for injury from an hypoxic-ischemic insult include supportive care to facilitate adequate cerebral perfusion and delivery of nutrients to the brain, efforts to control seizures, maintenance of glucose homeostasis, correction of anemia, and management of renal, hepatic, cardiac, and respiratory failure.

In recent years, it has become apparent that temperature can modify the extent of hypoxic-ischemic brain injury. There is an increasing body of experimental and clinical data showing a reduction in the extent of brain injury after intrapartum hypoxia-ischemia with induced hypothermia (a reduction of body temperature by about 3° C) initiated within 6 hours of birth.[57,58] Cooling preserves cerebral energy metabolism, reduces cerebral tissue injury, and improves neurological function. Conversely, there is experimental evidence indicating a worsening of cerebral injury during or after ischemia under conditions of elevations in temperature. Randomized trials in full-term and near full-term newborns suggest that treatment with mild hypothermia (either selective head or total body cooling) is safe and improves survival without developmental disabilities up to 18 months of age.[59] Meta-analysis of these trials suggests that for every six or seven infants with moderate to severe HIE who are treated with mild hypothermia, there will be one less infant who dies or has significant neurodevelopmental disability.[60] Nonetheless, mortality and severe morbidity still approaches 50% and additional strategies are needed. These include the use of oxygen-free radical inhibitors and scavengers, excitatory amino acid antagonists, and growth factors; prevention of nitric oxide formation; and blockage of apoptotic pathways. Other avenues of potential neuroprotection that have been studied in immature animals include xenon inhalation, platelet-activating factor antagonists, insulin-like growth factor-1, and erythropoietin. They have been evaluated experimentally but have not been rigorously tested in a systematic manner in the human neonate.

HYPERTHERMIA

Elevation of the deep body temperature may be caused by an excessive environmental temperature, infection, dehydration, or alterations of the central mechanisms of heat control associated with cerebral birth trauma or malformations and drugs.

The question of systemic infection is invariably raised in infants with elevated deep body temperatures. Due consideration should also be given to the environmental conditions that alter heat control. It is not uncommon to find an elevated core temperature following the increased heat input with the commencement of the use of phototherapy. This can also occur if the incubator is placed in the sun (see Fig. 6-6). A febrile baby overheated by the environment becomes vasodilated trying to lose heat, and the infant's extremities and trunk are at almost the same temperature. A septic baby is usually vasoconstricted, and the extremities become colder than the rest of the body.[61] Therefore, measuring the temperature difference between the abdominal skin (Tc) and the sole of the foot (Tp) is sometimes helpful clinically.

It is important that asphyxiated infants are not overheated. Relatively high temperatures during usual care after hypoxia-ischemia were associated with increased risk of adverse outcomes.[62] The odds of death or disability were increased 3.6 to 4-fold for each 1° C increase in the highest quartile of skin or esophageal temperatures. There were no associations between temperatures and

outcomes in the cooling-treated group. The results may reflect underlying brain injury and/or adverse effects of temperature on outcomes.

Regional heat loss and skin temperature changes in 25 healthy, full-term infants were studied under controlled conditions at environmental temperatures of 28° C to 32° C.[63] Mean regional skin temperatures measured at 11 body regions followed the changes in environmental temperatures (Fig. 6-9, *A*). The regional dry heat losses closely followed the external temperature gradient, defined as the difference between skin and environmental temperatures. In eight of the infants, lowering the environmental temperature 3° C to 4° C induced peripheral vasoconstriction only in the feet. Many clinicians are enamored with the concept of differences

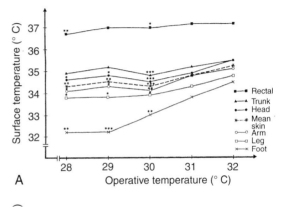

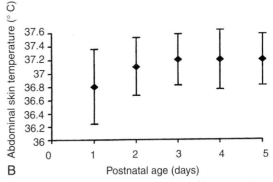

Figure 6-9. A, Rectal temperature, mean skin temperature, and regional skin temperatures for different body regions at different operative temperatures. Asterisk, *p* <.05; double asterisk, *p* <.01; triple asterisk, *p* <.001 compared with 32° C. **B,** Mean (standard deviation) abdominal skin temperature according to postnatal age. (*A, From Karlsson H, Hanel SE, Nilsson K, et al: Measurement of skin temperature and heat flow from skin in term newborn babies,* Acta Paediatr *84:605–612, 1995;* **B,** *From Lyon AJ, Pikaar ME, Badger P, et al: Temperature in very low birthweight infants during first five days of life,* Arch Dis Child *76:F47–F50, 1997.)*

in the toe-tummy temperature as an indication of sepsis. Although it is reasonable to consider sepsis, it is equally important to carefully evaluate the thermal environment if a gradient is detected between the abdominal and foot temperature.

ASPHYXIA

With newborn infants, prolonged resuscitative attempts often are carried out on a damp towel, with precipitous decreases in body temperature.

Temperature responses following delivery are sometimes a guide to the state of the infant during delivery.[64] If the infant was severely asphyxiated or hypoxic, temperature control is reflexively turned off, and body temperature is often not maintained immediately after delivery.

The following resuscitative procedures should be performed with due attention to heat control:

1. Evaporative losses may effectively be reduced by immediately drying the infant.
2. Conductive losses can be eliminated by laying the infant on a dry, warm towel or cloth.
3. A radiant source of heat in the form of a radiant warmer provides a heat-giving environment. This is ideal for resuscitation, because the infant can be maintained nude and is readily accessible. Abdominal skin temperature should be maintained.
4. Convection must be controlled; there should be no drafts in the room; and the oxygen must be warmed.

APNEA

Despite the beneficial effects of maintaining a warm environment, a possible disadvantage is its effect on respiratory control.

1. Immersing a normal infant in a bath equal to the maternal temperature sometimes stops respiration. Rapid warming is also associated with apneic episodes.
2. Observations in a group of low-birth-weight infants having apneic attacks revealed that lowering the servo-controlling temperature less than 1° C significantly reduced the number of episodes.[65]

It is suggested, therefore, that a premature infant having apneic attacks should be maintained closer to the low range of neutral thermal environment, and most importantly, temperature fluctuations should be kept to a minimum.[66]

WEANING FROM THE INCUBATOR

Weaning from the incubator[67,68] can typically be started when the infant is physiologically stable, at least 32 weeks' corrected gestational age, weighs at least 1500 g and takes 100 kcals/kg/day, provided there is no medical indication for continuing incubator/warmer care, such as the need for close observation.

Decrease incubator temperature by 1° C to 1.5° C daily until incubator temperature is 28° C. When skin temperature is maintained at 36° C to 37° C for at least 8 hours in an incubator at 28° C, attempt to transition to an open crib. The baby should be fully clothed and swaddled, and maintained in a room with normal ambient temperature (68° F to 75° F). If the baby fails an attempt to wean from the incubator/warmer, as evidenced by low body temperature or cessation of growth, the baby should be placed back in an incubator and weaning should be attempted again in 24 to 48 hours.

PRACTICAL ADVICE (FROM RAINBOW BABIES AND CHILDREN'S HOSPITAL NICU PROTOCOL)

1. Transition infant to open crib during the day or early evening hours to optimize success.
2. Do not swaddle infants in blankets in incubator.
3. If an infant drops body temperature, do not rewarm faster than 0.5° C to 1° C per hour.
4. Do not use warming lights during transition to open crib—if infant cannot maintain temperature greater than 36° C in open crib, return to isolette at 28° C.
5. Do not feed infant orally unless skin temperature is greater than 35.9° C. Monitor glucose if no IV is in place.
6. Do not bathe infant for first 24 hours in open crib or if demonstrating temperature instability later.

QUESTIONS

True or False

If the rectal temperature is maintained between 36.5° C and 37° C (97.7° F and 98.6° F), the infant can be considered to be in the "neutral thermal environment."

A single measurement of temperature is of little value in defining the neutral thermal environment. The infant may have an elevated metabolic rate and be "working" to maintain normal body temperature. Therefore, the statement is false.

True or False

When trying to produce a neutral thermal environment, take into account ambient air temperature, air flow, relative humidity, and temperature of surrounding objects.

The neutral thermal environment is that set of thermal conditions associated with minimal metabolic rate in a resting subject; thus, potential heat loss by conduction, convection, radiation, and evaporation must be considered. Therefore, the statement is true.

True or False

Swaddling the infant should not influence the temperature of the incubator when it is set to achieve neutral thermal environment.

The use of the Scopes tables to achieve the neutral thermal environment refers to a set of specific conditions—namely, that the incubator wall temperature is 1° C higher than the air temperature and that the infants are nude. All the processes of heat exchange are altered and reduced by clothing the baby. The ambient air temperature inside the clothing is warmer than ambient incubator air, and humidity is higher, too. Therefore, the statement is false.

True or False

Overheating the infant produces no noticeable clinical effects and can only be detected by monitoring deep body temperature.

Overheating is documented by monitoring deep body temperature. However, the infant would be flushed and panting, and the extremities and trunk would be at the same temperature. The infant would hyperventilate and initially show irritability and may have apnea. Sweating may occur but is reduced in immature infants. With prolonged hyperthermia, stupor, coma, and convulsions may occur, and brain damage may be irreversible. The statement is false.

True or False

The stimulus for an increased metabolic rate begins immediately after onset of cold stimulus, even before the deep body temperature has decreased.

Bruck has shown that it is not necessary for body temperature to decrease before there is an increase in metabolic rate. Therefore, the statement is true. Even mild cold stress (e.g., blowing cold air on the face) may result in a significant increase in oxygen consumption. This occurs when unwarmed oxygen is blowing over the infant's face.

True or False

Maintaining an infant with respiratory distress syndrome (RDS) in the neutral thermal environment plays an insignificant part in overall management.

Many infants with RDS have a limited capacity to transfer oxygen, and the maintenance of the neutral thermal environment is most important in their care.[69] Therefore, the statement is false.

True or False

The rate of growth in body weight and length can be influenced by environmental temperature.

Infants kept at a warmer environment showed a significantly greater increase in body weight and length over those maintained in a cooler environment when both groups had the same caloric intake. Infants in a cooler environment require more calories to regulate body temperature and thus have fewer calories available for growth. Therefore, the statement is true.

True or False

When a fever develops in an infant who is being monitored in a servo incubator, this is reflected by an increase in incubator temperature.

As the infant's temperature increases, the abdominal skin temperature that is controlling the infant also increases, resulting in a decrease in incubator temperature. Thus, a decrease in incubator temperature reflects an increase in the temperature of the infant and vice versa. Therefore, the statement is false.

True or False

An elevated temperature during the first month of life is common and no cause for concern.

Too often an elevated temperature in a newborn has been attributed to environmental conditions, with disastrous consequences—for example, sepsis overlooked. A temperature elevation, particularly in infants at home, should be carefully evaluated (see Chapter 14). The answer is false.

True or False

Radiant heat losses are similar in adults and immature infants because they are both homeotherms.

Radiant heat loss is of less significance in adults because they are clothed. Radiant heat loss has no bearing on the question of homeothermy. A homeotherm is an animal that attempts to maintain a constant body temperature despite alterations in environment—for example, metabolic rate increases in a cool environment. Therefore, the statement is false.

True or False

The newborn infant loses equal amounts of heat per unit of body mass compared with the adult.

Although at birth the infant's body mass is approximately 5% of that of the adult, the surface area is nearly 15%. There is also less subcutaneous tissue, resulting in a higher thermal conductance and a higher skin temperature at lower ambient temperatures. Bruck has estimated that, because of these facts, the heat loss of the newborn infant per unit of body mass is about four times that of the adult.[7] Therefore, the statement is false.

True or False

Full-term infants who have been cold stressed at birth may have a normal pH and low HCO_3.

A compensated metabolic acidosis probably secondary to lactic acid production is sometimes observed. Therefore, the statement is true.

True or False

The duration of sleep is markedly reduced when small nude infants are exposed to an environmental temperature of only 1° C to 2° C below the lower limit of the presumed range of thermal neutrality.

It has been suggested by some investigators that the temperature range in which the least amount of oxygen is consumed is also the temperature range of thermal comfort for the neonate. Therefore, the statement is true.

True or False

Swaddled full-term babies may not cry or otherwise call attention to the fact that they are under severe cold stress.

This statement is true and is particularly important because the upper limit of heat production is reached for cot-nursed, full-term infants when the room temperature declines to about 10° C (50° F). In some situations at night, bedrooms get colder, and the infants become hypothermic.

True or False

The signs and symptoms of hypothermia shortly after delivery may imitate the clinical picture of RDS.

The signs of RDS—notably grunting, acidosis, and an increased right-to-left shunt—can all be observed in a hypothermic infant. The statement is true.

True or False

The precipitous drop in temperature after delivery in preterm infants is inevitable, physiologic, and of no major consequence.

The body temperature of preterm babies can drop precipitously after delivery, and this hypothermia is associated with an increase in mortality and morbidity. Hypothermia on admission to neonatal units is an independent risk factor for mortality in preterm babies.

During the first few hours of life, extremely low-birth-weight infants may become hypothermic during umbilical or other venous line insertions, endotracheal intubation, other procedures, including x-rays and ultrasound, or even taking vital signs. Anticipating the need for heat preservation started at delivery by prewarming the delivery room, placing the baby in a plastic bag with a plastic head wrap and warming mattresses can assist the transition for these babies and avoid hypothermia. The statement is false.

True or False

The temperature in the delivery room should be set to the zone of thermal comfort for the staff.

The temperature in the delivery room should be set to minimize the chances of cooling the newborn baby—term or preterm. Suggested delivery room temperatures are tabulated in Table 6-3 displayed subsequently. These temperatures may be uncomfortable for obstetrical staff, but it is of crucial importance to the newborn. The statement is false.

AMERICAN ACADEMY OF PEDIATRICS POLICY FOR HYPOTHERMIA PREVENTION

- Radiant warmer to "full-on" prior to delivery.
- Delivery room temperature 72° F or higher.
- Deliver infant, hemostat cord, place in bag feet first to torso.
- Dry head, put on cap.
- Resuscitate as necessary per Neonatal Resuscitation Program Guidelines.
- Clamp cord, remove hemostat, transport to NICU in heated incubator.
- Do not place heating pad under infant (hyperthermia risk).

CASE 1

Baby D. O. is an 1160-g male delivered at 31 weeks' gestation. No problems are encountered in the immediate neonatal period, and the pregnancy is uncomplicated. Delivery is by cesarean section with the mother under caudal anesthesia. The Apgar score at 1 minute is 6. On the second day of life, the rectal temperature is noted to be 36.8° C (98.2° F). The incubator temperature at this time was 34.1° C (93.4° F).

What additional data is needed to define the neutral thermal environment?

To define the neutral thermal environment, one also requires the temperature of the mattress with regard to conductive heat loss, the air flow in the incubator, the relative humidity, and the temperature of the inner walls of the incubator to determine the radiant heat losses that can occur to the surrounding walls of the incubator. A continuous recording of the abdominal skin temperature would permit a rough idea of whether the infant is in the neutral thermal zone. When a servo incubator is controlled to maintain an abdominal skin temperature of 36.5° C (97.7° F), oxygen consumption has been found to be minimal. In this case, the abdominal skin temperature is 34.9° C (94.8° F), the side wall of the incubator is 32.5° C

(90.5° F), and the relative humidity is 80%. We can assume the temperature of the mattress to be the same as the incubator air temperature.

With these available data, is the infant in the neutral thermal environment?

No, the infant is not in the neutral thermal environment. Our indications of this are that the abdominal skin temperature is only 34.9° C (94.8° F) even with the incubator air at 34.1° C (93.4° F). In Table 6-2, the appropriate temperature for this infant to be in the neutral thermal environment is listed as an environmental temperature of 34° C to 35° C (93.2° F to 95° F), provided that the walls are 1° C higher than the air. Note that the side wall temperature is only 32.5° C (90.5° F). The infant is losing heat by radiation. Be aware that the baby exchanges heat with its environment through radiation, convection, conduction, and evaporation and all these modalities must be checked. Mechanisms of heat production are limited as is the ability to reduce heat loss by peripheral vasoconstriction. Furthermore, the immature baby, because of a high surface area-to-volume ratio and increased evaporation of fluid from the skin, easily loses heat and does not have the capacity to generate heat.

Table 6-3. Suggested Delivery Room Temperatures by Gestational Age and Birth Weight	
Estimated Gestational Age (EGA) and/or Estimated Birth Weight (EBW)	**Delivery Room Temperature**
≤26 wks EGA and/or ≤750 g EBW	76° F (24°C) or more; target: 78° F-80° F (25.5-26.5°C)
27-28 wks EGA and/or ≤1000 g EBW	74° F (23°C) or more; target: 78° F-80° F (25.5-26.5°C)
29-32 wks EGA and/or 1001–1500 g EBW	72° F (22°C) or more
33-36 wks EGA and/or 1501–2500 g EBW	72° F (22°C) or more
37-42 wks GA or ≥2501 g EBW	70° F (21°C) or more

CASE 2

Baby H is delivered after a 42-week pregnancy; she weighs 1600 g. No problems are noted in the immediate neonatal period. The neurologic examination is appropriate for an infant with a 42-week gestation, except that there is diminished neck flexor tone. Head circumference is 33 cm. The infant is assumed to be unable to increase her metabolic rate with cold stress.

How can the optimal thermal environment be found?

This is a difficult question to answer because no tables are available for this age and weight. The problem may best be managed by servo-control of the incubator and maintaining the abdominal skin temperature at 36.5° C (97.7° F). Another approach is to use the "warmest" incubator possible to maintain a normal temperature in the infant.

REFERENCES

The reference list for this chapter can be found online at www.expertconsult.com.

Nutrition and Selected Disorders of the Gastrointestinal Tract

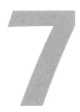

PART ONE

NUTRITION FOR THE HIGH-RISK INFANT

David H. Adamkin, Paula G. Radmacher, and Salisa Lewis

The goal of nutritional support for the high-risk infant is to provide sufficient nutrients postnatally to ensure continuation of growth at rates similar to those observed in utero. The preterm infant presents a particular challenge in that the nutritional intake must be sufficient to replenish tissue losses and permit tissue accretion. However, during the early days after birth, acute illnesses such as respiratory distress, patent ductus arteriosus, and hyperbilirubinemia preclude maximal nutritional support. Functional immaturity of the renal, gastrointestinal, and metabolic systems limits optimal nutrient delivery. Substrate intolerances are common, limiting the nutrients available for tissue maintenance and growth.

During the last trimester of pregnancy, nutrient stores are established in preparation for birth at 40 weeks' gestation. Fat and glycogen are stored to provide ready energy during times of caloric deficit. Iron reserves accumulate to prevent iron-deficiency anemia during the first 4 to 6 months of life. Calcium and phosphorus are deposited in the soft bones to begin mineralization, which continues through early adult life. However, the infant who is delivered before term has minimal nutrient stores and higher nutrient requirements per kilogram than the full-term infant.

Infants weighing less than 1.5 kg have a body composition of approximately 85% to 95% water, 9% to 10% protein, and 0.1% to 5% fat. The fat is primarily structural with only negligible amounts of subcutaneous fat; hepatic glycogen stores are virtually nonexistent. The growth of these infants lags considerably after birth.[1] Such infants, especially those less than 1000 g birth weight (extremely low birth weight [ELBW]), typically do not regain birth weight until 2 to 3 weeks of age. The growth of most less than 1500 g (very low-birth-weight [VLBW]) infants proceeds at a slower rate than in utero, often by a large margin.[1] Although many of the smallest VLBW infants are also born small for gestational age (SGA), both appropriate for gestational age (AGA), VLBW, and SGA infants develop "extrauterine growth restriction" (EUGR). Figure 7-1 from the National Institute of Child Health and Human Development (NICHD) Neonatal Research Network demonstrates the differences between normal intrauterine growth and the observed rates of postnatal growth in the NICHD study. These postnatal growth curves are shifted to the right of the reference curve in each gestational age category. This "growth faltering" is common in ELBW infants.

Nutrient intakes received by VLBW infants are much lower than what the fetus receives in utero—an intake deficit that persists throughout much of the infants' stay in the hospital and even after discharge.[2] Although nonnutritional factors (comorbidities) contribute to the slower growth of VLBW infants, suboptimal nutrient intakes are critical in explaining their poor growth outcomes. Considerable evidence exists that early growth deficits, which reflect inadequate nutrition, have long-lasting effects, including short stature and poor neurodevelopmental outcomes. The most convincing data concerning the neurodevelopmental consequences of inadequate early nutrition are those reported by Lucas et al.[3,4] They demonstrated that premature infants fed a preterm formula containing a

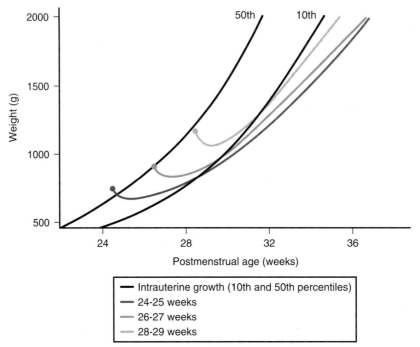

Figure 7-1. Mean body weight versus gestational age in weeks for infants with gestational ages at birth of 24 to 29 weeks.

higher content of protein and other nutrients over the first postnatal month of life had higher neurodevelopmental indices at both 18 months and 7 to 8 years of age compared with infants fed a term formula.[4]

Nutritional management of VLBW infants is marked by a lack of uniformity from one neonatal intensive care unit (NICU) to the next as well as within individual practices. This heterogeneity of practice persists from the first hours after birth to hospital discharge and beyond. Diversity of practice thrives where there is uncertainty. Because under-nutrition is, by definition, nonphysiologic and undesirable, any measure that diminishes it is inherently good, providing safety is not compromised. Avoiding inadequate nutrition is a priority in neonatal nutrition today.

This chapter addresses the nutrient needs of the sick and LBW infant, methods for provision of nutrients both parenterally and enterally, and methods for assessing nutritional status. Figure 7-2 provides an overview of the important aggressive nutrition strategies that will be reviewed in a timeline configuration based on a "typical" ELBW infant growth curve.[5]

FLUID

In the fetus at 24 weeks' gestation, the total body water (TBW) represents more than 90% of the total body weight, with approximately 65% in the extracellular compartment, 25% in the intracellular compartment, and 1% in fat stores. The TBW and extracellular fluid volumes decrease as gestational age increases; by term, the infant's TBW represents 75% of total body weight with extracellular and intracellular compartments comprising 40% and 35%, respectively.

Compared with the full-term infant, the preterm infant is in a state of relative extracellular fluid volume expansion with an excess of TBW. The dilute urine and negative sodium balance observed during the first few days after birth in the preterm infant may constitute an appropriate adaptive response to extrauterine life. Therefore, the initial diuresis should be regarded as physiologic, reflecting changes in interstitial fluid volume. This should be included in the calculation of daily fluid needs. As a result, a gradual weight loss of 10% to 15% in a VLBW infant and 5% to 10% in a larger baby during the first week of life is expected without adversely affecting urine output, urine osmolality, or clinical status. Provision of large volumes of fluid (160 to 180 mL/kg/d) to prevent this weight loss appears to increase the risk of the development of patent ductus arteriosus, cerebral intraventricular hemorrhage, bronchopulmonary dysplasia (BPD), and necrotizing enterocolitis (NEC).

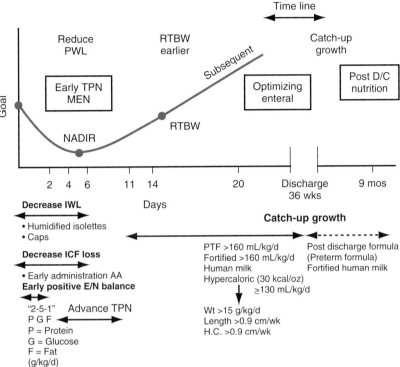

AGGRESSIVE NUTRITION:
PREVENTION OF EUGR

Figure 7-2. Aggressive nutrition and prevention of extrauterine growth restriction (EUGR). *AA,* Amino acid; *D/C,* discharge; *E/N,* enteral nutrition; *HC,* head circumference; *ICF,* intracellular fluid; *IWL,* insensible water loss; *MEN,* minimal enteral nutrition; *PTF,* preterm formula; *PWL,* postnatal weight loss; *RTBW,* [return to birth weight]; *TPN,* total parenteral nutrition. *(Adapted from Adamkin DH: Feeding the preterm infant. In Bhatia J, editor:* Perinatal nutrition: optimizing infant health and development, *New York, 2005, Marcel Dekker, pp 165-190.)*

Therefore, a careful approach to fluid management is currently appropriate. It appears that the preterm infant can adjust water excretion within a relatively broad range of fluid intake (65-70 mL/kg/d to 140 mL/kg/d) without disturbing renal concentrating abilities or electrolyte balance.

Estimation of daily fluid requirements includes insensible water losses (IWLs) from the respiratory tract and skin, gastrointestinal losses (emesis, ostomy output, and diarrhea), urinary losses, and losses from drainage catheters (chest tubes). IWL is a passive process and is not regulated by the infant. However, the environmental conditions in which the infant is nursed should be controlled to minimize losses (Box 7-1). The transepithelial losses are dependent on gestational age, the thickness of the skin and stratum corneum, and blood flow to the skin. The preterm infant has a high body surface area-to-body weight ratio with thinner, more permeable skin that is highly vascularized. These factors increase heat and fluid losses. In addition,

Box 7-1.	**Factors Affecting Insensible Water Loss in Preterm Neonates**

Severe prematurity
Open warmer bed
Forced convection
Phototherapy
Hyperthermia
Tachypnea

the use of open bed platforms with radiant warmers as well as phototherapy lights may increase the IWL by more than 50%. This excessive IWL may be reduced with the use of humidified isolettes to care for the infant.[6] The measurement of urine specific gravity is commonly used to predict urine osmolality. Although this is a reliable means of predicting hyperosmolality (urine osmolality of greater than 290 mOsm/kg water with a urine specific gravity 1.012 or greater), its reliability in predicting hypo-osmolality (urine osmolality of <270 mOsm/kg water with a urine specific gravity 1.008 or less) is variable, ranging from 71% to 95% accuracy, and in predicting iso-osmolality (urine osmolality of 270 to 290 mOsm/kg water with a urine specific gravity of 1.008 to 1.012), the accuracy is even less. In addition, glucose and protein in the urine may increase the urine specific gravity, giving a falsely high estimate of urine osmolality. Therefore, urine specific gravity should be checked only to rule out hyperosmolar urine; a test for sugars and proteins in the urine should be conducted at the same time. The maximal concentrating capabilities in the neonate are limited compared with those in adults; thus, an infant with a urine osmolality of approximately 700 mOsm/kg water (urine specific gravity of 1.019) may be dehydrated. One can estimate the urine osmolality by determining the potential renal solute load of the infant's feeding and the fluid intake (Box 7-2). Infants at risk for high urine osmolality are those who are receiving a concentrated formula and those whose fluid intake is restricted.

Water balance may be maintained with careful attention to input and output. Infants should be weighed nude and at approximately the same time of day. During the first week of life, VLBW infants should be weighed daily; ELBW infants should be weighed twice daily. Meticulous records of fluid intake (with the use of accurate infusion pumps and careful measurement of enteral feedings) and output (by weighing diapers and collecting urine, ostomy output, and drainage from any indwelling catheters) are necessary to compute fluid requirements. Serum glucose, electrolytes, blood urea nitrogen (BUN), and creatinine may be monitored two to three times per day during the first 2 days in critically ill ELBW infants and then daily or as needed thereafter. Urine glucose is routinely tested and urine specific gravity is measured as necessary.

Pauls et al. published data on 136 medically stable ELBW infants receiving early and aggressive parenteral and enteral nutrition.[7] From their data, they developed a series of weight-stratified growth curves of this population over the first months of life. The fluid and nutrient administration was uniform in these patients and included (1) initiation of fluid intake at 60 to 70 mL/kg/day on day 1 with 15 mL/kg daily increases up to a maximum of 160 to 180 mL/kg/day; (2) targeted postnatal weight loss of 10% below birth weight; (3) 1 g/kg/day intravenous (IV) amino acid intake started on

---

Box 7-2.   Renal Solute Load Calculation

Potential renal solute load (PRSL):
4 (g protein/L) + mEq sodium/L +
  mEq potassium/L + mEq chloride/L =
                           PRSL (mOsm/L)

Example:
  Preterm formula$_{24}$ (PT$_{24}$) contains:
  22 g protein/L × 4   = 88
  15.2 mEq sodium/L × 1   = 15.2
  26.9 mEq potassium/L × 1 = 26.9
  18.6 mEq chloride/L × 1 = 18.6
  _____
                    PRSL = 148.7 mOsm/L

Baby A is a 2-week-old former 32-week
  AGA infant weighing 1400 g now receiving
  150 mL/kg/d of PT$_{24}$.

  Estimated fluid losses are:
    Stool   10 mL/kg/d
    Insensible water loss 70 mL/kg/d
    _____
    Total water loss   80 mL/kg/d

150 mL/kg/d intake – 80 mL/kg/d output =
        70 mL/kg/d available for urine output

The PRSL of PT$_{24}$ is 148.7 mOsm/L:

$$\frac{148.7 \text{ mOsm}}{1000 \text{ mL}} \times \frac{X \text{ mOsm}}{150 \text{ mL}}$$
$$22.3 \text{ mOsm} = X$$

This infant has 70 mL/kg/d to excrete 22.3 mOsm of potential renal solute.

$$\frac{22.3 \text{ mOsm}}{70 \text{ mL}} \times 1000 = X \text{ mOsm}/\text{L}$$
$$318.6 \text{ mOsm} = X$$

Therefore, the estimated osmolality of the urine is 319 mOsm/L.

_____
AGA, Appropriate for gestational age.

---

day 1 and increased by 0.5 g/kg/day up to 3 g/kg/day; (4) IV lipid started 1 g/kg/day at day 2 and increased 0.5 g/kg/day up to 3 g/kg/day as long as triglyceride concentrations remained normal; and (5) initial total energy intakes of 27 kcal/kg/day, increasing by 10 kcal/kg/day to 100 kcal/kg/day. In addition, minimal enteral feedings were initiated on day 1 in the form of 24 calorie per ounce fortified human milk or preterm formula and were advanced as tolerated. In all groups, maximal weight loss averaged 10.1% ± 4.6% (SD), and occurred on day of life 5.4 ± 1.7. The age at which birth weight was regained was 11 ± 3.7 days. Small-for-gestational age infants had lower maximal weight loss and regained birth weight at a significantly earlier age. Mean weight gain after day 10 was 15.7 ± 7.2 g/kg/day, which is within the recommended in utero growth rates of 14 to 20 g/kg/day. Although this was a small study, it shows that aggressive nutritional strategies with higher earlier amino acid intakes are affecting the growth curves of these ELBW infants. However, the maximal fluid volumes may be excessive in this population. If possible, the maximal fluid volume should be limited to 140 mL/kg/day.

ELECTROLYTES

Often the electrolyte management of the infant is difficult due to the various sources of electrolyte input. For example, in a 600-g infant, the isotonic saline solution infused to maintain the patency of the umbilical arterial catheter may result in administration of sodium and chloride in excess of estimated daily requirements. Although VLBW infants are capable of regulating sodium balance by altering renal sodium excretion, this may not be sufficient to prevent changes in serum sodium and serum chloride concentrations. Because administration of high amounts of sodium may increase the risk of hypernatremia in the VLBW infant, careful calculation of total intake of sodium, potassium, chloride, glucose, and water from all sources (i.e., maintenance IV fluids, flushes, medications, and bolus injections) is necessary. As fluid requirements are adjusted, recalculation should be done frequently to ensure that appropriate quantities of nutrients are given (Table 7-1).

Sodium is required in quantities sufficient to maintain normal extracellular fluid volume expansion, which accompanies tissue growth. In animal studies, if insufficient amounts are provided, the extracellular fluid volume expansion is suppressed and there are subsequent alterations in quantitative and qualitative somatic growth.

Catheter flushes (using isotonic saline solution) may contribute significant quantities of electrolytes, including chloride, to the infant's total intake. Hyperchloremic metabolic acidosis in LBW infants has been associated with chloride loads greater than 6 mEq/kg/day. The intake can easily be decreased by substituting acetate or phosphate for chloride in the IV solution.

Hypochloremia has also been associated with poor growth. Supplementation with chloride to normalize serum chloride concentrations in infants with BPD resulted in improved growth. Hypochloremia has been noted in infants with BPD who did not survive; however, whether this is a predictor of poor outcome or a symptom of severe illness remains to be resolved.

Potassium chloride (2 mEq/kg/day) is added to the IV fluid within the first days of life as soon as urinary output is established and hyperkalemia is not present. The potassium dose may be adjusted dependent on urine output and use of diuretics. However, it is often difficult to obtain accurate determinations of serum potassium, especially when the blood samples are from heel-sticks, which may lead to excessive red blood cell hemolysis and spuriously high serum potassium levels. If an elevated potassium concentration is obtained, a second blood sample from venipuncture should be obtained for confirmation of the level. If infused via a peripheral vein, concentrations of potassium chloride up to 40 mEq/L are usually tolerated and do not cause localized pain. However, if higher concentrations are needed because of fluid restriction, a central vein should be used.

TOTAL PARENTERAL NUTRITION

Immaturity of the gastrointestinal tract in VLBW infants precludes substantive enteral nutritional support. Thus, nearly all of these infants are supported with total parenteral nutrition (TPN), which has been a huge success, particularly in the management of the ELBW infant.

Historically, the initiation of TPN has been delayed during the first week of life. Reasons for this delay have not been clear but probably have been related to metabolic derangements seen when solutions designed for adults were infused in the neonatal population. There were also concerns about VLBW infants' ability to catabolize amino acids. Data and clinical experience have defined the requirements for parenteral nutrients and led to the development of new products and new methods of delivery designed specifically for use in the neonate.[8] Guidelines for certain minerals and vitamins were published in 1988 and then updated (Table 7-2).[8] Tables 7-3 and 7-4 contain recommended vitamin and mineral intakes for parenteral and enteral nutritional support.

Table 7-1.	Characteristics of Intravenous Fluids					
	Cations			**Anions**		
Type of Fluid	Na (mEq/L)	K (mEq/L)	Ca (mEq/L)	Cl (mEq/L)	HCO$_3$* (mEq/L)	Osmolarity (mOsm/L)†
DEXTROSE IN WATER SOLUTIONS						
D$_5$W						252
D$_{10}$W						505
D$_{20}$W						1010
D$_{50}$W						2525
DEXTROSE IN SALINE SOLUTIONS						
D$_5$W and 0.2% NaCl	34			34		320
D$_5$W and 0.45% NaCl	77			77		406
D$_5$W and 0.9% NaCl	154			154		559
D$_{10}$W and 0.9% NaCl	154			154		812
SALINE SOLUTIONS						
½ NS (0.45% NaCl)	77			77		154
NS (0.9% NaCl)	154			154		308
NS (3% NaCl)	513			513		1026
MULTIPLE ELECTROLYTE SOLUTIONS						
Ringer's solution	147	4	5	155		309
Lactated Ringer's	130	4	3	109	28	273
D$_5$W in Lactated Ringer's	130	4	3	109	28	524
LIPID EMULSIONS						
Lipid emulsions (20%)						258-315

An easy way to approximate the osmolarity of an IV fluid is to consider that for each 1% dextrose, there are 55 mOsm/L; for each 1% amino acids there are 100 mOsm/L; and for each 1% NaCl there are 340 mOsm/L. Therefore:

D$_{10}$W and 0.45% NaCl (½ NS)	
D$_{10}$W = (10 × 55) =	550 mOsm/L
0.45% NaCl = (0.45 × 340) =	153 mOsm/L
Total	**703 mOsm/L**
12.5% dextrose and 17 g amino acids/L (or 1.7% amino acids)	
D$_{12.5}$W = 12.5 × 55 =	687 mOsm/L
1.7% AA = 1.7 ×100 =	170 mOsm/L
Total	**857 mOsm/L**

Parenteral nutrition solutions with an osmolarity >900 mOsm/L should be infused through a central line.

Adapted from Wolf BM, Yamahata WI: In Zeman FJ, editor: *Clinical nutrition and dietetics,* Lexington, Mass, 1983, DC Heath.
*Or its equivalent in lactate, acetate, or citrate.
†Osmolarity of the blood is 285-295 mOsm/L.

Supporting an infant on TPN is not without risk. This method of nutrient delivery should not be undertaken without knowledge of the potential metabolic and mechanical (or catheter-related) complications. Most complications can be avoided with careful monitoring and prompt intervention. Complication rates are minimized when parenteral nutrition is administered with strict adherence to established protocols.

ENERGY

Energy needs are dependent on age, weight, rate of growth, thermal environment, activity, hormonal activity, nature of feedings, and organ size and maturation (Table 7-5). Measurement of a true basal metabolic rate requires a prolonged fast and cannot ethically be determined in VLBW infants; therefore, resting metabolic rate (RMR) is used to estimate energy needs, dietary-induced thermogenesis, minimum energy expended in activity, and the metabolic cost of growth. The metabolic rate increases during the first weeks of life from an RMR of 40 to 41 kcal/kg/day during the first week to 62 to 64 kcal/kg/day by the third week of life. The extra energy expenditure is primarily due to the energy cost of growth related to various synthetic processes. The metabolic rate of

Table 7-2.	Parenteral Multivitamin Dosing Guidelines					
		Product Guidelines				
	ASCN Recommended Dose*	**30% Dose for Infants <1 kg**		**65% Dose for Infants 1-3 kg**		
Weight	≤2500 g	500 g	950 g	1000 g	2000 g	3000 g
Lipid-Soluble						
A (µg)	280	420	221	455	228	152
A (IU)	933	1380	726	1495	748	498
E (mg)	2.8	4.2	2.2	4.5	2.2	1.5
K (µg)	80	120	63	130	65	43
D (µg)	4	6	3.2	6.5	3.2	2.2
D (IU)	160	240	126	260	130	87
Water-Soluble						
Ascorbic acid (mg)	32	48	25	52	26	17
Thiamin (mg)	0.48	0.72	0.34	0.78	0.39	0.26
Riboflavin (mg)	0.56	0.84	0.44	0.91	0.46	0.30
Pyridoxine (mg)	0.4	0.6	0.32	0.65	0.33	0.22
Niacin (mg)	6.8	10.2	5.4	11.1	5.6	3.7
Pantothenate (mg)	2.0	3.0	1.4	3.3	1.6	1.1
Biotin (µg)	8.0	12.0	6.3	13.0	6.5	4.3
Folate (µg)	56	84	44	91	46	30
Vitamin B_{12} (µg)	0.4	0.6	0.32	0.65	0.33	0.22

From Groh-Wargo S, Thompson M, Cox JH, editors: *Nutritional care for high-risk newborns,* rev ed 3, Chicago, 2000, Precept Press, p 15.
*40% dose/kg body weight, maximum not to exceed term infant dose. The 1988 ASCN Subcommittee report suggested that until a preterm parenteral multivitamin is available, pediatric formulations meeting the 1975 AMA-NAG pediatric guidelines should be used at 40% of the standard dose per kg. The maximum dose should not exceed 100% of the term infant dose. Infants weighing >2500 g receive 100% of the standard dose.

the nongrowing infant is approximately 51 kcal/kg/day, which includes 47 kcal/kg/day for basal metabolism and 4 kcal/kg/day for activity.

The contribution of activity to overall energy expenditure is speculative but seems to be small, between 3 and 5 kcal/kg/day to the total energy expenditure. Because of the large amount of time spent in the sleep state, energy expenditure in muscular activity in immature infants is relatively small in comparison to their resting metabolism. As infants mature, they become more active; therefore, energy expenditure from activity increases.

The exposure of infants to a cold environment affects energy expenditure with small alterations in the thermal environment making a significant contribution to energy expenditure. Infants nursed in an environment just below thermal neutrality increase energy expenditure by 7 to 8 kcal/kg/day; any handling adds to this energy loss. A daily increase of 10 kcal/kg/day should be allowed to cover incidental cold stress in the preterm infant. Infants who are intrauterine growth restricted, particularly the asymmetrical type, have a higher RMR on a per

kilogram body weight basis because of their relatively high proportion of metabolically active mass. Other factors that may increase metabolic rate are speculative; the effects of fever, sepsis, and surgery on the infant's energy requirements are uncertain.

Caloric intake above maintenance is used for growth. On average, for each 1-g increment in weight, approximately 4.5 kcal above maintenance energy need are required. Therefore, to attain the equivalent of the third trimester intrauterine weight gain (10 to 15 g/kg/day), a metabolizable energy intake of approximately 45 to 70 kcal/kg/day above the 51 kcal/kg/day required for maintenance must be provided, or approximately 100 to 120 kcal/kg/day. Increasing metabolizable energy intakes beyond 120 kcal/kg/day with energy supplementation alone does not result in proportionate increases in weight gain. However, when energy, protein, vitamins, and minerals are all increased, weight gain with increases in rates of protein and fat accretion can be realized. The higher the caloric intake, the more energy that is expended through excretion, dietary-induced thermogenesis, and tissue synthesis. The energy cost of weight gain at 130 kcal/kg/day was

Table 7-3.	Recommended Intakes of Parenteral and Enteral Vitamins			
		ELBW and VLBW		
		Day 0 **per kg/day**	**Transition** **per kg/day**	**Growing** **per kg/day**
Vitamin A (IU)	Parenteral	700-1500	700-1500	700-1500
	Enteral	700-1500	700-1500	700-1500
Vitamin D (IU)	Parenteral	40-160	40-160	40-160
	Enteral	150-400	150-400	150-400
Vitamin E (IU)	Parenteral	2.8-3.5	2.8-3.5	2.8-3.5
	Enteral	6-12	6-12	6-12
Vitamin K (µg)	Parenteral	500 IM per child	10	10
	Enteral	500 IM per child	8-10	8-10
Thiamin (µg)	Parenteral	200-350	200-350	200-350
	Enteral	180-240	180-240	180-240
Riboflavin (µg)	Parenteral	150-200	150-200	150-200
	Enteral	250-360	250-360	250-360
Niacin (mg)	Parenteral	4-6.8	4-6.8	4-6.8
	Enteral	3.6-4.8	3.6-4.8	3.6-4.8
Vitamin B_6 (µg)	Parenteral	150-200	150-200	150-200
	Enteral	150-210	150-210	150-210
Folate (µg)	Parenteral	56	56	56
	Enteral	25-50	25-50	25-50
Vitamin B_{12} (µg)	Parenteral	0.3	0.3	0.3
	Enteral	0.3	0.3	0.3
Pantothenic acid (mg)	Parenteral	1-2	1-2	1-2
	Enteral	1.2-1.7	1.2-1.7	1.2-1.7
Biotin (µg)	Parenteral	5-8	5-8	5-8
	Enteral	3.6-6	3.6-6	3.6-6
Vitamin C (mg)	Parenteral	15-25	15-25	15-25
	Enteral	18-24	18-24	18-24
Taurine (mg)	Parenteral	0-3.75	1.88-3.75	1.88-3.75
	Enteral	0-9	4.5-9	4.5-9
Carnitine (mg)	Parenteral	0-2.9	0-2.9	0-2.9
	Enteral	0-2.9	0-2.9	0-2.9

Adapted from Tsang RC, Uauy R, Koletzko B, et al, editors: *Nutrition of the preterm infant*, ed 2, Cincinnati, 2005, Digital Educational Publishing, pp 415-416.
Day 0 = Day of birth.
Transition: The period of physiologic and metabolic instability following birth, which may last as long as 7 days.

reported to be 3.0 kcal/g of weight gain. However, at an intake of 149 kcal/kg/day and 181 kcal/kg/day, the energy cost of weight gain has been estimated to be 4.9 and 5.7 kcal/g of weight gain, respectively. In summary, to increase lean body mass accretion and limit fat mass deposition, an increase in protein-to-energy ratio in enteral diets is necessary.

The energy needs of the parenterally nourished infant differ from the enterally fed infant in that there is no fecal loss of nutrients. Preterm infants who are appropriately grown for gestational age are able to maintain positive nitrogen balance when receiving 50 nonprotein calories (NPCs)/kg/day and 2.5 g protein/kg/day. At an NPC intake of greater than 70 NPC/kg/day and a protein intake of 2.7 to 3.5 g/kg/day, preterm infants exhibit nitrogen accretion and growth rates similar to in utero levels.

The sources of energy for parenteral nutrition in infants are either as glucose or lipid, or a combination of the two. Although both glucose and fat provide equivalent nitrogen-sparing effects in the neonate, studies have demonstrated that a nutrient mixture using IV glucose and lipid as the nonprotein energy source is more physiologic than supplying glucose as the only nonprotein energy source. The amount of glucose required to meet the total energy needs approximates 7 mg/kg/min (10 g/kg/day). The excess glucose administered is converted to fat or triglycerides. A nutrient mixture with glucose

Table 7-4.	Recommended Mineral Intakes for Very Low Birth Weight Infants			
		ELBW and VLBW		
		Day 0 per kg/day	Transition per kg/day	Growing per kg/day
Sodium (mg)	Parenteral	0-23	46-115	69-115 (161*)
	Enteral	0-23	46-115	69-115 (161*)
Potassium (mg)	Parenteral	0	0-78	78-117
	Enteral	0	0-78	78-117
Chloride (mg)	Parenteral	0-35.5	71-178	107-249
	Enteral	0-35.5	71-178	107-249
Calcium (mg)	Parenteral	20-60	60	60-80
	Enteral	33-100	100	100-220
Phosphorus (mg)	Parenteral	0	45-60	45-60
	Enteral	20-60	60-140	60-140
Magnesium (mg)	Parenteral	0	4.3-7.2	4.3-7.2
	Enteral	2.5-8	7.9-15	7.9-15
Iron (mg)	Parenteral	0	0	0.1-0.2
	Enteral	0	0	2-4
Zinc (µg)	Parenteral	0-150	150	400
	Enteral	0-1000	400-1200	1000-3000
Copper (µg)	Parenteral	0	≤20	20
	Enteral	0	≤150	120-150
Selenium (µg)	Parenteral	0	≤1.3	1.5-4.5
	Enteral	0	≤1.3	1.3-4.5

Adapted from Tsang RC, Uauy R, Koletzko B, et al, editors: *Nutrition of the preterm infant,* ed 2, Cincinnati, 2005, Digital Educational Publishing, pp 415-416.
Day 0 = day of birth.
Transition: The period of physiologic and metabolic instability following birth, which may last as long as 7 days.
*May need up to 160 mg/kg/day for late hyponatremia.

Table 7-5.	Estimation of the Energy Requirement of the Infant with Low Birth Weight.*
	Average Estimation, kcal/kg/day
Energy expended	40-60
Resting metabolic rate	40-50*
Activity	0-5*
Thermoregulation	0-5*
Synthesis	15†
Energy stored	20-30†
Energy excreted	15
Energy intake	90-120

Adapted from the Committee on Nutrition of the Preterm Infant, European Society of Paediatric Gastroenterology and Nutrition, Bremer HJ, Wharton BA: *Nutrition and feeding of preterm infants,* Oxford, 1987, Blackwell Scientific and American Academy of Pediatrics: *Pediatric nutrition handbook,* ed 6, Elk Grove Village, Ill, 2009, p 83.
*Energy for maintenance.
†Energy cost of growth.

and lipids providing NPCs as well as essential fatty acids is suggested.

When 60% to 63% of the NPCs given to LBW infants are derived from lipids, nitrogen retention is decreased and temperature control is adversely effected.[9] A moderate IV fat intake comprising approximately 35% of the NPCs is preferred.

There is a paucity of studies available to examine energy expenditure in VLBW infants on assisted ventilation. Technical difficulties and methodologic limitations affect interpretation of data. Leitch and Denne reviewed 12 studies, with 29 of 75 patients studied in the first 2 to 3 days of life.[10] Early studies suggest a mean energy expenditure of approximately 54 kcal/kg/day.[11,12]

Carbohydrates

Carbohydrates are the main energy substrate for the preterm infant receiving parenteral nutrition. At least at the outset, lipids play a minor role in supplying energy, although they play an important role at all times in providing essential fatty acids. Clearly, the infant must eventually transition to enteral feedings, which provide about half the energy from fat. However, while receiving TPN, carbohydrate remains the dominant energy substrate.

Glucose intolerance, defined as inability to maintain euglycemia at glucose administration rates of less than 6 mg/kg/min, is a frequent problem in VLBW infants, especially those weighing less than 1000 g. Hyperglycemia in VLBW infants may also occur with nonoliguric hyperkalemia.[13] These two comorbid conditions were frequently observed in ELBW infants before the practice of early initiation of amino acids. Endogenous glucose production is elevated in VLBW infants compared with term infants and adults.[14] Also, high glucose production rates are found in VLBW infants who received only glucose compared to those receiving glucose plus amino acids and/or lipids.[15] Clinical experience with glucose intolerance suggests that glucose alone does not always suppress glucose production in VLBW infants. It is not clear what circumstances or metabolic conditions lead to glucose intolerance. It appears likely, however, that persistent glucose production is the main cause, fueled by ongoing proteolysis that is not suppressed by physiologic concentrations of insulin. There is uncertainty whether abnormally low peripheral glucose utilization is also involved.

The glucose infusion rate should maintain euglycemia. Depending on the degree of immaturity (<26 weeks), 5% glucose or 10% glucose may be used. Another objective becomes the achievement of higher energy intakes. Glucose intolerance can limit delivery of energy to the infant to a fraction of the resting energy expenditure, leaving the infant in negative energy balance. Several strategies are used to manage this early hyperglycemia in ELBW infants: (1) decreasing glucose administration until hyperglycemia resolves (unless the hyperglycemia is so severe that this strategy would require infusion of a hypotonic solution); (2) administering IV amino acids, which decrease glucose concentrations in ELBW infants, presumably by enhancing endogenous insulin secretion; (3) initiation of exogenous insulin therapy at rates to control hyperglycemia[16,17]; and (4) using insulin to control hyperglycemia and to increase nutrient uptake.[18] The first and third strategies prevent adequate early nutrition and the safety of the last has been questioned in this population because of the possible development of lactic acidemia. Several studies have shown that insulin, used as a nutritional adjuvant, successfully lowers glucose concentrations and increases weight gain in preterm infants without

significant risk of hypoglycemia.[17,18] However, excessive energy is associated with increased fat accretion, not accompanied by lean mass or increase in head circumference, and little is known about its effects on counterregulatory hormone concentrations. A study examined the effect of insulin using a hyperinsulinemic-euglycemic clamp in ELBW infants receiving only glucose. These infants were normoglycemic before the initiation of insulin. They demonstrated a significant elevation in plasma lactate concentrations and the development of significant metabolic acidosis.[19]

The administration of amino acids early after birth appears to prevent the need for IV insulin, perhaps through stimulation of insulin by amino acids (e.g., arginine and leucine).[20] Improved glucose tolerance enables appropriate energy intake for growth. Therefore, amino acids are administered aggressively from the first hours of life to avoid the period of early neonatal malnutrition.

The human placenta actively transports amino acids to the fetus, and animal studies indicate that fetal amino acid uptake greatly exceeds protein accretion requirements. Approximately 50% of the amino acids taken up by the fetus are oxidized and serve as a significant energy source. Urea production is a by-product of amino acid oxidation. Relatively high rates of fetal urea production are seen in human and animal fetuses compared with the term neonate and adult, suggesting high protein turnover and oxidation rates in the fetus. Therefore, a rise in blood urea nitrogen, which is often observed after the start of TPN, is not an adverse effect or sign of toxicity in the absence of other signs of renal compromise or severe dehydration. Several controlled studies have demonstrated the efficacy and safety of amino acids initiated within the first 24 hours of life.[21-23] There were no recognizable metabolic derangements, including hyperammonemia, metabolic acidosis, or abnormal aminograms.

A strong argument for the early aggressive use of amino acids is the prevention of "metabolic shock." Concentrations of some key amino acids begin to decline in the VLBW infant from the time the cord is cut. This metabolic shock may trigger the starvation response, of which endogenous glucose production is a prominent feature. Irrepressible glucose production may be the cause of the so-called "glucose intolerance"

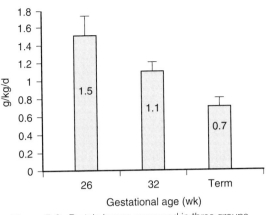

Figure 7-3. Protein losses measured in three groups of infants receiving glucose alone at 2 to 3 days of age. Protein losses are calculated from measured rates of phenylalanine catabolism. *(Adapted from Denne SC: Protein and energy requirements in preterm infants, Semin Neonatal 6:377, 2001.)*

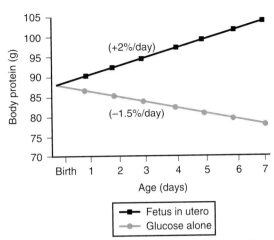

Figure 7-4. Change in body protein stores in a theoretical 26-week gestation, 1000-g premature infant receiving glucose alone with a fetus in utero. *(Adapted from Denne SC: Protein and energy requirements in preterm infants, Semin Neonatal 6:377, 2001.)*

that often limits the amount of energy that can be administered to the VLBW infant. It makes sense to smooth the metabolic transition from fetal to extrauterine life. Withholding TPN for days or even hours means unnecessarily sending the infant into a metabolic emergency. Thus, the need for parenteral nutrition may never be more acute than right after birth. It is noteworthy that Rivera et al. made the unexpected observation[24] that glucose tolerance was substantially improved in the group receiving early amino acids. Early amino acids may stimulate insulin secretion, consistent with the notion that forestalling the starvation response improves glucose tolerance. Recent data show that ELBW infants receiving earlier and higher dosages of amino acids (3 g/kg/day) had lower glucose levels than those receiving early amino acids but at lower dosages the first 5 days of life.[25]

Dose of Amino Acids

Figure 7-3 shows protein loss that occurs in mechanically ventilated, 26-week gestation 900-g–birth weight infants at 2 days of age who were receiving glucose alone.[26] Clinically stable 32-week gestation premature infants and normal term infants are also shown for comparison. It is clear that there is a significant effect of gestation on protein metabolism because the rate of protein loss in ELBW infants is twofold higher than in normal term infants.

The impact of this rate of protein loss is shown in Figure 7-4. At 26 weeks' gestation,

a 1000-g–birth weight infant begins with body protein stores of ~88 g. Without any protein intake, the infant loses more than 1.5% of body protein per day.[26] Compare this with the normal fetus who would accumulate body protein in excess of 2% per day. It is obvious that significant body protein deficits can accumulate rapidly in ELBW infants if early aggressive amino acid administration is not offered.

The first studies of early TPN used doses between 1 and 1.5 g/kg/day, an amount that will replace ongoing losses. Dosages have recently been increased toward 3 g/kg/day with initiation within hours of birth. Ultimate amino acid intake should be 3 g/kg/day; however, one can consider intakes of 3.5 to 4 g/kg/day for infants weighing less than 1200 g in situations where enteral feeds are extremely delayed or withheld for prolonged periods. A desirable protein to energy ratio is 25 kcal/kg for every gram of protein/kg or 2 to 3 mg/kg/min of glucose per gram of protein intake.

Protein quality, or amino acid composition, in parenteral nutrition can influence nitrogen utilization as well as the metabolic responses. Histidine is known to be necessary for protein synthesis and growth in the neonate but exact requirements are not known. Certain other amino acids are considered semi-essential or conditionally essential in that the capacity to synthesize them is limited in the preterm infant. Therefore, if these conditionally essential amino acids are not exogenously available or available only in limited amounts, the infant's requirements may not be met. Three of these semi-essential amino acids are cysteine, tyrosine, and taurine.

Cysteine is synthesized in vivo from methionine by the enzyme cystathionase. Because the hepatic activity of cystathionase has been found to be low or absent during fetal development and in the preterm and term neonate,[27] it has been considered an essential amino acid for the infant. Zlotkin and Anderson observed reduced hepatic cystathionase activity in preterm infants compared with full-term infants at the time of birth with the activity increasing in the preterm infant over the first month of life[28]; however, mature levels were not attained until approximately 8 months. When total cystathionase activity was estimated, which included the enzyme activity in the liver, kidneys, pancreas, and adrenal glands, they concluded that even the preterm infant has the capacity to endogenously produce adequate cysteine if adequate methionine is provided. In fact, increased parenteral methionine has been shown to increase urinary cysteine excretion. Supplementation of parenteral amino acid solutions with cysteine hydrochloride has not been shown to affect either nitrogen balance or growth in LBW infants. However, the two pediatric amino acid solutions, Trophamine (McGaw, Inc., Irvine, Calif) and Aminosyn-PF (Abbott Laboratories, Abbott Park, Ill), are low in methionine content, 81 and 45 mg/2.5 g of amino acids, respectively, and do not contain cysteine. Therefore, supplementation with cysteine hydrochloride is recommended.

Tyrosine, which is endogenously synthesized from phenylalanine through the activity of phenylalanine hydroxylase, has also been considered an essential amino acid; however, the enzyme activity is not low during development. The low plasma tyrosine concentrations seen in infants on tyrosine-free parenteral nutrition infusates appear to be independent of the plasma phenylalanine levels and not all infants on tyrosine-free parenteral nutrition solutions have low plasma tyrosine levels. In addition, extremely preterm infants have been shown to convert substantial quantities of phenylalanine to tyrosine.[29] Therefore, the requirement for an exogenous source of this amino acid remains uncertain.

Taurine, which is synthesized endogenously from cysteine, is a sulfur amino acid, which is not part of structural proteins but is present in most tissues of the body; it is particularly high in the retina, brain, heart, and muscle. The biological function of taurine in mammals includes neuromodulation, cell membrane stabilization, antioxidation, detoxification, osmoregulation, and bile acid conjugation; however, its conjugation with bile acids is the only adequately documented metabolic reaction in humans. Depletion of taurine during long-term parenteral nutrition has resulted in abnormal electroretinograms in children and auditory brainstem-evoked responses in preterm infants. Taurine supplementation of preterm infant formula has been shown to improve fat absorption, especially saturated fats, in LBW infants. Human milk is rich in taurine; infants fed human milk have higher plasma and urine concentrations of taurine than infants fed unsupplemented infant formula. Infant formulas and pediatric parenteral amino acid solutions are supplemented with taurine.

Currently, there are two kinds of crystalline amino acid solutions available for use in the neonate. The standard solutions originally designed for adults are often used for infants but are not ideal. The adult products contain little or no tyrosine, cysteine, or taurine, and contain relatively high concentrations of glycine, methionine, and phenylalanine. Because the plasma amino acid patterns reflect the amino acid composition of the amino acid solution infused, the resulting abnormal plasma amino acid levels could be potentially harmful. Hyperglycinemia, for example, may have adverse effects on the central nervous system because glycine is a potent neurotransmitter inhibitor. The pediatric amino acid solutions have a greater distribution of nonessential amino acids (particularly less glycine), greater amounts of branched-chain amino acids, less methionine and phenylalanine, and more tyrosine, cysteine, and taurine.

Studies of these products have demonstrated improved nitrogen retention and plasma aminograms resembling those of full-term breast-fed infants at 30 days of life.[27] However, studies of protein turnover and urea production (protein oxidation) have not shown any difference between Trophamine and other amino acid mixtures.[30] Because of the lower pH of the pediatric crystalline amino acid solutions, greater concentrations of calcium and phosphorous may be added without precipitation, which is an advantage particularly for the preterm neonate because the requirements for both minerals are quite high.[8]

Lipids

There are two roles for lipids as part of a TPN regimen. The first function is to serve as a source of linoleic acid. When used in small amounts, it can prevent or treat essential fatty acid deficiency. The second function is its use as an energy source. Larger quantities serve as a partial replacement for glucose as a major source of calories (Table 7-6).

The preterm neonate is especially susceptible to the development of essential fatty acid deficiency because tissue stores of linoleic acid are small and requirements for essential fatty acids are large because of rapid growth. The human fetus depends entirely on placental transfer of essential fatty acids. A VLBW infant with limited nonprotein calorie reserve must mobilize fatty acids for energy when receiving IV nutrition devoid of lipid. Studies in these infants confirm other studies that show essential fatty acid deficiency can develop in the VLBW infant during the first week of life on lipid-free regimens.

The importance of long-chain polyunsaturated fatty acids (LC-PUFAs) for the development of the brain and the retina has been recognized.[31,32] Infants are not capable of forming sufficient quantities of LC-PUFAs from the respective precursor fatty acids (linoleic and α-linolenic acids), and thus depend on an exogenous source of LC-PUFAs. Intravenous lipid emulsions contain small amounts of these fatty acids as part of the egg phospholipid used as a stabilizer.

The "routine" use of IV lipid emulsions has not been universally accepted in critically ill, ventilated VLBW infants because of potential complications. Hazards most pertinent to the ventilated VLBW infant include adverse effects on gas exchange and displacement of bilirubin from albumin. Both Brans and Adamkin found no difference in oxygenation between infants randomly assigned to various lipid doses (including controls without lipids) when using lower rates and longer infusion times of IV lipids.[33,34] The displacement of bilirubin from binding sites on serum albumin may occur even with adequate metabolism of infused lipid. In vitro, displacement of albumin-bound bilirubin by free fatty acids (FFAs) depends on the relative concentrations of all three compounds. An in vivo study has shown no free bilirubin generated if the molar FFA to albumin ratio is less than 6.[35] Data with lipid initiation at 0.5 g/kg/day of lipids in VLBW infants on assisted ventilation with respiratory distress syndrome showed a mean FFA to albumin ratio of less than 1. No individual patient value exceeded a ratio of 3 when daily doses were increased to 2.5 g/kg/day (in increments of 0.5 g/kg/day) over an 18-hour infusion time.[36] Other investigators found no adverse effect on bilirubin binding when lipid emulsion was infused at a dose of 2 g/kg/day over either 15 or 24 hours. Proper use includes slow infusion rates (≤0.15 g/kg/hr), slow increases in dosage, and avoidance of unduly high doses (e.g., >3 g/kg/day).

Concerns have been raised regarding the possible adverse effects of IV lipids on pulmonary function, but these have generally proved to be unfounded. For the late preterm infant with increased pulmonary vascular resistance (PVR) and respiratory disease, however, it appears that a more prudent approach with IV lipids should be taken. Significant concerns have been raised because of the high polyunsaturated fatty acid (PUFA) content of lipid emulsions as excessive omega 6 (linoleic acid, 18:2ω6)

Table 7-6.	Composition of Intravenous Lipid Emulsions				
Product	**Oil Base**	**Linoleic Acid (%)**	**Linolenic Acid (%)**	**Glycerin (%)**	**Osmolarity (mOsm/L)**
Intralipid*	100% Soybean	44-62	4-11	2.25	260
Nutrilipid†	100% Soybean	49–60	6-9	2.21	315
Soyacal‡	100% Soybean	49-60	6-9	2.21	315
Liposyn III§	100% Soybean	54.5	8.3	2.5	284

*KabiVitrum, Alameda, Calif. Data from product insert.
†McGaw, Inc., Irvine, Calif.
‡Alpha Therapeutic, Los Angeles, Calif.
§Abbott Laboratories, Abbott Park, Ill. Data from product insert.
Other sources: *Drug facts and comparisons*, St. Louis, 1990, JB Lippincott.

acids are required substrates for arachidonic acid pathways which lead to synthesizing prostaglandins and leukotrienes (Fig. 7-5).[37] It is speculated the IV lipid infusion may enhance thromboxane synthesis activity, which increases thromboxane production.[38] The prostaglandins may cause changes in vasomotor tone with resultant hypoxemia.[39,40] In addition, the production of hydroperoxides in the lipid emulsion also might contribute to untoward effects by increasing prostaglandin levels.[40-42]

Although there is no firm evidence of the effects of lipid emulsions in infants with severe acute respiratory failure with or without pulmonary hypertension, it appears prudent to avoid high dosages in these patients. For those with respiratory diseases without increased pulmonary vascular resistance, provide IV lipids at a dosage to prevent essential fatty acid deficiency. For those with elements of persistent pulmonary hypertension (PPHN), avoidance of lipids during the greatest labile and critical stages of their illness should be considered. When the infant is more stable, IV lipids at a modest dosage can be initiated.

Common practice is to begin IV lipids on the second day of life following initiation of amino acids shortly after delivery. Starting dose is 0.5 g/kg/day or 1.0 g/kg/day. Plasma triglycerides are monitored after each increase in dose and levels are maintained less than 200 mg/dL. A 20% lipid emulsion is used exclusively with an infusion rate less than or equal to 0.15 g/kg/hr. Therefore, a dose of 3 g/kg/day would be infused over 24 hours.

Lipid emulsions are supplied as either 10% or 20% solutions, providing 10 or 20 g of triglyceride/dL, respectively. Both contain the same amount of egg yolk phospholipid emulsifier (approximately 1.2 g/dL) and glycerol (approximately 2.25 g/dL). However, each contains more phospholipid than is required to emulsify the triglyceride. The excess is formed into triglyceride-poor particles with phospholipid bilayers called liposomes. For any given dose of triglyceride, twice the volume of 10% emulsion must be infused compared with the 20% emulsion. Therefore, for a fixed amount of triglyceride, the 10% emulsion provides at least twice and perhaps up to four times the amount of liposomes as the 20% emulsion. The 10% emulsion has been shown to be associated with higher plasma triglyceride concentrations and an accumulation of cholesterol and phospholipid in the blood of the preterm infant, probably because of the higher phospholipid content. LBW infants infused with lipids at 2 g/kg/day of 10% emulsion had significantly higher plasma triglycerides, cholesterol, and phospholipids than infants infused with 4 g lipid/kg/day as 20% emulsion. It is speculated that the excessive phospholipid liposomes in the 10% emulsion compete with the triglyceride-rich particles for binding to lipase sites, resulting in slow triglyceride hydrolysis. It is, therefore, recommended that 20% lipid emulsions be used for the LBW and VLBW infants.

Adverse side effects of IV lipid emulsions have been reported, including displacement of indirect bilirubin from albumin-binding sites, increasing the risk of kernicterus, suppression of the immune system, coagulase-negative staphylococcal and fungal infection,[43] thrombocytopenia, and accumulation of lipids in the alveolar macrophages and capillaries, subsequently altering pulmonary gas exchange.[44] As noted earlier, because FFAs compete with bilirubin for binding to albumin, the use of IV lipid emulsions in jaundiced newborns has been questioned. However, it is more a theoretical concern, in that FFA concentrations do not reach high enough levels to cause displacement of bilirubin and increase free bilirubin to a very high range. Careful monitoring of plasma triglycerides has been suggested when lipids are administered to babies with hyperbilirubinemia.

There may be a beneficial effect of infusing lipids. Infusion of lipid emulsion exerts

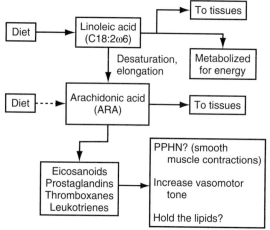

Figure 7-5. Metabolic derivatives of linoleic acid and ARA, *PPHN*, Persistant palmonary hypertension. *(Adapted from Adamkin DH: Nutrition in very very low birth weight infants,* Clin Perinatol *13[2]:419, 1986.)*

a beneficial effect on the vascular endothelium of peripheral veins leading to longer venous patency time. Malhotra et al. noted that hyperbilirubinemic infants given a lipid infusion of 1 to 2 g/kg/day had a significant increase in lumirubin,[45] a water-soluble structural isomer of bilirubin that can be excreted in the bile without hepatic conjugation. Therefore, IV lipid infusions may enhance the effect of, and may be a useful adjunct to, phototherapy.

Suppression of immune function and increased risk of sepsis have been associated with the use of IV lipid emulsions. Diminished motility and metabolic activity of polymorphonuclear (PMN) leukocytes exposed to fat emulsion in vitro have been reported. However, this could not be demonstrated in vivo in full-term and preterm infants given lipid 0.5 to 3 g/kg/day over 16 hours. On the contrary, some aspects of PMN migratory properties and their oxidative metabolism improved during the study period, most likely the result of chronologic and functional maturity.[46] There have been reports of fungal infections with *Malassezia furfur* and coagulase-negative staphylococci associated with lipid administration.[43] Freeman and colleagues have reported that 56.6% of all cases of nosocomial bacteremia in two neonatal intensive care units in Boston were highly correlated with lipid administration.[43] However, they stress that the benefits derived from the lipids outweigh the apparent risk of infection.

Carnitine
Carnitine is an essential cofactor required for the transport of long-chain fatty acids (LCFAs) across the mitochondrial membrane for β-oxidation. Because the preterm infant is born with limited carnitine reserves and low plasma carnitine levels develop when parenteral nutrition is not supplemented with carnitine, several investigators have suggested adding carnitine to parenteral nutrition with lipids for preterm infants.[47,48] Addition of supplemental carnitine does increase oxidation of fat and circulating ketone body levels and results in increased tolerance to IV lipids. However, data on increase in weight gain and nitrogen retention are not as convincing.[49] Therefore, carnitine is recommended only for LBW infants who require prolonged (over 2 to 3 weeks) parenteral nutrition. IV carnitine dosage has been used at 8 to 10 mg/kg/ without any observable side effects.[50]

PARENTERAL VITAMINS
The parenteral multivitamin guidelines proposed by the American Medical Association have been accepted for the pediatric formulation. A special committee of the American Society for Clinical Nutrition made recommendations for a new multivitamin preparation specifically for the preterm infant.[8] Although no preparation meets these guidelines, the committee recommends that MVI-Pediatric (Armour Pharmaceutical, Kankakee, Ill) should be used for preterm infants at 40% of a vial (or 2 mL) per kilogram body weight per day, not to exceed a total daily dose of one vial (5 mL); infants and children should receive one vial (5 mL) daily (see Table 7-2).

Intravenous vitamins, especially vitamin A, riboflavin, ascorbic acid, and pyridoxine, may be lost through adherence to the plastic tubing or through photodegradation caused by light exposure. There is often high light intensity in a special care nursery and the TPN fluid in the tubing moves slowly; therefore, it is exposed to light for prolonged periods. For these reasons, vitamins are added to the TPN shortly before infusing and some nurseries have the TPN bags and infusion tubings covered with foil or opaque material to minimize light exposure.

TRACE MINERALS
Because the infant has minimal endogenous stores, trace minerals are added to the TPN solution (see Table 7-4). The need for iron supplementation should be evaluated. Intravenous iron should be used with caution because excess iron can easily be given and may result in iron overload, increased risk of gram-negative septicemia, and an increase in the requirement for antioxidants, especially vitamin E.[8]

CALCIUM, PHOSPHORUS, MAGNESIUM, AND VITAMIN D
Preterm infants require increased intakes of calcium and phosphorus for optimal bone mineralization. The intrauterine accretion rates for calcium in the last trimester range from 104 to 125 mg/kg/day at 26 weeks' gestation to 119 to 151 mg/kg/day at 36 weeks' gestation; phosphorus accretion rate is 63 to 86 mg/kg/day. These levels of calcium and phosphorus intake cannot be attained with conventional TPN solutions because they would be insoluble. The pediatric crystalline amino acids solutions, however, have a lower pH, especially when cysteine

hydrochloride is added; therefore, greater concentrations of calcium and phosphorus can remain in solution.

VLBW infants should receive 60 to 80 mg/kg/day of calcium, 45 to 60 mg/kg/day of phosphorus, 4 to 7 mg/kg/day of magnesium, and 25 IU of vitamin D.[8] A calcium-to-phosphorus ratio of 1.3 to 1 is suggested, although others have noted improved mineral retention with a 1.7 to 1 ratio. These high calcium and phosphorus infusions should be given through a central venous line and not through a peripheral line.

PRACTICAL HINTS FOR FLUID AND TPN MANAGEMENT

- During the first few days of life, provide sufficient fluid to result in urine output of 1 to 3 mL/kg/hour, a urinespecific gravity of 1.008 to 1.012, checking urine for sugar and protein at the same time, and a weight loss of approximately 5% or less in full-term and approximately 15% or less in VLBW infants.
- Weigh infants twice a day the first 2 days of life, then daily thereafter to accurately monitor input and output.
- Use birth weight to calculate intake until birth weight is regained.
- Record fluid intake, output, and weight.
- If the infant is hyperbilirubinemic, provide lipids 0.5 to 1 g/kg/day, maintaining a serum triglyceride no greater than 150 mg/dL. Serum triglyceride should be checked before the start of the first lipid infusion, as lipids are being advanced, and weekly thereafter.
- Aim for a parenteral nutrition goal of 90 to 100 kcal/kg/day and 2.7 to 3 g protein/kg/day with a nonprotein caloric-to-nitrogen ratio (NPC:N) of 150 to 250. The NPC:N ratio can be calculated as follows:

$$\frac{\text{lipid calories} + \text{dextrose calories}}{(\text{grams of protein})(0.16)} = \frac{\text{NPC}}{1 \text{ g N}}$$

ENTERAL NUTRITION

When parenteral nutrition is used exclusively for the provision of nutrients, morphologic, and functional changes occur in the gut with a significant decrease in intestinal mass, a decrease in mucosal enzyme activity, and an increase in gut permeability. The changes are due primarily to the lack of luminal nutrients rather than the TPN. The timing of the initial feedings for the preterm infant has been debated for nearly a century and remains controversial.[51] As suitable TPN solutions designed for neonates became available, many physicians chose to use parenteral nutrition alone in the sick, ventilated, preterm infant because of concerns about necrotizing enterocolitis (NEC). Total parenteral nutrition was thought to be a logical continuation of the transplacental nutrition the infants would have received in utero. However, this view discounts any role that swallowed amniotic fluid may play in nutrition and in the development of the gastrointestinal tract. In fact, by the end of the third trimester, the amniotic fluid provides the fetus with the same enteral volume intake and approximately 25% of the enteral protein intake as that of a term, breast-fed infant. Parenteral nutrition does little to support the function of the gastrointestinal tract. Enteral feedings have direct trophic effects and indirect effects secondary to the release of intestinal hormones. Lucas et al. demonstrated significant rises in plasma concentrations of enteroglucagon,[52] gastrin, and gastric-inhibiting polypeptide in preterm infants after milk feeds of as little as 12 mL/kg/day. Similar surges in these trophic hormones were not seen in IV-nourished infants.

Clearly, one of the important benefits of using TPN is that it allows feedings to be advanced slowly, which probably increases the safety of enteral feedings. However, how neonatologists feed VLBW neonates has traditionally been based on local practices and not subjected to rigorous scientific investigation.[53] Regardless of feeding strategy, the advancement of feedings has been based on the absence of significant pregavage residuals or greenish aspirates. According to Ziegler and others, gastric residuals are very frequent in the early neonatal period and are virtually always benign when not accompanied by other signs of gastrointestinal abnormalities, that is not associated with NEC.[53,54] One study demonstrated that in ELBW infants, excessive gastric residual volume either determined by percent of the previous feed or an absolute volume (>2 mL or >3 mL) did not necessarily affect feeding success as determined by the volume of total feeding on day 14.[55] Similarly, the color of the gastric residual volume (green, milky, clear) did not predict feeding intolerance.[56] Nonetheless, the volume of feeding on day 14 did correlate with a higher proportion of episodes of zero gastric residual volumes and with predominantly milky gastric residuals. Thus, isolated findings related to gastric emptying alone should not be the sole criterion in initiating or advancing feeds. Stooling pattern, abdominal distention, and the nature of the stools should also be considered.[53]

The etiology of NEC remains unclear. Because NEC rarely occurs in infants who are not being fed, feedings have come to be seen as the cause of NEC. The pathophysiology of NEC is incompletely understood. However, intestinal immaturity, abnormal microbial colonization and a highly immunoreactive intestinal mucosa appear to be leading elements of a multifactorial cause. The association between feedings and NEC is likely to be explained by the fact that feedings act as vehicles for the introduction of bacterial or viral pathogens or toxins. They are more likely to survive the gastric barrier because of low acidity, against which the immature gut is poorly able to defend itself. Efforts aimed at minimizing the risk of NEC have focused on the time of introduction of feedings, on feeding volumes, and on the rate of feeding volume increments. One by one, the strategies that had been developed with the aim of reducing the risk of NEC were shown to be ineffective.

One of the main strategies involved the withholding of feeding for prolonged periods of time. Although it was never shown that the prolonged withholding of feedings actually prevented NEC, some form of the strategy was widely adopted in the 1970s and 1980s. The withholding of feedings eventually came under scrutiny and was compared in a number of controlled trials with early introduction of feedings.[57] A systematic review of the results of these trials concluded that early introduction of feedings shortens the time to full feeds, as well as the length of hospitalization, and does not lead to an increase in the incidence of NEC. A controlled study involving 100 VLBW infants confirmed these findings and found, in addition,[58] a significant reduction of serious infections when feedings were introduced early. Another strategy aimed at preventing NEC has been to keep the rate increments low. The strategy was based on the findings of Anderson and Kliegman,[58] who in their retrospective analysis of 19 cases of NEC, found that in infants who went on to develop NEC, feedings were advanced more rapidly than in control infants without NEC. Based on these findings, they recommended

that feedings not be advanced by more than 20 mL/kg each day.[58] This recommendation has found wide acceptance, although its validity has not been confirmed in randomized controlled trials. In a prospective randomized trial, Rayyis et al. compared increments of 15 mL/kg/day with increments of 35 mL/kg/day.[59] They found that with fast advancement, return to birth weight occurred earlier; full intakes were achieved sooner; weight gain set in earlier; and there was no difference in the incidence of NEC. Whether it protects against NEC or not, limiting feeding increments in VLBW infants to 20 mL/kg/day has become acceptable practice. It still permits achievement of full feedings in a reasonable period (about 8 days). When initiating early enteral feedings in infants with umbilical artery catheters (UACs) in place, safety is often a concern. The presence of a UAC has been associated with an increased risk for NEC, and it is a common nursery policy to delay feedings until catheters are removed. However, few data from controlled studies support this policy. Davey et al. examined feeding tolerance in 47 infants weighing less than 2000 g at birth who had respiratory distress and UACs.[60] Infants were assigned randomly to begin feedings as soon as they met the predefined criterion of stability or to delay feeding until their UACs were removed for 24 hours. Infants who were fed with catheters in place, started feeding significantly sooner and required half the number of days of parenteral nutrition. The incidence of NEC was comparable for infants fed with catheters in place and those whose catheters were removed before initiation of feedings. In addition, large epidemiologic surveys have not shown a cause-and-effect relation between low-lying umbilical artery catheters and NEC.[53,54]

The decision when to start these early enteral or trophic feeds may be influenced by what milk is available to feed the infant. Lucas and Cole,[61] in a multicenter feeding trial involving nearly 1000 preterm infants with birth weights less than 1850 g, demonstrated that the incidence of confirmed NEC was six times greater in formula-fed infants than in those receiving exclusive human milk. In addition, NEC was rare for infants greater than 30 weeks' gestation who were fed exclusively human milk, but this was not the case for formula-fed babies. A delay of feeding in the formula-fed group was associated with a reduced risk of NEC, whereas the use of early human milk feedings versus delaying had no correlation with the occurrence of NEC. Therefore, initiating feeds for individual patients should take into account individual risk factors and the milk available for the infant.

Feedings should be started within the first days of life. A frequently encountered problem is that breast milk takes at least 2 days to come in and often does not come in for 3, 4, or 5 days. During that time, only small amounts of colostrum are available, which is very beneficial to the infant and must be fed. Gastric residuals should not interfere with feeding. Initial feeding volumes should be kept low (1 to 2 mL/feed) and provided at 3-hour intervals. Incremental advances should be about 20 mL/kg/day when a decision is made to advance feedings.

For ELBW infants on life support with invasive monitoring, one may introduce trophic feedings with 1 mL/feed every 8 hours for a period of a few days and then proceed as above. Each nursery should establish criteria for feeding readiness. These may include normal blood pressure and pH, PaO_2 greater than 55, at least 12 hours from last surfactant or indomethacin dose, normal gastrointestinal exam, heme-negative stools, and fewer than two desaturation episodes (SaO_2 less than 80%) per hour. Collectively, these signs are a surrogate for establishing "physiologic" stability prior to feeding initiation.

CARBOHYDRATE

Carbohydrate provides 41% to 44% of the calories in human milk and most infant formulas. In human milk and standard infant formulas, it is present as lactose, which has been shown to enhance calcium absorption. In soy and other lactose-free formulas, the carbohydrate is in the form of sucrose, maltodextrins, and glucose polymers (corn syrup solids or modified starches). The three major disaccharidases responsible for the digestion of disaccharides are lactase, maltase, and sucrase-isomaltase. Maltase and sucrase-isomaltase first appear at 10 weeks' gestation, reaching approximately 70% of newborn levels at 28 weeks' gestation. However, by 28 to 34 weeks' gestation, lactase has only 30% of the activity found in the term infant; babies born before this time may have relative lactase deficiency, resulting in lactose intolerance.

When lactose is not hydrolyzed in the small intestine, bacterial fermentation of the undigested portion occurs in the colon, producing short-chain fatty acids, which enhance mineral and water absorption and may stimulate growth and cell replication in the gut lumen. Thus, colonic salvage is apparently important in disposal of unabsorbed lactose; however, its exact quantitative contribution remains unknown. Colonic bacterial fermentation of unabsorbed lactose to absorbable organic acids enables the infant to reclaim this carbohydrate energy and appears to prevent clinical symptoms of diarrhea.

Although pancreatic α-amylase, the major enzyme in starch hydrolysis, is either absent or in very low concentrations in the first 6 months of life, newborns are capable of tolerating small amounts of starch without side effects and preterm infants are able to hydrolyze glucose polymers. Several enzymes may compensate for the physiologic pancreatic amylase deficiency in infancy. Glucoamylase, an enzyme found in the brush border of the small intestine, is present in the neonate in concentrations similar to those in adults. Also, salivary and human milk amylases may provide additional pathways for glucose polymer digestion in infancy.

Because lactase is found only at the tip of the villus, it is very sensitive to mucosal injury; therefore, lactose intolerance may develop in infants with diarrhea, those suffering from undernutrition, or those recovering from NEC, necessitating temporary use of a lactose-free formula. In contrast, glucoamylase is able to survive partial intestinal atrophy because it is located at the base of the villi, thus enabling glucose polymers to be an alternative carbohydrate source when enteritis is present and lactase may be found in low concentrations.

In premature infant formulas, lactose has been partially replaced by glucose polymers, polysaccharides with chains of 5 to 10 glucose residues joined linearly by 1,4-α linkages to decrease the osmolality of the formula and to decrease the lactose load in the diet. Glucose polymers are well tolerated by preterm infants with glucose and insulin responses similar to those of a lactose feeding.

PROTEIN

The protein requirement of the preterm infant is estimated to be 3.2 to 4.2 g/kg/day for VLBW infants and 3.5 to 4.4 g/kg/day for ELBW infants (Table 7-7). The quality and quantity of protein that the infant

Table 7-7. Recommended Nutrient Intakes for Very Low Birth-Weight Infants

		ELBW		Growing		VLBW		Growing	
		Day 0 per kg/day	Transition per kg/day	per kg/day	per 100 cal	Day 0 per kg/day	Transition per kg/day	per kg/day	per 100 cal
Energy (Cal)	Parenteral	40-50	75-85	105-115	100	40-50	60-70	90-100	100
	Enteral	50-60	90-100	130-150	100	50-60	75-90	110-130	100
Fluid (mL)	Parenteral	90-120	90-140	140-180	122-171	70-90	90-140	120-160	120-178
	Enteral	90-120	90-140	160-220	107-169	70-90	90-140	135-190	104-173
Protein (g)	Parenteral	2	3.5	3.5-4	3-3.8	2	3.5	3.2-3.8	3.2-4.2
	Enteral	2	3.5	3.8-4.4	2.5-3.4	2	3.5	3.4-4.2	2.6-3.8
Carbohydrate (g)	Parenteral	7	8-15	13-17	11.3-16.2	7	5-12	9.7-15	9.7-16.7
	Enteral	7	8-15	9-20	6-15.4	7	5-12	7-17	5.4-15.5
Fat (g)	Parenteral	1	1-3	3-4	2.6-3.8	1	1-3	3-4	3-4.4
	Enteral	1	1-3	6.2-8.4	4.1-6.5	1	1-3	5.3-7.2	4.1-6.5
Linoleic acid (mg)	Parenteral	110	110-340	340-800	296-762	110	110-340	340-800	340-889
	Enteral	110	110-340	700-1680	467-1292	110	110-340	600-1440	462-1309
Docosahexaenoic acid (mg)	Parenteral	≥4	≥4	≥11	≥10	≥4	≥4	≥11	≥12
	Enteral	≥4	≥4	≥21	≥16	≥4	≥4	≥18	≥16
Arachidonic acid (mg)	Parenteral	≥5	≥5	≥14	≥13	≥5	≥5	≥14	≥16
	Enteral	≥5	≥5	≥28	≥22	≥5	≥5	≥24	≥22

Adapted from Tsang RC, Uauy R, Koletzko B, et al, editors: *Nutrition of the preterm infant: scientific basis and practical guidelines*, ed 2, Cincinnati, 2005, Digital Educational Publishing, pp 415-416.
Day 0 = Day of birth.
Transition: The period of physiologic and metabolic instability following birth, which may last as long as 7 days.
Linoleate: linolenate: 5-15 for all phases.

receives are important. Although weight gain and growth of LBW infants fed protein intakes of 2.2 to 4.5 g/kg/day of either a casein- or whey-predominant formula have been shown to be no different from those receiving pooled human milk, the metabolic responses can be significantly different. Serum BUN, ammonia, albumin, and plasma methionine and cysteine concentrations were higher in the infants receiving high-protein formulas. Elevated levels of phenylalanine and tyrosine were seen in infants fed the casein-predominant, high-protein formula and lower concentrations of taurine were noted in infants fed casein-predominant formulas regardless of quantity. Preterm infants fed soy protein formula supplemented with methionine exhibit slower weight gain and lower serum protein and albumin concentrations than infants fed a whey-predominant formula. Thus, premature infant formulas are whey-predominant with a 60 to 40 whey-to-casein ratio; soy protein-based formulas are not recommended for the preterm infant.[62]

Human milk is considered to have the ideal amino acid distribution for the human infant. Preterm infants fed their own mother's milk have more rapid growth than infants fed pooled, banked human milk with accretion of protein and fat similar to that of the fetus.[63] Human milk is lower in mineral content, especially magnesium, calcium, phosphorus, sodium, chloride, and iron. To attain intrauterine growth rates, large volumes (180 to 200 mL/kg/day) of human milk must be fed.

To improve growth and bone mineralization, human milk fortifiers have been developed; VLBW infants fed their own mother's milk with human milk fortifier added have improved growth and higher serum albumin, transthyretin (prealbumin), and phosphorus concentrations than those receiving their mothers' milk unfortified. Absorption and retention of nutrients is similar to that in infants fed preterm infant formula. The recommended dietary allowances for infants and children to age 12 months are listed in Table 7-8.

LIPIDS

Fat is a major source of energy for the infant, with approximately 50% of the calories in human milk derived from fat. The preterm infant has limited capacity to digest and absorb certain fats. Because of a limited bile salt pool and lower levels of pancreatic

Table 7-8.	Dietary Reference Intakes (DRIs): Recommended Intakes for Infants	
Nutrients	**0-6 Months**	**7-12 Months**
Protein, g/kg/day	1.52	**1.05**
Carbohydrate, g/day	60*	95*
Fat, g/day	31*	30*
Linoleic acid, g/day	4.4*	4.6*
Sodium, mg/day	120*	370*
Potassium, mg/day	400*	700*
Chloride mg/day	180*	570*
Calcium mg/day	210*	270*
Phosphorus, mg/day	100*	275*
Magnesium, mg/day	30*	75*
Iron, mg/day	0.27*	**11**
Zinc, mg/day	2*	**3**
Copper, mcg/day	200*	220*
Selenium, mcg/day	15*	20*
Vitamin A, mcg/day	400*	500*
Vitamin D, IU/day	200*	200*
Vitamin E, mg/day	4*	5*
Vitamin K, mcg/day	2*	2.5*
Thiamin, mcg/day	200*	300*
Riboflavin, mcg/day	300*	400*
Niacin, mg/day	2*	4*
Vitamin B_6, mcg/day	100*	300*
Folate, mcg/day	65*	80*
Vitamin B_{12}, mcg/day	400	500
Pantothenic acid, mg/day	1.7*	1.8*
Biotin, mcg/day	5*	6*
Vitamin C, mg/day	40*	50*

Source: http://www.iom.edu/CMS/3788/21370.aspx and American Academy of Pediatrics: *Pediatric nutrition handbook,* ed 6, Elk Grove Village, Ill, 2009, pp 1294-1296.
*The AI (Adequate Intake) represents the mean intake for healthy breast-fed infants.
Bold Type: RDAs (Recommended Dietary Allowances) RDAs are set to meet the needs of 97% to 98% of individuals in a group.

lipase, preterm infants malabsorb long-chain triglycerides (LCTs), the majority with chain lengths of 14 to 20 carbons.

Human milk contains a bile salt-activated lipase that enhances lipid digestion in the duodenum. Standard infant formulas contain LCTs, which may be poorly digested by the premature infant, producing calcium soaps in the gut that render the calcium unavailable for absorption.

Because of the relatively poor digestion of LCTs, a theoretically attractive alternative is use of medium-chain triglycerides (MCTs), oils with a carbon chain length of 8 to 12 carbons. Unlike LCTs, MCTs do not require bile for emulsification. MCTs are rapidly hydrolyzed in the gut and pass directly to the liver through the portal circulation, whereas LCFAs must be reesterified once absorbed and are transported via the lymph system into the blood circulation where they are hydrolyzed by lipoprotein lipase. Medium-chain fatty acid (MCFA) metabolism differs from that of LCFA in that it does not require carnitine for transport into the mitochondria and is not regulated by cytosolic acyl-CoA synthetase. MCFAs enter the mitochondria directly and are rapidly oxidized. Formulas with MCTs have been shown to improve nitrogen, calcium, and magnesium absorption. Preterm infant formulas have been developed with approximately half the fat as MCTs.

VITAMIN A

At birth, preterm infants less than 36 weeks' gestational age have been reported to have lower plasma retinol concentrations as compared with full-term infants, although the measured levels are quite variable. There is a further decrease in the plasma retinol and retinol-binding protein levels during the first 2 weeks after birth, particularly when sufficient amounts of vitamin A are not provided. The measured hepatic levels of retinol expressed as µmol/g in preterm infants are reported to be the same as in infants born at term gestation but lower than those in older children and adults. The recommended allowance for infants, based on the average retinol content of human milk (40 µg/100 mL) and average daily milk consumption, corresponds to 420 µg of retinol per day up to 6 months of age.

Retinol has been shown to be essential for the growth and differentiation of epithelial cells, has been suggested to have a role in prevention and repair of lung injury and vitamin A deficiency state, and is associated with histopathologic changes in the lung similar to those seen in bronchopulmonary dysplasia (BPD). Furthermore, infants dying of BPD were reported to have lower liver retinol ester levels. For these reasons, the impact of vitamin A supplementation on BPD in VLBW infants has been examined.[64,65] In a multicenter, blinded, randomized trial, the use of vitamin A 5000 IU (1.5 mg) administered intramuscularly three times per week for 4 weeks improved the biochemical vitamin A status and resulted in a modest advantage in relation to prevention of chronic lung disease.[65] Vitamin A in such large doses was shown to have no clinically measurable toxic effects. In a metaanalysis of seven randomized trials, results suggested that supplementation with vitamin A resulted in reduction of death or oxygen requirement at 1 month of age and oxygen requirement at 36 weeks post-menstrual age (chronic lung disease) as well as trends toward reduction in oxygen requirement in survivors at 1 month of age.[66]

VITAMIN E

Vitamin E, or tocopherol, serves as an antioxidant to protect double bonds of cellular lipids. Vitamin E requirements are increased with increasing polyunsaturated fatty acid (PUFA) intake and in the presence of oxidant stress, such as high iron intake. Vitamin E deficiency is rarely seen in infants because infant formulas are supplemented with vitamin E in proportion to the PUFA content. However, infants who are breastfed and receiving supplemental iron should be given additional vitamin E. Preterm infants have low serum vitamin E levels and may be at increased risk for oxidative damage to cell membranes. Studies to investigate the effectiveness of pharmaceutical doses of vitamin E on retinopathy of prematurity and BPD have not demonstrated benefits of this therapy. Supplemental vitamin E given during the first week of life may play a role in the prevention of intracranial hemorrhage in infants, especially those weighing 500 to 750 g.[67] Further studies need to be conducted before this becomes routine care for the ELBW infant. An increased risk of sepsis and NEC was seen in a group of VLBW infants whose serum vitamin E levels were maintained over 3 mg/dL.[68] According to the American Academy of Pediatrics, serum vitamin E concentrations should be maintained between 1 and 2 mg/dL.[69]

VITAMIN K

Vitamin K, an important cofactor in the activation of intracellular precursor proteins to blood clotting proteins, is synthesized endogenously by bacterial flora. However, because intestinal synthesis cannot be relied on because of a lack of gut colonization in the neonate, it is recommended that 0.5 to 1 mg of vitamin K be given to all newborns as protection against hemorrhagic disease of the newborn. Preterm infants may be at particular risk for vitamin K deficiency because of low stores and frequent use of broad-spectrum antibiotics. In addition, asphyxiated infants have been shown to have a reduction in vitamin K-dependent coagulant proteins.

Human milk is generally low in vitamin K, and intestinal flora of breast-fed infants may produce less vitamin K than formula-fed infants. Therefore, antibiotic therapy may increase the risk of vitamin K deficiency in breast-fed infants by decreasing endogenous synthesis.

CALCIUM, PHOSPHORUS, MAGNESIUM, AND VITAMIN D

The amount of enteral calcium, phosphorus, and magnesium intake required to match intrauterine accretion rates is high: calcium 185 to 200 mg/kg/day, phosphorus 100 to 113 mg/kg/day, and magnesium 5.3 to 6.1 mg/kg/day. VLBW infants with minimal illness may require lower intakes.[70] The American Academy of Pediatrics recommends intakes of calcium of 185 to 210 mg/kg/day, phosphorus 123 to 140 mg/kg/day, and magnesium 8.5 to 10 mg/kg/day. However, magnesium intake at this level with such high calcium and phosphorus intake results in negative magnesium balance; therefore, a higher intake of magnesium, approximately 20 mg/kg/day, may be needed.[71]

The recommendation for vitamin D, which is required for normal metabolism of calcium, phosphorus, and magnesium, has ranged from 200 to 2000 IU per day for the preterm infant. VLBW infants can maintain normal vitamin D status with 400 IU/day; high-dose vitamin D supplementation does not decrease the incidence of rickets in VLBW infants.

Human milk has concentrations of calcium and phosphorus that are appropriate for full-term infants. These amounts are inadequate for the VLBW infant. Breast milk should be supplemented with additional calcium, phosphorus, and vitamin D, which can easily be done with human milk fortifiers. Fortification yields better mineral accretion than breast milk alone, similar to that of VLBW infants fed a premature infant formula.[63]

Inadequate intakes of calcium, phosphorus, and vitamin D result in metabolic bone disease of prematurity, also called rickets of prematurity. This disease is characterized by reduced bone mineralization and, in severe cases, frank radiologic evidence of rickets and spontaneous fractures. The biochemical findings, although not highly sensitive, include an elevated alkaline phosphatase (>500 U/L), decreased serum phosphorus (<4 mg/dL), and normal serum calcium; 25-hydroxycholecalciferol (25-OH vitamin D)

level is usually normal, but 1,25 dihydroxycholecalciferol (1,25-OH vitamin D) levels may be elevated as a result of increased parathyroid hormone levels and low serum phosphorus levels. The incidence of rickets was high before institution of the current nutrient practice of higher calcium and phosphorus levels in parenteral nutrient solution and early enteral feedings. The etiology of rickets remains unclear but is thought to be primarily an inadequate intake of calcium and phosphorus. Risk factors for rickets are listed in Box 7-3. Confirming the diagnosis requires radiologic evidence of osteopenia.

Fortified human milk or premature infant formula is the preferred feeding for LBW infants. The use of soy formulas is not recommended for infants with birth weight less than 1800 g. If continuous infusion feeding of human milk is necessary, the syringe and the pump should be placed upright to prevent loss of calcium, phosphorus and milk fat by separation and adherence to the tubing.

WATER SOLUBLE VITAMINS

Vitamin B_{12} requires intrinsic factor for its absorption in the distal ileum; therefore, particular attention to this vitamin is necessary in infants who have had gastric resection or resection of the terminal ileum (e.g., NEC surgery). The potential neurologic complications of vitamin B_{12} deficiency are irreversible.

Serum folate levels may be low in the preterm infant. Folate is supplemented in the pediatric IV multivitamin preparation (MVI-Pediatric) and in infant formulas. It is not available in the infant multivitamin drops because of its instability in the liquid form. Folate plays an important role in DNA synthesis; deficiency of this vitamin may result in megaloblastic anemia, neutropenia, thrombocytopenia, and growth failure. Requirements for water-soluble vitamins

Box 7-3.	Risk Factors for Metabolic Bone Disease of Prematurity

Extremely low birth weight (≤1000 g)
Prolonged parenteral nutrition
Unsupplemented human milk
Use of elemental formulas and soy formulas
Chronic diuretic therapy (especially furosemide)
Chronic problems such as necrotizing enterocolitis, bronchopulmonary dysplasia, cholestasis, and acidosis

in VLBW and ELBW infants are shown in Table 7-3. Advisable intakes for infants 0 to 12 months are shown in Table 7-8.

IRON

There has been increased interest in iron deficiency, with the data suggesting that mental and developmental test scores are lower in infants with iron deficiency anemia and that iron therapy sufficient to correct the anemia is insufficient to reverse the behavioral and developmental disorders in many infants.[72,73] This indicates that certain ill effects are persistent depending on the timing, severity, or degree of iron deficiency anemia during infancy.

Iron stores in the preterm infant are lower than in the term baby because iron stores are relatively proportional to body weight.[74] Iron depletion occurs around the time the baby doubles her/his birth weight and thus iron therapy should begin by 4 weeks of life in the preterm infant when enteral feedings are tolerated. Smaller preterm infants may need as much as 4 to 6 mg/kg/day, with about 2 mg/kg/day provided by iron-fortified formula and the remainder as iron supplementation at 2 to 4 mg/kg/day. A higher dose is also necessary for infants being given erythropoietin. Oral iron supplementation can interfere with vitamin E metabolism in the LBW infant,[72] thereby further increasing the need for vitamin E in an infant who is at risk for low serum tocopherol levels. Although premature infant formulas, both with and without iron fortification, are manufactured with ample amounts of vitamin E and a PUFA-to-E ratio of 6 or greater, premature infants on human milk and receiving supplemental iron can be also supplemented with 4 to 5 mg (6 to 8 IU) of vitamin E per day. This can be readily accomplished by use of an oral multivitamin with iron.

The impression that low-iron formulas are associated with fewer gastrointestinal disturbances is not supported by controlled studies. Because the bioavailability of iron from iron-fortified infant cereals is somewhat low, it is recommended that iron-fortified formulas or daily iron supplements be continued through the first year of life.[72]

Among term infants, breast feeding usually provides adequate iron intake during the first 4 to 6 months of life and supplementation during this time is not necessary. Although the iron content of human milk is low, averaging 0.8 mg iron/L, the bioavailability is high, with term infants absorbing about 49% of the iron content compared with 10% to 12% from iron-fortified cow's milk formula. Infants who are breast fed exclusively can maintain normal hemoglobin and ferritin levels, and do not need iron supplementation until 4 to 6 months.

FLUORIDE

Due to reports of dental fluorosis in infants and toddlers, fluoride supplementation is no longer recommended in the infant younger than 6 months of age. The supplementation schedule (Table 7-9) recommended by the American Academy of Pediatrics and the American Dental Association should be followed according to the fluoride content of the local water supply.[75]

GROWTH IN THE NEONATAL INTENSIVE CARE UNIT INFLUENCES NEURODEVELOPMENTAL AND GROWTH OUTCOMES

A multicenter cohort study from the NICHD included 600 infants with birth weights from 501 to 1000 g. These infants were stratified by 100-g–birth weight increments and divided into quartiles based on in-hospital growth velocity rates.[76] As the rate of weight gain increased between quartile 1 and quartile 4, from 12 to 21.2 g/kg/day, the incidence of cerebral palsy, Bayley II Mental Developmental Index (MDI) scores of less than 70, Psychomotor Developmental Index (PDI)

Table 7-9.	Dietary Reference Intake for Fluoride	
Age Group	**Adequate Intake (mg/day)**	**Tolerable Upper Intake (mg/day)**
Infants 0-6 mo	0.01	0.7
Infants 7-12 mo	0.5	0.9
Children 1-3 yr	0.7	1.3
Children 4-8 yr	1	2.2
Children 9-13 yr	2	10
Boys 14-18 yr	2	10
Girls 14-18 yr	3	10
Males 19 yr and older	4	10
Females 19 yr and older	3	10

Data from Institute of Medicine: *Dietary reference intakes for calcium, phosphorous, magnesium, vitamin D, and fluoride,* Washington, DC, 1997, National Academies Press and American Academy of Pediatrics: *Pediatric nutrition handbook,* ed 6, Elk Grove Village, Ill, 2009, p 1050.

scores of less than 70, abnormal neurologic examination findings, neurodevelopmental impairment, and need for rehospitalization fell significantly at 18 to 22 months corrected age. Similar findings were observed as rate of head circumference growth increased from 0.67 to 1.12 cm/week. Also, higher inhospital growth rates were associated with a decreased likelihood of anthropometric measurements below the 10th percentile at 18 months' corrected age. The influence of growth velocity remained after controlling for variables known at birth or identified during the infants' neonatal intensive care unit hospitalizations that affect outcome including comorbid conditions such as NEC or BPD. This study emphasizes the importance of closely monitoring the rate of in-hospital growth when birth weight has been regained. Goals for growth including head circumference gain of more than 0.9 cm/week and weight gain of 18 g/kg/day from return to birth weight through discharge were associated with better neurodevelopmental and growth outcomes. If growth rates falter, the infants' diets should be reviewed to ensure adequate nutritional support including protein/energy ratios of feeds and the use of caloric dense milks (>24 kcal/ounce).

METHOD OF FEEDING

An important consideration in feeding the newborn is the development of sucking, swallowing, gastric motility, and emptying. Swallowing is first detected at 11 weeks' gestation and the sucking reflex is first observed at 24 weeks' gestation. However, a coordinated suck-swallow is not present until 32 to 34 weeks' gestation and even then, it is immature; the maturation of the swallowing reflex is related to postnatal age. Swallowing must be coordinated with respiration, in that the two processes share the common channels of the nasopharynx and laryngopharynx. The inability of the infant to coordinate this action results in choking, aspiration of feedings, and vomiting.

To evaluate the suck-swallow reflex, one should observe the number of swallows per second. An infant with a good suck-swallow reflex swallows approximately once per second. If greater than 2 per second are observed, the infant is probably not able to coordinate the swallowing. With a good suck, the temporal muscle will bulge.

When starting to introduce the nipple, a rule of thumb is to bottle feed for 20 minutes then gavage the remainder. At first, the infant may be offered nipple feeding once in a 24-hour period; the number of feedings is then increased as the infant becomes more able to nurse. Because of the additional work of sucking, the energy expenditure increases; therefore, an increased calorie intake may be required to maintain adequate rate of growth. Weight gain during the start of nipple feeding should be closely monitored. It is not necessary for an infant to be able to bottle feed before attempting to breast feed. Infants who will be breast feeding may actually be able to nurse from the breast sooner than they will be able to coordinate bottle feeding. If an infant's respiratory rate is 70 to 80 breaths per minute or more, he or she should be tube fed because of the increased risk of aspiration.

If an infant is unable to nipple feed, he or she needs to be fed through an orogastric or nasogastric tube or, rarely, transpylorically. Intragastric tube feedings are preferable in that it allows for normal digestive processes and hormonal responses. The acid content of the stomach may impart bactericidal effects; other benefits of intragastric tube feeding include ease of insertion of tube, tolerance of greater osmotic loads with less cramping, distention, and diarrhea, and less risk of development of dumping syndrome. Continuous transpyloric feeding is rarely used in infants who cannot tolerate feedings because of impaired gastric emptying or a high risk of aspiration. However, this route of infusion has a higher risk of perforation of the gut, may not enable delivery of a large volume of feedings, and may result in inefficient nutrient assimilation because bypassing the gastric phase of digestion limits the exposure of food to acid hydrolysis and the lipolytic effects of lingual and gastric lipases.

If tube feeding is used, the decision to feed intermittently or continuously must be made. There are differences seen in the endocrine milieu between infants fed continuously compared with those fed intermittently. The significance of these differences is unclear and it is not possible to state with certainty which method is best for the prematurely born neonate. It has been suggested that the cyclic changes in circulating hormones and metabolites as seen in intermittent-bolus feeding may have quite different effects on cell metabolism,[77] gall bladder emptying, and gut development. Continuous infusion of human milk is not recommended because there is a loss of fat and, therefore, calories, in the tubing of the pump. Additionally, at the end of the infusion, a large bolus of fat is delivered to the infant owing to the separation of the fat during the infusion period.

Gastrostomy feedings are chosen when it becomes apparent that there will be long-term tube feeding (e.g., for a neurologically impaired infant), when there is persistent gastroesophageal reflux that is unresponsive to medical treatment, or when esophageal anomalies prevent the use of an orogastric or nasogastric tube.

Positioning of the infant during feeding is important for more efficient stomach emptying. Infants with respiratory distress fed in the supine position have delayed gastric emptying. The stomach empties more rapidly in the prone or right lateral positions; thus, these positions are preferred especially in infants with respiratory distress and in those infants who have the potential for feeding intolerance.

The evaluation of an infant's feeding tolerance is an ongoing process to determine the appropriate feeding method, type of formula to feed, and increment of feeding advancement. Vomiting, abdominal distention, significant gastric residuals, abnormal stooling patterns, and presence of reducing substances or frank or occult blood in the stool are indicators of intolerance. Sepsis and NEC may first manifest with one or more of these signs of feeding intolerance. Vomiting or spitting in the high-risk infant increases the risk of aspiration.

NONNUTRITIVE SUCKING

Nonnutritive sucking, that is, placing a nipple or pacifier in the infant's mouth, has been related to accelerated weight gain and early hospital discharge in preterm infants. Reported benefits of nonnutritive sucking include improved oxygenation, accelerated maturation of sucking reflex, decreased intestinal transit time, and accelerated transition from gavage to oral feeding. Ernst and colleagues conducted a randomized trial in medically stable infants receiving tube feedings,[78] controlling for caloric intake, birth weight, and sex of the infant, and found no difference in growth, gastrointestinal transit time, fat excretion, or energy expenditure. Even so, providing a pacifier to a tube-fed infant may well give the infant great comfort and enable the infant to calm more quickly.

HUMAN MILK

Although breast milk is considered the ideal food for the term infant, for the preterm infant it provides inadequate amounts of several nutrients, especially protein, vitamin D, calcium, phosphorus, and sodium. If given in sufficiently large volume (180 mL/kg/day), the energy content of human milk is sufficiently great to enable nearly all LBW infants to gain weight at intrauterine rates (approximately 15 g/kg/day). However, the protein content is suboptimal, especially for VLBW infants weighing less than 1500 g, resulting in lower serum albumin and transthyretin (prealbumin) levels, which have been shown to be reliable indicators of protein nutriture in preterm infants.[79] The calcium and phosphorus content is low in unsupplemented human milk in comparison to that required to achieve intrauterine accretion rates, resulting in poor bone mineralization in VLBW infants. In addition, the sodium content of human milk results in less sodium retention than intrauterine estimates and may result in hyponatremia.

In a large multicenter study on the short- and long-term clinical and developmental outcomes of infants randomized to different diets, Lucas and colleagues found that, by the time infants weighing less than 1200 g at birth who were fed unfortified human milk reached 2 kg,[3,80] they were less than 2 standard deviations below the mean for weight for age. Infants weighing less than 1 kg at birth who were fed unfortified human milk would be expected to take 3 weeks longer to reach a weight of 2 kg than infants receiving formula. In a later nonrandomized study, Lucas et al. observed that infants receiving breast milk had a significantly higher intelligence quotient at 8 years than formula-fed infants.[4]

The probability that human milk may have certain nonnutritional advantages must also be considered. Human milk contains immunocompetent cellular components including secretory IgA, which has a protective effect on the intestinal mucosa.

Since the composition of preterm milk varies greatly from one mother to another and the concentration of nutrients in preterm milk changes over time, it is difficult to determine the actual macronutrient intake of an infant. However, new technology (infra-red spectrophotometry) allows accurate bedside analysis of the macronutrients in human milk. To confer the potential nonnutritional advantages yet provide optimal nutrient intake, human milk should be supplemented, or fortified, with protein, calcium, phosphorus, vitamin D, and sodium.

There are many practical considerations when feeding an LBW infant with his or her own mother's milk. One of the common concerns is to provide sufficient volumes of bacteriologically acceptable milk. The practice of culturing human milk before its first use and weekly thereafter remains controversial. Refrigerated breast milk actually decreases in bacterial content over a 5-day period, and fresh frozen milk inoculated with bacteria demonstrated significant inhibition of bacterial growth. Many mothers are unable to maintain adequate milk production even with frequent milk expression with an electric breast pump. The assistance of a health professional trained to counsel and support breast-feeding mothers may increase success rates within the hospital.

It is difficult for the mothers of ELBW infants to provide sufficient volumes of milk to meet their infant's needs over the entire hospitalization. Therefore, pasteurized human milk from donor milk banks and industry have become available as a potential proxy for the mother's own milk.[81] The studies showing a lower rate of NEC with donor milk were conducted before the use of human milk fortifiers. Many of these infants suffered growth failure and osteopenia of prematurity secondary to inadequate protein, calcium and phosphorous in donor milk.

Recently, a randomized controlled multicenter trial to evaluate an exclusively human milk diet in extreme premature infants (500 to 1250-g birth weight) was done and was the first to use a human milk-based fortifier.[83] Three study groups received on average 70% of their feeds as mother's own milk. One group of infants received mother's milk fortified with powdered bovine fortifier. When mother's milk was unavailable, these infants received preterm formula. The other two groups were fed donor pasteurized milk when the mother's own milk was not available and were fortified with human milk fortifier.[83] The rates of NEC (medical and surgical) were lower in the exclusively human milk fed infants, who only differed in the volume of human milk they were receiving at time of fortification. There was a 50% reduction in medical NEC and almost a 90% reduction in surgical NEC for the infants fed an exclusive human milk diet compared to a diet containing bovine milk-based products.[83]

Data like these and others suggest that exclusive human milk diets may exert protective effects,[84,85] rather than threshold effects with respect to NEC. Therefore, the feeding of a species-specific milk may be critical for protection against infection and NEC.

A new therapy under investigation is the use of lactoferrin in these VLBW infants to prevent late-onset sepsis and NEC. A recombinant human lactoferrin product is being evaluated for its safety and efficacy and is now in Phase 2 trials.

A multicenter, double-blind, placebo controlled, randomized trial was done in VLBW infants in Italy comparing administration of a bovine lactoferrin (BLF) alone or in combination with *Lactobacillus rhamnosus* GG (LGG) to placebo.[86] Invasive infections (blood or cerebrospinal fluid or peritoneal fluid) were significantly lower in the treatment groups (5.9% for BLF and 4.6% for BLF plus LGG versus 17% for placebo).[86] The incidence of NEC was decreased in the BLF plus LGG group (0% versus 6% in infants receiving placebo).[86]

FORMULA TYPES

To be able to select the proper formula for feeding a sick infant, a clear understanding of the differences between formulas and unique qualities of a given formula is necessary (Table 7-10).

PREMATURE INFANT FORMULAS

Providing optimal nutrition to a preterm infant is complicated by a lack of a natural standard. For the healthy full-term infant, human milk is considered the ideal food; therefore, it is used as the reference standard for the development of commercial infant formulas. Although early milk of mothers who deliver their infants prematurely is higher in nitrogen (early in lactation), fatty acid content, sodium, chloride, magnesium, and iron, it is still inadequate in other nutrients, especially calcium and phosphorus. It, therefore, cannot be used as a standard for the development of premature infant formula. The special premature infant formulas have been developed from knowledge of the accretion rates of various nutrients relative to the reference fetus, from studies of the development of the gastrointestinal tract that have defined absorptive efficiency and function, and from metabolic studies.

Premature infant formulas have a lower lactose concentration with approximately

Table 7-10. Comparison of Human Milk and Formula							
NUTRIENTS	**Preterm Human Milk***	**Premature Infant Formula**	**Premature Postdischarge Formula**	**Term Human Milk**	**Term Infant Formula**	**Term Infant Soy Formula**	**Term Infant Lactose-Free Formula**
Energy (kcal/oz.)	20-28	24	22	20	20	20	20
Protein (g/dL)	1.4-1.6	2.4	2.1	1.03	1.4-1.6	1.6-1.8	1.4-1.5
Source	Whey-predominant	60:40	60:40 or 50:50	Whey-predominant	60:40 or 18:82	Soy protein isolate	Milk protein isolate
Fat (g/dL)	2.9-4.3	4.1-4.4	3.9-4.1	4.4	3.4-3.7	3.4-3.7	3.6-3.7
Source	Human milk	MCT Soy Coconut	MCT SoyCoconut	Human milk	Palm Soy Coconut HOSO	Palm Soy Coconut HOSO	Palm Soy Coconut HOSO
Carbohydrate (g/dL)	6.3-7.1	8.4-9	7.7-7.9	6.9	7.1-7.4	7-7.4	7.2-7.4
Source	Lactose	Lactose, CSS, glucose polymers	Lactose, glucose polymers, maltodextrin, CSS'	Lactose	Lactose	CSS, sucrose	CSS, sucrose
Calcium (mg/dL)	24-34	134-146	78	32	52-55	70-71	55-57
Phosphorus (mg/dL)	6.8-11.8	67-81	46-49	14	28-31	42-51	31-38
Iron (g/dL)	0.03	1.4-1.5	1.3	0.03	1.2	1.2	1.2

From Tsang RC, Uauy R, Koletzko B, et al, editors: *Nutrition of the preterm infant: scientific basis and practical guidelines*, ed 2, Cincinnati, 2005, Digital Educational Publishing, p 336 and American Academy of Pediatrics: *Pediatric nutrition handbook*, ed 6, Elk Grove Village, Ill, 2009, Author, pp 1250-1265.
CSS: Corn syrup solids; HOSO: high oleic safflower oil; MCT: medium chain triglycerides.
*Preterm, mature milk (days 22-30).

50% of the carbohydrate as lactose to reduce the lactose load because of relative lactase deficiency. The remainder of the carbohydrate is provided as glucose polymers, which are readily hydrolyzed by glucoamylase and result in a product with low osmolality.

The premature infant formulas are whey-predominant, which has been shown to result in less metabolic acidosis in VLBW infants. The risk of lactobezoar formation is reduced when a whey-predominant formula is used. In addition, the concentration of protein per liter is approximately 50% greater than that of standard infant formula to provide 3.6 to 4.2 g protein/kg/day. The fat is approximately 50% LCTs and 50% MCTs. The vitamin concentration is higher because the volume of formula consumed is significantly less in the tiny baby. The calcium and phosphorus content is greater than standard formula with variation between formula manufacturers. The calcium-to-phosphorus ratio generally is 2 to 1 as compared to 1.4 to 1 to 1.5 to 1 with standard infant formulas. Too high of a concentration of calcium and phosphorus may result in intestinal milk bolus obstruction. As with all formulas, it is important to shake the formula before use, because precipitation may occur and the precipitate, containing high amounts of calcium and phosphorus, may remain in the bottom of the container.

Premature infant formulas have always been low in iron content (3 mg elemental iron/L) because these infants were often receiving transfusions and because the use of iron would increase the requirement for vitamin E. However, because some infants are receiving this type of formula for greater than 2 months and because the advantages of continuing a baby on premature infant formula after hospital discharge have been recognized, premature infant formulas have been available with low iron content (3 mg elemental iron/L) and with iron fortification (15 mg elemental iron/L).

The sodium content of premature infant formula is greater than human milk or standard infant formula. Because sodium requirements vary considerably between infants and are influenced by receipt of diuretics, this amount may be inadequate to maintain normal serum levels. Supplementation with 3% sodium chloride (0.5 mEq sodium and chloride/mL) may be necessary. Because this is a highly osmolar solution (see Table 7-4), the dose should be divided and administered several times throughout the day. One distinct advantage of premature infant formula is that, despite the high concentration of nutrients, the 24-calorie/oz. premature infant formula is iso-osmolar with osmolalities ranging from 280 to 300 mOsm/kg H_2O.

Preterm infants fed human milk have advanced neurodevelopmental outcome as compared to formula-fed infants, measured by electroretinograms, visual evoked potentials, and psychometric tests.[31,87-89] The better performance, in part, has been related to dietary docosahexaenoic (DHA) and arachidonic (ARA) acids because plasma and erythrocyte phospholipid, contents of ARA and DHA are higher in breast-fed infants than in infants fed formulas lacking these fatty acids.[90] Inadequate long-chain fatty acids in the diet may be related to performances on tests of cognitive function.[4,91] The inability to synthesize enough DHA and ARA from their precursors and the lack of preformed DHA may be the cause of lower content of these fatty acids in formula-fed infants. The addition of these fatty acids to formulas in the United States has led to renewed interest and debate about the effects of long-chain fatty acids on later neurodevelopmental outcome and has been reviewed elsewhere.[92]

STANDARD INFANT FORMULAS

The carbohydrate in standard infant formula is 100% lactose and the fat is all long-chain triglycerides of vegetable origin, usually soy and coconut oils. Most standard formulas are whey-predominant, with 60% of the protein whey and 40% casein. Standard formulas are available in iron-fortified and non–iron-fortified (or "low iron") forms. Iron-fortified formula contains elemental iron 12 mg/L or approximately 2 mg/kg/day for an infant receiving approximately 108 kcal/kg/day. Low-iron formula contains elemental iron 1.5 mg/L or 0.2 mg/kg/day.

Most standard infant formulas are available as ready-to-feed, liquid concentrate, and powder. The concentrate and the powder provide the option of concentrating the formula to a higher caloric density. Concentrations above 1 calorie per milliliter or 30 calories per ounce are not recommended because of the high renal solute load that results from the decrease in free water intake. As the formula is concentrated, the osmolality increases to approximately the same degree as the concentration. Thus, for a 20 kcal/oz formula with an osmolality of 300 mOsm/kg H_2O, if concentrated 135%, or to 27 kcal/oz formula, the osmolality increases to approximately 405 mOsm/kg H_2O. If formula is to be concentrated, a written recipe should be given to the caregiver because over-concentration may be hazardous to small preterm infants.

Caloric density of a formula may also be increased by the addition of glucose polymers, which increases the osmolality of the formula, or by adding fat (e.g., vegetable oil, MCT oil). However, when an infant formula is supplemented with calories only, the intake of nutrients must be calculated and compared with recommended guidelines (see Tables 7-3, 7-4 and 7-7) to ensure adequacy of intake. The distribution of calories will be affected using this method of increasing calories; therefore, the percent of calories from carbohydrate, protein, and fat should be determined. Approximately 35% to 65% of the total calories should be derived from carbohydrate, 30% to 55% from fat, and 8% to 16% from protein. LBW infants fed a formula contributing 7.8% of calories as protein grew at a significantly slower rate than infants fed formulas with either 9.4% or 12.5% of the calories from protein.

SOY FORMULAS

Soybean-based formulas with soy protein isolate or soybean solids with added methionine as the protein source are lactose-free and, therefore, are recommended for infants with galactosemia, with primary lactase deficiency, or recovering from secondary lactose intolerance. The carbohydrate is provided as sucrose or corn syrup solids, or as a combination of the two. The fat is provided as a vegetable oil (LCTs), usually soy and coconut oils. All soy formulas are iron-fortified. Although soy formulas have been used when cow's milk protein allergy is suspected, the American Academy of Pediatrics cautions that infants allergic to cow's milk may also develop an allergy to soy-based milk[62]; a protein hydrolysate formula should be the initial formula of choice. Infants with a family history of allergy who have not shown clinical manifestations may benefit from soy protein formula; however, such infants should be closely monitored for soy protein allergy. Soy protein formulas are appropriate for infants of vegetarian families who eat no animal products.

The use of soy protein formulas for VLBW infants is not recommended because of the low calcium and phosphorus content of these formulas. Preterm infants fed soy protein formulas have significantly lower serum phosphorus and serum alkaline phosphatase levels and an increased risk of development of osteopenia. Even when supplemented with additional calcium, phosphorus, and vitamin D, VLBW infants fed these formulas exhibit slower weight gain and lower serum protein and albumin concentrations than infants receiving a whey-predominant premature infant formula.

PROTEIN HYDROLYSATE FORMULAS

Protein hydrolysate formulas are designed for infants who are allergic to cow's milk or soy proteins. Some protein hydrolysate formulas are also elemental with the carbohydrate in easily absorbable forms, such as glucose polymers or monosaccharides, and the fat as both medium-chain and long-chain triglycerides. These are sometimes used in the management of infants with intestinal resection or intractable diarrhea.

FOLLOW-UP FORMULAS

Although considerable attention has been directed toward improving the nutrition of hospitalized VLBW infants with nutrient-enriched formulas and multinutrient fortifiers for human milk, only recently has attention been paid to nutrition support of such infants after hospital discharge. The first postnatal year may provide an important opportunity for human somatic and brain growth to compensate for earlier deprivation. A key question is whether VLBW infants have special nutrient requirements in the post-discharge period. In more biological terms, it is reasonable to ask whether this period is also critical for later health and development because it is common for human milk fortifiers to be stopped or term formulas to be substituted at hospital discharge. Available data suggest that preterm infants are in a state of suboptimal nutrition at the time of discharge from the hospital and beyond. Improving this situation would be beneficial in the short-term and, potentially, for longer-term health and development.

Nutrient-enriched formula for preterm infants after hospital discharge (post-discharge formula) is generally intermediate in composition between preterm and term formulas. Compared with term formula, preterm formula contains an increased amount of protein with sufficient additional energy to permit utilization. Post-discharge formula contains extra calcium, phosphorus, and zinc, all of which are necessary to promote linear growth. Additional vitamins and trace elements are included to support the projected increased growth. A pilot study of 32 preterm infants was the first to show that infants randomized to receive the post-discharge formula up to 9 months postterm showed significantly greater weight and length gains and had higher bone mineral content in the distal radius than infants who received a standard term formula.[93] Studies add additional insight into the role for post-discharge formula, suggesting that benefits may be related to birth weight,[94] gender,[2,95,96] and a "window of opportunity" (a critical growth epoch) when supplemental nutrients can promote catch-up and subsequent growth, even after discontinuation of post-discharge formula. The reports also raise the possibility that post-discharge nutrition may benefit long-term development.[95,96]

A total of 284 preterm infants received either term formula or post-discharge formula for the first 9 months postterm. At 9 months postterm, post-discharge formula-fed infants were significantly heavier (mean difference, 370 g) and longer (1.1 cm) than term formula-fed infants, and the length difference persisted to 18 months postterm or 9 months after post-discharge formula was discontinued. Differences between diet groups were significantly greater in boys, who had a length advantage of 1.5 cm at 18 months if they received post-discharge formula. There was no evidence that the post-discharge formula had made infants fat. Their mean weight percentile was still below the 50th percentile and skinfold thickness was not increased. Head circumference and developmental outcomes at 9 or 18 months did not differ significantly between groups, although post-discharge formula-fed infants had a 2.8 ± 0.25 point advantage in the Bayley MDI Score.[96] Carver found improved growth in preterm infants who were fed a post-discharge formula after discharge up to 12 months corrected age, with the significant differences in weight, length, or head circumference.[2] This was more pronounced for smaller infants (birth weight <1250 g) and male infants. The differences in growth produced by post-discharge formula occurred early (critical growth epoch) but did not increase appreciably over time, suggesting that the benefit of post-discharge formula with respect to catch-up occurred soon after discharge. The benefits persisted throughout the period of observation and, for infants whose birth weights were less than 1250 g, growth in head circumference was the most beneficial effect.

Another study examined the use of preterm formula after discharge in 129 preterm infants randomly assigned to one of three dietary regimens until 6 months postterm: term formula, preterm formula, or preterm formula until term followed by term formula to 6 months.[95] Males fed preterm formula after discharge showed significantly greater weight and length gain and larger head circumference by 6 months postterm than those fed term formula throughout the study period. Infants fed preterm formula consumed an average of 180 mL/kg/day, resulting in a protein intake of approximately 4 g/kg/day. Those fed term formula took more milk and increased consumption to about 220 mL/kg/day, but their protein intake still did not match that of the preterm formula group. At 18 months postterm, boys previously fed preterm formula were on average 1 kg heavier, 1 cm longer, and had 1 cm greater head circumference than those fed term formula. Body composition measurement using dual x-ray absorptiometry suggested that the additional weight gain was composed predominantly of lean tissue rather than fat.[97] There were no significant differences in neurodevelopment measured using Bayley Scales of Infant Development at 18 months.[95]

Randomized studies demonstrate that the use of either preterm formula or post-discharge formula after discharge in preterm infants results in improved growth, with differences in weight and length persisting beyond the period of intervention in two studies. Such findings raise the hypothesis that nutrition during the post-discharge period may have longer-term effects on growth trajectory. Evidence from three randomized trials suggests that the effect of a nutrient-enriched post-discharge diet is greatest in boys, possibly reflecting their higher growth rates and protein requirements. Whether the observed growth effects persist or have consequences for other aspects of health or development requires further investigation.

PRACTICAL HINTS FOR ENTERAL NUTRITION

- Start small breast milk or formula feedings (10 to 20 mL/kg/day) as soon as possible. It is unnecessary to start with 5% glucose water.

- Assess the infant's ability to nipple feed. Infants younger than 32 weeks' gestational age and infants with respiratory rates between 60 and 80 breaths per minute need to be tube fed.
- Use premature infant formula or fortified breast milk for infants weighing less than 1800 g. Encourage the mother to provide human milk. If breast milk is to be used, start feedings with unfortified breast milk until tolerance is established, then add fortifier.
- Intermittent gavage feedings are preferred; continuous feedings or "compressed" feedings over an hour or so may be helpful for infants with feeding intolerance.
- Monitor feeding tolerance. Vomiting, a sudden increase in abdominal girth, frank or occult blood in the stool, with large gastric residuals may be signs of infection or NEC. The feedings should be stopped, the stomach should be aspirated, and an #8 Fr nasogastric tube should be inserted for gastric decompression.
- Record fluid intake, output, weight, type of feeding given, and feeding tolerance.
- Reduce parenteral feedings proportionate to the increase of enteral feedings to prevent excess fluid intake.
- Increase feedings at a rate of 20 mL/kg/day and monitor tolerance to previous volume before increasing rate. Feed the infant in a prone position to facilitate gastric emptying and maintain better oxygenation. Once the infant is receiving 90 to 100 mL/kg/day enterally, the TPN should be discontinued; if greater fluid volume is required, provide it as an IV glucose-electrolyte solution.
- Aim for a goal of 110 to 130 kcal/kg/day and 3.5 to 4 g protein/kg/day with a weight gain of approximately 15 to 18 g/kg/day.
- Offer a pacifier to the infant, especially while being gavage fed.

- Encourage the parents to feed the infant after the infant is feeding well; it may be very frustrating for the parents to attempt feeding when the infant is resistant.

NUTRITIONAL ASSESSMENT

An in-depth nutritional assessment requires anthropometric, biochemical, dietary, and clinical data. However, interpreting anthropometric and biochemical measurements is difficult; therefore, nutritional assessment in neonates receiving intensive care treatment is often confined to detecting fluctuations in weight gain and in caloric intake. Nonetheless, it is necessary for the clinician to be able to assess the neonate's nutritional status because of the potentially serious sequelae of malnutrition on multiple organ systems and the importance of growth (especially brain growth) on developmental outcome.

In nutritional assessment, one must consider the length of gestation and adequacy of intrauterine growth and nutrient tolerance. There should be a static assessment (current balance between intake and output) as well as a dynamic assessment (evaluation of infant's growth over time or growth velocity) of each infant. Also, the non-nutritional factors such as disease state, medication, and stress (e.g., infection and surgery) must be considered.

Weight gain is the most frequently used anthropometric measure. It is important to use the same scale, obtain weight measurements at the same time each day to avoid diurnal changes, and indicate any equipment being weighed (especially arm boards and dressings); if equipment is not recorded, changes in weight may be spurious. In preterm infants, weight gain should be expressed on a gram per kilogram per day basis. Table 7-11 contains suggested weight gain goals.

When assessing weight, there are several problems to consider. In the first week

Table 7-11.	Growth Velocity of Preterm Infants from Term to 24 Months (Range includes ±1 SD)		
Age from Term (mo)	Weight (g/day^{-1})	Length (cm/mo^{-1})	Head Circumference (cm/mo^{-1})
1	26-40	3-4.5	1.6-2.5
4	15-25	2.3-3.6	0.8-1.4
8	12-17	1-2	0.3-0.8
12	9-12	0.8-1.5	0.2-0.4
18	4-10	0.7-1.3	0.1-0.4

Adapted from Theriot L: Routine nutrition care during follow-up. In Groh-Wargo S, Thompson M, Cox JH, editors: *Nutrition care for high risk newborns*, Chicago, 2000, Precept Press, p 570.

of life, all newborns lose weight as a result of loss of free water and low intake; however, most preterm infants are also calorie and fluid restricted during that period as a result of illness, so that it may be difficult to separate changes in growth measurements caused by diuresis from those caused by poor protein-calorie intake. Weight gain does not necessarily reflect growth, which is a deposition of new tissue of normal composition; weight increase may reflect excessive fat deposition or water retention, neither of which is truly growth.

Length measurements are the most inaccurate anthropometric measurement. Accurate technique is important in performing length measurements to detect small changes. Two trained individuals are needed to measure the infant on a measuring board containing a stationary head board, movable foot board, and a built-in tape measure. Skeletal growth is often spared relative to weight in mildly malnourished infants; therefore, initially, linear growth is often slow or stops. Serial length measures obtained weekly are helpful in assessing nutritional status when plotted over time; length measures are especially useful in infants, such as those with BPD, whose weight fluctuates greatly. A gain in length of 1 cm per week is expected.

Increase in head circumference (HC), the measurement of the largest occipitofrontal circumference, correlates well with cellular growth of the brain in normal infants. During acute illness, the velocity of head growth for the sick preterm infant is less than that of the normal fetus. During recovery, head growth parallels that of normal fetal growth and subsequently rapid "catch-up" growth in HC may occur. Normal growth does not occur until the acute illness has resolved, despite high energy intake. Preterm infants who were calorically deprived for the longest periods showed slower growth rates and longer duration of catch-up growth. In this respect, the longer these infants remain with suboptimal head size, the greater is their developmental risk.

HC is usually measured once a week using a paper tape; a new tape should be used for each infant. A goal of about 0.9 cm per week is to be expected. If hydrocephalus is of concern, more frequent measuring is warranted. The initial HC may differ from subsequent measurements because of molding of the head. Measuring HC may be difficult because of interfering equipment such as IV lines on the scalp. Serial weight, length,

and HC measurements should be plotted on an appropriate growth chart. Daily weights may be plotted on a number of charts.[98,99] The Fenton growth curve is used most often now.[100]

Skinfold measures of several sites have been used to estimate body fat stores and the percent of body fat in children and adults. These determinations are made by using a variety of formulas that are based on the assumption that the percent of total body water and fat distribution remains constant. In the neonate, these assumptions are not valid because the percent age of body water decreases with increasing gestational age and postnatal age and fat increases with increasing gestational age.

The biochemical assessment of nutritional status may be more specific than anthropometric measures and may be useful in combination with anthropometric indices for nutritional assessment of the sick neonate. Many routine tests may signal nutrition-related problems. For example, an elevated alkaline phosphatase level (>500 IU) and a low serum phosphorus level (<4 mg/dL) may occur during the active phase of rickets. This combination of biochemical findings indicates the need to obtain diagnostic x-ray studies. However, abnormal alkaline phosphatase levels may occur due to hepatic dysfunction; therefore, heat fractionation of the isoenzyme is suggested to determine its origin. As rickets begins to heal, the serum phosphorus levels normalize, whereas the alkaline phosphatase continues to be elevated during the radiographic picture of healing. Elevated alkaline phosphatase levels generally precede radiologic changes by 2 to 4 weeks.

Albumin is a serum protein commonly measured in routine laboratory tests. Although it has limited value for nutritional assessment, it may serve as an indicator of inadequate energy and protein intake. The average serum albumin concentration in infants younger than 37 weeks' gestation ranges from 2 to 2.7 mg/dL. This relative hypoalbuminemia of the preterm infant appears to be a result of a more rapid turnover of a small plasma pool versus a decreased rate of albumin synthesis; the half-life of albumin is approximately 7.5 days in the preterm infant versus 14.8 days in adults. Despite the relatively rapid turnover, serum albumin concentration changes slowly in response to nutrition rehabilitation.

To quickly assess response to nutrition support, a serum protein with a shorter half-life is necessary. Transthyretin (prealbumin), with a half-life of approximately 2 days in adults has been shown to be a suitable marker for evaluation of nutritional status in VLBW infants.[79] Because transthyretin increases with gestational age as well as with protein and energy intake, the direction of change in serial tests may be more useful than striving for absolute values.

Because of the various metabolic, renal, respiratory, and gastrointestinal abnormalities to which VLBW infants are subjected, close monitoring of blood gases, serum electrolytes, calcium, phosphorus, glucose, BUN, and creatinine is necessary. Ongoing nutritional assessment includes careful calculation of dietary intake relative to estimated requirements, determination of fluid balance and hydration status, and tolerance to feeding method. In combination with anthropometric, clinical, and biochemical data, adjustments in intake or method of nutrient delivery can be made to achieve effective nutritional support.

CASE A-1

M. J. is a former 1160-g, 28-week gestational age infant who is returning to the clinic at 5 months of age. He has gained weight at a rate of about 18 g/day over the past 2 months and currently weighs 4 kg. He is receiving 18 oz. of 24 calorie/oz. iron-fortified standard infant formula per day. His mother states he is a "good" eater; her friends advise her that he should be starting solid food. She wants to know what she should give him as his first feeding and how much she should give him.

Is this infant's growth appropriate?

Whenever assessing the growth of a former preterm infant, one must correct for gestational age at the time of birth. To correct, simply subtract the number of weeks preterm from the chronologic age. In this example, a former 28-week gestational age infant who is now 5 months old is, in fact, only 2 months corrected age (5 months chronologic age minus 3 months premature = 2 months corrected age).

If his weight is plotted on the Benda and Babson growth chart,[98] his weight of 4 kg at 2 months' corrected age places him 2 standard deviations below the mean or the third percentile. His average weight gain of 18 g/day would result in a weight gain to approximately 4.5 kg in 1 month, which, if plotted at 3 months' corrected age, would drop him below the third percentile.

What is his caloric intake? Is it sufficient?

M. J. is receiving 18 oz./day of 24-calorie/oz. formula, which provides a total daily caloric intake of 432 kcal or 108 kcal/kg/day. This is an appropriate intake for a former full-term infant; however, for M. J. it is inadequate to provide for catch-up growth. A weight gain of approximately 30 g/day, equivalent to the growth rate of a 2-month-old infant at the 50th percentile, would result in accelerated growth and weight gain of 900 g in the next month, which would place him above the 3rd percentile at 3 months. Additional calories and protein (i.e., use of post-discharge formula) need to be given to enable this kind of weight gain. Therefore, if the infant's intake can be increased to 21 oz. each day or the caloric concentration is increased to 27 calories/oz., an intake of 122 calories/kg/day would result, or an additional 56 calories/day. Because 1 g of mixed tissue growth requires approximately 4.5 extra calories,[55] in theory, it should result in an additional weight gain of 12 g/day. However, increasing protein is critical.

What other information would you like to know?

An accurate measure of linear growth using an infant measuring board and an occipitofrontal head circumference (HC) measurement is necessary for a more complete assessment of growth. HC should catch up by 8 months' corrected age, even if the weight and length are still suboptimal.

Information on vitamin supplementation also would be helpful. A vitamin supplement should be provided to infants whose enteral intake is less than 750 mL of 20-calorie/oz. formula or the equivalent in concentrated formula. This infant is receiving 540 mL/day of formula concentrated 120% (24 kcal/20 kcal = 1.2 × 100 = 120%) or the equivalent of the nutrients found in 648 mL of 20-kcal/oz. formula (18 oz. × 30 mL/oz. × 1.2 = 648 mL). If no vitamin supplements have been used, there may have been a period of inadequate vitamin intake; therefore, a supplement should be started and used over the next month. If a supplement has been used and if the formula is to be concentrated 135% to 27 kcal/oz. or the total volume per day is increased to 21 oz. of 24 kcal/oz. formula, this will provide the equivalent of approximately 750 mL of 20-kcal/oz. formula and the supplement may be stopped.

Should the mother start solid foods?

An infant at 2 months has low concentrations of pancreatic amylase and may not completely digest the starch present in cereal; the developmental readiness for solids is not yet present. The infant will still have a strong tongue thrust, which would push solid foods out of the mouth instead of to the back of the mouth in preparation for swallowing. Therefore, it should be recommended to this mother that she wait until the infant is 4 to 6 months' corrected age or 7 to 9 months' chronologic age before solids are begun. Some infants develop feeding aversions after extended periods of parenteral nutrition, tube feeding, and ventilatory support. In these infants, the introduction of solids should occur at 4 months' corrected age to provide the infant with ample time to learn to accept the spoon. An occupational or speech therapist may need to become involved to teach the caregivers techniques to use to stimulate feeding readiness.

PART TWO

SELECTED DISORDERS OF THE GASTROINTESTINAL TRACT

Avroy A. Fanaroff

Anomalies of the gastrointestinal tract may involve any part of the primitive tube from the hypopharynx to the anal dimple. The most common lesions are atresias, stenoses, duplications, and functional obstructions. Vascular occlusions, sometimes resulting from rotational anomalies and intussusceptions, may be in utero factors in atresias and stenoses. Presenting findings include the following:

- History of hydramnios
- Increased salivation, cyanosis, and choking with feedings
- Large gastric aspirate (>25 mL) in delivery room
- Vomiting, especially bile stained
- Abdominal distention with or without visible peristalsis
- Failure to pass a stool or delayed passage of stool

DEFINITIONS

Atresia is complete luminal discontinuity of the gastrointestinal tract, ranging from the shortest segment web to complete loss of a major segment of bowel and mesentery. Multiple atresias may occur throughout the intestinal tract, especially in the jejunoileal segments.

Stenosis is a narrowing that may involve the entire thickness of the bowel wall or may be merely a partial web.

Duplications may vary from simple cystlike projections into the mesentery to complete replication of any length of the gastrointestinal tube, with or without luminal continuity with the in-line segment. They may occur anywhere along the gastrointestinal tract and manifest as obstructions, as perforations, or simply as a palpable mass.

Functional obstructions are those that are not associated with anatomic malformation. They include achalasia, pyloric stenosis, and aganglionic megacolon, all of which have some component of myoneural dyscoordination in their etiologies. Other functional obstructions, such as meconium ileus and meconium plug syndrome, are caused by abnormalities of intraluminal contents.

Understanding of the basic entities and familiarity with some essential principles help to differentiate the lesions. The following basic principles are helpful when considering neonatal and infant bowel problems:

- Intestinal obstruction may be anticipated in 1 of every 1000 births. Multiple anomalies occur frequently.
- Lesions producing obstruction of the upper gastrointestinal tract may be associated with maternal polyhydramnios and large gastric aspirates at birth.
- Green vomitus is considered an indication of bowel obstruction until proven otherwise.
- Clinical features of intestinal obstruction include vomiting, abdominal distention, visible peristalsis, and delayed passage of meconium. With upper gastrointestinal obstruction, meconium may be passed but no transitional stool is seen.
- Gastrointestinal obstruction between the pylorus and the ligament of Treitz is considered malrotation until proven otherwise.
- When the continuity of the gastrointestinal tract is clearly demonstrated postnatally by the passage of transitional stools, air, or contrast medium, congenital atresia can be excluded as the cause of the obstruction. Meconium may be passed from the bowel distal to a complete obstruction, so passage of meconium does not exclude obstruction.

- Colonic obstruction may manifest with the same constellation of symptoms as upper gastrointestinal obstruction. Particular note is taken of delayed passage of meconium (Hirschsprung disease, meconium plug syndrome).
- In patients younger than 2 years, it is hazardous to attempt to differentiate large from small bowel on the basis of plain abdominal radiographs, particularly because the frequent errors in this evaluation may lead to delay in diagnosis and therapy for an obstructive bowel lesion.
- An entity that can obstruct the bowel may also lead to perforation and the resulting signs and symptoms of peritonitis. Thus, when peritonitis is the presenting symptom, an obstructing lesion must be sought and corrected.

Imaging plays a major role in most neonatal gastrointestinal emergencies. The role varies from helping to establish a diagnosis to evaluating associated abnormalities and planning surgical solutions or therapy for such conditions as meconium ileus and meconium plug syndrome. Plain radiographs and bowel contrast examinations serve as primary imaging modalities with ultrasound, computed tomography (CT) scan, and magnetic resonance imaging (MRI) playing roles in more complex cases.

Ultrasound can help correctly identify meconium ileus and meconium peritonitis and is useful in the diagnosis of enteric duplication cysts and intussusception. In malrotation and anorectal anomalies, CT and MRI can provide superb anatomic detail and added diagnostic specificity. Intestinal duplications manifest as an abdominal mass at radiography, contrast enema examination, or ultrasound. On CT scan, most duplications manifest as smoothly rounded, fluid-filled cysts or tubular structures with thin, slightly enhancing walls. On MRI scan, the intracystic fluid has heterogeneous signal density on T1-weighted images and homogeneous high signal intensity on T2-weighted images. Familiarity with these gastrointestinal abnormalities is essential for correct diagnosis and appropriate management.

Lilien et al. accumulated a series of 45 newborns[101] initially thought to be normal, who had green vomiting in the first 72 hours of life; 20% required surgical intervention, 11% had nonsurgical obstruction (meconium plug, left microcolon), and 60% had idiopathic bilious vomiting. The last group of infants had a benign course. Of note, 56% of infants with surgical lesions had negative plain films of the abdomen and required contrast studies to establish the diagnosis. They concluded that, whereas isolated green vomiting in an otherwise normal neonate is not always a surgical problem, a thorough investigation including contrast studies is warranted. With these principles in mind, the following illustrative cases deal with approaches to some serious and frequently seen gastrointestinal anomalies.

CASE B-1

A pregnancy is complicated by polyhydramnios. A full-term male infant presents with increased salivation and chokes with feedings. Vomitus is never bile stained. Subsequently, respiratory distress develops. On physical examination, the infant is noted to be blue when crying and salivating excessively. The abdomen is distended. No obvious external malformation is noted. The x-ray film from the referring hospital is reported to demonstrate aspiration pneumonia.

EDITORIAL COMMENT: With a history of polyhydramnios and increased salivation, the most likely diagnosis is esophageal atresia. The presence of abdominal distention suggests that atresia is associated with a fistula. The absence of bile staining of the vomitus indicates obstruction proximal to the entry of the common duct into the duodenum.

A baby with esophageal atresia plus or minus tracheoesophageal fistula classically manifests with respiratory distress, choking, feeding difficulties, and frothing in the first few hours after birth. Neonates are unable to swallow, which accounts for the overflow of saliva, and they are vulnerable to aspirate into their lungs. A nasogastric tube will stick and coil in the upper pouch.

The diagnosis may be suspected antenatally because of polyhydramnios and an absent fetal stomach bubble detected on ultrasound. In the absence of other anomalies, the prenatal detection rate approaches 50%. A karyotype should be obtained because of the high association with trisomy 18. Mortality is significantly higher in prenatally diagnosed infants and in infants with additional congenital anomalies. Isolated esophageal atresia is associated with good outcome.[102]

Diagnostic Maneuver

Pass a radiopaque nasogastric tube until it stops and obtain an x-ray film, including neck, chest, and upper abdomen. When passing a nasogastric tube for a diagnostic maneuver in suspected esophageal atresia, use as large a tube as will pass the nares. A small tube may enter the larynx and pass down the trachea, through the fistula to the esophagus, and into the stomach, giving the false impression of esophageal continuity. A large tube will not be tolerated in the larynx. If the tube passes through the esophagus to the stomach, esophageal atresia is ruled out.

Contrast medium should not be used in this evaluation until continuity of the esophagus has been demonstrated because the inhalation of contrast medium from a blind esophageal pouch may produce pneumonia.

X-Ray Findings in Esophageal Atresia with Tracheoesophageal Fistula

1. There is a wide, air-filled pouch in the neck or upper mediastinum.
2. The nasogastric tube is seen to stop in the upper mediastinum at about T3.
3. Aspiration pneumonia may be noted, usually in the right upper lobe.
4. Parts of the abdomen show air in the intestines (often as an excess amount). With atresia and no fistula there is a gasless abdomen.
5. Often skeletal anomalies are present (vertebrae/ribs).
6. The VATER association is a nonrandom association of **v**ertebral defects, imperforate **a**nus, **t**racheo**e**sophageal fistula, and **r**adial and **r**enal dysplasia. The association may be broadened by the inclusion of **c**ardiac defects, and **l**imb abnormalities (VACTERL).

MANAGEMENT CONSIDERATIONS IN ESOPHAGEAL ATRESIA[102-106]

More than 90% of all patients with esophageal atresia have the common variety of blind upper esophagus with the lower segment entering into the membranous posterior portion of the trachea above the carina as a fistula. This connects the acid-filled stomach to the tracheobronchial tree. A small percentage of cases have esophageal atresia without tracheoesophageal fistula, in which case the abdomen is airless. From the first suspicion that a fistula exists until complete separation of the esophagus from the trachea is achieved, proper management is essential to prevent the fatal complication of aspiration pneumonia. Aspiration from the proximal pouch into the larynx is prevented by withholding all feedings and continuously aspirating the pouch with a sump tube. Reflux of gastric juice into the fistula is more damaging and more difficult to prevent but can be offset by attention to optimal positioning and by early surgical intervention. The child should be maintained in the prone, head-elevated position, which allows the stomach to fall anteriorly away from the esophagus and provides an inclined esophagus as a retardant to reflux of gastric juice.

When the diagnosis is confirmed, rapid evaluation of the child for tolerance of surgical correction should be undertaken. Criteria for primary repair (transthoracic extrapleural fistula ligation and end-to-end esophageal anastomosis) include the following:

- Chest is clear to auscultation and on radiograph
- No life-threatening cardiac anomalies
- Pao_2 of 60 mm Hg or better in room air (usually from an established arterial catheter, such as umbilical)

If these criteria cannot be immediately satisfied, immediate gastrointestinal decompression by tube gastrostomy performed with the patient under local anesthesia should be achieved, and intensive respiratory care should be instituted. Established aspiration pneumonitis may require 2 to 3 weeks of intensive therapy to clear. If improvement is not rapid, tracheostomy may be an essential therapeutic component, because the fistula may interfere with effective coughing.

If prolonged preoperative care is required, nutritional support by TPN will be essential. Feedings by gastrostomy are rarely tolerated as long as the tracheoesophageal fistula remains.

Cervical esophagostomy in esophageal atresia when initial repair cannot be made makes sham feeding necessary. This teaches the child the mechanics of swallowing and supports the oral gratification so essential in this period for later motor development. An interposition procedure using colon or stomach will be required but is usually delayed until after 6 months of age.

EDITORIAL COMMENT: Spitz and associates reported on the outcome of 148 infants with esophageal atresia encountered over 5 years at the Hospital for Sick Children,[106] Great Ormond Street, the regional referral center in London. The results were outstanding, with deaths predominantly resulting from associated congenital cardiac anomalies. They reported that endoscopy provided valuable information in planning the surgery, which should be delayed if there is aspiration pneumonia. They recommended immobilization and mechanical ventilation of the infants for 5 days after the operative repair.

Choudhury and colleagues have confirmed these excellent results even in infants with birth weights less than 1500 g.[107] Death is associated with complex cardiac and chromosomal anomalies.

Overall survival now exceeds 90% in dedicated centers. Associated congenital heart defects and low birth weight can affect survival. Early mortality is usually due to cardiac and chromosomal abnormalities. Late mortality is usually due to respiratory complications.

The Spitz classification has been used prognostically[106]: group I—birth weight greater than 1500 g, no major cardiac disease (survival 97%); group II—birth weight less than 1500 g or major cardiac disease; group III—birth weight less than 1500 g plus major cardiac disease (survival 22%).(See also http://www.patient.co.uk/doctor/oesophageal-atresia .htm).

DUODENAL OBSTRUCTION

The diagnosis of gastrointestinal obstruction in the fetus is difficult with only half of the lesions identified. Sonographic findings suggestive of duodenal atresia include a dilated fluid-filled stomach adjacent to a dilated proximal intestinal segment (fetal "double bubble"). The diagnosis can be made in the early second trimester, but more commonly is made in the third trimester when the duodenum becomes more dilated. Polyhydramnios develops in up to 50% of cases.

EDITORIAL COMMENT: Fetal dilated or echogenic bowel is a marker for a variety of conditions including bowel obstruction, chromosomal and congenital infectious disorders, and cystic fibrosis. Jackson reported on 35 fetuses with echogenic bowel of whom 12 babies underwent surgery for intestinal atresia,[108] meconium ileus, and duplication cysts. Postoperative courses and outcomes were good. They concluded that echogenic bowel on antenatal ultrasound is a nonspecific marker for a variety of disorders including intestinal atresia. Although associated with higher rates of fetal loss, the majority of neonates are normal at delivery. Obstruction of the duodenum may be complete or partial and caused by extrinsic (malrotation, annular pancreas) or intrinsic lesions (duodenal atresia, duodenal stenosis). Malrotation is the most common extrinsic lesion obstructing the duodenum and, because of the potential for vascular compromise to the bowel, it constitutes a true emergency in the neonate. Vomiting is the predominant manifesting

symptom and, if the obstruction is below the second part of the duodenum, it will be bile stained. Duodenal atresia is commonly associated with trisomy 21.

The diagnosis of duodenal atresia is made with a plain x-ray film of the abdomen revealing a "double-bubble," that is, the air- and fluid-filled stomach and duodenum. The presence of air bubbles beyond the second part of the duodenum suggests incomplete obstruction. An upper gastrointestinal series is indicated if malrotation is suspected.

Killbride warned that infants with congenital duodenal obstruction,[109] particularly if breast fed, may not present with classic findings of upper gastrointestinal obstruction in the first days of life. Careful in-hospital evaluation of infants with persistent regurgitation, even low volume, is recommended to avoid missing this diagnosis.

St. Peter reported on 408 patients with duodenal atresia.[110] There was a 28% incidence of trisomy 21. Only two patients (0.5%) were identified as having a second intestinal atresia. In this, the largest series of duodenal atresia patients compiled to date, the rate of a concomitant jejunoileal atresia is less than 1%. This low incidence is not high enough to mandate extensive inspection of the entire bowel in these patients, and a second atresia should not be a concern during laparoscopic repair of duodenal atresia.

JEJUNOILEAL ANOMALIES

Atresia is more common than stenosis, and ileal lesions are more common than jejunal lesions.[111] It has been postulated that these lesions arise from intrauterine bowel ischemia. Anomalies that produce obstruction of the small intestine may manifest with bilious vomiting, abdominal distention, and obstipation. The combination of bilious vomiting and passage of blood by rectum signifies vascular compromise of the intestine, necessitating immediate operative intervention. Atresias and stenoses must be differentiated from meconium ileus and meconium peritonitis as described later.

Plain radiographic studies may show nonspecific bowel dilation. It is extremely difficult to distinguish small bowel from colon in the neonatal period. Contrast enemas may show a microcolon together with one or more focal small bowel stenoses.

Dalla Vecchia et al. encountered 277 neonates with intestinal atresia and stenosis between 1972 and 1997.[112] The level of obstruction was duodenal in 138 infants, jejunoileal in 128, and colonic in 21. Of the 277 neonates, 10 had obstruction in more than one site. Duodenal atresia was associated with prematurity (46%), maternal polyhydramnios (33%), Down syndrome (24%), annular pancreas (33%), and malrotation (28%). Jejunoileal atresia was associated with intrauterine volvulus (27%), gastroschisis (16%), and meconium ileus (11.7%). Operative mortality for neonates with duodenal atresia was 4%; with jejunoileal atresia, 0.8%; and with colonic atresia, 0%. Cardiac anomalies (with duodenal atresia) and ultrashort-bowel syndrome (<40 cm) requiring long-term total parenteral nutrition, which can be complicated by liver disease (with jejunoileal atresia), are the major causes of morbidity and mortality. The long-term survival rate for children with duodenal atresia was 86%; with jejunoileal atresia, 84%; and with colon atresia, 100%.

Infants with mild jejunal or ileal atresias have an excellent prognosis and long-term survival. Severe atresias are associated with longer parenteral nutrition support and secondary procedures for intestinal failure. Associated anomalies adversely affect outcomes in jejunoileal atresia.[113]

MALROTATION/VOLVULUS

Incomplete rotation and fixation of the embryonic intestine as it returns to the fetal abdominal cavity from its embryonic extracoelomic position is referred to as malrotation.[114] The normal alignment of the gut has the distal duodenum crossing to the left of the vertebral column to join the jejunum at a normally positioned ligament of Treitz with the cecum in the right lower quadrant. With malrotation, the cecum is undescended and situated in the right hypochondrium, abnormally fixed by bands crossing the second part of the duodenum.

Fetal bowel obstruction has a prevalence of 1 in 3000 to 5000 live births. Ultrasonographic diagnosis is made by demonstrating distended loops of bowel, fetal ascites, or echogenic bowel. Echogenic bowel, defined as small bowel more echogenic than liver or bone, in addition to bowel obstruction, has also been associated with congenital infections, cystic fibrosis, and chromosomal abnormalities.

Malrotation may be associated with other gastrointestinal lesions, including duodenal atresia, small intestinal atresia, gastroschisis, omphalocele, and congenital diaphragmatic hernia as well as cardiac, renal, and other major anomalies. Malrotation may manifest with bile-stained vomiting and abdominal distention. The obstruction may be intermittent. Alternatively, there may be a dramatic manifestation with bile-stained vomiting, abdominal distention, possibly an abdominal mass, shock, pallor, and bloody stools. This manifestation signifies a volvulus (i.e., a strangulation obstruction with occlusion of blood flow to the gut).

Plain films of the abdomen may reveal a double bubble, with air patterns visible beyond the duodenum. Malrotation or volvulus must be diagnosed with upper gastrointestinal contrast studies, because the diagnosis is missed on plain films. The major purpose of the study is to establish the anatomic relationships and that the duodenum crosses the midline. A sharp cutoff with curved narrowing of the distal duodenum is characteristic of an obstruction secondary to a volvulus. If there is any doubt concerning the diagnosis, an exploratory laparotomy is mandatory because the integrity of the bowel may be rapidly compromised by vascular occlusion.

> **EDITORIAL COMMENT:** Volvulus of the bowel can be a fulminant and even fatal condition. Rapid diagnosis and prompt surgical intervention are mandatory to maintain the integrity of the bowel. The traditional approach to a suspected volvulus was a barium enema examination; however, this only provided indirect evidence of a volvulus if the cecum was not in the right lower quadrant. Volvulus of the small bowel may occur with a normal rotation and position of the colon. Therefore, an upper gastrointestinal approach has been adopted to establish the diagnosis. Both the site of obstruction and often the cause can be identified in this manner. Concerns about the contrast medium above the obstruction are unfounded. If the obstruction is complete, surgery is indicated and the contrast can be removed during the operative procedure.

Ultrasound is an additional means of evaluating infants with suspected upper gastrointestinal obstruction. Cohen et al.[115] using a fluid-aided ultrasound evaluation of the stomach and duodenum, were able to obtain a dynamic view of duodenal rotation and anatomy and correctly identify a number of lesions.

> **EDITORIAL COMMENT:** Intestinal malrotation in neonates or infants requires urgent surgical treatment, especially when volvulus and vascular compromise of the midgut are suspected. Hagendoorn wished to determine whether laparoscopy for the treatment of malrotation has a success rate equal to that of open

surgery.[116] Successful laparoscopic treatment of intestinal malrotation could be performed in 75% of the cases (n = 28), and conversion to an open procedure was necessary in 25% of the cases (n = 9). Postoperative clinical relapse due to recurrence of malrotation, volvulus, or both occurred in 19% of the laparoscopically treated patients (n = 7). They concluded that "diagnostic laparoscopy is the procedure of choice when intestinal malrotation is suspected. If present, malrotation can be treated adequately with laparoscopic surgery in the majority of cases. Nevertheless, to prevent recurrence of malrotation or volvulus, a low threshold for conversion to an open procedure is mandated."

MECONIUM ILEUS

Meconium ileus is a luminal obstruction of the distal small intestine by abnormal meconium, in contrast to meconium plug syndrome, which is a colonic obstruction. Meconium ileus is seen predominantly in patients with cystic fibrosis. The infants present with bile-stained vomiting and abdominal distention and the meconium filled loops have a doughy feel. The sonographic findings associated with meconium peritonitis in utero include polyhydramnios, ascites, dilatation of the bowel, hyperechoic bowel, and the tell-tale sign of intraabdominal calcification, which is pathognomonic of meconium ileus.

Radiographic evidence exists of complete obstruction with a characteristic soap bubble appearance produced by the air trapped in the thick meconium. Intrauterine perforation (meconium peritonitis) with the passage of sterile meconium into the peritoneal cavity may be reflected by calcification and predisposes to intestinal obstruction from adhesive bands. The diagnosis may be confirmed with a water-soluble diatrizoate enema, which may also be therapeutic because it facilitates passage of the tenacious meconium. The study is contraindicated if signs of peritonitis or pneumoperitoneum are present.

Gorter published a series of 43 patients from Amsterdam.[117] Twenty-three of the patients (53.5%) were diagnosed as having cystic fibrosis. They concluded that the clinical entity of meconium ileus represents a spectrum of underlying pathologies.

MECKEL DIVERTICULUM

The omphalomesenteric duct usually obliterates spontaneously during embryonic development. Umbilical anomalies arise from fetal structures such as the omphalomesenteric duct or urachus, or from failure of closure of the umbilical fascial ring. Persistence of the omphalomesenteric duct may lead to several anomalies including umbilical sinus, umbilical cyst, Meckel diverticulum, or patent omphalomesenteric duct.[118] A patent omphalomesenteric duct is usually associated with the ileum; rarely, it may be associated with the cecum or appendix. If the duct remains patent at the umbilicus, the umbilicus is constantly moist from intestinal secretions, whereas persistence of a blind duct produces a "strawberry" tumor at the umbilicus. Persistence at the ileal end is noted in 2% of the population and results in Meckel diverticulum, which often also contains ectopic gastric and pancreatic tissue. Meckel diverticulum is rarely significant in the neonatal period but may manifest with painless rectal bleeding (the result of ulceration caused by gastric secretions) or obstruction. The diverticulum may also serve as the point for an intussusception.

COLONIC LESIONS

MECONIUM PLUG SYNDROME

Meconium plug syndrome is part of the spectrum of colonic hypomotility and is seen predominantly in preterm infants and infants of diabetic mothers. Infants with meconium plug syndrome fail to pass meconium in the first 24 hours of life and present with clinical and radiologic features of intestinal obstruction. Rectal examination may prompt passage of meconium with a characteristic white plug; otherwise, a radiographic contrast enema is indicated. This may serve the dual function of diagnosis and therapy. Inspissated meconium may be documented in the distal colon with dilation above. The contrast examination may precipitate passage of the meconium plug and relieve the symptoms. It is important to recognize that a meconium plug may be associated with cystic fibrosis and Hirschsprung disease. Hence, if the symptoms persist or recur, the infant should have a sweat chloride test and rectal mucosal biopsy.

Failure of a small premature newborn to adequately evacuate meconium for days or weeks has been attributed to probable necrotizing enterocolitis (NEC), or "microcolon of prematurity." Extremely premature infants may also present with intestinal obstruction and perforation secondary to inspissated meconium in the absence of cystic fibrosis.

Krasna reported a series of 20 babies with birth weights between 480 and 1500 g who appeared to have an unusual type of "meconium plug syndrome,"[119] which required a contrast enema or Gastrografin upper gastrointestinal series to evacuate the plugs and relieve the obstruction. Many of the mothers were on magnesium sulfate or had eclampsia. The plugs were diagnosed late rather than shortly after birth, and the plugs were significant, extending to the right colon.

Greenholz identified 13 patients who underwent treatment for intestinal obstruction secondary to inspissated meconium.[120] The average birth weight was 760 g. Prenatal and postnatal risk factors included intrauterine growth restriction, maternal hypertension, prolonged administration of tocolytic agents, patent ductus arteriosus, respiratory distress syndrome, and intraventricular hemorrhage. Stooling was absent or infrequent during the first 2 weeks of life. The infants had abdominal distention or perforation between days 2 and 17 of life. Twelve patients required operative intervention. Findings invariably included one or more obstructing meconium plugs with proximal distention, and the dilated segments were frequently necrotic. None of the patients had cystic fibrosis. The markedly premature infant is at risk for obstruction and eventual perforation secondary to meconium plugs, presumably formed in conjunction with intestinal dysmotility. This entity must be distinguished from spontaneous intestinal perforation, which occurs in the absence of plugs (see later text). Prompt diagnosis and timely intervention require a high index of suspicion, including close attention to stooling patterns, careful abdominal examinations, and screening radiographs when indicated. Patients with this disorder should be evaluated for cystic fibrosis and may need to undergo a rectal biopsy to rule out Hirschsprung disease.

NEONATAL SMALL LEFT COLON

Small left colon is a rare entity encountered predominantly among infants of diabetic mothers. The presenting features characteristically include delayed passage of meconium. Radiographic evidence includes dilation of the proximal colon, a clearly delineated transition zone, usually the splenic flexure, and narrowing of the distal colon. Resolution of the problem may be anticipated in the first month of life. Management is expectant.

CONGENITAL AGANGLIONIC MEGACOLON (HIRSCHSPRUNG DISEASE)

Congenital aganglionic megacolon occurs in approximately 1 in 5000 births and is the most common cause of large-bowel obstruction in the newborn. It can be life threatening and should be considered in any neonate with intestinal obstruction. It is more common in males, infants with trisomy 21, and siblings of children with the disorder. Hirschsprung disease is thought to result from defective migration of neural crest cells to the distal colon, leaving a segment of bowel aganglionic and dysfunctional.

Only 10% to 20% of patients with this disorder are first seen in the newborn period. In the infant, symptoms may manifest as acute obstruction, abdominal distention, vomiting, and delay in passing or failure to pass meconium (95% of normal term newborns pass meconium in the first 24 hours of life). Constipation is a prominent feature. Irritability, poor feeding, and failure to thrive are other presenting features. Rectal examination or rectal stimulation such as with a rectal thermometer may produce an explosive gush of gas, and meconium may obscure the diagnosis; however, in the absence of rectal stimulation, no stools are passed.

Radiographic findings include nonspecific obstructive features, such as dilated loops of bowel and multiple fluid levels with the absence of air in the rectum. Barium studies should be performed without prior cleansing enemas. The findings include proximal dilation and distal narrowing in the aganglionic segment. Note, however, that the transition zone may not be clearly defined in the neonate and the barium may be retained for more than 24 hours. The diagnosis is established by biopsy, which must be of adequate depth to confirm the absence of ganglia in the nerve plexus.

Surgical treatment is mandated in the newborn. Generally, a colostomy in a segment of normally innervated bowel is required. Definitive correction had usually been deferred until the end of the first year of life. Hirschsprung disease can now be successfully treated in the neonatal period with a one-stage pull-through. The short- and long-term results are as good as those with the three-stage procedure, with the child usually benefiting by having a shorter hospital stay and not requiring a stoma.

ABDOMINAL WALL DEFECTS

Omphalocele and gastroschisis are major defects of the abdominal wall resulting in parts of the gastrointestinal tract remaining outside the abdominal cavity. An omphalocele is covered by peritoneum and is frequently associated with other anomalies (congenital heart disease, trisomy 13 or 18, urinary tract anomalies, and Beckwith-Wiedemann syndrome, which includes macrosomia, macroglossia, omphalocele, and hypoglycemia;) (see Chapter 12). Malrotation is invariable with an omphalocele. The pentalogy of Cantrell refers to an omphalocele accompanied by defects in the diaphragm, sternum, heart, and pericardium.

Gastroschisis is a cleft in the abdominal wall to the right of the umbilicus. The extruded loops of bowel are thickened and covered by a fibrinous peel that develops in the latter part of the third trimester. Atresias, strictures, adhesions, and stenoses of the bowel accompany gastroschisis, but other malformation syndromes are unusual. The atretic areas are secondary to vascular insults.

Both lesions may be identified relatively early in gestation through alpha-fetoprotein screening (see Chapter 2) and the lesions can be accurately delineated with antenatal ultrasound. Delivery should take place at a tertiary center because these cases represent complex management problems. The mode of delivery is determined by obstetric factors; vaginal delivery has not been proved to increase morbidity, mortality risk, or length of stay. Thermal regulation, fluid and electrolyte management, nutritional support, and measures to prevent infection are needed to complement the surgical team.

EDITORIAL COMMENT: Gastroschisis and omphalocele are usually considered together because both are congenital abdominal wall defects, yet their anatomy, embryogenesis, clinical presentation, and associated problems are quite different. For gastroschisis, evidence points to environmental teratogens as the cause with little evidence for a genetic cause,[121] whereas for omphalocele, substantial data support genetic or familial factors as a cause, with little evidence for environmental factors. Omphalocele and gastroschisis are recognized as congenital malformations with a high mortality. Only 60% of children with such malformations survive until the end of the first year of age. It has been suggested that omphalocele and gastroschisis are associated with other congenital malformations, concerning the bones, the heart, and the kidney.

INGUINAL HERNIA

Inguinal hernias occur in 1% to 3% of all children, more often in premature infants, in boys much more frequently than girls, and more often on the right side than left, but can also occur on both sides. Hernias occur more often in children with a parent or sibling who had a hernia as an infant, cystic fibrosis, developmental dysplasia of the hip, as undescended testes or urethral abnormalities. They need to be differentiated from a hydrocele, although both may occur together. The prevalence of incarceration of the hernia in infants discharged home is very low. Inguinal hernia repair is one of the most common surgical procedures performed on premature infants. Improved survival rates in the NICU have led to an increase in the incidence of premature infants with inguinal hernias.

Murphy et al. reported on a 5-year, retrospective chart review of all premature infants undergoing inguinal hernia repair.[122] Because the literature suggested that postoperative apneas occurred in up to 49% of premature infants undergoing anesthesia for inguinal hernia repair, their practice is to monitor all of these babies in the intensive care unit (ICU) overnight after surgery. In addition to the considerable expense to the health care system, these cases are cancelled if no ICU bed is available. They reported that only 5 of 126 (4.7%) had apnea after the repair. All five had a previous history of significant apnea, and these babies were less mature with a more complicated hospital course. They concluded that selective use of postoperative ICU monitoring for high-risk patients could result in significant resource and cost savings to the health care system.

CASE B-2

An infant takes initial feedings and then vomits bile-stained material. He is otherwise asymptomatic. Examination may or may not reveal abdominal distention. The anus is patent, and meconium is usually passed.

Any gastrointestinal obstruction distal to the entry of the common duct into the duodenum can lead to bile-stained vomiting. As a general rule (but not an infallible one), the earlier the onset of bile-stained vomiting, the higher the level of obstruction. Lower-level obstructions usually manifest initially with distention and failure to pass meconium with bile-stained vomiting occurring hours to days later.

X-ray findings vary with the level and type of obstruction. They may be clearly diagnostic, as is the case with complete obstruction of the duodenum (double bubble; duodenal atresia, annular pancreas, occasionally malrotation), or they may be equivocal, as in meconium ileus or Hirschsprung disease.

Eventual diagnosis is forthcoming in every case, given enough time and persistence. In the interim, effective nasogastric decompression and parenteral fluid, electrolyte, and nutritional support by vein sustain most of these infants, even if significant time lapses before diagnosis and definitive therapy. Only those lesions that may lead to catastrophe require urgent diagnosis and treatment, so attention should be directed to recognizing these disorders rapidly. These disorders include malrotation, volvulus, bowel perforations, and aganglionic megacolon.

EDITORIAL COMMENT: Intestinal malrotation is a common cause of upper gastrointestinal obstruction and manifests with duodenal obstruction caused by volvulus of the midgut loop. Patients are at risk of catastrophic midgut infarction, and malrotation is a more frequent cause of duodenal obstruction in infants than duodenal atresia. Bilious vomiting and bloody stools are the two most common clinical presentations in neonates. Rectal bleeding is an ominous sign. Most patients manifesting such bleeding have a gangrenous bowel. Urgent upper contrast studies are necessary. Ultrasound studies may also be helpful as a characteristic pattern of echogenic ascites, thickened bowel wall; dilated, fluid-filled bowel lumen; and lack of peristalsis may be seen in children with gangrenous bowel.

Note that a less invasive laparascopic approach is successful 75% of the time.

CASE B-3

Bilious vomiting, usually with some abdominal distention, occurs in a baby who passed normal meconium and has an open anus. X-ray films may show duodenal obstruction and usually show some gas throughout the abdomen.

Diagnosis: Malrotation

Malrotation is the most malevolent lesion of infancy because of its propensity toward volvulus with resultant strangulation of the superior mesenteric artery. This catastrophe can lead to total destruction of the digestive-absorptive segment of the intestinal tract—the jejunoileum. Furthermore, compared with any other single anomaly, this lesion is quite common. It must, therefore, always be in the differential diagnostic forefront to be rapidly ruled in or out. The most direct method for doing so is by upper gastrointestinal contrast study, which demonstrates obstruction of the duodenum. If obstruction is incomplete, the study reveals that the duodenal C loop fails to complete its normal course to a position in the left upper quadrant behind the stomach—the ligament of Treitz.

Contrast enemas, frequently recommended for diagnosis of malrotation in the past, may be confusing. The high-riding cecum with malpositioned appendix is diagnostic if clearly present, but often the cecal position is equivocal and difficult to locate clearly. Reflux of dye into the ileum may mask the position of the cecum. Therapeutic delay is intolerable here. One should quickly intervene operatively in any duodenal obstruction not clearly caused by an entity other than malrotation.

BLOOD IN STOOL

Blood in the stool[123] is a frequent problem confronting the neonatal team. Whether gross blood is present, streaks of blood are on the outside of an otherwise normal-appearing stool, or only occult blood is present, a prompt and diligent search for the cause is mandatory. In many instances no cause will be found; however, major pathologic disorders accounting for the blood in the stool must be ruled out.

Disorders causing frank blood in the stool, range from swallowed maternal blood, an inconsequential problem, to life-threatening disorders, including NEC, malrotation with volvulus, disturbances of coagulation, ulcerative disorders, and infections. Blood-streaked stools are most commonly seen with an anal fissure or following trauma to the rectum with temperature probes and thermometers. Occult blood may signify blood swallowed during breast feeding, upper gastrointestinal disorders, milk intolerance, hemorrhagic disorders, or NEC.

Gastrointestinal bleeding in the newborn must be differentiated from swallowed maternal blood caused by antepartum hemorrhage, the episiotomy, or cracked, bleeding nipples. The Apt test distinguishes maternal from fetal red blood cells, in that the fetal cells are resistant to alkali denaturation (addition of sodium hydroxide). Hence, a solution containing maternal blood changes from pink to brown. Other laboratory tests include a complete blood count with a differential and smear; platelet count; coagulation studies such as partial thromboplastin time, prothrombin time, and fibrinogen level; blood culture; and a plain film of the abdomen. These tests should point to the cause of the bleeding, which can then be managed appropriately.

SPONTANEOUS INTESTINAL PERFORATION

Another disorder has emerged among the ELBW infants. It has been designated spontaneous intestinal perforation and may be indistinguishable from NEC. Spontaneous perforation, however, occurs much less frequently than NEC in preterm infants. The infants may have dramatic abdominal distention often associated with blue discoloration of the abdominal wall. Obvious clinical signs of bowel perforation are infrequent with spontaneous intestinal perforation.

Infants with spontaneous perforation are smaller and born more prematurely when compared with infants who had NEC.[124,125] The onset of illness was earlier and was associated with antecedent hypotension, leukocytosis, and a gasless appearance on abdominal radiograph. Infants with spontaneous perforations are more likely to have received postnatal steroids or to have systemic candidiasis. Conditions associated with fetal or neonatal hypoxia are important antecedents for this emerging distinct clinical entity. Other factors implicated in the etiology include indomethacin therapy, patent ductus arteriosus, and intraventricular hemorrhage. Peritoneal drainage alone may be considered definitive therapy for intestinal perforation in the majority of extremely immature infants. The prognosis for spontaneous intestinal perforation is better than for necrotizing enterocolitis (see later).

PART THREE

NECROTIZING ENTEROCOLITIS

Deanne Wilson-Costello,
Robert M. Kliegman, and Avroy A. Fanaroff

NEC remains the major gastrointestinal cause of morbidity and mortality among the neonatal intensive care population. The incidence varies among countries and among units. Uauy et al,[126] reporting on behalf of the National Institute of Child Health and Development Neonatal Multicenter Research Network, noted that 10% of 2681 infants with birth weights between 501 and 1500 g had proven NEC (Bell stage II and beyond) (Table 7-12). Approximately 7% of all babies with birth weights below 1500 g will develop necrotizing enterocolitis. Most infants with NEC have a low birth weight, are inappropriately grown, and are immature.[127-129]

Although patent ductus arteriosus, low Apgar scores, and umbilical catheters have been implicated in the etiology, matched studies did not identify these as risk factors. Nonetheless, the odds ratio for NEC increased with antepartum hemorrhage, prolonged rupture of membranes beyond 36 hours, and 5-minute Apgar scores below 7.

The age of onset for NEC varies inversely with gestation. In approximately half of the term infants with NEC, symptoms manifest in the first day of life. Specific risk factors for NEC among term infants include cyanotic heart disease, polycythemia, and twin gestation. Whereas sporadic cases of endemic NEC occur throughout the year, temporal and geographic epidemic clusters are associated with gastrointestinal illness among nursery staff.

Infection plays a prominent role and the disease occurs in clusters with various outbreaks reported from *Escherichia coli* and *Klebsiella, Salmonella,* and *Clostridium* species. Viruses have also been implicated. Recent reports suggest significant alterations in the gastrointestinal flora colonizing critically ill neonates. An altered intestinal microbiome coupled with an unbalanced proinflammatory response in a high-risk premature infant may lead to the final common pathway of intestinal necrosis.

A review of peritoneal cultures from infants undergoing surgery for NEC reveals a predominance of *Klebsiella* and *Enterobacter* species (63%), frequent *E. coli* (21%), coagulase-negative staphylococci (30%), occasional anaerobes (6%) and *Candida* isolates (10%). Clinical classifications and the pathogenesis of the disease are outlined in Tables 7-12 and Box 7-4 and Figure 7-6. The inciting event may be hypoxemia, sepsis, low cardiac output, or factors within the bowel such as hypertonic feeding. Although feeding precedes the onset of symptoms in most cases, delayed feeding does not lower

Table 7-12. Modified Bell's Staging Criteria for Neonatal Necrotizing Enterocolitis

Stage	Systemic Signs	Intestinal Signs	Radiologic Signs	Treatment
IA—Suspected NEC	Temperature instability, apnea, bradycardia, lethargy	Elevated pregavage residuals, mild abdominal distention, emesis, guaiac-positive stool	Normal or intestinal dilation, mild ileus	Nothing by mouth, antibiotics for 3 days pending cultures
IB—Suspected NEC	Same as above	Bright red blood from rectum	Same as above	Same as above
IIA—Definite NEC: mildly ill	Same as above	Same as above, *plus* diminished or absent bowel sounds with or without abdominal tenderness	Intestinal dilation, ileus, pneumatosis intestinalis	Nothing by mouth, antibiotics for 7-10 days if examination is normal in 24-48 hr
IIB—Definite NEC: moderately ill	Same as above *plus* mild metabolic acidosis and mild thrombocytopenia	Same as above *plus* definite abdominal tenderness, with or without abdominal cellulitis or right lower quadrant mass, absent bowel sounds	Same as stage IIA with or without portal vein gas, with or without ascites	Nothing by mouth, antibiotics for 14 days, $NaHCO_3$ for acidosis
IIIA—Advanced NEC: severely ill, bowel intact	Same as IIB *plus* hypotension, bradycardia, severe apneas, combined respiratory and metabolic acidosis, disseminated intravascular coagulation, neutropenia, anuria	Same as above *plus* signs of generalized peritonitis, marked tenderness, distention of abdomen, and abdominal wall erythema	Same as stage IIB, definite ascites	Same as above *plus* 200 mL/kg/day fluids, fresh frozen plasma, inotropic agents; intubation, ventilation therapy; paracentesis; surgical intervention if patient fails to improve with medical management within 24-48 hr
IIIB—Advanced NEC: severely ill, bowel perforation	Same as stage IIIA	Same as stage IIIA	Same as stage IIB *plus* pneumoperitoneum	Same as above *plus* surgical intervention

NEC, Necrotizing enterocolitis.

the incidence of NEC and, in fact, may promote its occurrence.[130] It remains unclear whether the major factor is the formula itself, the volume of formula, the rate at which feeding is advanced, or the effect of the bacteria on the formula.

Gut ischemia is a potential risk factor for NEC. Intrauterine growth-restricted infants with aberrant fetal Doppler blood flow velocity waveforms and infants born to cocaine-abusing mothers show increased rates of NEC.[131-133] In addition, cocaine-exposed infants with NEC are more likely to require surgical intervention, have massive gangrene, or die.[131]

EDITORIAL COMMENT: Michael Caplan MD: The search for predictive markers of NEC has been inconsistent, although some might have clinical utility, including C-reactive protein, hydrogen breath test, interleukin-8 (IL-8), platelet activating factor, and, most recently, complement 5a, cytosolic beta-glucosidase, serum amyloid A, and salivary H secretor phenotype.[134-136] In these studies, most markers were measured at the time of NEC diagnosis, and unfortunately patients will only benefit if a marker is discovered that predicts NEC before the diagnosis is made. Chabaan has identified inter-alpha inhibitor protein (Ialp) as a potential marker of necrotizing enterocolitis.[137] Inter-alpha inhibitor proteins are serine protease inhibitors that modulate endogenous protease activity and improve survival in adult models of sepsis. The beneficial effects of Ialp appear to be via suppression of proinflammatory cytokines such as TNF-α rather than augmentation of IL-10. The impact of Ialp may be significantly greater than that of a just as reliable predictive marker for NEC—Ialp may be useful in the treatment of this dreaded disease. It has been shown that serine proteases initiate a cell death pathway in epithelial cells, and this mechanism may contribute to the pathogenesis of NEC.[138] If so, low Ialp levels due to consumption or immaturity would lead to prolonged serine protease exposure and may contribute

Box 7-4.	**Clinical Classification of Neonatal Enterocolitis***

Classic NEC

Endemic

Epidemic

- Identifiable organism
- No organism identified

Benign NEC (Pneumatosis coli)

NEC following exchange transfusion

NEC following mucosal injury

Hypertonic feeding

Allergic enteritis

Nonspecific diarrhea

Polycythemia

Primary bowel pathologic findings

Spontaneous bowel perforation

Congenital intestinal obstruction

Neonatal appendicitis

Neonatal pseudomembranous colitis

Adapted from Kliegman RM, Fanaroff AA: Necrotizing enterocolitis, N Engl J Med 310:1093, 1984.
*Each category is a distinct clinical and pathologic entity. The inclusive heading of neonatal enterocolitis includes classic idiopathic NEC (I, II), NEC associated with other factors (III, IV), and those newborn diseases that clinically resemble NEC (V, VI, VII). These disease processes may be distinguished from each other by history, clinical course, laboratory tests, and pathologic examination.
NEC, Necrotizing enterocolitis.

to increased epithelial cell death. It seems plausible that exogenous Ialp could reduce serine protease effects, and in animals, Ialp treatment has reduced the risk of death in a neonatal sepsis model.[139] Additional studies are needed to explore the possible role of Ialp in the diagnosis and treatment of neonatal NEC.

In summary, NEC is a multifactorial disorder with a delicate balance between bowel perfusion, enteric organisms, and nutritional intake. The disorder was reduced by the prenatal administration of steroids,[140] although larger series have not confirmed this, or possibly by the postnatal administration of immunoglobulin A.[141] Breast milk is also protective, as shown by Lucas and Cole in a multicenter study addressing the role of diet in NEC.[61] Furthermore, pasteurizing the milk did not reduce its effectiveness and the combination of breast milk and formula was less likely to be associated with NEC than formula alone. Breast milk contains bifidus factor, which enhances gut colonization with *Lactobacillus*. Mothers

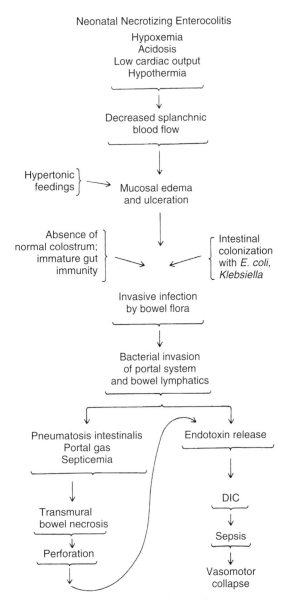

Figure 7-6. Possible factors in etiology and outcome of neonatal necrotizing enterocolitis. *DIC,* Disseminated intravascular coagulation. *(From Burrington JD:* Necrotizing enterocolitis in newborn infant, Clin Perinatol *5:29, 1978.)*

should, therefore, be encouraged to provide breast milk for their own infants during their sojourn in the intensive care unit.

Late-onset sepsis and NEC may result from bacterial translocation. Lactoferrin (LF) is a member of the transferring family and a multifunctional protein. It has antimicrobial, antiinflammatory, immunoregulatory, and growth-promoting properties. All of these contribute to the prevention of bacterial translocation in VLBW infants. Manzoni et al. observed a significant reduction in late-onset sepsis among VLBW infants fed bovine lactoferrin (BLF).[86] Incidence of late-onset sepsis was significantly lower in the BLF and BLF plus *Lactobacillus rhamnosus* GG (LGG) groups (5.9% and 4.6%, respectively), compared to the control group receiving placebo (17.3%). The decrease occurred for both bacterial and fungal sepsis. No adverse effects or intolerances to treatment occurred. When BLF and *L. rhamnosus* GG were given enterally to the infants, NEC was significantly decreased compared to controls.

Deshpande included 15 trials and nearly 3000 infants in a metaanalysis that demonstrated significant reduction in death or necrotizing enterocolitis (30%) without any significant side effects.[142] However, probiotics have not been available in the United States for use in preterm infants because of problems in obtaining a standardized probiotic acceptable to the U.S. Food and Drug Administration (FDA).

CLINICAL FEATURES

The clinical features of NEC are variable, and the signs and symptoms may not be specific.[143] Most often, temperature instability, lethargy, abdominal distention, and retention of feedings develop. Occult blood is present in the stools, which may sometimes reveal frank blood. Reducing substances are often detected before the onset of NEC. Apnea may be a prominent feature as well as bilious vomiting, increased abdominal distention, acidosis, and disseminated intravascular coagulation. The characteristic x-ray features are pneumatosis intestinalis, with bubbles or layers of gas in the wall of the bowel as well as portal venous gas. Free air within the peritoneum is associated with perforation of a viscus. Engel et al. demonstrated that about 30% of the gas in the wall of the bowel is hydrogen,[144] the product of bacterial fermentation of formula.

Medical management includes nasogastric suction, IV fluids, and broad-spectrum systemic antibiotics (Appendix A-2). Frequent abdominal examinations as well as determination of abdominal girth and cross-table lateral x-ray films are important to detect free air. Infants should be maintained on a regimen of nothing per os for up to 2 weeks while they receive all nutritional support intravenously. The main indication for surgery is perforation, which is demonstrated by free air in the peritoneum. However, surgery may also be considered for infants with worsening clinical status, refractory disseminated intravascular

coagulation, or acidosis. The discovery of an abdominal mass and gas in the portal venous system is not necessarily an indication for surgery. Some infants may require surgery at a later stage because of the development of strictures. With present vigorous medical and surgical management as outlined earlier, 75% of infants with birth weights above 1 kg should survive.

Perforated necrotizing enterocolitis is a major cause of morbidity and mortality in premature infants, and the optimal treatment is uncertain. Blakely documented that survival to hospital discharge after operation for necrotizing enterocolitis (NEC) or isolated intestinal perforation (IP) in ELBW (<1 kg) neonates was only 51%. Among the 156 enrolled infants, 80 underwent initial peritoneal drainage and 76 had initial laparotomy.[145,146] Patients with a preoperative diagnosis of NEC have a relative risk for death of 1.4 compared with those with a preoperative diagnosis of isolated intestinal perforation. They could distinguish on the basis of radiologic findings and age at surgery preoperatively between NEC and isolated intestinal perforation. The overall incidence of postoperative intestinal stricture was 10.3%, wound dehiscence 4.4%, and intraabdominal abscess 5.8%, and did not significantly differ between groups undergoing initial laparotomy versus initial drainage. By 18 to 22 months, 78 (50%) had died; 112 (72%) had died or were shown to be impaired. Outcome was worse in the subgroup with NEC.

Subsequently, Moss reported from a multicenter randomized trial that compared outcomes of primary peritoneal drainage with laparotomy and bowel resection in preterm infants with perforated necrotizing enterocolitis.[147] At 90 days postoperatively, 19 of 55 infants assigned to primary peritoneal drainage had died (34.5%), as compared with 22 of 62 infants assigned to laparotomy (35.5%, $P = 0.92$). They concluded that the type of operation performed for perforated necrotizing enterocolitis does not influence survival or other clinically important early outcomes in preterm infants.[147] Among ELBW infants, surgical NEC, which is likely to be associated with a greater severity of disease, is associated with significant growth delay and adverse neurodevelopmental outcomes at 18 to 22 months' corrected age compared with infants who did not have NEC.[148] Medically treated NEC does not seem to confer additional risk and the outcomes are similar to very low-birth-weight babies without NEC.

The incidence of surgical short bowel syndrome in a cohort of 12,316 VLBW infants (<1.5 kg) was 0.7%.[149] Necrotizing enterocolitis was the most common diagnosis associated with surgical short bowel syndrome. More VLBW infants with short bowel syndrome (20%) died during initial hospitalization than those without NEC or short bowel syndrome (12%), but fewer than the infants with surgical NEC without short bowel syndrome (53%). Among 5657 ELBW infants (<1 kg birth weight) the incidence of surgical short bowel syndrome was 1.1%. At 18 to 22 months, ELBW infants with short bowel syndrome were more likely to still require tube feeding (33%) and to have been rehospitalized (79%). Moreover, these infants had growth delay with shorter lengths and smaller head circumferences than infants without necrotizing enterocolitis or short bowel.

CASE C-1

C. K. weighs 1300 g at 32 weeks' gestation. His Apgar scores were 4 at 1 minute and 6 at 5 minutes. Respiratory distress syndrome (RDS) develops on the first day of life, an arterial catheter is placed at the level of T10, and 60% oxygen but no assisted ventilation is used. The RDS resolves by 48 hours of life, and the catheter is removed. Standard formula is first fed on the third day of life. On the eighth day, abdominal tenderness and distention are observed, and the nurses reported guaiac-positive stools, 5 mL residual from the last feeding, and a higher incubator temperature required to maintain body temperature.

What is the most likely preliminary diagnosis?

1. Meconium plug syndrome
2. Necrotizing enterocolitis
3. Septicemia
4. Malrotation
5. Hirschsprung disease

Any neonate with a triad of abdominal distention, Hematest or guaiac-positive stools, and retention of gastric formula should be suspected of having NEC and should be immediately evaluated for it. The initial manifestation of NEC may be indistinguishable from septicemia, and a positive blood culture is obtained from 30% of infants with NEC. The answer is 2, necrotizing enterocolitis.

Initially, how should this patient be evaluated?

1. Culture of blood, urine, cerebrospinal fluid, and stool
2. Complete blood count and clotting profile

3. Barium swallow
4. Gastrografin enema
5. Anteroposterior and lateral film of abdomen
6. Blood gases and serum electrolytes

1. Because sepsis is present in many if not all of these patients and many investigators believe that infection is directly related to the pathogenesis of the disease, blood, urine, stool, and cerebrospinal fluid cultures should be obtained.
2. A complete blood count, blood smear, and clotting profile should be ordered and the type and cross-match sent to the blood bank. Take specific note of fragmented red blood cells (disseminated intravascular coagulation), neutropenia (margination of white blood cells), and thrombocytopenia.
3. Barium swallow is not indicated immediately. If there is evidence of obstruction without pneumatosis intestinalis on the flat film, then a barium swallow may be necessary to exclude malrotation.
4. Gastrografin enema may be curative if there is a meconium plug but is contraindicated in this case because the hyperosmolar contrast medium may produce further damage to already compromised bowel and result in perforation.
5. Abdominal x-ray films, both KUB (kidney, ureter, and bladder) and cross-table lateral, should be obtained to detect the presence of pneumatosis intestinalis, hepatic portal gas, or free intraabdominal gas, indicating a perforated viscus. If no free air is seen initially but there is pneumatosis intestinalis present, the cross-table lateral x-ray film should be repeated every 4 to 6 hours or sooner if there is clinical deterioration.
6. It is important to evaluate acid-base status and serum electrolytes in infants with suspected gastrointestinal disturbances. Correction of these metabolic derangements is crucial before submitting these precarious infants to major surgery.

The x-ray films reveal pneumatosis intestinalis with no air in the liver or free intraperitoneal air. The blood pressure is 55/35; blood gases pH 7.32, Pao_2 65 and Pco_2 40; bicarbonate 20; serum sodium 132; potassium 4.8; chloride 105; BUN 10; hematocrit 38%; white blood cell count 14,900 with 70% segmented cells; platelets adequate and clotting profile normal. Pediatric surgeons were consulted and, together with the nursery staff, they managed the case.

The following treatments should be instituted (True or False):

1. Nasogastric suction, IV fluids, and nothing per os (NPO)
2. Systemic and orogastric antibiotics
3. Laparotomy

4. Exchange transfusion
5. Placement of central hyperalimentation line

1. True. It is imperative to decompress the abdomen with a large oral or nasogastric tube. Carefully record all intake and output, weigh the baby twice daily, and measure abdominal girth frequently. IV fluid therapy must take into consideration significant third-space losses. Patients with documented NEC should be managed with NPO for at least 7 to 10 days.
2. True. The patient was started on appropriate doses of IV piperacillin and an aminoglycoside. Antibiotics via nasogastric tube has not proved to be efficacious.
3. False. There is no clear-cut indication for laparotomy at this stage. Whereas surgery is clearly indicated for intestinal perforation, some centers operate when medical management fails to correct the shock-acidosis; if there is persistent cellulitis of the anterior abdominal wall; or if radiologically a single dilated loop of bowel persists.
4. False. With normal clotting studies and no evidence of bleeding or significant hyperbilirubinemia, exchange transfusion is not indicated.
5. False. TPN is going to be necessary for this infant. However, with septicemia likely, it is advisable to wait until the sepsis has been controlled and the general condition is stabilized before placing a central line for IV nutrition. Some centers provide all nutritive support with peripheral lines using glucose-amino acid mixtures supplemented with IV lipid.

Four hours later, the blood pressure drops from 55/35 to 40/0. The urine output decreases to less than 1 mL/hour, and the abdomen is more distended, edematous, and tender. On physical examination, the infant is pink with a wide pulse pressure, tachycardia, and warm extremities. Repeat complete blood count reveals white blood cell count of 3.1, with 10% segmented cells and 10% bands.

These data should be interpreted as (True or False):

1. Septic shock
2. Perforated abdominal viscus
3. Patent ductus arteriosus with congestive heart failure
4. Pneumothorax
5. Third-space loss

1 and 5, True. The patient as described—pink with wide pulse pressure, tachycardia, and warm extremities—has the classic features of warm shock. When such cases are untreated, the blood pressure decreases further and vasoconstriction predominates, transforming the "warm" shock to "cold" shock. A major factor contributing to shock in patients with NEC is the massive third space

that develops in the abdomen, which results from the inflammatory response and bowel necrosis. These large fluid and protein losses result in hypovolemia and require urgent therapy. The mainstay of treatment is to elevate the blood pressure by supporting the intravascular space with sufficient blood, plasma, or crystalloid to maintain the blood pressure and urine output. Whole blood is preferred because it remains in the intravascular space, whereas other fluids leak through the damaged capillaries and contribute to intestinal edema. Large volumes of crystalloid may be required. Neutropenia may be documented in NEC without bacteremia. Margination of neutrophils is assumed because marrow reserves are not depleted.

2. False. Although the sudden deterioration is suggestive of perforation and evaluation by transillumination and an x-ray film is certainly indicated, no perforation was present at the time. The wide pulse pressure is not usually detected at the time of perforation.
3. False. Tachycardia, edema, and wide pulse pressure are present with patent ductus arteriosus and congestive heart failure. However, the striking abdominal findings, together with the diminished blood pressure, suggest that this is not the primary problem. Patent ductus arteriosus, however, is found frequently in infants with NEC.
4. False. This is unlikely, given the complete picture, particularly with a pink baby and wide pulse pressure.

Two hours later, x-ray films show increased distention and no evidence of free air but the appearance of bowel "floating" in the abdomen.

What is the significance of this finding?

Bowel floating in the abdomen in a patient with sepsis and a distended tender abdomen indicates ascites caused by peritonitis. Because many cases of "intraabdominal sepsis" are caused by anaerobic bacteria, anaerobic antimicrobial coverage should be started following paracentesis. (Clindamycin is instituted for infants with suspected NEC and perforation.)

On surgically introducing a drain into the left lower quadrant, 10 mL of purulent fluid is removed. The cell count shows 90,000 white blood cells with 75% PMN leukocytes. Gram stain shows both gram-positive and gram-negative rods.

The patient is noted to have blood oozing from venipuncture sites, with petechiae and a falling hematocrit despite multiple blood transfusions.

Laboratory Data

CBC: Hct-28; platelets 5000; smear shows fragmented red blood cells and burr cells

Prothrombin time: patient, 50 seconds; control, 10 seconds

Partial thromboplastin time: patient, 180 seconds; control, 30 seconds

Fibrinogen: 50 mg/dL (normal 200 mg/dL)

Fibrin split products: 4+ (normal not present)

Disseminated intravascular coagulation has complicated the picture, and therefore an exchange transfusion with fresh blood is performed (see Chapter 17).

Blood pressure, urine output, and activity are normal for 3 days. The abdomen is softer, but there is still some edema of the abdominal wall. Repeated x-ray films fail to reveal free intraabdominal air. After 5 days of relative stability, the patient becomes acutely distended with signs of respiratory embarrassment.

Which of the following management options is appropriate?

1. Repeat clotting profile and exchange transfusion.
2. Percuss abdomen and then transilluminate while awaiting x-ray film.
3. Repeat blood cultures and change antibiotics.
4. Measure blood gas and increase environmental oxygen.

1. This acute episode following a period of stability cannot entirely be attributed to disseminated intravascular coagulation.
2. This acute change is probably due to intestinal perforation. Abdominal percussion used to demonstrate the absence of hepatic dullness and positive transillumination may confirm suspicions before the cross-table lateral x-ray film has been developed. The film in this instance demonstrated free air.
3. Blood culture should be repeated, but there is no reason to change antibiotics at this time.
4. This is only symptomatic management. The basic cause for the abdominal distention and respiratory embarrassment must be determined. The blood gas will indicate the need for ventilatory support.

The child is brought to the operating room where the perforated area of ileum is resected and an ileostomy and colostomy are performed. Two days postoperatively a central line is placed in the NICU operating room and TPN is administered via this route for 21 days. After 14 days of being NPO, he was started on breast milk and did well.

CASE C-2

M. P. is born at 34 weeks' gestation, weighing 1200 g. His perinatal course is complicated by intrauterine growth restriction, hyperbilirubinemia, and polycythemia, requiring a single volume exchange transfusion done through an umbilical venous catheter. At 8 days of age, abdominal distention, hematochezia, acidosis, and hypotension develop. NEC is

diagnosed and is treated with medical management. He recovers and begins enteral feedings 14 days after the onset of acute NEC.

M. P. is discharged home at 6 weeks of age, having tolerated full volume enteral feedings for 2 weeks. Three weeks after discharge, he has acute abdominal distention, vomiting, and hematochezia. Abdominal examination reveals guarding and tenderness.

What is the most likely diagnosis?

1. *Clostridium difficile* infection
2. Intestinal stricture
3. Anal fissure
4. Milk protein allergy

Strictures are one of the most common complications of NEC, occurring in 10% to 35% of all survivors.[150,151] They result from healing and cicatricial scarring of an ischemic area of bowel.[152] Signs include hematochezia, vomiting, abdominal distention, and sudden bowel obstruction. Strictures usually manifest in the first 2 months following acute NEC, but may occur as late as 6 months afterward.

Which of the following management options is appropriate?

1. Perform stool culture and start oral antibiotics.
2. Change infant to soy formula feedings.
3. Obtain abdominal x-ray, do barium enema, and consult pediatric surgery.
4. Reassure the mother that rectal bleeding is common; send child home with office follow-up in 1 to 2 days.

1, 2, and 4, False. Any neonate with history of NEC followed by the onset of hematochezia and vomiting should undergo evaluation to rule out strictures. Recent reports have suggested that clinical observation alone is associated with significant morbidity in this population. Failure to rapidly detect and manage stricture complications has resulted in intestinal perforation and life-threatening sepsis.[153]

3, True. Proper management includes abdominal x-rays, barium enema, and pediatric surgical evaluation.

Abdominal x-rays reveal acute intestinal obstruction. Barium enema demonstrates multiple strictures of the ileum, transverse and descending colon, and rectosigmoid region, as well as perforation with intraperitoneal contrast extravasation.

Emergency ileostomy is performed. Postoperatively, M. P. has a rocky course, complicated by multiple episodes of sepsis and feeding intolerance. He is given several courses of antibiotics and nearly 3 weeks of total parenteral nutrition.

Approximately 1 month after surgery, M. P. is noted to have direct hyperbilirubinemia, poor growth, hepatomegaly, and elevated liver function tests.

Work-up includes a negative hepatitis panel, normal hepatic and gallbladder ultrasound, negative sepsis, TORCH (*to*xoplasmosis, *r*ubella, *c*ytomegalovirus, and *h*erpes simplex) work-ups, and a normal newborn screen.

What is the most likely diagnosis?

1. Biliary atresia
2. TPN cholestasis
3. α_1-Antitrypsin deficiency
4. Cystic fibrosis

Although all of the above are possible, the most likely diagnosis is TPN cholestasis. It typically develops after 2 or more weeks of enteral fasting with TPN providing the sole nutritional support. With initiation of trophic feeding to enhance bile flow, TPN cholestasis gradually resolves over 1 to 3 months. If symptoms persist despite enteral feeding, a full diagnostic work-up is indicated.

By 6 weeks after operation, M. P. has advanced to full-volume enteral feedings with slow resolution of the TPN cholestasis. However, he continues to demonstrate poor growth and develops increasing stool output through the ileostomy. He undergoes a second surgery to reanastomose the bowel. Following reanastomosis, M. P.'s nutritional status improves and he is discharged to home. At 10 months of age, he is tolerating a normal diet, although he remains at the third percentile for all growth parameters.

REFERENCES

The reference list for this chapter can be found online at www.expertconsult.com

Care of the Parents

Marshall H. Klaus, John H. Kennell, and Jonathan M. Fanaroff

Unfortunately…a certain number of mothers abandon the babies whose needs they have not had to meet, and in whom they have lost all interest. The life of the little one has been saved, it is true, but at the cost of the mother.[1]

Pierre Budin, *The Nursling*

A renewed interest in the first minutes, hours, and days of life has been stimulated by several provocative behavioral and physiologic observations in both mother and infant. These assessments and measurements have been made during labor, birth, the immediate postnatal period, and the beginning breast feedings. They provide a compelling rationale for major changes in care in the perinatal period for both mother and infant. Surprisingly, these findings form a novel way to view the mother-infant dyad.

To understand how these observations fit together, it is necessary to appreciate that the period of labor, birth, and the ensuing several days can probably best be defined as a "sensitive period." During this time, the mother and probably, the father, are especially open to changing their later behavior with their infant depending on the quality of their care during the sensitive period.

Winnicott also described this period.[2] He reported a special mental state of the mother in the perinatal period that involves a greatly increased sensitivity to, and focus upon, the needs of her baby. He indicated that this state of "primary maternal preoccupation" starts near the end of pregnancy and continues for a few weeks after the birth of the baby. A mother needs nurturing support and a protected environment to develop and maintain this state. This special preoccupation and the openness of the mother to her baby is probably related to the bonding process. Winnicott wrote that "Only if a mother is sensitized in the way I am describing, can she feel herself into her infant's place, and so meet the infant's needs." In the state of "primary maternal preoccupation," the mother is better able to sense and provide what her new infant has signaled, which is her primary task. If she senses the needs and responds to them in a sensitive and timely manner, mother and infant will establish a pattern of synchronized and mutually rewarding interactions. It is our hypothesis that as the mother-infant pair continues this dance pattern day after day, the infant will more frequently develop a secure attachment, with the ability to be reassured by well-known caregivers and the willingness to explore and master the environment when caregivers are present.

This chapter describes studies of the process by which a parent becomes attached to the infant, and the physiologic and behavioral components in the newborn, and suggests applications of these findings to the care of the parents of a normal infant, a premature or malformed infant, and a stillbirth or neonatal death.

PREGNANCY

A mother's and father's actions and responses toward their infant are derived from a complex combination of their own genetic endowment, the way the infant responds to them, a long history of interpersonal relations with their own families and with each other, past experiences with this or previous pregnancies, the absorption of the practices and values of their cultures, and probably most importantly, how each was raised by his or her own mother and father. The parenting behavior of each woman and man, his or her ability to tolerate stresses, and his or her need for special attention differ greatly and depend on a mixture of these factors. Figure 8-1 is a schematic diagram of the major influences on paternal and maternal behavior and the resulting disturbances that we hypothesize may arise from them.

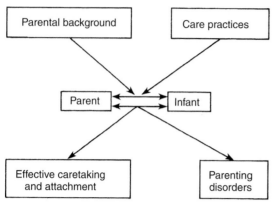

Figure 8-1. Algorithm of major influences on parent-infant attachment and resulting outcomes.

Included under parental background are the parent's care by his or her own mother, genetics of parents, practices of their culture, relationships within the family, experiences with previous pregnancies, and planning, course, and events during pregnancy. Strong evidence for the importance of the effect of the mother's own mothering on her caretaking comes from an elegant 35-year study by Engel et al. that documented the close correspondence between how Monica (an infant with a tracheoesophageal fistula) was fed during the first 2 years of life,[3] how she then cared for her dolls, and how as an adult she fed her own four children.

Included under care practices are the behavior of physicians, nurses, and hospital personnel, care and support during labor, first days of life, separation of mother and infant, and rules of the hospital.

Included under parenting disorders are the vulnerable child syndrome,[4] child abuse,[5,6] failure to thrive,[7] and some developmental and emotional problems in high-risk infants.[8] Other determinants—such as the attitudes, statements, and practices of the nurses and physicians in the hospital, whether the mother is alone for short periods during her labor, whether there is separation from the infant in the first days of life, the nature of the infant, his or her temperament, and whether he or she is healthy, sick, or malformed—will affect parenting behavior and the parent-child relationship.

The most easily manipulated variables in this scheme are the separation of the infant from the mother and the practices in the hospital during the first hours and days of life. It is here, during this period, that studies have in part clarified some of the steps in parent-infant attachment. A diversity of observations are beginning to piece together some of the various phases and times that are helpful for this process (Box 8-1). Pregnancy for a woman has been considered a process of maturation,[9,10] with a series of adaptive tasks, each dependent on the successful completion of the preceding one.

Many mothers are initially disturbed by feelings of grief and anger when they become pregnant, because of factors ranging from economic and housing hardships to interpersonal difficulties. However, by the end of the first trimester, the majority of women who initially rejected pregnancy have accepted it. This initial stage as outlined by Bibring is the mother's identification of the growing fetus as an "integral part of herself."[9]

The second stage is a growing perception of the fetus as a separate individual, usually occurring with the awareness of fetal movement. After quickening, a woman generally begins to have some fantasies about what the baby may be like; she attributes some human personality characteristics, and develops a sense of attachment and value toward the baby. At this time, further acceptance of the pregnancy and marked changes in attitude toward the fetus may be observed; unplanned, unwanted infants may seem more acceptable. Objectively, the health worker usually finds some outward evidence of the mother's preparation in such actions as the purchase of clothes or a crib, selecting a name, and arranging space for the baby.

The increased use of amniocentesis and ultrasound has appeared to affect parents' perceptions of babies in a rather unexpected fashion. Many parents have discussed the

Box 8-1.　Steps in Attachment

Before pregnancy
Planning the pregnancy

During pregnancy
Confirming the pregnancy
Accepting the pregnancy
Experiencing fetal movement
Beginning to accept the fetus as an individual

Labor

Birth

After birth
Touching and smelling
Seeing the baby
Breast feeding
Caring for the baby
Accepting the infant as a separate individual

disappointment they experienced when they discovered the sex of the baby. Half of the mystery was over. Everything was possible, but once the amniocentesis was done and the sex of the baby known, the range of the unknown was considerably narrowed. However, the tests have the beneficial result of removing some of the anxiety about the possibility of the baby having an abnormality. We have noted that, following the procedure, the baby is sometimes named, and parents often carry around a picture of the very small fetus. This phenomenon requires further investigation to understand the significance of these reactions to the bonding process.

Cohen suggests the following questions to learn the special needs of each mother[11]:

- How long have you lived in this immediate area, and where does most of your family live?
- How often do you see your mother or other close relatives?
- Has anything happened to you in the past (or do you currently have any condition) that causes you to worry about the pregnancy or the baby?
- What was the father's reaction to your becoming pregnant?
- What other responsibilities do you have outside the family?

When planning to meet the needs of the mother, it is important to inquire about how the pregnant woman was mothered—did she have a neglected and deprived infancy and childhood or grow up with a warm and intact family life?

LABOR AND DELIVERY

Newton and Newton noted that those mothers who remain relaxed in labor,[12] who are supported, and who have good rapport with their attendants, are more apt to be pleased with their infants at first sight.

A recent Cochrane review looked at the importance of continuous support for women during childbirth. Looking at 21 trials involving 15,061 mothers, the results showed that women who had continuous social support during labor and birth had labors that were significantly shorter, were more likely to have a spontaneous vaginal birth, and less likely to have intrapartum analgesia.[13] They also were less likely to have a cesarean section or instrumented vaginal birth, regional anesthesia, or a baby with a low 5-minute Apgar score. This low-cost intervention may be a simple way to reduce the length of labor and perinatal problems for women and their infants during childbirth.

EFFECTS OF SOCIAL AND EMOTIONAL SUPPORT ON MATERNAL BEHAVIOR

This short, but highly significant time in a woman's life, has been explored in depth because the care during labor appears to affect a mother's attitudes, feelings, and responses to her family, herself, and especially her new baby to a remarkable degree. In a well-conducted trial of continuous social support in South Africa, both mothers with and without doula support were interviewed immediately after delivery and 6 weeks later.[14,15] Women who had doula support during labor had significantly increased self-esteem, believed they had coped well with labor, and thought the labor had been easier than they had imagined. Women who received this support reported being less anxious 24 hours after birth compared with mothers without a doula. Doula-supported mothers were significantly less depressed 6 weeks postpartum, as measured on a standard depression scale, than mothers who had no doula. Also, doula-supported mothers had a significantly greater incidence of breast feeding without supplements (52% versus 29%), and they breast fed for a longer period.

The supported mothers said it took them an average of 2.9 days to develop a relationship with their babies compared with 9.8 days for the nonsupported mothers. This feeling of attachment and readiness to fall in love with their babies made them less willing to leave their babies alone. They also reported picking up their babies more frequently when they cried than did nonsupported mothers. The doula-supported mothers were more positive in describing the special attributes of their babies than were the nonsupported mothers. A higher percentage of supported mothers not only considered their babies beautiful, clever, healthy, and easy to manage, but also believed their infants cried less than other babies. The supported mothers believed that their babies were "better" when compared with a "standard baby," whereas the nonsupported mothers perceived their babies as "almost as good as" or "not quite as good as" a "standard baby." "Support group mothers also perceived themselves as closer to their babies, as managing better, and as communicating better with their babies than control-group mothers did," the study reported. A higher percentage of the doula-supported mothers indicated that they were pleased to have their babies, found becoming a mother was easier than expected, and thought that they could look after their babies better than any other person could. In contrast, the nonsupported mothers perceived their adaptation to motherhood as more difficult and believed that others could care for their baby as well as they could.

A most important aspect of emotional support during childbirth may be the most unexpected internalized one—that of the calm, nurturing, accepting, and holding model provided for the parents by the doula during labor. Maternal care needs modeling; each generation is influenced from the care received by the earlier one. Social support appears to be an essential ingredient of childbirth that was lost when birthing moved from home to hospital.

THE DAY OF DELIVERY

Mothers after delivery appear to have common patterns of behavior when they begin to care for their babies in the first hour of life. Filmed observations reveal that when a mother is presented with her nude,[16] full-term infant in privacy, she begins with fingertip touching of the infant's extremities and within a few minutes proceeds to massaging, encompassing palm contact of the infant's trunk. Mothers of premature infants also follow this sequence, but proceed at a much slower rate. Fathers go through some of the same routines.[17]

A strong interest in eye-to-eye contact has been expressed by mothers of both full-term and premature infants. Tape recordings of the words of mothers who had been presented with their infants in privacy revealed that 73% of the statements referred to the eyes. The mothers said, "Let me see your eyes" and "Open your eyes and I'll know you love me." Robson has suggested that eye-to-eye contact appears to elicit maternal caregiving responses.[18] Mothers seem to try hard to look "en face" at their infants—that is, to keep their faces aligned with their baby's so that their eyes are in the same vertical plane of rotation as the baby's. Complementing the mother's interest in the infant's eyes is the early functional development of the infant's visual pathways. The infant is alert, active, and able to follow during the first hour of life if maternal sedation has been limited and the administration of eye drops or ointment is delayed.

Additional information about this early period was provided by Wolff,[19] who described six separate states of consciousness in the infant, ranging from deep sleep to screaming. The state in which we are most interested is state 4, the quiet, alert state. In this state, the infant's eyes are wide open, and he or she able to respond to his or her environment. The infant may only be in this state for periods as brief as a few seconds. However, Emde et al. observed that the infant is in a wakeful state on the average for a period of 38 minutes during the first hour after birth.[20] It is currently possible to demonstrate that an infant can see, has visual preferences, has a memory for the mother's face at 4 hours of age, will turn his or her head to the spoken word, and moves in rhythm to the mother's voice in the first minutes and hours of life—a beautiful linking and synchronized dance between the mother and infant. After this, however, the infant goes into a deep sleep for 3 to 4 hours.

Therefore, during the first 60 to 90 minutes of life, the infant is alert, responsive, and especially appealing. In short, the infant is ideally equipped to meet his or her parents for the first time. The infant's broad array of sensory and motor abilities evokes responses from the mother and begins the communication that may be especially helpful for attachment and the initiation of a series of reciprocal interactions.

Observations by Condon and Sander reveal that newborns move in rhythm with the structure of adult speech.[21] Interestingly, synchronous movements were found at 16 hours of age with both of the two natural languages tested, English and Chinese.

Mothers also quickly become aware of their infant. Kaitz et al. demonstrated that after only 1 hour with their infants in the first hours of life,[22,23] mothers are able to discriminate their own baby from other infants. Parturient women know their infant's distinctive features after minimal exposure using olfactory and tactile cues (touching the dorsum of the hand), whereas discrimination based on sight and sound takes somewhat longer to develop. Fathers are good at quickly recognizing their newborn through visual-facial cues, though not quite as good as mothers at recognizing olfactory cues.[24]

WHEN DOES LOVE BEGIN?

The first feelings of love for the infant are not necessarily instantaneous with the initial contact.

MacFarlane et al. helped to answer this question by asking 97 mothers, "When did you first feel love for your baby?"[25] The replies were as follows: during pregnancy—41%; at birth—24%; first week—27%; and after the first week—8%.

In another study of two groups of primiparous mothers ($n = 112$ and $n = 41$), 40% recalled that their predominant emotional reaction when holding their babies for the first time was one of indifference.[26] The same response was reported by 25% of 40 multiparous mothers. In both groups, 40% felt immediate affection.

CARE OF THE NORMAL INFANT AND PARENTS FOLLOWING BIRTH

After birth, the newborn should be thoroughly dried with warm towels so as not to lose heat, and once it is clear that he has good color and is active and appears normal (usually within 5 minutes), he can go to his mother. At this time, the warm and dry infant can be placed between the mother's breasts or on her abdomen or, if she desires, next to her. The new NRP guidelines emphasize that babies who do not need resuscitation should not be separated from their mother.[27]

When newborns are kept close to their mother's body or on their mother, the transition from life in the womb to existence outside the uterus is made much easier for them. The newborn recognizes his mother's voice and smell,[28,29] and her body warms his to just the right temperature.[30] In this way, the infant can experience sensations somewhat similar to what he felt during the last several weeks of uterine life.

In the past, many caretakers believed that the newborn needs help to begin to nurse. So often, immediately after birth, the baby's lips are placed near or on the mother's nipple. In that situation, some babies do start to suckle, but most babies just lick the nipple or peer up at the mother. They appear to be much more interested in the mother's face, especially her eyes, even though the nipple is right next to their lips. They most commonly begin, when left on their own,

to move toward the breast 30 to 40 minutes after birth.

THE BREAST CRAWL

One of the most exciting observations made is the discovery that the newborn has the ability to find her mother's breast all on her own and to decide for herself when to take her first feeding. In order not to remove the taste and smell of the mother's amniotic fluid, it is necessary to delay washing the baby's hands. The baby uses the taste and smell of amniotic fluid on her hands to make a connection with a certain lipid substance on the nipple related to the amniotic fluid.

The infant usually begins with a time of rest and quiet alertness, during which he rarely cries and often appears to take pleasure in looking at his mother's face. Around 30 to 40 minutes after birth, the newborn begins making mouthing movements, sometimes with lip smacking, and shortly after, saliva begins to pour down onto his chin.[31] When placed on the mother's abdomen, babies maneuver in their own ways to reach the nipple. They often use stepping motions of their legs to move ahead, while horizontally moving toward the nipple, using small push-ups and lowering one arm first in the direction they wish to go. These efforts are interspersed with short rest periods. Sometimes babies change direction in the midst of their journey. These actions take effort and time. Parents find patience worth every minute if they wait and observe their infant on his first journey.

In Figure 8-2, one newborn is seen successfully navigating his way to his mother's breast. At 10 minutes of age, he first begins to move toward the left breast, but 5 minutes later, he is back in the midline. Repeated mouthing and sucking of the hands and fingers is commonly observed. With a series of push-ups and rest periods, he makes his way to the breast completely on his own, placing his lips on the areola of the breast. He begins to suckle effectively and closely observes his mother's face.

In one group of mothers who did not receive pain medication and whose babies were not taken away during the first hours of life for a bath, vitamin K administration, or application of eye ointment, 15 of 16 babies placed on their mother's abdomen were observed to make the trip to their mother's breast, latch on their own, and begin to suckle effectively.[32]

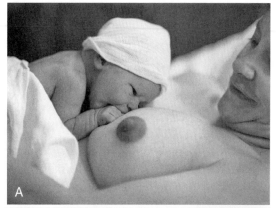

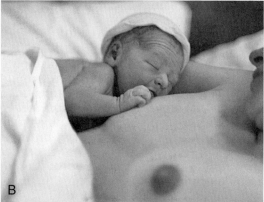

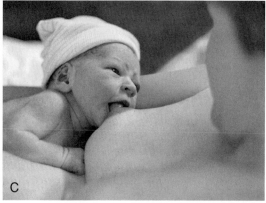

Figure 8-2. A, Infant about 15 minutes after birth, sucking on the unwashed hand and possibly looking at mother's left nipple. **B,** An arm push-up, which helps the infant to move to mother's right side. **C,** At 45 minutes of age, the infant moved to the right breast without assistance and began sucking on the areola of the breast. The infant has been looking at the mother's face for 5 to 8 minutes. *(Photographed by Elaine Siegel. From Klaus PH:* Your amazing newborn, *Cambridge, Mass, 1998, Perseus, pp 13, 16, 17.)*

This sequence is helpful to the mother as well, because the massage of the breast and suckling induce a large oxytocin surge into her bloodstream, which helps contract the uterus, expelling the placenta and closing off many blood vessels in the uterus,

thus reducing bleeding. The stimulation and suckling also helps in the manufacture of prolactin, and the suckling enhances the closeness and new bond between mother and baby. Mother and baby appear to be carefully adapted for these first moments together.

To allow this first intimate encounter, the injection of vitamin K, application of eye ointment, washing, and any measuring of the infant's weight, height, and head circumference may be delayed for at least 1 hour. More than 90% of all full-term infants are normal at birth. In a few minutes, they can be easily evaluated to ensure that they are healthy. They can then, after thorough drying, be safely placed on their mother's chest if the parents wish.

The odor of the nipple appears to guide a newborn to the breast.[29,33] If the right breast is washed with soap and water, the infant will crawl to the left breast, and vice versa. If both breasts are washed, the infant will go to the breast that has been rubbed with the amniotic fluid of the mother. The special attraction of the newborn to the odor of *his* mother's amniotic fluid may reflect the time in utero when, as a fetus, he swallowed the liquid. Although it is not breast milk, amniotic fluid probably contains a substance that is similar to a secretion of the breast. Amniotic fluid on the infant's hands probably also explains part of the interest in sucking the hands and fingers seen in the photographs. This early hand-sucking behavior is markedly reduced when the infant is bathed before the crawl. With all these innate programs, it almost seems as if the infant comes into life carrying a small computer chip with these instructions.

At a moment such as childbirth, we come full circle to our biological origins. Many separate abilities enable a baby to do this. Stepping reflexes help the newborn push against his mother's abdomen to propel him toward the breast. Pressure of the infant's feet on the abdomen may also help in the expulsion of the placenta and in reducing uterine bleeding. The ability to move his hand in a reaching motion enables the baby to claim the nipple. Taste, smell, and vision all help the newborn detect and find the breast. Muscular strength in the neck, shoulders, and arms helps newborns to bob their heads and do small push-ups to inch forward and side to side. This whole scenario may take place in a matter of minutes; it usually occurs within 30 to 60 minutes, but it is within the capacity of the newborn. It appears that young humans, like other baby mammals, know how to find their mother's breast.

When the mother and infant are resting skin-to-skin and gazing eye-to-eye, they begin to learn about each other on many different levels. For the mother, the first minutes and hours after birth are a time when she is uniquely open emotionally to respond to her baby and to begin the new relationship.

A SENSITIVE PERIOD?

Many studies have focused on whether additional time for close contact of the mother and infant alters the quality of attachment.[16,34,35] These studies have addressed the question of whether there is a sensitive period for parent-infant contact in the first minutes, hours, and days of life that may alter the parents' later behavior with their infant. In many biological disciplines, these moments have been called *sensitive periods*. However, in most of the examples of a sensitive period in biology, the observations are made on the young of the species rather than on the adult. Evidence for a sensitive period comes from the following series of studies. Note that in each study, increasing mother-infant time together or increased suckling improves caretaking by the mother.

In six of nine randomized trials of only early contact with suckling (during the first hour of life), both the number of women breast feeding and the length of their lactation were significantly increased for early contact mothers compared with women in the control group.

In addition, studies of Brazelton and others have shown that if nurses spend as little as 10 minutes helping mothers discover some of their newborn infant's abilities,[36] such as turning to the mother's voice and following the mother's face, and assisting mothers with suggestions about ways to quiet their infants, the mothers become more appropriately interactive with their infants face-to-face and during feedings at 3 and 4 months of age.

O'Connor et al. carried out a randomized trial with 277 mothers in a hospital that had a high incidence of parenting disorders.[37] One group of mothers had their infants with them for 6 additional hours on the first and second day, but no early contact. The routine care group began to see their babies at the same age but only for 20-minute

feedings every 4 hours, which was the custom throughout the United States at that time. In follow-up studies, 10 children in the routine care group experienced parenting disorders, including child abuse, failure to thrive, abandonment, and neglect during the first 17 months of life compared with two children in the experimental group who had 12 additional hours of mother-infant contact. A similar study in North Carolina that included 202 mothers during the first year of life did not find a statistically significant difference in the frequency of parenting disorders[7]; 10 infants failed to thrive or were neglected or abused in the control group compared with seven in the group that had extended contact. When the results of these two studies are combined in a metaanalysis ($P = .054$), it appears that simple techniques, such as adding additional early time for each mother and infant to be together and continuous rooming-in, may lead to a significant reduction in child abuse. A much larger study is necessary to confirm and validate these relatively small studies.

Swedish researchers have shown that the normal infant,[30] when dried and placed nude on the mother's chest and then covered with a blanket, will maintain his or her body temperature as well as when elaborate, high-tech heating devices that usually separate the mother and baby are used. The same researchers found that when the infants are skin-to-skin with their mothers for the first 90 minutes after birth, they cry hardly at all compared with infants who were dried, wrapped in a towel, and placed in a bassinet. It is likely that each of these features—the crawling ability of the infant, the decreased crying when close to the mother, and the warming capabilities of the mother's chest—are adaptive features that have evolved to help preserve the infant's life.

When the infant suckles from the breast, it stimulates the production of oxytocin in both the mother's and the infant's brains, and oxytocin in turn stimulates the vagal motor nucleus, releasing 19 different gastrointestinal hormones, including insulin, cholecystokinin, and gastrin. Five of the 19 hormones stimulate growth of the baby's and mother's intestinal villi and increase the surface area and the absorption of calories with each feeding.[38] Stimuli for this release are touch on the mother's nipple and the inside of the infant's mouth. The increased gut motility with each suckling may help remove meconium with its large load of bilirubin.

These research findings may explain some of the underlying physiologic and behavioral processes and provide additional support for the importance of 2 of the 10 caregiving procedures that the United Nations International Children's Emergency Fund (UNICEF) is promoting as part of its Baby Friendly Initiative to increase breast feeding: (1) early mother-infant contact, with an opportunity for the baby to suckle in the first hour, and (2) mother-infant rooming-in throughout the hospital stay.

Following the introduction of the Baby Friendly Initiative in maternity units in several countries throughout the world, an unexpected observation was made. In Thailand,[39] in a hospital where a disturbing number of babies are abandoned by their mothers, the use of rooming-in and early contact with suckling significantly reduced the frequency of abandonment from 33 in 10,000 births to 1 in 10,000 births a year. Similar observations have been made in Russia, the Philippines, and Costa Rica, where early contact and rooming-in were also introduced.

These reports are additional evidence that the first hours and days of life are a sensitive period for the human mother. This may be due in part to the special interest that mothers have shortly after birth in hoping that their infant will look at them and to the infant's ability to interact in the first hour of life during the prolonged period of the quiet alert state. There is a beautiful interlocking at this early time of the mother's interest in the infant's eyes and the baby's ability to interact and to look eye-to-eye.

A possible key to understanding what is happening physiologically in these first minutes and hours comes from investigators who noted that, if the lips of the infant touch the mother's nipple in the first hour of life, a mother will decide to keep her baby 100 minutes longer in her room every day during her hospital stay than another mother who does not have contact until later.[40] This may be partly explained by the small secretions of oxytocin (the "love hormone") that occur in both the infant's and mother's brains when breast feeding occurs. In sheep,[41] dilation of the cervical os during birth releases oxytocin within the brain which, acting on receptor sites, is important for the initiation of maternal behavior and for the facilitation of bonding

between mother and baby. In humans, there is a blood-brain barrier for oxytocin, and only small amounts reach the brain via the bloodstream. However, multiple oxytocin receptors in the brain are supplied by de novo oxytocin synthesis in the brain. Increased levels of brain oxytocin result in slight sleepiness, euphoria, increased pain threshold, and feelings of increased love for the infant. It appears that, during breast feeding, elevated blood levels of oxytocin are associated with increased brain levels; women who exhibit the highest plasma oxytocin concentration are the most sleepy.

Measurements of plasma oxytocin levels in healthy women who had their babies skin-to-skin on their chests immediately after birth reveal significant elevations compared with the prepartum levels and a return to prepartum levels at 60 minutes. For most women, a significant and spontaneous peak concentration was recorded about 15 minutes after delivery, with expulsion of the placenta.[42] Most mothers had several peaks of oxytocin up to 1 hour after delivery. The vigorous oxytocin release after delivery and with breast feeding not only may help contract the uterine muscle to prevent bleeding, but may also enhance bonding of the mother to her infant. These findings may explain an observation made in France in the 19th century when many poor mothers were giving up their babies. Nurses recorded that mothers who breast fed for at least 8 days rarely abandoned their infants. We hypothesize that a cascade of interactions between the mother and baby occurs during this early period, locking them together and ensuring further development of attachment. The remarkable change in maternal behavior with just the touch of the infant's lips on the mother's nipple, the effects of additional time for mother-infant contact, and the reduction in abandonment with early contact, suckling, and rooming-in, as well as the elevated maternal oxytocin levels shortly after birth in conjunction with known sensory, physiologic, immunologic, and behavioral mechanisms all contribute to the attachment of the parent to the infant.

EARLY AND EXTENDED CONTACT FOR PARENTS AND THEIR INFANT

Although debate continues on the interpretation and significance of some of the research studies regarding the effects of early and extended contact for mothers and fathers on bonding with their infants, both sides agree that all parents should be offered such contact time with their infants. A recent Cochrane Review looked at 30 studies involving 1925 participants (mother-infant dyads) and concluded that early skin-to-skin contact for mothers and their healthy newborns reduced crying, improved mother-baby interaction, kept the baby warmer, and helped women to breast feed successfully.[43]

On the basis of observations and the reports of parents, every parent has a task to perform during the postpartum period. The mother, in particular, must look at and "take in" her real live baby and then reconcile the fantasy of the infant she imagined with the one she actually delivered.

Evidence suggests that many of these early interactions also take place between the father and his newborn child. Parke has demonstrated that when fathers are given the opportunity to be alone with their newborns,[44] they spend almost exactly the same amount of time as mothers in holding, touching, and looking at them.

How strongly should physicians and nurses emphasize the importance of parent-infant contact in the first hour and extended visiting for the rest of the hospital stay? Despite a lack of early contact experienced by many parents in hospital births in the past, almost all these parents became bonded to their babies. The human is highly adaptable, and there are many fail-safe routes to attachment. Parents who miss the bonding experience can be assured that their future relationship with their infant can still develop as usual. Mothers who miss out on early and extended contact are often those at the limits of adaptability and who may benefit the most—the poor, the single, the unsupported, and the teenage mothers.

At least 60 minutes of early contact in privacy should be provided, if possible, for parents and their infant to enhance the bonding experience. If the health of the mother or infant makes this impossible, then discussion, support, and reassurance should help the parents appreciate that they can become as completely attached to their infant as if they had the usual bonding experience. The infant should only be with the mother and father if she is known to be physically normal and if appropriate temperature control is used. The baby should remain with the mother as long as desired throughout the hospital stay so that the mother and the baby can get to know each other. This permits both mother and father more time to learn about their baby and to gradually develop a strong tie in the first weeks of life.

From these many findings are the following recommendations for changing the perinatal period for mother and infant.

- Every mother should have continuous physical and emotional support during the entire labor by a knowledgeable, caring woman (e.g., doula, obstetric nurse, or midwife) in addition to her partner.
- Childbirth educators and obstetric caregivers should discuss with every pregnant woman the advantages of an unmedicated labor to avoid interference with the infant's ability to interact, self-attach, and successfully breast feed.
- Immediately after birth and a thorough drying, an infant who has good Apgar scores and appears normal should be offered to the mother for skin-to-skin contact, with warmth provided by her body and a light blanket covering the baby. The baby should not be removed for a bath, footprinting, or administration of vitamin K or eye medication until after the first hour. The baby thus can be allowed to decide when to begin his first feeding.
- The central nursery should be used infrequently. All babies should room-in with their mothers throughout the short hospital course unless this is prevented by illness of mother or infant.
- Early and continuous mother-infant contact appears to decrease the incidence of abandonment and increase the length and success of breast feeding. All mothers should begin breast feeding in the first hour, nurse frequently, and be encouraged to breast feed for at least the first 2 weeks of life, even if they plan to return to work. Early, frequent breast feeding has many advantages, including earlier removal of bilirubin from the gut as well as aiding in mother-infant attachment.

THE SICK OR PREMATURE INFANT

Although parental visiting has been permitted in the intensive care nursery, a number of studies have revealed that most parents continue to suffer severe emotional stress.[45-48] Harper et al. noted that,[46] even when parents have close contact with their infants in the intensive care nursery, they experience prolonged stress.

Newman described "coping through commitment" as an intense yet variable involvement in the care of a low-birth-weight infant.[48] In contrast, "coping through distance" was a slower acquaintance process in which the parents expressed fear, anxiety, and at times denial before they accepted the surviving infant.

Highly interacting mothers visit and telephone the nursery more frequently while the infants are hospitalized and stimulate their infants more at home. Mothers who stimulate their infants very little in the nursery also visit and telephone less frequently and provide only minimal stimulation to them at home. Most perceptively, Minde et al. noted that mothers who touched and fondled their infants more in the nursery had infants who opened their eyes more often.[49] He and his associates observed the contingency between the infant's eyes being open and the mother's touching and between gross motor stretches and the mother's smiling. They could not determine to what extent the sequence of touching and eye opening was an indication of the mother's primary contribution or whether it was initiated by the infant. Thus, Newman and Minde et al. predict that mothers who become involved with,[49,48] interested in, and anxious about their infants in the intensive care nursery will have an easier time when the infant is taken home.

Field has demonstrated the close connection between what a mother does and her infant's arousal level.[50] Whereas most mothers of full-term babies adopt a moderate level of activity that is associated with optimal arousal in their babies, some mothers of "preemies" either overreact or underreact. Field found that mothers of premature infants who were overreactive during early face-to-face interactions were more likely to be overprotective and over-controlling during interactions with their infants 2 years later.[50]

EDITORIAL COMMENT: Recent studies have found an alarmingly high rate of psychologic pathology and traumatic stress in parents of infants in the NICU. Lefkowitz et al. had 86 mothers and 41 fathers complete measures of acute stress disorder (ASD) and found that 3 to 5 days after the infant's NICU admission,[10] 35% of mothers and 24% of fathers met diagnostic criteria for acute stress disorder. Additionally, 30 days later, 15% of mothers and 8% of fathers actually met diagnostic criteria for posttraumatic stress disorder. In some units, a psychiatrist is available to regularly meet with parents who wish to speak with him/her; this is an extremely helpful and necessary program.[51]

INTERVENTIONS FOR FAMILIES OF PREMATURE INFANTS

TRANSPORTING THE MOTHER TO BE NEAR HER SMALL INFANT

With the development of high-risk perinatal centers, an increasing number of mothers are transported to the maternity division of hospitals with a neonatal intensive care nursery just before delivery or shortly after. If there is not sufficient time to arrange for her transport before she gives birth, it is strongly recommended that the mother be moved as soon as possible.

ROOMING-IN FOR THE PARENT OF A PREMATURE INFANT

When Tafari and Ross in Ethiopia permitted mothers to live within their crowded premature unit 24 hours each day,[52] they were able to care for three times as many infants in their premature nursery, and at the end of 1 year, the number of surviving infants had increased 500%. Mother-infant pairs were discharged when the infants weighed an average of 1.7 kg, and most infants were breast fed. Before this, most of the infants had gone home and were bottle fed, and usually died of intercurrent respiratory and gastrointestinal infections. When the cost of prepared milk amounts to a high proportion of the parents' weekly income, policies in support of the mother rooming-in and breast feeding in premature nurseries have a direct impact on infant mortality. In several other countries throughout the world, including Argentina, Brazil, Estonia, and South Africa, mothers of premature infants live in a room adjoining the premature nursery or they room in. This arrangement appears to have multiple benefits. It allows the mother to continue producing milk, permits her to take on the care of the infant more easily, greatly reduces the caregiving time required of the staff for these infants, and allows a group of mothers of premature infants to talk over their situation and gain from discussion and mutual support. This procedure is probably appropriate for 50% of the world.

Torres,[53] in a special care unit in the slums of Santiago, Chile, achieved excellent, low perinatal mortality and morbidity rates by placing special care units for low-birth-weight infants in the maternity unit, thus maintaining babies under professional observation for only as long as necessary.

Technological improvements and the resulting ability to continuously monitor sick premature infants even from a distance has allowed single-room neonatal intensive care units (NICUs) to become a reality, and parents are encouraged to room-in with their babies in the NICU.

NESTING

In the United States, James and Wheeler first described the successful introduction of a care-by-parent unit to provide a homelike caretaking experience.[54] Parents of premature infants received nursing support before discharge.

For several years "nesting" has been studied—namely, permitting mothers to live in with their infants before discharge. When babies reached 1.72 to 2.11 kg, each mother was given a private room with her baby where she provided all caregiving. Impressive changes in the behavior of these women were observed clinically. Even though the mothers had fed and cared for their infants in the intensive care nursery on many occasions before living-in, eight of the first nine mothers did not sleep during the first 24 hours so they could learn more about their infant's behavior. However, in the second 24-hour period, the mothers' confidence and caretaking skills improved greatly. At this time, mothers began to discuss the proposed early discharge of their infants and, often for the first time, began to make preparations at home for their arrival. Several mothers insisted on taking their babies home earlier than planned.

Early discharge, preceded by a period of isolation of the mother and infant, may help to normalize mothering behavior in the intensive care nursery. Encouraging the increasing possibilities for mother-infant interaction and total caretaking may reduce the incidence of mothering disorders among mothers of small or sick premature infants.

PARENT GROUPS

A number of NICUs have formed groups of parents of premature infants who meet once each week or more often for 1- to 2-hour discussions. Documented clinical reports from these centers suggest that parents find support and considerable relief in being able to talk with each other and to express and compare their inner feelings.

Minde et al.[47] in a controlled study of a self-help group, reported that parents who participated in the group visited their infants in the hospital significantly more often than did parents in the control group.

The self-help parents also touched, talked, and looked at their infants more in the en face position and rated themselves as more competent than the control group on infant care measures. The mothers in the group continued to show more involvement with their babies during feedings and were more concerned about their general development 3 months after their discharge from the nursery.

KANGAROO BABY CARE

Allowing a mother to hold the infant skin-to-skin for prolonged periods in the hospital is known as kangaroo care and it has salutary effects (Fig. 8-3). Several trials have noted that, if the usual precautions are taken, such as hand washing, there is no increase in the infection rate or problems in oxygenation, apnea, or temperature control. A significant medical benefit appears to be a significant increase in the mother's milk supply and success at nursing.[55,56] A recent randomized controlled trial in Madagascar also found a significantly increased proportion of exclusive breast feeding at 6 months of age with earlier initiated continuous kangaroo mother care.[57] Several studies noted that the mother's own confidence

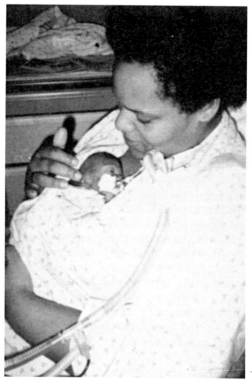

Figure 8-3. Small immature infant (on ventilator) skin-to-skin with his mother.

in her caretaking improved along with an eagerness for discharge, and many women reported feeling an increased closeness to the infant compared with a control group of mothers. At the first skin-to-skin experience, the mother is usually tense, so it is best for the nurse to stay with her to answer questions and make any necessary adjustments in position and ensure that warmth is maintained. A few mothers find that one such experience is enough. However, most mothers find repeated kangaroo care experiences especially pleasurable. However, there is not adequate information to support discharge of appropriate-for-gestational-age (AGA) infants weighing less than 1700 g on solely kangaroo care without daily nursing visits.

EARLY DISCHARGE

Derbyshire and associates have studied discharging premature infants when they weighed about 2 kg and found no deleterious effects associated with this early discharge.[58] To make this workable and to prevent complications, experienced personnel should visit the home to organize the families and, after discharge, to help supervise infant care. Studies of early discharge have not revealed any adverse effects on the physical health of the infants.

Another approach for the mother with emotional distress after the birth of a small premature infant is to alter the responses of the developing infant, an area of intense study by Als et al.[59] In a series of creative studies, they demonstrated that individualized nursing care plans for high-risk, low-birth-weight infants involving their behavioral and environmental needs remarkably altered their outcome. Their requirements for light, sound, position, and detailed nursing were only developed after a sensitive, detailed behavioral assessment.

In randomized trials using the preceding procedure, infants receiving individualized behavioral management required shorter stays on a respirator and fewer days on supplemental oxygen; their average daily waking time increased; they were discharged earlier; and they had a lower incidence of intraventricular hemorrhage. In addition, following discharge, their behavioral development progressed more normally and their parents more easily developed ways of sensing their needs and responding and interacting with them in a pleasurable fashion. Parents have an easier time

adapting to premature infants who are more responsive.

Further emphasizing the importance of the home and family in the final result is a very large, randomized, well carried out trial (985 premature infants) in eight centers in the United States.[60] The study demonstrated that a comprehensive program with weekly home visits in the first year of life; group meetings for mothers during all 3 years; and daily attendance by the child at a developmental center from 1 to 3 years of age resulted in a significant improvement in intelligence quotient (IQ) scores, as well as reports by mothers of fewer developmental problems.

In assessing the effects of any intervention following discharge from the hospital, it is important to remember that more than one half the variance in IQ can be accounted for by social conditions that include parental occupation, education, minority status, anxiety, and mental illness. As the social conditions for the population are improved, so will the outcome for the low-birth-weight infant.

FAMILY-CENTERED CARE IN THE NICU

Providing the optimal hospital environment for a critically ill newborn clearly involves a great deal of care and consideration for the needs of the family as well. Modern NICU design and planning ideally incorporate features such as healing art, family/social spaces, and respite areas for staff.[61] One randomized, controlled trial in Stockholm found that allowing parents to stay in the NICU reduced the total length of hospital stay by 5.3 days.[62] Every facility, no matter what level of resources, can take steps to improve the environment for infants and their families by developing a unit vision and philosophy that promotes the principles of family-centered care. Multidisciplinary groups have created tools and lists of potentially better practices for family-centered care.[63]

Some practices that may be considered for implementing family-centered care include the following[64]:

- The unit vision and philosophy should clearly articulate the principles of family-centered care.
- Leaders at the center and the unit level should clearly promote the principles of family-centered care.
- Parents are not "visitors." Rather, parents should be treated as essential components

of the care team. Policies should be revised to reflect this view. "Visiting Policies" should be revised to address nonparent family members and friends, whereas policies related to parents should be more appropriately addressed as participants in care.

- Neonatal care is multidisciplinary and based on mutual respect among providers for their roles and expertise. Parents are integral to care and should be encouraged to participate in patient care rounds, communication with personnel at the change of shifts, and in the bedside care of their infant. Parents should have access to information in their infant's medical record, and many units have initiated parent documentation into the record.
- The physical environment should provide for the needs of parents. Parents' needs for accessing information, rest, nutrition, privacy, childcare for siblings, and support for their infants by breast milk pumping are often inadequately addressed.
- Nursery staff should receive the support they need to provide optimal family-centered care. This support includes an environment that allows staff a time to rest to meet their own needs and ongoing education and resources to support family-centered care.

Families should be incorporated at various levels as advisors. The perspective of experienced families should be integral to the unit administrative activities. These could include parents as teachers during orientation and continuing education of staff, and parent advisory committees to collaborate in planning of new policies or space and ongoing quality improvement activities.

PRACTICAL HINTS FOR PARENTS OF SICK OR PREMATURE INFANTS

- The obstetrician of a high-risk mother should consult the pediatrician early and continue to involve him or her in decisions and plans for the management of the mother and baby.
- If the baby must be moved to a hospital with an intensive care unit, it is always helpful to give the mother a chance to see and touch her infant, even if the baby has respiratory distress and is in an oxygen hood. The house officer or the attending physician should stop in the mother's room with the transport incubator and encourage her to touch her baby and look at her at close hand. A comment about the baby's strength and healthy features may be long remembered and appreciated.
- The father should be encouraged to follow the transport team to the hospital so he can see what is happening with his baby. He uses his own transportation so that he can stay in the premature unit for 3 to 4 hours. This extra time allows him to get to know the nurses and physicians in the unit, to find out how the infant is being treated, and to talk with the physicians about what they expect will happen with the baby in the succeeding days. He can help by acting as a link between the NICU and his family by carrying information back to the mother. He should visit the baby in the NICU before visiting the mother so that he can let her know how the baby is doing. Taking pictures, even if the infant is on a respirator, allows him to show and describe to the baby's mother in detail how the baby is being cared for. Mothers often tell us how valuable the picture is in allowing them to maintain some contact with the infant, even while physically separated.
- Transporting the mother and baby together to the medical center that contains the intensive care nursery should be encouraged for its immediate and long-term benefits.
- The intensive care nursery should be open for parental visiting 24 hours each day and should be flexible about visits from others such as grandparents, supportive relatives, and sometimes siblings. If proper precautions are taken, infection transmission will not be a problem.
- Communication is essential. The health care workers should communicate with the mother about her condition and about the baby's condition. This is important before, during, and after the birth of the baby, even if the information is brief and incomplete. Clinically, there may be devastating and lasting untoward effects on the mothering capacity of women who have been frightened by a physician's pessimistic outlook about the chance of survival and normal development of an infant. For example, when the newborn premature baby is doing well, but the mother is told by a physician that there is a likelihood that the baby may not survive, the mother will often show evidence of mourning (as if the baby were already dead) and reluctance to "become attached" to her baby. Such mothers may

refuse to visit or will show great hesitation about any physical contact. When discussing such a situation with the physician who has spoken pessimistically with the mother, it is important to share all concerns with her so that she will be prepared in case of a bad outcome. This may be acceptable once there is a close and firm bond between the mother and infant (which may only occur after an infant has been home for several months). However, while the ties of affection are still fragile and forming, they can be easily inhibited, altered, or possibly permanently damaged. Physicians should be truthful because parents will quickly sense their true feelings, but statements must be based on the facts of the current situation, not on improbable outcomes that are causing concern for the physician. The physician should be forthright about all the medical conditions and express appropriate concern related to these problems. Describe what the infant looks like to the medical team and how the infant will appear physically to the mother. Rather than talk about chances of survival and giving percentages, stress that most babies survive despite early and often worrisome problems. Do not emphasize problems that may occur in the future. Try to anticipate common developments (e.g., the need for bilirubin reduction lights for jaundice in small premature infants).

- It is useful to talk with the mother and father together. When this is not possible, it is often wise to talk with one parent on the telephone in the presence of the other. At least once each day discuss how the child is doing with the parents; talk with them at least twice each day if the child is critically ill. It is essential to find out what the mother believes is going to happen or what she has read about the problem. Move at her pace during any discussion.

- The physician should not relieve his anxiety by burdening the family with unnecessary concerns. For example, if there is a possibility that the child has Turner syndrome, it is not necessary to share this with the parents while the infant is still acutely ill with other problems and while affectional bonds are still weak. If the physician is worried about a slightly elevated bilirubin level that would respond promptly to phototherapy, it is not necessary to dwell on kernicterus. Once mentioned, the possibility of death or brain damage can never be completely erased. Remember, words are like a sword, and families remember forever the remarks of their caregivers. Remember too, nonverbal communication is also important and the demeanor of the caregivers will affect the response to information.

- Before the mother comes to the neonatal unit, the nurse or physician should describe in detail what the baby and the equipment will look like. When she makes her first visit, it is important to anticipate that she may become distressed when she looks at her infant. Always have a stool nearby so that she can sit down, and a nurse stays at her side during most of the visit, describing in detail the procedures being carried out, such as the monitoring of respiration and heart rate. The nurse should be nearby so questions may be answered and support given during the difficult period when the mother first sees her infant.

- It is important to remember that feelings of love for the baby are often elicited through contact. Therefore, turn off the lights and remove the eye patches from an infant under phototherapy lights, so that the mother and infant can see each other.

- When the immature infant has passed the acute phase, both the father and the mother should be encouraged to touch, massage, and interact with their infant. This helps the parents get to know the baby, reduces the number of breathing pauses (if this is a problem), increases weight gain, and hastens the infant's discharge from the unit. Initially, if the infant is acutely ill, touching and fondling sometimes results in a decrease in the level of blood oxygen; therefore, parents should begin this contact when the infant is stable and the nurse or physician agrees that the infant is ready. Firm massage of preterm infants 15 minutes three times a day results in markedly improved growth, less stress behavior, improved performance on the Brazelton Neonatal Behavior Assessment scale, and better performance on a developmental assessment at 8 months.[65]

- The mother and father can receive feedback from their baby in response to their caregiving. If the infant looks at their eyes, moves in response to them, quiets down, or shows any behavior in response to their efforts, the parents' feeling of attachment is encouraged. Practically speaking, this means that the mother must catch the baby's glance and be able to note that some maneuver on her part, such as picking up the baby or making soothing sounds, actually triggers a response or quiets the baby. Suggest to parents, therefore, that they think in terms of trying to send a message to the baby and of picking one up from them in return. Small premature infants do see and are especially interested in patterned objects, can hear, and evidence suggests they will benefit greatly from receiving messages.

- Continue to study interventions such as rooming-in, nesting, and early discharge as well as transporting a healthy premature infant to be with his mother. It is necessary to test these various interventions in different hospital settings and to evaluate their ability to reduce the severe anxiety that many parents experience during the prolonged hospitalization and the early days following discharge.

- Nurses should support and encourage mothers during these early days and weeks.[1] The nurse's guidance in helping a mother with simple caregiving tasks can be extremely valuable in helping her to overcome anxiety. In this sense, the nurse assumes the role of the mother's own mother and contributes much more than teaching her basic techniques of caregiving.

- To begin an intervention with parents early, it is necessary to identify high-risk parents who are having special difficulties in adapting. Generally, these parents visit rarely and for short periods,[18] appear frightened, and do not usually engage the medical staff in any questioning about the infant's problems. Sometimes the parents are hostile or irritable and show inappropriately low levels of anxiety.

- As a further understanding of the process by which normal mothers and infants interact with each other during the first months and year of life is developed, it appears that some recommendations for stimulation may be detrimental to normal development. Rather than suggesting stimulation, it may be important for a mother naturally and unconsciously to use imitation to learn about and get to know her own infant.

CONGENITAL MALFORMATIONS

The birth of an infant with a congenital malformation presents complex challenges to the physician who will care for the affected child and his family. Although previous investigators agree that the child's birth often precipitates major family stress,[66] relatively few have described the process of family adaptation during the infant's first year of life.[66] Solnit and Stark's conceptualization of parental reactions emphasized that a significant aspect of adaptation is the mourning that parents must undergo for the loss of the normal child they had expected.[67] Observers have also noted pathologic aspects of family reactions, including the chronic sorrow that envelops the family of a defective child.[68] Less attention has been given to the more adaptive aspects of parental attachment to children with malformations.

Parental reactions to the birth of a child with a congenital malformation appear to follow a predictable course. For most parents, initial shock, disbelief, and a period of intense emotional upset (including sadness, anger, and anxiety) are followed by a period of gradual adaptation, which is marked by a lessening of intense anxiety and emotional reaction (Fig. 8-4). This adaptation is characterized by an increased satisfaction with and ability to care for the baby. These stages in parental reactions are similar to those reported in other crises, such as those that occur with terminally ill children. The shock, disbelief, and denial reported by many parents seem to be an understandable attempt to escape the traumatic news of the baby's malformation, news so at variance with their expectations that it is impossible to register except gradually.

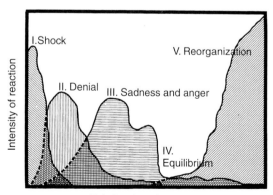

Figure 8-4. Hypothetical model of normal sequence of parental reactions to birth of malformed infant. *(Adapted from Drotar D, Baskiewicz A, Irwin N, et al: Pediatrics 51:710, 1975. Reproduced by permission of Pediatrics.)*

The intense emotional turmoil described by parents who have produced a child with a congenital malformation corresponds to a period of crisis (defined as "upset in a state of equilibrium caused by a hazardous event that creates a threat, a loss, or a challenge for the individual"). A crisis includes a period of impact, an increase in tension associated with stress, and finally a return to equilibrium. During such crisis periods, a person is at least temporarily unable to respond with his or her usual problem-solving activities to solve the crisis. Roskies note a similar "birth crisis" in her observations of mothers of children with limb defects caused by thalidomide.[66]

With the birth of a child with a malformation, the mother must mourn the loss of her expected normal infant.[67] In addition, she must become attached to her actual living, damaged child (Fig. 8-5). However, the sequence of parental reactions to the birth of a baby with a malformation differs from that following the death of a child in another respect. Because of the complex issues raised by the continuation of the child's life and hence the demands of his physical care, the parents' sadness, which is initially important in their relationship with the child, diminishes in most instances when they take over the physical care. Most parents reach a point at which they are able to care adequately for their child and to cope effectively with disrupting feelings of sadness and anger. The mother's initiation of the relationship with her child is a major step in the reduction of anxiety and emotional upset associated with the trauma of the birth. As with normal children, the parents' initial experience with their infant seems to release positive feelings that aid the mother-child relationship following the stresses associated with the news of the child's anomaly and, in many instances, the separation of mother and child in the hospital. Lampe et al. noted a significantly greater amount of visiting if an infant with an abnormality had been at home for a short while before surgery for a cleft lip repair.[69]

PRACTICAL SUGGESTIONS FOR PARENTS OF MALFORMED INFANTS

- If medically feasible, it is far better to leave the infant with the mother and father for the first 2 to 3 days or to discharge them. If the child is rushed to the hospital where special surgery will eventually be done, the mother and father will not have enough opportunity to become attached to her. Even if immediate surgery is necessary, as in the case of bowel obstruction, it is best to bring the baby to the mother first, allowing her to touch and handle her, and to point out to her how normal her baby is in all other respects.
- The parents' mental picture of the anomaly may often be far more alarming than the actual problem. Any delay greatly heightens their anxiety and causes their imaginations to run wild. Therefore, it is helpful to bring the baby to both parents when they are together as soon after delivery as possible.
- Parents should not be given tranquilizers, which tend to blunt their responses and slow their adaptation to the problem. However, a sedative at night is sometimes helpful.
- Parents who are adapting reasonably well often ask many questions and indeed at times appear to be almost over-involved in clinical care. There is more concern about the parents who ask few questions and who appear stunned or overwhelmed by the problem. Parents who become involved in trying to find out what procedures are best and who ask many questions about care are sometimes frustrating, but often adapt best in the end.
- It best to move at the parents' pace. It is beneficial to be a good listener, ask the parents how they view their infant, and to express their concerns, which can then be addressed.
- Each parent may move through the process of shock, denial, anger, guilt, and adaptation at a different pace. If the parents are unable to talk with each other about the baby, their own relationship

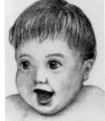

Mother's mental image (during pregnancy)

Real baby

Happy, beautiful active boy (blue-eyed)

Figure 8-5. Change in mental image that mother with malformed baby must make following delivery. Normal mental portrait must be changed to that of her real baby.

may be disrupted. Use the process of early crisis intervention and meet several times with the parents. During these discussions, ask the mother how she is doing, how she feels the father is doing, and how he feels about the infant. Then reverse the questions and ask the father how he is doing and how he thinks the mother is progressing. Many times a parent is surprised by the responses of his or her partner. The hope is that the parents not only will think about their own reactions, but also will begin to consider each other's. For further discussion on this subject, see Case 2.

- One of the major goals of postpartum discussions is to keep the family together during this early period and in subsequent years. This is best done by working hard to bring out issues early and by encouraging the parents to talk about their difficult thoughts and feelings as they arise. It is best for them to share their problems with each other. Some couples who do not seem to be close previously may move closer together as they work through the process of adaptation. As with any painful experience, the parents may be much stronger after they have gone through these reactions together. It is helpful when the father stays with his partner during the hospitalization. Sometimes the stresses of having a malformed, sick baby will ultimately disrupt the relationship of the parents.

STILLBIRTH OR DEATH OF A NEWBORN

Despite the advances in obstetrical and neonatal care, many mothers encounter a great disappointment with an early abortion or the perinatal loss of an infant. A mourning reaction in both parents after the death of a newborn is universal.[70] Whether the baby lives 1 hour or 2 weeks, whether the baby is a nonviable 400 g, or weighs 4000 g, whether or not the baby was planned, and whether or not the mother has had physical contact with her baby, clearly identifiable mourning will be present. Mothers and fathers who have lost a newborn show the same mourning reactions as those reported by Lindemann,[71] who studied survivors of the Coconut Grove fire. Lindemann concludes that normal grief is a definite syndrome. It includes the following aspects:

- Somatic distress with tightness of the throat, choking, shortness of breath, need for sighing, and an empty feeling in the abdomen; lack of muscular power; and an intense subjective distress described as tension or mental pain
- Preoccupation with the image of the deceased infant
- Feelings of guilt and preoccupation with one's negligence or minor omissions
- Feelings of hostility toward others
- Breakdown of normal patterns of conduct

Originally it was believed that loss of an infant was similar to the loss of a close relative; however, based on clinical studies and observations, it fits far more closely with the concepts proposed by Furman[72] and Lewis.[73] Furman eloquently notes these reactions:

Internally, the mourning process consists of two roughly opposing mechanisms. One is the generally known process of detachment, by which each memory that ties the family to the person who is deceased has to become painfully revived and painfully loosened. This is the part of the process that involves anger, guilt, pain, and sadness. The second process is commonly called "identification." It is the means by which the deceased or parts of him are taken into the self and preserved as part of the self, thereby soothing the pain of loss. In many instances, a surviving marriage partner takes over hobbies and interests of the deceased spouse. These identifications soothe the way and make the pain of detachment balanced and bearable.

For the surviving parents, the death of a newborn is special in several ways. Because mourning is mourning of a separate person, the process can apply only to that small part of the relationship to the newborn that was characterized by the love of a separate person, but there has not been time to build up strong ties and memories of mutual living. It is also not possible for parents—adults functioning in the adult world—to take into themselves any part of a helpless newborn and make it adaptively a part of themselves; the mechanism of identification does not work. But what about the part of the newborn that was still part of the self and that cannot be mourned? To understand this part, one has to look at the different process by which individuals cope with a loss of a part of the self (e.g., amputation or loss of function). Insofar as the newborn remains a part of the parent's self, the death has to be dealt with as would the amputation of a limb or the loss of function of the parent's body. Detachment is the mechanism with which the victim deals with such tragedies, but it is detachment of a different kind. Acceptance that one will never ever again have that part of oneself is very different from the detachment that deals with the memories of living together with a loved one. The feelings that accompany this detachment are similar in kind and intensity: anger, guilt, fury, helplessness, and horror. In the case of the loss of a part of the self, however, they are quite unrelieved by identification.

Next, with such a tragedy there must be a readjustment in one's self-image. It is, however, altogether different to have to readjust to thinking of oneself as an imperfect human being, a human being that cannot walk or cannot see. That is a pain of a different kind, and the feelings that accompany it are emptiness, loss of self-esteem, and feeling low. Because the internal self never materialized in those arms and has not had a chance to be detached, it is very different from the process of mourning.

These feelings are made particularly difficult because people around the parents are not there to help. At a conscious level, people say they simply do not understand about losing part of the self, and, indeed, they do not. Subconsciously, they understand it all too well. It fills them with fear and anxiety and makes them turn away. Parents of a dead newborn often experience this isolation. They quite often are shunned, and they may not rely on the sympathy that is usually accorded the bereaved.

This grief syndrome may appear immediately after a death or may be delayed or apparently absent. Those who have studied mourning responses have indicated that a painful period of grieving is a normal and necessary response to the loss of a loved one and the absence of a period of grieving is not a healthy sign but rather a cause for alarm.

Without any therapeutic intervention, a tragic outcome for the mother has been shown in one third of the perinatal deaths. Cullberg found that 19 of 56 mothers studied 1 to 2 years after the deaths of their neonates had developed severe psychiatric disease (psychoses, anxiety attacks, phobias, obsessive thoughts, and deep depressions).[74] Because of the disastrous outcome in such a high proportion of mothers, it is necessary to examine in detail how to care for the family following a neonatal death.

In observations of parents who have lost newborns, the disturbance of communication between the parents has been a particularly troublesome problem. A father and mother who have communicated well before the birth of a baby often have such strong feelings after an infant's death that they are unable to share their thoughts and, therefore, have an unsatisfactory resolution to their grieving. In the United States, it is expected that men will be strong and not show their feelings, so a physician should encourage a father and mother to talk together about the loss and advise them not to hold back their responses—"Cry when you feel like crying." Unless told what to expect, their reactions may worry and perplex them, and this may tend further to disturb the preexisting father and mother relationship.

At the time of the baby's death, it is important to tell the parents *together* about the usual reactions to the loss of a child and the length of time these last. It is desirable to meet a second time with both parents before discharge to go over the same suggestions, which may not have been heard or may have been misunderstood under the emotional shock of the baby's death. The pediatrician or social worker should plan to meet with the parents together again 3 or 4 months after the death to check on the parents' activities and on how the mourning process is proceeding. The autopsy findings may be discussed and any further questions asked by the parents may be addressed. At this visit, the pediatrician or social worker should be alert for abnormal grief reactions, which, if present, may guide the physician to refer the parents for psychiatric assistance. It is important that these recommendations do not become an exact prescription for every parent. As noted by Leon,[75] "Such protocols can lead to a regimented assembly-line approach—which impedes attempts to attune to parents individually and empathetically—the very essence of providing support."

Lindemann noted that pathologic mourning reactions represent distortion of normal grief. On the basis of his observations, he lists 10 such reactions.[71]
- Overactivity without a sense of loss
- Acquisition of symptoms belonging to the last illness of the deceased
- Psychosomatic reactions such as ulcerative colitis, asthma, or rheumatoid arthritis
- Alterations in relation to friends and relatives
- Furious hostility against specific persons
- Repression of hostility against specific persons

- Repression of hostility, leading to a wooden and formal manner resembling schizophrenic pictures
- Lasting loss of patterns of social interaction
- Activities detrimental to one's own social and economic existence
- Agitated depressions

For further discussion on this subject, see Case 4.

Cullberg's report about severe psychiatric reactions following stillbirth or neonatal death in Swedish mothers was published in 1966, when the field of neonatology was in its infancy. Following other reports about parents' turbulent and prolonged mourning reactions, changes in the care of bereaved families were introduced.

In a systematic study of 380 women following a stillbirth, Rädestad observed that mothers of stillborn infants had a diminished risk of symptoms 3 years after the death if there was a short time between diagnosis of death and initiation of the delivery,[76] if the mother was allowed to meet and say farewell to her child as long as she wished, and if there was a collection of tokens of remembrance (hand or footprints, lock of hair, and photograph). They noted that mothers living alone may have special needs for support.

EDITORIAL COMMENT: Katherine Shear and Harry Shair have written about the concept of "Complicated Grief" which may occur with ineffective coping after the death of a loved one. They note as follows[77]:

Bereavement is a highly disruptive experience that is usually followed by a painful but time-limited period of acute grief. An unfortunate minority of individuals experience prolonged and impairing complicated grief, an identifiable syndrome that differs from usual grief, major depression, and other *DSM-IV* diagnostic entities. Underlying processes guiding symptoms are not well understood for either usual or complicated grief. We propose a provisional model of bereavement, guided by Myron Hofer's question: "What exactly is lost when a loved one dies?" We integrate insights about biobehavioral regulation from Hofer's animal studies of infant separation, research on adult human attachment, and new ideas from bereavement research. In this model, death of an attachment figure produces a state of traumatic loss and symptoms of acute grief. These symptoms usually resolve following revision of the internalized representation of the deceased to incorporate the reality of the death. Failure to accomplish this integration results in the syndrome of complicated grief.[2]

The clinical relevance of this subject can best be appreciated by the following case examples and the questions they raise. The words chosen in any discussion depend on the needs and problems of individual patients at that moment. Answers are not given as a specific formula, but to show the reader how parents are approached.

CASE 1

Mrs. W had a normal pregnancy until 24 weeks' gestation, when she unexpectedly went into labor and delivered a 2 lb, 15 oz (1332 g) female infant in a community hospital. The baby cried promptly, but then moderate respiratory distress developed, requiring arterial catheterization, intubation, surfactant administration, and ventilator care up to and during transfer to a tertiary level NICU at the medical center.

The following questions should be answered when caring for this mother, father, and infant.

What is the ideal method of communicating with both parents?

The best method of communicating with both parents is to have them sit down with you in a quiet, private room. You will be most effective if you can listen to the parents, let them express their worries and feelings, and then give simple, realistically optimistic explanations.

How should advice be given when discussing the situation with the parents? What should they be told about their infant and her chances for survival?

When first discussing the situation with the parents, advice should be given promptly, simply, and optimistically. As soon as possible after the birth, the mother and father can be told that the baby is small but well formed. When it is clear that the baby has respiratory distress, you can explain to the parents that the baby has a common problem of premature infants ("breathing difficulty") caused by the complex adjustments she must make from life in utero to life outside. This is called respiratory distress syndrome (RDS). In addition, it should be stated that because this condition is common, the neonatologists at the tertiary NICU in a medical center know best how to treat it, and their results with infants who are this weight infant are very good.

What should the mother and father be told about the ventilator?

Some of the parents' anxiety can be relieved by pointing out that the ventilator is augmenting the baby's breathing; that is, the baby is still able to breathe, but this is helping. Explaining that the baby is not able to cry audibly when an endotracheal tube is present relieves another common concern.

Can the parents see the baby before transfer?

Yes, you can explain that the mother, father, and siblings will be given time and an opportunity to see and touch the baby in the transport incubator with a nurse or neonatologist present to monitor and support the baby, siblings, and parents. Pictures of the baby will be obtained before the transfer.

Is it wise to discuss breast feeding and the value of breast milk for a baby that will be transferred?

Yes, emphasizing the importance of pumping milk right away will increase the odds that Mrs. W will be able to provide breast milk for her baby. Discussing breast feeding at this time when the parents are extremely anxious about their baby conveys to the parents that you expect their baby to do well. You can explain that the staff will help the mother start pumping her breasts because her breast milk will be an essential part of the treatment for her daughter, not only for her nutrition, but also to decrease the risk of infection and to improve the baby's brain development. It will also enhance the mother's bonding with her daughter, particularly when Mrs. W begins to directly breast feed her daughter and repeatedly experiences the let-down reflex.

What other arrangements should be made before the baby is transferred?

Communication with both the referring and receiving centers and the obstetrician is necessary. Most obstetricians want to know when a baby is transferred. They can help the family by arranging for the early discharge of the mother, when medically appropriate, so she can go to her baby in the medical center. Sometimes mother and baby can both be transferred.

Baby Girl W is transported to the NICU at the medical center. She receives surfactant and gradually begins to wean off the ventilator. After 4 hours, the ventilator settings have decreased to FiO_2 27%, peak inspiratory pressure 22 mm Hg, positive end-expiratory pressure 5 mm Hg, and pulse rate 25. An arterial blood gas (ABG) reveals pH 7.33, $PaCO_2$ 41 mm Hg, and PaO_2 62 mm Hg. When the mother and father arrive, the neonatologist meets with them in her office.

The physician asks "Would you please tell me what the doctors at the community hospital told you and what you understand about your daughter's condition?" After hearing the answer, the physician explains that the baby tolerated the transfer well and that they are beginning to wean their daughter

off the ventilator. She agrees with the diagnosis of RDS and comments that "RDS often runs a course of increasing symptoms for a day or two and then the breathing gradually becomes easier. With RDS there is stress on the whole baby, so as the lungs improve, other organs such as the intestines, may show problems. Distention or fullness of the abdomen may develop, and it may be necessary to progress slowly with feedings. Throughout the first few days, routine blood tests, ultrasound, x-rays, and other studies may be obtained repeatedly to be certain that the diagnosis and treatment are correct and to check that no other problem such as infection has developed. The overall outlook for your daughter is good."

The physician says that she will be giving their daughter routine care for a premature infant. She says, "When I have had time to complete more tests and observations, if there is any change in what I have told you, I will call you. I will keep you posted on the baby's progress. I would like you to call at other times if you have questions. I am pleased that you both came in together. In the next days, if one of you is here and I have something new to report, I will plan to talk to one of you on the telephone while the other is in the office with me. I would like you to come to the nursery as often as you can. I want you to become well acquainted with your daughter and her care. Your milk will be a very important part of her treatment and you may find your milk flows more abundantly when you are with your baby, particularly when you are skin-to-skin in kangaroo care. I will tell you more about this when I think the baby is ready."

Can the nurses help the mother adapt to the premature infant?

The nurses can aid the mother in adapting to the premature infant by standing with her and explaining the equipment being used for the baby, by welcoming the mother by name, and with personalized comments at each visit and encouraging her to come back soon, by carefully considering the mother's concerns and feelings, by explaining to her that the baby will benefit from her visits, and by showing her how she can gradually assume more of the baby's care, and do the mothering better than the nurses. Together, they may identify events such as loud noises and bright lights that appear to be stressful to the baby, as well as environmental changes that appear to relax her. Then they can plan modifications in positioning, feeding, and times for medications as well as environmental adjustments to increase the amount of time when the baby appears to be free of stress.

What are the normal processes that a mother goes through when she delivers

a premature infant and how can the physicians and nurses assist her?

The premature delivery often occurs before a mother is thoroughly ready to accept the idea that she is going to have an infant. Such a mother is faced with a baby who is thin, scrawny, and very different from the ideal full-sized baby she has been picturing in her mind. She may have to grieve the loss of this anticipated ideal baby as she adjusts to the reality of the premature baby with all her problems and special needs.

All of the equipment and activities of a premature nursery are new and may be frightening to a mother. The tubes, the flashing lights, the alarms, and other instruments used in a premature nursery are disturbing. If the functions of these items are explained to the mother, her concerns will decrease. For example, "The two wires on the baby's chest and the beeping instrument tell us if the baby slows down in her respirations so we can rub her skin to remind her to keep breathing. This is frequently necessary during the first few days with a tiny infant." It may be helpful for the mother and infant to be together as much as possible in the early days. The mother's guilt and anxiety, and the fear that touching the infant will harm her, sometimes leads her to turn down an offer to visit the infant. No mother should be forced to visit her infant against her wishes; however, it is important for the hospital personnel to reassure her and encourage her visits, but always to move at the mother's pace.

What should the mother be told when she asks, "How is the baby doing?"

It is a common reflex in physicians and nurses to prepare patients for a possible poor outcome and to think in a problem-oriented manner. It is of great importance to provide encouragement to the mother so that mother-infant affectional ties develop as easily as possible, so it is desirable to approach this question in an optimistic but realistic manner. It is wise to start out by asking the mother how *she* thinks the baby is doing.

When should these parents take the baby home?

At 2 weeks, Baby Girl W developed an episode of suspected sepsis with abdominal distention that responded to nothing-by-mouth and antibiotics. The cultures were negative. At 4 weeks, Baby Girl W weighs 3 lb, 14 oz (1758 g).

The baby has been breast feeding one or two times a day for the past 4 days and taking breast milk from the bottle. She is gaining weight and has good temperature control without an incubator. There is no infection in the home. Shortly after the baby responded to the sepsis treatment, Mrs. W called to say she was sick with the flu and would not come to the NICU. She called each day for 10 days and her husband brought in the breast milk she had pumped. In this case, the timing of going home depended on the mother, whose visiting pattern was regular until the last week. At that time, Baby Girl W's nurse suggested that the mother spend 3 or 4 hours with her baby, give her a bath, and feed her. Mrs. W agreed, enjoyed this, and spent 6 to 8 hours caring for her baby girl over the next 3 days. Mrs. W has a bassinet and equipment to care for her daughter at home and her husband has canceled his out-of-town trips for the next 3 weeks.

Baby Girl W went home in the winter so the parents were advised to avoid contact with children with colds. Because she has a sibling younger than 5 years of age, Baby Girl W was given the first injection of Synagis (palivizumab) to be followed by two more injections to protect her against respiratory syncytial virus infection.

CASE 2

Mrs. J, a 25-year-old primiparous mother, delivered a full-term infant after a 12-hour uneventful labor. The infant was found to have a cleft lip and palate. The following questions should be answered concerning the care of this infant and mother.

Should the father be told about this before the mother has returned to her room?

Every effort should be made to tell the mother and father together about this problem; however, this is such an obvious defect that the father will notice it and the mother will at least sense that something is wrong. If this is the case, the doctor should indicate that there is a problem, but that he wants to check the baby over thoroughly and will then tell both parents about the problem and what will be done about it. It is popularly believed that the father is in much better condition to learn about difficulties right after delivery than the mother, but often a woman is better able to accept news about an illness or abnormality in her baby—in an emotional sense—than the father. Any plan to give one bit of news or a different shading about the prognosis to one parent and not the other interferes with the communication between the parents. It is extremely important to support and encourage communication. The infant should be brought to the parents as soon as the mother and the infant are in satisfactory condition and after the caregiving physician (obstetrician or pediatrician) has the details of the baby's problem clearly in mind and is aware of the baby's health status. The baby should be kept in the delivery room for the examinations and then brought to the mother's bed. The appearance of a baby with an uncorrected cleft palate and lip is grotesque and shocking for anyone who has not seen this before. Allowing the parents time to observe, react, and ask questions will be necessary. The experienced physician or nurse will point out the underlying structures, emphasize that they are normal, and demonstrate how the surgeon will pull the skin edges of the cleft together to cover the exposed underlying tissue. Before and after pictures of surgically repaired infants are helpful and may enable parents to appreciate why the physician has been so optimistic about the baby's future appearance and normal developmental potential. It is worthwhile to repeat and emphasize the general good health and well-being of the baby.

Who should tell the mother: the obstetrician, the pediatrician, the nurse, or the father?

The obstetrician, whom the mother has known for many months, is usually the best person to tell the mother. He or she needs information from a pediatrician about the nature of the problem and the general health of the baby. Even better, the obstetrician and the pediatrician may go together to tell the parents about the problem. If the obstetrician can speak briefly and calmly to the mother, then the pediatrician can continue with a brief explanation about the problem. Under most circumstances, neither the nurse nor the father will be in a position to provide enough reassurance to the mother to make this first encounter progress optimally.

How should the problem be presented to the parents?

It is desirable whenever possible to emphasize to the parents the normal healthy features of the baby. For example, "Mr. and Mrs. Jones, you have a strong 8-pound baby boy who is kicking, screaming, and carrying out all the normal functions of a healthy baby. There is one problem present that fortunately we will be able to correct, so it will not be a continuing problem for your son. As far as I can tell, the baby is completely well otherwise. I would like to show the baby and this problem to you."

Should the baby be present?

Yes. As ugly as a cleft palate and lip may appear to a mother, exposure to the reality of the problem is important and is usually less disturbing than the mother's imagination.

CASE 3

At birth, the male infant of a white 28-year-old mother was scrawny with decreased subcutaneous fatty tissue and axillary and gluteal skinfolds. At 35 weeks' gestational age, the weight was 3 lb, 4.5 oz (1480 g), more than 2 standard deviations below the mean and fiftieth percentile for 31 weeks. The length was in the low normal range and the head circumference was at the 2nd percentile line. The baby breathed and cried promptly. The mother was upset with his thinness, saying her two previous babies were full term and "filled out." When blood was drawn and an intravenous (IV) line with glucose started, the infant was noted to be jittery. Glucose, calcium, electrolytes, and blood counts were normal. Examination showed no malformations.

What other causes should be considered?

The previous record of the mother was not found. When asked about prenatal care, she indicated that she had attended two prenatal visits with an obstetrician at the medical center. She said she had planned to deliver there but when labor pains started, she had thought it best to go to the nearby community hospital. This was an unusual course of action. Obstetric patients do not often change obstetrician and hospital with onset of labor.

Shortly after delivery, a well-dressed, polite father arrived and immediately inquired which laboratory tests had been sent on his wife and son. The father remained with his wife during all postnatal care, often answering questions for her. Upon seeing his newborn son attached to an IV line, he insisted, "My child is perfectly well, just small and cold. I want both my wife and son discharged today."

Perplexed by the excessive anxiety of the family as well as the continued jitteriness of the baby, the neonatologist sent infant urine and stool toxicology screens, which were positive for cocaine. At this point, the father picked up the baby, and with his wife, started to leave. Security personnel were called and stopped the father. He had a gun in his pocket. Emergency custody for the baby was obtained.

What other concerns should be checked when a baby is positive for cocaine?

This is often just the tip of an iceberg. Spousal abuse, human immunodeficiency virus infection, and the safety of other children in the home must be seriously considered.

When the mother was examined, there were large bruises on her trunk. When asked in privacy, she said her husband hit her. She agreed to go into treatment for her cocaine addiction. As an adult, she could not be kept in the hospital if she did not wish to stay. Photographs of the mother and her bruises were taken before she left, and she was told that these and the records of what she said would be kept if she needed them in the future. Custody of the baby was given to the maternal grandmother. Later, the mother said she came to this community hospital because she thought there would be no testing for cocaine.

Because of this incident, the hospital has installed surveillance cameras. Some hospitals have coded bracelets for the baby's arms or ankles, or umbilical tags that set off an alarm if a baby is taken. Others have a hospital public address code for a missing baby, e.g., "Baby White."

CASE 4

A 1 lb, 15-oz (880 g) infant of a 29-year-old mother with a 2-year-old and a 4½-year-old child died suddenly at 26 hours. The pregnancy was planned. The mother had not held or touched her baby.

What are the processes this mother and father will go through?

The parents in this situation will go through intense mourning reactions. It will help the parents to see and hold the baby after the death. They may wish to bathe or undress and dress the baby. There should be no restriction on the time with their infant. The mother and father may desire to have a nurse with them or to be alone and may want relatives or friends or the two siblings to see the baby. If the parents can cry together, they themselves can best help each other. The use of drugs, except for a night's sleep, is, therefore, not indicated. Even though the mother did not handle the infant, she and the father will be expected to show strong mourning responses, which will be intense for 1 or 2 months, and under optimal circumstances will be decreased by 6 months. In the United States, where the expression of emotion is not encouraged, the father will often force himself to hold back his emotions to provide "strong support" for the mother. This is actually harmful, because a free and easy communication between the parents about their feelings is highly desirable for the resolution of mourning. On the basis of the studies that have been carried out, the stronger the mourning reaction in the early days and weeks, the more favorable the outcome.

How can the physician help them?

It is important for the physician to describe the details of the baby's death to both parents together within a few hours of the death of the baby. At that time, he should explain the type of mourning reaction they will go through. Then, at a minimum, the physician should again meet with the parents 3 or 4 days later, or after the funeral, to find out how

they are managing, to go over the details once more, and to indicate availability for any questions or problems. At the postpartum checkup, the obstetrician should take time to ask how the parents are managing and should evaluate the normality of their mourning and their communication. When there are other children in the family, the pediatrician should inquire about their responses. Parents are in emotional pain and are distracted with their own thoughts after a perinatal loss. It is desirable to have someone else—a grandparent or a friendly neighbor—be attentive to the surviving children and to listen to their questions and concerns. It should be explained (if appropriate) that changes in the appearance or behavior of their parents are because they feel so badly about the death. This "surrogate parent" should reassure the siblings that the baby died because of its premature birth and that nothing they thought or did caused the baby to be sick or to die.

About 3 or 4 months after the death of the baby, the physician should set aside a time to meet with both parents to present and discuss the autopsy results, review the present status of the parents and their children, and go over what has occurred since the death, their understanding of the death, and the normality of their reactions. If the mourning response is pathologic, the physician should then refer the parents for additional assistance. Using these procedures, Forrest et al. noted significantly less depression and anxiety in parents compared with control subjects.[78] Also, they noted that an early pregnancy (<6 months after the loss) was strongly associated with high depression and anxiety scores at 14 months.

This short enumeration of guidelines may incorrectly convey the impression of a mechanical quality to these discussions, which is not at all our intent. Parents appreciate evidence of human concern and reactions in a physician at times such as these, so it is appropriate for physicians to show the sadness they feel and to allow the parents to express their pent-up feelings by making a statement such as "I know you both must feel very sad and upset."

SUMMARY

In most instances, the hospital determines the events surrounding birth and death, stripping these two most important events in life of the long-established traditions and support systems established over centuries to help families through these transitions.

Because the newborn baby completely depends on his or her parents for survival and optimal development, it is essential to understand the process of attachment.

Although we are only beginning to understand this complex phenomenon, those responsible for the care of mothers and infants would be wise to reevaluate the hospital procedures that interfere with early, sustained parent-infant contact and to consider measures that promote parents' experiences with their infant.

REFERENCES

The reference list for this chapter can be found online at www.expertconsult.com.

Nursing Practice in the Neonatal Intensive Care Unit

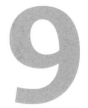

9

Linda Lefrak and Carolyn Houska Lund

The planning and delivery of nursing care to critically ill neonates is a complex process that necessitates thorough, ongoing evaluation to determine effectiveness of both nursing and medical therapies. This unique evaluation takes into account (1) the frequent introduction of new treatment modalities, (2) the lack of verbal communication with the patient, (3) the narrow margin between safe and adverse responses to therapy, (4) the lack of disease-specific symptoms because of immature development, and (5) the patient's extreme vulnerability, particularly in the most premature or sick infants.

Neonatal nursing involves a variety of unique functions, skills, and responsibilities that are essential in assessing, understanding, and safely supporting the newborn infant and family during this critical time. Neonatal intensive care unit (NICU) nurses must anticipate problems and systematically evaluate the infant and all the support systems to identify any new problems as early as possible. Each nurse completes the following head-to-toe assessment and prepares the associated documentation at least every 8 to 12 hours:

1. Observes physical characteristics such as color, tone, skin integrity, perfusion, and edema
2. Assesses organ systems, including chest auscultation, peripheral pulses, heart sounds, urine output, bowel sounds, and presence of reflexes
3. Checks patency and function of all intravascular devices and security of endotracheal tubes and other invasive devices
4. Verifies presence and appropriate function of all respiratory equipment and monitors
5. Assesses neurobehavioral activity, including level of pain or discomfort in relation to treatment

6. Describes parental contact and attachment behaviors

Thorough assessment by the NICU nurse is followed by the identification of specific patient problems that require either nursing or medical intervention. Once problems are identified, the process of planning and implementing of interventions is undertaken. The signs and signals that nurses perceive may be the first indication that a major problem is beginning.

The nurse is also responsible for the safe and appropriate use of technical equipment in the care of these critically ill newborns. Since the 1970s, the number of electrical devices used for a single patient has steadily increased, beginning with the use of a single warming device (the incubator) and progressing to the current standard use of 10 to 12 devices per patient. The nurse is responsible for using these devices with a level of expertise such that problems can be recognized. An essential component of the nursing role involves the relationship between the nurse and the parents and family of each infant. Because initial phases of attachment develop during this time of crisis, the whole family is in a vulnerable position as members begin to establish their relationship with the baby. The neonatal nurse assists the parents in beginning to know and appreciate their baby in a highly technical environment where touching and holding are sometimes difficult to accomplish (see Chapter 8). The modeling of communication and interaction with fragile newborns is a particularly effective method of assisting parents with this process. The explanation of the treatments and continual reinforcement of information provided by the infant's physicians regarding current condition and prognosis are necessary during this crisis. Nurses often become a major source of social support, especially during long or complicated hospitalizations.

Neonatal nurses play a major role as protector, advocate, and, at times, nurturer to the infant in the NICU. Because the nurse's scope of responsibility is limited to a small number of patients at any given time (generally two to three), and because of the need to be almost constantly present at the bedside of these patients, the nurse's observations and evaluations often guide any interventions. For example, an observation regarding an infant's adverse reaction to noise or handling may guide the team to alter interventions or physical examination. Nurses provide a vital link between the patient and the health care team through their knowledge, proximity to the patient, and skill at interpreting physiologic, behavioral, and technical information. The following discussion provides an overview of nursing practice that currently exists in the NICU, touching on four areas: developmental care, skin care, venous access, and iatrogenic complications.

DEVELOPMENTAL CARE

A significant aspect of providing nursing care to infants in the NICU is to create an environment that reduces noxious stimuli, promotes positive development, and minimizes the negative effects of illness, early delivery, and separation from parents. Neonatal nurses have become increasingly concerned about the negative effects of the NICU environment and have begun to identify preventive strategies and integrate changes in this highly technical, over-stimulating environment.

Developmental care is the term used to describe interventions that can minimize the stress of the NICU environment. These include elements such as control of external stimuli (vestibular, auditory, visual, tactile),

clustering of nursing and medical interventions, and positioning the infant using swaddling or containment techniques. The Newborn and Infant Developmental Care and Assessment Program (NIDCAP) was designed to combine these elements in a way that is specific to individual infants, using a detailed assessment system.

Studies using NIDCAP methodology have reported improved developmental and medical outcomes for premature infants cared for in a developmentally supportive environment with caregivers specially educated in assessing premature infant behavior and modifying care practices to reduce negative or stressful responses.[1-3] A Cochrane Systematic Review of 36 randomized controlled trials involving four major groups of developmental care reported limited benefit to preterm infants in the following areas: decreased moderate to severe chronic lung disease,[4] decreased incidence of necrotizing enterocolitis, and improved family outcome. An increase in mild chronic lung disease and length of stay with developmental care compared to controls was also reported. There is limited evidence of improved neurodevelopmental behavioral performance. Reviewers identified a significant methodologic concern with these studies, in that the assessments were performed by non-blinded staff.

Despite ongoing skepticism and critique of developmental research, the modern NICU appears quite different than its predecessor: for example, dimmed lights, crib covers, swaddling and supported positioning, and dB meters are becoming familiar sights. The reactions of staff to reduced noise are reported to be positive, although reduced light levels are not as favorable.[5]

Future research to better understand the effects and contributions of each intervention for the infant and NICU staff may provide more information about the impact of these interventions. The following section addresses the effects of noise, light, positioning, and handling during routine care, and it suggests modifications in each area that can reduce the detrimental effects.

NOISE IN THE NEONATAL INTENSIVE CARE UNIT

Much of the technology used to support the newborn in the NICU generates a significant amount of noise and activity. Excessive noise can over-stimulate the premature or ill term newborn and lead to agitation and crying.

This agitation has been shown to cause decreased oxygenation, increased intracranial pressure, elevated heart and respiratory rates, and increased apnea.[6] Autonomic nervous system arousal using skin conductance measurements in response to a noise stimuli has been reported in premature infants, and correlates with increases in heart rate.[7] Noise also disrupts the sleep-wake cycle and may delay recovery and the ability to have positive interactions with parents and caregivers because of fatigue and overwhelming overstimulation.[8] Noise levels in the NICU range from 50 to 80 dB. Inside the incubator even higher levels are reached. Damage to delicate auditory structures has been associated with prolonged exposure to greater than 90 dB in adults. In neonates, the dB levels that result in hearing damage have not been identified.

Incubator motors generate an average of 55 to 60 dB; equipment and activity inside or around the incubator can add an additional 10 to 40 dB. Routine care activities such as placing glass formula bottles on the bedside table, closing storage drawers, or opening packaged supplies have been recorded at sound levels from 58 to 76 dB; alarms from intravenous (IV) pumps and cardiorespiratory monitors have also measured 57 to 66 dB.[9] Noise from respiratory therapy equipment, monitors, staff talking, and infant fussiness also contribute to higher sound levels.[10] The American Academy of Pediatrics Committee on Environmental Health expressed concern that exposure to environmental noise in the NICU may result in cochlear damage and may disrupt normal growth and development. The Committee to Establish Recommended Standards for Newborn ICU Design advises that average noise levels not exceed 45 dB,[11] and intermittent high levels not reach 65 dB or greater. However, several studies report levels that are consistently higher despite renovations and other measures to address noise levels.[10,12,13] Noise awareness educational programs may improve staff knowledge about the problem of noise in the NICU and result in strategies that improve environmental modifications.[14]

Interventions to Reduce Noise Levels
1. Modify staff behaviors such as loud talk and playing radios near radiant warmers and incubators.
2. Institute "quiet hours" several times each day when noise-producing activities are curtailed and lights are dimmed.

3. Measure dB levels to identify baseline sounds as well as any problem areas and times.
4. If possible, avoid overhead paging systems.
5. Remove loud devices from patient care areas.
6. Observe carefully individual infant's responses to auditory stimulation such as music boxes and tape recorders.
7. Consider offering only one sensory stimulus at a time, such as talking or singing without visual, tactile, or vestibular stimuli.
8. Gently open and close isolette doors.
9. Pad doors and drawers of storage closets.
10. Design NICUs with noise-absorbing materials.

EDITORIAL COMMENT: The intensity of sound is expressed in dB and measured on a semi-logarithmic scale, which means that an increase of about 10 dB represents a doubling of the sound intensity. The 2006 Recommended Standards for Newborn ICU Design calls for NICU sound levels to remain below 50 dB the majority of the time.[15] Infant sleep is usually not disturbed at this level. Much of the "background" noise in a typical NICU comes from the building itself — audible sound or vibrations from activity outside the hospital and from machinery within the hospital, and sounds generated by airflow through the heating, ventilation, and air conditioning system (HVAC). Without sufficient attention to these sources, the background noise in a NICU, even before any equipment or personnel are brought in, can be greater than 40 dB. Ventilators, CPAP, and compressed air all add to the noise levels as do monitors, alarms, telephones, and the staff talking and carrying out their duties. Hence, the recommended hourly loudness equivalent (Leq) of 45 dB of acceptable noise (dBA), L10 of 50 dBA and Lmax of 65 dBA remains an elusive goal.[16]

LIGHT IN THE NEONATAL INTENSIVE CARE UNIT

The effect of continuous light exposure is another topic of interest when providing an environment that is developmentally supportive for babies in the NICU. Premature infants have thin, translucent eyelids that are ineffective in blocking light transmission, and have limited capacity for pupil constriction to modulate light; both of these deficits can interfere with sleep and rest.

Cycled lighting, involving periods of time with greater light intensity with periods of dim light, has been studied in the NICU population, and findings include increased organization of physiologic functions such as heart rate, respiratory rate, and energy expenditure.[17,18] Thus, cycling of light periods should be considered in nurseries to help infants begin their regulation of sleep-wake periods.

Safe levels of light in the NICU have not yet been established and further research is needed to define the optimal approaches for lighting the immediate environment for the NICU patient. However, shielding infants from light in incubators or on warming tables is relatively easy and may prove beneficial in promoting rest, behavioral stability, and recovery. The use of fabric incubator and crib covers is common practice in today's NICU, although the type of cover may be an important factor in reducing the light levels. One study found that covers made with dark fabrics are more effective than those made from light-colored or bright-patterned fabrics.[19]

Interventions to Reduce Light Levels

1. Shade head of table, crib, or incubator whenever possible using cloth crib covers, blankets, or quilts; tenting over the head can be used if constant visual observation of the infant is needed.
2. When infants are stable, consider markedly reducing nursery light levels for 12-hour periods each day.
3. Consider individual lighting over each bedside with a dimmer switch to control light intensity and individualize lighting needs.

POSITIONING

Because body alignment is known to affect many physiologic and neurobehavioral parameters, the positioning of neonates is important. Proper positioning can prevent postural deformities such as hip abduction and external rotation, ankle eversion, retracted and abducted shoulders, increased neck hyperextension and shoulder elevation, cranial molding, or dolichocephaly, and can improve neuromuscular development. Positioning can also alter respiratory physiology. Placing an infant in the prone position increases oxygenation, tidal volume, and lung compliance, and reduces energy expenditure when compared with the supine position.[20,21]

Body position affects gastric emptying and skin integrity as well as neurobehavioral development. Activities such as hand-to-mouth

ability, midline orientation, flexion, and self-soothing and self-regulatory abilities can be enhanced through facilitating body positions.

Head shape is also affected by positioning. Premature infants in particular are prone to develop dolichocephaly (narrow head shape) or plagiocephaly (asymmetrical head shape). These conditions can be avoided to some extent, or minimized by careful positioning.[22] All infants should be placed in supine position for sleep before discharge from the NICU. This may require an adjustment period for some infants before they are comfortably sleeping in the supine position, so this is best undertaken before discharge from the NICU. Positioning a sleeping infant with rolls, nests and other containment devices are not appropriate for unmonitored infants, and should be discontinued well before discharge.[23] Implementation of these recommendations remains inconsistent in NICUs because of knowledge deficits about the guidelines, and routines such as prone position for sleeping.[24] Gestational age, degree of illness, and use of neuromuscular blocking medications all influence positioning decisions. Global hypotonia in infants younger than 30 weeks' gestation requires significant intervention. Critically ill premature and term infants cannot expend any energy to move and require assistance to attain any body position. Infants receiving neuromuscular blocking agents, such as pancuronium, must receive positioning assistance to maintain basic physiologic stability. Thus, selecting an appropriate body position and assisting the patient into it are important considerations for nurses in the NICU.

Interventions to Position Neonates

1. Change the infant's position every 2 to 3 hours for extremely ill or immature infants.
2. Promote hand-to-mouth behavior by allowing the hands to be free when the caregiver is present; side-lying positioning also assists in this goal.
3. Attempt to "nest" the infant with blanket rolls or other positioning aids (Fig. 9-1).
4. Place rolls under the infant's hips when the infant is prone to prevent hip abduction.
5. Roll the infant's shoulders gently forward with soft rolls when both prone and supine to prevent shoulder extension.

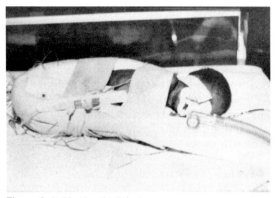

Figure 9-1. Nesting the infant.

6. Use water- or air-filled pillows under the infant's head to minimize cranial molding; frequent position changes (every 2 to 3 hours) from side to side and midline also facilitate this goal.
7. Support the infant's soles of the feet with rolls to prevent ankle extension.
8. Swaddle the infant with blankets or buntings when the infant is stable to promote flexion and self-regulatory behavior.
9. Consider gentle massage to promote skin blood flow in infants on neuromuscular blocking agents; reposition the infant every 2 hours to prevent pressure sores.
10. Position infants with right side down or prone to promote gastric emptying. Prone position is best for minimizing effects of gastroesophageal reflux. In preterm infants, it improves oxygenation.
11. Elevate head of bed after feedings to reduce pressure of full stomach against the diaphragm and improve respiratory capacity.
12. Hold stable infants, even when on the ventilator; holding may be soothing and provides vestibular stimulation similar to fetal experience.

SKIN CARE

Protection and preservation of the skin of term and premature newborns are significantly important, because this organ acts as a barrier against infection and is a major contributor to temperature control. It is a challenge to maintain the integrity of this delicate organ when providing care to premature infants in the NICU. Trauma to skin can occur when life support or monitoring devices that have been securely attached to the skin are removed or replaced, or when procedures such as blood sampling and chest tube insertion penetrate the skin's barrier. Repair of the skin after tissue injury also requires a large consumption of energy. When the skin is damaged, evaporative heat loss and the risk of toxicity from topically applied substances are increased. In addition, there is an increased portal of entry for microorganisms including common skin flora such as coagulase-negative *Staphylococcus* and *Candida*. Thus, significant morbidity and even death can potentially be attributed to practices that cause trauma or alterations in normal skin function.

DEVELOPMENTAL VARIATIONS IN PREMATURE SKIN

The term infant has a well-developed epidermis, although structurally different from adult skin; the stratum corneum, the uppermost layer of the epidermis, is 30% thinner and contains keratinocyte cells that are smaller.[25] As measured by transepidermal water loss (TEWL) techniques, full-term newborns have been shown to have similar barrier function compared to adult skin. However, there is now some evidence that the stratum corneum does not function as well as adult skin throughout the first year of life.[26] The premature infant has fewer layers of stratum corneum and is histologically thinner, with the cells of all strata more compressed. This results in increased permeability and transepidermal water loss. Clinical implications of these differences include increased evaporative heat loss, increased fluid requirement, and risk of toxicity from topically applied substances. Despite acceleration in the maturation of the stratum corneum during the first 10 to 14 days of life in premature infants, higher transepidermal water losses, and decreased barrier function may last up to 28 days. In infants of 23 to 25 weeks' gestation, skin barrier function reaches mature levels more slowly, taking as long as 8 weeks after birth, or until the infants reaches 30 to 32 weeks' postconceptional age, regardless of the postnatal age.

In premature infants, the numerous fibrils connecting the epidermis to the dermis are fewer and more widely spaced than in the term infant. Thus, premature infants are more vulnerable to blistering and a tendency toward stripping of the epidermis when adhesives are removed because the adhesives may be more firmly attached to the epidermis than the epidermis is to the dermis.

The functional capacity of the skin to form an "acid mantle" also differs. Normally in both adults and children, skin surface pH is less than 5. In the term newborn, the pH immediately after birth is alkaline, with a mean pH of 6.34, with a decline to 4.95 within 4 days. Premature infants have been shown to have a pH greater than 6 on the first day of life, decreasing to 5.5 over the first week and gradually declining to 5 by the fourth week. Bathing and other topical treatments transiently affect the skin pH,[27] and diapered skin has a higher pH due to the combined effects of urine contact and occlusion.[28] An acid skin surface is credited with bacteriocidal qualities against some pathogens and serves in the defense against infection. A shift in skin surface pH from acidic to neutral can result in an increase in total numbers of bacteria, a shift in the species present, and an increase in transepidermal water loss.

Another developmental variation affecting newborn skin is the presence of vernix caseosa. Vernix is a protective fetal skin covering, unique to humans, that acts as a chemical and mechanical barrier in utero and facilitates postnatal adaptation to the extrauterine, dry environment. Production of vernix begins at the end of the second trimester, accumulating on the skin in a cephalocaudal manner.[29] Vernix detaches from the skin as levels of pulmonary surfactant rise, resulting in progressively more turbidity of the amniotic fluid. Vernix contains antimicrobial peptides and proteins that may be protective against bacteria, assist in pH development, and assist in cleansing.[30,31] Studies about this important substance are generating interest in the possibility of using vernix as a prototype of a new barrier cream to facilitate the development of the stratum corneum in premature neonates.[32]

SKIN CARE PRACTICES

Skin care practices performed daily by nurses in the NICU include bathing, moisturizing with emollients, antimicrobial skin preparation, umbilical cord care, and affixation of adhesives for life support and monitoring devices. These activities have the potential for causing trauma and altering the skin pH, thereby disrupting the barrier function of the skin. In 2001, two national nursing organizations in the United States, the Association of Women's Health, Obstetric and Neonatal Nurses (AWHONN) and the National Association of Neonatal Nurses (NANN) collaborated on the formulation of evidence-based neonatal skin care guidelines that encompass these and other aspects of providing skin care to newborns. In 51 nurseries, the overall skin condition of 2820 newborn infants was evaluated in terms of skin dryness, erythema, and breakdown using the Neonatal Skin Condition Score (NSCS), and was found to be improved after each nursery implemented the evidence-based practices.[33] The Neonatal Skin Care Guideline has recently been revised to include new studies pertinent to neonatal skin and skin care practices.[34]

Bathing

The daily bath is traditionally administered to all hospitalized patients, including newborns in the NICU. Newborns are bathed to remove waste materials, improve general aesthetic qualities, and reduce microbial colonization. Bathing full-term infants immediately after delivery can potentially compromise temperature regulation and cardiorespiratory stability, and should be delayed until the infant has achieved thermal and cardiorespiratory stability, and has had time for skin-to-skin contact with the mother.[34]

Cleansers that are used for routine bathing include alkaline soaps, neutral pH synthetic detergents, and deodorant-type cleansers that contain antimicrobial properties. Bathing infants has been shown to cause an increase in the skin's pH and a decrease in its fat content, most significantly with alkaline soap. Skin surface pH is enhanced if vernix is retained and not mechanically removed, even after bathing with a mild cleanser.[32] Although some studies involve bathing with water alone in the first week of life,[35] a comparison of four different bathing regimens including water alone, water plus washing gel, and water plus moisturizer—with or without the wash gel—fail to show significant influences on skin parameters, although the use of the moisturizer did transiently improve barrier function measurements.[36] Water hardness, pH, and osmolarity are also potential irritants. In addition, washing with water alone may not remove some substances that soil the skin, are not water soluble but fat soluble, and there may be benefit from using a mild cleanser.[27] Routine bathing should be no more frequent than every other day, as bathing does not reduce skin colonization with pathogenic microorganisms,[37] leads to drier skin surfaces,[28] and may lead to behavioral and physiologic instability.[38] Premature infants less than 32 weeks are recommended to have water bathing only for the first 2 weeks of life due to considerations for their overall skin immaturity, as well as the potentially physiologic instability that may occur as a result of bathing.[34]

Although the first and subsequent baths in many hospitals are sponge baths, tub or immersion bathing may be beneficial. Immersion bathing places the infant's entire body, except the head and neck, into warm water (100.4° F), deep enough to cover the shoulders. A randomized controlled trial of immersion versus sponge bathing in 102 newborns for their first bath and subsequent baths showed that the immersion-bathed infants had significantly less temperature loss, appeared more content, and their mothers reported more pleasure with the bath; there was no difference in umbilical cord healing scores between immersion or sponge bathing.[39] Bathing is also an opportunity to educate parents about how to physically care for their babies as well as integrating information about neurobehavioral status and social characteristics. Infants who may benefit from immersion bathing include healthy, full-term newborns with the umbilical clamp in place, and stable preterm infants after umbilical catheters are discontinued.[34]

Moisturizers

The degree of hydration in the stratum corneum is related to the capacity of this layer to absorb and retain water. Moisturizers improve skin function by restoring intercellular lipids in dry or injured stratum corneum. These are products such as emollients, creams, lanolin, mineral oil, or lotions; many include petrolatum as an ingredient because of its excellent hydrating and healing qualities.[40]

Although there may be beneficial effects of routine emollient use in premature infants younger than 33 weeks' gestation, an association has been shown between routine (twice daily) applications of petrolatum-based emollient and *S. epidermidis* blood stream infections in a randomized, controlled trial of 1191 premature infants less than 1000 grams.[41]

Routine use of an emollient to prevent or treat excessive drying, skin cracking, or fissures is not recommended. However, dry, scaling, or cracking skin will benefit from an emollient that is free of perfumes or dyes; products containing perfumes or dyes that can be absorbed and may result in later sensitization or toxicity are not recommended.[41]

Skin Disinfectants

Use of skin disinfectants before invasive procedures is commonplace in hospitalized full-term and premature newborns. The most common disinfectants that are used in newborns include 70% isopropyl alcohol, povidone-iodine, and chlorhexidine gluconate, both an aqueous solution and one combined with 70% isopropyl alcohol. There have been anecdotal reports of skin blistering, burns, and sloughing from isopropyl alcohol and chlorhexidine gluconate products in premature infants.[42,43] Povidone-iodine has been associated with case reports of high iodine levels, iodine goiter, and hypothyroidism. Several prospective studies of routine povidone-iodine use in neonatal intensive care units found elevated urinary iodine levels and alterations in thyroid function in premature infants because of iodine absorption through the skin.

A sequential study of 254 premature and term infants in the NICU found IV catheter colonization to be reduced in sites prepared with 0.5% chlorhexidine in alcohol solution compared with povidone-iodine.[44]

Because of the risk of skin injury from isopropyl alcohol and methanol-containing chlorhexidine gluconate products,[43] there is currently no single disinfectant that can be recommended for all neonates.[34] Aqueous 2% chlorhexidine gluconate is available in 4 ounce bottles and must be poured onto a sterile gauze sponge for application, and 2% chlorhexidine gluconate in 70% isopropyl alcohol is available in single-use products but is approved by the U.S. Food and Drug Administration (FDA) only in infants older than 2 months of age. Although some nurseries elect to use this product "off-label," there is significant risk of skin injury in prematures infants. Many nurseries continue to use 10% povidone-iodine. When any of the skin disinfectant solutions are used, it is necessary to remove the preparation completely when the procedure is finished. Water or saline is preferred for removing disinfectants to reduce the risk of further skin injury from these caustic preparations.

Adhesive Application and Removal

Traumatic effects of adhesive removal for premature infants include reduced barrier function, increased transepidermal water loss, increased permeability, erythema, and skin stripping. Solvents have been used in hospitals for a number of years to remove tape and adhesives. Although effective, these products should not be used in the premature infant because of the risk of toxicity from absorption and because of the potential for skin irritation and injury. Bonding agents that increase the adherence of adhesives may also cause more skin stripping and damage because they form a stronger bond between the adhesive and the epidermis than the fragile bond between epidermis and dermis, especially in the premature infant. Plastic polymer skin protectants are available to protect skin from adhesives and do not increase adhesive aggressiveness.[45] Products that do not contain isopropyl alcohol are preferred because the alcohol can also irritate newborn skin.

Skin barriers made from pectin and methylcellulose are used between skin and adhesive; they mold well to curved surfaces, and maintain adherence in moist areas. Although there is less visible trauma to skin with pectin barriers, evaporimeter measurements of skin barrier function shows that pectin causes a similar degree of trauma as commonly used plastic tape. Even more mature newborns are at risk for trauma from adhesive removal. However, hydrocolloid products continue to be helpful in the hospitalized newborn owing to improved adherence as the product warms to skin temperature, and the ability to mold to surfaces better than many other products. These adhesives do require care on removal, similar to adhesive tapes.

Transparent adhesive dressings made from polyurethane are impermeable to water and bacteria but allow the free flow of air, thereby enabling the skin to "breathe." Uses for transparent dressings include securing IV catheters, percutaneous catheters, and central venous lines, nasogastric tubes, and nasal cannulas. They can also be used to prevent skin breakdown over areas that have the potential for friction burns or pressure sores, such as the knees, elbows, or sacrum, or as a dressing over surface injuries. Semipermeable dressings have proven to be very beneficial for selective taping procedures, such as IV and central venous catheter dressings, nasogastric tubes, and chest tubes. The potential for skin damage when removed is similar to other adhesive tapes.

Preventing trauma from adhesives can be accomplished by minimizing use of tape when possible, dabbing cotton on tape to reduce adherence, using hydrogel adhesives for electrodes, and delaying tape removal for more than 24 hours when the adhesive attaches less well to skin. Removal can be facilitated by applying warm water or an emollient or mineral oil if reapplication of adhesives at the site is not necessary. Slowly pulling adhesives at a very low angle, parallel to the skin surface, while holding the surrounding skin in place may reduce epidermal stripping.[46] Silicone-based adhesives are primarily used in wound care products, although silicone tapes are also available and have been shown to improve adherence to wounds and reduce discomfort when removed.[47] This technology holds promise for developing future adhesive products for newborns.

Skin Care Recommendations

Bathing: Use neutral pH cleansers on infants. Bathe the infant with cleansers infrequently—two to three times per week; at other times, use warm water baths. For infants with very immature skin, less than 32 weeks' gestation, clean with warm water and cotton balls for the first week.

Moisturizers: Use a petrolatum-based, water-miscible emollient that does not contain perfume or dyes. Apply moisturizer sparingly to cracked or fissured areas on an as-needed basis. If the infant's skin is colonized with *Candida*, use antifungal ointment instead of petrolatum-based ointment. Routine use of emollients in infants less than 1000 grams is not recommended.

Antimicrobial skin preparation: Use aqueous chlorhexidine or povidone-iodine solution before any invasive procedure that penetrates the skin surface; remove the solution completely with water or saline. Avoid the use of isopropyl alcohol to remove skin disinfectants.

Adhesives and adhesive removal: Limit the amount of tapes and adhesives used to secure equipment. Do not use solvents, but remove tape with water-soaked cotton balls. Tincture of benzoin and other bonding agents are not routinely recommended for very immature infants because this can create a stronger bond of adhesive to the epidermis than the bond between epidermis and dermis. Consider use of hydrocolloid adhesives, such as pectin barriers, between tape and skin for better adherence. Use hydrogel adhesives for electrodes, soft gauze wraps for pulse oximeter probes, and transparent adhesive dressings to secure IV catheters, central venous catheters, nasogastric tubes, or oxygen cannulas.

PAIN MANAGEMENT IN THE NEONATE

Nurses collaborate with medical and surgical staff to assess and treat pain in neonates related to disease processes, invasive treatments, and surgical procedures. The attitudes of staff and parents continue to have an impact on the use of pharmacologic interventions. Barriers include, but are not limited to, the following: (1) lack of clinical trials for pain assessment and treatment in the neonate, (2) fear of side effects of the treatment, (3) concern over dependence and or neurologic sequelae with the use of pain medications, (4) pharmacologic and individual differences of the drug used to treat pain, (5) lack of agreement about the adverse effects of pain, and (6) shortcomings of all tools in the nonverbal patient.[48,49] Even the most immature infant perceives pain and there are real and ongoing physiologic and potentially neurodevelopmental consequences of inadequately treated pain.[48,49]

Significant advances have been made in the assessment and treatment of neonatal pain since The Joint Commission (TJC) made this a survey standard. Pain treatment has improved significantly in the past decade for neonatal patients. Successful pain management is best facilitated by (1) staff orientation on pain assessment and treatment, (2) use of a neonatal pain tool, (3) development of pain management standards that address procedural, postoperative and disease-related pain, (4) ongoing efforts to reduce painful procedures that are not necessary, and (5) interdisciplinary collaboration with surgery, anesthesia, neonatology, nursing, and other ancillary personnel about the standards of pain management.

Currently, many neonatal units are using tools such as the PIPP (Premature Infant Pain Profile) or N-PASS (Neonatal Pain, Agitation, and Sedation Scale) that assess differences in the premature infant who may not mount a vigorous behavioral response to pain.[50] Most neonatal tools use a combination of behavioral and physiologic indicators to help assess pain. Behavioral indicators include, but are not limited to, crying, grimacing, brow bulge, eye squeeze, gaze aversion, clenched fingers and toes, arching, kicking, inconsolability, or lack of movement and decreased tone. Physiologic indicators include, but are not limited to, increased heart rate and blood pressure, mottled or pale skin color, increased oxygen requirements, palm sweating, and decreased or labile oxygen saturations. The *FLACC* (*f*ace, *l*egs, *a*rms, *c*rying, and *c*onsolability) is a behavioral tool that can be used in settings where monitoring is not available, such as a newborn nursery.

Pain should be assessed using all of the information available to the bedside nurse including the biochemical indicators of stress such as elevated blood glucose and metabolic acidosis, as well as the context of the infant's current condition. In infants who have undergone a surgical procedure or invasive procedure, pain is clearly present regardless of the pain tool score. Additionally, waiting for an increase in scores may not be reasonable for pain medication administration in the postoperative infant. Pain is more efficiently treated if "preempted." Many neonatal units have written postoperative pain protocols that start with regularly scheduled or "around-the-clock" dosing when pain source is clear and scoring remains the most difficult. Pain assessment should be comprehensive, multidimensional, and include the contextual, behavioral, and physiologic indicators available to bedside nurses.[51]

Postoperative pain protocols have been developed through teams working together to develop consensus on appropriate medications, dosing, and method of administration. These protocols should include an initial postoperative dose based on last operative opiate dose and then an "around-the-clock" dosing schedule. Continuous opiate infusions have the advantage of steady-state dose delivery, less opening of IV lines, and fewer opportunities for error in calculation. There is some concern that tolerance develops more rapidly with opiate infusions, but tolerance can be handled by tapering the drug dose if the drip exceeds a 5-day course. Many postoperative pain protocols advise drip opiates for 48 to 72 hours for major thoracic and abdominal procedures with a transition to as-required (p.r.n.) opiate dosing and introduction of acetaminophen. Morphine has advantages over fentanyl in that it has a longer duration of action. When given slowly and in appropriate doses, there is minimal to no effect on blood pressure, CO_2 response, or oxygen requirements.

Postoperative Pain Management Protocol for Infants After a Major Abdominal or Thoracic Procedure

1. Give a 0.02 to 0.1 mg/kg IV bolus of morphine sulfate within 1 hour of last intraoperative opiate dose.
2. Begin continuous drip of morphine sulfate at 0.01 to 0.02 mg/kg/hour, adjust drip rate as needed based on pain assessment, and source.

3. Acetaminophen rectally 15 mg/kg around the clock for 48 hours to potentiate opiates; frequency is based on gestation (term infants every 6 hours, >32 weeks every 8 hours, <32 weeks every 12 hours), then p.r.n. as pain intensity lessens.

The pharmacokinetics of analgesia and opiate clearance and tolerance are extremely variable based on gestation, and opiate experience. Infants who have had recent or repeated opiate doses may require higher doses than infants who are opiate "naïve" and very immature. Premature infants have prolonged clearance times of opiates and sedatives which improve with postconceptual age. Clearance reaches adult values at about 1 month of age. Unlike other medications, both opiates and sedatives can be readily reversed or partially reversed if adverse side effects occur. It is important to remember that there are significant adverse effects of inadequately treated pain, such as reduced gut motility, urinary retention, hypercoagulation, decreased tidal volume, increased splinting, hypoxia, atelectasis, hypermetabolism, protein catabolism, and exaggerated stress response. Infants treated on a protocol are likely to be extubated faster, have less postoperative fluid retention, and need less drug overall than infants who were not on a protocol.[52]

The success of postoperative pain management requires that the nurse consult with the neonatologist, surgeon, and anesthesiologist. It is essential to determine the relative pain potential based on similar procedures in verbal children or adults and to determine any intraoperative procedures that may lessen postoperative pain such as a caudal anesthetic or local instillation of an anesthetic. For surgical procedures such as ventricular-peritoneal shunt placement, simple colostomy for imperforate anus, or laparoscopic gastrostomy, the postoperative pain medication of choice is less clear. An option for low-dose opiate by intermittent bolus infusion with acetaminophen is a good starting point with pain assessment and tool scores to guide the management.

Procedural pain management requires group consensus from medical and nursing staff. Most units begin by evaluating all invasive procedures to see if they are essential to care or if they can be modified or reduced. This process includes reviewing all procedures and protocols that require blood sampling, suctioning, tape removal, or tube insertion. Many units have improved procedural pain management by reducing the number of painful procedures to which each infant is exposed. Laboratory blood draws are coordinated and tests "batched" to avoid multiple punctures. Many units have eliminated routine suctioning and only suction when there are clinical indications. Examples of procedural pain management are (1) oral sucrose for heel sticks, tape removal, eye examinations, nasogastric tube insertion, intramuscular injections, and other minor painful procedures, (2) subcutaneous or topical anesthetics (4% lidocaine) for starting IVs and as an adjunct to a local anesthetic for lumbar punctures, chest tube insertion, and peripheral arterial catheter insertion, (3) systemic opiates for intubations, chest tube insertion, and peritoneal taps.

Oral sucrose has been used for many years for minor pain management and the efficacy and safety has been confirmed in multiple studies. A recent study was unable to demonstrate a difference in nociceptive brain activity after a heel lance, but did demonstrate a significant difference in pain scores in infants who received sucrose versus sterile water.[53]

Current practice should evaluate pain behaviors after a pharmacologic intervention, with preprocedural sucrose to reduce crying and pain scores. Sucrose is most effective when dipped on a pacifier prior to the

EDITORIAL COMMENT: Pain management is an integral part of modern neonatal intensive care. However, there are still many unanswered questions. Stevens et al. completed a Cochrane review that included forty-four studies enrolling 3496 infants.[54] Results from only a few studies could be combined in metaanalyses. Sucrose significantly reduced duration of total crying time, but did not reduce duration of first cry. Although true pain perception cannot be measured in nonverbal populations, neural activity in nociceptive pathways is a more direct measure than behavioral and physiologic assessment. Slater et al. found that sucrose does not change neural activity,[53] which strongly suggests that pain perception is not affected by this intervention. Nonetheless, Lasky and van Drongelen noted,[55] "… until we better understand pain pathways and the short-term and long-term sequelae of painful procedures, it seems premature to conclude that sucrose might not be an effective analgesic for newborn babies."

procedure. It does not reach the stomach, and can therefore be used in infants who are receiving nothing by mouth. It has not been associated with a rise in blood glucose when administered by pacifier dipping. It should be used with caution in very low-birth-weight intubated infants due to concerns of choking. [52,56,57]

Topical lidocaine (4%) has also been shown to be safe and efficacious and requires only a 20-minute application to achieve effect to about 4-mm depth.[58] It does need to be used sparingly to just the area of the pain source. Data are sparse in very premature infants.

It is important to use a combination of the pharmacologic interventions available with the nonpharmacologic measures such as swaddling, containment, nonnutritive sucking, and massage. Nonpharmacologic measures do not replace the need for topical and subcutaneous anesthetics, nerve blocks, or systemic opiates. Many procedures in the NICU have been completed with a higher success rate and less morbidity when pain management is successful. One example is the use of premedication for intubation, with a 50% reduction in time to intubation, success on the first attempt, and minimal or no bradycardia or hypoxia being reported.[59] Intubation induction protocols include a systemic opiate such as fentanyl, atropine, and a fast-acting neuromuscular blockade agent. Procedural pain management in the NICU remains variable and surveys show that many units continue not to premedicate infants for the same procedures where premedication is a standard for older children or infants in Pediatric Intensive Care Units of the same age.[60-62]

There are many practical aspects of improving the safety of pain management. They include staff education on medication dosing and side effects used in pain management. Medication references should be readily available for dosing ranges and strategies. Protocols should be written and agreed on by nursing and medical staff to guide pain treatment. Staff should be familiar with the reversal agents for adverse opiate and sedative effects, naloxone and flumazenil. Consultation with a pain service and/or anesthesia practitioner should be available for difficult cases. Finally, nurses and physicians should use an opiate-weaning protocol when the use of opiates equals or exceeds 5 days. Infants, as adults, may become tolerant or dependent to the opiate and may have an adverse response if the medication is abruptly discontinued. Opiates should be tapered with abstinence scoring every 4 hours—or more often—to reduce the adverse effects of withdrawal. The length of the taper depends on the length of drug use or exposure. For example, for an infant undergoing a staged abdominal wall defect closure the opiate exposure from the first surgical procedures through the second procedure may be 6 to 8 days. The dose should then be tapered by no more than 10% to 25% every 24 to 48 hours depending on scores. The Finnegan Scoring Tool (Fig. 9-2) can be used for this purpose, with a score of less than 8 being used to reduce dose. Pain must also continue to be scored during the tapering process.

Concerns about the long-term developmental effects of using opiates and sedatives in neonates and young infants are ongoing.[55,63] Pain medications should be used for the treatment of pain and tapered or discontinued when the pain source is no longer present. No absolute test determines if pain is being experienced in a neonate. Nurses need to develop knowledge and skill at assessing pain behaviors, continue to advocate for their patients, and provide the nonpharmacologic and pharmacologic interventions to treat pain. Barriers to treatment include difficulties of assessment, attitudes about the competing goals of postoperative care, and knowledge of pain treatment options in the neonate.

VASCULAR ACCESS

IV access is used in the NICU to deliver medications, therapeutic agents, nutritional support, and hydration. There are numerous options for IV access that need to be evaluated for risk and benefit on a patient-by-patient basis. Peripheral access is predominately provided by Teflon "intracath" devices. Stainless steel needles are available but the dwell time is short and they are not the preferred method if IV catheters are available. When IV access is needed, the duration of therapy, size of the infant, skill of the bedside caregivers, type of IV fluid and/or medication required, and number of veins available should be taken into consideration. For short-term therapy (3 to 5 days), peripheral therapy is usually, but not always, adequate. In infants requiring 7 to 10 days of antibiotics, medications known to be associated with vein irritation, total parenteral nutrition, high

Analgesia/sedation orders (drug/dose/frequency) **Addressograph**

Date													
Drug													
Administration time													
Dose ↑ or ↓ or frequency													

Time:

Choose one: Crying/agitated 25%-50% of interval	2													
Crying/agitated >50% of interval	3													
Choose one: Sleeps ≤25% of interval	3													
Sleeps 26%-75% of interval	2													
Sleeps >75% of interval	1													
Choose one: Hyperactive Moro	2													
Markedly hyperactive Moro	3													
Choose one: Mild tremors, disturbed	1													
Moderate/severe tremors, disturbed	2													
Increased muscle tone	2													
Temperature 37.2°C-38.4°C	1													
Temperature >38.4°C	2													
Respiratory rate >60 (extubated)	2													
Suction > twice/interval (intubated)	2													
Sweating	1													
Frequent yawning (>3-4/interval)	2													
Sneezing (>3-4/interval)	1													
Nasal stuffiness	1													
Emesis	2													
Projectile vomiting	3													
Loose stools	2													
Watery stools	3													
Total score														
Adjusted score														
Initials of person scoring														

Directions: Score every 2-4 hours per guideline. Score greater than 8-12 may indicate withdrawal.

Figure 9-2. Assessment form for drug withdrawal: Opiate weaning flow sheet. *(Adapted from Finnegan LP, Connaughton JF Jr, Kron RE, et al: Neonatal abstinence syndrome: assessment and management,* Addict Dis *2:141, 1975. Version 1/94.)*

glucose infusions, or IV calcium therapy, it is often reasonable to consider central venous access. For those infants with a peripheral IV, management and assessment of the IV line are essential for patient safety. The following recommendations may reduce complications:

1. Select an IV catheter that is of high quality and smooth; Teflon, silicone, or polyurethane
2. Develop a staff training program that includes education on vein selection, procedural pain management, IV insertion, stabilization, and documentation.
3. Experienced nurses should train and supervise new employees.
4. Use IV models for skill practice (available from companies who manufacture IV devices).
5. Have written procedures for inserting, securing, and assessing hourly.
6. Limit the glucose concentration to D12.5%, amino acids to 2%, and calcium gluconate to 200 mg/100 mL. Avoid IV calcium if possible for older infants with normal calcium levels.
7. Use infusion pumps that have safety options or air detection, no runaway option, and occlusion alarms.
8. Instruct on the signs of infiltration that include swelling, redness, blanching, larger size than contralateral extremity, crying or grimacing with flushing, lack of blood return, and skin temperature difference.
9. Use a second opinion from an experienced nurse when there is doubt.
10. Use an IV infiltration scale to guide treatment and reporting.
11. Use an infiltration protocol that involves hyaluronidase (Vitrase) or (phentolamine Regitine) with hydrogel treatment for residual tissue injury.
12. Report and track all adverse effects of IV therapy, such as infiltrates resulting in tissue injury and loss of access.

Hyaluronidase is a protein enzyme that helps diffuse IV infiltrates by modifying the permeability of the connective tissue. The needle used to give the drug around the circumference of the swelling also has the effect of allowing the fluid to drain from the puncture sites; this multiple puncture technique has also been shown to be effective if hyaluronidase is not available. Both the drug and the punctures will decrease the swelling, allow the infiltrated fluid to leak from the puncture sites and improve tissue perfusion.

Vitrase, a hyaluronidase-containing formulation, does not contain preservatives and comes as 200 mg/mL that requires a 1:10 dilution before administration of the 20-mg dose in five divided injections of 0.2 mL aliquots around the swelling. Phentolamine is used when a vasoactive drug has infiltrated and directly counteracts the drug and improves skin perfusion.[64-66] The dose is 0.25-0.5 mg diluted to 1 mL. When the infiltration includes vasoactive drugs and maintenance fluids such as TPN, the phentolamine should be administered first until the color improves and then the hyaluronidase should be administered. Using a 23-gauge needle for the injection of the drugs can also allow the infiltrated fluid to leak out. Placing the site on a clean surface and dripping warm saline will keep the puncture sites open and allow more fluid to be drained.

CENTRAL VENOUS ACCESS

Central venous access can be achieved using umbilical venous catheters (UVCs), surgically placed catheters, tunneled, such as Broviac (Bard Access Systems, Salt Lake City, Utah) or, non-tunneled such as a Cook (Cook Medical, Bloomington, Ind), or percutaneously placed central catheters (PICCs). The adoption of standardized, evidence-based central line insertion and maintenance bundles significantly reduces NICU central-line-associated bloodstream infection rates (Box 9-1). These catheters can be placed in high-flow, large vessels such as the superior vena cava (SVC) or inferior vena cava (IVC). The advantages are less risk of infiltration for high concentration glucose and protein and irritating medications (vesicants) such as acyclovir and calcium salts, provision of a steady system for infusion, and reduction in the number of painful procedures that may be required for peripheral IVs. The risks of central venous access include thrombus, infection, and rarely, pleural and pericardial effusion. These risks can be reduced with the use of the small-sized silicone or polyurethane catheters that are placed percutaneously through a peripheral vein (PICC).[67]

PICC catheters come in multiple sizes that can be used in neonates ranging from 1.2 to 3 Fr. They are threaded through a variety of introducer needles to achieve a central venous tip location and then the introducer is removed from the system. Catheter tips should be in the SVC or IVC to reduce effusion risk. These small catheters made from silicone and polyurethane reduce the risk of

Box 9-1.	**Central-Line Insertion and Maintenance Bundle Elements**

Insertion bundle

Establish a central line kit or cart to consolidate all items necessary for the procedure.

Perform hand hygiene with hospital-approved alcohol-based product or antiseptic-containing soap before and after palpating insertion sites and before and after inserting the central line.

Use maximal barrier precautions (including sterile gown, sterile gloves, surgical mask, hat, and large sterile drape).

Disinfect skin with appropriate antiseptic (e.g., 2% chlorhexidine, 70% alcohol) before catheter insertion.

Use either a sterile transparent semipermeable dressing or sterile gauze to cover the insertion site.

Maintenance bundle

Perform hand hygiene with hospital approved alcohol-based product or antiseptic-containing soap before and after accessing a catheter or before and after changing the dressing.

Evaluate the catheter insertion site daily for signs of infection and to assess dressing integrity.

At a minimum, if the dressing is damp, soiled, or loose change dressing aseptically and disinfect the skin around the insertion site with an appropriate antiseptic (e.g., 2% chlorhexidine, 70% alcohol).

Develop and use standardized intravenous tubing set-up and changes.

Maintain aseptic technique when changing intravenous tubing and when entering the catheter including "scrub the hub".

Daily review of catheter necessity with prompt removal when no longer essential.

From Schulman J, Stricof R, Stevens TP, et al: Statewide NICU central-line-associated bloodstream infection rates decline after bundles and checklists, Pediatrics 127:436, 2011.

reduce complications and infections.[68,69] New split septum "ports" have been shown to reduce the contamination of the fluid path if a 15-second scrub with alcohol precedes any catheter entry. Dwell time can be weeks to months and, therefore, reduce painful procedures for IV starts, provide uninterrupted vascular access, and allow for hyperosmolar IV solutions to be used. When frequent blood sampling or blood product administration is needed, then a surgical line, tunneled or non-tunneled, or a 3 Fr PICC should be considered. Tunneled catheters (such as a Broviac are available in 2.7 and 4.2 Fr sizes and can be used for blood draws and blood product administration. These catheters can be used for long-term access in cases of short bowel syndrome or other complicated surgical conditions. Cook catheters can be placed percutaneously in the subclavian or femoral vein, are available in 3 and 4 Fr, and have double lumen options for critical infants. Units using PICCs should consider the following recommendations for standards of care that include:

1. Place lines early before peripheral veins are damaged.
2. Safe insertion sites include the basilic, cephalic, saphenous, or preauricular vein in the scalp. The axillary vein can be used, but is technically more difficult to stabilize, and is close to the artery. The jugular veins should be avoided due to high bacterial counts found at that site and the technical difficulties with dressings.
3. Maximize barrier precautions for insertion; cover site after x-ray confirmation with a transparent dressing.
4. Change dressings only when soiled or adhesion is lost to minimize skin injury with adhesive removal and potential loss of line during the process.
5. Confirm tip location using an injection of radiopaque contrast such as Optiray (Covidien, Mansfield, Mass) to better visualize tip, have arm or leg in flexed position during the film because extremity position affects the tip location.[70]
6. Minimize opening of the line to reduce introduction of bacteria.
7. Change IV medications to oral as soon as possible.
8. Avoid use for blood samples or blood product administration.
9. Avoid the use of small-bore syringes (1 and 3 mL), which will increase the pressure in the catheter and may lead to catheter rupture.

thrombus. The catheter is soft and flexible and can be maintained without arm boards, sutures, or limits of patient positioning. They are made by several manufacturers and now come in a double lumen option.

Infections can be reduced by standardizing the insertion technique, the dressing, the procedure for changing the tubing, and the procedure for administering medications. Research has also shown that a small dedicated team of inserters will also

10. Track all complications and nonelective removal to identify staff knowledge and skill deficits or systems problems that need to be addressed to improve safety and dwell time.
11. Educate nursing and medical staff about complications, troubleshooting, and line repair.
12. Train a core group of nurses to insert PICCs in adequate numbers to ensure a high skill level and to meet patient needs.
13. Standardize all insertion, dressings, line changes, and medication delivery into a procedure and checklist.

All venous access is monitored and maintained by nurses. Nurses should actively participate in the selection of appropriate IV devices for patients' needs. Practice should be standardized with procedures, protocols, and policy to reduce related risks and improve patient safety.

> **EDITORIAL COMMENT:** Nosocomial infections occur worldwide and are among the major causes of death and increased morbidity among hospitalized patients. Neonatal hospital-acquired infections add to functional disability and emotional stress of the family and may lead to neuro-cognitive impairment. The financial costs are considerable with the increased length of stay contributing most to the added costs. Efficient progress in decreasing neonatal nosocomial infection rates can be achieved when statewide quality-improvement collaboratives using structured interventions ("tool kits") are augmented with brief interactions that introduce, orient, and motivate potential users.[71-73] These interventions are simple and require maintaining a checklist of the steps in the procedure. Ensuring sterility, making certain that all items necessary to complete the placement of the line are present before starting the procedure, and providing routine care of the dressings and tubing must be a priority. Careful care of the hub when the line is in place and asking the question daily as to the need for the central line are all important elements of the "bundle" to prevent central line infections.
>
> Key elements of the bundle to prevent nosocomial infection include:
>
> 1. Use a central line associated blood stream infections (CLABSI) insertion bundle (e.g., chlorhexidine for skin antisepsis, maximal sterile barrier precautions, and hand hygiene). A properly applied and maintained PICC dressing is the first line of defense to minimize the risk of complications such as dislodgement, migration, and infection.
> 2. All needed supplies are "bundled" in one area (e.g., a cart or kit) to ensure items are available for use before starting the procedure.
> 3. A checklist is used to ensure all insertion practices are followed.
> 4. There is a policy or program to empower staff to stop a nonemergent central line insertion if proper procedures are not followed.
> 5. There is an education or training program for staff responsible for insertion and maintenance of catheters.
> 6. Chlorhexidine is the preferred agent for skin cleansing for central line insertion and/or maintenance.

COMPLICATIONS OF CARE

In light of the serious emotional, biological, and social burdens to which complications of therapy can lead, it is imperative that nurses collaborate with members of the medical team to identify and reduce these complications.[74] Reducing errors can only occur through comprehensive programs that address the spectrum of what can go wrong with the systems and human aspects that contributed to the error. It is also clear that patient safety is best achieved when errors can be reported in a nonpunitive environment. The concept of psychological safety fosters the belief by staff that "well intended actions will not lead to punishment or rejection by others." Staff will report their errors and ask for help if the likelihood of rejection or embarrassment is low. This "no blame" environment does not stop managers from evaluating staff practice. Individuals continue to have the responsibility to be knowledgeable and skilled in medication preparation and administration, and to follow the rules. Individuals who engage in recurrent unsafe practices need to be given a plan for practice improvement and a time frame to meet a knowledge or skill deficit. NICUs should consider creating staff competencies that test and review for knowledge, skill, and safe practice guidelines.

All nursing care delivery should be organized in a systematic way that includes staff orientation and education, written policies, protocols and procedures, education, and staff development for all employees, and a method of audits and safety checks to ensure that practice standards are met. Staff education requires a combination of skill training, knowledge of pathophysiology, periodic review of the evidence for practice, and interpersonal relationship skills. Policies state what the standard is, such as "two identifiers will be used for all patient testing and reports and they are the name and medical record number." Procedures are the psychomotor skills required to complete a task such as performing a bladder catheterization. Procedures can incorporate policy (e.g., what type of preparation is used for an invasive procedure or how many attempts one nurse can try before asking for assistance). Protocols are sets of instructions or information about how to care for a patient receiving a particular therapy such as phototherapy or total parenteral nutrition. These documents set standards, clarify practice, and can be used for reference by new staff or in unusual circumstances. Nursing care that differs from the identified standard can be justified and, at times, in the patient's best interest, modified with team discussion and supportive documentation. All of these documents should be readily available electronically for ease of access and evaluated at intervals to include new evidence and practice change. Recently, the use of checklists has been recommended to provide a shortened version of a long protocol or procedure. These checklists help define critical steps, reduce the reliance on short-term memory, and have been shown to improve patient safety.

Nursing staff should participate in all equipment and supply selection and evaluation. Nurses should be clear about how to handle equipment or supplies that malfunction or break. The Safe Medical Device Act (SMDA) requires that equipment or supplies that cause patient harm, or could have caused patient harm, must be reported. These reports provide a database for product recalls and directs intervention with the manufacturer from the FDA (MedSun, Medical Product Safety Network) for investigation about the product problem. For example, if a new IV pump is marketed and in setting the rate it is possible to get a double entry if the button is pressed for too long, an overinfusion of fluids may occur. Through SMDA reporting the FDA can quantify the problem and work with the manufacturer to make design changes to reduce this risk. The reports are traditionally done through a hospital safety officer or the biomedical engineering department and nurses only need to send basic information to an individual who then collects all of the details. All problem reporting should be designed to be clear, simple, and efficient. Nurses should focus their time on patients and families and have support staff work on risk reduction from their reports.

Nurses should also be encouraged to inspect all supplies before they are used on patients and save the packaging for tracking if the device is defective or broken. Lot numbers and identifying information is essential in the problem solving process. Cost containment, participation in buying cooperatives, and the push for standardization often places supplies and equipment at the NICU bedside that is substandard or not suited for infants. Manufacturing problems can occur in a previously reliable product. Timely reporting of adverse patient impact resulting from a product can facilitate prompt removal from the area and change to a product that meets patient needs and safety requirements.

Other new concepts in patient safety include the use of forcing functions. Designs or steps have been established that make it less likely or impossible for the error to be made. An example is the use of specialized tubing for infused enteral feeds that cannot be connected to an IV line. Redundancies are double, triple, and quadruple checks of critical processes that can identify an error. These checking processes have been used for the calculations of high-risk drugs such as opiates, anticoagulants, potassium, and digoxin. Double checks have also been successfully used to check breast milk feedings. Confirmation bias is a concept that leads to errors. The category of "look-alike, sound-alike" medication or formula errors occur because the first few letters are the same. Nurses may be performing a task that they have done many times and can go through the process and not read the label correctly; they see what is familiar or what they want to see, rather than what is actually there. These errors can be reduced by putting in place a process that slows the individual down, reduces distractions, and creates labeling that is clearer. Lastly, creating areas where the nurse performing critical procedures such as preparing medications, mixing feedings, or reporting of patient information is protected from distractions that can lead to an omission or error.[75] It is a concept taken from the airline industry where pilots are only allowed to talk about landing at 10,000 feet or below. See also Box 9-2.

The introduction of new technology has also helped reduce errors related to medication administration. Computerized Physician Order Entry (CPOE) systems have been introduced in NICUs since around 2002. These systems provide several advantages

---

Box 9-2. Medication Errors

Types of errors
Adverse drug event
Adverse reaction causing injury from a drug-related intervention

Administration
Wrong
- Drug
- Patient
- Dose
- Technique
- Time
- Route
- Documentation
Omission errors

Pharmacy-related
Dispensing error
Labeling error (instructions or information)
Education deficit

Human factors
Communication errors, phone or verbal
Education deficit
Order errors
- Ambiguous or incomplete
- Illegible handwriting
- Misplaced/missing zeros and decimal points
- Confirmation bias (errors induced by familiarity with procedures and materials)

Error reduction
User friendly, non–punitive-based error reporting system
Rate collection method
Access to national reporting database, problems and solutions
Documentation of event
Planning for intervention when error occurs
Intradisciplinary error review process
Identification of causes
Improvement or change in contributing factors
Evaluation of intervention

Adapted from Cohen MR, editor: Medication errors, ed 2, Washington, DC, 2007, American Pharmacists Association.

---

including legibility, electronic interface with the pharmacy, reduced turnaround time for dispensing, a decrease in "rule (formal policy, department-specific procedures, or informal understandings) violations," and an option to customize order screens to prompt safe dose and lock out doses that are too high or too low. Smart pump technology is now available to calculate critical drug doses, and has allowed nurseries to use standardized concentrations instead of the "rule of six" (mathematical formula used in the preparation of infusions for pediatric intensive care units and neonatal intensive care units, stating that the number of milligrams of drug to be added to 100 mL of IV fluid is equal to the weight (in kilograms) of the child multiplied by six; when the fluid is infused at 1 mL per hour, it will deliver 1 μg/kg per minute).

Smart pumps incorporate computer technology for storing drug information, making calculations, and checking entered patient information (weight and dose/kg/hour) against dosing parameters. These pumps have reduced calculation errors and utilize premixed bags. Bar coding technology has reduced administration errors in that the drug, patient, and nurse are scanned at the time of administration and electronically checked against the medical record order. Neonatal-specific medication information is now also available electronically and can be loaded onto computer desktops for staff access or downloaded into handheld devices for personal use. *Neofax* and the *Pediatric Dosage Handbook* provide the most up-to-date accurate information. The Institute for Safe Medication Practice (ISMP) provides monthly safety alerts, and nurse advice alerts online. This publication includes articles about labeling problems, sound-alike, look-alike drug (SALAD) errors, and recommendations on safe practice based on national trends and safety initiatives, research, and practical implementation guidelines for safety measures. A strong relationship with the pharmacy is essential in reducing medication errors.[76-78] A NICU pharmacy liaison has a profound effect on the safety of medication dosing and monitoring. They have also been successfully employed to monitor drug use when concerns of overuse or misuse have been identified. Similar liaisons should be developed with biomedical engineering, the safety officer, infection control nurse, and risk management. These disciplines can provide safety-specific consultations when needed by NICU staff.

It is essential to patient safety that teams representing the NICU disciplines meet regularly to review reported errors in a systematic way. Even though reports indicate only a fraction of actual errors made, they provide a representation of the types of errors that occur. Each error or "near miss" should be seen as an opportunity to make changes that would decrease the probability of it being made again. The changes should be planned, assigned, and then evaluated to see if they had the desired effect. This process requires time, dedication, and a certain aptitude for the investigative process. These teams operate under names such as practice improvement, quality improvement, safety, and leadership. Practice improvement teams also improve safety by utilizing the failure mode effect analysis (FMEA) process. This process in used to discover the potential risks in a product or a system by examining ways that it might fail. It can be used for introducing new equipment, procedures, medications, and treatments. Once identified, systems can be put into place to reduce these risks. Including a bedside nurse on this team is essential to the process.

Serious complications and sentinel events should be reviewed using the Root Cause Analysis (RCA) process. This can be downloaded from The Joint Commission website for a template of steps. This process includes selecting a team of disciplines involved in the event and selecting a leader who was not involved in the incident and has experience in the process. The steps leading to the event are flow-charted. Once the steps are charted, there is discussion about the contributing factors, both systems and human. A list of "root causes" is agreed on and action plans are created to address each root cause. NICUs require dedicated teams to look at systems and human factors to keep patients safe and to provide an environment for staff that reduces their chance of making a mistake.

"There are some patients we cannot help, but none that we cannot harm."
                              Florence Nightingale

CASE 1

An infant born at 26 weeks' gestation weighing 680 g is admitted to the neonatal intensive care unit. His skin is extremely translucent in appearance, and there is already an area of skin excoriation on the right side of the chest where an electrocardiogram (ECG) electrode has been removed.

What is the recommended treatment for the area of excoriation?

This area can be covered with a transparent adhesive dressing to promote healing and reduce the risk of infection through the site, or coated with petrolatum-based emollient. The combination of a silicone dressing (such as Mepitel, Mölnlycke Healthcare, Norcross,

Ga) and ointment works well. The best option for the ECG electrodes is hydrogel adhesive.

What are the best ways to approach bathing and moisturizing?

Areas of the skin that become soiled (with blood or stool) can be cleansed with warm water and cotton balls for the first 2 weeks. After this time, twice weekly baths with neutral pH cleanser are begun, with warm water baths given on alternating days. Twice daily application of petrolatum-based emollient promotes better skin barrier function.

What is the safest way to prepare the skin surface before invasive procedures?

The skin is prepped with povidone-iodine or aqueous chlorhexidine solution before any procedure and the disinfectant is then removed entirely with sterile saline water after the procedure. Isopropyl alcohol alone or disinfectants that contain isopropyl alcohol are to be avoided until the skin matures because it causes drying and can be absorbed. It has been reported to cause burns in the very low-birth-weight infant.

CASE 2

B. N. is born at 32 weeks' gestation after an uncomplicated delivery. She recovers from her respiratory distress syndrome (RDS) and is on room air by 5 days of age. At 12 days, she is taking full enteral feeds, but necrotizing enterocolitis (NEC) develops and she requires resection of 13 cm of terminal ileum. Postoperatively, she is managed on peripheral total parenteral nutrition (TPN). An IV infiltrate is found, and the site, the left foot, is white and cool to the touch.

What is the recommended treatment of the site?

Treatment is with hyaluronidase (Vitrase, Alliance Medical Products, Irvine, Calif), 20 U injected subcutaneously in four or five sites surrounding the area of infiltrate. The 20 U is divided into 0.2 mL injections.

Within what time frame should the treatment occur?

The treatment should occur as soon as possible, but is thought to be of benefit if instituted within 1 hour of identifying the extravasation.

What is a logical alternate IV access in this infant?

For this preterm infant needing TPN until the bowel has rested and feedings are established, a percutaneous central venous line is recommended. This access would allow the infant to receive a high-calorie, high-protein solution that would optimize wound healing and growth. It would also provide long-term access that would reduce time and pain associated with intermittent IV insertion. This method has additional benefits in that it does not require an incision, does not require vein ligation, and costs less to insert than surgically placed venous catheters.

REFERENCES

The reference list for this chapter can be found online at www.expertconsult.com.

Respiratory Problems

10

Richard J. Martin and Moira A. Crowley

When one considers the complexity of the pulmonary and hemodynamic changes occurring after delivery, it is surprising that the majority of infants make the transition from intrauterine to extrauterine life so smoothly and uneventfully. Nonetheless, the staff working in the intensive care nursery spends a lion's share of their time caring for neonates with respiratory problems that are responsible for much of the morbidity and mortality in this period.

PHYSIOLOGIC CONSIDERATIONS

NORMAL DEVELOPMENTAL CHANGES

Before birth, the lung is a fluid-filled organ receiving 10% to 15% of the total cardiac output. Within the first minutes of life a large portion of the fluid is absorbed or expelled, the lung fills with air, and the blood flow through the lung increases eight- to tenfold. This considerable increase results from a decrease in pulmonary arterial tone and other physiologic changes that convert the circulation from a parallel arrangement to a series circuit.

The high vascular resistance in the fetal lung is caused by pulmonary arterial vaso-constriction. The pulmonary arterial vaso-dilation observed following delivery results, in part, from the large increase in oxygen tension, from the small decrease in CO_2 tension, and the corresponding increase in pH, biochemical changes, such as elevated prostaglandins, and from the mechanical effect of lung inflation.

At the same time, an adequate functional residual capacity (FRC = volume of air in the lungs at end expiration) is quickly attained. In healthy term infants, the first breaths are characterized by short deep inspirations and prolonged expirations through a partially closed glottis to ensure lung inflation. In preterm infants, continuous positive airway pressure (CPAP) enhances lung inflation.[1] By 1 hour, the distribution of air with each breath in the newborn is already similar to that observed in later life. Specifically, lung compliance (change in lung volume expressed in mL of air/cm of H_2O pressure change/mL of lung volume) and vital capacity increase briskly in the first hours of life, reaching values proportional to those in the adult.

Chemical control of respiration is, in general, similar in the newborn infant and the adult. As inspired (and arterial) Pco_2 is increased, both infants and adults increase their ventilation, although the neonatal ventilatory response is smaller. The ventilation of the newborn is also transiently increased when inspired gas mixtures contain less than 21% oxygen; this response suggests that the carotid body chemoreceptors are active at birth. The infant, however, differs from the adult in that if hypoxic exposure continues beyond about 1 minute, respiration is depressed during the first weeks of life. Hypoxia thus appears to depress the respiratory center, negating the hypoxic stimulation via peripheral chemoreceptors. This hypoxic respiratory depression in the newborn appears to depend on the presence of suprapontine structures in the brain. Even though hypoxic respiratory depression may be useful to the fetus (who maintains a normal Pao_2 of 20 to 25 mm Hg), persistence of this phenomenon into postnatal life may enhance vulnerability of neonatal respiratory control.

The effects of pulmonary stretch receptor activity on the timing of respiration (Hering-Breuer reflex) are more readily elicited in the newborn than in the adult. In infants, a sustained increase in FRC causes a marked slowing of respiratory rate by prolonging expiratory time.[2] In the first days of life, a brisk lung inflation causes a deep gasp (Head's paradoxical gasp reflex) followed by apnea, which is, again, a manifestation of the Hering-Breuer inflation reflex. The deep gasp observed in the first day of life with low inflation pressures may explain the clinical observation that very low pressures

(10 to 15 cm H_2O) are often effective in resuscitating the apneic newborn at birth by stimulating a gasp reflex.

The partial pressure of carbon dioxide (Pco_2) reflects the ability of the lung to remove CO_2. The HCO_3 concentration is controlled by the kidney. When the pH and CO_2 are determined, the HCO_3 can be calculated by using the Henderson-Hasselbalch equation:

$$pH = 6.1 + \log \frac{HCO_3}{Pco_2 \times 0.03}$$

If only the pH is measured, the cause of the acidosis or alkalosis cannot be determined. With metabolic acidosis, HCO_3 is decreased. To compensate for this, the infant hyperventilates, lowering arterial Pco_2. With respiratory acidosis caused by pulmonary disease, apnea, or hypoventilation, the arterial Pco_2 increases. The kidney attempts compensation by retaining HCO_3 and excreting hydrogen ions. Only by measuring the Pco_2 and pH and calculating HCO_3 can the cause of an abnormality in acid-base balance be determined. The normal newborn quickly regulates his or her pH to near adult values, although HCO_3 may be lower than normal adult values.

OXYGEN DELIVERY

Oxygen is carried in the blood in chemical combination with hemoglobin and also in physical solution. The oxygen taken up by both processes depends on the partial pressure of oxygen (PO_2).

At ambient pressures, the amount of dissolved oxygen is only a small fraction of the total quantity carried in whole blood (0.3 mL O_2/dL plasma/100 mm Hg at 37° C). Most of the oxygen in whole blood is bound to hemoglobin (1 g of hemoglobin can maximally bind to 1.34 mL of oxygen at 37° C). The quantity of oxygen bound to hemoglobin depends on the partial pressure and is described by the oxygen dissociation curve (Fig. 10-1). The blood is almost completely saturated* at an arterial oxygen tension (Pao_2) exceeding 90 mm Hg.

As an example, if the arterial PO_2 is 50 mm Hg, saturation is 90%, and hemo-

*The arterial oxygen saturation is the actual oxygen bound to hemoglobin divided by the capacity of hemoglobin for binding oxygen.

$$\% \, sat. = \frac{mL \, O_2 \, bound \, to \, Hb}{Hb \, (g) \times 1.34} \times 100$$

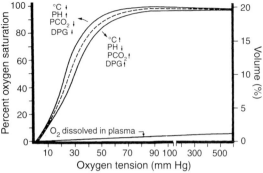

Figure 10-1. Factors that shift oxygen dissociation curve of hemoglobin. Fetal hemoglobin is shifted to left as compared with that of adult. *DPG,* Diphosphoglycerate. *(From Fanaroff AA, Martin RJ, Walsh MC, editors: Neonatal-perinatal medicine, ed 9, Philadelphia, 2011, Elsevier.)*

globin (Hb) is 10 g/dL, then 9 g Hb is bound to oxygen. Thus, the oxygen content of this 100 mL sample is 12.06 mL O_2 bound to Hb (1.34 × Hb 9) + 0.15 mL O_2 (0.3 × Hb 50/100) dissolved in plasma for a total of 12.21 mL O_2. Naturally, if the hemoglobin is doubled, then for the same saturation, the O_2 transported by hemoglobin is also doubled (1.34 × Hb 18 = 24.12 mL O_2) without changing the amount dissolved. The dissociation curve of fetal blood is shifted to the left and, at any Pao_2 less than 100 mm Hg, fetal hemoglobin binds to more oxygen compared to adult hemoglobin. The shift is the result of the lower affinity of fetal Hb for diphosphoglycerate (DPG). In contrast, the dissociation curve is shifted to the right by increasing acidosis and temperature. The clinical significance of the shift to the left for fetal Hb is that fetal blood will take up more oxygen at a given O_2 tension (PO_2). However, tissue PO_2 will need to decrease to a lower level to unload adequate oxygen. Thus, oxygen delivery to the tissues is determined by a combination of cardiac output, total hemoglobin concentration, and hemoglobin oxygen affinity in addition to arterial PO_2.

The shift in dissociation curve induced by fetal hemoglobin makes clinical recognition of hypoxia (insufficient amount of oxygen molecules in the tissues to cover the normal aerobic metabolism) more difficult, because cyanosis is observed at a lower oxygen tension. Cyanosis is first observed at saturations from 75% to 85%, which correspond to oxygen tensions of 32 to 42 mm Hg on the fetal dissociation curve. Cyanosis in the adult is observed at higher tensions. The flattening of the upper portion of the S-shaped dissociation curve makes it almost impossible to monitor oxygen tensions above 60 to 80 mm Hg by following arterial oxygen saturation. Although the shape of the oxygen dissociation curve limits the usefulness of pulse oximetry to detect high Pao_2 values, keeping saturation measured via pulse oximeter between 92% and 95% is one of the most effective and practical ways of reducing the risk of hyperoxemia.

The partial pressure of oxygen in arterial blood not only depends on the ability of the lung to transfer oxygen, but also is modified by the shunting of venous blood into the systemic circulation through the heart or lungs. Breathing 100% oxygen for a prolonged time partially corrects desaturation resulting from alveolar hypoventilation, diffusion abnormalities, or ventilation/perfusion inequality. Measurements of Pao_2 while breathing 100% oxygen are, therefore, useful diagnostically in determining whether arterial desaturation is caused by an anatomic right-to-left shunt, in which case oxygenation will fail to improve the condition (hyperoxia testing).

After birth, Pao_2 increases to between 60 and 90 mm Hg. During the first days of life, 20% of the cardiac output is normally shunted from right to left, in either the heart or lungs. When the normal adult breathes 100% oxygen, Pao_2 increases to 600 mm Hg as compared with approximately 300 to 500 mm Hg in healthy neonates, which results from the substantial shunting in infants.

At the end of the first hour of life, perfusion of the lung is distributed in proportion to the distribution of ventilation. In the healthy newborn baby, oxygen saturations rise slowly over the initial few minutes of life, however, they do not reach 90% in the first five minutes. The postductal oxygen saturation levels are usually lower than the preductal measurements for as long as 15 minutes, indicating a persistence in elevated pulmonary vascular resistance for a significant period of time after birth[3] (Fig. 10-2). The speed with which pulmonary ventilation and perfusion is uniformly distributed is an indication of the remarkable adaptive capacities of the newborn infant for the maintenance of homeostasis.

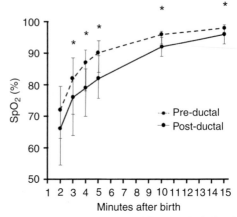

Figure 10-2. Pre- and postductal Spo_2 levels during the first 15 minutes after birth (median; IQR), inter quartile ranges Postductal Spo_2 levels were significantly lower than preductal Spo_2 levels at 3, 4, 5, 10, and 15 minutes($*p <$ .05). *(From Mariani G, Dik PB, Ezquer AJ, et al: Preductal and post-ductal O_2 saturation in healthy term neonates after birth, J Pediatr 150[4]:418, 2007.)*

EDITORIAL COMMENT: Dawson et al. defined the reference ranges for pulse oxygen saturation (Spo_2) values in the first 10 minutes after birth for 468 infants who received no medical intervention in the delivery room. For all 468 infants, the 3rd, 10th, 50th, 90th, and 97th percentile values at 1 minute were 29%, 39%, 66%, 87%, and 92%, respectively; those at 2 minutes were 34%, 46%, 73%, 91%, and 95%; and those at 5 minutes were 59%, 73%, 89%, 97%, and 98%. It took a median of 7.9 minutes (interquartile range: 5 to 10 minutes) to reach an Spo2 value of >90%. Spo_2 values for preterm infants increased more slowly than those for term infants (see also Chapter 3).

Dawson JA, Kamlin CO, Vento M, et al: Defining the reference range for oxygen saturation for infants after birth, Pediatrics 125:e1340, 2010.

PRACTICAL CONSIDERATIONS

OXYGEN THERAPY

Oxygen supplementation is critical for the survival of many infants with respiratory problems. Previous restricted use resulted in an increase not only in mortality rate, but also in neurologic handicaps. Additionally, recognition of the toxic effects of excessive or prolonged oxygen therapy is imperative when treating newborn infants. This has resulted in curtailed use of supplemental oxygen during neonatal resuscitation of both term and preterm infants (see Chapter 3). Therefore, oxygen administration must be performed with great precision, while carefully monitoring arterial oxygen tension or assessing oxygenation via noninvasive techniques.

OXYGEN ADMINISTRATION

For spontaneously breathing infants, a small hood to provide supplemental oxygen prevents fluctuations in inspired oxygen when opening the incubator. This has been largely replaced by low flow nasal cannulae to deliver gas mixtures. Because improper oxygen administration can be detrimental, the following practical considerations should be highlighted:

1. Peripheral cyanosis may be present in a neonate with a normal or high arterial oxygen tension.
2. Inspired oxygen concentration should be continuously monitored in all infants receiving supplementary oxygen or assisted ventilation.
3. Oxygen therapy without concurrent assessments of arterial oxygen tension is dangerous. A noninvasive monitoring device to measure oxygen saturation by pulse oximetry or transcutaneous PO_2 should be used continuously in preterm infants receiving any supplemental oxygen. In the presence of an arterial line during the acute phase of illness, measure Pao_2 at least every 4 hours if the infant is receiving oxygen.
4. In preterm infants, arterial oxygen tension should be maintained between 50 and 80 mm Hg during the acute phase of respiratory failure. In the absence of available Pao_2 monitoring, SaO_2 should be kept in the 90% to 95% range,[4] although this remains a subject of intense investigation.
5. The development of retinopathy of prematurity (ROP) is related to high arterial oxygen tension levels, and these may rise above the normal range even with relatively low inspired oxygen concentrations. Whereas initial hyperoxia stunts retinal vascular development, later hypoxia appears to stimulate damaging vascular proliferation.
6. When infants receiving supplemental oxygen require mask-and-bag ventilation, both oxygen concentration and inflating pressures must be monitored closely.
7. Use of a nasal cannula for prolonged oxygen therapy allows greater mobility for the infant and enables oral feeding without manipulating oxygen concentration. Both inspired oxygen concentration and flow rate are precisely adjusted and the infant's oxygenation is closely monitored, typically via pulse oximetry. Administration of oxygen by nasal cannula requires close monitoring because in active infants, the cannula is easily displaced from the nose. Also, changes in respiratory pattern and oral breathing may entrain different amounts of room air around the prongs, changing the true inspired oxygen concentration. Finally, high gas flows via nasal prongs are under evaluation, although safety concerns remain.
8. When the infant with respiratory distress syndrome (RDS) is improving, environmental oxygen should be lowered in small decrements while continuously monitoring oxygenation.
9. Any inspired oxygen concentration above room air can be damaging to pulmonary tissue if maintained over several days. Oxygen therapy is continued only if necessary.
10. All premature infants 30 weeks' gestation or less, or older if they had an unstable course or need for significant supplemental oxygen, receiving additional oxygen for extended periods of time should be examined by an experienced ophthalmologist by the later of 31 weeks' postmenstrual age (PMA) or four weeks after birth for treatable retinopathy of prematurity (ROP).[5]

Carlo et al. performed a randomized trial with a 2-by-2 factorial design to compare target ranges of oxygen saturation of 85% to to 89% or 91% to to 95% among 1316 infants who were born between 24 weeks 0 days and 27 weeks 6 days of gestation.[4] The primary outcome was a composite of severe retinopathy of prematurity (defined as the presence of threshold retinopathy, the need for surgical ophthalmologic intervention, or the use of bevacizumab), death before discharge from the hospital, or both. All infants were also randomly assigned to CPAP or intubation and surfactant. The rates of severe retinopathy or death did not differ significantly between the lower oxygen saturation group and the higher oxygen saturation group. However, death before discharge occurred more frequently in the lower oxygen saturation group (in 20% of infants versus 16%; relative risk, 1.27; 95% CI, 1.01 to 1.60; $P = .04$), whereas severe retinopathy among survivors occurred less often in this group (8.6% versus 17.9%;

relative risk, 0.52; 95% CI, 0.37 to 0.73; *P* <.001). There were no significant differences in the rates of other adverse events. These results have been replicated in another trial that terminated prematurely. Hence, because of concerns regarding the increased mortality in the lower oxygen saturation group, despite the better retinopathy outcome, the recommendation has been to maintain the oxygen saturation between 90% and 95%.

NEONATAL PROBLEMS

DIAGNOSIS

The initial objective is to establish an etiologic diagnosis for any observed respiratory symptoms. A major error in care can easily be made if other organ systems are not considered initially. Not every rapidly breathing infant has respiratory distress syndrome or even respiratory disease. Hypovolemia, hyperviscosity (polycythemia), anemia, hypoglycemia, congenital heart disease, hypothermia, metabolic acidosis of any etiology, or even the effects of drugs or drug withdrawal may all mimic primary respiratory disorders. Appropriate care depends on the diagnosis. For example, rewarming should rapidly relieve respiratory symptoms in a mildly hypothermic infant; otherwise, sepsis must be strongly considered.

A working classification of some of these disorders is presented in Box 10-1. Whenever faced with these respiratory symptoms, the next steps (following a history and physical examination) should be to obtain the following:
- Chest x-ray
- White blood cell count with differential and hematocrit (Peripheral hematocrits can be higher than intravascular hematocrits.)
- Blood sugar
- Assessment of blood gas status via an arterial stick or capillary blood gas. A capillary blood gas reliably estimates $Paco_2$ and pH, but not Pao_2.
- Pulse oximetry to assess oxygenation

The decision to catheterize the umbilical artery (see Appendix D) depends on the infant's condition. The umbilical artery and/ or vein may need to be catheterized if significant metabolic acidosis or blood loss is suspected or if the infant remains severely distressed (as defined by continued hypoxemia and severe respiratory distress). On the other hand, if the infant has tachypnea and grunting with retractions but is active and pink, it is possible to withhold catheterization

Box 10-1.	**Differential Diagnosis of Neonatal Respiratory Distress**

Pulmonary disorders
Respiratory distress syndrome
Transient tachypnea
Meconium aspiration syndrome
Pneumonia
Air leak syndromes
Pulmonary hypoplasia

Systemic disorders
Hypothermia
Metabolic acidosis
Anemia/polycythemia
Hypoglycemia
Pulmonary hypertension
Congenital heart disease

Anatomic problems of the respiratory system
Upper airway obstruction
Airway malformations
Space-occupying lesions
Rib cage anomalies
Phrenic nerve injury
Neuromuscular disease

unless there is deterioration as manifested by marked respiratory distress and an oxygen requirement exceeding 40% to 50%.

Although the newborn has a relatively larger cardiac output and a lower peripheral resistance and blood pressure than the older child and adult, measurements of blood pressure must be routine. It has been shown that hypotension in sick preterm infants need not be associated with hypovolemia. Hypothermia or acidemia results in severe peripheral vasoconstriction and will confound blood volume estimates from measurement of blood pressure. In a hypovolemic infant, blood pressure often declines only after acidemia and hypoxemia are corrected. Blood pressure can be measured with a blood pressure cuff of correct size placed on one or all extremities (if coarctation of the aorta is suspected), employing either oscillometric or Doppler ultrasound techniques. Alternatively, direct arterial measurements may be made via indwelling catheters. Normal blood pressures and ranges may be found in Appendix C.

If the initial hematocrit is less than 30% without blood incompatibility or if the blood pressure is reduced, it is reasonable to assume blood loss (e.g., an acute fetomaternal hemorrhage) and consider immediate correction of blood volume. With acute blood loss, hypotension prevails over anemia, whereas after chronic blood loss, anemia dominates the clinical picture and perfusion is less compromised. Saline is initially used and blood is requested, starting with a push infusion of 10 mL/kg, observing blood pressure, heart rate, and the infant's general condition. One must be extremely careful with rapid infusions of any solution in the critically ill premature infant because of the risk of increasing the incidence of intraventricular hemorrhage (IVH) by rapid volume expansion. Once a diagnosis has been made, it is necessary to determine whether the neonatal unit has all of the facilities that might be needed during the course of the illness. The following section discusses RDS in great depth because this has been the primary model for understanding pathophysiology and management of neonatal respiratory disease.

RESPIRATORY DISTRESS SYNDROME

RDS is still probably the most common initial problem in the intensive care nursery among premature infants, weighing less than 1500 g. However, in preterm infants whose mothers have received antenatal steroids, and after postnatal intratracheal surfactant therapy, the characteristic clinical course for RDS may not be apparent. The following lists give the common symptoms, the physiologic abnormalities, and the pathologic findings.

SIGNS AND SYMPTOMS

- Difficulty in initiating normal respiration. The disease should be anticipated if the infant is premature, the mother has diabetes, or if the infant has suffered perinatal asphyxia.
- Expiratory grunting or whining (caused by closure of the glottis), is a most important sign that sometimes may be the only early indication of disease; this maintains air in the immature lungs during expiration, and a decrease in grunting may be the first sign of improvement.
- Sternal and intercostal retractions (secondary to decreased lung and increased rib cage compliance)
- Nasal flaring
- Cyanosis (if supplemental O_2 is inadequate)
- Respirations—rapid (or slow when seriously ill)
- Extremities edematous—after several hours (altered vascular permeability)
- X-ray film showing reticulogranular, ground-glass appearance with air bronchograms

PHYSIOLOGIC ABNORMALITIES

- Lung compliance reduced to as much as one fifth to one tenth of normal (Fig. 10-3)
- Large areas of lung not ventilated (right-to-left shunting of blood)[6]
- Large areas of lung not perfused
- Decreased alveolar ventilation and increased work of breathing
- Reduced lung volume

These changes result in hypoxemia, often hypercarbia, and, if hypoxemia is severe, metabolic acidosis.

PATHOLOGIC FINDINGS (ANATOMIC, BIOPHYSICAL, BIOCHEMICAL)

- Gross—the lung is collapsed, firm, dark red, and liver-like.
- Microscopic—alveolar collapse, with overdistention of the dilated alveolar ducts, pink-staining membrane on alveolar ducts (composed of products of the infant's blood and destroyed alveolar cells); hence the earlier term *hyaline membrane disease.*
- Electron microscopic—damage and loss of alveolar epithelial cells (especially type II cells); disappearance of lamellar inclusion bodies.
- Biophysical and biochemical—deficient, or absent pulmonary surfactant,[7] especially phospholipid (surface-tension lowering) component; abnormal pressure volume curve, as shown in Figure 10-3.

ETIOLOGY

The distal respiratory epithelium responsible for gas exchange features two distinct

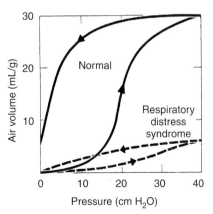

Figure 10-3. Air pressure volume curves of normal and abnormal lung. Volume is expressed as milliliters of air per gram of lung. Lung of infant with respiratory distress syndrome (RDS) accepts smaller volume of air at all pressures. Note that deflation pressure volume curve closely follows inflation curve for the RDS lung.

cell types in the mature infant lung. Type I pneumocytes cover most of the alveolus, in close proximity to capillary endothelial cells. Type II cells have been identified in the human fetus as early as 22 weeks' gestation, but become prominent at 34 to 36 weeks of gestation. These highly metabolically active cells contain the cytoplasmic lamellar bodies that are the source of pulmonary surfactant. Surfactant synthesis is a complex process that requires an abundance of precursor substrates, such as glucose, fatty acid, and choline, and a series of key enzymatic steps that are regulated by various hormones, including corticosteroids.

Phosphatidylcholine is the dominant surface tension-lowering component of surfactant. In addition, surfactant-specific proteins have been characterized and their functions partially elucidated. Of particular interest is surfactant protein B (SP-B), which is critical for minimizing surface tension and whose absence results in the phenotypic expression of lethal RDS at term.[8] Following secretion from lamellar bodies within the type II alveolar cells, the key phospholipid and protein components of surfactant are conserved by recycling and subsequent regeneration of surfactant. Exogenously administered surfactant appears to contribute to this recycling program by increasing surfactant pool size without inhibiting endogenous surfactant production.[7]

It is widely accepted that RDS is the result of a primary absence or deficiency of this highly surface-active alveolar lining layer (pulmonary surfactant). Surfactant, a complex lipoprotein rich in saturated phosphatidylcholine molecules, binds to the internal surface of the lung and markedly lessens the forces of surface tension at the air-water interphase, thereby reducing the pressure tending to collapse the alveolus. By equalizing the forces of surface tension in alveolar units of varying size, it is a potent anti-atelectasis factor and is essential for normal respiration. Alteration or absence of the pulmonary surfactant would lead to the sequence of events shown in Figure 10-4. This results in decreased lung compliance (stiff lung) and thus an increase in the work of breathing. The additional work would soon tire the infant, leading to a sequence of reduced alveolar ventilation, atelectasis, and alveolar hypoperfusion.

Asphyxia would induce pulmonary vasoconstriction; blood would bypass the lung through the fetal pathway (patent ductus arteriosus, foramen ovale), lowering pulmonary blood flow; and a vicious circle would be promoted. The resulting ischemia would be an added insult and may further reduce lung metabolism and surfactant production.

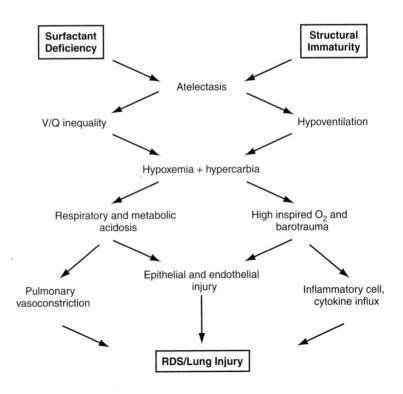

Figure 10-4. Pathophysiology of neonatal respiratory distress syndrome (RDS). $\dot{V}/\dot{Q}$, Ventilation-perfusion ratio.

GENERAL PREVENTIVE MEASURES

A major effort in treating this disease should continue to focus on its prevention, including elective cesarean deliveries performed without adequate documentation of pulmonary maturity from amniotic fluid testing. The prolongation of pregnancy with bed rest or drugs that inhibit premature labor, as well as the induction of pulmonary surfactant with maternally administered steroids, plays an important role in reducing the incidence of this disease (see Chapter 2).

Antenatal steroids not only enhance surfactant production but also may improve pulmonary function (e.g., tissue elasticity) by non-surfactant mechanisms.[9] Therefore, the combined use of prenatal corticosteroids and postnatal surfactant therapy is complementary.[10] Antenatal steroids also reduce the incidence of periventricular hemorrhage in preterm infants, possibly secondary to enhanced vascular integrity in the germinal matrix. Concern about the possibility of increased infection with antenatal steroids in mother or infant appears unfounded. Therefore, antenatal steroids are now standard of practice for pregnancies at risk of preterm delivery, although precise limits are still being defined. Thyroid hormones enhance surfactant production; however, maternally administered thyrotropin-releasing hormone (TRH) combined with antenatal steroids failed to offer any advantage over glucocorticoid therapy alone.[11]

SURFACTANT THERAPY

Since the discovery that surfactant deficiency was a prominent feature of the pathophysiology of RDS, investigators have attempted to administer artificial aerosolized phospholipids to these infants.[12] Limited therapeutic success was encountered in these early studies. In contrast, animal models, in which natural surfactant compounds were used, yielded promising results. This stimulated Fujiwara et al. to develop a mixture of both natural and synthetic surface-active lipids for use in humans.[13] The goal was to achieve alveolar stability with less potential risk for a reaction to foreign protein than would be the case with exclusively natural surfactant. When administered to an initial group of 10 preterm infants with severe RDS who were not improving despite artificial ventilation, a single 10-mL dose of surfactant instilled into the endotracheal tube resulted in a dramatic decrease in inspired oxygen and ventilator pressures. Other studies confirmed this initial success, employing calf and pig lung extract, pooled human surfactant obtained from amniotic fluid, and purely synthetic phospholipid preparation.[14]

Subsequent collaborative multicenter trials employed multiple doses of purely synthetic and mixed natural/synthetic preparations and confirmed clinical efficacy, leading in the 1990s, to the widespread introduction of exogenous surfactant therapy into neonatal care. The most efficacious mixed surfactant products are all protein-containing preparations derived from bovine or porcine tissue. Both prevention (delivery room administration) and rescue (administration for established RDS) protocols have their advocates.[15] Of particular interest, as summarized in Box 10-2, is the ability of surfactant to decrease

---

Box 10-2. Surfactant Therapy for Respiratory Distress Syndrome

Resolved

Greatest benefit when combined with antenatal corticosteroids

Major surface tension-lowering ingredient: phosphatidylcholine

Administration of fluid suspension requires endotracheal tube

Improvement in arterial oxygenation

Surfactant proteins enhance speed of action

Exogenous surfactant enhances rather than inhibits endogenous surfactant synthesis

Decrease in incidence of air leaks

Improved mortality rate

Prevention more effective than rescue up to <29 weeks

Unresolved

Ideal preparation: role of surfactant proteins in improving respiratory function

Role of ventilatory strategy in optimizing surfactant response-rapid wean to nasal CPAP

Effect on incidence and severity of chronic lung disease

Role of surfactant therapy in other neonatal respiratory disorders: meconium aspiration, pneumonia, pulmonary hypoplasia, congenital diaphragmatic hernia, pulmonary hemorrhage

---

Adapted from Hamvas A: Pathophysiology and management of respiratory distress syndrome. In Martin RJ, Fanaroff AA, Walsh MC, editors: Neonatal-perinatal medicine, *ed 9, St. Louis, 2011, Elsevier.*

the number of deaths in low-birth-weight infants without significantly reducing the incidence of bronchopulmonary dysplasia (BPD) in the smallest infants. The latter may be a consequence of the enhanced survival caused by surfactant administration to very preterm infants or to the multifactorial etiology of BPD.

Surfactant therapy currently requires the presence of an endotracheal tube, although less invasive techniques of administration are under study. Multiple doses may be needed for optimal benefit. The dramatic improvement in oxygenation is not accompanied by an immediate improvement in $Paco_2$ or lung compliance unless ventilator settings are rapidly weaned.[16] Data suggest that the increase in lung volume, induced by surfactant, needs to be accompanied by ventilator and supplemental oxygen weaning. Hypotension and bradycardia may occur acutely during surfactant therapy; therefore, caution must be exercised when using this treatment to avoid potential iatrogenic complications.

Since the genes that code for the surfactant proteins have been characterized, recombinant DNA technology will make production of modified human surfactant proteins possible. In combination with synthetic phospholipids, this will allow the widespread availability of a protein-containing artificial surfactant. Although no adverse immunologic consequences of foreign tissue protein administration have yet been reported in the recipients of natural surfactant therapy, close follow-up of these high-risk survivors of neonatal intensive care is always imperative.

EDITORIAL COMMENT: There are limited data to inform the choice between early treatment with CPAP and early surfactant treatment as the initial support for extremely low-birth-weight infants. Finer et al. randomly assigned 1316 immature infants to intubation and surfactant treatment (within 1 hour after birth) or to CPAP treatment initiated in the delivery room, with subsequent use of a protocol-driven limited ventilation strategy. Infants were also randomly assigned to one of two target ranges of oxygen saturation.[4] The primary outcome was death or BPD as defined by the requirement for supplemental oxygen at 36 weeks (with an attempt at withdrawal of supplemental oxygen in neonates who were receiving less than 30% oxygen). The rates of the primary outcome did not differ significantly between the CPAP group and the surfactant group (47.8% and 51.0%, respectively). Infants who received CPAP treatment, as compared with infants who received surfactant treatment, less frequently required intubation or postnatal corticosteroids for BPD ($P < .001$), required fewer days of mechanical ventilation ($P = .03$), and were more likely to be alive and free from the need for mechanical ventilation by day 7 ($P = .01$). The rates of other adverse neonatal outcomes did not differ significantly between the two groups. These data support consideration of CPAP as an alternative to intubation and surfactant in preterm infants.

SUPPORT Study Group of the Eunice Kennedy Shriver NICHD Neonatal Research Network, Finer NN, Carlo WA, Walsh MC, et al: Early CPAP versus surfactant in extremely preterm infants, N Engl J Med 362:1970, 2010.

GENERAL CLINICAL MANAGEMENT

The same principles of basic care for RDS can be applied to infants with many other neonatal pulmonary problems. During the acute phase, every maneuver is directed toward ensuring the infant's survival with minimal risk of chronic morbidity. The infant is placed in a neutral thermal environment (see Chapter 6) to reduce oxygen requirements and CO_2 production. To meet fluid and partial caloric requirements (dependent on environmental conditions, maturity, renal function, risk for patency of the ductus arteriosus, and hydration), the infant is typically begun at 60 to 80 mL/kg/day of a 10% dextrose solution. This is increased to 120 to 160 mL/kg/day by the fifth day, recognizing that there is a high risk for either fluid overload or dehydration if clinical status, fluid balance, and electrolytes are not closely monitored in the smallest infants with RDS, who may require much more than 160 mL/kg/day. Administration of an amino acid solution should begin the first day, supplemented with small volume feeds as respiratory status stabilizes. Respiration, heart rate, blood pressure, and oxygenation (via noninvasive techniques) are monitored continuously and complemented by blood gas sampling at least every 4 to 6 hours during the acute phase of illness.

Most important in the prescription is skilled nursing and physician management. Vital signs must be noted and observations made in such a fashion as not to disturb the infant continually, yet the patient must always be observed. Modern electronic monitoring of heart rate, respiration, temperature, and oxygenation makes gentler care easier to administer. Noninvasive monitoring of oxygenation has confirmed the importance of minimizing simple maneuvers such as taking a rectal temperature, vigorous oral, pharyngeal, or endotracheal suctioning, and vigorous auscultation of the chest. The real skills of a unit can be tested by noting attentiveness to small details in neonatal respiratory management. Is the environmental oxygen at the correct percentage and flow rate? Is the arterial oxygen permitted to go too high or too low for a prolonged period? Does the unit anticipate future needs of the infant or does it always treat complications? As an example, if during the acute phase, an infant with RDS has increasing apneic episodes, it usually signifies that the infant's condition is deteriorating and additional intervention is indicated. Waiting for a Pao_2 of 30 mm Hg and a severe respiratory and metabolic acidosis before beginning ventilatory therapy is not adequate anticipation. While basic care is being arranged (metabolic rate minimized, fluid and electrolyte needs met), the essentials of care involve maintaining an adequate Pao_2 and pH and closely observing for changes in the infant's state.

A general plan is to maintain the $Paco_2$ in the abdominal aorta between 50 and 80 mm Hg, $Paco_2$ in the 40 to 55 mm Hg range, and pH above 7.25. Because clinical differentiation from group B streptococcal (or other bacterial) pneumonia is not possible, a blood culture should be obtained and antibiotics should be administered for at least 48 hours. It is equally important to discontinue broad-spectrum antibiotics as soon as the possibility of infection is ruled out to prevent nosocomial fungal and bacterial infections.

Correction of severe metabolic acidosis with alkali has many theoretical physiologic benefits. With normalization of pH, myocardial contractility is increased, pulmonary vascular resistance is reduced, and the length of survival with asphyxia is prolonged. However, the rapid injection of hypertonic solutions such as $NaHCO_3$ is associated with a marked change in osmolality. Studies have revealed that excessive and rapid $NaHCO_3$ administration may be associated with an increased incidence of intracranial hemorrhage.[17,18] Current consensus is that $NaHCO3$ administration is of very limited benefit.[19] Because administered $NaHCO_3$ is converted to CO_2 and is dependent on the lung for its removal, $NaHCO_3$ is contraindicated in the presence of respiratory acidosis without some form of controlled or assisted ventilation if it is to be administered.

Almost all infants with RDS require ventilatory support in the form of CPAP. Some of these infants do not stabilize on CPAP and require ventilator support and surfactant therapy (Fig. 10-5). Indications for placing an infant on a ventilator include: respiratory acidosis with a pH of less than 7.20, apnea, and/or a need for a high concentration of inspired oxygen (i.e., ≥40%).

Other criteria for a ventilator include a respiratory acidosis with a pH of less than 7.20 (and possibly 7.25) and apnea complicating the course of RDS.

After 72 hours of age (or earlier after surfactant therapy), most infants with classic RDS start the recovery phase. Respiratory rate and retractions decrease, and Pao_2 increases without evidence of further CO_2 retention.

EDITORIAL COMMENT: This recovery phase is preceded by a period of spontaneous diuresis during which there is improved gas exchange, lung compliance, and functional residual capacity. Since the improved pulmonary function occurs after diuresis, it is important that the clinician anticipate the recovery phase and reduce ventilatory support to prevent barotrauma.

Waldemar Carlo

During this phase, expertise in oxygen management is required. Oxygen saturation via pulse oximetry is the mainstay of assessing oxygenation during recovery of respiratory distress. Levels are typically maintained between 90% and 95%,

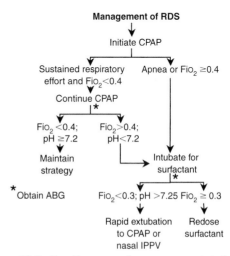

Figure 10-5. Algorithm suggesting management strategy of respiratory distress syndrome (RDS). *ABG,* Arterial blood gas; *CPAP,* continuous positive airway pressure; *Fio₂,* fraction of inspired oxygen; *IPPV,* intermittent positive-pressure ventilation.

although determination of the optimal saturation within this range is still under study.

In infants of very low-birth-weight, even in the absence of severe RDS over the first few days, recovery may be prolonged. This may be attributed to impaired respiratory drive or respiratory muscle failure, persistent atelectasis not related to surfactant deficiency, nutritional compromise, intercurrent infection, congestive heart failure, or some combination of these interrelated factors.

Enteral feedings can begin during the recovery phase, when bowel sounds are present, and respiratory status has stabilized. Many very low-birth-weight infants require prolonged assisted ventilation and prolonged supplemental oxygen. Small volume gavage feeds, preferably of breast milk, can begin, despite continuing ventilatory support. This is a valuable adjunct to amino acid-glucose IV alimentation. As the infant recovers, apneic periods may be observed, but they do not have the ominous significance as when observed in the acute phase.

The complications of RDS may occur spontaneously or result from well-intended therapeutic interventions. Major problems may be a consequence of arterial catheter placement, oxygen administration, mechanical ventilation, and the use of endotracheal tubes, as discussed in Chapter 11. As the number of very low-birth-weight survivors grows, the time and effort devoted to preventing and treating respiratory morbidity in this population steadily increases.

During or following the recovery phase of RDS, cardiac failure secondary to a large left-to-right shunt through the patent ductus arteriosus may occur as pulmonary vascular resistance declines. This may initially manifest as inability to wean oxygen or ventilator support. Bounding pulses, a wide pulse pressure, and a systolic murmur are most useful in making a clinical diagnosis. In most cases, conservative medical management with cautious fluid administration and diuretics will control the congestive heart failure, and the patent ductus arteriosus will close as the infant grows. Although the patent ductus arteriosus will close spontaneously in most cases, intervention to close it may reduce the risk of chronic pulmonary overflow, edema, and prolonged ventilator dependence.

Although cardiomegaly is often noted on x-ray examination, an enlarged liver and edema are not usually found with cardiac failure. Evaluation of the magnitude of shunting by echocardiography is usually indicated before initiating either pharmacologic or surgical closure of the ductus arteriosus (see Chapter 15). (Table 10-1). Although prophylactic indomethacin administration appears to reduce the frequency of large left-to-right ductal shunts, there is no clear evidence that routine early indomethacin therapy reduces longer-term morbidity in susceptible infants. An additional benefit of prophylactic indomethacin may be to decrease the incidence of IVH. Ibuprofen therapy also promotes ductal closure and is less likely to impair renal blood flow and renal function when compared to indomethacin. Surgical closure should be a last resort as infants subject to ductal ligation may be at greater risk for later neurodevelopmental impairment. The case problems and questions in this chapter further illustrate the care of these infants.

PERSISTENT PULMONARY HYPERTENSION

Persistent pulmonary hypertension (PPHN), rather than the previous nomenclature, persistent fetal circulation (PFC), more aptly describes the syndrome characterized by pulmonary hypertension resulting in severe hypoxemia secondary to right-to-left shunting through the foramen ovale and ductus arteriosus in the absence of structural heart disease. Pulmonary hypertension in these infants is thought to result from pulmonary vasospasm, presumably because of altered pulmonary vasoreactivity and, at times, it may be accompanied by an increase in muscle mass in the pulmonary vascular bed. The increase in pulmonary arterial smooth muscle tone may develop in response to intrauterine stress and can be associated with a decrease of a circulating (or local) pulmonary vasodilator such as nitric oxide (NO) or an increase in the amount of circulating (or local) pulmonary vasoconstrictors such as endothelin. This syndrome was initially described in term infants with respiratory distress and cyanosis without demonstrable cardiac, pulmonary, hematologic, or central nervous system (CNS) disease. However, this same hemodynamic pattern can occur in preterm and term infants with primary pulmonary disease (e.g., surfactant deficiency, pneumonia, or meconium aspiration syndrome), polycythemia, or pulmonary hypoplasia (e.g., congenital diaphragmatic hernia) or following neonatal asphyxia. Among preterm infants, pulmonary hypoplasia and sepsis appear to be associated with a higher incidence of pulmonary hypertension.[20] Sometimes no clear etiology for the PPHN or underlying lung disease can be assigned. The result is cyanosis, tachypnea, and acidemia, which can superficially resemble cyanotic congenital heart disease, primary pulmonary disease, or cardiomyopathy. The initial roentgenographic descriptions of PPHN stressed the absence of pulmonary parenchymal disease and decreased vascular markings; however, the chest x-ray study may, instead, reflect the concurrence of underlying pulmonary disease such as meconium aspiration or pneumonia. Echocardiography is invaluable as a guide to assessing elevated pulmonary artery pressure and pulmonary vascular resistance and, more importantly, as a means of excluding most anatomic cardiac malformations (see Chapter 15) and demonstrating right-to-left shunting at the level of the foramen ovale and ductus arteriosus.

The management of PPHN can be complex and very difficult, because the severe hypoxemia may be poorly responsive to high oxygen therapy or pulmonary vasodilators. Every attempt should be made to anticipate, and possibly prevent, the development of PPHN in patients with severe meconium aspiration syndrome or neonatal pneumonia, and early and aggressive treatment of hypoxemia should be provided. These babies are exquisitely sensitive to changes in environmental oxygen. Most require an environmental oxygen approaching 100% and may show little improvement without mechanical ventilation. Some infants have benefited from modest alkalinization, brought about by hyperventilation or the administration of $NaHCO_3$, which may relieve the intense pulmonary vasospasm and allow oxygenation to improve. This approach has mainly been abandoned with the focus on improving

Table 10-1. Supportive Care for Infants with Respiratory Distress Syndrome

Treatment	Logic
Trained staff nurses, respiratory therapists, and monitoring equipment	Early management of complications and notification of change in course (e.g., apnea, bleeding from catheter)
Available trained physicians, nurse practitioners	
Precise temperature control to maintain infant in neutral temperature	Maintains minimal oxygen consumption and carbon dioxide production
pH, Pao_2, $Paco_2$, and HCO_3 measurements at least every 4-6 hr. Maintain Pao_2 at 50-80 mm Hg. Continuous Pao_2 or Sao_2 is optimal.	Permits continual assessment of infant's condition and limits toxic effects of oxygen or hypoxic injury
Monitor blood pressure.	Recognizes hypoperfusion, hypovolemia, patent ductus arteriosus
Attempt to keep pH >7.25. If $Paco_2$ >60 or Pao_2 <50 mm Hg, change treatment.	Permits continual assessment of infant's condition and limits toxic effects of oxygen or hypoxic injury
Lower environmental oxygen slowly when RDS infant is still ill.	Prevents greater than expected decrease in Pao_2 when environmental oxygen is reduced (right-to-left shunt etiology?)
Surfactant therapy (requires endotracheal tube)	Therapeutic approach to underlying etiology of RDS
Glucose-containing IV fluid 60 mL/kg first day, 80-100 mL/kg second day with body weight determination for small infants to calculate if larger amounts of H_2O required. May require 150 mL/kg or more.	Need to balance fluid and partial caloric requirements while minimizing the risk of fluid overload problems (e.g., patent ductus arteriosus)
Controlled oxygen administration: via ventilatory support, cannula, or hood	Prevents large swings in environmental oxygen concentration
Continually monitor respiration, heart rate, and temperature as well as blood pressure.	Prevents hypoxemia and acidemia with apneic episodes
Frequent determinations of blood sugar, hematocrit and electrolytes (Na, K, and Cl)	Necessary for calculating general metabolic requirements
Transfuse if central hematocrit <35 during acute phase of illness	For adequate oxygen-carrying capacity
Record all observations (laboratory, nurse's notes, etc.) on single form.	Permits immediate correlation of many variables
Urinary output, blood urea nitrogen, creatinine, and when indicated, urinary pH, electrolytes, and osmolality	Evaluation of renal function and blood flow to the kidney. An increase in output occurs as the infant starts to improve.
Obtain blood culture; treat with ampicillin and gentamicin until cultures are available.	Cannot radiographically separate RDS from group B streptococcal (or other) pneumonia
Minimize routine procedures such as suctioning, handling, and auscultation.	Prevents iatrogenic decreases in Pao_2

RDS, Respiratory distress syndrome.

oxygenation and decreasing pulmonary vascular resistance with inhaled nitric oxide. Similarly, Pao_2 is maintained at the upper recommended levels (80 to 100 mm Hg) to minimize hypoxic pulmonary vasoconstriction while minimizing barotrauma. Polycythemia, hypoglycemia, hypocalcemia, and hypotension should be treated if present. In fact, maintenance of systemic blood pressure at the high range of normal is often required to exceed excessively high pulmonary artery pressures and thereby counteract right-to-left shunting. Pharmacologic pressor support (e.g., dopamine or dobutamine) may be preferable to volume expansion, because excessive fluids are poorly tolerated. Adequate sedation and, at times muscle paralysis, may be necessary to combat the hypoxemia associated with agitation.

A major breakthrough in the treatment of PPHN has been the use of inhaled nitric oxide (NO) at doses of 20 ppm or less to produce pharmacologic selective pulmonary vasodilation without producing significant systemic hypotension. Among preterm infants, the likelihood of a successful response to inhaled NO increases with advancing gestational age.[20] Inhaled NO, together with other therapeutic approaches such as surfactant therapy and high frequency ventilation, has been reported to significantly reduce the need for ECMO.[21]

More data suggest that sildenafil, an inhibitor of cGMP-specific phosphodiesterase, may effectively induce pulmonary vasodilation by increasing endogenously released cGMP.[22] Nonetheless, ECMO remains a lifesaving treatment modality in infants who fail to respond to ventilatory and pharmacologic management of severe PPHN.[23]

MECONIUM ASPIRATION SYNDROME

Meconium is present in the amniotic fluid in 10% of all births, and its presence suggests that the infant may have suffered some asphyxial episode in utero. Evidence of this is derived from studies such as postmortem data demonstrating severe structural abnormalities in the muscular walls of the pulmonary arterial vascular bed, suggesting chronic in utero hypoxia in infants with fatal meconium aspiration.[24] It is doubtful that amniotic fluid alone can produce any airway obstruction. However, pulmonary disease is definitely observed in infants who have aspirated meconium (Fig. 10-6), and mortality and morbidity are significant without immediate aggressive management. Interestingly, the passage and subsequent aspiration of meconium are almost never seen before 34 weeks' gestation.

In order to prevent significant morbidity and mortality associated with meconium aspiration, traditional practice has been that

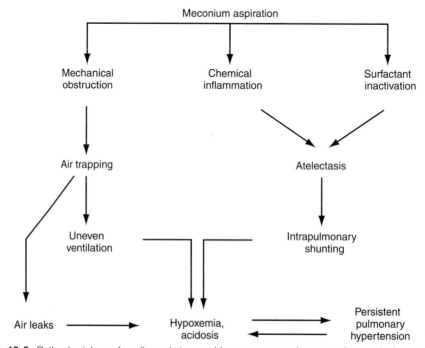

Figure 10-6. Pathophysiology of cardiorespiratory problems accompanying meconium aspiration syndrome.

every infant with frank meconium staining of the amniotic fluid requires the following preventive measures:

1. Immediate suctioning of the nasopharynx by the obstetrician as soon as the head appears on the perineum. Interestingly, this practice of routine intrapartum suctioning of the upper airway may not decrease the incidence of meconium aspiration syndrome.[25]

2. If there is cardiorespiratory depression immediately after delivery, visualization of the cords by laryngoscopy and direct suctioning of the trachea through an endotracheal tube. This endotracheal suctioning should be done before stimulation of the infant or positive pressure ventilation, although this population has not been subjected to a well-designed randomized trial.

Because asphyxia is often the basis for the presence of meconium in the amniotic fluid, the infant who aspirates meconium at birth is often depressed and requires some resuscitation. Positive pressure resuscitation should be delayed in these infants if possible until adequate laryngotracheal toilet has been performed, to prevent pushing meconium farther into the small airways. Current recommendations do not include aggressive laryngotracheal suctioning in vigorous infants (see Chapter 3). In support of a conservative approach to such infants, a multicenter, multinational trial to assess whether intubation and suctioning of apparently vigorous, meconium-stained neonates would reduce the incidence of meconium-aspiration syndrome (MAS) enrolled 2094 neonates. Compared with expectant management, intubation and suctioning of the apparently vigorous meconium-stained infant did not result in a decreased incidence of MAS or other respiratory disorders. There were few and only short-lived complications of intubation. Obstetricians have applied transcervical amnioinfusion in labor when meconium-stained amniotic fluid is present; however, a conclusive positive effect on neonatal outcome remains to be demonstrated.[26]

Meconium aspiration syndrome is characterized by respiratory distress ranging from tachypnea to gasping respirations. Rales and wheezing may be heard. The infant may appear barrel-chested with an increase in the anteroposterior diameter of the chest. A chest radiograph shows areas of increased density and areas of overexpansion irregularly distributed throughout the lung; differentiation from pneumonia and retained lung fluid may be difficult.

The lung can remove meconium rapidly. Infants with mild cases usually recover after 48 hours of life. However, in sicker infants, respiratory compromise may be severe, with mechanical obstruction, hyperinflation, and atelectasis producing severe gas maldistribution with ventilation-perfusion mismatching. One complication of partially blocked, over-expanded areas of lung, occurring in 20% to 50% of infants with MAS, is the development of air leaks, such as pneumothorax. Pneumothorax should be suspected if the clinical status of the infant deteriorates suddenly. Additional pulmonary pathology caused by meconium aspiration includes chemical pneumonitis, interstitial edema, and surfactant inactivation. Frequently, PPHN with severe superimposed hypoxemia develops in infants with significant meconium aspiration syndrome (see Fig. 10-6). Respiratory failure is associated with a significant mortality rate in these infants. Several studies have demonstrated that surfactant replacement therapy improves oxygenation, reduces pulmonary air leaks, reduces the need for ECMO, and improves outcome in infants with meconium aspiration syndrome.[27] Nevertheless, severe respiratory failure and hypoxemia may require additional treatment modalities such as high frequency ventilation and nitric oxide administration, with ECMO therapy for those who fail to respond.

EDITORIAL COMMENT: Dargaville et al. conducted a randomized controlled trial that enrolled 66 ventilated infants with meconium aspiration syndrome. Infants randomized to lavage received two 15-mL/kg aliquots of dilute bovine surfactant instilled into, and recovered from, the lung. Control subjects received standard care, which in both groups included high-frequency ventilation, nitric oxide, and where available and necessary, ECMO. Fewer infants who underwent lavage died or required ECMO: 10% (3 to 30) compared with 31% (11 to 35) in the control group. Lavage transiently reduced oxygen saturation without substantial heart rate or blood pressure alterations. Mean airway pressure was more rapidly weaned in the lavage group after randomization. Thus, lung lavage with dilute surfactant does not alter duration of respiratory support, but may reduce mortality, especially in units not offering ECMO.

Dargaville PA, Copnell B, Mills JF, et al: Less MAS Trial Study Group: Randomized controlled trial of lung lavage with dilute surfactant for meconium aspiration syndrome, J Pediatr 158:383-389.e2, 2011.

PNEUMOTHORAX

Pulmonary air leaks comprise a spectrum of disorders that includes pneumomediastinum, pneumopericardium, pulmonary interstitial emphysema, and pneumothorax. An asymptomatic pneumothorax is found in approximately 1% of all routine newborn chest radiographic examinations. Considering the high negative intrathoracic pressures recorded during the first minutes of life, it is surprising that pneumothorax does not occur more frequently. When air leak occurs, air from the ruptured alveolus dissects up the vascular sheath into the mediastinum and from there into the pleural space. In some series, as many as half of the symptomatic patients had aspirated meconium or blood. This suggests that obstruction with a ball-valve action may be the basis for the rupture. A pneumothorax frequently develops in infants with pulmonary interstitial emphysema, in whom there is a tracking of air from ruptured alveoli into the perivascular pulmonary tissues, usually during prolonged assisted ventilation. Multiple studies of various exogenous surfactant preparations have demonstrated a significant reduction in pneumothorax among surfactant-treated infants.[28,29] Pneumothorax, manifesting with concurrent hypotension, is associated with increased risk of IVH, probably via impairment of venous return.

Pneumothorax should be suspected in any newborn with respiratory distress or in a baby on a respirator whose condition suddenly worsens. In infants with RDS, a pneumothorax may develop when the severity of disease is decreasing and lung compliance is increasing. Bilateral pneumothoraces are often observed in infants with hypoplastic lungs accompanying renal agenesis (Potter syndrome), other forms of renal dysplasia, or congenital diaphragmatic hernia. In fact, the presence of otherwise unexplained extrapulmonary air in the early neonatal period should raise the question of an underlying renal or pulmonary malformation.

A high-intensity transilluminating light, using a fiberoptic probe, is especially helpful in quickly diagnosing a pneumothorax. If the infant's clinical condition is relatively stable, it is wise to check the diagnosis radiographically before treatment. An anteroposterior film may underestimate the size of a large anterior pneumothorax, in which case a horizontal-beam lateral film of the supine infant is helpful. A cross table lateral film with the suspected pneumothorax side up will differentiate a pneumothorax from a pneumomediastinum.

Clinical findings include cyanosis, tachypnea, grunting, nasal flaring, or intercostal retractions. If the pneumothorax is unilateral and under tension, the cardiac impulse may be shifted away from the affected side and ipsilateral breath sounds may be decreased. A distended abdomen with an easily palpable liver or spleen pushed down by the diaphragm is often a useful clinical feature signifying a tension pneumothorax. This may be useful in differentiating a left-sided tension pneumothorax manifesting in the delivery room from a (typically left-sided) congenital diaphragmatic hernia. Both are characterized by mediastinal shift to the right hemithorax; however, in the hernia patient, a scaphoid (rather than distended) abdomen is a presenting feature.

If the pneumothorax causes only minor symptoms, no specific therapy is necessary, but the infant's color, heart rate, respiratory rate, blood pressure, and oxygenation should be monitored. If severe respiratory distress is noted or the infant has underlying pulmonary disease, a thoracostomy tube should be placed. Lung perforation has been described following chest tube placement, and care should be exercised when guiding the catheter into the pleural space. Traumatic events may be reduced with a pigtail catheter. The catheter should be placed in the pleural space anterior to the lung. This is best achieved by insertion near the third intercostal space just lateral to the anterior axillary line. Occasionally, with a large area of rupture or bronchopleural fistula, chest tube placement may be required for several days. Pneumomediastinum does not require intervention, and asymptomatic pneumopericardium should be managed conservatively. Pneumopericardium may manifest with profound hypotension if there is accompanying gas tamponade, and pericardiocentesis will be lifesaving. Both pneumopericardium and pulmonary interstitial emphysema (PIE) are almost invariably complications of assisted ventilation. In an attempt to avoid air leak and to manage air leak when present, mechanical ventilatory pressures should be kept at a safe minimum. The use of high-frequency ventilation appears to be effective in treating air leak and may actually reduce the risk of development of air leak in preterm infants with severe respiratory failure[30] (see also Chapter 11).

TRANSIENT TACHYPNEA OF THE NEWBORN

Transient tachypnea of the newborn (TTN) often follows an uneventful delivery at (or close to) term. The major presenting symptom is a persistently high respiratory rate. Cyanosis may be present but is usually not of great significance, with few infants requiring more than 35% to 40% oxygen to remain pink. Air exchange is good and, therefore, rales and rhonchi, expiratory grunting, and intercostal retractions are minimal; arterial pH and $Paco_2$ measurements are usually within normal limits. The chest x-ray reveals central perihilar streaking because fluid remains in the periarterial tissue, often with fluid in the interlobar fissure, and occasionally there is a small pleural effusion; the cardiac silhouette may be slightly enlarged. If the radiologic picture includes patchy infiltrates, which probably reflect liquid-filled lobes, then TTN probably cannot be initially distinguished from infiltrates associated with meconium aspiration or bacterial pneumonia. The clinical picture of increased respiratory rate improves gradually during the first 5 days of life.

The pathogenesis appears to involve delayed resorption of fetal lung fluid, a process that requires activation of airway epithelial sodium channels.[31] In experimental situations, catecholamines have been found to stimulate fetal lung fluid resorption. Infants delivered by cesarean section without antecedent labor are found to have decreased catecholamine levels and an increased likelihood of development of transient tachypnea.[32] In fact, the respiratory morbidity associated with elective repeat cesarean delivery before 39 weeks is typically TTN.[33] Infants of diabetic mothers are also at increased risk of transient tachypnea, thought to be due to the interference by insulin on the β-adrenergic response of the lung.[34]

The presence of unabsorbed lung fluid produces decreased lung compliance, whereas the infant's increased respiratory rate attempts to minimize respiratory work. Ultrasound has been reported to demonstrate a unique difference in lung echogenicity between upper and lower lung areas in TTN.[35] The syndrome appears to be self-limited, and there have been no reported complications. The use of diuretics such as furosemide has not been found to be effective in decreasing the symptoms or duration of illness.[36]

EDITORIAL COMMENT: Neonatal respiratory distress is associated with changes in β-epithelial sodium channel (β-ENaC) and aquaporin (AQP_5) expression. The various roles of β ENaC and aquaporin in respiratory distress and transient tachypnea of the newborn (TTN) serve as a reminder that it is not only surfactant, oxygen, and CPAP or mechanical ventilation that must be considered in the delivery room, but also the shift in the function of the lung from secretion to absorption of fluid. AQP_5 expression enhances reabsorption of postnatal lung liquid, and aids in the rapid recovery of infants with transient tachypnea of the newborn.[*] Transition for the fetus from a liquid environment with gas exchange through the placenta to air breathing must occur efficiently and effectively. Given all the physical and biochemical switching, it is a miracle that most babies accomplish this seemingly without effort. A key element in this transition is the clearance of lung fluid. This is accomplished by a combination of decreased secretion, increased absorption, and to a lesser extent, excretion accompanying the big squeeze of the thorax during the birth process. The bulk of this fluid clearance is mediated by transepithelial sodium reabsorption through amiloride-sensitive sodium channels in the alveolar epithelial cells with only a limited contribution from mechanical factors and Starling forces. Disruption of this process can lead to retention of fluid in air spaces, setting the stage for alveolar hypoventilation. When infants are delivered near-term, especially by cesarean section (repeat or primary) before the onset of spontaneous labor, the fetus is often deprived of these hormonal changes, making the neonatal transition more difficult.

Barker noted that the mechanisms for lung liquid clearance during the neonatal period develop gradually during the latter part of the third trimester of pregnancy,[†] but the phenotypic switch of the lung epithelium from net secretion to net absorption triggered by events at birth, is sudden. Although lung liquid absorption at birth is "a performance without rehearsal," the lung may be called on for an encore in later life when these same mechanisms are activated to clear accumulated edema liquid.

Bioelectrical studies of human infants' nasal epithelia demonstrate that transient tachypnea of the newborn and RDS have defective amiloride-sensitive Na^+ transport. Neonatal respiratory distress syndrome has, in addition to a relative deficiency in surfactant, defective Na^+ transport, which plays a mechanistic role in the development of the disease.

---

*Li Y, Marcoux MO, Gineste M, et al: Expression of water and ion transporters in tracheal aspirates from neonates with respiratory distress, Acta Paediatr 98:1729, 2009.

†Barker PM, Olver RE: Lung edema clearance: 20 years of progress. Invited review, J Appl Physiol 93:1542, 2002.

PULMONARY HEMORRHAGE

The signs of pulmonary hemorrhage range from blood-tinged tracheal or pharyngeal secretions to massive intractable bleeding. Most studies define significant pulmonary hemorrhage as bright red blood from the endotracheal tube in amounts that increase the need for ventilatory support or produce chest x-ray changes. Historically, pulmonary hemorrhage was associated with intrapartum asphyxia, infection, hypothermia, and defective hemostasis. Although occasionally manifesting in low-birth-weight infants who have previously appeared well, it more often affects infants who are already suffering from other life-threatening abnormalities or illnesses. The composition of the lung effluent in infants with massive pulmonary hemorrhage in most cases is a filtrate of plasma with a small admixture of whole blood, producing a hemorrhagic edema fluid, presumably formed because of increased pulmonary capillary pressure. Factors that might predispose infants to development of hemorrhagic pulmonary edema includes those favoring filtration of fluid (hypoproteinemia, overtransfusion), those causing damage to lung tissue (infection, RDS, and mechanical ventilation in high inspired oxygen), and abnormalities of coagulation.

In a retrospective cohort study, pulmonary hemorrhage was associated with the presence of a clinically significant patent ductus arteriosus before, or at the time of, the hemorrhage.[37] In fact, left-to-right shunting through a patent ductus arteriosus should be considered the primary etiology for pulmonary hemorrhage in a preterm infant who is often recovering from RDS. Surfactant therapy, by improving lung mechanics and decreasing pulmonary vascular resistance, may enhance the process. Pulmonary hemorrhage is probably not an indication to withhold surfactant therapy because the blood products in the lung parenchyma may inactivate surfactant.[38] On rare occasions, aspiration of blood around the time of delivery may simulate pulmonary hemorrhage as a cause of neonatal respiratory distress when other risk factors for pulmonary hemorrhage are absent.[39] Pulmonary hemorrhage has also been seen in several neonates following treatment with extracorporeal life support.[40]

Pulmonary hemorrhage occurs most commonly on the second to fourth days of life. The usual mode of presentation is the development of bradycardia, apnea, or slow gasping respirations and peripheral vasoconstriction. Blood-stained hemorrhagic edema is then seen welling from the trachea. Pulmonary hemorrhage can often be successfully treated by mechanical ventilation employing extra positive end-expiratory pressure (PEEP) and transfusion of fresh blood; occasionally, high-frequency ventilation may be required.

BRONCHOPULMONARY DYSPLASIA/ NEONATAL CHRONIC LUNG DISEASE

In 1967, Northway et al. first described BPD as a clinical syndrome associated with the use of assisted ventilation and high concentrations of oxygen.[41] Their patients had been on respirators using greater than 70% oxygen for longer than 5 to 6 days. During the prolonged recovery, the infants exhibited persistent respiratory difficulty and a characteristic radiographic progression that resulted in cystic lung changes. Increased concentrations of oxygen were required for several weeks before slow improvement was noted. Autopsy revealed that their lungs were diffusely involved with areas of emphysema and collapse, interstitial fibrosis, and changes in the epithelium of the airway.

The radiographic sequence initially described by Northway et al. is no longer commonly seen, and stage I is essentially indistinguishable from uncomplicated RDS. Dense parenchymal opacification, as seen in stage II BPD, may commonly simulate another process, such as congestive heart failure from a patent ductus arteriosus or an infection. The bubbly pattern of stage III BPD is not necessarily seen, and when it does appear, it may not follow a period of parenchymal opacity. Finally, roentgenographic development of bronchopulmonary dysplasia (BPD) (stage IV) may be more insidious than originally described. The characteristic picture of BPD ultimately appears at around 20 or 30 days of age. The major features of stage IV disease include hyperinflation and nonhomogeneity of pulmonary tissues, together with multiple fine, lacy densities extending to the periphery.

Since the original description of BPD by Northway et al., the problem of chronic respiratory disease in infants has steadily increased because of aggressive respiratory management and increased survival of very low-birth-weight infants. In the absence of clear diagnostic criteria for BPD, the following definitions for BPD are in current use: (1) oxygen dependence beyond 28 days of age with persistent chest x-ray changes after mechanical ventilation; and (2) oxygen dependence beyond 36 weeks' corrected postnatal gestational age.[42,43] BPD has been correlated with subsequent abnormal pulmonary findings at follow-up. It has been proposed that the more nonspecific term, *neonatal chronic lung disease*, be employed; however, BPD is still most widely used. Most very low-birth-weight infants who develop BPD may never have had severe RDS with high inspired oxygen or ventilator requirements. Laughon found that 68% of infants who develop BPD never required more than an Fio_2 of 30% in the first 7 days of life.[44]

PATHOPHYSIOLOGIC AND CLINICAL FEATURES

Controversy surrounds the individual contributions of immaturity, inhaled oxygen, ventilator pressures, endotracheal tube injury,

infection, and nutritional deficiencies to the overall pathologic picture of BPD (Fig. 10-7). Recent attention has focused on the role of a dysmorphic vascular structure that is prominent in animal models of BPD and the resultant marked decrease in alveolarization, as well as a role for genetics in contributing to BPD.[45]

Oxygen Toxicity

The lung is the organ exposed directly to the highest partial pressure of inspired oxygen. Although oxygen itself is essentially nonreactive, its potential for toxicity is derived from the formation of reactive oxygen species during normal cell metabolism, and even more so during exposure to high concentrations of oxygen. These oxygen-free radicals are cytotoxic because of their potential for interaction with all of the principal cellular components, resulting

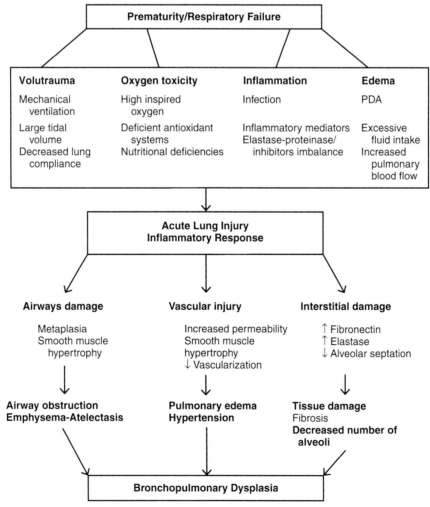

Figure 10-7. Pathogenesis of bronchopulmonary dysplasia. *PDA,* Patent ductus arteriosus.

in inactivation of enzymes, lipid peroxidation in cellular and organelle membranes, and damage to DNA. The precise concentration of oxygen that is toxic to the lung probably depends on a large number of variables, including maturation, nutritional and endocrine status, and duration of exposure to oxygen and other oxidants. A safe level of inspired oxygen has not been established; it is even possible that exposure of the extremely immature lung to 21% oxygen may represent a cytotoxic challenge.

To combat the detrimental effects of oxygen toxicity, cells have evolved a complex system of antioxidant defenses to scavenge and detoxify reactive oxygen-free radicals. These antioxidant defenses include both chemical antioxidants, such as vitamin E, ascorbate, and glutathione, and the antioxidant enzyme system, consisting mainly of superoxide dismutase, catalase, and glutathione peroxidase. Studies have demonstrated a late gestational developmental pattern of pulmonary antioxidant enzyme maturation in numerous species. Therefore, experimental animals, and presumably the human infant as well, if delivered prematurely, would be denied late gestational increases in antioxidant enzyme activities. This could partially explain the vulnerability of the premature infant to oxidant lung damage. Similarly, studies in rabbits have shown that the preterm rabbit is not capable of inducing a protective increase in antioxidant enzymes in response to hyperoxia exposure,[46] which may offer an additional explanation for the vulnerability of the premature infant to hyperoxic exposure.

Additional factors may contribute to the negative influence of hyperoxia on the neonatal lung. When the lung is continuously exposed to high oxygen, an influx of polymorphonuclear leukocytes containing proteolytic enzymes, such as elastase, occurs, resulting in proteolytic damage of structural elements in alveolar walls. Loss of mucociliary function may be an additional pathogenetic component, in that exposure to 80% oxygen has resulted in a cessation of ciliary movement after 48 to 96 hours in cultured human neonatal respiratory epithelium. Finally, lung growth and development appear to be highly sensitive to oxygen exposure with reduced total alveolar number and lung internal surface area, as well as abnormal alveolar architecture in BPD infants.

Studies designed to enhance antioxidant capabilities in the human infant have yet to show any sustained benefit in terms of lung protection, although some show considerable promise. Clinical trials of vitamin E failed to demonstrate a lung protective effect; more recently, however, vitamin A (which may enhance lung development and repair via multiple mechanisms) has been shown to modestly reduce the primary outcome variable, death or BPD.[47] In addition, administration of antioxidant enzymes, particularly superoxide dismutase, might provide protection of the lung from oxidant damage.[48] Other agents that could potentially be protective include such iron-binding agents as deferoxamine or transferrin, which could function via reduction of iron-catalyzed free radical formation.

Epidemiologic data suggest that BPD may not primarily relate to oxidant lung damage. Specifically, BPD has been found to occur with significant frequency in very low-birth-weight infants without preceding RDS, and with minimal early supplemental oxygen exposure. Therefore, antioxidant augmentation alone may not be adequate to completely eradicate BPD from premature infant populations.

Abnormal pulmonary function is characterized by decreased lung compliance resulting from areas of fibrosis, overdistention, and atelectasis and increased pulmonary resistance caused by airway damage.[49] Wheezing may be episodic and markedly contribute to the increased work of breathing and oxygen requirement. Increased airway reactivity is a major problem at follow-up of preterm infants, especially those with BPD.[50,51] Chronic respiratory acidosis is accompanied by elevated bicarbonate and close-to-normal pH. This increase in serum bicarbonate is frequently exaggerated by chronic diuretic therapy.

Pulmonary edema is a prominent complication of BPD, largely caused by the increased pulmonary vascular pressure and permeability. Hypoxic pulmonary vasoconstriction and injury to the pulmonary vascular bed appear to be involved. Exacerbations of congestive heart failure may manifest with wheezing, fluid retention, and hepatomegaly. The underlying disease may mask the chest x-ray changes of pulmonary edema including cardiomegaly.

Infection and the resultant inflammatory response frequently complicate the clinical course of chronic neonatal lung injury. Inflammatory mediators released by either infection or high inspired oxygen may aggravate the bronchoconstriction and vasoconstriction to which the lungs of these infants are predisposed.

Nutritional deficiencies and inadequate caloric intake can interfere with normal alveolar development and with the repair process of injured lung tissue. It can also negatively affect the antioxidant mechanisms. The problem is compounded because contributes to the increased work of breathing these infants' elevated oxygen consumption[52]

MANAGEMENT

With skillful and patient management, most of these infants will recover, although abnormalities in pulmonary function may persist into childhood. Prolonged need for supplemental oxygen over several months is associated with a greater incidence of neurodevelopmental disorders when compared with infants with less severe lung disease.[53] The key to survival for infants with severe lung disease depends on close attention to details such as vigorous treatment of right-sided heart failure, precise fluid balance, use of diuretics, and gradual weaning from mechanical ventilation and raised environmental oxygen. The latter may need to occur in decrements of 1% to 2% of inspired oxygen. Oxygenation is typically monitored via pulse oximetry, and oxygen saturation is maintained in the low to mid-90s. Furosemide (Lasix), 1 to 2 mg/kg/day, is the most widely used diuretic, although prolonged use has been associated with nephrocalcinosis.

These infants need to be closely watched for early signs of infection because pneumonia generally results in a setback. Bronchodilators are of benefit, especially when there are clinical signs of acute bronchospasm. They may be administered as systemic theophylline or as β-agonist inhalation therapy.[54] Controlled trials of both diuretic therapy and bronchodilator inhalation have revealed encouraging short-term improvements in airway resistance, even in the absence of wheezing.[55]

Steroids administered systemically or by inhalation have also been used to ameliorate BPD or to assist in weaning these infants from the ventilator[56]; however, reports of an increased incidence of cerebral palsy after postnatal systemic steroid use for BPD are of concern. This has led to considerable controversy as to the role, duration, and timing of postnatal systemic steroid therapy for BPD. Of particular concern is evidence that postnatal dexamethasone therapy may be associated with reduced cerebral tissue volumes as determined by follow-up MRI.[57] Therefore, hydrocortisone therapy has been proposed as an alternative to dexamethasone because hydrocortisone treatment for BPD may not be associated with the adverse neurobehavioral effects seen on follow-up of dexamethasone treatment.[58] An additional concern is a reported relationship between gastrointestinal perforation and indomethacin treatment for patent ductus arteriosus in hydrocortisone-treated infants.[59] Current recommendations for postnatal steroid use in BPD include taking a cautious approach, avoidance of treatment in the first week of life or for a prolonged period, and tapering therapy over approximately 1 week.[60]

Inhaled nitric oxide has emerged as an alternative approach for treatment of BPD by inhalation over approximately 21 days. This therapy appears to enhance several parameters of lung maturation resulting in a reduction in BPD rate in some, but not all, studies.[61-63] Caution is also advised with this approach pending longer term respiratory and neurodevelopmental outcome data.

Many of these infants require prolonged hospitalization, and a well-organized program of infant stimulation may help the child achieve maximum potential. Parents must be encouraged to assume some of the responsibility for medical procedures, such as chest physiotherapy, and, where possible, a consistent medical team should oversee the infant's care and be available for continuing parental support. Finally, adequate nutritional management is very important because malnutrition delays somatic growth and the development of new alveoli in these high-risk, labile infants.

APNEA IN THE IMMATURE INFANT

Periodic breathing (short, recurring pauses in respiration) of 5 to 10 seconds' duration is common in the immature infant and should be considered a normal respiratory pattern at this age. Apnea, however, has been defined as either (1) a given time period with complete cessation of respiration (typically >15 to 20 seconds) or (2) the time without respiration after which functional changes are noted in the infant, such as a decrease in heart rate to about 80 beats per minute or oxygen saturation to about 80%. Although the use of a standard apneic duration appears to simplify routine nursery management, some small infants (usually <1000 g) appear to have oxygen desaturation if the apneic period extends beyond as little as 10 seconds. The problem increases substantially in incidence and severity with decreasing gestational age.

The relationship between apnea, desaturation, and bradycardia is not simple, as summarized in Figure 10-8. Decreased central respiratory drive is the usual initiating event, with reflex bradycardia presumably triggered by the resultant desaturation. Excitation of inhibitory reflexes occasionally precipitate apnea and bradycardia.[64] A particularly perplexing problem is the frequent occurrence of oxygen desaturation and bradycardia in intubated, ventilated, very low-birth-weight infants. In such infants, hypoventilation is probably the initiating event associated with impaired lung function and ineffective ventilation.[65,66]

Hypoglycemia, fluid and electrolyte imbalance, temperature fluctuations, sepsis, anemia with or without a patent ductus arteriosus, and severe brain lesions can be heralded by apneic spells and should be ruled out when apneic episodes first begin. In a small number of infants, usually close to term, apneic spells may be the manifestation of a seizure disorder. However, the majority of apneic periods occur in infants who are immature and have no organic disease. An exception is an apneic episode in an infant with severe RDS, which usually indicates the presence of hypoxia and acidemia or sepsis, and is a clear indication for immediate intervention, such as assisted ventilation.

The premature infant in whom specific causes for apnea have been reasonably excluded may be considered to have true idiopathic apnea of prematurity. Although no single physiologic or neurochemical explanation completely describes these apneic spells, Table 10-2 lists factors that singly or together make the immature infant more susceptible to apnea.[80-83]

TREATMENT

Because prolonged apnea may cause clinically significant hypoxemia, and because these spells occur so commonly, hospitalized premature infants are typically continuously monitored until no clinically significant apneic episode has occurred for up to 5 to 7 days. Because apnea with an obstructive

Table 10-2.	Factors Related to Apnea in the Immature Infant
Observation	**Explanation**
Hypoxemia causes respiratory depression and results in hypoventilation in neonate instead of sustained hyperventilation as in adult.	Hypoxemic depression of respiration in young infant is centrally mediated and appears to override stimulation from peripheral chemoreceptors.*
Hypercapnia causes hyperventilation as in adult, with diminished response in apneic versus non-apneic infants.	Decreased hypercapnic ventilatory response in apneic infants is probably secondary to immature central neural mechanisms.*
Obstructed inspiratory efforts may occur during apnea and may be misdiagnosed as primary bradycardia when breathing movements persist.[82]	Pharyngeal hypotonia and failure of upper airway respiratory muscles (genioglossus, alae nasi) to contract during inspiration may compromise upper airway patency.*
Apnea is more common during active sleep.	During active sleep, respiration is irregular, lung volume and oxygenation may decrease.

*Data from references 80, 81, 83.

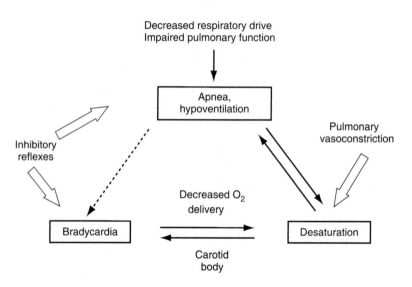

Figure 10-8. Neonatal apnea, bradycardia, and desaturation.

component (so-called *mixed apnea*) may not trigger a respiration alarm, simultaneous heart rate must always be monitored. In these infants, oxygen saturation is a useful adjunct to cardiorespiratory monitoring. Most episodes of 15 to 20 seconds' duration of apnea resolve spontaneously. Most of the remainder cease with gentle diffuse cutaneous stimulation. However, a mask and bag should be available near every monitored infant, to be used if breathing does not begin promptly after stimulation. Inspired oxygen concentration depends on the infant's prior oxygen requirement.

A marked reduction in apnea has been noted with a low CPAP and respiratory stimulants such as theophylline or caffeine.[67-69] Box 10-3 illustrates principles in the management of idiopathic apnea. The order in which these therapeutic steps are undertaken is based on the assessment of each individual patient.

A reasonable principle is to commence with a therapy that carries a low potential for short- or long-term side effects. Nasal CPAP at 3 to 5 cm H_2O is particularly effective in treatment of apneic episodes with an obstructive component.[69] The most probable mechanisms for the beneficial effect of CPAP include maintenance of upper airway patency, increase in FRC and Pa_{O_2}, and stabilization of the chest wall. The use of xanthine therapy (theophylline, caffeine) is widespread in the management of neonatal apnea. Theophylline is metabolized to caffeine in substantial amounts in neonates; their precise mechanism whereby either of these xanthine

agents decreases apnea remains unclear.[70] Proposed mechanisms include generalized enhancement of central respiratory drive via adenosine receptor antagonism, more efficient diaphragmatic contraction, and reversal of hypoxic respiratory depression. Although long-term sequelae from xanthine use have not appeared, care must be taken to avoid short-term side effects such as tachycardia and diuresis, probably more so with theophylline than with caffeine because the latter appears to have a greater margin of safety. Caffeine therapy does significantly shorten duration of supplemental oxygen administration and assisted ventilation.[71] Its use is associated with a transient increase in metabolic rate and impaired weight gain. Data suggest longer term neurodevelopmental benefit from caffeine therapy.[72] Caffeine therapy will require longer term follow-up and improved understanding of the mechanism underlying this benefit.

RESOLUTION OF NEONATAL APNEA

Apnea may persist longer in preterm infants than was generally acknowledged. Such episodes may be accompanied by desaturation and/or bradycardia and often persist beyond 40 weeks of age in infants delivered before 28 weeks' postconceptional age.[73,74] Persistent apnea may also be asymptomatic in a large proportion of very low-birth-weight infants.[75] Prolonged apnea, often manifesting as bradycardia in these very low-birth-weight infants, is often associated with chronic neonatal lung disease. Persistence of symptomatic apnea and bradycardia prolongs the hospitalization of very premature infants and raises questions about the margin of safety for their discharge as well as about the indications for,[76] and utility of, home apnea monitoring.

What is the overall significance of these events in former preterm infants? Evidence does not link the persistence of these events to sudden infant death syndrome (SIDS). Persistence of these cardiorespiratory events may be part of the spectrum of normal postnatal maturation. However, the possibility exists that they represent a subtle marker for neurodevelopmental or sleep disturbances, or other disorders of childhood. Data from several sources suggest that persistence of apnea of prematurity and accompanying bradycardia may be a risk factor for later impairment in neurodevelopmental outcome.[77-79] However, establishment of a causal, rather than associative, relationship between these events and later outcome remains problematic.

Box 10-3. **Management of Idiopathic Apnea**

Diagnosis and treatment of specific causes (e.g., hypoglycemia, anemia, sepsis)
Nasal continuous positive airway pressure (4 cm H_2O)*
Xanthine (caffeine or theophylline) therapy, commencing with a loading dose followed by maintenance therapy, and serum level monitoring, especially for theophylline
Increased environmental oxygen as necessary to maintain adequate baseline oxygen saturation; often associated with treatment of anemia
Assisted ventilation if all else fails

---

*From Miller MJ, Carol WA, Martin RJ: Continuous positive airway pressure selectively reduces obstructive apnea in preterm infants, J Pediatr 106:91, 1985.

QUESTIONS

True or False

As long as the arterial Pao_2 remains less than 100 mm Hg, there will be no retinal damage when using high concentrations of oxygen (>40%) for the treatment of RDS.

The answer is false. When Pao_2 is closely monitored and remains less than 100 mm Hg, retinal damage still develops in some very low-birth-weight infants. There are several possible explanations: (1) blood from a large right-to-left ductal shunt is directed to the sampling site in the lower aorta, while the retinal vessels receive unmixed blood with a higher Pao_2; (2) Pao_2 constantly fluctuates between arterial measurements; and (3) factors other than Pao_2 are involved in retinal injury. Continuous monitoring should help detect the Pao_2 fluctuations. Placing a skin Po_2 electrode or pulse oximeter on the right upper extremity to measure the saturation in the preductal blood should help detect any large right-to-left shunts and is useful to guide management in these situations. Nevertheless, even with continuous monitoring of the oxygen level, retinopathy of prematurity still occurs. Any infant born at less than 30 weeks of gestation or having a birth weight less than 1500 g, or infants who do not fit those categories but have had a significant exposure to supplemental oxygen during their early life should be examined by an experienced pediatric ophthalmologist at 4 weeks of age or a corrected age of 31 weeks' postmenstrual age, whichever is later, for retinopathy of prematurity.

True or False

You are taking care of a 2-day-old, 1200-g male infant with moderate RDS. During the first 2 days of life, he has not been apneic and has maintained a reasonable pH, $Paco_2$, and Pao_2 on 40% oxygen. However, the most recent Pao_2 measurement has decreased to 45 mm Hg (still on 40% oxygen). This environmental oxygen concentration should be left the same because raising it beyond 40% predisposes the infant to oxygen toxicity.

The answer is false. A decrease in Pao_2 to 45 mm Hg suggests worsening of the infant's condition. His condition may deteriorate rapidly if he remains on 40% oxygen. If the arterial oxygen is monitored closely (continually or at least every 4 hours), elevating the inspired oxygen concentration to maintain the Pao_2 between 50 and 80 mm Hg should not predispose the infant to lung or retinal injury as appropriate readjustments to the inspired oxygen content can be made in response to an improved condition. Alternatively, the infant could be placed on CPAP, or if the infant is already on CPAP, the flow can be increased—to increase the mean airway pressure—which, in turn, would lead to improved oxygenation. Also, evaluation of the underlying reason for the deterioration in Pao_2 would be important so the derangement can be rectified.

True or False

Maintaining the Pao_2 between 50 and 80 mm Hg will prevent pulmonary oxygen toxicity and lung injury.

The answer is false. Pulmonary oxygen toxicity is related to the inspired concentration of oxygen, not the arterial oxygen concentration, and any oxygen concentration more than room air can be damaging to pulmonary tissue. It should be noted, however, that oxygen toxicity is not the only contributor to neonatal lung injury. Other factors such as volutrauma, barotrauma, atelectrauma, and lung inflammation also play important roles in injury to the developing lung.

True or False

Your sister is 36 weeks pregnant and is scheduled for an elective cesarean section next week. You are concerned because you believe that the infant may be at risk for developing respiratory distress.

The answer is true. Respiratory distress syndrome is the result of a primary absence of surfactant production and affects most premature infants; however, in certain circumstances it can affect term and near-term infants as well. Surfactant is produced by type II pneumocytes, which become a prominent cell in the alveolus at ~34 to 36 weeks of gestation. In general, surfactant secretion is increased during labor, and therefore, if an infant is born via cesarean section before the onset of labor, they are at risk for decreased production and therefore, respiratory distress after delivery. If a cesarean section is to be pursued prior to 39 weeks' gestation, an explanation of the indication for the delivery must be documented in the chart and documentation of lung maturity should be done prior to delivery.

For each of the following cases, the blood gas information will be given in the following format: pH/ $Paco_2$/ Pao_2/HCO_3. All information necessary will be given to you within the question.

full-term infant in CPAP is done with extreme caution, and some would argue that intubation is the better choice of the two when treating a term infant with significant lung disease.

CASE 1

Baby A is a 3900-kg female with meconium aspiration syndrome. She is transferred to the NICU soon after birth and umbilical venous and arterial catheters are placed. She is initially placed in an oxyhood for oxygen desaturation, and by 8 hours of age, she requires 70% oxygen.

At 8 hours of age, the baby's left leg turns dusky. What should be done?

Initially, try warming the opposite extremity which should cause a reflexive vasorelaxation in the extremity of interest. If the blanching does not improve quickly, then the umbilical arterial catheter must be removed immediately.

If the catheter is removed, how should the infant's oxygenation be managed?

There is no substitute for the combination of continuous oxygen monitoring (via pulse oximetry) and intermittent arterial blood sampling via an indwelling arterial catheter in an acutely ill neonate. Placement of a peripheral arterial line (e.g., radial artery line) should be attempted to continue arterial sampling in this patient to monitor pH, $Paco_2$, and Pao_2.

When arterial catheterization is impossible, heelstick or venous blood sampling can be used to monitor pH and $Paco_2$, but not Pao_2. In that case, noninvasive oxygen monitoring is needed to control supplemental oxygen delivery.

The arterial gas obtained at 8 hours of age is: pH 7.16, $Paco_2$ 60, Pao_2 50, and HCO_3 17. How should this infant's ventilation and oxygenation be managed at this time?

Given this infant's respiratory acidosis and borderline oxygenation at a relatively high inspired oxygen concentration, the infant requires endotracheal intubation with mechanical ventilation. Arterial blood gases should continue to be monitored every 2 to 4 hours to adjust both ventilator and oxygen support required by the infant to resolve the respiratory acidosis and hypoxia. If the hypoxia is not resolving and it is thought that the infant has developed pulmonary hypertension, inhaled nitric oxide should be added to the therapy. If this was a preterm infant with RDS, placing the infant on CPAP would be an alternative to intubation. However, in a full-term infant, CPAP is not always well tolerated and could lead to a worsening of respiratory status and possibly cause a pneumothorax; placing a

CASE 2

Baby B is a 2100-g, small-for-gestational-age, term male who has been grunting since birth. A chest x-ray shows no significant lung disease. The results of a blood gas at 30 minutes of life are: pH 7.14, $Paco_2$ 35, Pao_2 30, and HCO_3 11.4. At that time, the infant is also noted to have a core body temperature of 34° C, heart rate of 140, respiratory rate of 60, and a mean arterial blood pressure of 39 mm Hg.

What are this infant's obvious problems?

This infant is hypothermic, hypoxemic, and has metabolic acidosis. The hypoxemia and acidosis may be the result of hypothermia due to inadequate thermoregulation after delivery. Infants, especially those who are small for gestational age, are at particular risk of hypothermia during the first hours of life because of their relatively large head-to-body surface area. However, sepsis must be a first consideration in the differential diagnosis of a hypothermic, acidotic infant.

How should these problems be handled?

The infant should be warmed by being placed under a radiant warmer or in an incubator. While the infant's body temperature is improving, the acidosis and hypoxemia should also be addressed. The infant should be placed on supplemental oxygen to treat the hypoxemia. Appropriate cultures should be obtained and antibiotics begun to treat the potential diagnosis of neonatal sepsis. Treating the infant's acidosis initially with bicarbonate is somewhat controversial. First, one could consider giving this infant a normal saline bolus (10 mL/kg) in anticipation of possible hypovolemia, and if the acidosis does not improve, repeat the bolus and then consider giving bicarbonate (2 mEq/kg). In addition, many would feel more comfortable intubating this hypoxic infant before giving bicarbonate to provide a controlled manner in which to ensure CO_2 elimination. The placement of an umbilical arterial catheter should be considered so that frequent blood gas samples can be drawn to monitor the infant's response to the interventions that have been made.

At 1 hour of age, after the infant has been in an incubator, placed on a nasal cannula at 1 liter per minute (LPM) with an Fio_2 of 40%, and given a normal saline bolus of 10 mL/kg, the repeat arterial blood gas is: pH 7.28, $Paco_2$ 36, Pao_2 90, and HCO_3 16.4. At this time, the core body temperature is

36° C, HR 120, RR 70, and the mean arterial blood pressure is 22. What problem(s) does the infant have now?

Hypoxemia or acidemia alone or in conjunction with one another can result in an elevation of blood pressure due to their effect on peripheral vasoconstriction. In this patient, partial correction of the metabolic acidosis and increasing the Pao_2 probably caused a decrease in peripheral vascular resistance, reflected as a decrease in the mean arterial blood pressure. The low blood pressure suggests a severely reduced blood volume, which should be expanded with isotonic fluid and/or blood products, if necessary. Of note, acidosis can worsen initially after fluid resuscitation as the build-up of lactate in the tissue is now mobilized into the circulation and large fluid replacement volumes may be necessary.

CASE 3

Baby C is a 900-g female delivered at 27 weeks' gestation. Her Apgar scores are 1 and 7 at 1 and 5 minutes, respectively. She is initially placed on CPAP in the delivery room and transferred to the NICU for further management. A chest x-ray is consistent with the diagnosis of RDS. Umbilical lines are placed, and an initial arterial blood gas result is: pH 7.19, $PaCO_2$ 55, Pao_2 60, HCO_3 19.5 on CPAP 5, and Fio_2 is 50%. There have been no apneic episodes noted.

Should surfactant therapy be administered?

Over recent years, there has been a shift in neonatology practice from automatically intubating very low and extremely low-birth-weight infants for surfactant administration to an approach of initially starting some of these infants on noninvasive modes of ventilation (i.e., CPAP, noninvasive positive pressure ventilation, etc.) in the delivery room. The question then becomes when, if ever, should these infants be treated with surfactant. Surfactant has improved survival, reduced the incidence of air leaks, and probably reduced the severity and incidence of CLD in infants with respiratory distress. In infants who have RDS and are not initially intubated, there are some guidelines available to help decide when and if a preterm infant should be intubated for surfactant, which takes into account gestational age, respiratory drive, and inspired oxygen concentration (see Fig. 10-5). In the case of this patient, although the infant has a strong respiratory drive, given the need for supplemental oxygen of 50%, it would be recommended to administer surfactant to this infant.

At 5 hours of age, the infant is weaned from an Fio_2 of 60% to 27% and the blood gas is: pH 7.28, $Paco_2$ 55, Pao_2, 62, and HCO_3 22. Should surfactant be repeated?

There has been a great deal of flexibility with regard to the redosing of surfactant. However, given the fact that her pH is greater than 7.25 and her Fio_2 is less than 30%, it would be reasonable to extubate this infant to either CPAP or another form of noninvasive ventilation and not to administer another dose of surfactant.

What are the complications of surfactant therapy?

Significant oxygen desaturation occurs in a small percentage of infants shortly after receiving surfactant therapy, which is usually quick to resolve as the surfactant is absorbed and ventilation and perfusion improve. There have also been concerns about pulmonary hemorrhage associated with surfactant administration. This appears to be a more significant problem in the most immature infants (those weighing <750 g and <25 weeks' gestation) and is likely due to changes in lung compliance in the face of an open ductus arteriosus. Also, there is a risk of developing a pneumothorax after surfactant administration as lung compliance improves if the inspiratory pressure used to inflate the less compliant lungs before surfactant administration is not decreased appropriately.

CASE 4

Baby D is a 2000-g male who has been grunting since birth. His chest x-ray reveals questionable RDS. He is placed in 70% oxygen.

At 3 hours, a blood gas is obtained: pH 7.36, $Paco_2$ 40, Pao_2 280, and HCO_3 22.2. What should be done, if anything?

This infant is hyperoxic on 70% Fio_2, thus the oxygen concentration should be decreased to 60% immediately, and pulse oximetry should be placed (if it has not been already) for rapid weaning of oxygen. Plan to decrease the Fio_2 by 2% to 5% every 5 to 10 minutes while maintaining a pulse oximeter reading of 92% to 96%. A repeat blood gas should be obtained in 2 to 4 hours or earlier if desaturation occurs.

At 5 hours of age, the repeat blood gas is: pH 7.36, $Paco_2$ 43, Pao_2 45, and HCO_3 24 on an Fio_2 of 40%. What happened and how should it be addressed?

The patient demonstrated a greater than expected decrease in Pao_2 when the oxygen concentration was weaned and is now hypoxic. This can generally be avoided with continuous monitoring. To resolve the problem, first, return the Fio_2 to 60% to 70%. Second, transilluminate the chest to rule out the possibility of a pneumothorax, which can manifest as a sudden drop in the Pao_2; if transillumination is inconclusive, an x-ray should be obtained. Fifteen to

20 minutes after the Fio_2 has been increased, repeat the blood gas to determine what effect increasing the oxygen concentration has made.

The repeat blood gas after increasing the Fio_2 to 60% is: pH 7.37, $Paco_2$ 45, Pao_2 70, and HCO_3 22. What is the explanation for what happened between our first and last blood gases?

There is not a complete physiologic explanation underlying this phenomenon. It is assumed that, in some infants, the pulmonary vessels are particularly sensitive to changes in oxygen tension, and lowering the environmental oxygen results in pulmonary vasoconstriction and an increased right-to-left shunt. Under these circumstances, the Pao_2 decreases out of proportion to what might ordinarily be expected when the inspired oxygen concentration is reduced, thus explaining the decrease in the Pao_2 seen at 5 hours of age, which improved after increasing the oxygen.

CASE 5

Baby D is a 3000-g infant born at 41 weeks' gestation and is covered with thick meconium. Labor was complicated by late deceleration. Apgar scores are 2, 5, and 7 at 1, 5, and 10 minutes, respectively. The infant is immediately intubated and suctioned for meconium below the cords. After, the infant is bradycardic with poor respiratory effort and requires positive pressure ventilation and intubation to improve the heart rate, and is transported to the NICU for further care. Chest x-ray shows bilateral patchy infiltrates. Umbilical lines are placed and the infant is maintained on a ventilator and 100% oxygen.

At 6 hours of life, a blood gas is obtained: pH 7.35, $Paco_2$ 34, Pao_2 32, and HCO_3 19. What is the infant's main problem at this time?

The infant is markedly hypoxemic on 100% oxygen; however, the infant is not hypercarbic. It is unusual for such a degree of hypoxemia without CO_2 retention to be attributable solely to meconium pneumonitis. It appears that this infant's condition is compounded by persistent pulmonary hypertension secondary to neonatal asphyxia.

How should this be treated?

The response of the hypoxemia to ventilator support in such an infant is variable. Nonetheless, assisted ventilation should be continued with the goal to normalize the pH without maintaining the $Paco_2$ below 40. The goal is to improve any acidemia because this can cause pulmonary vasoconstriction that will worsen hypoxia, which can be achieved by administering bicarbonate. If oxygenation fails to improve, other therapies such as increasing peripheral arterial blood pressure, sedation, surfactant, and inhaled nitric oxide should be employed. ECMO should be reserved for those infants who do not respond to maximal medical therapy.

REFERENCES

The reference list for this chapter can be found online at www.expertconsult.com.

Assisted Ventilation

11

Waldemar A. Carlo and Namasivayam Ambalavanan

But that life may, in a manner of speaking, be restored to the animal, an opening must be attempted in the trunk of the trachea, into which a tube or reed or cane should be put; you will then blow into this so that the lung may rise again and the animal take in air. Indeed, with a single breath in the case of this living animal, the lung will swell to the full extent of the thoracic cavity and the heart become strong and exhibit a wondrous variety of motions...when the lung long flaccid has collapsed, the beat of the heart and arteries appears wavy, creepy, twisting, but when the lung is inflated, it becomes strong again and swift and displays wondrous variations...as I do this, and take care that the lung is inflated at intervals, the motion of the heart and arteries does not stop.

Andreas Vesalius
De Humani Corporis Fabrica (1543)

The primary objective of assisted ventilation is to support gas exchange until the patient's ventilatory efforts are sufficient. Ventilation may be required during immediate care of the depressed or apneic infant, before evaluation and during treatment of an acute respiratory disorder, or for prolonged periods of treatment for respiratory failure. Trained personnel and equipment for emergency ventilation should be available in every delivery room and newborn nursery. Positive pressure ventilation effectively stabilizes most infants who require resuscitation.

This chapter is an introduction to assisted ventilation. Before undertaking assisted ventilation of any form, it must be recognized that the techniques demand time, resources, and experienced personnel. Prolonged ventilation should only be used in units where expert nurses, respiratory therapists, and medical personnel are continuously available.

RESPIRATORY FAILURE

Hypercapnic respiratory failure is the inability to remove CO_2 by spontaneous respiratory efforts and results in an increasing arterial P_{CO_2} (Pa_{CO_2}) and a decreasing pH. Assisted ventilation is most commonly needed to treat hypercapnic respiratory failure. Hypoxemia is usually (but not invariably) present; in many instances, arterial oxygenation can be normalized if the inspired oxygen is increased. Infants with hypoxemic respiratory failure have a predominant problem of oxygenation, usually the result of right-to-left shunt or severe ventilation-perfusion mismatch. Respiratory failure can occur because of disease in the lungs, or in other organs and systems (Figure 11-1). Assisted ventilation is usually required when severe respiratory failure ensues (Box 11-1). Depending on many clinical considerations (e.g., extreme prematurity), assisted ventilation may be initiated earlier.

CLINICAL MANIFESTATIONS OF RESPIRATORY FAILURE IN THE NEWBORN

The following are findings that should make the clinician suspect respiratory failure:
- Worsening hypercapnia and/or hypoxemia
- Increase or decrease in respiratory rate
- Increase or decrease in respiratory efforts (grunting, flaring, retractions)
- Periodic breathing with increasing prolongation of respiratory pauses
- Apnea
- Decreasing blood pressure with tachycardia associated with pallor, circulatory failure, and ultimately bradycardia

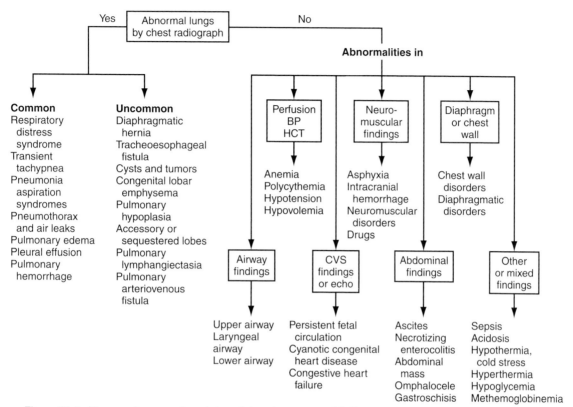

Figure 11-1. Diagram of causes of respiratory distress in neonates. *BP,* Blood pressure; *CVS,* cardiovascular system; *echo,* echocardiogram; *HCT,* hematocrit.

Box 11-1. **Indications for Assisted Ventilation**

Respiratory acidosis with pH less than 7.20 to 7.25

Hypoxemia while on 100% oxygen or continuous positive airway pressure with 60% to 100% oxygen

Severe apnea

CARDIAC VERSUS PULMONARY DISEASE

The clinician may frequently need to distinguish between cardiac and pulmonary disease in the sick newborn infant. Cyanotic heart disease may mimic respiratory disease. One possible way to differentiate between the two is to perform a hyperoxia test: place the infant in 100% oxygen for 10 minutes and then obtain an arterial Po_2 (Pao_2). In infants with pulmonary disease, Pao_2 usually increases to more than 100 mm Hg, whereas infants with cyanotic heart disease show little change in Pao_2. The hyperoxia test, although useful diagnostically, may also be misleading. In infants with severe pulmonary hypertension and right-to-left shunt, Pao_2 may not elevate with 100% oxygen. Alternatively, Pao_2 may increase more than 100 mm Hg early in life in infants with forms of cyanotic heart disease with high pulmonary blood flow (e.g., total anomalous pulmonary venous return). Echocardiography should be used to distinguish between cardiac and pulmonary disease when hypoxemia is unresponsive to ventilatory support.

ENDOTRACHEAL INTUBATION

Most infants should receive positive pressure ventilation before attempting endotracheal intubation. This improves oxygenation and decreases $Paco_2$, thereby decreasing the likelihood of bradycardia during endotracheal intubation. Positive pressure ventilation is impractical for prolonged periods but can be used for the following:
- Immediate resuscitation
- Stabilization before and after endotracheal intubation

- Ventilation in infants whose condition is deteriorating without obvious cause
- Ventilation during transport to intensive care facilities when mechanical ventilation is unavailable

Mechanical ventilation is a highly invasive therapy and is indicated only when the benefits outweigh the burdens. In situations where there is little reasonable chance of survival, there should be honest discussions with the family regarding of the appropriateness of aggressive measures such as intubation.

ENDOTRACHEAL TUBE SIZE

It is preferable to use relatively small endotracheal tubes to prevent tracheal damage. The endotracheal tube should fit loosely enough to allow a leak of gas between tube and trachea when 10 cm H_2O inspired pressure is generated. Tube size can be related to infant size or gestational age. Recommended sizes are as follows:

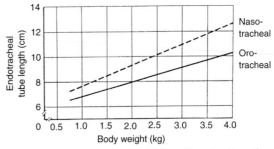

Figure 11-2. Graph for determination of length of insertion of endotracheal tubes. The tip of the endotracheal tube is aimed at the midtrachea. *(From Lough MD, Carlo WA: Clinical care techniques. In Carlo WA, Chatburn RL, editors: Neonatal respiratory care, Chicago, Year Book, 1988, p 122.)*

be placed midway between the carina and the glottis. The length of insertion of the endotracheal tube is shown in Figure 11-2. The following measurements can be used for endotracheal tube placement:

Gestational Age (wk)	Birth Weight (g)	Endotracheal Tube Size (mm internal diameter)
Below 28	Below 1000	2.5
28-34	1000-2000	3.0
35-38	2000-3000	3.5
Above 38	Above 3000	3.5-4.0

Infant Weight (g)	Endotracheal Tube Insertion Length (tip to lip, cm)
1000	7
2000	8
3000	9
4000	10

INTUBATION

Insertion of an endotracheal tube should be performed with universal precautions under a radiant heat source to keep the infant warm. Free-flow oxygen should be administered as necessary.

Intubation can be a painful procedure and so premedication with an analgesic agent (morphine, fentanyl, or remifentanil) should be used for all non-emergent intubations in neonates.[4] A muscle relaxant (paralytic agent) should only be used with analgesia. Other agents which may be considered include sedatives (midazolam) and vagolytic agents (atropine). The ideal combination and sequence of premedications in neonates has not yet been established. Each unit should develop protocols and lists of preferred medications to maximize safety.

The infant should receive positive pressure ventilation and oxygen as needed between attempts. The tip of the tube should

At these lengths, the distal end of the endotracheal tube should be at the midtrachea. It is easy to inadvertently pass the tube into the right mainstem bronchus, but using these insertion length guidelines prevents this complication. Breath sounds should be equal bilaterally. A CO_2 detector should be used to confirm endotracheal placement. The tube should be secured so that movement of the head and neck will not dislodge it. Lightweight plastic connectors can be used to prevent kinking the tube. The endotracheal tube position should be checked radiographically.

ORAL INTUBATION

The advantages of oral intubation are the relative ease of insertion and that a stylet can be used to aid insertion. Oral tubes should always be used in emergencies. The disadvantages of oral intubation are the increased tube mobility if the tube is inadequately secured and the greater difficulty in keeping the tube in position.

A laryngoscope with a Miller number 0 or 1 blade inserted in the vallecula is used to pull upward to visualize the glottis while leaving the head in a neutral position. It is important not to traumatize the gums and tooth buds. The heart rate should be monitored continuously with auditory and visual signals during attempts at intubation. Continuous O_2 saturation or transcutaneous Po_2 monitoring is invaluable because oxygenation can worsen abruptly. It is helpful if the tube has been previously curved. To stiffen the tube for orotracheal intubation, a stylet may be used or it may be cooled.

NASAL INTUBATION

The advantage of nasal intubation is the improved stability with the reduced likelihood of slippage into the right mainstem bronchus or accidental extubation. The disadvantages are trauma to the nares and nasal septum, greater difficulty in insertion of the tube, possibility of an increased number of gram-negative nasal superinfections, and potential trauma to the developing eustachian tubes and sinuses. Nasotracheal intubation should always be performed as an elective procedure and should not be done in emergencies.

Using a laryngoscope blade, the lubricated endotracheal tube is inserted through the nares until it is visualized in the oropharynx. The McGill forceps are used to guide the tube into the glottis. It is helpful if the endotracheal tube has been previously lubricated with a nontoxic, water-soluble lubricant. A stylet is never used for nasotracheal intubation.

SUCTIONING

Suctioning can be done if there are copious amounts of secretions or suspicion of endotracheal tube occlusion by secretions, but routine suctioning is not necessary. Strict sterile technique with disposable gloves and suction tubes is necessary. The infant should be allowed to recover between episodes of suctioning by maintaining stable O_2 saturations with increases in inspired oxygen concentrations as needed and by reexpanding the lung with 10% to 20% more pressure than used for routine ventilation. Saline instillation is done to facilitate removal of secretions when secretions are thick.

Although sometimes necessary, suctioning is potentially dangerous; it may cause a hypoxic episode owing to discontinuation of ventilation, extraction of gas from small airways, or atelectasis. It may also produce lesions in the trachea at the site of the suction catheter tip. Use of a special endotracheal tube connector allows mechanical ventilation during suctioning and prevents the catheter tip from going beyond the endotracheal tube.

> **EDITORIAL COMMENT:** Suctioning of the endotracheal tube will decrease oxygenation and pulmonary function. I would advocate being guided by pulse oximetry during the procedure, which may require transiently increasing inspired oxygen concentration by 10% to 15% immediately before and following the period of suctioning. I would also advocate avoiding the practice of "routine" suctioning except as secretions warrant.
>
> *John Kattwinkel*

CHANGING AN ENDOTRACHEAL TUBE

An endotracheal tube change is required only if the tube becomes dislodged or occluded or if the infant outgrows it. Routine change is not indicated.

APPLIED PULMONARY MECHANICS

The following principles are helpful in understanding mechanical ventilation. A pressure gradient between the airway opening and alveoli must exist to drive the flow of gases during both inspiration and expiration. The pressure gradient required to inflate the lungs is determined largely by the compliance and the resistance of the lungs.

COMPLIANCE

Compliance is a property of distensibility (i.e., of the lungs and chest wall) and is calculated from the change in volume per unit change in pressure:

$$Compliance = \frac{\Delta\ Volume}{\Delta\ Pressure}$$

The higher the compliance, the larger the delivered volume per unit of pressure. Compliance in babies with normal lungs ranges from 3 to 6 mL/cm H_2O. Compliance in infants with respiratory distress syndrome (RDS) ranges from 0.1 to 1 mL/cm H_2O.

RESISTANCE

Resistance is a property of the inherent capacity of the gas-conducting system (i.e., airways, endotracheal tube, and lung tissue) to oppose airflow and is expressed as the change in pressure per unit change in flow:

$$Resistance = \frac{\Delta\ Pressure}{\Delta\ Flow}$$

Resistance in babies with normal lungs ranges from 25 to 50 cm H_2O/L/second. Resistance is not dramatically altered in infants with RDS but is increased in intubated infants and ranges from 50 to 150 cm H_2O/L/second.

TIME CONSTANT

Time constant is a measure of the time (expressed in seconds) necessary for 63% of a step change (e.g., airway pressure gradient) toward equilibration. A step change in airway pressure occurs between the beginning and the end of a machine-delivered inspiration (during pressure-limited, time-cycled ventilation). The product of compliance and resistance determines the time constant of the respiratory system:

$$\text{Time constant} = \text{Compliance} \times \text{Resistance}$$

For example, in an infant with normal lungs:

$$\begin{aligned} \text{One time constant} &= 0.005 \text{ L/cm } H_2O \\ &\quad \times 25 \text{ cm } H_2O\text{/L/second} \\ &= 0.125 \text{ second} \end{aligned}$$

In an intubated infant with RDS:

$$\begin{aligned} \text{One time constant} &= 0.001 \text{ L/cm } H_2O \\ &\quad \times 50 \text{ cm } H_2O\text{/L/second} \\ &= 0.050 \text{ second} \end{aligned}$$

It takes three time constants to achieve 95% of the pressure change to be equilibrated throughout the lungs; it takes five time constants for 99% equilibration. Thus, to allow for a fairly complete inspiration and expiration, inspiratory and expiratory times set on the ventilator should last about three to five time constants. In this example of an intubated infant with RDS, the duration of three to five time constants is 0.150 to 0.250 second. A very short inspiratory time can lead to inadequate tidal volume because ventilatory pressures may not equilibrate throughout the lungs (Fig. 11-3). A very short expiratory time can lead to gas trapping because exhalation may not be completed. Very long inspiratory or expiratory times are also not beneficial.

CONTINUOUS POSITIVE AIRWAY PRESSURE

Respiration can also be assisted by expansion of the lungs with continuous distending pressure. This technique is valuable

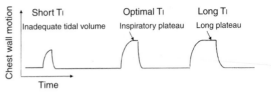

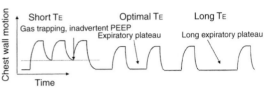

Figure 11-3. Estimation of optimal inspiratory (T_I) and expiratory (T_E) times. Inspiratory and expiratory times are optimal when inspiration and expiration are complete but the times are not too prolonged. (See text for further details) *PEEP*, Positive end-expiratory pressure.

when respiratory drive is normal and pulmonary disease is not overwhelming. Continuous distending pressure can be applied with continuous positive airway pressure (CPAP) or continuous negative pressure around the chest wall. Because of the ease of delivery, CPAP is the usual mode of delivery of continuous distending pressure.

Surfactant deficiency in infants with RDS predisposes to alveolar collapse. The resulting atelectatic areas of the lungs are the sites of right-to-left shunting. When alveoli are prevented from closing by maintaining a continuous positive transpulmonary pressure throughout the respiratory cycle, functional residual capacity increases. In addition, ventilation of perfused areas of the lung increases, which reduces intrapulmonary shunt.

A simple system for CPAP was described by Gregory et al. in 1971[1] (Fig. 11-4). A suitable air-oxygen mixture passes through a humidifier. Gas passes through the tubing, which is attached to an endotracheal tube. The screw clamp on the reservoir controls the flow of gas and maintains a constant positive pressure within the system, as indicated on the pressure manometer. The side arm acts as an underwater safety valve by ending under a column of water. Nasal CPAP is simple and effective; it is usually applied with nasal or nasopharyngeal prongs, although other techniques for delivery can be used (Table 11-1). Problems with CPAP generally revolve around feeding difficulties, maintaining a good seal, and nasal trauma. Nursing and medical care are

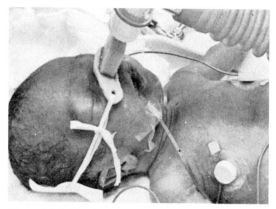

Figure 11-4. Nasal continuous positive airway pressure (CPAP) unit in place on infant.

Table 11-1.	Techniques of Applying Continuous Positive Airway Pressure		
Method	**Advantages**	**Disadvantages**	
Nasal prongs	Simple	Trauma to turbinates and septum; excessive crying; variation in Fio_2; increased work of breathing	
Nasopharyngeal prongs	Relatively simple, fixation easy	May become blocked or kinked	
Endotracheal	Effective	Requires intubation; nursing and medical skills as for ventilator	
Head box	Noninvasive	Neck seal a problem; suction difficult; nerve palsies	
Face mask	Simple, inexpensive	Abdominal distention, pressure on face and eyes; CO_2 retention; cerebellar hemorrhage	
Face chamber	Good seal, minimal trauma to face	Expensive; baby inaccessible	

similar to those undertaken during mechanical ventilation.

Trials performed before the era of surfactant showed that CPAP decreased death and the need for mechanical ventilation, but increased the risk for pneumothorax.[2] Subsequent surfactant trials showed that surfactant treatment in the first 2 hours after birth decreased mortality, air leaks, and death or bronchopulmonary dysplasia (BPD).[3]

However, the control infants in these trials received mechanical ventilation, and it is possible that mechanical ventilation without surfactant causes lung injury. Recent trials have compared the effects of CPAP to mechanical ventilation with surfactant administration. A large trial showed that in very immature infants CPAP resulted in less need for intubation, fewer days of mechanical ventilation, and less need for postnatal steroid treatment for BPD than treatment with surfactant.[5] In addition, there was a trend for less BPD and/or death in the CPAP group. Similar trends in reduction of BPD and/or death with early CPAP have been reported in other clinical trials and meta-analyses show significant reductions in BPD and/or death. In bigger preterm infants, CPAP results in benefits comparable to that of surfactant.[6] Together, these studies indicate that CPAP is an effective alternative to intubation and surfactant in the treatment of RDS in most preterm infants.

EDITORIAL COMMENT: In a multicenter randomized trial, Dunn et al. compared approaches to the initial respiratory management of preterm neonates (26 to 29 weeks' gestation): prophylactic surfactant followed by a period of mechanical ventilation (prophylactic surfactant [PS], prophylactic surfactant with rapid extubation to bubble nasal continuous positive airway pressure (intubate-surfactant-extubate [ISX], or initial management with bubble nasal continuous positive airway pressure and selective surfactant treatment (nCPAP).[7] Forty-eight percent were managed without intubation and ventilation and 54% without surfactant treatment. The primary outcome was death or BPD. Preterm neonates who were initially managed with either nCPAP or PS with rapid extubation to nCPAP had similar clinical outcomes to those treated with PS followed by a period of mechanical ventilation. An approach that uses early nCPAP leads to a reduction in the number of infants who are intubated and given surfactant. These results reinforce the SUPPORT date.[5]

Dunn Ms, Kaempf J, de Klerk A et al, Vermont Oxford Network DRM Study Group: Randomized trial comparing 3 approaches to the initial respiratory management of preterm neonates. Pediatrics 128:e1069, 2011.

GENERAL GUIDELINES FOR CONTINUOUS POSITIVE AIRWAY PRESSURE

1. CPAP should be initiated soon after birth in the most immature infants (less than ~29 weeks' gestation) with presumed RDS. In more mature infants, CPAP can be initiated when the infant requires

more than 40% to 50% oxygen or when the infant has recurrent apnea.

2. Initially, nasal CPAP of 5 to 6 cm H_2O can be used. If there is no improvement, the pressure can be increased in increments of 2 cm H_2O up to 8 to 10 cm H_2O. Very high CPAP levels may overdistend the lungs, decrease their compliance, and increase the risk for pneumothorax. Nasal synchronized intermittent mechanical ventilation can be added to augment the benefits of CPAP.

3. Continuous measurement of transcutaneous Po_2 and Pco_2, and oxygen saturation with a pulse oximeter are of great value and can decrease the need for frequent blood gas measurements.

4. Because these positive pressures are not completely transmitted to the pleural space due to reduced lung compliance, venous return and cardiac output are usually not compromised. However, if $Paco_2$ increases and Pao_2 decreases, a reduction in CPAP pressure should be considered.

EDITORIAL COMMENT: Thoracic wall elastic recoil is almost nonexistent in extremely preterm babies (e.g., 29 weeks' gestation or less), so that the resting volume of the lung is very close to the collapsed volume. Also, the compliant chest wall tends to collapse as the diaphragm descends, resulting in an ineffective tidal volume. Early use of CPAP may improve the efficiency of ventilation in these very immature babies.

John Kattwinkel

WEANING FROM CONTINUOUS POSITIVE AIRWAY PRESSURE

1. Inspired oxygen can be reduced in steps of 2% to 5% when the O_2 saturation exceeds 93% to 95%.

2. CPAP can be reduced when the O_2 saturation is more than 93% to 95% and the inspired oxygen is less than 30% to 40%.

EDITORIAL COMMENT: With small babies (<1500 g), if recurrent apneic spells are a problem, we may continue low-pressure CPAP (<5 cm H_2O) until inspired oxygen concentrations have been reduced to 21% to 30%.

John Kattwinkel

See Chapter 10 for a discussion of the use of CPAP for apnea of prematurity.

MECHANICAL VENTILATION

Mechanical ventilation is one of the most important breakthroughs in the history of neonatal care. Mechanical ventilation allows the survival of previously nonviable infants, stimulating the development of a new era in neonatology.

Conventional mechanical ventilators achieve a pressure gradient between the airway opening and lungs, producing a flow of gas into the lung. This is usually created by intermittently building up a positive pressure in the proximal airway. Ventilators for infants are usually one of the following types:

1. *Pressure-controlled ventilators.* These ventilators deliver a preset peak inspiratory pressure (PIP), thus delivering a variable tidal volume depending largely on lung compliance. A constant flow of gas passes through the ventilator. Intermittently, the expiratory relief valve closes and the gas flows to the infant. Pressure is limited to the desired magnitude. When the expiratory relief valve has been closed for the preset time, the valve opens, and inspiration ceases. Pressure-controlled ventilation is usually used with the technique of synchronized intermittent mandatory ventilation, which allows spontaneous breathing between ventilator breaths.

PIP depends largely on the desired tidal volume and the compliance of the lungs. Suggested initial ventilator settings are as follows:

	Normal Lungs	RDS Lungs
PIP (cm H_2O)	10-15	15-20
PEEP (cm H_2O)	2-3	4-5
Rate (per min)	10-20	40-80
I/E ratio	1:2-1:10	1:1-1:2

I/E, Inspiratory/expiratory; *PEEP,* positive end-expiratory pressure; *PIP,* peak inspiratory pressure; *RDS,* respiratory distress syndrome.

2. *Volume-controlled ventilators.* These ventilators deliver a preset tidal volume with a variable PIP depending largely on lung compliance. When this gas has been delivered by the piston, inspiration is terminated.

The tidal volume delivered by the ventilator must be adequate to normalize arterial oxygen and carbon dioxide. Important considerations are as follows:

• Infant's tidal volume (4 to 8 mL/kg)
• Compression loss in the ventilator tubing (if ventilator tubing volume is large, this may be appreciable)
• Volume losses by leaks from the tubing around the endotracheal tube

Pressure-controlled ventilators have been the most frequently used types in neonates, but volume-controlled neonatal ventilators are being used increasingly because recent evidence suggests that lung injury is most likely related to volutrauma.[7] Theoretical advantages of volume ventilation include consistency of delivered tidal volume, ability to prevent excessive volume delivery, and automatic weaning of pressure as lung compliance improves. Volume ventilation results in reductions or trends for reductions in duration of ventilation, pneumothorax, intracranial hemorrhage, and BPD. The clinician should learn about and understand one or two types of ventilators versus trying to be an expert in many types.

- Independent of the type of ventilator used, Fio_2 should initially correspond to the Fio_2 necessary to maintain an adequate Pao_2 (40 to 60 mm Hg) or oxygen saturation (90% to 95%). The clinician should watch for elevated oxygen saturation after starting mechanical ventilation because effective mechanical ventilation may result in a sudden reduction in oxygen requirement. Ventilators have the following features:

1. Gas mixer (blender)—to allow easy adjustment of the inspired oxygen concentration between 21% and 100%.
2. Time adjustment—to allow altering of the inspiratory and expiratory times. This permits prolongation of inspiratory time in patients with a long inspiratory time constant or widespread atelectasis as well as its shortening if the time constant is short (see Fig. 11-3). Expiratory time should be prolonged when gas trapping is present or when the expiratory time constant is long. Expiratory time can be shortened when the respiratory time constant is short.
3. Expiratory relief valve—to limit the PIP. When used in combination with the inspiratory time adjustment, it allows the peak pressure to be held, generating a pressure plateau (see Fig. 11-3). A very long plateau is not beneficial. This valve also allows one to limit the peak pressure to reduce the likelihood of volutrauma or barotrauma.
4. Pressure gauge—to measure the applied airway pressures accurately. An adequate pressure monitor must be placed close to the endotracheal tube to measure correct peak inspiratory and positive end-expiratory pressures.
5. Alarms—to warn of inadvertent disconnections, pressure loss, high pressures, and failure of the ventilator to cycle at the proper time.
6. Humidification or nebulization—to saturate the inspired gases with water. The temperature of the inspired gas close to the endotracheal tube should be measured continuously and used to servo-control the humidification system.
7. Positive end-expiratory pressure (PEEP)—to maintain functional residual capacity.
8. Exhalation assist—to reduce the end-expiratory pressure to desired levels when rapid rates are used. Inadvertent PEEP can be a problem with some pediatric ventilators because of a high expiratory resistance.

ALTERNATIVE MODES OF MECHANICAL VENTILATION

Technologic advances, including improvement in flow delivery systems, breath termination criteria, guaranteed tidal volume delivery, stability of PEEP, air leak compensation, prevention of pressure overshoot, pulmonary function monitoring, and triggering systems, have resulted in better ventilators.[8] Patient-initiated mechanical ventilation, patient-triggered ventilation, synchronized intermittent mandatory ventilation, and noninvasive ventilation are increasingly being used in neonates.

1. *Patient-triggered ventilation/synchronized intermittent mandatory ventilation.* Patient-triggered ventilation uses spontaneous respiratory efforts to trigger the ventilator. Airflow, chest wall movements, airway pressures, esophageal pressures, or diaphragmatic electrical activity are used as indicators of the onset of the inspiratory effort. When the ventilator detects an inspiratory effort, it delivers a ventilator breath of predetermined settings (PIP, inspiratory duration, flow). Synchronized intermittent mandatory ventilation achieves synchrony between the patient and the ventilator breaths. Synchrony occurs easily in most neonates because strong respiratory reflexes during early life elicit relaxation of respiratory muscles at the end of lung inflation. Furthermore, inspiratory efforts usually start when lung volume is decreased at the end of exhalation. Synchrony may be achieved by nearly matching the ventilator frequency to the spontaneous respiratory rate or by simply ventilating at relatively high rates (60 to 120 breaths/minute). Triggering systems can be used to achieve

synchronization when synchrony does not occur with these maneuvers.

2. *Proportional assist ventilation.* These ventilators reduce work of breathing. Both modes of patient-initiated mechanical ventilation discussed earlier (patient-triggered ventilation, synchronized intermittent mandatory ventilation) are designed to synchronize the onset of the inspiratory support. In contrast, proportional assist ventilation matches the onset and duration of both inspiratory and expiratory support and provides ventilation in proportion to the volume or flow of the spontaneous breath. Thus, the ventilator can selectively decrease the elastic or resistive work of breathing. The magnitude of the support can be adjusted depending on the patient's needs. When compared with conventional and patient-triggered ventilation, proportional assist ventilation may reduce ventilatory pressures while maintaining or improving gas exchange.[9] Randomized clinical trials are needed to determine whether proportional assist ventilation leads to major benefits when compared with conventional mechanical ventilation.

3. *Combination modes.* Many of the newer generation ventilators offer combinations of volume and pressure ventilation. Often these modes use pressure ventilation with a guarantee of a certain volume. No agreement among different ventilator manufacturers on terminology has been established, so similar modes have different names. To date, these combination modes have not been proven superior to the traditional modes.

4. *Noninvasive ventilation.* Noninvasive ventilation delivered nasally is being increasingly used to supplement nasal CPAP. Noninvasive ventilation has been shown to reduce apnea and the need for ventilation. Further research is needed to determine efficiency and safety of this mode of ventilation.

CARBON DIOXIDE ELIMINATION

CO_2 elimination largely depends on the amount of gas that passes in and out of the alveoli (Fig. 11-5). The total amount of gas that passes in and out of the lungs (including alveoli and airways) is called *minute ventilation*. Minute ventilation may be calculated from the product of the tidal volume and respiratory frequency. Thus, increases in tidal volume or frequency increase minute ventilation, increase CO_2 elimination, and decrease Pa_{CO_2}. Some of the tidal volume distributes to parts of the lungs (dead space) that are not involved in gas exchange (e.g., airways).

Tidal volume may be increased by increasing the pressure gradient between inspiration and expiration. This may be accomplished by increasing PIP or by decreasing PEEP. Tidal volume is usually independent of inspiratory and expiratory times. However,

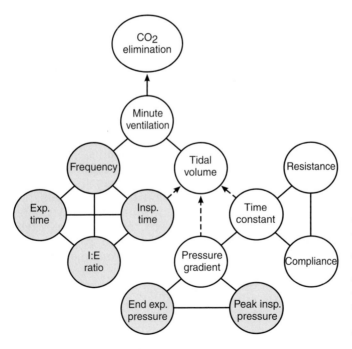

Figure 11-5. Determinants of CO_2 elimination during pressure-limited, time-cycled ventilation. Ventilator-controlled variables are shaded. The relations between the circles that are joined by *solid lines* are described by simple mathematical equations. *Exp,* Expiration; *insp,* inspiration. *(Adapted from Chatburn RL, Lough MD: Mechanical ventilation. In Lough MD, Doerschuck C, Stern R, editors: Pediatric respiratory therapy, ed 3, Chicago, Mosby Year Book, 1985, p 161.)*

depending on the time constant of the respiratory system, very short inspiratory times may limit tidal volume delivery.

Frequency is the other major determinant of minute ventilation. In addition to the frequency set on the ventilator, the infant may take spontaneous breaths because neonatal ventilators provide a continuous flow of gas during the expiratory phase.

Hypercapnia can be caused by hypoventilation or ventilation-perfusion ($\dot{V}/\dot{Q}$) mismatch. Hypoventilation is a very important cause of hypercapnia. Hypercapnia occurs when alveolar ventilation decreases. Hypercapnia caused by hypoventilation is easily managed with mechanical ventilation. Hypercapnia secondary to severe $\dot{V}/\dot{Q}$ mismatch may be more difficult to manage with mechanical ventilation. Optimal $\dot{V}/\dot{Q}$ matching occurs when the ratio of alveolar ventilation and alveolar perfusion is approximately 1. $\dot{V}/\dot{Q}$ mismatch is probably the most important mechanism of gas-exchange impairment in infants with respiratory failure of various causes, including RDS.

OXYGENATION

Hypoxemia can be due to $\dot{V}/\dot{Q}$ mismatch, shunting, diffusion abnormalities, and hypoventilation.[10] $\dot{V}/\dot{Q}$ mismatch is a major cause of hypoxemia in infants with RDS and in neonates with other causes of respiratory failure. In these patients, the alveoli are poorly ventilated relative to their perfusion. In neonates with persistent pulmonary hypertension or cyanotic congenital heart disease, shunting is the predominant mechanism that leads to hypoxemia. Diffusion abnormality, typical of interstitial lung disease and other diseases that affect the alveolar-capillary interface, is not prominent in neonates with RDS and does not cause severe hypoxemia. Hypoventilation usually causes mild hypoxemia unless severe hypercapnia ensues.

Unlike other causes of hypoxemia, shunting usually is unresponsive to oxygen supplementation and mechanical ventilation unless the shunt is reversed. Hypoxemia resulting from $\dot{V}/\dot{Q}$ mismatch can be difficult to manage, but may be resolved if an increase in airway pressure reexpands atelectatic alveoli. Hypoxemia caused by impaired diffusion or hypoventilation usually responds to oxygen supplementation and mechanical ventilation.

In infants with RDS, oxygenation depends largely on the inspired oxygen concentration and the mean airway pressure (Fig. 11-6). Oxygenation increases linearly with increases in mean airway pressure, largely because functional residual capacity can be optimized with mean airway pressure adjustments resulting in improved $\dot{V}/\dot{Q}$ match. Mean airway pressure is a measure of the average pressure to which the lungs are exposed during the respiratory cycle. Mean airway pressure may be calculated from the area under the curve divided by the duration of the cycle (Fig. 11-7). The equation is as follows.

Mean airway pressure $=$

$$K(PIP - PEEP)\frac{(T_I)}{(T_I + T_E)} + PEEP$$

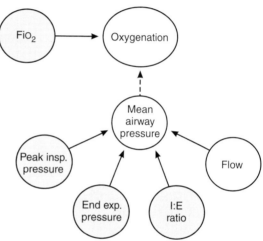

Figure 11-6. Determinants of oxygenation during pressure-limited, timed-cycle ventilation. *Circles* depicting ventilation-controlled variables are shaded. *Solid arrows* represent mathematical relationships.

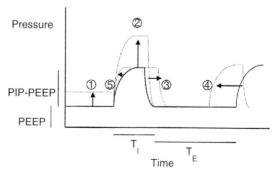

Figure 11-7. Methods to increase airway pressure. Interventions: *1.* Increase PEEP; *2.* Increase PIP; *3.* Increase I/E or T_i; *4.* Increase rate; *5.* Increase flow. *I/E,* Inspiratory-to-expiratory ratio; *PEEP,* positive end-expiratory pressure; *PIP,* peak inspiratory pressure; *T_E,* expiratory time; *T_I,* inspiratory time.

where K is a constant that depends on the rate of increase of the airway pressure curve, PIP is peak inspiratory pressure, PEEP is positive end-expiratory pressure, T_I is inspiratory time, and T_E is expiratory time. Therefore, mean airway pressure is increased by increasing any of the following (see Fig. 11-7):

1. PEEP
2. PIP
3. Inspiratory to expiratory (I/E) ratio or inspiratory time
4. Rate
5. Inspiratory flow (increases K)

Although a direct relationship usually exists between mean airway pressure and oxygenation, several limitations follow:

1. For the same change in mean airway pressure, increases in PIP and PEEP enhance oxygenation more than increases in I/E ratio.
2. Increases in PEEP are not as effective when an elevated level (more than 5 to 6 cm H_2O) is reached.
3. Very high mean airway pressure may cause lung overdistention, right-to-left shunting in the lungs (by redistribution of blood flow to poorly ventilated areas), or decreased cardiac output.
4. Long inspiratory times increase the risk for pneumothorax.

VENTILATOR SETTING CHANGES AND GAS EXCHANGE

From the earlier discussion, the effects of the changes in individual ventilator settings on blood gases can be extrapolated. The major effects are summarized in Table 11-2. Although effects may vary, these basic principles should serve as guidelines. However, when faced with an abnormal blood gas result, several alternative ventilator setting changes may be acceptable. Controversy still exists as to the optimal way to ventilate infants. It is generally preferred to provide an adequate tidal volume and then adjust the frequency to achieve sufficient CO_2 elimination. Mean airway pressure can then be changed to optimize oxygenation. The use of very high frequencies, in which short inspiratory time decreases tidal volume delivery or short expiratory time causes gas trapping and inadvertent PEEP, is not advocated.

In summary, major concepts of gas exchange in infants with RDS are that CO_2 elimination is proportional to minute ventilation and that oxygenation is related directly to mean airway pressure. Based on these concepts, ventilatory strategies have been developed[11] that should provide an organized, logical, and consistent means of achieving desired blood gas results, thereby supporting the clinician in ventilator management decisions. Studies in neonates with RDS, who were managed with such an algorithm, revealed more frequent correction of blood gas derangements and more appropriate efforts to wean the infant from ventilatory assistance.[10]

MONITORING THE INFANT DURING MECHANICAL VENTILATION

During mechanical ventilation, the clinician undertakes the responsibility for the

Table 11-2.		Effect of Ventilator Setting Changes on Blood Gases			
	Change	Paco$_2$	Pao$_2$	Comments	
PIP	↑	↓	↑	Use of high PIP increases risk of barotrauma (e.g., pneumothorax, interstitial emphysema)	
	↓	↑	↓		
PEEP	↑	↑	↑	An increase in PEEP prevents alveolar collapse and improves ventilation/perfusion relationship. A PEEP of 2 to 3 cm H$_2$O is physiologic. A higher PEEP is indicated in babies with RDS.	
	↓	↓	↓	A decrease in PEEP may improve compliance and may improve CO$_2$ retention. Very high PEEP (e.g., >6 cm H$_2$O) is not very effective in increasing Pao$_2$.	
Frequency	↑	↓	—	High ventilator frequencies may allow the use of low PIP and reduce the risk of pneumothorax. If I/E ratio is kept constant, frequency changes do not alter mean airway pressure and do not substantially affect Pao$_2$.	
	↓	↑	—		
I/E Ratio	↑	—	↑	I/E ratio changes do not usually alter tidal volume or CO$_2$ elimination unless inspiratory time or expiratory time, or both, are too short.	
	↓	—	↓		
Flow	↑	± ↓	± ↑	The effects of flow changes on blood gases have not been well studied in infants.	
	↓	± ↑	± ↓		

I/E ratio, Inspiratory to expiratory ratio; *PEEP,* positive end-expiratory pressure; *PIP,* peak inspiratory pressure; *RDS,* respiratory distress syndrome.

infant's gas exchange. Hence, monitoring the patient's condition is vital and requires continuous observation.

The goal should be to maintain Pao_2 between 40 and 60 mm Hg, $Paco_2$ at more than 40 mm Hg, and pH between 7.25 and 7.40. Continuous monitoring with a pulse oximeter and transcutaneous Pco_2 and Po_2 electrodes or a catheter electrode is invaluable during intubation, stabilization procedures, or weaning because blood gases can change abruptly. Because arterial CO_2 equilibrates with alveolar CO_2, quantitative end-tidal CO_2 monitoring can be used to estimate arterial CO_2. However, in patients with alveolar disease, there is incomplete equilibration of arterial and alveolar CO_2; therefore, end-tidal CO_2 can underestimate arterial CO_2. Neonatal qualitative exhaled CO_2 monitoring is extremely useful in determining endotracheal tube placement because the diagnostic accuracy approximates 100%.[12]

CHANGES IN BLOOD GAS STATUS

A Practical Approach

1. *A sudden decrease in* Pao_2 *accompanied by an increase in* $Paco_2$ *associated with rapid clinical deterioration of the infant.* To differentiate whether the problem is with the ventilator or the infant, disconnect the ventilator from the infant and manually inflate the infant's lungs.

If the infant's condition improves, the problem is with the ventilator. Check the following:
- Concentration of inspired oxygen going to the ventilator
- Presence of leaks or disconnected tubing
- Mechanical or electrical failure

If the infant shows no clinical improvement with manual inflation, the problem is with the infant. Check gas entry bilaterally by auscultation, listen over the stomach, and determine the position of the heart and trachea. If gas entry is diminished bilaterally, look for the following causes:
- Tube displaced into nasopharynx. There may be gas entry heard over the stomach, and gas may be visibly escaping at the mouth or via a nasogastric tube with the end placed under water. Action—Replace the tube.
- Tube blocked. Tube blockage occurs especially after a few days of ventilation and afterward because of the increased accumulation of secretions. Action—Suction tube briefly. If this has no effect, replace the tube.

- Tension pneumothorax. Diminished breath sounds are heard on the affected side and there may also be abdominal distention and an easily palpable liver and spleen; the condition is usually critical. Action—Emergency relief of tension pneumothorax by inserting a chest tube or a 22-gauge catheter attached to a three-way stopcock and a 20-mL syringe into the third intercostal space at the midclavicular line or the fourth or fifth intercostal space at the anterior axillary line. Remove gas until the condition improves. If the infant has deteriorated do NOT wait for a chest radiograph to perform the procedure. After stabilizing the infant, obtain a chest radiograph and consider inserting a chest tube.

If gas entry is diminished unilaterally, check for the following causes:
- Tube in mainstem bronchus. It is usually in the right mainstem bronchus, producing decreased gas entry on the left. Action–Verify endotracheal tube measurement at the lip level. Withdraw tube 0.5 to 1 cm. Immediate improvement in gas entry will result. Recheck position by chest x-ray.
- Unilateral pneumothorax. Radiologic confirmation of clinical diagnosis is obtained if the condition of the infant warrants a delay in initiating therapy. If not, treat as for tension pneumothorax.

If gas entry is not diminished and the infant does not improve with manual lung inflation, this suggests a nonrespiratory cause such as intraventricular hemorrhage, pneumopericardium, convulsions, hypoglycemia, hypotension, or overwhelming sepsis. The incidence of intraventricular hemorrhage is greatly increased in infants who have a pneumothorax. The occasional occurrence of pneumoperitoneum, owing to forcing gas through the diaphragm in the periaortic spaces, can seriously mislead the clinician into the assumption that a ruptured viscus has occurred and abdominal surgery is indicated.

EDITORIAL COMMENT: Airway sounds are easily transmitted across a small chest, and therefore evaluation of breath sounds can be terribly misleading in small infants. Even with "adequate" breath sounds, I would transilluminate the chest, check the placement of the endotracheal tube with a laryngoscope, and perhaps replace the endotracheal tube before attributing the problem to a nonrespiratory etiology.

John Kattwinkel

2. *Gradual decrease in Pao_2 accompanied by an increase in $Paco_2$ associated with gradual deterioration of the infant.* This suggests inappropriate ventilator settings. A decrease in Pao_2 suggests increasing intrapulmonary shunting resulting from progressive atelectasis.

To improve Pao_2, consider the following measures:
- Increase PIP
- Increase PEEP
- Increase tidal volume by 1 to 2 mL/kg (increases PIP; volume ventilator)
- Increase the I/E ratio or the inspiratory time
- The responses to these maneuvers may vary, and blood gas analyses must be obtained.

3. *Gradual increase in $Paco_2$ without gross changes in Pao_2.* A gradual increase in $Paco_2$ is usually due to insufficient alveolar ventilation (insufficient tidal volume or frequency, or both). A gradual increase in $Paco_2$ can also be due to increased "anatomic" (i.e., airways, tubing) or "physiologic" (i.e., nonventilated but perfused alveoli) dead space. An increase in $Paco_2$ is an indication for an increase in alveolar ventilation by increasing PIP or decreasing PEEP during pressure ventilation, by increasing tidal volume during volume ventilation, or by increasing cycling frequency. A reduction of anatomic dead space (e.g., shortening the endotracheal tube) may relieve hypercapnia.

To improve $Paco_2$, increase minute ventilation by the following measures:
- Increase PIP by 2 to 5 cm H_2O (pressure ventilator)
- Increase tidal volume by 1 to 2 mL/kg (increases PIP; volume ventilator)
- Increase ventilator rate by 5 to 10 breaths/minute

4. *A decrease in $Paco_2$ caused by overventilation.* A decrease in $Paco_2$ is potentially dangerous because alkalosis is associated with decreases in cerebral blood flow and tissue oxygen delivery. Hypocarbia is also associated with periventricular leukomalacia as well as deafness. The lungs may be subjected to volutrauma if the low $Paco_2$ is the result of ventilation with large tidal volumes. Hence, a low $Paco_2$ is an indication for a reduction in overall alveolar ventilation.

5. *Increase in Pao_2 unaccompanied by changes in $Paco_2$.* This suggests a decrease in intrapulmonary shunting and reduction in degree of atelectasis. Because of the toxic effect of high inspired oxygen on lung tissue but the benefits of maintaining lung inflation, it is generally better to reduce the concentration of inspired oxygen to less than 40% to 70% before attempting to markedly reduce ventilator parameters.

ROUTINE CARE OF THE INFANT

Monitoring of blood gases and respiratory status is an important aspect of supportive treatment, but attention must also be paid to temperature control, caloric and fluid intake, and metabolic balance. Clinicians should avoid excessive and unnecessary handling of the infant. Measures such as elevating the head of the bed 15 to 30 degrees, mouth care, daily assessments of readiness for extubation, and strict attention to hand hygiene may decrease the incidence of ventilator associated pneumonia.

SPECIAL CIRCUMSTANCES

PULMONARY INTERSTITIAL EMPHYSEMA

Infants with severe RDS and those who have pulmonary interstitial emphysema (PIE) on chest x-ray may respond better to a rapid ventilating rate (60 to 150 breaths/minute), low peak pressure, low PEEP, and high-frequency ventilation.

PULMONARY HYPERTENSION/ MECONIUM ASPIRATION SYNDROME

Infants with severe pulmonary hypertension with or without meconium aspiration syndrome may benefit from inhaled nitric oxide, a selective pulmonary vasodilator. Nitric oxide reduces the need for extracorporeal membrane oxygenation (ECMO) in neonates with pulmonary hypertension.[13] Other therapies include oxygen, surfactant, sedation, analgesia, and inotropic support, but there are limited data to support their clinical efficacy.

NEONATAL SURGERY

Intubation of the very low-birth-weight infant in the intensive care nursery and use of a ventilator during surgery are preferable. In this way, inspired oxygen and inspired gas temperature can be carefully controlled, as can pain management. Continuous oxygen saturation and intermittent arterial blood gas analyses are monitored throughout surgery to maintain the infant with adequate blood gases.

DRUG THERAPY

The use of muscle paralysis may be invaluable in infants who "fight" the ventilator when Pa_{CO_2} is increasing and Pa_{O_2} is decreasing on "maximum" ventilation. A marked improvement in oxygenation may be observed, particularly in infants with pulmonary hypertension.

> **EDITORIAL COMMENT:** Muscle paralysis for babies on ventilators must be viewed with caution. The histamine-releasing effect of competitive neuromuscular blocking agents (particularly curare) can cause hypotension and, rarely, bronchospasm. Some patients may require higher ventilator settings after paralysis as their own respiratory efforts are eliminated. Also, a system failure (e.g., extubation, tubing disconnection) in a paralyzed patient will be rapidly fatal.
>
> *John Kattwinkel*

Sedatives and analgesics are increasingly being used in the care of neonates requiring assisted ventilation. These agents may be used in combination with muscle paralysis. However, when it is desirable to preserve the patient's own respiratory effort, sedatives or analgesics may be used without muscle paralysis. Fentanyl and morphine sulfate are commonly used sedatives/analgesics. Sedatives and analgesics may decrease respiratory drive and should be used carefully. Routine opiate administration during conventional ventilation in neonates has not been shown to improve outcomes.[14]

Antibiotics should be used whenever a bacterial infection is suspected.

Preextubation systemic corticosteroids and postextubation racemic epinephrine reduces airway resistance when there is laryngeal edema. However, if the endotracheal tube is not too large, is well positioned, and is not mobile during ventilation, problems with the glottis following extubation are rarely observed.

WEANING FROM VENTILATOR

Ventilator weaning can be attempted when the concentration of inspired oxygen is approximately 50% or less. The PIP is gradually reduced as is the ventilator rate to allow the patient to contribute more to his or her ventilation. When the ventilator breaths elicit minimal chest rise, ventilator frequency is minimal (~10/minute), and the infant has adequate blood gases, the infant should be accomplishing almost all of the minute ventilation spontaneously. At this point, most infants can be successfully extubated to CPAP.

HIGH-FREQUENCY VENTILATION

Although conventional mechanical ventilation has contributed to a substantial reduction in neonatal mortality, air leaks or BPD occurs in about 20% to 40% of ventilated infants. Although the precise pathophysiologic mechanisms underlying these forms of lung injury have not been determined, high ventilatory pressures and the resultant volutrauma are thought to be contributing factors.

High-frequency ventilation encompasses modes of assisted ventilation that employ smaller tidal volumes and higher frequencies than conventional techniques. The characteristics of the various high-frequency ventilators overlap (Table 11-3). Furthermore, clinicians may employ widely varying ventilatory strategies. High-frequency ventilation may improve blood gases because, in addition to the gas transport by convection, other mechanisms may become active at high frequencies (for example, variable velocity profiles of gas during inspiration and exhalation, gas exchange between parallel lung units, increased turbulence, and diffusion may improve blood gases).

High-frequency positive-pressure ventilators employ standard ventilators modified with low-compliance tubing and connectors so that an adequate tidal volume may be delivered despite very short inspiratory times. High-frequency jet ventilation is characterized by the delivery of gases from a high-pressure

Table 11-3.	Techniques for High-Frequency Ventilation			
	HFPPV	**Jet Ventilation**	**Flow Interruption**	**Oscillatory Ventilation**
Tidal volume	> Dead space	> or < Dead space	> or < Dead space	< Dead space
Expiration	Passive	Passive	Passive	Active
Airway pressure waveform	Variable	Triangular	Triangular	Sine wave
Frequency	60-150/min	60-600/min	300-900/min	300-900/min

HFPPV, High-frequency positive pressure ventilation; >, larger than; <, smaller than.

source through a small-bore injector cannula. It is possible that the fast flows out of the cannula produce areas of relative negative pressure that entrain gases from their surroundings. High-frequency flow interruption also delivers small tidal volumes by interrupting a flow of pressure source, but in contrast to jet ventilation, it does not use an injector cannula. High-frequency oscillatory ventilation can exchange gas adequately with small volumes (even smaller than dead space at times) at extremely high frequencies. Oscillatory ventilation is unique because exhalation is actively generated, as opposed to other forms of high-frequency ventilation, in which exhalation is passive.

RESPIRATORY DISTRESS SYNDROME

There has been extensive clinical use of the various high-frequency ventilators in neonates with RDS. High-frequency positive pressure using rates of 60 breaths/minute (with inspiratory times less than 0.5 seconds) versus 30 to 40 breaths/minute for conventional mechanical ventilation with inspiratory times longer than 0.5 seconds) decreases air leaks.[15] High-frequency oscillator ventilation does not offer important advantages over conventional ventilation. High frequency oscillator ventilation may decrease BPD but it may increase air leaks.[16]

AIR LEAKS

High-frequency ventilation has been used to treat established air leaks. Jet ventilation in neonates with pulmonary interstitial emphysema may accelerate resolution of the air leak.[17] However, air leaks may be increased with oscillatory ventilation.[16]

Table 11-4.	Complications of Assisted Ventilation
Pulmonary air leaks	Pneumothorax, pneumomediastinum, pneumoperitoneum, pulmonary interstitial emphysema, pneumopericardium, pulmonary venous air embolism
Airway injury	Erosion, granuloma, palatal groove, subglottic stenosis, necrotizing tracheobronchitis
Endotracheal tube related	Dislodgement, extubation, atelectasis, occlusion, tracheal stenosis, vocal cord paralysis
Infection	Pneumonia, septicemia, meningitis
Miscellaneous	Volutrauma, bronchopulmonary dysplasia, hyperinflation, impaired cardiac output, intracranial hemorrhage, patent ductus arteriosus, retinopathy of prematurity

EDITORIAL COMMENT: The technique of high-frequency ventilation requires major changes in the concept of gas flow in the lung. Currently it is believed that by vibrating the gas column, gas exchange is promoted by setting up asymmetric flow within the airways rather than by convection, which is the predominant mechanism of conventional ventilation. Studies suggest that high-frequency ventilation may improve ventilation/perfusion matching throughout the respiratory cycle, thus permitting lower peak inflation pressures and lower inspired oxygen concentrations. High pressure, high volume and high oxygen have all been implicated in the development of bronchopulmonary dysplasia.

John Kattwinkel

COMPLICATIONS OF ASSISTED VENTILATION

Despite major improvements in equipment and increased expertise in the applications of assisted ventilation, the care of smaller and sicker infants may result in many complications (Table 11-4). Pulmonary air leaks are one of the most common complications and occur in approximately 5% to 10% of ventilated patients. Pneumothorax may occur due to the lung disease or may result from the use of high PIP and inspiratory time, particularly in infants who "fight" the ventilator. However, spontaneous pneumothoraces are commonly observed, even in healthy neonates without lung disease. Transillumination of the chest is extremely useful for immediate diagnosis, but radiographic confirmation should be obtained if the patient's status is not life threatening. PIE, an air leak usually secondary to the use of high airway pressures, is associated with gas trapping and impaired gas exchange.

Bronchopulmonary dysplasia, a form of chronic lung disease that occurs in neonates, is one of the most important complications associated with assisted ventilation. BPD was initially defined as an oxygen requirement and characteristic chest x-ray at 28 days of life. With the increasing survival of ELBW infants, the definition was changed to an oxygen requirement at 36 weeks' postmenstrual age. The chest x-ray of infants with BPD often shows opacification of the lung fields, atelectasis, fibrosis, and overdistention. Although its precise pathophysiology remains obscure, volutrauma appears to be a contributing factor. The increasing incidence of BPD is largely due to improved survival rates of infants with immature or ill lungs. The incidence of BPD varies widely and may be as high as 50% in infants weighing less than 1000 g who require assisted ventilation from birth. Management of these patients must be multidimensional, with particular emphasis on prevention of further lung injury, maintenance of adequate oxygenation and nutrition, and prevention of infection and fluid overload. The effect of differences in care practices on the incidence of BPD suggests that optimal respiratory management of very low-birth-weight infants may decrease the incidence of BPD.[18] As discussed previously, clinical trials of early CPAP and minimal ventilation strategies have shown moderate reductions in the incidence of death and/or BPD.

EXTRACORPOREAL MEMBRANE OXYGENATION

ECMO is a technique whereby blood drains from the patient; then the blood passes through a membrane for extracorporeal exchange of oxygen and carbon dioxide; and is then routed back to the patient. ECMO is particularly useful in neonates with transient pulmonary artery hypertension and severe hypoxemia resulting from a right-to-left shunt. Common conditions associated with pulmonary hypertension include meconium aspiration syndrome, RDS, idiopathic pulmonary hypertension of the neonate, pneumonia/sepsis, asphyxia, and congenital diaphragmatic hernia. Neonates with these and other conditions are considered candidates for ECMO if they have severe impairment of oxygenation. The alveolar-to-arterial oxygen gradient (A/aDO_2) is frequently used to evaluate impairment of oxygenation. An alveolar-arterial oxygenation gradient of 600 to 620 for 8 to 12 hours despite maximal therapy is usually considered an indication for ECMO. In the past, predicted survival rate for infants with such severe respiratory failure was as low as 20%. In marked contrast, following the introduction of ECMO, survival currently approximates 90% in these infants.

Complications during ECMO may be related to the primary disease or to technical aspects of the circuit. Intracranial hemorrhage and infarction, hemodynamic alterations, and hematologic disturbances occur occasionally. The improved survival rate has not been accompanied by an increase in permanent morbidity.

INHALED NITRIC OXIDE

High pulmonary artery resistance is common in infants with pulmonary disease.

Pulmonary artery vasodilators have been used in treatment of these infants, but the systemic vasodilatory effects have precluded efficacy and widespread use. Nitric oxide, a molecule produced endogenously by endothelial cells and other cell types, regulates pulmonary artery tone in utero and after birth. Exogenous nitric oxide reduces pulmonary vascular resistance during the perinatal period. Inhaled nitric oxide has been shown to improve oxygenation and reduce the need for ECMO in well-designed, large, randomized, controlled trials in term and late preterm neonates with severe hypoxemic respiratory failure.[19] However, inhaled nitric oxide has not been shown to have consistent benefits in preterm infants with RDS.[20]

SUMMARY

Survival of infants with severe pulmonary disease has dramatically improved with the introduction of techniques of assisted ventilation. Meticulous care is necessary with the following: strategies to optimize conventional ventilation; placement of endotracheal tubes; frequent blood gas determinations; continuous monitoring of oxygen saturation, transcutaneous Po_2, and transcutaneous Pco_2; and, fluid, caloric, and thermal balance. However, most of the difficulty with adequately ventilating small infants resides not in the ventilator, but in the infant's lungs and airways. The clinician should identify and correct atelectasis, increased dead space, and gas trapping and treat the patient's pulmonary problems with appropriate ventilatory strategies rather than look for a better ventilator to solve the problems. Long-term morbidity associated with mechanical ventilation is still a major problem. Because assisted ventilation is a critical part of neonatal intensive care, a thorough understanding of pulmonary mechanics and gas exchange, as well as knowledge of the techniques and alternative modes of ventilation, is essential to optimize its use.

QUESTIONS

True or False

If you set a pressure-limited safety valve on a volume-controlled ventilator at 30 cm H_2O, a pneumothorax will not occur.

Although pneumothorax is particularly associated with high inflation pressures, it can occur at any time during either mechanical or spontaneous ventilation—even at low PIP. The statement is false.

The larger the volume of ventilator tubing, the less the compression volume at any given pressure.

During ventilation, a proportion of the gas delivered by the pump ("compression volume") does not reach the alveoli. The larger the volume of ventilator tubing, the greater the compression volume. Hence, ventilator tubing should be low volume and nondistensible. The statement is false.

Condensation of water in ventilator inspiratory tubing can be reduced by placing as much tubing as possible inside the incubator.

A temperature gradient exists between air outside and inside the incubator. Water vapor condenses at lower temperatures, and droplets appear in tubing exposed to low temperatures. If water condensation occurs in the tubing, the gas delivered to the infant will have a water saturation lower than gas coming out of the humidifier. Heated ventilator tubing can also reduce condensation. The statement is true.

If a small leak develops between the trachea and the endotracheal tube during pressure-controlled ventilation, there will be adequate compensation by the ventilator.

A pressure-controlled ventilator delivers gas until a preset pressure is attained. Although it is possible to compensate for a small leak (e.g., around the endotracheal tube); a large leak may cause failure to reach the desired PIP. The statement is true.

During mechanical ventilation with 80% oxygen (for RDS), an increase in PIP may increase the Pa_{O_2} to 200 mm Hg without altering Pa_{CO_2} significantly.

When breathing a high concentration of oxygen, a low Pa_{O_2} indicates venous admixture or shunting. This shunting is thought to occur primarily through areas of atelectatic lung. Effective ventilation may open some of these atelectatic areas, reducing the degree of shunting, with an ensuing increase in Pa_{O_2}. However, a large right-to-left shunt may not increase Pa_{CO_2} markedly because the arteriovenous difference for CO_2 is only 4 mm Hg. Resolution of the shunt may not decrease Pa_{CO_2}, so the statement is true.

During mechanical ventilation, pH remains constant as long as the Pa_{CO_2} does not change.

The pH depends on the Pa_{CO_2} and the bicarbonate level. Metabolic and respiratory factors are often closely associated (e.g., a period of apnea is associated with an increase in Pa_{CO_2} and a decrease in Pa_{O_2}, the latter leading to tissue anoxia and anaerobic metabolism). However, metabolic and respiratory factors may operate quite independently. The statement is false.

CASE 1

You are called to attend the delivery of a 26 weeks' gestational-age infant whose mother received a full course of antenatal steroids.

After resuscitation with bag and mask ventilation, the infant requires 30% F_{IO_2}. A trial of CPAP is indicated in this infant. True or false?

CPAP used early in preference of mechanical ventilation reduces lung injury. The statement is true.

Surfactant should be given as soon as possible to this infant because it has been shown to improve outcomes. True or false?

Surfactant prophylaxis and early surfactant were shown to reduce mortality and air leaks when compared to intubation without surfactant. However, the new trials of CPAP versus early surfactant have shown no benefits of prophylactic or early surfactant. The statement is false.

CASE 2

Before mechanical ventilation using a pressure-limited ventilator, the Pa_{O_2} is 30 mm Hg and the Pa_{CO_2} is 60 mm Hg in 100% oxygen in a preterm baby. Thirty minutes after initiating therapy, a blood gas analysis is performed.

Pa_{O_2} has risen to only 35 mm Hg, and Pa_{CO_2} is still 60 mm Hg. It is advisable to switch to a volume-controlled ventilator because the lungs are too stiff to be adequately

ventilated by a pressure-controlled machine. True or false?

The statement is false. The initial ventilator settings were probably somewhat subjective and should be adjusted to the infant's requirements. The high $Paco_2$ indicates hypoventilation, and an attempt should be made to increase minute ventilation by increasing PIP. The increase in PIP should also improve oxygenation. Adjustments should be made every 10 minutes, checking blood gases until oxygen saturation is higher than 85% and $Paco_2$ is less than approximately 50 mm Hg.

Pao_2 is only 35 mm Hg and $Paco_2$ is 35 mm Hg. It might be helpful to increase PEEP before increasing PIP further. True or false?

A positive end-expiratory pressure of 5 to 6 cm H_2O will help to prevent small airway closure. This may prevent atelectasis and reduce the degree of right-to-left shunt. The statement is true.

The Pao_2 has risen to 140 mm Hg. This is a dangerous level, and the concentrations of inspired oxygen should be reduced at once. True or false?

In immature infants, arterial oxygen tensions in that range have been associated with retinopathy of prematurity. The statement is true. Priority should be given to reducing the concentration of inspired oxygen in this situation versus altering other ventilator settings. Decrease inspired oxygen concentrations frequently and continuously monitor oxygen saturation.

CASE 3

A blood gas analysis is performed during mechanical ventilation on 80% oxygen. There has been no change in the clinical condition of the infant since the previous estimation.

It is found that $Paco_2$ has changed from 36 to 24 mm Hg and pH has risen from 7.38 to 7.56. This is a sign that the infant is recovering and ventilator settings should remain unchanged. True or false?

A $Paco_2$ of 24 mm Hg suggests overventilation. The resulting alkalosis is dangerous because it causes a reduction in oxygen delivery and cerebral blood flow and may be associated with lung injury. The $Paco_2$ should be brought back to a more physiologic range by reducing minute ventilation (i.e., by reducing PIP, tidal volume, or frequency). The statement is false.

The arterial oxygen tension is 30 mm Hg; pH is 7.30; and $Paco_2$ is 45 mm Hg. The ventilator should not be changed. True or false?

$Paco_2$ and pH are satisfactory, but oxygenation is too low. PEEP can be increased to increase mean airway pressure. The statement is false.

The arterial oxygen tension is 56 mm Hg; pH is 7.23, and $Paco_2$ is 26 mm Hg on low ventilator settings. Although the pH is within normal range, there is severe metabolic acidosis, which should be corrected with intravenous sodium bicarbonate. True or false?

Spontaneous hyperventilation on the ventilator may be due to compensation for a metabolic acidosis. Correction of severe metabolic acidosis is indicated with intravenous bicarbonate. However, search should be made for the etiology of the acidosis, such as reduced cardiac output, anemia, sepsis, or pneumothorax, and the underlying cause corrected.

CASE 4

During mechanical ventilation, an infant becomes cyanotic. He is noted to be making very vigorous respiratory efforts with considerable intercostal and sternal retractions out of phase with the ventilator.

This is a good indication for sedation and adjusting the ventilator to accommodate the infant's respiratory pattern. True or false?

Although "out of phase" respiration could account for this clinical picture, an obstructed endotracheal tube, a pneumothorax, or other major problem must first be excluded. The statement is false.

Gas entry is diminished over the left lung field. The diagnosis is pneumothorax, which should be relieved immediately. True or false?

Diminution of gas entry over the left lung field may be due to (1) the endotracheal tube slipping into the right mainstem bronchus or (2) pneumothorax. The steps should be to check the endotracheal tube length of insertion (at the lip) and, if necessary, to withdraw the endotracheal tube slightly. If this fails to improve the infant's condition, a chest x-ray is indicated unless the infant is deteriorating rapidly and the left side of the chest is tympanic, transillumination is positive, and the heart is displaced. Emergency relief of a pneumothorax is then indicated. The statement is false.

A sample for blood gas estimation is obtained immediately and resuscitative measures are started. When the blood sample is analyzed 1 hour later, the results show Pao_2 to be 127 mm Hg and $Paco_2$ to

be 8 mm Hg. This suggests that the infant had been crying before this cyanotic spell. True or false?

The most likely explanation for these bizarre blood gas findings is that an air bubble was left in the syringe and equilibration has occurred between gas in the blood and gas in the air. The values tend to approximate the Pao_2 and $Paco_2$ of room air. Samples drawn for blood gases must be bubble free, capped, iced, and analyzed immediately. The statement is false.

Following prolonged mechanical ventilation and extubation, an infant may have some stridor and copious secretions. The stridor usually decreases spontaneously. True or false?

Despite the use of nontoxic endotracheal tubes, there can be some laryngeal edema. This, together with large quantities of secretions and lack of tracheal cilia, may lead to some degree of upper airway obstruction, which decreases in 2 to 3 days. The statement is true.

CASE 5

A 1500-g male infant delivered precipitously after 31 weeks' gestation, whose mother had not received antenatal steroids, had signs of respiratory distress at birth. Apgar scores were 4 and 7 at 1 and 5 minutes, respectively. At initial assessment, the infant was tachypneic (60 breaths/minute) and had nasal flaring and retractions. Breath sounds were equal but diminished bilaterally. Dubowitz examination was consistent with maternal dates. Immediate chest x-ray showed diffuse granularity and air bronchograms. Blood sugar was 45 mg/dL, hematocrit 43%, blood pressure 50/32 (mean 40 mm Hg), and temperature 36.3° C. In 55% oxygen by CPAP, arterial blood gas values from an umbilical catheter were as follows: pH 7.15, Pco_2 55, and Po_2 40. The infant was intubated, given surfactant, and placed on a pressure-limited ventilator at PIP of 15 cm H_2O, PEEP of 4 cm H_2O, frequency (rate) of 50 breaths/minute, I/E ratio of 1:5, and Fio_2 of 50%. The patient initially responded well, but 2 hours later, arterial blood gas values were as follows: pH 7.30, Pco_2 46, and Po_2 35.

NOTE: There may be several arterial blood gases and ventilator changes between each situation presented. Assume good breath sounds, chest rise, and blood pressure throughout, unless otherwise stated. Attempting to answer questions by looking at data subsequently presented is only confusing.

Select the **best** answer, although more than one answer may be acceptable.

What is the most appropriate ventilator setting change at this time?

1. Increase PIP
2. Increase PEEP
3. Increase frequency
4. Decrease I/E ratio (e.g., 1:3 to 1:3.5)
5. Increase Fio_2

The patient has hypoxemia with adequate ventilation and relatively low Fio_2. The best answer is to increase Fio_2.

At 12 hours of age, the ventilator settings and arterial blood gas values are pressure 20/4 cm H_2O, frequency 50 breaths/minute, I/E ratio 1:1.5, Fio_2 80%, pH 7.16, $Paco_2$ 55 mm Hg, and Pao2 135 mm Hg. What is the most appropriate change at this time?

1. Decrease PIP and decrease Fio_2
2. Increase PEEP and decrease Fio_2
3. Increase frequency and decrease Fio_2
4. Increase I/E ratio and decrease Fio_2
5. Decrease I/E ratio and decrease Fio_2

The patient has hyperoxemia and mild respiratory acidosis. Of the alternatives given, increasing frequency is the most effective way to increase minute ventilation and resolve the respiratory acidosis. Fio_2 should be decreased.

At 18 hours of age, the ventilator settings and arterial blood gas values are pressure 20/5 cm H_2O, frequency 70 breaths/minute, I/E ratio 1:1, Fio_2 90%, pH 7.19, $Paco_2$ 52 mm Hg, and Pao_2 35 mm Hg. What is the most appropriate change at this time?

1. Increase PIP
2. Increase PEEP
3. Increase frequency
4. Increase I/E ratio
5. Increase Fio_2

Respiratory acidosis is still present but is now accompanied by hypoxemia. Increasing peak PIP is the best choice because the resultant increase in minute ventilation and mean airway pressure should improve $Paco_2$ and Pao_2. Increasing frequency is also an acceptable alternative.

REFERENCES

The reference list for this chapter can be found online at www.expertconsult.com.

Glucose, Calcium, and Magnesium

12

Michael R. Uhing and Robert M. Kliegman

These infants are remarkable not only because like foetal versions of Shadrach, Meshach and Abednego, they emerge at least alive from within the fiery metabolic furnace of diabetes mellitus, but because they resemble one another so closely that they might well be related. They are plump, sleek, liberally coated with vernix caseosa, full-faced and plethoric. … They convey a distinct impression of having had such a surfeit of both food and fluid pressed upon them by an insistent hostess that they desire only peace so that they may recover from their excesses. And on the second day their resentment of the slightest noise improves the analogy while their trembling anxiety seems to speak of intrauterine indiscretions of which we know nothing.

*James W. Farquhar** *

The newborn emerges from a uterine environment in which glucose, calcium, and magnesium have been continuously provided and fetal plasma levels are closely regulated, in part by maternal metabolic homeostasis and placental exchange, as well as by fetal regulatory mechanisms. Abrupt termination of nutrient supply at birth requires profound changes in energy and mineral metabolism, depending on the provision of exogenous nutrients and the mobilization of endogenous fuel and mineral stores. The result is the potential for rapid changes in plasma glucose and calcium levels during the first days of life. The infant who is premature, growth restricted, stressed, or born to a diabetic mother is at increased risk for problems with homeostasis, and hypoglycemia or hypocalcemia can develop.

Broad surveys using modern analytic methods demonstrated that glucose and calcium problems are common, are frequently asymptomatic, and thus often go unrecognized in high-risk infants. Since that time, changing routines of care to include prevention, early identification, and metabolic support of the sick newborn has made severe hypoglycemia and hypocalcemia infrequent problems.

GLUCOSE

FETAL AND NEONATAL ENERGY METABOLISM

A composite picture of fetal and neonatal fuel metabolism has emerged from studies in animals and humans.[1] Fetal energy consumption is high, deriving from growth needs and energy storage as well as metabolic maintenance. Maternal glucose crosses the placenta via facilitated diffusion (primarily by the glucose transporters GLUT1 and GLUT3) and serves as the principal energy source for the fetus. There is a linear relationship between maternal and fetal glucose concentrations, with fetal concentrations 60% to 80% of maternal concentrations.[2] This linear relationship is present even during episodes of maternal hyperglycemia secondary to maternal diabetes or glucose infusions.

Under normal circumstances, fetal gluconeogenesis is negligible; however, fetal gluconeogenesis may occur during episodes of prolonged maternal hypoglycemia or starvation. Glucose alone cannot account for the total oxygen consumption of the fetus. Other substrates such as lactate, free fatty acids, ketones, and amino acids cross the placenta and are potential energy sources for the fetus.

---

*Farquhar JW: The child of the diabetic woman, Arch Dis Child 34:76, 1959.

Energy is stored rapidly near term. Fat storage exceeds 100 kcal/day in the ninth month and accounts for 14% of total body weight at term.[3] Glycogen stores, a vital source of energy in the first hours of life, increase toward term to reach about 5% by weight in liver and muscle and up to 4% in heart muscle. These energy stores are compromised by prematurity and by intrauterine growth restriction. Acute perinatal distress or chronic fetal hypoxia can particularly diminish glycogen stores and predispose the infant to hypoglycemia after birth.

Insulin and glucagon do not cross the placenta and are present in the fetus by 12 and 15 weeks, respectively. The fetal insulin response to glucose infusion is poor very early in gestation. At the end of gestation, the insulin response is improved but remains blunted. Fetal blood insulin levels gradually rise toward term, whereas fetal glucagon levels remain low. The resulting high insulin-to-glucagon ratio promotes the accumulation of hepatic glycogen stores and suppresses gluconeogenesis.

Insulin is an important hormone for fetal growth. The presence of maternal hyperglycemia and fetal hyperinsulinemia as seen in the infant of a diabetic mother is associated with macrosomia with elevated liver glycogen and total body fat stores.[4,5] Macrosomia in the presence of fetal hyperinsulinemia without maternal hyperglycemia is seen in infants with Beckwith-Wiedemann syndrome and in the rare infant with hyperinsulinemic hypoglycemia, which suggests that fetal insulin and *not maternal hyperglycemia* may be the important growth-promoting factor. Furthermore, infants born with pancreatic aplasia and those with transient neonatal diabetes mellitus have little or no insulin present and demonstrate severe intrauterine growth restriction.

At birth, cold stress, work of respiration, and muscle activity cause increased energy demands. Because of the interrupted supply of maternal glucose, the newborn must call on stored fuels to maintain blood glucose levels. This transition at birth is facilitated by increased catecholamine and glucagon levels, which promote lipolysis and glycogenolysis. Decreased insulin levels and increased cortisol levels also facilitate glucose homeostasis at birth. Rapid glycogenolysis causes hepatic glycogen to fall to low levels within 24 hours in a fasted neonate. Because the newborn has a twofold greater basal fasting glucose utilization than the adult, gluconeogenesis must supplement glycogenolysis. Lipolysis begins at birth, with the respiratory quotient decreasing from 1.0 in the fetus to less than 0.8 during the first day as most tissues switch to burning fat. Metabolism of free fatty acids and ketones stabilizes blood glucose levels by (1) sparing glucose utilization in heart, liver, muscle, and brain (ketones) and (2) supporting hepatic gluconeogenesis by producing the reduced form of nicotinamide adenine dinucleotide (NADH).

In the newborn, basal glucose production and utilization is 4 to 6 mg/kg/min. This high glucose utilization compared with the adult is primarily due to the higher ratio of brain weight to body weight in the newborn infant. During euglycemic conditions most of the brain's metabolic needs are met by oxidation of glucose. When the availability of glucose is limited, alternative cerebral fuels such as lactate and ketone bodies may by used. Although these alternative fuels provide some protection to reduce the risk of hypoglycemia-induced brain injury in the newborn, the brain requires a continuous glucose supply; thus, these alternative substrates are unable to completely replace glucose as a fuel for brain metabolism.

Blood glucose level at birth is 60% to 80% of the simultaneous maternal plasma concentrations. Glucose concentrations normally decrease over 1 to 2 hours, stabilize at a minimum of 40 to 45 mg/dL, and then increase by 6 hours to 50 to 60 mg/dL in healthy unstressed newborns (Fig. 12-1). The current practice of early oral or intravenous alimentation avoids the many instances of neonatal hypoglycemia previously reported when neonates fasted for 24 hours (Fig. 12-2).

METHODOLOGY

Sampling Problems

Several factors need to be considered when interpreting glucose concentrations. First, blood glucose concentrations are 10% to 15% lower than simultaneous plasma concentrations. This is particularly pronounced when the hematocrit is very high.[6] Second, use of capillary samples from unwarmed heels may lead to an underestimation of venous glucose concentration because of stasis. Finally, glucose concentrations decline as much as 18 mg/dL/hr at room temperature while analysis is awaited. Thus, all samples should be analyzed immediately or placed on ice.

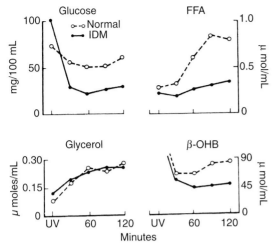

Figure 12-1. Fuel metabolism in infants of "controlled" diabetic mothers. Glucose, free fatty acid (FFA), β-hydroxybutyrate (βOHB) in normal infants *(open circles)* and infants of diabetic mothers (IDMs) *(filled circles)*. Note that not only does blood glucose level decline more abruptly in the IDMs, but FFA and ketones increase less. The blood glucose concentration spontaneously increases over the next 4 to 6 hours. *(From Persson B, Gentz J, Kellum M, et al: Metabolic observations in infants of strictly controlled diabetic mothers. II. Plasma insulin, FFA, glycerol, β-hydroxybutyrate during intravenous glucose tolerance test,* Acta Paediatr Scand *65:1,1976.)*

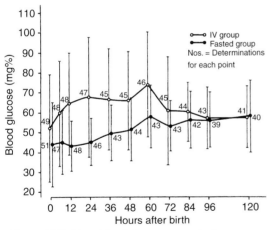

Figure 12-2. Mean blood glucose concentration as a function of age in infants receiving early intravenous (IV) feedings and in fasted infants. Bars indicate ±1 standard deviation. *(From Mamunes P, Baden M, Bass J, et al: Early intravenous feeding of low birth weight neonate,* Pediatrics *43:241,1969. Reproduced by permission of* Pediatrics. *Copyright 1969.)*

Point-of-Care Testing

Although plasma glucose determination in the laboratory using the glucose oxidase reaction is the optimum method, point-of-care (POC) testing using reflectance glucometers offers the advantage of speed. The sensitivity for detecting hypoglycemia ranges from 80% to 100% and the negative predictive values ranges from 80% to 96% depending on the device and parameters used.[7,8] Therefore, confirmatory plasma glucose concentrations should be measured if hypoglycemia is detected using a POC device or if the infant has symptoms consistent with hypoglycemia even if the POC test value shows a normal blood glucose concentration.[6]

EDITORIAL COMMENT: Accurate measurement of blood glucose levels in the newborn is important, but although POC glucose testing provides rapid results with small sample volumes and permits quick clinical responses, the common thresholds for the diagnosis of hypoglycemia in the newborn (blood glucose concentration of <2.0 mmol/L or <2.6 mmol/L, 35 to 45 mg/dL) and hyperglycemia (blood glucose concentration of >10 mmol/L, 170 mg/dL) are at the limits of accuracy for many POC glucose analyzers. Therefore, although useful for screening, such devices cannot be relied upon for accurate diagnosis of hypoglycemia. Also, with intermittent blood sampling there may be many hours between measurements when both hypoglycemia and hyperglycemia may be undetected clinically. Continuous glucose monitoring has the potential to help improve glucose assessment and management in the high-risk neonate. Harris et al used a continuous glucose monitoring system (CGMS) in 102 infants of 32 weeks' gestation or less who were at risk for hypoglycemia.[9] The babies received routine treatment, including intermittent blood glucose measurement using the glucose oxidase method, and blinded continuous interstitial glucose monitoring. The investigators documented 265 episodes of low interstitial glucose concentrations, 215 (81%) of which were not detected with blood glucose measurement. One hundred seven episodes in 34 babies lasted longer than 30 minutes, and 78 (73%) of these were not detected with blood glucose measurement. Platas et al also studied continuous glucose monitoring.[10] Hyperglycemia was detected in 22 of 38 patients (58%) and lasted a mean of 20 ± 30 hours. Hypoglycemia was detected in 14 (37%) and lasted a mean of 2.45 ± 2.3 hours. However, the CGMS was not able to provide real-time glucose concentration data. Continuous glucose monitoring via a subcutaneous sensor gives a safe and useful estimate of glucose levels in very low-birth-weight infants, revealing abnormal glucose levels at a much higher rate than expected by usual sampling. The physiologic significance of these previously undetected episodes is unknown. A CGMS may be very useful in providing information on the influence of hyperglycemia and hypoglycemia on short- and long-term outcomes in very low-birth-weight infants.

HYPOGLYCEMIA

Definition

The definition of *hypoglycemia* is controversial.[11-13] Several factors contribute to this controversy, including the poor correlation between glucose concentrations and symptoms; the nonspecific nature of the symptoms of hypoglycemia; the performance of epidemiologic studies under differing conditions (i.e., fed versus fasted states, formula feeding versus breast feeding); and the poor correlation between low glucose values and adverse long-term outcome. Rather than making the diagnosis of hypoglycemia when the plasma glucose concentration is below a specific value, a consensus statement recommends the use of an "operational threshold" that defines the glucose concentration below which clinical intervention to raise the plasma glucose should be considered.[14] These threshold values are pragmatic rather than diagnostic and recognize the uniqueness of each individual's physiologic characteristics while providing an adequate safety margin to prevent long-term sequelae. The recommended thresholds for asymptomatic and symptomatic infants are plasma glucose concentrations of less than 36 mg/dL (2.0 mmol/L) and less than 45 mg/dL (2.5 mmol/L), respectively. The diagnosis of hypoglycemia can be made when all components of the Whipple triad have been observed: (1) low plasma glucose concentration, (2) signs and symptoms consistent with hypoglycemia, and (3) resolution of these signs and symptoms when the glucose concentration is normalized. As a practical matter, most nurseries use a screening blood glucose level of 40 mg/dL or less or the presence of signs and symptoms consistent with hypoglycemia as a threshold for obtaining a plasma glucose measurement and evaluating the need for further intervention. Because blood glucose values are 10% to 15% below plasma glucose values, this allows for a safety margin when using POC test devices.

EDITORIAL COMMENT: In 2011, a position statement issued by the Committee of the Fetus and Newborn (COFN)[12] of the American Academy of Pediatrics (AAP) discussed the challenge of defining clinically significant hypoglycemia based on blood glucose concentrations. "This report provides a practical guide and algorithm for the screening and subsequent management of neonatal hypoglycemia. Current evidence does not support a specific concentration of glucose that can discriminate normal from abnormal or can potentially result in acute or chronic irreversible neurologic damage.[15] Early identification of the at-risk infant and institution of prophylactic measures to prevent neonatal hypoglycemia are recommended as a pragmatic approach despite the absence of a consistent definition of hypoglycemia in the literature." This report noted that the generally adopted level used to define neonatal hypoglycemia is less than 47 mg/dL (2.6 mmol/L) and proposed an operational threshold of 45 mg/dL (2.5 mmol/L) as a target glucose level before routine feeds.

Symptoms

Hypoglycemia in newborns is often asymptomatic. The most frequent symptoms are jitteriness and cyanosis. Other symptoms include convulsions, hypotonia, coma, poor feeding, apnea, congestive heart failure, high-pitched cry, abnormal eye movements, and temperature instability with hypothermia. In small sick infants, symptoms may easily be missed. When symptoms are present, the age of onset is most commonly between 24 and 72 hours.

Because these symptoms are nonspecific, they often occur in newborns who are normoglycemic and have other problems. For example, jitteriness, the most common symptom, is found in up to 44% of normal newborns as well as in infants with a variety of other conditions (Box 12-1). Hypoglycemia must therefore always be confirmed by chemical analysis and by response to treatment.

Transient Neonatal Hypoglycemia

Transient neonatal hypoglycemia is the most common type of hypoglycemia in a well-baby nursery and an intensive care nursery. It may occur within 1 to 2 hours of birth and resolves within hours to days. Asymptomatic patients exceed those with symptoms by about 10 to 1. Transient hypoglycemia typically occurs in "high-risk" infants in association with either alterations in maternal metabolism or other neonatal problems (Box 12-2).[16]

The pathogenesis involves multiple factors affecting glucose supply and demand, including hyperinsulinism; inadequate total body energy reserves; high energy requirement—particularly a large, glucose-requiring brain; and inordinate energy demands imposed by disease. There is an association with central nervous system (CNS) injury or anomaly, which may reflect a subtle control problem.

Box 12-1.	**Differential Diagnosis of Jitteriness and Tremors in the Newborn**

Metabolic disorders
- Hypoglycemia
- Hypocalcemia
- Hypomagnesemia
- Hyponatremia
- Hypernatremia

Neonatal drug withdrawal
- Opiates
- Selective serotonin reuptake inhibitors (SSRIs)
- Cocaine

Central nervous system disorders
- Malformations
- Hypoxic-ischemic encephalopathy
- Intracranial hemorrhage

Polycythemia

Sepsis, meningitis

Box 12-2.	**Classification of Transient Neonatal Hypoglycemia**

Hyperinsulinism
- Infant of diabetic mother (IDM)
- Intrapartum glucose administration
- Erythroblastosis fetalis
- Maternal use of β-sympathomimetics
- Maternal use of oral hypoglycemic agents
- Large for gestational age (non-IDM)

Decreased substrate
- Prematurity
- Small for gestational age
- Asphyxia
- Discordant twins
- Intrauterine growth restriction

Altered metabolism
- Polycythemia
- Hypothermia
- Severe illness, respiratory distress syndrome
- Sepsis, infection

Healthy term infants do not require routine screening for hypoglycemia if they do not have clinical manifestations.[17] "At-risk" infants (see Box 12-2), including all infants admitted to the intensive care nursery or those with clinical manifestations, should undergo screening blood glucose determination. Providing caloric support with early feeding or intravenous glucose by 1 to 2 hours of age and maintaining a continuous energy supply throughout the neonatal period dramatically reduce the incidence of hypoglycemia. High-risk infants should be screened for hypoglycemia as soon as possible after birth at intervals of 1 to 2 hours initially and then every 2 to 4 hours until their condition is definitely stabilized.

Infants of Diabetic Mothers

Hypoglycemia occurs in infants of diabetic mothers soon after birth, with a nadir at 1 to 2 hours of age that may be as low as 10 mg/dL (see Fig. 12-1). A spontaneous increase in glucose concentration usually follows, with acceptable levels reached by 4 to 6 hours of age. Few infants of diabetic mothers become symptomatic. Infants of mothers with gestational diabetes have a less dramatic decline in glucose level.

Fluctuating maternal hyperglycemia results in fetal hyperglycemia, pancreatic beta cell hyperplasia, and hyperinsulinism. After birth, hyperinsulinemia persists, as evidenced by accelerated use of exogenous glucose and diminished endogenous glucose production. Furthermore, levels of free fatty acids and ketones are low (see Fig. 12-1). In addition to having increased insulin levels, infants of diabetic mothers have increased concentrations of leptin, insulin-like growth factor I, and insulin propeptides.[18-20] Infants of diabetic mothers have multiple problems in addition to hypoglycemia (Box 12-3).[21-27] Congenital anomalies occur in 4.2% to 12.1% of infants of mothers with type 1 diabetes.[21,23,27] The rate of anomalies decreases with improved preconceptual glycemic control.[21,28] Infants of mothers with gestational diabetes do not have an increased risk of congenital anomalies but continue to have a high rate of the other morbidities (see Box 12-3). Achieving tight metabolic control in pregnant diabetic women during pregnancy and preventing hyperglycemia in labor ameliorates excess fetal weight and helps prevent perinatal deaths and reduces the incidence of neonatal hypoglycemia and hypocalcemia.[29] Early oral feeding is both prophylactic and therapeutic. Poor feeding, respiratory distress, or additional problems (congenital anomalies) may require intravenous glucose administration.

Maternal Drugs (e.g., β-Sympathomimetics, β-Blockers, Oral Antidiabetic Agents)

β-Sympathomimetics (e.g., terbutaline, ritodrine) are used as tocolytic agents and may cause maternal hyperglycemia and fetal hyperinsulinism leading to neonatal

Box 12-3.	**Morbidities of Infants of Diabetic Mothers**

Fetal demise
Prematurity
Macrosomia
Birth injury
Hyperbilirubinemia
Hypoglycemia
Hypocalcemia
Hypomagnesemia
Polycythemia
Respiratory distress syndrome
Thrombosis (renal vein)
Cardiac malformations and abnormalities
- Intraventricular septal hypertrophy
- Ventricular septal defect
- Dextrocardia
- Transposition of the great arteries
- Truncus arteriosus
- Tricuspid atresia
- Pulmonary valve abnormalities
Genitourinary malformations
- Renal agenesis or dysgenesis
- Obstructive lesions
- Hypospadias
Central nervous system malformations
- Anencephaly
- Spina bifida
- Hydrocephaly
Limb abnormalities
- Caudal regression
Small left colon syndrome

hypoglycemia. Use of β-blockers may lead to hypoglycemia by blocking catecholamine release at birth, which results in decreased lipolysis and glycogenolysis.

First-generation sulfonylurea oral antidiabetic agents (e.g., chlorpropamide, tolbutamide) cross the placenta and have a long half-life in the newborn. These agents cause increased insulin release and may cause prolonged hypoglycemia.[30] Newer oral antidiabetic agents do not lead to significant neonatal hypoglycemia, either because they do not cross the placenta in significant concentrations (second-generation sulfonylureas such as glipizide and glyburide) or because they do not enhance insulin production (biguanides and α-glucosidase inhibitors).[31]

Intrauterine Growth Restriction, Small Size for Gestational Age, Prematurity

Infants with intrauterine growth restriction, small size for gestational age, and prematurity have inadequate glycogen stores, which leads to decreased glucose production after birth. Glucose homeostasis is further complicated in these infants by reduced fat stores, increased brain-to-body weight ratios, immature hepatic enzymes, and an inadequate cortisol response.[32] Infants who are small for gestational age or experienced intrauterine growth restriction have inadequate stores due to fetal malnutrition, which is often associated with placental insufficiency, maternal preeclampsia, maternal hypertension, and severe maternal diabetes with vascular disease.[33] Premature infants fail to undergo the normal deposition of glycogen and fat that occurs during the third trimester of pregnancy.

A subset of infants with intrauterine growth restriction and small size for gestational age have prolonged hypoglycemia associated with hyperinsulinism. These infants are most often male, are born by cesarean section, and have a history of perinatal stress.[34]

Hyperviscosity-Polycythemia

Hypoglycemia occurs in approximately 13% to 40% of infants with polycythemia. An increased rate of glucose disposal without hyperinsulinemia is part of the syndrome of hyperviscosity; it responds to exchange transfusion to reduce the hematocrit.

Erythroblastosis Fetalis

Infants with erythroblastosis show islet cell hyperplasia, increased cord blood insulin levels, and hypoglycemia both shortly after birth and reactively following exchange transfusion. It is speculated that glutathione release from severe hemolysis stimulates insulin production.[35] The severity of the problem relates inversely to cord hemoglobin level and is decreased by intrauterine transfusion.[35]

Other Causes of Transient Hypoglycemia

Excess intrapartum glucose administration leads to acute maternal and fetal hyperglycemia. The subsequent transient hyperinsulinemia can lead to rebound neonatal hypoglycemia.

Hypoglycemia is also associated with infection, asphyxia, and hypothermia. The cause of hypoglycemia in these conditions is multifactorial but is most often due to increased glucose utilization. Perinatal asphyxia may occasionally be associated with hyperinsulinism requiring high glucose infusion rates.

Infusion of glucose through an umbilical artery catheter located above the celiac axis may lead to hyperinsulinemic hypoglycemia from direct infusion of glucose into the pancreatic artery with resulting beta cell overstimulation.

Persistent or Recurrent Hypoglycemia

Persistent or *recurrent hypoglycemia* refers to conditions in which the hypoglycemia persists for more than several days. Many of these conditions require prolonged therapy and may continue beyond the neonatal period (Box 12-4). In contrast with infants with transient hypoglycemia, the majority of these infants are symptomatic.

Persistent Hyperinsulinemic Hypoglycemia of Infancy

Persistent hyperinsulinemic hypoglycemia of infancy (PHHI) is caused by abnormalities in the regulation of insulin secretion. This condition was previously known as *nesidioblastosis,* in reference to a histopathologic finding that implied abnormal islet formation; however, this histologic pattern has been found to be common in the developing pancreas of infants without hypoglycemia in the first year of life.[36,37]

PHHI occurs in both sporadic and familial patterns. The majority of cases involve mutations on chromosome band 11p14-15.1, leading to abnormalities in one of the two components of the islet beta cell adenosine triphosphate–sensitive potassium channel (K_{ATP} channel), either the sulfonylurea receptor (SUR1) or the inward rectifier K^+ channel (Kir6.2).[38,39] The inability to open the islet beta cell K_{ATP} channel causes membrane depolarization and calcium influx resulting in inappropriate insulin release. Usually these mutations are autosomal recessive and associated with diffuse beta cell hyperplasia.

Milder autosomal dominant forms of the disease are caused by mutations in the glutamate dehydrogenase gene or the glucokinase gene.[40,41] These mutations cause an increase in the ratio of ATP to adenosine diphosphate (ADP) in the beta cell, which inappropriately closes the structurally normal K_{ATP} channels. These forms of PHHI are also usually associated with diffuse beta cell hyperplasia.

Focal beta cell hyperplasia is found when abnormalities of the beta cell K_{ATP} channel are associated with unbalanced expression of one or more growth suppression

---

Box 12-4. Classification of Persistent Neonatal Hypoglycemia

Hyperinsulinemia
Persistent hyperinsulinemic hypoglycemia of infancy
- Sporadic
- Familial
- Focal beta-cell adenoma
- Hyperammonemic hyperinsulinism

Beckwith-Wiedemann syndrome

Endocrine disorders
Panhypopituitarism
Growth hormone deficiency
Adrenocorticotropic hormone deficiency
Adrenal insufficiency
Glucagon deficiency
Epinephrine deficiency

Glycogen storage disease (GSD)
Glucose-6-phosphatase deficiency (GSD type I)
Debrancher deficiency (GSD type III)

Disorders of gluconeogenesis
Fructose 1,6-diphosphatase deficiency
Pyruvate-carboxylase deficiency
Phosphoenol pyruvate-carboxykinase deficiency

Disorders of fatty acid oxidation
Carnitine-acylcarnitine translocase deficiency
Very long-chain acyl-CoA dehydrogenase deficiency
Long-chain acyl-CoA dehydrogenase deficiency
Medium-chain acyl-CoA dehydrogenase deficiency
Multiple acyl-CoA dehydrogenase deficiency

Disorders of amino acid and organic acid metabolism
Maple syrup urine disease
Propionic acidemia
Methylmalonicacidemia
Isovalericacidemia
Multiple carboxylase deficiency
3-Hydroxy-3-methylglutaryl CoA lyase deficiency

Mitochondrial disorders
3-Methylglutaconicaciduria

Glycosylation disorders

Systemic disorders
Hepatic failure
Congestive heart failure

CoA, Coenzyme A.

Box 12-5.	**Clinical Features of Beckwith-Wiedemann Syndrome**

Macrosomia
Abdominal wall defects
  • Omphalocele
  • Diastasis recti
  • Umbilical hernia
Craniofacial features
  • Macroglossia
  • Ear lobe creases
  • Posterior helical pits
  • Nevus flammeus
  • Prominent occiput
  • Metopic ridge
Neonatal hypoglycemia
Neonatal polycythemia
Visceromegaly
Congenital heart defects
Hemihypertrophy
Clitorimegaly
Cryptorchidism
Embryonal malignancies

genes due to focal loss of the maternal DNA on chromosome band 11p15.[42,43] Other genetic mutations associated with PHHI have been described but occur less frequently.[44]

Infants with PHHI are large for gestational age with profound, symptomatic hypoglycemia. Plasma insulin and C-peptide concentrations are inappropriately elevated during episodes of hypoglycemia.[45] Plasma free fatty acid and ketone concentrations are low. Ketonuria is absent. Glucagon infusion results in a glycemic response in the presence of hypoglycemia.[45] Mutation in the glutamate dehydrogenase gene also causes elevated ammonia concentrations.[46] Hyperinsulinemia may be temporarily managed with diazoxide (which opens the K_{ATP} channel) or the long-acting somatostatin analog octreotide (which opens rectifier K channels).[45,47] These therapies are most effective when the K_{ATP} channel is intact but is closed due to altered ATP/ADP concentrations. Other potential therapies include nifedipine, which inhibits insulin release, and glucagon, which increases gluconeogenesis.[45]

The majority of neonates do not respond to medical management and require either a partial pancreatectomy (for focal lesions) or a 95% pancreatectomy (for diffuse disease).[48-50] Previously, selective pancreatic arterial calcium stimulation with hepatic venous and portal venous insulin sampling using interventional radiology was used to identify focal or diffuse disease preoperatively. Positron emission tomography, a less invasive technique, has now been shown to be more accurate in diagnosing whether the disease is focal or diffuse.[51] Neurodevelopmental impairment secondary to frequent and severe episodes of hypoglycemia is common in PHHI.[52,53] Complications of pancreatectomy include diabetes mellitus and pancreatic exocrine insufficiency.

Beckwith-Wiedemann Syndrome (Hyperplastic Fetal Visceromegaly)

Beckwith-Wiedemann syndrome (BWS) is an overgrowth syndrome associated with macrosomia (88% of cases), macroglossia (97% of cases), abdominal wall defects (80% of cases), usually an omphalocele, hypoglycemia in the neonatal period, and embryonal cancers of infancy and early childhood (4% of cases). Other clinical features of BWS are listed in Box 12-5. The frequency of hypoglycemia in BWS is between 30% and 63%, and the hypoglycemia is caused by hyperinsulinism.[54] The hypoglycemia may be asymptomatic and usually resolves within the first 3 days of life. Fewer than 5% of infants will have hypoglycemia beyond the neonatal period requiring either continuous feeding or, in rare cases, partial pancreatectomy.[55] The genetics of BWS is complex and involves defects in imprinted gene expression in the 11p15 region.[56,57] The majority of cases are sporadic but 10% to 15% occur in an autosomal dominant pattern, with maternal transmission associated with increased penetrance. The risk of BWS is higher after the use of assisted reproductive therapies.[58] Seventy percent of cases can be detected by DNA methylation analysis at the differentially methylated regions 1 (regulating insulin-like growth factor II) and 2.[59] The similarity of affected gene regions in BWS and PHHI may provide a molecular basis for hypoglycemia in BWS, particularly for the occasional patient with hypoglycemia requiring a partial pancreatectomy.[60]

Endocrine Deficiencies

Hypopituitarism with deficiencies in growth hormone and adrenocorticotropic hormone (ACTH) is often associated with facial and genital abnormalities (microphallus).

Cortisol deficiency secondary to congenital adrenal hyperplasia or adrenal hemorrhage is associated with hypoglycemia. These disorders may cause electrolyte abnormalities and cardiovascular collapse. Congenital adrenal hyperplasia causes virilization in female infants.

Metabolic Diseases

Metabolic disorders associated with persistent neonatal hypoglycemia are all very rare.[61,62] Box 12-4 lists the disorders that manifest in the neonatal period. Many other metabolic syndromes are associated with hypoglycemia but present later in infancy or childhood. Clues to the diagnosis include lactic acidosis, excessive or reduced ketonuria, persistent emesis and coma despite correction of hypoglycemia, hepatomegaly, family history, and elevated values on liver function tests (e.g., ammonia, direct bilirubin).

Glycogen storage diseases result in impaired ability of hepatic glucose release. Neonatal presentation is most common with glycogen storage disease type I (glucose-6-phosphatase deficiency). Glycogen storage disease type III (Debrancher deficiency) may be detected after prolonged fasting. These diseases also are associated with lactic acidosis, ketosis, and hepatomegaly.

Disorders of fatty acid oxidation, particularly disorders of very long-chain and long-chain fatty acid metabolism, may occur in the neonatal period. These disorders are often accompanied by hyperammonemia, liver disease, and cardiac disease. Usually ketosis is absent. Medium-chain acyl–coenzyme A (CoA) dehydrogenase deficiency is the most common disorder of fatty acid oxidation but only rarely presents in the neonatal period.

Amino acid and organic acid disorders are also associated with hypoglycemia but often ketosis, lactic acidosis, and hyperammonemia are present.

Treatment of Hypoglycemia

Prevention is key and consists of early oral or enteral tube feeding of breast milk or formula if appropriate. For those infants who are not able to be fed enterally, early initiation of intravenous fluids with 10% dextrose at a glucose infusion rate of 4 to 8 mg/kg/min is indicated. Glucose infusion should be continuous and steady, by pump, and should be continued until replaced calorically by enteral feeding.

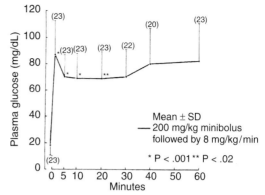

Figure 12-3. Minibolus therapy for neonatal hypoglycemia achieves euglycemia without excessively high glucose levels, which may further stimulate insulin release and later result in rebound hypoglycemia. Numbers in parentheses indicate the number of determinations at each point. *(From Lilien L, Pildes R, Srinivasan G, et al: Treatment of neonatal hypoglycemia with minibolus and intravenous glucose infusion,* J Pediatr *97:295, 1980.)*

Treatment is indicated for all hypoglycemic infants (plasma glucose level of <36 mg/dL if asymptomatic, <45 mg/dL or higher if symptomatic). Asymptomatic infants with transient hypoglycemia and *no* other medical illness may be given enteric formula or breast milk. Blood glucose concentration should be monitored every 30 minutes to determine adequacy of response. If glucose concentrations do not increase or if enteric alimentation is contraindicated, intravenous glucose, 4 to 8 mg/kg/min, should begin. If hypoglycemia is severe (plasma glucose level of <20 to 25 mg/dL) or if symptoms are present, intravenous glucose should be initiated starting with a bolus of 200 mg/kg glucose (2 mL/kg of 10% dextrose in water) followed by a continuous infusion of 6 to 8 mg/kg/min of glucose (Fig. 12-3).[63] The bolus of glucose should be no greater than 200 mg/kg to prevent excessive hyperglycemia and rebound hypoglycemia. Blood glucose concentrations should be monitored every 30 to 60 minutes until stable. This bolus and infusion is adequate for most infants; however, if plasma glucose concentrations remain low the glucose infusion should be increased in increments of 2 mg/kg/min. On rare occasions, refractory hypoglycemia may require as much as 20 mg/kg/min.

For those infants with persistent hypoglycemia requiring high glucose infusion rates (>12 to 14 mg/kg/min), additional laboratory studies should be considered. These studies should be performed during episodes of hypoglycemia and include plasma insulin, cortisol, and growth hormone concentrations. For severe persistent hypoglycemia additional therapies may be required, including hydrocortisone, diazoxide, octreotide, or glucagon.

Prognosis

Symptomatic, prolonged, or recurrent hypoglycemia may cause neurologic impairment.[64] Although the degree of neurologic injury correlates with the severity and duration of hypoglycemia, scientific analysis does not allow one to define a specific level or duration of hypoglycemia at which harm occurs.[64-67] Infants with asymptomatic, transient hypoglycemia do well.[68] Infants with hypoglycemic seizures have the poorest outcome. Neurologic impairment is also more likely when other risk factors such as asphyxia and intrauterine growth restriction are present. Infants with hyperinsulinemic hypoglycemia or with inborn metabolic errors have a prognosis related to their primary illness.

In infants of diabetic mothers, long-term neurologic outcome is also related to maternal metabolic factors independent of postnatal glucose concentrations.[69]

> **EDITORIAL COMMENT:** To define the relationship between magnetic resonance imaging (MRI) findings and hypoglycemia, Burns et al studied 35 term infants who underwent early brain MRI scanning after symptomatic neonatal hypoglycemia (median glucose level: 1 mmol/L) without evidence of hypoxic-ischemic encephalopathy and assessed neurodevelopmental outcome at a minimum of 18 months.[70] White matter abnormalities occurred in 94% of infants with hypoglycemia and was severe in 43%, with a predominantly posterior pattern in 29% of cases. Cortical abnormalities occurred in 51% of infants; 30% had white matter hemorrhage; 40% had basal ganglia/thalamic lesions; and 11% had an abnormal posterior limb of the internal capsule. Three infants had middle cerebral artery territory infarctions. At 18 months, 23 infants (65%) demonstrated impairments, which were related to the severity of white matter injury and involvement of the posterior limb of the internal capsule.
>
> Patterns of injury associated with symptomatic neonatal hypoglycemia were more varied than described previously. White matter injury was not confined to the posterior regions; hemorrhage, middle cerebral artery infarction, and basal ganglia/thalamic abnormalities were seen, and cortical involvement was common. Surprisingly, early MRI findings were more instructive than the severity or duration of hypoglycemia for predicting neurodevelopmental outcomes.

Boluyt et al attempted to assess the effect of episodes of neonatal hypoglycemia on subsequent neurodevelopment.[65] A comprehensive search revealed 18 eligible studies. The overall methodological quality of the included studies was considered poor in 16 studies and high in 2 studies. None of the studies provided a valid estimate of the effect of neonatal hypoglycemia on neurodevelopment. Boluyt et al concluded, "Recommendations for clinical practice cannot be based on valid scientific evidence in this field. To assess the effect of neonatal hypoglycemia on subsequent neurodevelopment, a well-designed prospective study should be undertaken."

HYPERGLYCEMIA

Hyperglycemia (glucose concentration of >150 mg/dL) is a common, serious problem of very immature infants. Risk factors include low birth weight (especially when <1000 g), earlier gestational age, administration of intravenous glucose infusions (especially glucose infusion rates of >6 mg/kg/min), high illness severity, and glucocorticoid therapy (Box 12-6). Factors contributing to hyperglycemia in premature infants are reduced glucose-induced insulin secretion, immature insulin processing, and increased ratio of GLUT1 to GLUT2 in tissues.[71,72] Hepatic glucose release may fail to decrease when exogenous glucose is given. Stress from illness increases catecholamine release, which may further elevate glucose levels by inhibiting glucose use and insulin release.

Box 12-6. **Risk Factors for Neonatal Hyperglycemia**

Preterm birth
Intrauterine growth restriction (IUGR)
Increased stress hormone levels
- Increased catecholamine infusions
- Increased glucocorticoid concentrations (from use of antenatal steroids, postnatal glucocorticoid administration, and stress)
- Increased glucagon concentrations
Early intravenous (IV) lipid infusion and high rates of infusion
Higher-than-needed rates of IV glucose infusion
Insufficient pancreatic insulin secretion (preterm and IUGR)
Absence of enteral feedings, leading to diminished "incretin" secretion and action, which limits potential to promote insulin secretion

Hyperglycemia has been associated with increased length of hospitalization, risk of death, and incidence of intraventricular hemorrhage.[18,73] The mechanism of injury may involve increases in plasma osmolarity (a glucose level of 450 mg/dL is equivalent to an additional 24 mOsm/L) and glucosuria leading to renal water and electrolyte losses and vascular fluid shifts.

Treatment and prevention are accomplished by adjusting the glucose infusion rate to that tolerated by each individual infant. Rates of 4 to 8 mg/kg/min are *usually* tolerated; however, lower glucose infusion rates may be needed. Glucose infusion rates should be expressed as milligrams per kilogram per minute, because variations in either the volume or glucose content of the fluid result in alterations in actual delivery of glucose to the infant. Along with improving nitrogen balance, early amino acid administration at the time of birth in low-birth-weight infants decreases the incidence of hyperglycemia, possibly due to improved insulin release.[74,75] Occasionally, an insulin infusion starting at 0.01 U/kg/min but increasing to 0.1 U/kg/min if needed is indicated in those infants in whom decreasing the glucose infusion rate is inadequate or improved caloric intake is desired. Frequent monitoring of blood glucose concentration is crucial both to determine the adequacy of therapy and to avoid episodes of hypoglycemia.

EDITORIAL COMMENT: Among very low-birth-weight infants, early neonatal hyperglycemia is common and is associated with increased risk of death and major morbidities. Sinclair et al wished to assess effects on clinical outcomes of interventions for preventing hyperglycemia in very low-birth-weight neonates receiving full or partial parenteral nutrition.[76] They searched for randomized or quasi-randomized controlled trials of interventions for prevention of hyperglycemia in neonates with a birth weight of less than 1500 g or a gestational age of less than 32 weeks. They found *only* four eligible trials. Two trials compared lower and higher rates of glucose infusion in the early postnatal period. These trials were too small to assess effects on mortality or major morbidities. Two trials, one a moderately large multicenter trial,[77,78] compared insulin infusion with standard care. Insulin infusion therapy reduced hyperglycemia, but increased death before 28 days and was complicated by hypoglycemia. Reduction in hyperglycemia was not accompanied by significant effects on major morbidities; effects on neurodevelopment are awaited. The authors concluded,

"There is insufficient evidence from trials comparing lower with higher glucose infusion rates to inform clinical practice. Large randomized trials are needed, powered on clinical outcomes including death, major morbidities, and adverse neurodevelopment." With regard to insulin infusion, they noted that "the evidence reviewed does not support the routine use of insulin infusions to prevent hyperglycemia in very low-birth-weight neonates. Further randomized trials of insulin infusion may be justified. They should enroll extremely low-birth-weight neonates at very high risk for hyperglycemia and neonatal death."

Neonatal Diabetes

Neonatal diabetes is a rare disorder. Most infants with neonatal diabetes are born at or near term, with marked intrauterine growth restriction reflecting low levels of insulin and insulin-like growth factor I. Weight loss, dehydration, hyperglycemia, and occasional ketosis usually appear in the first month of life. Seventy to eighty percent of cases involve an abnormality on chromosome band 6q24 caused by uniparental disomy of chromosome 6, duplication of paternal 6q24, or loss of methylation at the differentially methylated region at the 6q24 locus.[79,80] Treatment is with insulin, with a usual daily dose of 2 to 6 U.

The transient form of the disease usually resolves within a few months. However, many infants subsequently develop diabetes later in childhood or early adulthood. Approximately 50% of patients have permanent neonatal diabetes and remission never occurs.[81] Permanent neonatal diabetes is associated with activating mutations to the K_{ATP} channel in the pancreatic beta cell, causing the channel to remain open and preventing insulin secretion. Some of these patients are responsive to sulfonylurea, which binds to the sulfonylurea receptor and helps to close the K_{ATP} channel.[81,82]

CALCIUM

FETAL AND NEONATAL CALCIUM METABOLISM

The placenta actively transports calcium to the fetus and maintains fetal total and ionized calcium levels at about 1 mg/dL above the respective maternal levels. Between 28 weeks' gestation and term, fetal weight triples, but calcium content quadruples as bone mineral density progressively increases (Fig. 12-4). Fetal acquisition of

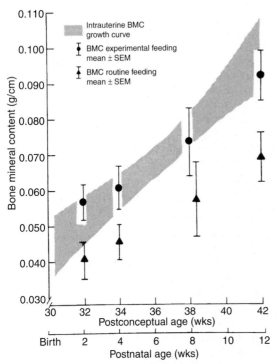

Figure 12-4. Bone mineral content (BMC) in premature infants compared with intrauterine bone mineralization. Hatched area is the in utero rate of BMC increase and shows progressive bone mineralization during gestation until term. Premature infants fed Similac 20 *(triangles)* have diminished bone mineral accumulation; in contrast, infants fed formula with calcium (1260 mg/L), phosphorus (630 mg/L), and vitamin D (1000 U/L) *(circles)* have intrauterine rates of bone mineralization. These latter infants received calcium, 220 to 250 mg/kg/day, and phosphorus, 110 to 125 mg/kg/day. This calcium intake exceeds the in utero rate of calcium accumulation (150 mg/kg/day); the failure of BMC to exceed intrauterine rates in this group is possibly a result of fecal losses. *SEM,* Standard error of the mean. *(From Steichen J, Gratton T, Tsang R, et al: Osteopenia of prematurity: the cause and possible treatment,* J Pediatr *96:528, 1980.)*

calcium averages 150 mg/kg/day throughout this period.

Placental active transport allows fetal bone calcification to proceed normally. The calcium drain causes a modest decrease in maternal calcium levels near term. Maternal parathyroid activity, 1,25-dihydroxyvitamin D level, calcium absorption, and calcium mobilization from bone are all increased.[83] Parathyroid hormone (PTH) and calcitonin do not cross the placenta, whereas 25-hydroxyvitamin D does.

At birth, the constant placental calcium supply is interrupted. Although the premature baby has skeletal reserves of calcium,

the maintenance of serum calcium concentration requires rapid changes in endocrine function and in the equilibrium between serum and bone. The factors affecting calcium in the neonate can be summarized as follows:

1. PTH mobilizes calcium from bone, promotes calcium absorption from the gut, and increases renal phosphate excretion. Levels are low in cord blood, suppressed by the mild hypercalcemia caused by placental transport. Postnatally, PTH concentrations rise for the first 48 hours, decreasing by the end of the first week. A similar pattern occurs in preterm infants.[83] Parathyroid secretion and function require magnesium.

2. Vitamin D is required for effective PTH action on both bone and gut. Fetal concentrations of 25-hydroxyvitamin D and 24,25-dihydroxyvitamin D vary directly with gestational age and maternal plasma concentrations. Newborn stores are usually adequate unless there is significant maternal dietary inadequacy or poor exposure to sunlight. Levels of 1,25-dihydroxyvitamin D depend on both maternal plasma concentrations and synthesis in the fetal kidney. Concentrations of 1,25-dihydroxyvitamin D are elevated in term and preterm infants.[83]

3. Calcitonin inhibits calcium mobilization from bone. Levels are high in neonates and are further elevated by asphyxia and prematurity.

4. Serum phosphate level increases after birth, and even more so after birth asphyxia.

5. The calcium-sensing receptor (CaSR) is present in the parathyroid chief cells and renal tubular cells. The *CaSR* gene is located on chromosome band 3q13.3-21. The CaSR monitors extracellular Ca^{2+} concentrations, allowing appropriate PTH secretion and renal tubular handling of calcium.[84] Several clinical disorders that result from molecular abnormalities of the CaSR leading to either loss or gain of function have been described. Loss of function causes the hypercalcemic disorders, familial benign hypocalciuric hypercalcemia and neonatal severe hyperparathyroidism. Autosomal dominant hypocalcemia with calciuria results from gain in function.[85]

There is normally a decrease in the serum calcium level in the first hours after birth that continues for 24 to 48 hours; serum calcium then rises to stable levels by 5 to 10 days of age. In healthy full-term infants, mean total calcium levels fall from 2.3 to 2.9 mmol/L (9.0 to 11.4 mg/dL) at birth to 1.9 to 2.6 mmol/L (7.8 to 10.2 mg/dL) at 24 hours. Mean ionized calcium levels fall from 1.3 to 1.6 mmol/L (5.2 to 6.4 mg/dL) at birth to 1.1 to 1.36 mmol/L (4.4 to 5.4 mg/dL) at 24 hours. Levels rise gradually, so that by 1 week of age mean ionized calcium levels reach 1.4 mmol/L (5.6 mg/dL). Healthy premature infants 33 to 36 weeks of age have lower calcium levels at 24 to 48 hours but otherwise are not different from term infants. Reference values for smaller preterm infants have not been well characterized.

METHODOLOGY

Serum total calcium level, as routinely reported by clinical laboratories, represents the sum of protein-bound calcium (40%), diffusible but complexed calcium (e.g., citrate bound, 10%), and free ionized calcium (50%). Only the ionized calcium fraction, normally 1.10 to 1.36 mmol/L (4.4 to 5.4 mg/dL), is physiologically active, transported across membranes, and regulated homeostatically.

Variations in the two inert calcium fractions occur commonly due to alterations in serum protein level, albumin level, and pH; thus, correlation of total and ionized calcium is difficult. Various formulas have been used to estimate ionized calcium from total calcium by correcting for these alterations in serum albumin level, total protein level, and pH.[86] In general, these formulas have a low sensitivity and a high false-negative rate for predicting hypocalcemia in critically ill patients. Because most laboratories are currently able to measure ionized calcium in small blood volumes, direct determination of ionized calcium is the method of choice for evaluating calcium homeostasis in critically ill patients.[87]

HYPOCALCEMIA

Symptoms and Definition

Hypocalcemia has traditionally been defined as total calcium levels below 2 mmol/L (8.0 mg/dL) in term infants and 1.75 mmol/L (7.0 mg/dL) in preterm infants. In term infants, ionized calcium concentrations below 1.1 mmol/L (4.4 mg/dL) should be considered abnormal. Although ionized calcium concentrations are not as well defined,

---

> **Box 12-7. Causes of Neonatal Hypocalcemia**
>
> **Early onset**
> Prematurity
> Infant of diabetic mother
> Asphyxia
>
> **Late onset**
> Secondary hypoparathyroidism
> - Maternal hyperparathyroidism
> - Maternal hypercalcemic hypocalciuria
> - Hypomagnesemia
> Primary hypoparathyroidism
> - Transient congenital hypoparathyroidism
> - DiGeorge syndrome
> - Familial X linked
> - Familial autosomal dominant
> - Pseudohypoparathyroidism
> Vitamin D deficiency
> - Maternal anticonvulsant therapy
> - Diet
> - Malabsorption
> - Renal insufficiency ($\downarrow$ 1,25-dihydroxyvitamin D)
> - Hepatic disease ($\downarrow$ 25-hydroxyvitamin D)
> Hyperphosphatemia
> - Cow's milk–based formulas
> - Excessive phosphate administration

---

levels below 1.0 mmol/L (4.0 mg/dL) are abnormal in preterm infants.

Early neonatal hypocalcemia occurs in the first 3 days of life. Late-onset hypocalcemia occurs after 3 days of age. Although overlap occurs, the age of onset is often helpful in determining the cause of neonatal hypocalcemia (Box 12-7).

Hypocalcemia is often asymptomatic but may cause twitching, "hyperalertness," increased tone, hyperreflexia, jitteriness, and convulsions. Cyanosis, vomiting or intolerance of feedings, and a high-pitched cry have also been noted. Late-onset hypocalcemia frequently presents with seizures. Like hypoglycemia, seizures secondary to hypocalcemia may be either focal, unilateral, or general. The Chvostek sign does not have value in premature infants and occurs in only 20% of hypocalcemic term or older infants. Because the symptoms of hypocalcemia are nonspecific and are commonly found in other high-risk infants as well as in those with hypoglycemia and other electrolyte abnormalities, hypocalcemia must be confirmed both by the laboratory and by response to specific treatment (see Box 12-1).

Serum calcium concentration should be determined daily for all infants at risk of hypocalcemia, and supportive treatment should be considered when low levels are encountered. The differential diagnosis of hypocalcemia is noted in Box 12-7.

Early Neonatal Hypocalcemia

Early neonatal hypocalcemia represents an exaggeration of the physiologic decrease in serum calcium level during the first 2 days of life. In 30% to 40% of low-birth-weight infants, chemical hypocalcemia develops. A smaller number of infants become symptomatic. The following factors identify infants at high risk:

- Male sex
- Delivery in early spring (low maternal vitamin D level)[83]
- Prematurity
- Neonatal asphyxia and fetal distress[88]
- Neonatal illness—respiratory distress syndrome, cerebral injury, hypoglycemia, and sepsis
- Maternal diabetes[89]

The pathogenesis is a failure of homeostatic control of the calcium partition between bone and serum. Interruption of placental calcium supply, transient parathyroid hypofunction, hypercalcitoninemia, and increased endogenous phosphate loading contribute to the hypocalcemia in each of the aforementioned conditions. Bicarbonate therapy may aggravate hypocalcemia by decreasing calcium release from bone. In premature infants, resistance to 1,25-dihydroxyvitamin D action may exist. In infants of diabetic mothers, a low magnesium concentration with associated hypoparathyroidism has been proposed as a contributing factor.[89]

Classic Neonatal Tetany/ Hyperphosphatemia

Classic neonatal tetany occurs typically at 5 to 7 days of age. It is most commonly seen in infants fed cow's milk or evaporated milk with a high phosphate content. Cow's milk contains approximately 956 mg/L of phosphorus (molar Ca/P ratio of 1.0) compared with 150 mg/L in breast milk (molar Ca/P ratio of 1.5 to 1.6). The resulting hyperphosphatemia is aggravated by immaturity of the parathyroid, vitamin D metabolism, and renal function, which leads to hypocalcemia. Because current commercial formulas contain 280 to 360 mg/L of phosphorus (molar Ca/P ratio of 1.4 to 1.6), classic neonatal tetany has become rare. With breast-milk feeding, it should not occur.

Secondary Hypoparathyroidism

Maternal Hyperparathyroidism
Maternal hypercalcemia leads to fetal hypercalcemia and suppression of neonatal PTH secretion.[90] The mother's disease is frequently clinically silent. Vague maternal symptoms, a history of pancreatitis or renal stones, or a history of having a previous infant with neonatal tetany may be present. Calcium and phosphorus determinations should be obtained for the mother whenever neonatal hypocalcemia is prolonged or resistant to treatment.

Maternal Hypercalcemic Hypocalciuria
Loss of function of the CasR results in familial benign hypocalciuric hypercalcemia, an autosomal dominant disease. Unaffected infants born to mothers with this condition may develop hypocalcemia secondary to high fetal calcium concentrations.

Hypomagnesemia
Magnesium deficiency causes impaired PTH secretion and also causes resistance to PTH action. Hypocalcemia cannot be corrected with calcium therapy until hypomagnesemia has first been corrected.

Primary Hypoparathyroidism

Transient Congenital Idiopathic Hypoparathyroidism
Transient congenital idiopathic hypoparathyroidism is a benign, self-limited hypoparathyroid state persisting from 1 to 14 months and responding to calcium or moderate-level vitamin D supplements. The mother is euparathyroid.

Permanent Hypoparathyroidism
DiGeorge syndrome is classically characterized by conotruncal cardiac anomalies (truncus arteriosus, interrupted aortic arch, tetralogy of Fallot), thymic dysplasia, and hypocalcemia.[91] Approximately 60% of patients develop hypocalcemia. Hypoparathyroidism may be transient in the neonatal period, permanent, or latent.[92] Other associated features include dysmorphic facies and velopharyngeal incompetence. Many affected infants do not have congenital

heart disease, which often results in a delay in the diagnosis until later infancy or childhood.[93] Severe immunodeficiency occasionally occurs due to thymic aplasia.[94] The majority of patients have a microdeletion in the chromosome 22q11 region.

CATCH 22 is a medical acronym for cardiac defects, abnormal facies, thymic hypoplasia, cleft palate, hypocalcemia, and a variable deletion on chromosome band 22q11. Catch 22 includes three syndromes with overlapping phenotypes: DiGeorge syndrome, velocardiofacial syndrome, and conotruncal anomaly face syndrome.[95]

Several other familial forms of hypoparathyroidism have been described, including X-linked, autosomal dominant, and autosomal recessive forms. Autosomal dominant hypocalcemia with calciuria results from a gain in function in the CasR causing inappropriate PTH response to hypocalcemia.[85]

Other Hypocalcemic Syndromes

Severe maternal calcium and vitamin D deficiency can cause rickets in infants and neonatal hypocalcemia.[83] Maternal anticonvulsant therapy alters vitamin D metabolism, potentially leading to neonatal hypocalcemia. Pseudohypoparathyroidism is a condition in which peripheral response to PTH is inadequate.

Treatment of Hypocalcemia

Prevention

Supportive treatment may be given to asymptomatic infants at risk. If possible, early enteral feedings should be initiated. For infants requiring intravenous fluids, calcium may be added to the solution (18 to 36 mg/kg/day of elemental calcium). Alternatively intravenous bolus injections may be given every 6 to 8 hours. Calcium cannot be mixed with bicarbonate in intravenous solutions. Cardiac monitoring is required during calcium infusions. Calcium infusions should preferably be given through a central line whenever possible. Peripheral administration may result in skin sloughs from infiltration of intravenous solution.

Symptomatic Hypocalcemia

A slow intravenous calcium push is potentially hazardous but is indicated in infants with seizures or extreme irritability as a therapeutic trial while laboratory confirmation of hypocalcemia is awaited. An established intravenous line should be used. Continuous cardiac monitoring for bradycardia is required. An infusion of 1 to 2 mL/kg of 10% calcium gluconate (9 to 18 mg/kg of elemental calcium) is administered over 10 minutes.[96] The dose may be repeated in 10 minutes if there is no response. The hazards of intravenous calcium injection include bradycardia, cardiac arrest, cutaneous necrosis, cerebral calcifications, and intestinal gangrene. Care should be taken to ensure the patency of intravenous lines, with labels used to avoid inadvertent flushing. Intraarterial calcium administration should be avoided. Failure of hypocalcemia to respond to parenteral therapy suggests hypomagnesemia.

Continued Treatment

Following the bolus infusion, continuous calcium infusion at a rate of 75 mg calcium/kg/day is indicated. If the infant is in stable condition and can tolerate enteral feedings, oral calcium therapy can be initiated and intravenous therapy tapered. Oral calcium salts, calcium gluconate (9 mg/mL elemental calcium) or calcium glubionate (23 mg/mL elemental calcium), can be initiated at 75 mg/kg/day of elemental calcium divided equally into 4 to 6 doses. In infants at risk of necrotizing enterocolitis or malabsorption, calcium gluconate is preferred to calcium glubionate because of its lower osmolarity (700 mOsm/L versus 2500 mOsm/L). After normocalcemia is achieved, treatment should be tapered. Often, therapy can be discontinued by 2 to 4 weeks.

In patients with hyperphosphatemia, the phosphate load needs to be reduced. Low-phosphorus formula (Similac PM 60/40 [Abbott Nutrition, Columbus, Ohio], phosphorus 190 mg/L, molar Ca/P ratio of 1.5) or breast milk should be used. Additional oral calcium supplementation (10 to 20 mg elemental calcium/kg/day) helps to further increase the relative absorption of calcium to phosphorus. Oral calcium supplementation can usually be discontinued beginning in 1 week and routine formula started in 2 to 4 weeks.

In patients with hypoparathyroidism, both oral calcium supplementation and vitamin D supplementation, usually in the form of calcitriol (1,25-dihydroxy vitamin D), is required.

Prognosis

Hypocalcemia with seizures may present an immediate threat to life in an infant with other problems with which to contend. Unlike with hypoglycemia, however, there

---

Box 12-8. **Causes of Hypercalcemia**

Neonatal hyperparathyroidism (transient vs. permanent)
Maternal hypoparathyroidism
Excessive calcium supplementation
Excessive vitamin D supplementation
Williams syndrome ($\uparrow$ 1,25-dihydroxyvitamin D)
Familial hypocalciuric hypercalcemia
Phosphate depletion
Hypervitaminosis A
Use of thiazide diuretics
Hyperthyroidism
Adrenal insufficiency
Subcutaneous fat necrosis
Aluminum toxicity
Hypophosphatasia
Primary chondrodystrophy (metaphyseal dysplasia)

---

seems to be no structural damage to the central nervous system.[97] Thus, hypocalcemia alone has a good prognosis. If hypocalcemia is complicating other serious conditions such as asphyxia, the prognosis is determined by the other problems.[97]

HYPERCALCEMIA

Hypercalcemia is most often iatrogenic secondary to excessive calcium administration, excessive vitamin D administration, use of thiazide diuretics that reduce renal calcium excretion, or phosphate depletion usually caused by poorly constituted hyperalimentation solutions or human milk feedings.[98] Primary neonatal hyperparathyroidism occurs both sporadically and by autosomal recessive inheritance. It is due to abnormalities in CasR function resulting in increased PTH levels.[85] Familial hypocalciuric hypercalcemia is a related disorder also caused by abnormalities in the CasR but is benign and inherited in an autosomal dominant pattern.[85,99] PTH levels are normal with low to normal urinary calcium excretion in familial hypocalciuric hypercalcemia.[100] Individuals who are homozygous for the familial hypocalciuric hypercalcemia gene mutation develop severe neonatal hyperparathyroidism.[99] Secondary hyperparathyroidism occurs due to chronic maternal hypocalcemia (usually caused by maternal hypoparathyroidism), which leads to transient neonatal parathyroid overstimulation. The hypercalcemia associated with subcutaneous fat necrosis and Williams syndrome may be related to increased 1,25-dihydroxyvitamin

D synthesis.[101] Other causes are listed in Box 12-8.

Hypercalcemia may present with nonspecific symptoms including poor feeding, ileus, failure to thrive, polyuria, dehydration, lethargy, and irritability. Chronic hyperparathyroidism may be associated with bone demineralization and fractures.

Initial treatment includes discontinuation of all calcium and vitamin D supplementation, and hydration with furosemide to increase calcium excretion. Other therapies include calcitonin, glucocorticoids, and dialysis. Specific treatment is directed to the underlying disorder.

MAGNESIUM

FETAL AND NEONATAL MAGNESIUM METABOLISM

Magnesium is actively transported from mother to fetus. Unlike with calcium, this transfer is adversely affected both by placental insufficiency and by maternal magnesium deficiency caused by poor diet or disease. Approximately 65% of total body magnesium (versus 99% of calcium) is contained in bone, 34% in the intracellular space, and 1% in the extracellular space. Because the fraction of magnesium in the extracellular fluid is low, plasma magnesium concentrations do not adequately reflect total body magnesium content.

Parathyroid function has a small direct effect on serum magnesium levels. Magnesium, on the other hand, is critically necessary for normal parathyroid function.

Normal newborn serum magnesium concentration is 1.5 to 2.8 mg/dL (0.62 to 1.16 mmol/L) and relates directly to the mother's level.[102] Through the first week of life, magnesium levels show small variations, correlating directly with changes in serum calcium level and inversely with phosphorus level.

EDITORIAL COMMENT: Fetal exposure to magnesium sulfate in women at risk of preterm delivery significantly reduces the risk of cerebral palsy without increasing the risk of death.[103]

HYPOMAGNESEMIA

Magnesium levels of less than 1.5 mg/dL are encountered in the following conditions:

- In intrauterine growth restriction of any cause, including multiple gestation, or in association with maternal malnourishment or hypomagnesemia

- In association with maternal gestational diabetes and diabetes mellitus, in which it correlates with the severity of the mother's disease[89]
- With hyperphosphatemia and after exchange transfusion (magnesium, like calcium, is subject to citrate complexing)
- In hypoparathyroidism
- Secondary to diarrhea or malabsorption states in older infants
- In a specific magnesium malabsorption syndrome that is secondary to mutations in the transient receptor potential channel 6 (TRPM6) protein mapping to chromosome band 9q22.[104,105]
- Secondary to renal losses (primary or induced by drugs, e.g., amphotericin B)

Hypomagnesemia can cause symptoms similar to those caused by hypocalcemia but is unresponsive to calcium therapy.

Coexistence of Hypomagnesemia and Hypocalcemia

Hypomagnesemia and hypocalcemia, two metabolic problems, frequently coexist. They have common antecedents, such as maternal diabetes, hypoparathyroidism, malabsorption, exchange transfusion, and excess dietary phosphorus.

Magnesium deficiency causes failure of PTH release and of PTH's effect on serum calcium level. Treatment with calcium will not correct hypocalcemia until hypomagnesemia is corrected. Magnesium appears crucial for normal bone-serum calcium homeostasis.

Treatment of Hypomagnesemia

Hypomagnesemia with tetany is treated with 25 to 50 mg/kg of magnesium sulfate administered intravenously or intramuscularly every 6 to 8 hours. Serum magnesium concentration should be rechecked every 24 hours. Hypermagnesemia with hypotonia may occur with overtreatment. Alternatively, magnesium may be given with feedings. The sulfate, gluconate, chloride, or citrate salt may be used in an initial dosage of 100 to 200 mg magnesium per kilogram per day given in divided doses every 6 hours. Excessive dosages have a laxative effect.

HYPERMAGNESEMIA

Magnesium that crosses the placenta after treatment for toxemia or preterm labor may produce hypotonia, flaccidity, respiratory depression, poor suck, and decreased gastrointestinal motility. Prolonged maternal magnesium administration has been associated with abnormal bone mineralization.[106] Hypermagnesemia may also occur during excessive magnesium administration with total parenteral nutrition. Treatment is expectant, because magnesium levels decline by 48 hours. If severe symptoms are present, administration of calcium may reverse these effects, and forced saline diuresis may speed magnesium excretion.

METABOLIC BONE DISEASE OF PREMATURITY (FORMERLY OSTEOPENIA–RICKETS OF PREMATURITY)

Although *osteopenia* and *rickets* have been the traditional terminology, *metabolic bone disease of prematurity* is now the preferred nomenclature.

The major factor in metabolic bone disease and rickets of prematurity is mineral deficiency.[107,108] Bone mineralization in utero increases to term (see Fig. 12-4). Premature infants miss the large accumulation of calcium and phosphorus that occurs during the last trimester in pregnancy and are therefore very susceptible to mineral deficiency. The most susceptible infants are those that have very low birth weight (<1000 g) and have chronic problems, such as bronchopulmonary dysplasia and necrotizing enterocolitis, that preclude adequate intake or require treatment with calciuric drugs (e.g., furosemide). In one study of extremely low-birth-weight infants, 33% had low bone mineral content. Hepatic and renal disease may contribute by impairing vitamin D metabolism.

Metabolic bone disease may be asymptomatic or manifest as classic rickets at 1 to 4 months of age with undermineralized bone, pathologic fractures, craniotabes, rachitic rosary, hypocalcemia, hypophosphatemia, and elevated levels of PTH, alkaline phosphatase, and 1,25-dihydroxyvitamin D levels (if not caused by vitamin D deficiency).

Prevention begins with achieving adequate calcium and phosphorus intake. Recommended minimum parenteral intakes of calcium, phosphorus, and vitamin D are 500 to 600 mg/L (12.5 to 15 mmol/L), 400 to 450 mg/L (12.9 to 14.5 mmol/L), and 160 IU/kg/day (maximum 400 IU/day), respectively.[109,110] Smaller infants may require higher intakes, but care must be taken to ensure the solubility of calcium and phosphorus in the parenteral fluid.

Early enteral feeding is key to prevention. Bone mineralization improves with increasing calcium and phosphorus supplementation. Term formulas and unsupplemented human milk provide inadequate calcium and phosphorus for premature infants. Preterm formulas and human milk supplemented with fortifiers at recommended dosages provide enough calcium (1000 to 1460 mg/L) and phosphorus (550 to 850 mg/L) to prevent rickets in most infants.[109] Calcium and phosphorus intake is also improved through the use of premature discharge formulas, which have higher calcium and phosphorus content than term infant formulas. Adequate protein intake is also important for calcium retention.

For infants at risk, calcium, phosphorus, and alkaline phosphatase levels should be monitored. If results are consistent with developing metabolic bone disease, additional calcium and phosphorus supplementation may be required. Only infants with cholestasis or renal disease may require additional vitamin D beyond the recommended 400 IU/day.[109]

QUESTIONS

Match the clinical scenarios with the following conditions and state the reasons for selection (more than one condition may be correct):

1. Hypoglycemia
2. Hyperglycemia
3. Hypocalcemia
4. Hypercalcemia

A 3400-g 7-day-old infant with a large ventricular septal defect becomes jittery. Earlier in the day, the child's intravenous fluids were decreased from 20 mL/hr to 11 mL/hr because of congestive heart failure. The concentration of dextrose in the total parenteral nutrition was increased from 12.5% to 15%.

Although the concentration of dextrose in the intravenous fluids was increased, this did not offset the decrease in the rate of fluid administration. Therefore, the glucose infusion rate decreased from 12.3 mg/kg/min to 8.1 mg/kg/min. An acute decrease in the glucose infusion rate may lead to hypoglycemia. Although patients with DiGeorge syndrome often have cardiac disease, usually the lesions are conotruncal defects (e.g., interrupted aortic arch, truncus arteriosus, tetralogy of Fallot). Patients with isolated ventricular septal defects are unlikely to have DiGeorge syndrome. Therefore the answer is 1 (hypoglycemia). This highlights the need to calculate glucose infusion rates in milligrams per kilogram per hour, and not to be seduced by the concentration, when assessing patients with hypoglycemia or hyperglycemia.

A 1800-g male infant is born at 40 weeks' gestation.

Infants with intrauterine growth restriction can have hypoglycemia, hyperglycemia, or hypocalcemia (answers 1, 2, and 3). Hypoglycemia may occur because of inadequate glycogen stores or hyperinsulinism. Infants with neonatal diabetes are hyperglycemic and growth restricted because of low intrauterine insulin concentrations. Intrauterine growth–restricted infants can be hypocalcemic secondary to low magnesium concentrations or fetal distress. Hypercalcemia is not usually associated with intrauterine growth restriction.

A 5-day-old infant shows jerking movements of the left arm and leg. On close evaluation, the child is also found to have an abnormal-appearing facies with mild hypertelorism, short philtrum, mildly low-set ears, micrognathia, and downslanting palpebral fissures.

This infant has features consistent with DiGeorge syndrome. Hypoplasia of the parathyroid gland leads to hypoparathyroidism and hypocalcemia. Therefore the answer is 3 (hypocalcemia). Many patients with DiGeorge syndrome do not have cardiac disease and are therefore not diagnosed immediately after birth.

A 2600-g newborn has a hemoglobin level of 26 g/dL.

Hypoglycemia is frequent in plethoric infants. A high hemoglobin level may be a factor in hypoglycemia in infants of diabetic mothers and in those with Beckwith-Wiedemann syndrome. The answer is 1 (hypoglycemia).

A newborn exhibits jitteriness and seizures.

These symptoms are present with hypoglycemia and hypocalcemia. The answer is 1 and 3 (hypoglycemia and hypocalcemia).

Box 12-1 lists many other conditions that have similar symptoms.

May be a clue to undiagnosed disease in the mother.

In a large-for-date infant, early hypoglycemia should be sought and may indicate unsuspected maternal diabetes. Neonatal hypocalcemia may be a clue to maternal hyperparathyroidism or familial hypocalciuric hypercalcemia (FHH). Neonatal hyperparathyroidism with hypercalcemia may be present when both parents have FHH and the infant is homozygous for the FHH gene mutation. The answer is 1, 3, and 4.

Associated with iatrogenic excessive administration of Vitamin D or A.

Excess vitamin D or vitamin A administration leads to hypercalcemia. The answer is 4 (hypercalcemia).

Cannot be corrected if hypomagnesemia is present.

Normal magnesium concentrations are necessary for normal parathyroid function. Hypocalcemia cannot be corrected in the presence of hypomagnesemia. Therefore, the answer is 3 (hypocalcemia).

True or False

Prematurity is the single most important risk factor for the development of metabolic bone disease.

The frequency of metabolic bone disease is inversely related to gestational age and birth weight. Other factors include prolonged total parenteral nutrition with delayed enteral feeding, and the failure to fortify human milk. The statement is true.

CASE 1

A 3900-g infant born at 38 weeks' gestation after an uncomplicated pregnancy has a plasma glucose concentration of 30 mg/dL at 1 hour of age. The infant is asymptomatic.

What is your initial management?

Because the infant is asymptomatic and the glucose concentration is higher than 25 mg/dL, the infant should be fed and a repeat glucose determination ordered in 30 minutes. The infant most likely has transient hypoglycemia, which is usually asymptomatic. The presence of macrosomia indicates that the infant is probably

hyperinsulinemic. This may occur in infants of diabetic mothers (diagnosed and undiagnosed) or in large-for-gestational age infants without maternal diabetes.

The plasma glucose concentration 1 hour later is 25 mg/dL.

What is your management now?

Despite early feeding, the plasma glucose level fell; therefore, prompt intravenous therapy is indicated. The infant should be given a minibolus of dextrose (2 mL/kg 10% dextrose in water, 200 mg/kg of glucose) followed by a continuous glucose infusion starting at 6 to 8 mg/kg/min. Enteral feeding may be continued if tolerated. Glucose concentrations should be measured at least hourly until values are stable.

The infant continues to have intermittent episodes of hypoglycemia requiring an increase in the glucose infusion to 18 mg/kg/min over the next 72 hours.

What additional laboratory studies should be performed?

The prolonged hypoglycemia, need for a high rate of glucose infusion, macrosomia, and lack of other congenital anomalies (e.g., abdominal wall defect, macroglossia) make persistent hyperinsulinemic hypoglycemia of infancy most likely. Plasma insulin concentrations should be measured when the infant is hypoglycemic. Although the early onset of hypoglycemia and lack of midline facial defects (i.e., cleft palate) make metabolic and endocrine disorders unlikely, cortisol, growth hormone, blood pH, and ammonia concentrations should be obtained. Ammonia concentrations also need to be measured to evaluate for hyperammonemic hyperinsulinism caused by mutation of the glutamate dehydrogenase gene.

This case shows the need for continued reevaluation of infants. Initially, when a patient like this is encountered, the most common diagnosis is transient hyperinsulinemic hypoglycemia. The persistence of hypoglycemia and the lack of improvement should prompt one to perform further evaluation and consider other potential diagnoses.

EDITORIAL COMMENT: Hyperinsulinism/hyperammonemia (HI/HA) syndrome is the second most common form of congenital hyperinsulinism.[17] Children affected by this syndrome have both fasting and protein-sensitive hypoglycemia combined with persistently elevated ammonia levels. The disorder is identified in infancy when the child experiences hypoglycemic seizures after brief periods of fasting or the ingestion of a high-protein meal. Gain-of-function mutations in the mitochondrial enzyme glutamate dehydrogenase are responsible for HI/HA syndrome. Glutamate dehydrogenase is expressed in the liver, kidney, brain, and pancreatic beta cells.

Patients with HI/HA syndrome have an increased frequency of generalized seizures, especially absence-type seizures, in the absence of hypoglycemia. The hypoglycemia of HI/HA syndrome is well controlled with diazoxide, a K_{ATP} channel agonist.

Glutamate dehydrogenase has also been implicated in another form of hyperinsulinism, short-chain 3-hydroxyacyl-CoA dehydrogenase (SCHAD) deficiency–associated hyperinsulinism.

HI/HA syndrome provides a rare example of an inborn error of intermediary metabolism in which the effect of the mutation on enzyme activity is a gain of function.[111]

CASE 2

You are called to see a 5-day-old infant because of irritability and jerking movements of the left arm and leg. He was the product of a full-term pregnancy and had a birth weight of 2800 g. Pregnancy was complicated by third-trimester bleeding. Delivery was by cesarean section because of placenta previa. One-minute Apgar score was 6; 5-minute Apgar score was 9. Feeding with evaporated milk formula was begun at 16 hours of age, and he did very well until a few hours ago when he became tremulous and fed poorly. Intermittent convulsions were noted. Examination reveals irritability but no other abnormalities. However, as the examination ends, the child has another seizure.

What diagnostic tests and procedures would you perform initially?

The symptoms shown by this baby are nonspecific. Central nervous system injury or infection is possible, and a lumbar puncture must be done. There is nothing in the case history to suggest hypoglycemia as a *probable* cause of the seizures, but some less common hypoglycemic syndromes (inborn error of metabolism, islet adenoma) may present this way, and glucose testing should be performed. Serum should be drawn for determination of electrolyte, calcium, blood urea nitrogen, and glucose levels.

Several features of this case suggest the possibility of hypocalcemia, notably stormy obstetric course, milk feedings, the age of onset of symptoms after the initially benign course, and irritability and tremulousness as cardinal symptoms. These features justify a trial with parenteral calcium after initial studies are done.

The therapeutic infusion is 2 mL/kg of 10% calcium gluconate over 10 minutes into an established intravenous line with ECG monitoring. Subsequent to immediate evaluation and treatment, the laboratory reports an ionized calcium level of 0.5 mmol/L and a phosphorus level of 11.5 mg/dL.

What factors may be important in the pathogenesis of the hypocalcemia?

The high serum phosphorus concentration indicates that dietary phosphorus load, relative hypoparathyroidism, and renal immaturity with retention of phosphate are important factors in the hypocalcemia.

What management should be instituted?

A low-phosphorus formula or formula with a favorable Ca/P ratio (Similac PM 60/40 or human milk) should be fed. Additional calcium supplementation (elemental calcium 20 to 80 mg/kg/day) can be used to increase the Ca/P ratio in the feedings to further decrease phosphate absorption.

What is the prognosis?

The prognosis is excellent. Supplemental calcium may be tapered and withdrawn at 3 to 4 weeks of age. Serum calcium level should be monitored at this time to be sure hypocalcemia does not recur. There should be no long-term sequelae.

CASE 3

A 2-month-old infant has increasing respiratory distress and an "incidental" finding on chest radiograph. He was a 27-week, 800-g infant at delivery and has had respiratory distress syndrome necessitating 1 month of mechanical ventilation via respirator and 1 month of continuous positive airway pressure therapy. Multiple episodes of cor pulmonale requiring long-term diuretic therapy and failure to establish enteral alimentation have necessitated total parenteral alimentation. Direct reacting hyperbilirubinemia was evident at 1 month.

Figure 12-5 shows what important findings?

In addition to chronic lung disease and cardiomegaly, metabolic bone disease is evident. Poorly mineralized bone, rachitic rosary, and pathologic fractures are present.

What common deficiency may be present?

In preterm infants, acquired nutritional rickets is usually due to deficiencies in calcium and phosphorus intake. In this patient, cholestasis contributes to the problem by leading to vitamin D deficiency, and long-term diuretic therapy (i.e., furosemide) may potentiate renal calcium losses.

What therapy should be started?

Maximize calcium intake by oral and parenteral routes. If hypophosphatemia is present, maximize intake of phosphorus. In the presence of hepatic dysfunction (cholestasis) or suspected malabsorption, vitamin D (1000 U/day) should be added. The use of drugs that increase renal calcium loss (e.g., furosemide) should be minimized.

Why did this patient have pulmonary deterioration?

Rachitic muscle weakness or rib cage dysfunction may result in pulmonary insufficiency.

A similar patient also demonstrates periosteal bone elevation, anemia, and neutropenia. What rarer nutritional deficiency is present?

In infants receiving prolonged hyperalimentation, trace mineral deficiency may occur. In this particular infant, copper intake was deficient.

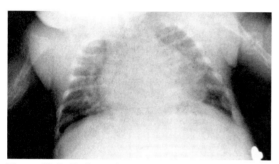

Figure 12-5. Radiographic findings in a 2-month-old, 800-g-birth-weight infant with respiratory distress (Case 3).

CASE 4

You attend the delivery of an infant at 37 weeks' gestation. The mother has preeclampsia and has received magnesium sulfate for the last 24 hours. At the time of delivery the infant is hypotonic and apneic, and requires intubation and positive pressure ventilation.

What is the most likely diagnosis and management?

Magnesium crosses the placenta, with fetal plasma concentrations directly correlating with maternal plasma concentrations. Maternal magnesium sulfate therapy leads to hypermagnesemia in the newborn infant. The diagnosis is most consistent with hypermagnesemia secondary to maternal therapy. Treatment is supportive. As long as urine output is adequate, magnesium levels will fall without further intervention.

CASE 5

A 1-day-old 1900-g infant born at 33 weeks' gestation to a diabetic mother has a focal seizure. Initial laboratory testing reveals an ionized calcium level of 0.5 mmol/L.

What is your initial treatment?

The initial treatment is 1.9 to 3.8 mL of 10% calcium gluconate infused intravenously over 10 minutes. Calcium should be added to the intravenous fluids to provide 75 mg/kg/day of elemental calcium.

A repeat ionized calcium concentration is 0.5 mmol/L. What is the most likely reason for the lack of response to therapy?

Premature infants and infants of diabetic mothers are at risk for hypomagnesemia. Magnesium is necessary for proper PTH secretion; therefore, calcium concentrations will not increase if hypomagnesemia is present. Magnesium concentration should be checked, and if it is low the infant should be treated with 25 to 50 mg/kg of magnesium sulfate.

True or False

The primary nutritional deficiency associated with metabolic bone disease in preterm infants is phosphorus deficiency.

The statement is factually correct. Risk factors for metabolic bone disease include prematurity and feeding practices as enunciated in the answer to the preceding question as well as drugs that deplete calcium from bone (corticosteroids, diuretics such as furosemide, and methylxanthines). Other factors include lack of movement, vitamin D deficiency, and aluminum toxicity. The statement is true.

REFERENCES

The reference list for this chapter can be found online at www.expertconsult.com.

Neonatal Hyperbilirubinemia

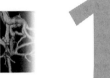

13

M. Jeffrey Maisels and Jon F. Watchko

Care of the high-risk neonate usually refers to care of the low-birth-weight infant or the sick term newborn. Although hyperbilirubinemia is certainly a matter of concern in these infants, the decisions that must be made regarding jaundice in the high-risk neonate are, in general, less complex than those that must be made in the healthy full-term infant. For the term and late preterm infant, shorter hospital stays, the need for outpatient surveillance and management, and the occasional disturbing case of extreme hyperbilirubinemia and even kernicterus raise new issues in the management of neonatal jaundice. Bilirubin has both salutary and toxic effects. At physiologic levels it exerts important antioxidant effects.[1] Although its toxic effects are well documented, there are also some concerns that aggressive use of phototherapy in very low-birth-weight infants may not be entirely innocuous.[2]

Most neonatal jaundice is the result of a combination of events—an increase in the rate of bilirubin production, reabsorption of bilirubin into the plasma from the gut (the enterohepatic circulation), and inability of the liver to clear sufficient bilirubin from the plasma.

FORMATION, STRUCTURE, AND PROPERTIES OF BILIRUBIN

Bilirubin is the end product of the catabolism of iron protoporphyrin, or heme, which comes predominantly from circulating hemoglobin (Fig. 13-1). Bilirubin is a tetrapyrrole compound with specific substitutions in the side chains of the four pyrrole rings. The outer pyrrole rings are linked to the inner ones by methene bridges (containing one double bond each), but the two central rings are joined by a methane bridge (no double bond). Normally, the methene bridge oxidized in heme is in the α-position, and the resultant isomer is bilirubin IX-α (see Fig. 13-3), the predominant isomer of bilirubin in the body. Although

its structure is conventionally represented in linear fashion as shown in Figure 13-2, the actual structure of bilirubin revealed by x-ray crystallography is similar to that shown in Figure 13-3, in which the bilirubin molecule is stabilized by the presence of intramolecular hydrogen bonds (indicated by the dashed lines). In this conformation, the hydrophilic, polar COOH and NH groups are not available for the attachment of water, whereas the hydrophobic hydrocarbon groups are on the perimeter, which makes the molecule insoluble in water but soluble in nonpolar solvents such as chloroform. The addition of methanol or ethanol interferes with hydrogen bonding and results in an immediate diazo reaction—the basis for measurement of indirect bilirubin by the van den Bergh reaction.

In the jaundiced newborn in whom the primary problem is excessive bilirubin formation or limited hepatic uptake and conjugation, unconjugated (i.e., indirect) bilirubin appears in the blood. When bilirubin glucuronide excretion is impaired (i.e., in cholestasis), conjugated bilirubin monoglucuronide and diglucuronide (direct reacting bilirubin) accumulate in the plasma and, because of their solubility, also appear in the urine. A fourth bilirubin fraction, known as *delta bilirubin*, is formed nonenzymatically from conjugated bilirubin, is covalently bound to albumin, and reacts directly with the diazo agent.

NEONATAL BILIRUBIN METABOLISM

Heme degradation leads to bilirubin production from two major sources (Fig. 13-4). Approximately 75% of the daily bilirubin production in the newborn comes from senescent erythrocytes (the catabolism of 1 g of hemoglobin yields 35 mg of bilirubin), but 25% is contributed by nonhemoglobin heme contained in the liver (in enzymes such as cytochromes and catalyses and in free heme) and in muscle myoglobin, or comes from ineffective erythropoiesis in the

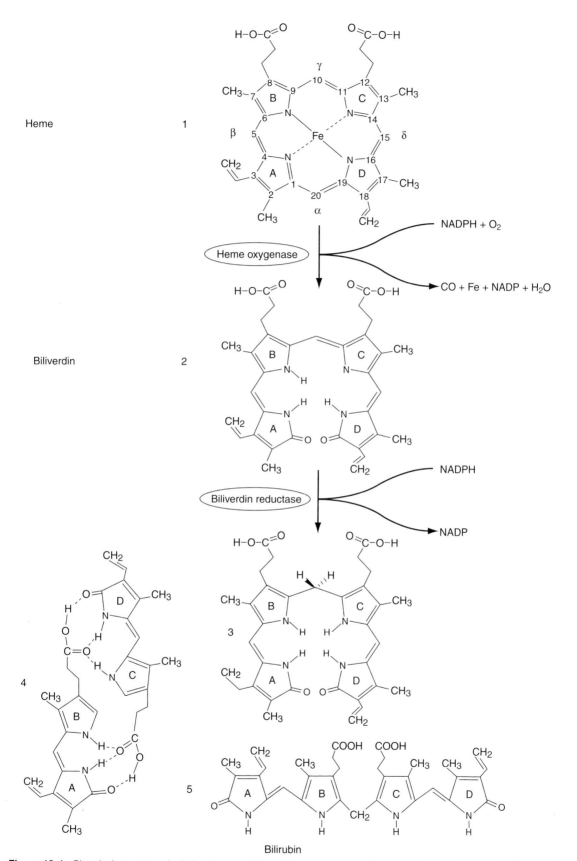

Figure 13-1. Chemical structures depicting the conversion of heme to bilirubin. Bilirubin is frequently represented by any of the three structures (*3* to *5*) shown at the bottom. *NADP,* Nicotinamide adenine dinucleotide phosphate; *NADPH,* reduced form of nicotinamide adenine dinucleotide phosphate. *(Redrawn from Gourley GR: Neonatal jaundice and disorders of bilirubin metabolism. In Suchy FJ, Sokol RJ, Balistreri WF, editors:* Liver disease in children, *ed 3, New York, 2007, Cambridge University Press.)*

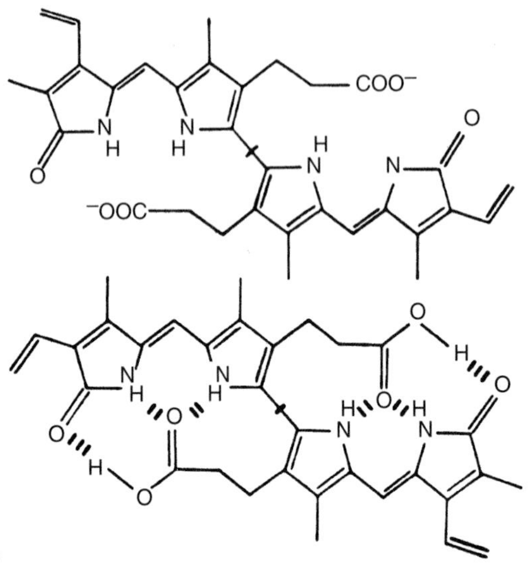

Figure 13-2. Chemical structure of bilirubin. **A,** Bilirubin dianion, with two free carboxyl groups; bilirubin monoanion has one free carboxyl group. **B,** Bilirubin diacid, the predominant form of free bilirubin in plasma at physiologic pH. *(From Brodersen R: Bilirubin transport in the newborn infant, reviewed in relation to kernicterus, J Pediatr 96:349–356, 1980.)*

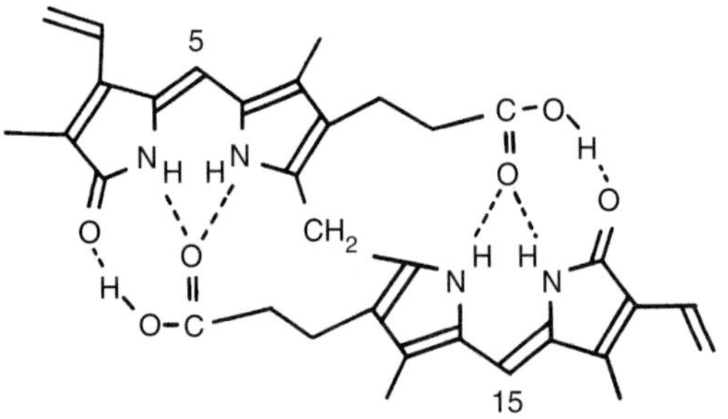

Figure 13-3. X-ray crystallographic structure of bilirubin IX-α. Dashed lines indicate hydrogen bonding.

bone marrow. Once it leaves the reticuloendothelial system, bilirubin is transported in the plasma, bound tightly to albumin, so that at physiologic pH the solubility of bilirubin is very low (about 4 nm/L [0.24 mg/dL]). When the bilirubin-albumin complex comes into contact with the hepatocyte, a proportion of the bilirubin, but not albumin, is transported into the cell, where it is bound to ligandin and then transported to the smooth endoplasmic reticulum for conjugation.

Conversion of unconjugated bilirubin to its water-soluble conjugate must occur before it can be excreted; this is achieved when bilirubin is combined enzymatically with a sugar, glucuronic acid, which produces bilirubin monoglucuronide and diglucuronide pigments that are more water soluble and sufficiently polar to be excreted into the bile or filtered through the kidney. The enzyme catalyzing this reaction is uridine diphosphate glucuronosyltransferase, a single form of which (UGT1A1) accounts for almost all of the bilirubin glucuronide in the human liver. The enzyme arises from the UGT1A1 gene complex situated on chromosome 2 at 2q37. Mutations and amino acid substitutions at different loci on this gene are responsible for the inherited unconjugated hyperbilirubinemias: Crigler-Najjar syndrome types I and II, and Gilbert syndrome. Data suggest a role for another bilirubin transporter, the hepatic solute carrier organic anion transporter 1B1 (SLCO1B1).[3] Gene polymorphisms of SLC1B1 may lead to hyperbilirubinemia by limiting hepatic bilirubin uptake. Once conjugated, bilirubin is excreted via the bile canaliculi into the small intestine. A detailed review of the chemistry and metabolism of bilirubin can be found elsewhere.[4,5]

NORMAL SERUM BILIRUBIN LEVELS AND THE NATURAL HISTORY OF NEONATAL JAUNDICE

Unconjugated bilirubin is transported efficiently via the placenta from fetal blood into the maternal circulation by passive diffusion.[6] The mean total serum bilirubin (TSB) levels in cord blood range from 1.4 to 1.9 mg/dL (24 to 32 μmol/L), whereas maternal TSB levels are less than 1 mg/dL (17.1 μmol). For years it has been taught that the TSB concentration in normal term infants increases from birth, reaches its apex on about the third or fourth day of life, and then declines, reaching normal levels by 7 to 10 days. When bilirubin levels are studied in large populations using transcutaneous bilirubin (TcB) measurements, however, it is clear that in those at or above the 50th percentile, the peak does not occur until about 96 hours and remains at that level through 120 hours (Fig. 13-5).[7] On the other hand, there are significant differences in the natural history in term and late preterm infants for each week of gestation.[8] In those with a gestational age of 40 weeks or longer, the peak TcB occurs at about 60 hours, whereas in those with a gestational age of 35 to 39½ weeks it does not occur until 96 hours or later (Fig. 13-6).[7,8] Because of intervention with phototherapy, no recent data are available on the natural history of bilirubinemia in infants of 34 weeks' gestation or less.

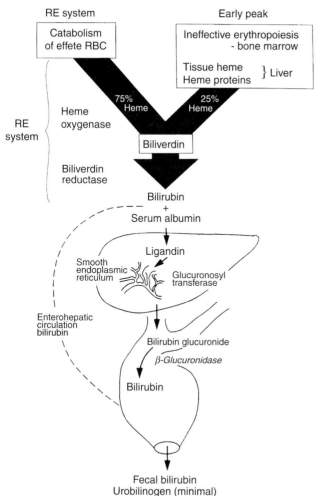

Figure 13-4. Neonatal bile pigment metabolism. *RBC*, Red blood cell; *RE*, reticuloendothelial. *(From Maisels MJ: Jaundice. In Avery GB, Fletcher MA, MacDonald MG, editors:* Neonatology: pathophysiology and management of the newborn, *Philadelphia, 1999, JB Lippincott, pp 765–819).*

DEVELOPMENTAL JAUNDICE

The normal increase of TSB levels in the newborn has been termed *physiologic jaundice,* but there is good reason to consider abandoning this term.[9] Depending on ethnic characteristics, breast feeding, and other factors, there are significant differences in TSB levels in different populations, so that what is physiologic for one infant may well be nonphysiologic for another. Particularly for low-birth-weight infants being cared for in the neonatal intensive care unit (NICU), the term *physiologic jaundice* has little meaning and is potentially dangerous. If no treatment is given, low-birth-weight infants have prolonged and exaggerated hyperbilirubinemia—the lower the birth weight, the higher the peak bilirubin level. A TSB of 10 mg/dL (171 μmol/L) on day 4 in a 750-g neonate is a normal bilirubin level for that infant and requires no investigation to identify a cause for the jaundice. Nevertheless,

most neonatologists would treat this bilirubin level with phototherapy. Thus, TSB levels well within the physiologic range are considered potentially hazardous and are commonly treated with phototherapy. The natural history of hyperbilirubinemia in this population is never observed, and defining these bilirubin levels as physiologic in such infants seems illogical and potentially dangerous. A better term for this phenomenon is *developmental jaundice.*[9]

The jaundice seen in almost every newborn results from a combination of mechanisms:

- The normal neonate produces about 6 to 8 mg/kg/day of bilirubin, which is about 2.5 times the rate of bilirubin production in the adult.[10]
- The newborn reabsorbs significant amounts of unconjugated bilirubin from the intestine (the enterohepatic circulation). Unlike the adult, newborns have few

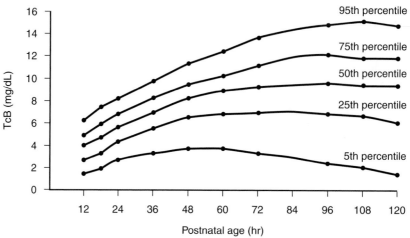

Figure 13-5. Smoothed curves from 14,035 transcutaneous bilirubin (TcB) measurements in 2646 newborns (gestational age ≥35 weeks and birth weight ≥2000 g). *(From Fouzas S, Mantagou L, Skylogianni E, et al: Transcutaneous bilirubin levels for the first 120 postnatal hours in healthy neonates,* Pediatrics 125:e52, 2009).

bacteria in the small and large bowel and they have greater activity of the deconjugating enzyme β-glucuronidase. As a result, conjugated bilirubin (which cannot be reabsorbed), is not converted to urobilinogen but is hydrolyzed to unconjugated bilirubin. This can be reabsorbed and increases the bilirubin load on the liver.

• There is a decrease in clearance of bilirubin from the plasma. This is the result of a deficiency in ligandin, the predominant bilirubin-binding protein in the hepatocyte, and a deficiency of UGT1A1, which, at term, has approximately 1% of the activity found in the adult.

AN APPROACH TO THE JAUNDICED INFANT

The overwhelming majority of both preterm and term infants who are jaundiced are not jaundiced as a result of any pathologic process. Their jaundice is the result of the mechanisms described earlier, and the relevant clinical and laboratory risk factors for the development of severe hyperbilirubinemia in the term and late preterm infant are well documented.[11] The pathologic causes of indirect hyperbilirubinemia are listed in Box 13-1.

WHO IS JAUNDICED?

Jaundice is a clinical sign, and for years clinicians have assessed the intensity of jaundice and used this assessment to decide whether to obtain a serum bilirubin measurement. But the ability of clinicians to

diagnose "clinically significant" jaundice varies widely, and this can lead to important errors in management.[12-14] In addition, whether the TSB level is "clinically significant" depends both on the actual TSB level and the infant's age, in hours (Figs. 13-5 to 13-7). Currently, experts recommend that before discharge, TSB or TcB should be measured in all newborns.[15,16]

NONINVASIVE BILIRUBIN MEASUREMENTS

TcB measurements are being used with increasing frequency in hospital nurseries, in outpatient settings, and in the preterm population.[7,17-25] They reduce significantly the number of TSB measurements needed in both the term nursery and the NICU, and they are invaluable in the outpatient setting.[19,22,26] TcB measurements provide instantaneous information while reducing the likelihood that a clinically significant TSB will be missed. There is good evidence that TcB measurements provide excellent estimates of the TSB level, although they are not a substitute for TSB values.[27]

The TcB value is a measurement of the yellow color of the blanched skin and subcutaneous tissues, not the serum bilirubin level, and should be used as a screening tool to help determine whether the TSB level should be measured. Because TcB measurements are noninvasive, they can be repeated several times during the birth hospitalization and provide useful information about the rate of rise of the bilirubin level. When plotted on a nomogram (see Figs. 13-5 to 13-7), TcB levels

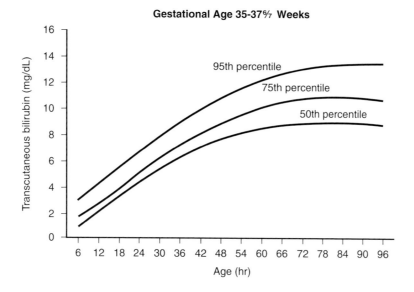

Gestational Age 35-37⁶⁄₇ Weeks

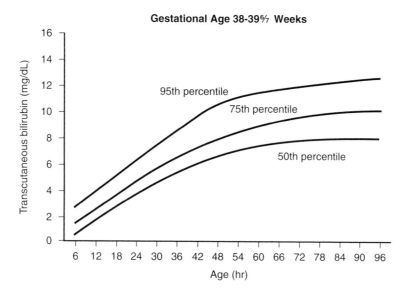

Gestational Age 38-39⁶⁄₇ Weeks

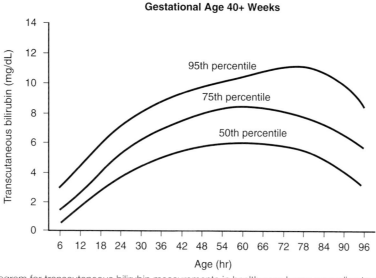

Gestational Age 40+ Weeks

Figure 13-6. Nomogram for transcutaneous bilirubin measurements in healthy newborns according to gestational age. *(From Maisels MJ, Kring E: Transcutaneous bilirubin levels in the first 96 hours in a normal newborn population of 35 or more weeks' of gestation, Pediatrics 117:1169, 2006.)*

Box 13-1.	Causes of Indirect Hyperbilirubinemia in Newborn Infants

Increased bilirubin production or load on the liver

Hemolytic disease

Immune mediated

- Rh alloimmunization
- ABO and other blood group incompatibilities

Heritable

Red cell membrane defects

- Spherocytosis,* elliptocytosis, stomatocytosis, pyknocytosis

Red cell enzyme deficiencies

- Glucose-6-phosphate dehydrogenase deficiency,* pyruvate kinase deficiency, and other erythrocyte enzyme deficiencies

Hemoglobinopathies

α-thalassemia, γβ-thalassemia

Unstable hemoglobins

Heinz body hemolytic anemia

Other causes of increased production

Sepsis*†

Disseminated intravascular coagulation

Extravasation of blood; hematoma; pulmonary, cerebral, or other occult hemorrhage

Polycythemia

Macrosomic infants of diabetic mothers

Increased enterohepatic circulation of bilirubin

Breast milk jaundice

Pyloric stenosis

Small or large bowel obstruction or ileus

Decreased clearance

Prematurity

Glucose-6-phosphate dehydrogenase deficiency

Metabolic

Crigler-Najjar syndrome types I and II, Gilbert syndrome

Tyrosinemia†

Hypermethioninemia†

Hypothyroidism

Hypopituitarism†

Modified from Watchko JF: Indirect hyperbilirubinemia in the neonate. In Maisels MJ, Watchko JF, editors: Neonatal jaundice, London, 2000, Harwood Academic Publishers, p 52.

*Decreased clearance is also part of the pathogenesis of indirect hyperbilirubinemia.

†Elevation of direct-reacting bilirubin also occurs.

Table 13-1.	Discharge Diagnosis in 306 Infants Admitted with Severe Hyperbilirubinemia*		
Diagnosis		**Number**	**Percentage**
Hyperbilirubinemia of unknown cause or breast milk jaundice		290	94.8
Cephalhematoma or bruising		3	1.0
ABO hemolytic disease†		11	3.6
Anti-E hemolytic disease		1	0.3
Galactosemia		1	0.3
Sepsis		0	

From Maisels MJ, Kring E: Risk of sepsis in newborns with severe hyperbilirubinemia, *Pediatrics* **90:741, 1992.**
*Infants were readmitted after discharge as newborns. Mean age at admission was 5 days (range: 2-17 days), and mean bilirubin level was 18.5 ± 2.8 mg/dL (range: 12.7-29.1 mg/dL).
†Mother was type O, infant was type A or B, direct Coombs test result was positive.

that are crossing percentiles indicate the need for additional observation and evaluation.

LABORATORY EVALUATION—SEEKING A CAUSE FOR JAUNDICE

In the NICU, many neonates are jaundiced simply because they were born prematurely and have extremely limited UGT1A1 activity (0.1% of adult levels at 30 weeks' gestation). Even among term and late preterm infants who are readmitted to the hospital in the first 2 weeks of life with TSB levels of 18 to 20 mg/dL (308 to 340 μmol/L), only about 5% have an identifiable pathologic cause for jaundice (Table 13-1).[28]

The guideline of the American Academy of Pediatrics (AAP) recommends laboratory evaluation for the cause of hyperbilirubinemia in infants of 35 weeks' gestation or more whose TSB levels exceed the 95th percentile or in whom the rate of increase appears to be crossing percentiles.[11] In preterm infants, laboratory evaluation is indicated in any infant who meets the criteria for phototherapy. Table 13-2 provides an approach to the clinical and laboratory evaluation of the jaundiced newborn, and Box 13-1 lists the causes of indirect hyperbilirubinemia in the newborn.

The timing of the onset of jaundice is important; jaundice that appears within the first 24 hours or increases rapidly and crosses percentiles is due to excessive bilirubin production (hemolysis) until proven otherwise. Most newborns whose TSB levels

Table 13-2.	Laboratory Evaluation of the Jaundiced Infant
Indications	**Assessments**
Jaundice in first 24 hr	Measure TcB and/or TSB
Infant meets criteria for phototherapy* or TSB rising rapidly (i.e., crossing percentiles [see Fig. 13-5])	Perform blood typing and Coombs test, if not done on cord blood. Perform complete blood count, reticulocyte count, and smear examination. Measure direct or conjugated bilirubin. Consider G6PD testing. Repeat TSB in 4-24 hr. depending on infant's age and TSB level.
TSB concentration approaching exchange levels or not responding to phototherapy	Perform investigations as above and G6PD testing and albumin level.
Elevated direct (or conjugated) bilirubin level	Do urinalysis and urine culture; evaluate for sepsis if indicated by history and physical examination.
Jaundice present at or beyond age 2-3 wk, or sick infant	Measure total and direct (or conjugated) bilirubin level. If direct bilirubin elevated, evaluate for causes of cholestasis. Check results of newborn thyroid and galactosemia screen, and evaluate infant for signs or symptoms of hypothyroidism.

*Because phototherapy is used at low TSB levels in low-birth-weight infants (see Table 13-9), these investigations are often unnecessary in low-birth-weight infants who meet the criteria for phototherapy.
G6PD, Glucose-6-phosphate dehydrogenase; *TcB*, transcutaneous bilirubin; *TSB*, total serum bilirubin.

exceed the 75th percentile on the Bhutani nomogram (see Fig. 13-7) have evidence of hemolysis.[11,29]

PATHOLOGIC JAUNDICE

HEMOLYTIC DISEASE

Immune-Mediated Hemolytic Disease

The combination of antepartum and postpartum prophylaxis with Rh(D) immunoglobulin has dramatically reduced the incidence of erythroblastosis fetalis resulting from the Rh9 (D) antigen, and the incidence of Rh hemolytic disease is currently estimated to be about 1 in 1000 live births. Approximately half of affected newborns require little or no treatment.[30]

ABO hemolytic disease generally occurs in infants of blood group A or B born to group O mothers. Because approximately 45% of Americans of Western European descent have type O blood and a similar percentage are type A, A-O incompatibility is the most common form of ABO incompatibility encountered in the United States.[31] Although about one of every three group A or B infants born to a group O mother has anti-A or anti-B antibodies attached to their red cells, only one in five of those with a positive result on a direct antibody test (DAT) develops a modest to significant degree of hyperbilirubinemia. In an Israeli population of 162 DAT-positive group A or B newborns born to group O mothers, 52% developed a TSB higher than the 95th percentile on the Bhutani nomogram.[32] Forty-eight percent of O-B babies developed hyperbilirubinemia in the first 24 hours compared with 26% of O-A babies.[33] Of 258 Canadian infants who developed TSB levels of more than 425 µmol/L (24.9 mg/dL), 48 (16.7%) had ABO hemolytic disease.[34] There appears to be considerable variation in the frequency with which ABO hemolytic disease is responsible for severe hyperbilirubinemia (see Table 13-1).

The diagnosis of *ABO hemolytic disease* as opposed to *ABO incompatibility* should generally be reserved for infants who have a positive DAT finding *and* clinical jaundice within the first 12 to 24 hours of life (icterus praecox). Reticulocytosis and the presence of microspherocytes on the smear support the diagnosis (Box 13-2). Underscoring the importance of a positive DAT result in support of the diagnosis of ABO hemolytic disease, Herschel et al concluded that in DAT-negative newborns of ABO-incompatible mother-infant pairs who have significant hyperbilirubinemia, a cause other than isoimmunization should be sought.[35] On the other hand, Kaplan and associates[36] found that 43% of DAT-negative, ABO-incompatible infants who were homozygous for the variant UGT promoter associated with Gilbert syndrome had a TSB level of 15 mg/dL (256 µmol/L) or higher compared with none of the ABO-incompatible DAT-negative infants who were homozygous normal (for the promoter element) (Fig. 13-8). There was no difference between ABO-incompatible and ABO-compatible DAT-negative newborns, as long as the ABO-incompatible neonates did not have Gilbert syndrome. This observation confirms that if another icterogenic factor is present, then ABO-incompatible newborns are at risk for hyperbilirubinemia even if they

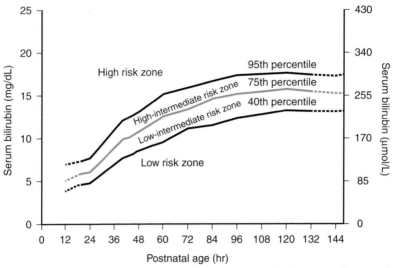

Figure 13-7. Risk designation of term and near-term well newborns based on their hour-specific serum bilirubin values. (Dotted extensions are based on <300 total serum bilirubin values per epoch.) *(From American Academy of Pediatrics, Subcommittee on Hyperbilirubinemia: Management of hyperbilirubinemia in the newborn infant 35 or more weeks of gestation,* Pediatrics *114:4, 2004.)*

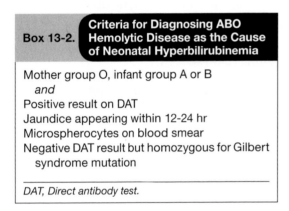

Box 13-2.	**Criteria for Diagnosing ABO Hemolytic Disease as the Cause of Neonatal Hyperbilirubinemia**

Mother group O, infant group A or B
   and
Positive result on DAT
Jaundice appearing within 12-24 hr
Microspherocytes on blood smear
Negative DAT result but homozygous for Gilbert
   syndrome mutation

DAT, Direct antibody test.

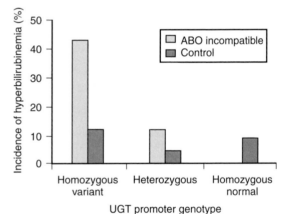

Figure 13-8. Incidence of hyperbilirubinemia defined as total serum bilirubin level of 15 mg/dL (256 μmol/L) in ABO-incompatible direct antibody test (DAT)-negative and ABO-compatible (control) infants according to the uridine diphosphate glucuronosyltransferase (UGT) promoter genotype. ABO-incompatible DAT-negative infants who were also homozygous for the variant UGT promoter (Gilbert syndrome) had a significantly higher incidence of hyperbilirubinemia than did ABO-incompatible DAT-negative infants who were homozygous normal for the UGT promoter. The former subgroup also had a significantly greater incidence of hyperbilirubinemia than any of the three UGT promoter genotype subgroups in the control (ABO-compatible) infants. *(From Kaplan M, Hammerman C, Renbaum P, et al: Gilbert's syndrome and hyperbilirubinaemia in ABO incompatible neonates,* Lancet *356:652, 2000.)*

are DAT negative.[36] There are other possible explanations for the finding of ABO hemolytic disease in the absence of a positive DAT result. Some cases may reflect the insensitivity of the DAT or may occur in infants who have a paucity of A and B antigens on their red cells or unusually efficient absorption of serum antibody by A and B antigen epitopes present in body tissues and fluids.

Heritable Causes of Hemolysis

Defects in the red cell membrane include hereditary spherocytosis, elliptocytosis, stomatocytosis, and infantile pyknocytosis. Although these conditions can occur in the newborn period, newborns frequently exhibit substantial variations in red cell size and shape, and it is not always easy to establish one of these diagnoses. Spherocytes are not usually seen on red cell smears and, when present, suggest the diagnosis of hereditary spherocytosis or ABO hemolytic disease. A recent observation suggests that a mean corpuscular hemoglobin concentration of 36 g/dL or more is a useful marker to identify neonates who might have sphe-rocytosis.[37] Because hereditary spherocyto-sis has an autosomal dominant inheritance pattern, a family history can often be elic-ited. In addition, the presence of severe jaundice in neonates with hereditary sphe-rocytosis is closely related to an interaction with the Gilbert syndrome allele, a phe-nomenon also observed (as noted earlier) in infants with glucose-6-phosphate dehy-drogenase (G6PD) deficiency.[38]

Red Cell Enzyme Deficiencies

G6PD deficiency is a problem that affects hundreds of millions of people around the world. Nevertheless, most neonatologists in the United States do not (but should) think about this enzyme deficiency as a likely cause of significant hyperbilirubinemia. Although G6PD deficiency occurs in approximately 12% of African American males and 4% of African American females,[39] severe hyperbil-irubinemia does not develop in most G6PD-deficient newborns. Nevertheless, extreme hyperbilirubinemia and kernicterus have been described in G6PD-deficient infants of African American descent.[40] In the ker-nicterus registry, G6PD deficiency was the cause of the hyperbilirubinemia in 21% of cases.[40] G6PD deficiency is an X-linked dis-order, and hemolysis can occur following exposure to an oxidative challenge. Agents potentially involved include naphthalene (a component of mothballs), dyes, and infec-tion, but more often than not, no offending agent is identified. Interestingly, in some, but not all, G6PD-deficient infants in whom severe hyperbilirubinemia develops, there are no signs of overt hemolysis (anemia and reticulocytosis),[41] and significant hyperbili-rubinemia associated with G6PD deficiency is primarily the result of abnormal biliru-bin clearance rather than hemolysis. Other researchers disagree with this view and sug-gest that overt signs of hemolysis are not found because the hemolysis is self-limited and extravascular, and involves an older fraction of the red cell population.[42]

The identification of a molecular marker for Gilbert syndrome in the promoter region of the *UGT1A1* gene has demonstrated a remarkable association between hyper-bilirubinemia, G6PD deficiency, and Gil-bert syndrome. The most common genetic polymorphism encountered in whites with Gilbert syndrome is an additional TA inser-tion in the TA TAA box of the *UGT1A1* gene promoter. Affected individuals are

homozygous for the variant promoter and have 7 repeats—(TA)$_7$ TAA (7/7) instead of the more usual 6 repeats—(TA)$_6$ TAA (6/6). Heterozygotes have 1 allele each of the wild-type and variant promoter (6/7). In Israel, G6PD-deficient infants with TSB levels of 15 mg/dL (257 μmol/L) more, only 10% were homozygous for the normal *UGT1A1* promoter (6/6), whereas 50% were homo-zygous for the variant Gilbert *UGT1A1* pro-moter (7/7). TSB levels ≥15 mg/mL did not develop in either the neonates with G6PD deficiency alone or in those with only the variant *UGT1A1* promoter (7/7).[38]

Pyruvate kinase deficiency is an autoso-mal recessive disorder that is less common than G6PD deficiency but may present with significant jaundice, anemia, and reticulo-cytosis. In particular, pyruvate kinase defi-ciency should be considered in neonates of Amish descent with marked neonatal hyperbilirubinemia.

Unstable Hemoglobins

The term *unstable hemoglobins* is applied to hemoglobins exhibiting reduced solubil-ity or higher susceptibility to oxidation of amino acid residues within the individual globin chains.[43] More than 100 structur-ally different unstable hemoglobin mutants have been documented, and the clinical syndrome associated with unstable hemo-globin disorders is often called *congenital Heinz body hemolytic anemia*. Some of these infants can manifest severe hemolytic ane-mia and hyperbilirubinemia.

OTHER CAUSES OF INCREASED BILIRUBIN PRODUCTION OR LOAD ON THE LIVER

The hemoglobinopathies rarely manifest themselves as jaundice in the neonatal period, although such cases have been described occasionally. Cephalhematomas, intracranial or pulmonary hemorrhage, or any occult bleeding may lead to an elevated TSB level from breakdown of the extravascular eryth-rocytes. In some studies, the presence of periventricular-intraventricular hemorrhage has been associated with an increase in TSB levels in very low-birth-weight infants, but others have not found this association. Poly-cythemia is usually listed as a cause of hyper-bilirubinemia, because the catabolism of 1 g of hemoglobin produces 35 mg of bilirubin. Nevertheless, mean bilirubin levels and the incidence of hyperbilirubinemia are simi-lar in polycythemic infants receiving partial exchange transfusion and in those receiving symptomatic treatment.

Any small or large bowel obstruction, ileus, or delayed passage of meconium exaggerates the enterohepatic circulation of bilirubin (this is also thought to be the mechanism for hyperbilirubinemia associated with pyloric stenosis). In any of these conditions, correction of the obstruction produces a prompt decline in bilirubin levels. Macrosomic infants of mothers with insulin-dependent diabetes are at an increased risk of hyperbilirubinemia, probably as a result of increased bilirubin production.

DECREASED BILIRUBIN CLEARANCE

Inherited Unconjugated Hyperbilirubinemia—Inborn Errors of Bilirubin UGT1A1 Activity

UGT1A1 accounts for almost all of the bilirubin glucuronidation activity in the human liver, and three degrees of inherited UGT1A1 deficiency are recognized. Crigler-Najjar syndrome type I is inherited in an autosomal recessive pattern with marked genetic heterogeneity, and more than 30 different genetic mutations have been identified. Infants with this condition have virtually complete absence of bilirubin UGT1A1 activity, severe jaundice develops in the first 2 to 3 days of life, and intensive phototherapy and, often, exchange transfusions are required.[44] Unless these children receive a liver transplant, which is curative, they are committed to lifelong phototherapy, which becomes less and less effective as they get older.

Type II Crigler-Najjar disease, also known as *Arias syndrome,* has a pattern of inheritance that is usually autosomal recessive, but it may also be autosomal dominant. The disorder is characterized by low but detectable activity of bilirubin UGT1A1, and the hyperbilirubinemia usually shows some response to phenobarbital therapy. Although jaundice is generally less severe than in patients with Crigler-Najjar syndrome type I, marked hyperbilirubinemia develops in some children with Crigler-Najjar syndrome type II, and kernicterus can also occur.[44]

At one time the diagnosis of Gilbert syndrome was never made until adolescence, when it manifests as a mild, benign, chronic unconjugated hyperbilirubinemia with no evidence of liver disease or overt hemolysis. Gilbert syndrome affects approximately

9% of the population, and both autosomal dominant as well as recessive inheritance patterns have been found. The identification of the genetic basis for this disorder (a variant promoter for the gene encoding UGT1A1) has permitted its identification in the newborn. Newborns who are homozygous for the A(TA)7TAA polymorphism have somewhat higher TSB levels in the first days of life than do heterozygous or normal infants, although the effect is modest.[45] The Gilbert syndrome genotype is also an important contributor to the prolonged indirect hyperbilirubinemia found in some breast-feeding infants. Twenty-seven percent of breast-fed infants who had TSB levels of more than 5.8 mg/dL (100 µmol/L) at age 28 days had the Gilbert syndrome genotype, and 16 of 17 breast-fed Japanese infants with prolonged jaundice had at least 1 mutation of the *UGT1A1* gene,[46] primarily of the G7IR type.[47] The association of the Gilbert genotype with significant jaundice in G6PD-deficient infants, ABO-incompatible DAT-negative infants (see Fig. 13-8), and infants with hereditary spherocytosis has been discussed earlier.

Other Inborn Errors of Metabolism

Jaundiced infants who have vomiting, excessive weight loss, hepatomegaly, and splenomegaly should be suspected of having galactosemia. In galactosemia, the hyperbilirubinemia during the first week of life is almost exclusively unconjugated, but the conjugated fraction tends to increase during the second week, which probably reflects liver damage. A test of the urine for reducing substances using alkaline copper sulfate reagent tablets (Clinitest, Bayer Corp., Elkhart, Ind.) helps to make the diagnosis. Infants with tyrosinemia and hypermethioninemia are jaundiced primarily as a result of the presence of neonatal liver disease, so that indirect hyperbilirubinemia is generally accompanied by some evidence of cholestasis. Prolonged indirect hyperbilirubinemia is one of the clinical features of congenital hypothyroidism, a condition that should be identified by routine metabolic screening programs currently used for newborns. Other causes of prolonged indirect hyperbilirubinemia are listed in Box 13-3.

Breast Feeding and Jaundice

A strong association between breast feeding and an increased incidence of neonatal hyperbilirubinemia has been found in

Box 13-3.	**Causes of Prolonged Indirect Hyperbilirubinemia**

Breast milk jaundice
Hemolytic disease
Hypothyroidism
Extravascular blood
Pyloric stenosis
Crigler-Najjar syndrome
Gilbert syndrome genotype in breast-fed infants

Box 13-4.	**Most Likely Causes of Cholestasis in Infants 2 Months of Age or Younger**

Obstructive cholestasis
Biliary atresia
Choledochal cyst
Gallstones or biliary sludge
Alagille syndrome
Inspissated bile
Cystic fibrosis
Congenital hepatic fibrosis/Caroli disease

Hepatocellular cholestasis
Idiopathic neonatal hepatitis
Viral infection
 • Cytomegalovirus
 • HIV
Bacterial infection
 • Urinary tract infection
 • Sepsis
 • Syphilis
Genetic/metabolic disorders
 • α1-antitrypsin deficiency
 • Tyrosinemia
 • Galactosemia
 • Hypothyroidism
 • Progressive familial intrahepatic cholestasis (PFIC)
 • Cystic fibrosis
 • Panhypopituitarism
 Toxic/secondary disorders
 • Parenteral nutrition-associated cholestasis

From Moyer V, Freese DK, Whitington PF, et al: Guideline for the evaluation of cholestatic jaundice in infants: recommendations of the North American Society for Pediatric Gastroenterology, Hepatology and Nutrition, J Pediatr Gastroenterol Nutr *39:115, 2004.*

most[40,48-50] but not all studies.[51] The primary contributors to jaundice associated with breast feeding are a decreased caloric intake in the first few days of life and an increased enterohepatic circulation.[52] Breast-fed infants usually receive fewer calories in the first days after birth than do those fed formula, and caloric deprivation itself appears to enhance the enterohepatic circulation of bilirubin. Increasing the frequency of breast feeding significantly reduces the risk of hyperbilirubinemia, which provides further support for the important role of caloric deprivation and the enterohepatic circulation in the pathogenesis of breast-feeding jaundice. The stools of breast-fed infants weigh less, and the cumulative wet and dry stool output of breast-fed infants is lower than that of formula-fed infants.[53]

MIXED FORMS OF JAUNDICE

Sepsis
Jaundice is one sign of bacterial sepsis, but septic infants almost always have other signs and symptoms. Unexplained indirect hyperbilirubinemia as the *only* sign of sepsis is rare (see Table 13-1), and lumbar punctures or blood and urine cultures in jaundiced infants who otherwise appear well are not recommended.[28] On the other hand, those who appear sick or have direct hyperbilirubinemia or other findings in the physical examination or laboratory evaluation that are out of the ordinary should be evaluated for possible sepsis. Other causes of mixed forms of jaundice include congenital syphilis, the TORCH (*t*oxoplasmosis, *o*ther infections *r*ubella, *c*ytomegalovirus infection, *h*erpes simplex) group of intrauterine infections, and Coxsackie B virus infection.

Cholestatic Jaundice
Cholestasis refers to a reduction in bile flow and is the term used to describe a group of disorders associated with conjugated (or direct reacting) hyperbilirubinemia. Such jaundice indicates inadequate bile secretion or biliary flow. Although it is frequently transient in sick low-birth-weight infants, particularly those receiving parenteral nutrition, a pathologic cause must always be ruled out. For a detailed discussion of the causes and management of cholestatic jaundice, refer to a review of this subject.[54]

Conditions most likely associated with conjugated hyperbilirubinemia in the neonatal period are listed in Box 13-4. Cholestasis occurs in about 1 in 2500 infants and can be categorized as obstructive or hepatocellular. Most cases of conjugated hyperbilirubinemia in early infancy are the

Table 13-3.	Recommended Approach to the Identification and Evaluation of Cholestasis in Infants	
Recommendation		**Level of Evidence**
It is recommended that any infant noted to be jaundiced at 2 weeks of age be clinically evaluated for cholestasis with measurement of total and direct serum bilirubin. However, breast-fed infants who can be reliably monitored and who have an otherwise normal history (no dark urine or light stools) and physical examination may be asked to return at 3 weeks of age, and if jaundice persists, total and direct serum bilirubin are measured at that time.		C
Retest any infant with an acute condition or other explanation for jaundice whose jaundice does not resolve with appropriate management of the diagnosed condition.		D
Ultrasonography is recommended for infants with cholestasis of unknown cause.		A
Liver biopsy is recommended for most infants with cholestasis of unknown cause.		A
Measurements of γ-glutamyl transpeptidase and lipoprotein X are not routinely recommended in the evaluation of cholestasis in young infants.		C
Scintigraphy and analysis of duodenal aspirate are not routinely recommended but may be useful in situations in which other tests are not readily available.		A
Magnetic resonance cholangiopancreatography and endoscopic retrograde cholangiopancreatography (ERCP) are not routinely recommended, although ERCP may be useful in experienced hands.		C

From Moyer V, Freese DK, Whitington PF, et al: Guideline for the evaluation of cholestatic jaundice in infants: recommendations of the North American Society for Pediatric Gastroenterology, Hepatology and Nutrition, *J Pediatr Gastroenterol Nutr* 39:115, 2004.
Level A, Recommendation based on two or more studies that compared the test with a criterion standard in an independent, blind manner in an unselected population of infants similar to those addressed in the guideline.
Level B, Recommendation based on a single study that compared the test with a criterion standard in an independent, blind manner in an unselected population of infants similar to those addressed in the guideline.
Level C, Recommendation based on lower quality studies or studies for which inadequate information is provided to assess quality, together with expert opinion and consensus of the committee.
Level D, No studies available; recommendation based on expert opinion and consensus of the committee.

result of neonatal hepatitis or biliary atresia. Neonatal hepatitis is characterized by prolonged conjugated hyperbilirubinemia without any obvious evidence of bacterial or viral infection or the other causes listed in Box 13-4. Extrahepatic biliary atresia occurs when there is obliteration of the lumen of part of the biliary tract or absence of some or all of the extrahepatic biliary system. Extrahepatic biliary atresia occurs in 1 in 10,000 to 19,000 newborn infants, and it is important to make the diagnosis expeditiously before irreversible sclerosis of the intrahepatic ducts occurs,[54] particularly if the biliary atresia is a component of the biliary atresia splenic malformation syndrome or is the cystic form of biliary atresia (see later discussion). The identification of cholestatic jaundice and initiation of the necessary diagnostic investigations will occur in a timely fashion if every infant who is clinically jaundiced beyond the age of 2 to 3 weeks undergoes measurement of direct-reacting bilirubin (Tables 13-2 and 13-3, and Fig. 13-9).[54] Earlier laboratory investigations are mandatory in any jaundiced infant who has pale stools or dark urine (the urine

of most newborns is nearly colorless). This simple approach ensures timely evaluation and treatment of infants with extrahepatic biliary atresia.

The initial treatment of extrahepatic biliary atresia is a portoenterostomy or Kasai procedure in which a loop of small intestine is anastomosed to the porta hepatis following excision of the atretic ducts. About one third of patients who undergo the Kasai procedure survive for longer than 10 years without liver transplantation.[55] About one third have adequate bile drainage, but complications of cirrhosis develop and liver transplantation is necessary before the age of 10 years. The remaining one third require earlier liver transplantation because bile flow is inadequate following portoenterostomy and progressive fibrosis and cirrhosis develop. Overall survival of these children, including those undergoing liver transplantation, is now about 90% at age 4 years.[56] Portoenterostomy must be done before there is irreversible sclerosis of the intrahepatic bile ducts, but the effect of the timing of the Kasai procedure on outcome remains controversial.[55,57] Although recent

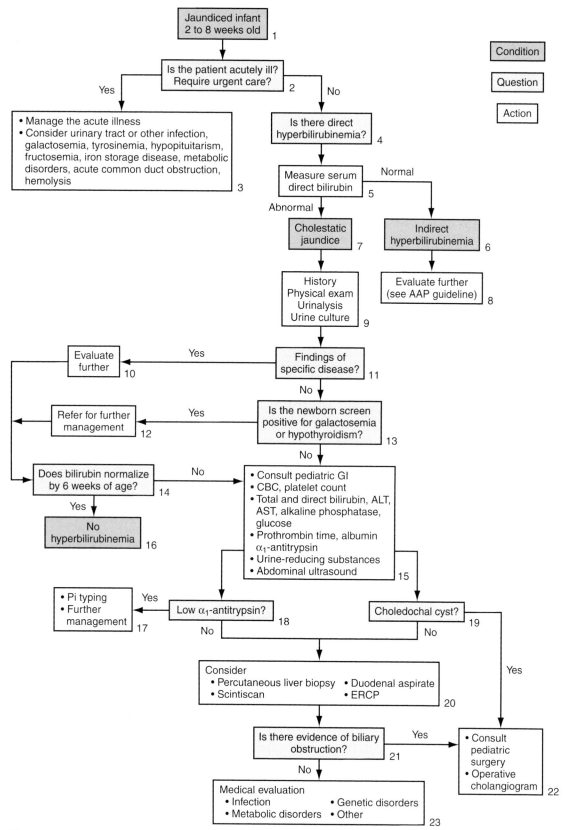

Figure 13-9. Cholestasis clinical practice guideline. Algorithm for a 2- to 8-week-old-infant. *AAP,* American Academy of Pediatrics; *ALT,* alanine aminotransferase; *AST,* aspartate aminotransferase; *CBC,* complete blood count; *ERCP,* endoscopic retrograde cholangiopancreatography; *GI,* gastroenterology; *Pi,* protease inhibitor. *(From Moyer V, Freese DK, Whitington PF, et al: Guideline for the evaluation of cholestatic jaundice in infants: recommendations of the North American Society for Pediatric Gastroenterology, Hepatology and Nutrition,* J Pediatr Gastroenterol Nutr *39:115, 2004.)*

data from France suggest that the outcome following this procedure is best when the procedure is performed before age 31 days,[55] data from the United Kingdom show no difference in outcome of isolated biliary atresia regardless of whether the Kasai procedure is performed before 40 days or between 41 and 60 days.[57] On the other hand, there is a major deleterious effect of delaying surgery in those infants whose biliary atresia is a component of the biliary atresia splenic malformation syndrome (splenic malformation, situs inversus, preduodenal portal vein, absence of the vena cava) and in those with cystic biliary atresia.[57]

By far the most common association with cholestasis in the NICU is prolonged use of intravenous alimentation. When total parenteral nutrition (TPN) is used for 2 weeks or longer, and particularly when such use is exclusive of enteral feedings, cholestatic jaundice may appear. Cholestasis develops in as many as 80% of infants who receive TPN for longer than 60 days, and 50% of those with birth weights of less than 1000 g are affected. The pathogenesis of TPN-associated cholestasis is not clear, but it is thought to be related to a combination of factors, including immaturity of bile secretion in preterm infants, a decrease in bile flow that occurs with no enteral feeding, the use of omega-6 poly unsaturated fatty acids, and potential toxicity of both trace elements and amino acids.

The term *neonatal hepatitis,* which implies an inflammatory or infectious process, is a misnomer. The term *transient neonatal cholestasis* is preferred because the clinical and biopsy findings are the result of a combination of factors, including (1) immaturity of bile secretion associated with prematurity; (2) chronic or acute ischemia-hypoxia of the liver following intrauterine growth restriction, acute perinatal distress, or lung disease; (3) liver damage caused by perinatal or postnatal sepsis; and (4) decrease in bile flow resulting from delays in enteral feeding.

An approach to the evaluation of infants with cholestatic jaundice is provided in Figure 13-9. Imaging findings may permit some shortcuts and even avoid the necessity for liver biopsy in some cases. Magnetic resonance cholangiography provides visualization of the extrahepatic bile ducts. Failure to see the bile ducts is highly suggestive of biliary atresia. Other studies suggest that identification of the "triangular cord" (a triangular or tube-shaped echogenic density just cranial to the portal vein bifurcation on a transverse or longitudinal ultrasound scan) can distinguish infants with extrahepatic biliary atresia (in whom the triangular cord is present) from those who have other causes of cholestasis.[58,59] The cord represents the fibrous remnant in the porta hepatis, and when it is seen, the authors recommend prompt laparotomy without further investigation. When it is absent, hepatic scintigraphy is done.[58,59]

Treatment of Cholestasis

The treatment of neonatal cholestasis involves treating the cause, although some pharmacologic agents have been used in an attempt to stimulate bile flow. Phenobarbital increases the uptake of bilirubin by the liver, induces conjugation, enhances bile acid synthesis, and increases bile flow. The administration of phenobarbital before performance of hepatic scintigraphy has helped to improve the reliability of this diagnostic test, but the therapeutic use of phenobarbital to improve bile flow and lower serum bilirubin concentrations in conditions such as TPN-associated cholestasis has been disappointing.

The use of ursodeoxycholic acid (UDCA) appears to offer more promise. UDCA is a hydrophilic bile acid with a significant choleretic effect. It appears to be a relatively safe agent when used in children who do not have a fixed obstruction to bile flow. It has been used in the treatment of cholestatic jaundice in infants with cystic fibrosis, as well as in erythroblastosis fetalis. UDCA may also be of value in the treatment of extreme hyperbilirubinemia in older children with Crigler-Najjar syndrome.[60] The mechanism of action of UDCA is not well understood, but it may affect the enterohepatic circulation of endogenous bile salts and increase hepatic bile flow.

BILIRUBIN TOXICITY

The presence of bilirubin pigment at autopsy in the brains of infants who were severely jaundiced was observed more than 100 years ago, and the term *kernicterus* was applied to infants who died and demonstrated bilirubin staining of the "kern," or nuclear region of the brain. The areas of the brain most commonly affected are the basal ganglia, particularly the subthalamic nucleus and the globus pallidus (Fig. 13-10); the hippocampus; the geniculate

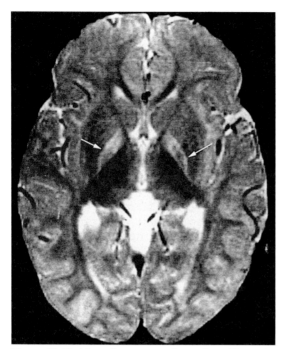

Figure 13-10. Magnetic resonance image for a 21-month-old male infant who had erythroblastosis fetalis and manifested extreme hyperbilirubinemia and clinical signs of kernicterus at age 54 hours. Note the symmetric, abnormally high-intensity signal from the area of the globus pallidus on both sides *(arrows). (From Grobler JM, Mercer MJ: Kernicterus associated with elevated predominantly direct-reacting bilirubin,* S Afr Med J *87:146, 1997.)*

body; various brain stem nuclei, including the inferior colliculus, oculomotor, vestibular, cochlear, and inferior olivary nuclei; and the cerebellum, especially the dentate nucleus and vermis.[61] Neuronal necrosis is the dominant histopathologic feature after 7 to 10 days of postnatal life.

The areas of neuronal injury explain the clinical sequelae of bilirubin encephalopathy. In classic kernicterus, markedly jaundiced infants pass through three clinical phases. Initially, the infant becomes lethargic and hypotonic, and sucks poorly. Subsequently, hypertonia, fever, and a high-pitched cry develop. The hypertonia is characterized by backward arching of the neck (retrocollis) and trunk (opisthotonos). After about a week, the hypertonia subsides and is replaced by hypotonia. In those who survive, extrapyramidal disturbances (choreoathetosis), auditory abnormalities (sensorineural hearing loss most severe in the high frequencies), gaze palsies, and dental enamel hypoplasia develop. The presence of retrocollis and opisthotonos (the acute intermediate phase of bilirubin encephalopathy)

was thought to represent irreversible damage, but with urgent intervention using phototherapy and exchange transfusion, a normal outcome is possible in some cases.

The diagnosis of kernicterus can be confirmed by magnetic resonance imaging (MRI).[62,63] (see Fig. 13-10). The characteristic image is a bilateral, symmetric, high-intensity signal in the globus pallidus seen on both T_1- and T_2-weighted images. High signal intensity may also be found in the hippocampus and thalamus, with the subthalamic nucleus commonly involved.[62] In addition, hyperechogenicity on cranial ultrasonography has been seen in the basal ganglia and globus pallidus in term and preterm infants who subsequently manifested signs of kernicterus.[62]

Although there is no doubt about the relationship between extremely high bilirubin levels and acute bilirubin encephalopathy, it is possible that this outcome is only the most obvious and extreme manifestation of a spectrum of bilirubin toxicity. At the other end of the spectrum might lie more subtle forms of neurodevelopmental impairment (NDI) that occur at lower bilirubin levels and in the absence of any obvious clinical findings in the neonatal period.[64,65] Nevertheless, prospective studies of large populations of hyperbilirubinemic infants have not found evidence of subtle NDI.[66]

KERNICTERUS IN THE TERM AND LATE PRETERM NEWBORN

Kernicterus remains a significant problem in the developing world and still occurs in the United States, Canada, and Western Europe.[40,67-74] Contrary to the experience in the 1940s and 1950s, however, these are not infants with Rh hemolytic disease; rather, most are term and late preterm newborns who are apparently healthy at the time of discharge but who subsequently develop extreme hyperbilirubinemia (usually a TSB level of >30 mg/dL).[40] Such bilirubin levels occur in only about 1 in 10,000 infants, and the risk of kernicterus at these TSB levels is about 1 in 7, or 14%.[75] Some of the factors that appear to have contributed to this situation are short hospital stays and inadequate follow-up for newborns; increased incidence of hyperbilirubinemia related to an increase in breast feeding; less concern by pediatricians about jaundice; and failure to interpret bilirubin levels according to the baby's age in hours, not days.

Short Hospital Stays for Newborns

There is evidence that early discharge is associated with an increased risk of significant hyperbilirubinemia. The AAP recommends that infants discharged at less than 72 hours be seen within 2 days of discharge unless the risk of hyperbilirubinemia is very low.[16] A recent commentary provides detailed guidelines for risk assessment and follow-up (see later discussion).[16] Figures 13-5 to 13-7 make one thing clear: If newborns leave the hospital before they are 36 hours old, their peak bilirubin level will occur after they are discharged. Thus, jaundice is now primarily an outpatient problem, and monitoring and surveillance following discharge are essential if extreme hyperbilirubinemia is to be prevented.[16]

HEMOLYTIC DISEASE AND OUTCOME

Initial observations in the late 1940s and early 1950s showed a strong relationship between increasing TSB levels (particularly levels of >20 mg/dL [>342 μmol/L]) and the risk of kernicterus in infants with Rh hemolytic disease. Hsia et al reported that the incidence of kernicterus in their erythroblastotic population was 8% for those with TSB levels of 19 to 24 mg/dL (325 to 410 μmol/L),[77] 33% for those with TSB levels of 25 to 29 mg/dL (428 to 496 μmol/L), and 73% for those with levels higher than 30 mg/dL (513 μmol/L). Subsequent studies, however, found strikingly different outcomes. In a study of 129 infants born between 1957 and 1958, all of whom had indirect bilirubin levels of more than 20 mg/dL (342 μmol/L), neurodevelopmental damage was seen in only 2 of 92 (2%) who underwent detailed psychometric, neurologic, and audiologic evaluations at 5 to 6 years of age.[78] The presence of hemolysis is considered to be a risk factor for bilirubin encephalopathy, although the reason for this is not clear. Recent studies have shown that infants with TSB levels of 25 mg/dL (428 μmol/L) or more and a positive DAT result are at greater risk for low IQ scores at ages 5 to 8 years.[66,79]

OUTCOME IN INFANTS WITHOUT HEMOLYTIC DISEASE

The relationship between hyperbilirubinemia and poor developmental outcome in full-term and late preterm infants who do not have hemolytic disease has been studied extensively.[80-83] When analyzed as a whole, the data tend to demonstrate that, in otherwise healthy neonates without hemolytic disease, TSB levels that do not exceed approximately 25 mg/dL (428 μmol/L) do not place these infants at risk of NDI. In such infants, there has been no convincing demonstration of any adverse affect of these bilirubin levels on IQ, definite neurologic abnormalities, or sensorineural hearing loss.[66,84]

A relationship has been described between neurologic and psychometric abnormalities and the duration of exposure to elevated TSB levels. In a Turkish study, exposure to TSB levels of more than 20 mg/dL (342 μmol/L) for fewer than 6 hours was associated with a 2.3% incidence of neurologic abnormality. The incidence increased to 18.7% if exposure lasted 6 to 11 hours and to 26% with 12 or more hours of exposure.[85] In the large National Institute of Child Health and Human Development (NICHD) collaborative phototherapy trial, a 6-year follow-up of 224 control group infants who did not receive phototherapy and who had birth weights of less than 2000 g show no association between IQ and duration of exposure to elevated bilirubin levels.[86]

HYPERBILIRUBINEMIA AND THE PRETERM INFANT

Compared with term infants, sick very low-birth-weight infants are at greater risk of developing kernicterus and autopsy-proven "low bilirubin kernicterus" at TSB levels of 5 to 7 mg/dL. Although pathologic kernicterus in premature newborns is now rare, it has not disappeared completely, and whether or not modest elevations of TSB cause brain damage in preterm infants is controversial.[87] Two studies of large populations of extremely low-birth-weight infants suggest an association between NDI and small increases in TSB.[2,88] Higher peak TSB levels were associated with an increased risk of death, hearing loss, and NDI in extremely low-birth-weight infants (<1000 g birth weight) born between 1994 and 1997.[88] In a randomized controlled trial of aggressive versus conservative phototherapy for extremely low-birth-weight infants, there was no difference between treatment groups in the primary outcome of death or NDI at 18 to 22 months of corrected age.[2] Among survivors, however, aggressive phototherapy produced a significant decrease in NDI, hearing loss, profound impairment, and athetosis compared with conservative phototherapy (see Table 13-4 for the details of how phototherapy was used in this study). Mean

Table 13-4.	Criteria for Initiating Phototherapy and Exchange Transfusions in the National Institute of Child Health and Human Development Neonatal Research Network Trial							
BIRTH WEIGHT	**AGGRESSIVE MANAGEMENT**				**CONSERVATIVE MANAGEMENT**			
	Phototherapy Begins	Exchange Transfusion			Phototherapy Begins		Exchange Transfusion	
		mg/dL	μmol/L		mg/dL	μmol/L	mg/dL	μmol/L
501-750 g	ASAP after enrollment	≥13.0	≥222		≥8.0	≥137	≥13.0	≥257
751-1000 g	ASAP after enrollment	≥15.0	≥257		≥10.0	≥171	≥15.0	≥257

From Morris BH, Oh W, Tyson JE, et al: Aggressive vs conservative phototherapy for infants with extremely low birth weight, *N Engl J Med* 359:1885, 2008.
Enrollment is expected within the period 12-36 hr after birth, preferably between 12 and 24 hr.

TSB levels in infants with hearing loss were 6.5 ± 1.7 mg/dL versus 5.5 ± 1.5 mg/dL in those with no hearing loss ($P < .001$). Peak TSB levels in infants with NDI were 8.6 ± 2.3 versus 8.3 ± 2.3 in unimpaired survivors ($P = .02$). Whether these small differences in TSB levels or the use of aggressive phototherapy was responsible for the outcomes is difficult to say.

Sugama et al documented hypotonia and choreoathetosis, together with the classical MRI findings of kernicterus at follow-up, in two preterm infants of 31 and 34 weeks' gestation.[89] Neither of these infants was acutely ill in the newborn period, and their peak TSB levels were 13.1 mg/dL (224 μmol/L) and 14.7 mg/dL (251 μmol/L). In a study from the Netherlands, classical MRI findings of kernicterus were found in five sick preterm infants (25 to 29 weeks' gestation) with peak TSB levels ranging from 8.7 to 11.9 mg/dL (148 to 204 μmol/L).[63] Serum albumin levels in these infants were strikingly low (1.4 to 2.1 g/dL).

Unbound or Free Bilirubin

Recognition that a peak TSB level, by itself, is a rather poor predictor of the likelihood of NDI or kernicterus raises the question of whether measurements of unbound or "free" bilirubin (B_f) or the ratio of bilirubin to albumin to predict hyperbilirubinemia risk should be used.[83,90] Bilirubin (B) is transported in the plasma as a dianion bound tightly but reversibly to serum albumin (A):

$$B^{2-} + A \leftrightarrow AB^{2-}$$

Most bilirubin in the circulation is bound to albumin, and a relatively small fraction remains unbound. The concentration of B_f is believed to dictate the biological effects of bilirubin in jaundiced newborns, including its neurotoxicity. Elevations of B_f have been associated with kernicterus in sick preterm infants. In addition, elevated B_f concentrations are more closely associated than TSB with transient abnormalities in the brain stem auditory evoked potential in both term and preterm infants. Although a B_f level of more than 1.0 mg/dL may predict the presence or absence of NDI in preterm neonates with high sensitivity and specificity, there is no agreement about what constitutes the neurotoxic B_f threshold[91]; that is, the threshold at which B_f produces changes in cellular function culminating in permanent cell injury and cell death. In addition, clinical laboratory measurement of B_f is not generally available.

The ratio of bilirubin (in milligrams per deciliter) to albumin (in grams per deciliter) does correlate with measured B_f in newborns and has been used as an approximate surrogate for the measurement of B_f, and the AAP has endorsed this approach.[76] A randomized controlled trial in the Netherlands (the BARTrial) is testing the use of the bilirubin-to-albumin ratio in conjunction with the TSB to determine when phototherapy and/or exchange transfusion should be used and will evaluate neurodevelopmental outcomes at 18 to 24 months' corrected age.[92] It must be recognized, however, that albumin-binding capacity varies significantly among newborns, is impaired in sick infants, and increases with increasing gestational age and postnatal age. A recent study of very low-birth-weight infants at one NICHD Neonatal Network institution confirmed that bilirubin-binding capacity was lower and unbound bilirubin higher in unstable neonates than in stable neonates.[93] An increase in unbound bilirubin was associated with higher rates of death or NDI. TSB levels were also associated with an increased risk of death or NDI but only in unstable and not in stable infants.[93] In fact, in stable infants, an increase in TSB levels was associated with a decrease in death or cerebral palsy, a puzzling and currently unexplained finding.[93] In the NICHD phototherapy trial involving 224 infants who were born between 1974 and 1976 with birth weights of less than 2000 g and who were evaluated at age 6 years, no relation was seen between measures of bilirubin-albumin binding and IQ scores at follow-up.[94] It will be instructive to see how the bilirubin-to-albumin ratio correlates with neurodevelopmental outcome in the BARTrial.[92]

Crucially important in the measurement of B_f is the bilirubin-albumin binding constant k, a term whose numeric value actually may vary considerably depending on conditions, including, among other factors, sample dilution, albumin concentration, and the presence of competing compounds.[83,90,91] Moreover, the risk of bilirubin encephalopathy is likely not simply a function of the B_f concentration alone or the TSB level but of a combination of several factors—namely, the total amount of bilirubin available (the miscible pool of bilirubin), the tendency of bilirubin to enter the tissue (the B_f concentration), and the susceptibility of the cells of the central nervous system to be damaged by bilirubin.[95] The bilirubin-to-albumin ratio can therefore be used together with, but not in lieu of, the TSB level as an additional factor in determining the need for exchange transfusion. Clarifying and defining clinically germane B_f concentrations, bilirubin-to-albumin ratios, exposure conditions, and exposure durations, as well as improving, standardizing, and validating B_f measurements, are important lines of clinical and translational research.

In calculating the risks of bilirubin toxicity, factors that affect the binding of bilirubin to albumin should be taken into account. One of these factors is the concentration of free fatty acids that compete with bilirubin for its binding to albumin, although this does not occur until the molar ratio of free fatty acids to albumin exceeds 4:1. Such ratios are generally not achieved with doses of up to 3 g/kg of intralipid given over 24 hours. The binding of bilirubin to albumin is not affected by changes in serum pH, but a decrease in pH does increase the binding of bilirubin to cells in the central nervous system.

Drugs can affect bilirubin-albumin binding both singly and in combination. Because of their bilirubin-displacing capabilities, drugs that should be avoided in the period immediately after birth, or at least until serum bilirubin levels are less than 5 mg/dL (85 µmol/L), include ethacrynic acid, azlocillin, carbenicillin, cefotetan, ceftriaxone, moxalactam, sulfisoxazole, and ticarcillin.

ENTRY OF BILIRUBIN INTO THE BRAIN

Under normal circumstances, there is a constant influx and efflux of bilirubin in and out of the brain, and changes in the brain stem auditory evoked response can be demonstrated at modest elevations of serum bilirubin. These changes reverse as the bilirubin level decreases. Bilirubin also enters the brain when there is a marked increase in the serum level of unbound bilirubin. Even bilirubin bound to albumin can enter the brain when the blood-brain barrier is disrupted, and in all of these situations, acidosis increases deposition of bilirubin in brain cells.

NEUROTOXICITY OF BILIRUBIN

It is not known exactly how bilirubin exerts its toxic effects, and no single mechanism of bilirubin intoxication has been demonstrated in all cells. Bilirubin lowers membrane potential, decreases the rate of tyrosine uptake and dopamine synthesis in dopaminergic striatal synaptosomes, and impairs substrate transport, neurotransmitter synthesis, and mitochondrial functions in neurons.[96] Unconjugated bilirubin also activates glial cells with the release of proinflammatory cytokines such as tumor necrosis factor, interleukin-1β, and interleukin-6, which suggests that inflammatory processes can contribute to the toxic effects of bilirubin on nerve cells.[97]

CLINICAL MANAGEMENT

PREVENTION OF SEVERE HYPERBILIRUBINEMIA IN THE TERM AND LATE PRETERM NEWBORN

Risk Assessment

Because severe hyperbilirubinemia in the term and late preterm newborn now occurs predominately, but not exclusively,

Exclusive breast feeding, particularly if nursing, is not going well and/or weight loss is excessive (>8%-10%)

Isoimmune or other hemolytic disease (e.g., glucose-6-phosphate dehydrogenase deficiency, hereditary spherocytosis)

Previous sibling with jaundice

Cephalhematoma or significant bruising

East Asian race

From Maisels MJ, Bhutani VK, Bogen D, et al: Hyperbilirubinemia in the newborn infant >35 weeks' gestation: an update with clarifications, Pediatrics 124(4):1193, 2009.

The gestational age and the predischarge TSB or TcB level are the most important factors that help to predict the risk of hyperbilirubinemia. The risk increases with each decreasing week of gestation from 42 to 35 weeks (see Fig. 13-11).

TcB, Transcutaneous bilirubin; TSB, total serum bilirubin.

in infants who have been discharged following birth, a systematic evaluation of the potential risk of subsequent severe hyperbilirubinemia should be carried out before discharge for all term and late preterm newborns. Box 13-5 lists factors that are most consistently associated with an increase in the risk of severe hyperbilirubinemia and should be used in conjunction with Figure 13-11 in performing a risk assessment before discharge.

Universal Newborn Bilirubin Screening

First described by Bhutani et al in 1999,[32] measurement of a predischarge TSB or TcB level has been shown in different populations to be a good predictor of the risk of an infant's subsequently developing or not developing hyperbilirubinemia.[98-101] Evidence suggests that combining predischarge measurement of the TSB or TcB with evaluation of clinical risk factors will improve the accuracy of this prediction.[102,103] In addition, measurement of the TSB or TcB, when interpreted using the hour-specific nomogram (see Fig. 13-7), provides a quantitative assessment of the degree of hyperbilirubinemia and indicates the need (or lack of) for additional testing to identify the cause of hyperbilirubinemia

and for additional TSB measurements (see Table 13-2).[11]

Because the measurement of predischarge TSB or TcB combined with assessment of clinical risk factors currently provides the best prediction of the risk of subsequent hyperbilirubinemia, a predischarge TSB or TcB value should be obtained for every infant.[16] The TSB can be measured on the same sample that is drawn for the metabolic screen, which saves an additional heel stick. The TSB or TcB is plotted on the nomogram to determine the risk zone and combined with the previously determined and relevant clinical risk factors (see Box 13-5) to assess the risk of subsequent hyperbilirubinemia and to formulate a plan of management and follow-up (see Fig. 13-11).[16] When combined with the risk zone, the factors that are most predictive of hyperbilirubinemia risk are lower gestational age and exclusive breast feeding. The lower the gestational age, the greater the risk of hyperbilirubinemia.[102,103] When two or more successive TSB or TcB measurements are obtained, it is helpful to plot these data on the nomogram to assess the rate of rise. Hemolysis is likely if the TSB or TcB is crossing percentiles on the nomogram, and further testing and follow-up are needed (see Table 13-2 and Fig. 13-11). Note that even with a low predischarge TSB or TcB value, the risk of subsequent hyperbilirubinemia is not zero, so that appropriate follow-up should always be provided (see Fig. 13-11).[102]

RESPONSE TO PREDISCHARGE TSB MEASUREMENTS AND FOLLOW-UP AFTER DISCHARGE

Figure 13-11 provides a guideline for management and follow-up according to predischarge screening and also provides suggestions for evaluation and management at the first follow-up visit.[16]

MEASURING BILIRUBIN PRODUCTION

When heme is catabolized, carbon monoxide (CO) is produced in equimolar quantities with bilirubin, and measurements of blood carboxyhemoglobin levels or end-tidal CO, corrected for ambient CO ($ETCO_c$), provide the only available methods for quantifying hemolysis.[104] Unfortunately neither of these techniques is currently available for routine clinical use. Routine measurement of $ETCO_c$ at 30 ± 6 hours of life does not improve the prediction of subsequent

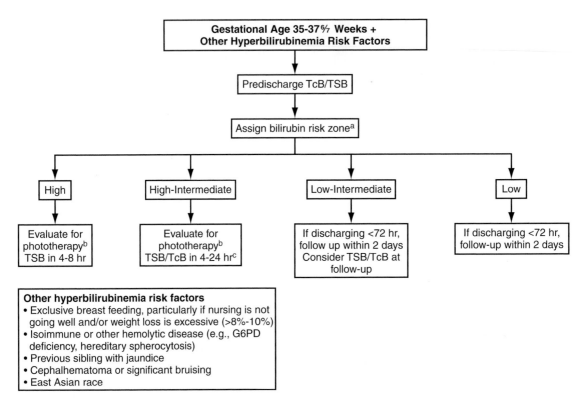

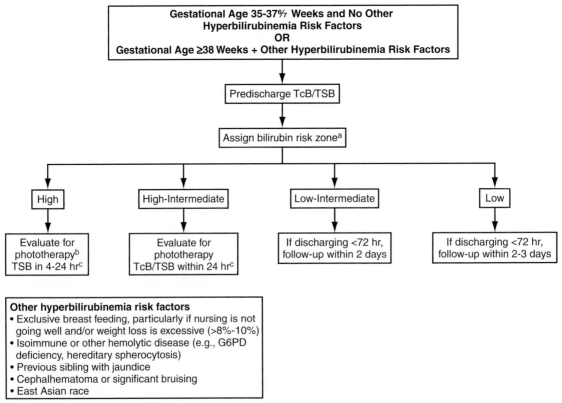

Figure 13-11. For legend see following page.

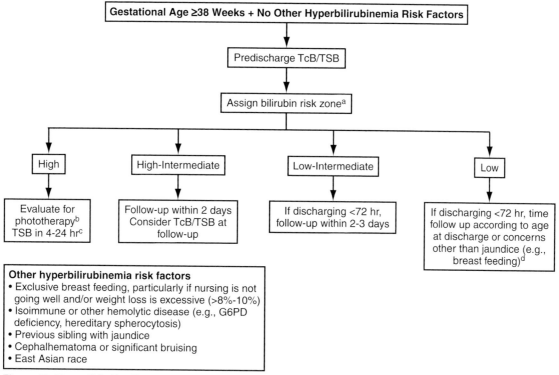

Figure 13-11, cont'd. Algorithm providing recommendations for management and follow-up according to predischarge bilirubin measurements, gestational age, and other risk factors for subsequent hyperbilirubinemia.
- Provide lactation evaluation and support for all breast-feeding mothers.
- Recommendation for timing of repeat TSB measurement depends on age at measurement and how far the TSB level is above the 95th percentile (see Fig. 13-7). Higher and earlier initial TSB levels require an earlier repeat TSB measurement.
- Perform standard clinical evaluation at all follow-up visits.
- For evaluation of jaundice see Table 13-3.

[a]See Figure 13-7. [b]See Figure 13-12. [c]In hospital or as outpatient. [d]Follow-up recommendations can be modified according to level of risk for hyperbilirubinemia; depending on the circumstances, in infants at low risk later follow-up can be considered. *G6PD*, Glucose-6-phosphate dehydrogenase; *TcB*, transcutaneous bilirubin; *TSB*, total serum bilirubin. (*From Maisels MJ, Bhutani VK, Bogen D, et al: Hyperbilirubinemia in the newborn infant ≥35 weeks' gestation: an update with clarifications, Pediatrics 124[4]:1193, 2009.*)

hyperbilirubinemia, but measurements of $ETCO_c$ and carboxyhemoglobin have proven very useful in research studies, where they can identify infants who have increased bilirubin production.

TREATMENT

TERM AND LATE PRETERM NEWBORNS

The AAP guidelines for the use of phototherapy and exchange transfusion in infants of 35 weeks' gestation or more are provided in Figures 13-12 and 13-13. These guidelines have achieved widespread acceptance and are used throughout the United States and in many other countries. Nevertheless, a recent analysis of the phototherapy guidelines suggests that they are not internally consistent and could be modified to decrease the number of infants who need

treatment.[105] There is little doubt, however, that if significantly jaundiced infants were identified and these guidelines were followed, kernicterus would be extremely rare. Effective use of phototherapy in these infants is described later (see "Phototherapy: Effective Use of Phototherapy").

BREAST-FED INFANTS

Of infants who have TSB levels high enough to require phototherapy and who do not have evidence of isoimmunization or other obvious hemolytic disease, 80% to 90% are fully or partially breast fed.[28] Much of this hyperbilirubinemia is associated with inadequate breast feeding, and attention to increasing the frequency of breast feeding during the first few days after birth will decrease TSB levels. Supplemental feedings of water or dextrose water should not be

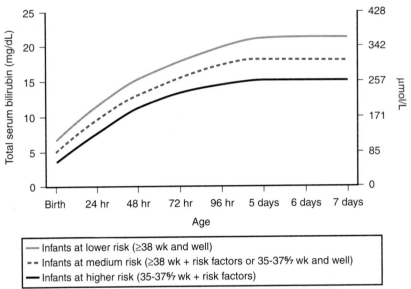

Figure 13-12. Guidelines for phototherapy in hospitalized infants of 35 or more weeks' gestation.
- Use total bilirubin level. Do not subtract direct reading or conjugated bilirubin.
- The lines for lower, medium, and higher risk refer to risk of neurotoxicity.
- Risk factors for neurotoxicity are isoimmune hemolytic disease, glucose-6-phosphate dehydrogenase deficiency, asphyxia, significant lethargy, temperature instability, sepsis, acidosis, and albumin level of less than 3.0 mg/dL (if measured).
- For well infants of 35 to 37⁶⁄₇ weeks' gestation, one can adjust total serum bilirubin (TSB) levels for intervention around the medium risk line. It is an option to intervene at lower TSB levels for infants closer to 35 weeks and at higher TSB levels for those closer to 37⁶⁄₇ weeks.
- It is an option to provide conventional phototherapy in hospital or at home at TSB levels of 2 to 3 mg/dL (35 to 50 µmol/L) below those shown, but home phototherapy should not be used for any infant with risk factors.
    Note: These guidelines are based on limited evidence and the levels shown are approximations. The guidelines refer to the use of intensive phototherapy, which should be used when the TSB level exceeds the line indicated for each category. Infants are designated as "higher risk" because of the potential negative effects of conditions affecting albumin binding of bilirubin, the blood-brain barrier, and the susceptibility of the brain cells to damage by bilirubin.
    "Intensive phototherapy" implies irradiance in the blue-green spectrum (wavelengths of approximately 430 to 490 nm) of at least 30 µW/cm²/nm (measured at the infant's skin directly below the center of the phototherapy unit) and delivered to as much of the infant's surface area as possible. Note that irradiance measured below the center of the light source is much greater than that measured at the periphery. Measurements should be made with the spectroradiometer specified by the manufacturer of the phototherapy system.
    A TSB level that does not decrease or continues to rise in an infant who is receiving intensive phototherapy strongly suggests the presence of hemolysis. *(From American Academy of Pediatrics, Subcommittee on Hyperbilirubinemia: Management of hyperbilirubinemia in the newborn infant 35 or more weeks of gestation, Pediatrics 114:297, 2004.)*

provided to breast-fed infants, because this does not lower their TSB levels. If supplementation is deemed necessary in an infant with hyperbilirubinemia, formula should be provided. It is always undesirable to interrupt nursing, and when the TSB level in a breast-fed infant reaches a level at which intervention is being considered, breast feeding may be continued while the infant undergoes treatment with intensive phototherapy (see "Phototherapy").

LOW-BIRTH-WEIGHT INFANTS

Over the last 2 to 3 decades, there has been a remarkable decrease in the incidence of kernicterus found at autopsy in infants who died in the NICU. Some of this could be the result of liberal use of phototherapy. Phototherapy has dramatically decreased the necessity for exchange transfusion in low-birth-weight infants, so that these procedures are becoming increasingly rare in the NICU.[2,106] In the recent NICHD Neonatal Research Network study,[2] only 5 of 1974 extremely low-birth-weight infants (0.25%) required an exchange transfusion. Table 13-4 provides an approach to the use of phototherapy and exchange transfusion based on birth weight. There is no solid evidence base for the recommendations provided. The recommended treatment levels are based on operational thresholds or therapeutic

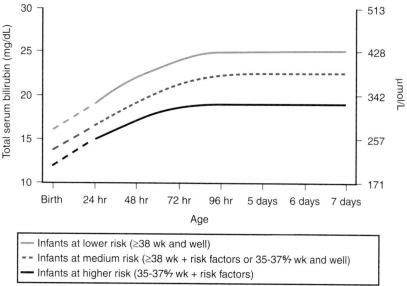

Figure 13-13. Guidelines for exchange transfusion in infants of 35 or more weeks' gestation.

- The dashed lines for the first 24 hours indicate uncertainty caused by a wide range of clinical circumstances and a range of responses to phototherapy.
- Immediate exchange transfusion is recommended if the infant shows signs of acute bilirubin encephalopathy (hypertonia, arching, retrocollis, opisthotonos, fever, high-pitched cry) or if total serum bilirubin level (TSB) is ≥5 mg/dL (85 μmol/L) above these lines.
- The lines for lower, medium, and higher risk refer to risk of neurotoxicity.
- Risk factors for neurotoxicity are isoimmune hemolytic disease, glucose-6-phosphate dehydrogenase deficiency, asphyxia, significant lethargy, temperature instability, sepsis, and acidosis.
- Measure serum albumin level and calculate the ratio of bilirubin to albumin (see table).
- Use total bilirubin level. Do not subtract direct reacting or conjugated bilirubin.
- If the infant is well and of 35 to 37⁶⁄₇ weeks' gestation (median risk) one can individualize TSB levels for exchange based on actual gestational age.

Note: These guidelines are based on limited evidence and the levels shown are approximations. During birth hospitalization, exchange transfusion is recommended if the TSB rises to these levels despite intensive phototherapy. For readmitted infants, if the TSB level is above the exchange level, repeat TSB measurement every 2 to 3 hours and consider exchange if the TSB remains above the levels indicated after intensive phototherapy for 6 hours.

The following bilirubin-to-albumin ratios can be used together with, but in not in lieu of, the TSB level as an additional factor in determining the need for exchange transfusion.

Risk Category	Ratio of Bilirubin to Albumin at Which Exchange Transfusion Should Be Considered	
	TSB (mg/dL)/Alb (g/dL)	TSB (μmol/L)/Alb (g/L)
Infants ≥38⁶⁄₇ wk	8.0	137
Infants 35⁶⁄₇ -36⁶⁄₇ wk and well or ≥38⁶⁄₇ wk if higher risk or isoimmune hemolytic disease or G6PD deficiency	7.2	123
Infants 35⁶⁄₇ -37⁶⁄₇ wk if higher risk or isoimmune hemolytic disease or G6PD deficiency	6.8	116

If the TSB is at or approaching the exchange level, send blood for immediate typing and cross matching. Blood for exchange transfusion is modified whole blood (red cells and plasma) cross-matched against the mother and compatible with the infant.[136] *Alb,* Albumin; *G6PD,* glucose-6-phosphate dehydrogenase; *TSB,* total serum bilirubin.

(Modified from American Academy of Pediatrics, Subcommittee on Hyperbilirubinemia: Management of hyperbilirubinemia in the newborn infant 35 or more weeks of gestation, Pediatrics 114:297, 2004.)

normal levels (a level beyond which specific therapy will likely do more good than harm).[107] In the NICHD Neonatal Research Network, 1974 extremely low-birth-weight infants were randomly assigned at age 12 to 36 hours to receive either aggressive or conservative phototherapy. The protocol used in that study is shown in Table 13-4. In infants assigned to the aggressive phototherapy group, the mean TSB levels were lower

Table 13-5	Suggested Use of Phototherapy and Exchange Transfusion in Preterm Infants Less Than 35 Weeks' Gestational Age		
	Phototherapy		**Exchange Transfusion**
Gestational Age (wk)	**Initiate Phototherapy Total Serum Bilirubin (mg/dL)**		**Total Serum Bilirubin (mg/dL)**
<28	5-6		11-14
28%-29%	6-8		12-14
30%-31%	8-10		13-16
32%-33%	10-12		15-18
34%-34%	12-14		17-19

From Maisels MJ, Watchko JF, Bhutani VK, et al: An approach to the management of hyperbilirubinemia in the preterm infant less than 35 weeks of gestation, *J Perinatol* 2012, in press.

- This table reflects recommendations for operational or therapeutic TSB thresholds—bilirubin levels at, or above which, treatment is likely to do more good than harm.[58] These TSB levels are not based on good evidence and are lower than those suggested in recent UK[11] and Norwegian[5] guidelines.
- The wider ranges and overlapping values in the exchange transfusion column reflect the degree of uncertainty in making these recommendations.
- Use the lower range of the listed total serum bilirubin (TSB) levels for infants at greater risk for bilirubin toxicity, e.g., lower gestational age; serum albumin levels <2.5 g/dL; rapidly rising TSB levels, suggesting hemolytic disease; and those who are clinically unstable.[31] When a decision is being made about the initiation of phototherapy or exchange transfusion, infants are considered to be clinically unstable if they have one or more of the following conditions: blood pH <7.15; blood culture-positive sepsis in the previous 24 hours; apnea and bradycardia requiring cardiorespiratory resuscitation (bagging and or intubation) during the previous 24 hours; (d) hypotension requiring pressor treatment during the previous 24 hours; and (e) mechanical ventilation at the time of blood sampling.[31]
- Recommendations for exchange transfusion apply to infants who are receiving intensive phototherapy to the maximal surface area but whose TSB levels continue to increase to the levels listed.
- For all infants, an exchange transfusion is recommended if the infant shows signs of acute bilirubin encephalopathy (e.g., hypertonia, arching, retrocollis, opisthotonos, high-pitched cry), although it is recognized that these signs rarely occur in VLBW infants.
- Use total bilirubin. Do not subtract direct reacting or conjugated bilirubin from the total.
- For infants ≤26 weeks' gestation, it is an option to use phototherapy prophylactically starting soon after birth.
- Use postmenstrual age for phototherapy (e.g., when a 29%-week infant is 7 days old, use the TSB level for 30% weeks.
- Discontinue phototherapy when TSB is 1-2 mg/dL below the initiation level for the infant's postmenstrual age.
- Discontinue TSB measurements when TSB is declining and phototherapy is no longer required.
- Measure the serum albumin level in all infants.
- Measure irradiance at regular intervals with an appropriate spectroradiometer.
- The increased mortality observed in infants ≤1000 g who are receiving phototherapy [17,25,37] suggests that it is prudent to use less intensive levels of irradiance in these infants. In such infants, phototherapy is almost always prophylactic—it is used to prevent a further increase in the TSB, and intensive phototherapy with high irradiance levels usually is not needed. In infants ≤1000 g, it is reasonable to start phototherapy at lower irradiance levels. If the TSB continues to rise, additional phototherapy should be provided by increasing the surface area exposed (phototherapy above and below the infant, reflecting material around the incubator). If the TSB, nevertheless, continues to rise, the irradiance should be increased by switching to a higher intensity setting on the device or by bringing the overhead light closer to the infant. Fluorescent and LED light sources can be brought closer to the infant, but this cannot be done with halogen or tungsten lamps because of the danger of a burn.

than those in the conservative phototherapy group (4.7 ± 1.1 versus 6.2 ± 1.5 mg/dL). There was no difference between the groups in the primary outcome (death or NDI), but in survivors at 18 to 20 months of corrected age, aggressive phototherapy was associated with a significant decrease in NDI, profound impairment (mental or psychomotor developmental index of ≤50 or severe gross motor impairment), severe hearing loss, and athetosis. The authors noted that the reduction in NDI was "attributable almost entirely to there being fewer infants with profound impairment in the aggressive phototherapy group." These results suggest that aggressive phototherapy, as used in this trial, significantly reduced the risk of neurodevelopmental handicap in surviving infants.

On the other hand, in the aggressive phototherapy group, there was a 5% increase in mortality in the infants with birth weights of 501 to 750 g. Although this difference was not statistically significant, a post hoc Bayesian analysis estimated an 89% probability that aggressive phototherapy increased the rate of deaths in the subgroup. The reasons for these findings are not clear, but these tiny infants have gelatinous, thin skin through which light will penetrate readily, reaching more deeply into the subcutaneous tissue. There is some evidence that phototherapy can produce oxidative injury to cell membranes, and such injury could have a negative effect on these tiny infants.[108] The investigators planned to use a "target irradiance level" of 15 to 40 µW/cm²/nm, and the mean irradiance levels achieved were 22 to 25 µW/cm²/nm.[2] Because phototherapy in this study, and in almost all infants of this birth weight, is used in a prophylactic mode (with the goal of preventing further elevation of the TSB level), it is quite likely that lower irradiance levels could be equally effective and perhaps less harmful. In view of the observed increase in mortality it seems prudent, at least in infants with birth weights of less than 750 g, to initiate phototherapy at lower irradiance levels and to increase these levels, or to increase the surface area of the infant exposed to phototherapy, only if the TSB level continues to rise.

Should all NICUs adopt prophylactic phototherapy from birth for extremely low-birth-weight infants? This question cannot be answered with confidence, but in many units, phototherapy is initiated in infants of less than 1000 g when the TSB level reaches 5 mg/dL. Because the TSB level at the start of phototherapy in the aggressive group in the NICHD study was 4.8 mg/dL, it is likely that this approach will achieve similar outcomes.

INFANTS WITH ELEVATED DIRECT-REACTING OR CONJUGATED BILIRUBIN LEVELS

There are no good data to guide the clinician in dealing with the occasional infant who has a high TSB level as well as a significant elevation in direct-reacting bilirubin. Kernicterus has been described in infants with TSB levels of more than 20 mg/dL (340 μmol/L) but in whom, because of significant elevations in direct bilirubin levels, the indirect bilirubin levels were well below 20 mg/dL (340 μmol/L).[109,110] Elevated direct bilirubin levels may decrease the infant's albumin-binding capacity. The magnetic resonance image shown in Figure 13-10 was obtained from an infant with Rh erythroblastosis fetalis in whom a TSB level of 45.2 mg/dL (773 μmol/L) developed, of which 31.6 mg/dL (514 μmol) was direct reacting.[110] It is commonly recommended that the direct bilirubin concentration not be subtracted from the total bilirubin level unless it exceeds 50% of the TSB concentration.[11] This seems reasonable but would not have benefitted the aforementioned infant with Rh erythroblastosis.[110] It has been suggested, but not confirmed, that infants with bronze baby syndrome are at an increased risk of developing bilirubin encephalopathy.[111]

INFANTS WITH HEMOLYTIC DISEASE

Infants with hemolytic disease are generally considered to be at a greater risk for the development of bilirubin encephalopathy than are nonhemolyzing infants with similar bilirubin levels, although the reasons for this are not clear. In Rh hemolytic disease, phototherapy should be used early, as soon as there is evidence of a rapidly increasing bilirubin level. The AAP guidelines (Figs. 13-12 and 13-13) provide for earlier institution of phototherapy and exchange transfusion in the presence of isoimmunization.[11] Recent studies have confirmed the wisdom of this approach.[66,79] In infants with TSB concentrations of less than 25 mg/dL, the presence of isoimmunization (a positive DAT result) significantly increases the risk of a low IQ score. The use of intravenous γ-globulin (IVIG) has been shown to reduce the need for exchange transfusions in both Rh and ABO hemolytic disease,[112] although a recent randomized controlled trial involving several affected infants with Rh disease did not show any benefit from IVIG administration, and a Cochrane review concluded that the routine use of IVIG cannot currently be recommended.[113,114] Tin-mesoporphyrin will decrease TSB levels in infants with Coombs-positive ABO incompatibility and in G6PD deficiency (see "Pharmacologic Treatment").[115]

INFANTS WITH HYDROPS FETALIS

The pathogenesis of hydrops fetalis is not fully understood. In the fetal sheep model, acute severe anemia leads to hydrops associated with increased venous pressure and placental edema, whereas the same degree of anemia produced over a longer period does not. Thus, high-output failure resulting from anemia is probably not the primary mechanism for hydrops. Profound extramedullary hematopoiesis occurs in the fetus with erythroblastosis fetalis, and this leads to both portal hypertension and disruption of normal liver function. It is likely that these are the primary mechanisms responsible for the development of hydrops in isoimmune hemolytic disease. Infants with hydrops are commonly hypoxic and severely anemic, and they demand immediate treatment. Exchange transfusion of 50 mL/kg of packed cells soon after birth increases the hematocrit to about 40%. Phlebotomy should not be performed routinely on these infants because they are usually normovolemic and may even be hypovolemic, and their blood volume should not be manipulated without appropriate measurements of central venous and arterial blood pressures. To measure central venous pressure accurately, the umbilical venous catheter must enter the inferior vena cava via the ductus venosus. If the catheter is in a portal vein or the umbilical vein, the pressures so measured are meaningless and preclude interpretation of the infant's circulatory status. In addition, before therapeutic decisions are made based on measurements of central venous pressure, acidosis, hypercarbia, hypoxia, and anemia (all of which can affect the measured central venous pressure) must be corrected. Serum glucose levels must be monitored carefully, because hypoglycemia is common.

PHOTOTHERAPY

Phototherapy works in much the same way as do drugs: the absorption of photons of light by bilirubin molecules in the skin produces a therapeutic effect similar to the binding of drug molecules to a receptor. Whereas drug doses are conveniently measured in units of weight, photon doses are more difficult to measure and are expressed in less familiar terms. Table 13-6 defines the radiometric quantities used in assessing the dose of phototherapy, and Table 13-7 lists the major factors that influence the dose, and therefore the efficacy, of phototherapy.

LIGHT SPECTRUM

Bilirubin absorbs light most strongly in the blue region of the spectrum near 460 nm, and the penetration of tissue by light increases markedly with increasing wavelength.[116] The optical properties of bilirubin and skin determine the light wavelengths that most effectively lower bilirubin level; these are wavelengths that are predominately in the blue-green spectrum.[116] Note that none of the light systems used in phototherapy emit any significant amount of

ultraviolet (UV) radiation, and UV light is never used for phototherapy. A small amount of UV light is emitted by fluorescent tubes, but this UV light is of longer wavelengths (>320 nm) than those that cause erythema, and in any case, almost all UV light produced is absorbed by the glass wall of the fluorescent tube and by the Plexiglas cover of the phototherapy unit. Light-emitting diodes do not emit UV light.

IRRADIANCE

There is a direct relationship between the efficacy of phototherapy and the irradiance used (Fig. 13-14), and irradiance is inversely related to the distance between the light source and the infant (Fig. 13-15). The irradiance in a certain wavelength band is called the *spectral irradiance* and is expressed as $\mu W/cm^2/nm$ (see Table 13-6). As shown in Figure 13-15, there is a strong inverse relationship between the light intensity (measured as spectral irradiance) and the distance from the light source. Thus, the closer the phototherapy lamp is to the infant, the more effective it is. Note that halogen or tungsten lamps cannot be put close to the infant because of the risk of burn.

SPECTRAL POWER

The spectral power is the product of the skin surface irradiance and the spectral irradiance across this surface area. Calculations of spectral power permit comparisons of the dose of phototherapy received by infants using different phototherapy systems.

MECHANISM OF ACTION

The conversion of bilirubin to photoisomers during phototherapy probably does not take place in skin cells but most likely takes place in bilirubin bound to albumin in the blood vessels or in the interstitial space. Although it is not known exactly where phototherapy takes place, a biological response to light

Table 13-6. Radiometric Quantities Used		
Quantity	**Dimensions**	**Usual Units of Measure**
Irradiance (radiant power incident on a surface per unit area of the surface)	W/m^2	W/cm^2
Spectral irradiance (irradiance in a certain wavelength band)	$W/m^2/nm$ (or W/m^2)	$\mu W/cm^2/nm$
Spectral power (average spectral irradiance across a surface area)	W/m	mW/nm

From Maisels MJ: Why use homeopathic doses of phototherapy? *Pediatrics* 98:283–287. Copyright 1996 by the American Academy of Pediatrics.

Table 13-7. Factors That Affect the Dose and Efficacy of Phototherapy

Factor	Technical Terminology	Rationale	Clinical Application
Type of light source	Spectrum of light (nanometers)	Blue-green spectrum is most effective at lowering total serum bilirubin (TSB); light at this wavelength penetrates skin well and is absorbed strongly by bilirubin.	Use special blue fluorescent tubes or light-emitting diodes or another light source with output in blue-green spectrum for intensive PT.
Distance of light source from patient	Spectral irradiance (a function of both distance and light source) delivered to surface of infant	↑ Irradiance leads to ↑ rate of decline in TSB. Standard PT units deliver 8-10 μW/cm²/nm; intensive PT delivers ≥30 μW/cm²/nm.	If special blue fluorescent tubes are used, bring tubes as close as possible to infant to increase irradiance. (Do *not* do this with halogen lamps because of danger of burn.) Positioning special blue tubes 10-15 cm above infant will produce an irradiance of at least 35 μW/cm²/nm.
Surface area exposed	Spectral power (a function of spectral irradiance and surface area)	↑ Surface area exposed leads to ↑ rate of decline in TSB.	For intensive PT, expose maximum surface area of infant to PT. Place lights above and below* or around† the infant. For maximum exposure, line sides of bassinet, warmer bed, or incubator with aluminum foil.
Cause of jaundice		PT is likely to be less effective if jaundice is caused by hemolysis or if cholestasis is present (direct bilirubin is increased).	When hemolysis is present, start PT at a lower TSB level and use intensive PT. Failure of PT suggests that hemolysis is the cause of the jaundice. When direct bilirubin is elevated, watch for bronze baby syndrome or blistering.
TSB level at start of PT		The higher the TSB, the more rapid the decline in TSB with PT.	Use intensive PT for higher TSB levels. Anticipate a more rapid decrease in TSB when TSB >20 mg/dL.

From Maisels MJ, Watchko JF: Treatment of hyperbilirubinemia. In Buonocore G, Bracci R, Weindling M: *Neonatology: a practical approach to neonatal diseases,* Milan, 2009, Springer-Verlag.
*Commercially available sources for light below include special blue fluorescent tubes available in the Olympic Bili-Bassinet (Natus Medical, San Carlos, Calif.), BiliSoft fiberoptic LED mattress (GE Healthcare, Wauwatosa, Wisc.), NeoBLUE Cozy mattress (Natus Medical).
†The Mediprema Cradle 360 (Mediprema, Tours Cedex, France) provides 360-degree exposure to special blue fluorescent light.
PT, Phototherapy.

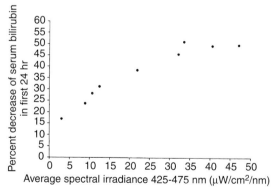

Figure 13-14. Relationship between average spectral irradiance and decrease in serum bilirubin concentration. Full-term infants with nonhemolytic hyperbilirubinemia were exposed to special blue light (Phillips TL52/20W) of different intensities. Spectral irradiance was measured as the average of readings at the head, trunk, and knees. *(From Maisels MJ: Why use homeopathic doses of phototherapy? Pediatrics 98:283, 1996. Copyright 1996 by the American Academy of Pediatrics.)*

can occur only if the light is absorbed by a photoreceptor molecule.

Phototherapy detoxifies bilirubin by converting it to photoproducts that are more lipophilic than bilirubin and can bypass the conjugating system of the liver and be excreted without further metabolism.[116] Absorption of light by dermal and subcutaneous bilirubin induces a fraction of the pigment to undergo several photochemical reactions that occur at very different rates. These reactions generate yellow stereoisomers of bilirubin and colorless derivatives of lower molecular weight.

BILIRUBIN PHOTOCHEMISTRY

During phototherapy, bilirubin absorbs light, and photochemical reactions occur.[116] The relative contributions of the various reactions to the overall elimination of bilirubin are unknown, although in vitro and in vivo studies suggest that photoisomerization is

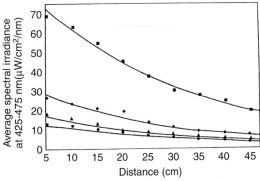

Figure 13-15. Effect of light source and distance from the light source to the infant on average spectral irradiance. Measurements were made across the 425- to 475-nm band using a commercial radiometer (Olympic Bilimeter Mark II). The phototherapy unit was fitted with eight 24-inch fluorescent tubes. ■, Special blue, General Electric 20-W F20T12/BB tube; ◆, blue, General Electric 20-W F20T12/B blue tube; ▲, daylight blue, four General Electric 20-W F20T12/D blue tubes and four Sylvania 20-W F20T12/D daylight tubes; •, daylight, Sylvania 20-W F20T12/D daylight tube. Curves were plotted using linear curve fitting (True Epistat, Epistat Services, Richardson, Tex.). The best fit is described by the equation $y = Ae^{BX}$. *(From Maisels MJ: Why use homeopathic doses of phototherapy? Pediatrics 98:283, 1996. Copyright 1996 by the American Academy of Pediatrics.)*

more important than photodegradation. Bilirubin elimination depends on the rates of formation as well as the rates of clearance of the photoproducts. Photoisomerization occurs rapidly during phototherapy, and isomers appear in the blood long before the level of plasma bilirubin begins to decline. The radiometric quantities used and the important factors that influence the dose and efficacy of phototherapy are listed in Table 13-7.

CLINICAL USE AND EFFICACY

Phototherapy is an effective mechanism for the prevention and treatment of hyperbilirubinemia and dramatically reduces the need for exchange transfusion. There are more than 50 published controlled trials confirming the efficacy of phototherapy.[48] Some idea of the magnitude of the effect of phototherapy can be gauged from the following: when phototherapy was not used, 36% of infants with birth weights of less than 1500 g required an exchange transfusion. In the recent NICHD Neonatal Research Network study, 5 of 1974 infants (0.25%) with birth weights of 1000 g or less required an exchange transfusion.[2]

DOSE-RESPONSE RELATIONSHIP

Figure 13-14 shows that there is a clear relationship between the dose of phototherapy and the decline in the TSB level, and Table 13-7 lists the factors that determine the dose. The initial TSB level is also an important factor that influences the rate of decline of serum bilirubin level, with the rate being proportional to the initial bilirubin concentration. Because configurational isomers formed during light treatment revert to natural unconjugated bilirubin in the intestine after hepatic excretion, reabsorption of natural bilirubin occurs via the enterohepatic circulation and contributes to the bilirubin load to be cleared by the liver. Both of these phenomena account for the fact that light treatment is most effective during the first 24 hours of therapy, after which the efficacy decreases.

TYPES OF LIGHT

Fluorescent Tubes

Daylight, white, and blue fluorescent tubes are widely used fluorescent light sources, but they are less effective than special blue fluorescent tubes, which provide significantly more irradiance in the blue spectrum (see Fig. 13-15). Special blue tubes are labeled F20T12/BB (General Electric, Westinghouse) or TL52/20W (Phillips). These are different from regular blue tubes (F20T12/B), which provide only slightly more irradiance than daylight or white tubes (see Fig. 13-15). Compact special blue fluorescent bulbs (Osram 18W) are also effective and are cheaper than standard fluorescent bulbs.[117] Systems have been developed that provide special blue fluorescent light above and below the infant as well as a 360-degree configuration (see footnote to Table 13-7).

Halogen Lamps

High-pressure mercury vapor halide lamps provide reasonably good output in the blue range and have the advantage of being much more compact than lamps containing standard fluorescent tubes. An important disadvantage, however, is that, unlike fluorescent lamps, they cannot be brought close to the infant (to increase the irradiance) without incurring the risk of a burn. Furthermore, the surface area covered by most halogen lamps is small, and the spectral power is, therefore, less than that produced by a bank of fluorescent lamps.

Fiberoptic Systems

Fiberoptic phototherapy systems contain a tungsten-halogen bulb that delivers light via a fiberoptic cable to be emitted by the sides and ends of the fibers inside a plastic pad. These systems provide a convenient way of delivering phototherapy above and below the infant simultaneously. But the original fiberoptic pads covered only a small surface area, which significantly reduced the spectral power achieved. New designs that combine an LED light source with fiberoptic pads have overcome this problem (see footnote to Table 13-7).

Light-Emitting Diodes

The use of high-intensity gallium nitride light-emitting diodes (LEDs) permits higher irradiance to be delivered in the spectrum of choice (e.g., blue, blue-green) with minimal heat generation.

An LED unit is a low-weight, low-voltage, low-power, portable device that provides an effective means of delivering intensive phototherapy.[118] An LED light source and a fiberoptic pad have recently been combined to create pads that are much larger than the original fiberoptic pads and have a high irradiance (GE Healthcare, Wauwatosa, Wisc.) (see footnote to Table 13-7).

EFFECTIVE USE OF PHOTOTHERAPY

Term and Late Preterm Infants

In the NICU, phototherapy is used primarily as a prophylactic measure to prevent slowly increasing serum bilirubin concentrations from reaching levels that might require an exchange transfusion. In the days when full-term infants remained in the hospital for 3 to 5 days, phototherapy was also commonly used to treat modestly jaundiced infants. Currently, full-term and late pre-term infants who need phototherapy are often those who have left the hospital and are readmitted on days 4 to 7 for treatment of severe hyperbilirubinemia. Such infants need a therapeutic dose of phototherapy (sometimes termed *intensive phototherapy*) to diminish the bilirubin level as soon as possible.[11] One effective way of delivering intensive phototherapy is to use special blue fluorescent tubes and to bring them as close as possible to the infant (see Fig. 13-15). To do this, a term or late preterm infant must be in a bassinet, not an incubator (the top of the incubator prevents the light from being brought sufficiently close to the infant). When necessary

in low-birth-weight infants or infants in the NICU, the special blue fluorescent lights can be placed between the radiant warmer and the warmer bed. In either case, the light should be no further than 10 to 15 cm from the infant. At this distance, special blue fluorescent tubes provide an average spectral irradiance of 40 to 50 $\mu W/cm^2/nm$ (see Fig. 13-15). This configuration does not produce significant warming of naked full-term infants, and if slight warming does occur, the lamps can be elevated slightly. Halogen phototherapy lamps cannot be positioned closer to the infant than recommended by the manufacturers without incurring the risk of burn.

LED lights are also effective for intensive phototherapy.[118] Their only potential disadvantage is that they produce almost no heat, so that most naked infants will need to be placed in an incubator or under a radiant warmer.

The use of fiberoptic or LED-fiberoptic pads has made it easy to increase the surface area of the infant exposed to phototherapy, and this type of "double phototherapy" is approximately twice as effective as single phototherapy in low-birth-weight infants and almost 50% better in full-term infants. The better response of low-birth-weight infants is likely the result of the fact that, at similar levels of irradiance, the fiberoptic pad covers more of a small infant than of a large one. With the newer LED-fiberoptic pads this difference might disappear.

Using these techniques, a decline of 30% to 40% in TSB concentrations can be achieved within 24 hours.[119]

Low-Birth-Weight Infants

Use of phototherapy in low-birth-weight infants is described earlier (see "Treatment: Low-Birth-Weight Infants").

MEASUREMENT OF PHOTOTHERAPY DOSE

Because phototherapy is a drug, like all drugs the dose should be measured to ensure that a therapeutic level is being achieved and that excessive levels of irradiance are not being used when they are not required. The radiometric quantity most commonly reported in the literature is the spectral irradiance (see Table 13-6). In the nursery, spectral irradiance can be measured by using commercially available spectroradiometers. These instruments take a single measurement across a band of wavelengths, typically 425 to 475 or 400 to 480 nm, and provide a readout in microwatts per square centimeter per nanometer. Unfortunately, there is no standardized method for reporting phototherapy doses in the clinical literature, so it is difficult to compare published studies on the efficacy of phototherapy. In addition, different radiometers and spectroradiometers produce markedly different results when measuring irradiance from the same phototherapy system.[108] Thus it is important to use the spectroradiometer recommended by the manufacturer for use with a given phototherapy system.

The measured irradiance varies widely depending on where the measurement is taken. Irradiance measured below the center of the light source is much greater than that measured at the periphery, but the recommendations issued by the AAP and given in this chapter refer to irradiance levels measured directly below the center of the light source.[11]

In the past, it was not thought necessary to measure spectral irradiance on a daily basis, but there is no longer any reason why this should not be done. It is recommended that irradiance from all phototherapy units be measured at least daily and documented in the medical record, as should the type of phototherapy system being used and the surface area of the infant being exposed.

Intermittent versus Continuous Therapy

Because light exposure increases bilirubin excretion (compared with darkness), continuous phototherapy should be more efficient than intermittent phototherapy. However, clinical studies comparing these two methods have produced conflicting results.[120] If bilirubin levels are very high, intensive phototherapy should be administered continuously until a satisfactory decline in the TSB level has occurred. On the other hand, in most circumstances, phototherapy does not need to be continuous. It should certainly be interrupted during feeding or parental visits, and eye patches must be removed to allow appropriate parent-infant contact.

HYDRATION

Because some of the lumirubin produced during phototherapy is excreted in urine, maintaining adequate hydration and a good urine output helps to improve the efficacy of phototherapy. However, supplementation (with dextrose water) is not necessary for an infant receiving phototherapy unless there is evidence that the infant is dehydrated. In such infants it makes more sense to provide both supplemental calories and fluids using a milk-based formula, because formula inhibits the enterohepatic circulation of bilirubin and helps to lower the bilirubin level.

BIOLOGICAL EFFECTS AND COMPLICATIONS

Even though phototherapy has been used on millions of infants for more than 30 years, reports of significant toxicity are exceptionally rare. Bilirubin is a photosensitizer and, in some circumstances, can act as a photodynamic agent in the presence of light and produce damage. In infants with congenital erythropoietic porphyria, phototherapy produces severe blistering and photosensitivity, and congenital porphyria is an absolute contraindication to the use of phototherapy. All of the affected infants had significant direct hyperbilirubinemia and elevated plasma porphyrin levels. Significant accumulation of coproporphyrin has also been described in infants with bronze baby syndrome, which occurs exclusively in phototherapy-exposed infants who also have cholestasis. In bronze baby syndrome, dark grayish brown discoloration develops in the skin, serum, and urine in infants with cholestatic jaundice who are exposed to phototherapy.[121] The pathogenesis of this syndrome is not fully understood. If phototherapy is necessary, an elevated direct-reacting bilirubin level is not a contraindication to its use, even if bronzing results.

Complications associated with the use of fiberoptic phototherapy blankets have been reported in extremely premature infants (≤25 weeks' gestation) who had conditions that might reduce skin integrity, such as birth trauma, hypotension, poor perfusion of the skin, or bacterial contamination of the incubator or bed, and have included extensive erythematous denuded areas of skin resembling a partial-thickness burn as well as purplish red necrotizing lesions.[122,123] It is important to note that the skin of extremely premature infants is remarkably fragile.

Because light can be toxic to the retina, the eyes of infants receiving phototherapy should be protected with appropriate eye patches.

Conventional phototherapy can produce an acute change in the infant's thermal environment, leading to an increase in peripheral blood flow and insensible water loss.[124] This issue has not been studied for

LED lights, but because of their relatively low heat output, they should be much less likely to cause insensible water loss. In term infants who are nursing or feeding adequately, additional intravenous fluids are usually not required.

Phototherapy decreases the expected postprandial increase in blood flow velocity in the superior mesenteric artery and might also increase cerebral blood flow velocity in preterm infants of 32 weeks' gestation or less. Phototherapy also increases the likelihood of a patent ductus arteriosus in very low-birth-weight infants.

In a recent randomized, controlled study there was a 5% increase in mortality in infants with birth weights of 501 to 750 g in the "aggressive phototherapy" group[2] (see "Treatment: Low-Birth-Weight Infants" discussed earlier).

A 6-year follow-up of children in the NICHD cooperative phototherapy study showed no differences between the phototherapy and control groups in any aspect of growth or developmental outcome.[86]

EXCHANGE TRANSFUSION

Exchange transfusion removes bilirubin-laden blood from the circulation and replaces it with donor blood (usually packed red blood cells reconstituted with plasma). In addition to removing bilirubin, when used in the treatment of immune-mediated hemolytic disease, it also accomplishes the following goals:
- Removal of antibody-coated red blood cells
- Correction of anemia
- Removal of maternal antibody
- Removal of other potential toxic byproducts of the hemolytic process

A double-volume exchange transfusion (approximately 170 mL/kg) removes about 85% of the infant's red blood cells and 110% of the circulating bilirubin (extravascular bilirubin enters the blood during the exchange), but because at least 50% of the infant's bilirubin is in the extravascular compartment, only 25% of the total body bilirubin is removed.[125] Postexchange bilirubin levels are about 60% of preexchange levels, and the reequilibration that occurs between the vascular and extravascular bilirubin compartments produces a rapid rebound of serum bilirubin levels (within 30 minutes) to 70% to 80% of preexchange levels. A detailed description of the basic indications for, and contraindications to,

performing exchange transfusions as well as the technique for and complications of the procedure has been provided elsewhere.[125,126]

As discussed previously, very few exchange transfusions are currently being done. The prevention of Rh hemolytic disease with Rh immunoglobulin and the effective use of phototherapy has led to a dramatic decline in the number of exchange transfusions performed.[2] As fewer of these procedures are done, it is likely that the risks and complications will increase. A list of potential complications is provided in Box 13-6. An overall mortality rate of 0.3 in 100 procedures has been reported, but in term and near-term infants who are relatively well, the risk of death is low.[127] Jackson reported a 15-year experience of exchange transfusion (1980 to 1995) in 106 infants.[128] Eighty-one infants were healthy, and there were no deaths in these infants, although severe necrotizing enterocolitis requiring surgery did develop in one child. There were 25 sick infants, of whom 3 (12%) experienced serious complications from the exchange transfusion and 2 (8%) died. There were three additional deaths that were considered "possibly" to be the result of the exchange transfusion. Thus, the total number of deaths in sick infants, possibly as the result of the exchange, was 5 of 25 (20%). Adverse events associated with exchange transfusions were reviewed at two perinatal centers in Cleveland, Ohio, between 1992 and 2002.[127] Over a 10.5-year period, only 67 infants were identified and had exchange transfusions for hyperbilirubinemia—an average of about three exchange transfusions per year in each institution. The gestational ages ranged from less than 32 weeks (*n* = 15) to term (*n* = 22). Adverse events occurred in 74% of the exchanges, with thrombocytopenia (44%), hypocalcemia (20%), and metabolic acidosis (24%) being the most common. There were only two serious adverse events, both in infants who had other preexisting, serious neonatal morbidities. The one infant who died was a critically ill 25-week gestation infant with a birth weight of 731 g. The investigators also found that exchange transfusions performed using umbilical venous and arterial catheters were significantly more likely to be associated with adverse events than those done through the umbilical vein alone or via other routes.[127]

Box 13-6.	**Potential Complications of Exchange Transfusion**

Cardiovascular
Arrhythmias
Cardiac arrest
Volume overload
Embolization with air or clots
Thrombosis
Vasospasm

Hematologic
Sickling (donor blood)
Thrombocytopenia
Bleeding (overheparinization of donor blood)
Graft-versus-host disease
Mechanical or thermal injury to donor cells

Gastrointestinal
Necrotizing enterocolitis

Biochemical
Hyperkalemia
Hypernatremia
Hypocalcemia
Hypomagnesemia
Acidosis
Hypoglycemia

Infectious
Bacteremia
Virus infection (hepatitis, cytomegalovirus infection)
Malaria

Miscellaneous
Hypothermia
Perforation of umbilical vein
Drug loss
Apnea

From Watchko JF: Exchange transfusion in the management of neonatal hyperbilirubinemia. In Maisels MJ, Watchko JF, editors: Neonatal jaundice, London, 2000, Harwood Academic Publishers, pp 169–176.

Exchange transfusion also carries the usual risk of infection associated with any blood transfusion, although this risk is currently very low.

PHARMACOLOGIC TREATMENT

For a recent detailed review of this topic please see Cuperus et al.[129]

ACCELERATION OF NORMAL METABOLIC PATHWAYS FOR BILIRUBIN CLEARANCE

Phenobarbital induces conjugation and excretion and increases bile flow and, when given to mothers and infants, can lower TSB levels in the first week of life. However, because of concerns about long-term toxicity, it is rarely used.

DECREASING BILIRUBIN PRODUCTION

The metalloporphyrins are inhibitors of heme oxygenase, the enzyme necessary for the conversion of heme to biliverdin, one of the first steps in the formation of bilirubin from hemoglobin. In a series of controlled clinical trials, the use of tin-mesoporphyrin was shown to be effective in reducing TSB levels and the requirement for phototherapy in full-term and preterm infants as well as in infants with G6PD deficiency.[130-133] The only side effect seen has been a transient, non–dose-dependent erythema that disappeared without sequelae in infants who received phototherapy after administration of tin-mesoporphyrin.[133] A multicenter randomized controlled trial of tin-mesoporphyrin is currently in progress in the United States.

Controlled trials have confirmed that the administration of IVIG to infants with Rh and ABO hemolytic disease significantly reduces the need for exchange transfusion.[85,112,134] The dosages usually range from 500 mg/kg given over 2 hours soon after birth to 800 mg/kg given daily for 3 days. The mechanism of action of IVIG is unknown, but it is possible that it might alter the course of hemolytic disease by blocking Fc receptors and thus inhibiting hemolysis. A recent observational study suggests an association between the use of IVIG in term and late preterm infants with Rh and ABO hemolytic disease and the diagnosis of necrotizing enterocolitis.[135]

BINDING OF BILIRUBIN TO DETERGENTS

Ursodeoxycholic acid, a bile salt, has been used to treat cholestatic jaundice and, under some circumstances, could be beneficial in ameliorating indirect hyperbilirubinemia as well.[60] The mechanism for this is not fully understood, although bile salts might capture unconjugated bilirubin in the intestinal lumen and decrease the enterohepatic circulation.[129]

CASE 1

A 37²⁄₇-week gestation male infant is born following an uncomplicated pregnancy and delivery. He is breast fed by his mother and appears to be nursing adequately. At age 40 hours, a physical examination reveals no jaundice and the TcB concentration is 6.7 mg/dL (low-risk zone). He is discharged home at the age of 42 hours, and the mother is instructed to bring him back to the pediatrician's office in 10 days. On the morning of the sixth day, he is brought to the office because the mother has noticed that he was increasingly jaundiced over the previous 2 days and had nursed poorly. He had refused the breast completely for the past 12 hours, was lethargic, and had a weight loss of 14% of his birth weight. On closer questioning, the mother acknowledges that he had never nursed very well. Upon examination, the infant appears extremely jaundiced but is otherwise alert and responsive and had no posturing or arching of hid back. A stat serum bilirubin level is 29.4 mg/dL (50 µmol/L) and he is admitted to the hospital. The attending pediatrician asks the resident to start phototherapy and requests that a repeat bilirubin level be obtained in 8 hours. The infant is placed under daylight phototherapy lamps that produce an irradiance of 9 µW/cm²/nm in the blue spectrum (420 to 480 nm). The resident asks about sending blood for typing and cross matching for a possible exchange transfusion, and the attending pediatrician responds, "Unless we find evidence of hemolytic disease, this sounds like typical breast milk jaundice, and these babies never get into trouble. But let's get a type and Coombs anyway." The resident complies. The baby's blood type is A Rh-positive with a weakly positive result on direct Coombs test. The mother's blood type is group O Rh-positive.

Do you agree with the attending pediatrician's orders?

There are several problems with the way this baby is being treated. The attending pediatrician's assertion that these infants "never get into trouble" is not true. Kernicterus is well described in apparently healthy term (≥37 weeks' gestation) and late preterm (34 to 36⁶⁄₇ weeks' gestation) breast-fed newborns. A bilirubin level of 29.4 mg/dL (503 µmol/L) is a medical emergency and demands immediate and intensive phototherapy. Under these circumstances, standard phototherapy lights are inadequate, and intensive phototherapy must be used. A phototherapy source that delivers light in the 460- to 490-nm blue region of the spectrum and that can deliver an irradiance of at least 30 µW/cm²/nm should be used, and lights should be placed above and below the infant (see Table 13-12 for a list of commercially available sources). The sides of the bassinet can be lined with aluminum foil to further optimize the surface area of the infant exposed to phototherapy. Typing and cross matching for blood for exchange transfusion must be performed immediately, because the cause of this extreme hyperbilirubinemia is unknown, and if a subsequent TSB level remains the same or even increases despite appropriate phototherapy, an exchange transfusion should be performed immediately. Because it is essential to know which way the bilirubin level is moving, a repeat TSB level should be obtained within 2 to 3 hours and certainly no later than 4 hours. In addition, the baby should be given formula in an attempt to reduce the enterohepatic circulation. Because the rate of decline of the TSB level with phototherapy is directly related to the initial TSB level (the higher the level, the more rapid the decline), a decrease of at least 2 to 3 mg/dL (and often more) can be expected in the first 4 hours. In addition to limiting the enterohepatic circulation, formula gives needed calories as well as additional fluid. Because the structural isomer lumirubin is excreted in the urine, maintaining a good urine output helps to lower the TSB level more rapidly.

Does this infant have ABO hemolytic disease?

It is hard to be sure. He was not at all jaundiced at age 40 hours, and although there is A-O incompatibility with a positive DAT result, if this were truly ABO hemolytic disease, clinical jaundice should have been seen within the first 24 hours and certainly by 36 hours. It is quite likely that this infant has a combination of increased bilirubin production from ABO incompatibility together with breast-feeding–associated hyperbilirubinemia related to a low caloric intake and exaggeration of the enterohepatic circulation.

A major error in the care of this infant was scheduling a follow-up visit at age 10 days in a newborn discharged at age 42 hours. As emphasized earlier, such infants should always be seen within 2 days of discharge, particularly if the baby is breast fed and younger than 38 weeks' gestation as was the case here.

What other tests should be ordered for this infant?

In addition to the blood typing and Coombs test, a complete blood count with smear, reticulocyte count, and G6PD determination should be performed. Measurement of serum albumin level would be helpful. In selected infants with very low serum albumin levels and therefore less ability to bind bilirubin, earlier exchange transfusion might be considered.

How could this extreme hyperbilirubinemia have been prevented?

Follow-up of this infant within 2 days of discharge would likely have identified an infant who was becoming progressively jaundiced. A TSB level would have been obtained, the mother would have been counseled to improve breast feeding efforts, and, if necessary, phototherapy would have followed.

CASE 2

A healthy full-term female infant is brought to the pediatrician's office at age 3 weeks. The baby is being breast fed, has had an excellent weight gain, and has perfectly normal examination results except that she is slightly jaundiced.

What questions should be asked of the mother?

The most important information needed is the color of the baby's stool and urine. If the urine is pale yellow and nearly colorless and the stool is a normal brownish color, the likelihood of cholestatic jaundice is slim.

The mother reports that the baby's stools and urine are normal. What should be done?

For any infant who is jaundiced at 3 weeks of age or older a total *and* direct-bilirubin level *must* be measured to rule out cholestatic jaundice and the possibility of extrahepatic biliary atresia.

The TSB level is 8.2 mg/dL and the direct bilirubin level 0.5 mg/dL. Do you need to do anything else?

Although it is overwhelmingly likely that this baby has breast milk jaundice, any baby with prolonged indirect hyperbilirubinemia should undergo an evaluation of thyroid function, because hypothyroidism is one cause of prolonged indirect hyperbilirubinemia. This can easily be accomplished without further testing by referring to the hospital chart (or the state laboratory results) and confirming that the metabolic screen was done and that the thyroid function was normal.

The mother comes back when the baby is 10 weeks old and the baby is still jaundiced. The TSB level is 7.5 mg/dL (130 μmol/L) and the direct bilirubin level is 0.4 mg/dL (7 μmol/L). What should the mother be told?

Indirect hyperbilirubinemia up to age 12 weeks is well within the limits of the breast milk jaundice syndrome; reassure the mother that she need not be concerned.

Are there additional questions that should be asked of the mother?

Ask the mother whether there is any history of mild, unconjugated hyperbilirubinemia in her family (Gilbert syndrome). There is a strong association between prolonged indirect hyperbilirubinemia in breast-fed infants and the (TA) [*UGT1A1*28*] dinucleotide variant allele within the A(TA)$_n$TAA repeat element of the *UGT1A1* TATAA box promoter[3], which differs from the more prevalent wild-type A(TA) TAA promoter. Individuals with Gilbert syndrome are homozygous for the *UGT1A1*28* allele.

CASE 3

A 40-week gestation African American female breast-fed infant, birth weight 3400 g, was discharged home at 36 hours of age with no evidence of jaundice and a predischarge TcB value of 7.6 mg/dL (low intermediate risk zone). The mother is a 26-year-old O Rh-positive, antibody screen–negative, multiparous woman who breast fed her two previous children. The infant was seen in the pediatrician's office 2 days after discharge and during that visit was noted to show marked signs of jaundice, including scleral icterus. The mother reported that her daughter had fed poorly that morning and has been less active. A TSB concentration is 24.7 mg/dL. The infant is directly admitted to a local NICU for further evaluation, and intensive phototherapy is started on arrival. The infant's admission weight is 3200 g and she is noted to be lethargic but otherwise neurologically intact. On admission, the TSB level is 28.8 mg/dL, and the infant's blood type is O Rh-positive and the DAT result is negative. The hemoglobin and hematocrit are 14 g/dL and 42%, respectively; the reticulocyte count is 2%; and red blood cell morphology on smear is unremarkable.

What is the most likely explanation for this infant's extreme hyperbilirubinemia?

Of the major risk factors for subsequent severe hyperbilirubinemia, only breast milk feeding is evident. However, by report the infant had been feeding well until the morning of admission and the infant's weight has declined only approximately 6% from birth. The blood type and DAT result rule out an immune-mediated hemolytic process. The TSB level is rising quickly, and an alternative cause must be sought.

The most likely cause of this infant's extreme hyperbilirubinemia is G6PD deficiency. Although the disorder is X-linked and is more prevalent in male infants, homozygous and heterozygous females may be affected. The prevalence of G6PD deficiency in African American females is 4.1%. The absence of overt anemia, reticulocytosis, and abnormal red cell morphology on smear do not exclude this diagnosis.

What would you anticipate the TSB trajectory to be in response to phototherapy?

Although hyperbilirubinemia in the context of G6PD deficiency is often responsive to intensive phototherapy, one cannot be assured of this. The marked increase in TSB from 24.7 mg/dL to 28.8 mg/dL in the period between the drawing of the bilirubin sample at the office visit and the measurement of TSB on NICU admission suggests active hemolysis, which may not be responsive to phototherapy alone. Appropriately, a blood sample is sent to the blood bank on NICU admission for typing and cross matching of blood for a possible double-volume exchange transfusion. Indeed, a repeat TSB measurement 3 hours after admission is 31.2 mg/dL despite intensive phototherapy, and the infant undergoes a double-volume exchange transfusion. A G6PD assay and genotyping are performed on the first aliquot of the infant's blood removed during the double-volume exchange transfusion.

After the exchange transfusion, the TSB level is 21.2 mg/dL, but the infant is noted to have posturing, both retrocollis and opisthotonos. What should be done?

The infant should undergo a second double-volume exchange transfusion. The presence of advanced clinical signs of acute bilirubin encephalopathy is an indication for immediate exchange transfusion irrespective of the TSB level.

Prompt institution of the second double-volume exchange transfusion is associated with a further decrease in TSB to 16.7 mg/dL and resolution of bilirubin encephalopathy signs. Magnetic resonance imaging results and auditory brain stem response before discharge are both normal.

The pediatric resident states that the infant is most likely a homozygous G6PD-deficient female given the infant's hyperbilirubinemia course. The attending neonatologist is not so sure.

The results of the quantitative G6PD enzyme assay is 7.6 IU/g hemoglobin (normal: 7.0 to 20.5 IU/g hemoglobin) and the infant is heterozygous for the *G6PD A* mutation. Female neonates heterozygous for the *G6PD* mutations represent a unique at-risk group. X inactivation results in a subpopulation of G6PD-deficient red blood cells in *every* female heterozygote; that is, each heterozygous female is a mosaic with two red blood cell populations including one that is G6PD deficient. A heterozygous female may be reported as enzymatically normal yet harbor a sizable population of G6PD-deficient, potentially hemolyzable red blood cells that represent a substantial reservoir of bilirubin. When this pool undergoes acute hemolysis, hazardous hyperbilirubinemia can evolve rapidly, as seen in this infant. There is no reliable biochemical assay to detect G6PD heterozygotes; only DNA analysis can provide this information. No apparent trigger for hemolysis (e.g., naphthalene in mothballs, sepsis) was identified as is frequently the case.

It should be noted that in the presence of acute hemolysis, the G6PD level can be normal, even in homozygotes, because older red blood cells are destroyed and the remaining younger cells have higher levels of G6PD. In such a case, if G6PD deficiency is suspected, the G6PD level should be measured again in 2 to 3 months. In a homozygous G6PD-deficient infant, the G6PD level will then be low.

REFERENCES

The reference list for this chapter can be found online at www.expertconsult.com

Infections in the Neonate

14

Jill E. Baley and Ethan G. Leonard

EPIDEMIOLOGY, RISK FACTORS, AND PRESENTATION

The fetus and the newborn are extremely susceptible to infections. This susceptibility stems from maternal risk factors, obstetrical complications, the postnatal environment, and the immature host defenses of the newborn. *Neonatal sepsis* is defined as a systemic inflammatory response syndrome secondary to infection. The age of onset of sepsis reflects the likely mode of acquisition, microbiologic features, mortality rate, and presentation of the infection. Meningitis is usually a sequela of sepsis. The incidence of neonatal sepsis ranges from 1 to 8 cases per 1000 live births, whereas meningitis may occur in 1 of every 6 septic infants.[1] Epidemiologically, neonatal sepsis is divided into the following categories: early-onset sepsis, late-onset sepsis, and very late-onset sepsis.

Early-onset sepsis (EOS) is a systemic, multiorgan disease that presents in the first week of life and usually on the first day of life. Infection is most often acquired before delivery. Obstetrical complications contribute to the development of infection and include rupture of membranes prematurely (before onset of labor) or a prolonged period (>18 hours) before delivery, chorioamnionitis, maternal fever, maternal urinary tract infection, and infant prematurity or low birth weight. These infants have a fulminant onset of respiratory symptoms, usually due to pneumonia; shock or poor perfusion; and temperature instability. Mortality may be as high as 30% to 50%. The microbiologic features of EOS reflect maternal genitourinary and gastrointestinal colonization. Before the adoption of intrapartum antibiotic prophylaxis (IAP) against group B *Streptococcus* (GBS), this pathogen caused the overwhelming majority of EOS. Today, GBS still causes most cases of EOS; however, enteric bacilli such as *Escherichia coli* have become more prevalent in term infants and are as likely as

GBS to cause EOS in very low-birth-weight premature infants.[2,3] Although GBS and enteric bacilli cause the preponderance of EOS, a third pathogen, *Listeria monocytogenes,* can cause EOS. Unlike GBS and the gram-negative pathogens, which usually are acquired through asymptomatic maternal colonization, *L. monocytogenes* generally causes a flulike or gastrointestinal illness in the mother. This organism is mostly acquired from animal products: unpasteurized milk, cheese, delicatessen meats, and hot dogs. The importance of this organism will become clear in the discussion of empiric antibiotic therapy.

Late-onset sepsis is defined as the infections that occur beyond the first week of life but before 30 days of life. Very late-onset sepsis occurs beyond 30 days of life. Although obstetrical complications may be identified, these are not typical. Late-onset disease is more likely to reflect infection with gram-positive organisms acquired in the nursery: coagulase-positive staphylococci, *Staphylococcus aureus,* and enterococci. Very late-onset disease includes infections caused by GBS, gram-negative bacilli, and *Streptococcus pneumoniae.*

The high incidence of gram-positive infection in the hospitalized infant reflects the combination of usually lower gestational age and low-birth-weight, and the consequent need for the insertion of central venous catheters for supportive care.[3] Although many of these infants will manifest poor feeding, temperature instability, and lethargy, they are more likely to have localized disease: urinary tract infection, osteoarthritis, or soft tissue infection. Meningitis is common. Presentation may be slowly progressive or fulminant. Mortality is lower than with EOS but may still be 20% to 40%.

The widespread use of IAP in the United States has been shown to have decreased the incidence of EOS by 70%, to 0.44 cases per 1000 live births, an incidence equivalent to that of late-onset sepsis.[4] Of importance is that the improved survival of very low-birth-weight infants has put them at increased risk of systemic nosocomial infection. In a multicenter trial of prophylactic intravenous immunoglobulin administration involving more than 2400 very low-birth-weight infants, 16% of the infants developed sepsis at a median age of 17 days. Compared with the infants who did not develop sepsis, these infants not only had increased morbidity, but their mortality rose from 9% to 21% (not always directly due to sepsis) and their average length of hospital stay increased from 58 to 98 days.[5]

The most important risk factors for the development of neonatal sepsis are low birth weight and prematurity. Sepsis conversely is also the most common cause of death in infants under 1500 g.[6] The incidence of sepsis is inversely proportional to the gestational age or birth weight of the infant. Other risk factors include immature immune function, exposure to invasive procedures, hypoxia, metabolic acidosis, hypothermia, and low socioeconomic status—all factors associated with low birth weight and prematurity. In a multicenter survey of GBS disease carried out by the Centers for Disease Control and Prevention (CDC), 13.5 cases per 1000 live births were diagnosed among black infants compared with 4.5 cases among 1000 white infants, and EOS was twice as common among black infants as among white infants.[7] Although males have a higher incidence of sepsis, once respiratory distress syndrome is accounted for, they are not at a significantly higher risk of sepsis, contrary to the results of older studies.[1,8] It is generally felt that sepsis is more common among the firstborn of twins. Infants with galactosemia are more likely to become infected with gram-negative organisms, in particular *E. coli*. The administration of iron for anemia appears to increase risk because iron may be a growth factor for a number of bacteria. Finally, the widespread use of broad-spectrum antibiotics may cause a shift in the nursery to a higher prevalence of resistant bacteria that are also more invasive.

EVALUATION AND MANAGEMENT OF NEONATAL SEPSIS

Definitive diagnosis of bacterial infection is predicated on the recovery of a pathogen from a normally sterile body site such as blood, urine, or cerebrospinal fluid (CSF). Although many indirect indices of infection have been identified and studied, including total white blood cell count, absolute neutrophil count, C-reactive protein level, procalcitonin level, and levels of a variety of inflammatory cytokines, these tests are nonspecific and are not adequately sensitive to confirm or exclude systemic infection.

In any infant with suspected EOS cultures of blood should be drawn and, if the infant is in hemodynamically stable condition, spinal fluid should be obtained, and the infant should be started on intravenous antibiotics. The need for lumbar puncture in the first 24 to 72 hours of life has been a topic of some controversy.[9] Data suggesting that lumbar puncture is unnecessary in these infants comes primarily from retrospective studies of asymptomatic infants. The poor correlation between the results of neonatal blood cultures and CSF cultures underscores the need for lumbar puncture. Several studies report that bacterial meningitis would be missed in approximately one third of neonates on the basis of blood culture results alone.[10,11] Antibiotic regimens should cover GBS, gram-negative bacilli, and *L. monocytogenes.* The most commonly used regimens are ampicillin and cefotaxime or ampicillin and gentamicin. Both regimens are quite effective against GBS. Unfortunately, *E. coli* has increasingly become resistant to ampicillin. In many institutions, more than half of the *E. coli* isolates are resistant to ampicillin. A search of the Cochrane database for evidence suggesting that one regimen is superior to another does not yield a conclusion.[12] Regardless of the regimen used, ampicillin should be included, because the cephalosporins have no activity against *L. monocytogenes,* and gentamicin monotherapy would be ineffective.

The data for empirical therapy in late- and very late-onset disease are not definitively in favor of any one regimen.[13] Given the prevalence of staphylococcal species, many clinicians would include vancomycin in the empiric treatment of a hospitalized neonate with signs of sepsis beyond the seventh day of life. If the infant is being admitted from the community, the regimen should include coverage for GBS, *E. coli,* and *S. pneumoniae.* Commonly cited guidelines for the evaluation of febrile children without a focus of infection who are between 30 and 60 days of life include obtaining blood and urine samples for culture and performing a lumbar puncture before administration of antibiotics.

GROUP B *STREPTOCOCCUS* INFECTION

Streptococcus agalactiae, or group B *Streptococcus* (GBS), is the most common cause of vertically transmitted neonatal sepsis, a significant cause of maternal bacteriuria and endometritis, and a major cause of serious bacterial infection in infants up to 3 months of age. Nine serotypes of GBS have been identified on the basis of differing polysaccharide capsules: Ia, Ib, II, and III through VIII. Traditionally, neonatal disease is considered early onset (EOGBS) if it occurs in the first 7 days of life and late onset if it occurs from 8 days through 3 months of life. Epidemiologically, the serotypes responsible for neonatal disease shifted significantly in the 1990s. Type Ia, type III, and type V cause 35% to 40%; 25% to 30%; and 15% of cases of EOGBS, repectively.[14-16] Type III still causes the majority of late-onset disease and neonatal meningitis.[17] Antibodies against specific serotypes of GBS are protective but not cross-reactive.

Although GBS can cross the placenta, the primary mode of transmission is after rupture of membranes and during passage through the birth canal. Approximately 20% to 40% of women are colonized in their genital tract, but the primary reservoir of GBS is the lower gastrointestinal tract. High genital inoculum at delivery increases the likelihood of transmission and the consequent rate of EOGBS. Half of infants born to colonized women will themselves be colonized with GBS. Before the use of IAP targeted against GBS, the incidence of EOGBS ranged from 1 to 3 cases per 1000 live births. By definition, EOGBS presents in the first 6 days of life, and close to 90% of cases present within 24 hours of life. The vast majority of these infants demonstrate systemic illness by 12 hours.

In 1986 Boyer and Gotoff published the first randomized controlled trial showing the effectiveness of IAP in reducing neonatal colonization and EOGBS.[18] In 1996 the CDC published the first set of guidelines for the prevention of perinatal GBS disease. The guidelines endorsed two approaches to IAP: (1) women with vaginal or rectal cultures positive for GBS should receive IAP; or (2) women with any of the following risk factors—delivery before 37 weeks' gestation, membrane rupture 18 hours or longer before delivery, or maternal fever of 38° C or higher—should receive IAP. In addition, any woman who had a history of GBS bacteriuria or who had previously delivered an infant with EOGBS was to receive IAP. In addition to the administration of IAP, the guidelines provided for the evaluation of the infant after delivery. These strategies reduced the incidence to 0.6 cases per 1000 live births in 1998.[19,20] Ongoing active surveillance of GBS demonstrated that the screening-based approach was superior to the risk-based approach in preventing EOGBS.[21] In 2002 the CDC published revised guidelines that promoted the universal screening of all pregnant women between 35 and 37 weeks' gestation using rectovaginal cultures and recommended that all women with positive culture results receive IAP.[19] The guidelines also recommended IAP for mothers who had any history of GBS bacteriuria during the pregnancy, who had suspected amnionitis, or who had previously delivered an infant with EOGBS. These guidelines also clarified the antibiotic dosages for IAP, alternatives for mothers with penicillin allergy, and the management of an exposed newborn (Fig. 14-1).

As of 2003, the incidence of EOGBS was down to 0.3 cases per 1000 live births.[22] Although effective, the screening-based approach incurs the costs of testing, IAP, and management of the exposed infant. Although, to date, no studies have shown an association between penicillin and ampicillin IAP and the emergence of antibiotic resistance in other bacteria, this risk remains a concern. An immunization-based strategy targeting pregnant women has the potential to prevent EOGBS, late-onset disease, and some maternal disease and to be more cost effective. A multivalent protein conjugate vaccine has proved effective in a murine model, and several human trials of individual serotype conjugate vaccines have shown promise.[23-26]

For documented GBS infection, penicillin is the drug of choice and is the most narrow-spectrum agent. Ampicillin is an acceptable alternative agent. No penicillin resistance has been reported to date. The dosages and intervals depend on the postgestational age of the infant. The duration of therapy is 10 days for bacteremia without a focus, 14 days for uncomplicated meningitis, and up to 4 weeks for septic arthritis, endocarditis, or ventriculitis.[27]

COAGULASE-NEGATIVE *STAPHYLOCOCCUS* INFECTION

For several decades, coagulase-negative staphylococci have been the most common cause of nosocomial blood stream infections

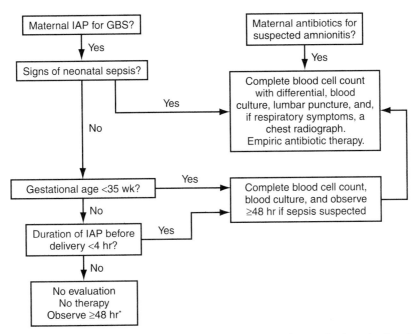

Figure 14-1. Algorithm for management of neonates exposed to intrapartum antibiotic prophylaxis (IAP). *GBS*, Group B *Streptococcus*.

in the neonatal intensive care unit and are responsible for the majority of cases of late-onset sepsis in preterm neonates. Infections with these gram-positive bacteria are most often associated with indwelling central venous catheters. These bacteria are part of normal human skin flora. *Staphylococcus epidermidis* is the most common species of coagulase-negative staphylococci recovered from human skin and mucous membranes. Most infants are colonized within the first week of life from passage through the birth canal and repeated exposure from colonized caregivers.

The major virulence factor for coagulase-negative staphylococci is its ability to adhere to plastic and other foreign bodies by producing a biofilm. The biofilm consists of multiple layers of bacteria surrounded by an exopolysaccharide matrix or slime. This biofilm protects the bacteria from host phagocytic cells and interferes with the ability of many antimicrobial agents to effectively eliminate infection. This affinity for plastic foreign bodies explains the high recovery rate of these organisms from infected catheters, ventricular shunts, endotracheal tubes, and artificial vascular grafts and cardiac valves.

Neonatal infections with coagulase-negative staphylococci typically present without localizing signs with fever, new-onset respiratory distress, or a deterioration in respiratory status. Other common nonspecific signs of coagulase-negative staphylococcus sepsis include apnea, bradycardia, poikilothermia, poor perfusion, poor feeding, irritability, and lethargy. Indolent infection is more common than fulminant disease, with mortality generally under 15%. Coagulase-negative staphylococci infections, however, are a major source of morbidity leading to increased antibiotic exposure, length of stay, and hospital costs.

Treatment of coagulase-negative staphylococci often requires the use of vancomycin. More than 80% of strains acquired in the hospital are resistant to β-lactam antibiotics.[28] Resistance is typically attributable to altered penicillin-binding proteins and β-lactamase production. Unfortunately, these types of resistance can be inducible and therefore may not be detected by routine microdilutional methods. If a strain is reported as penicillin sensitive, consultation with the hospital microbiologist is recommended to confirm testing for inducible resistance. More than 50% of coagulase-negative staphylococci are resistant to clindamycin, trimethoprim-sulfamethoxazole, gentamicin, and ciprofloxacin. Coagulase-negative staphylococci isolated from hospitalized patients show varying rates of resistance to the tetracyclines, chloramphenicol, rifampin, and newer-generation quinolone antibiotics. Some *S. epidermidis* isolates have been recovered that show resistance to vancomycin; however, these species have been susceptible to the newer agents for gram-positive organisms: linezolid, quinupristin-dalfopristin, and daptomycin.[29,30] Pharmacokinetic data and clinical experience with these agents in neonates are limited, and these drugs should be used only in consultation with a physician with expertise in infectious diseases.

The most effective management of coagulase-negative staphylococci infections is the combination of systemic antimicrobial therapy and, whenever possible, the removal of the foreign body. When a foreign body cannot be feasibly removed, the combination of vancomycin with rifampin, and/or an aminoglycoside, may be used. In the case of ventricular shunt infections, antibiotics may be administered both systemically and intraventricularly. If an attempt is made to manage an infection without foreign body removal, consultation with an infectious disease expert would be advised to determine the best antimicrobial agents and duration of therapy.

Although many groups have proposed different strategies to prevent neonatal catheter infections, few studies have yielded promising results. Several groups have studied the use of prophylactic antibiotics in neonates with indwelling catheters. The Cochrane Neonatal Group found no evidence to support this practice for neonates with umbilical arterial or venous catheters,[31,32] nor did they find evidence to support routine use of vancomycin in preterm infants to prevent nosocomial sepsis.[33] The use of a vancomycin-heparin lock solution to prevent nosocomial blood stream infection showed promise in a small randomized, controlled, double-blinded study in critically ill neonates with peripherally inserted central venous catheters[34]; however, larger studies are needed. The use of antibiotic- or silver-impregnated catheters has not been studied in neonates. In 2002, the CDC recommended against the routine use of antimicrobial prophylaxis for patients with central venous catheters.[35] In 2006, the Cochrane Neonatal Group began

a systematic review of the use of systemic antibiotics to reduce morbidity and mortality in neonates with central venous catheters. Results are not yet available.

STAPHYLOCOCCUS AUREUS INFECTION

Staphylococcus aureus is a gram-positive bacteria that is morphologically indistinguishable from the coagulase-negative staphylococci by light microscopy. *S. aureus* is part of normal skin flora. This organism causes a much wider and potentially more invasive spectrum of disease than that caused by coagulase-negative species. This pathogen is a common cause of superficial pustular disease and localized cellulitis, and is the most frequent cause of surgical site infection in infants and adult patients. The production of numerous toxins, enzymes, and binding proteins facilitates its ability to establish aggressive, life-threatening pyogenic infection. Small-inoculum colonization or infection can produce catastrophic, toxin-mediated disease such as scalded skin syndrome or toxic shock.

Over the last two decades, *S. aureus* has shown an increasing resistance to β-lactam antibiotics, as documented by methicillin susceptibility testing[36]; these methicillin-resistant strains (MRSA) are resistant to all penicillins, penicillin–β-lactamase inhibitor combination drugs, cephalosporins, and carbapenems. Most hospital-acquired strains are resistant to clindamycin. Until recently, these resistant strains were not inherently more virulent. Unfortunately, however, over the last several years community MRSA strains have acquired an additional virulence factor, Panton-Valentine leukocidin. This factor has contributed to a significant increase in invasive, pyogenic infection by MRSA. Several outbreaks in preterm and term neonates, as well as nosocomial transmission from caregivers, equipment, and toys in neonatal intensive care units, have been reported.[37-41] In an ill, hospitalized neonate who develops suspected or documented infection with gram-positive cocci, vancomycin should be included in the empirical antibiotic regimen. As discussed earlier, blood stream infections caused by coagulase-negative species are much more prevalent than bacteremias from *S. aureus;* however, many clinicians would elect to start vancomycin for any gram-positive blood stream infection in a hospitalized neonate because of the high rate of resistance to β-lactam antibiotics in the coagulase-negative strains and the potential consequences of not treating MRSA. Other drugs are available with activity against MRSA, including older drugs like tetracyclines and trimethoprim-sulfamethoxazole, but these drugs are typically avoided in neonates. Several newer drugs—quinupristin-dalfopristin, linezolid, and daptomycin—have activity against MRSA. MRSA infections in neonates should be managed by an individual with expertise in the pharmacodynamics and pharmacokinetics of these drugs.

CANDIDIASIS

The survival of fragile, very low-birth-weight neonates has led to increased infections due to candidiasis in the nursery. *Candida* species are responsible for 2.4% of early-onset infections in newborns but, more importantly, they cause 10% to 12% of late-onset infections. Overall, infections with these fungi are among the three most common infections in the neonatal intensive care unit.[6,42,43]

Although *Candida albicans* once caused 75% of invasive candidal infections, infections involving non-albicans species are now becoming more common, approaching 40% to 45% of infections. The incidence of *Candida parapsilosis* infection, unique to the newborn, has risen more than tenfold, and this species now causes 25% of fungal infections in the newborn. Also of note, the incidence of *Candida tropicalis* and *Candida glabrata* infection has nearly doubled during the same time period.[44,45] The reported mortality attributable to *C. albicans* infection varies widely but may be as high as 20% to 40%.[46,47] The mortality from *C. parapsilosis* is certainly significant but tends to be lower than that attributable to *C. albicans*.

Vertical transmission from mother to infant usually occurs during passage through the birth canal, especially in the presence of vaginitis. This is most often seen with *C. albicans* and *C. glabrata*. Congenital infections may rarely be seen and have been attributed both to ascending infection from the vagina and transplacental infection. *C. parapsilosis,* however, is frequently transmitted horizontally and is the most common fungal organism isolated from the hands of health care workers. This fungus is not commonly found in the genitourinary tracts of mothers. Colonization appears to occur more readily among very low and extremely low-birth-weight infants

than among term infants and occurs in up to 25% of these infants in the first week of life.[48] One fourth of intubated infants demonstrate respiratory colonization.

A large number of predisposing factors have influenced the rate of dissemination. One of the primary factors is the prolonged and frequent use of broad-spectrum antibiotics that suppress the growth of bacteria in the gastrointestinal tract and allow candidal overgrowth. Eventually, penetration of the epithelial barrier leads to disseminated disease. Mucosal penetration and dissemination are more likely the denser the colonization, and *C. albicans* has been shown to adhere to the mucosa of the preterm infant better than to that of the term infant. In particular, the use of third-generation cephalosporins seems to increase the risk of gastrointestinal colonization and subsequent candidemia.[46,49] Dense colonization of the gastrointestinal tract increases the chances of translocation of the yeast across the mucosa. Intestinal ischemia, necrotizing enterocolitis, and spontaneous perforation of the intestine, common in the preterm infant, are all highly associated with candidemia. Delayed enteral feeding has also been associated with infection.[49] The use of histamine 2 blockers raises the pH of the stomach and increases colonization, particularly of *C. parapsilosis*.[50] Abdominal and cardiac surgeries are greater risks in term infants. In a similar fashion, candidal organisms readily penetrate the relatively poor barrier provided by the immature skin of the preterm infant, and that skin also readily breaks down during ordinary care. Colonized infants are more likely to be delivered vaginally than by cesarian section.[48,51] The use of topical petrolatum for skin care of extremely low-birth-weight infants may increase the risk. Catheters, as well as all other indwelling tubes (endotracheal, chest, urinary, ventriculoperitoneal), may become infected. The longer the duration of an indwelling catheter, particularly if used for total parenteral nutrition or infusion of intravenous lipids, the greater the risk is to the infant.[50] Immature immune defenses provide yet another set of risk factors. Neutrophils ingest and kill *Candida* intracellularly, but neutropenia is also common in very low-birth-weight infants. Theophylline, frequently used in preterm infants, may inhibit the candidacidal activity of neutrophils. Steroids inhibit the immune response, induce hyperglycemia, and, in the mouse, increase the adherence of the yeast to the intestinal mucosa.

Congenital candidiasis is extremely rare. In the term infant, infection results in an erythematous, macular eruption that then becomes pustular and desquamates.[52] These same skin infections become burnlike in the preterm infant and then develop either a branlike or sheetlike desquamation, becoming superficial erosions. Intrauterine infection is highly associated with the presence of genital tract foreign bodies, in particular, cerclage, but have not been associated with maternal diabetes or urinary tract infections. The diagnosis in the newborn can be made with skin scrapings and blood and cerebrospinal fluid cultures. In the term infant with only cutaneous infection, survival is the rule. These infants do not require treatment, although many will administer topical therapy to relieve symptoms and to decrease the mass of organisms the infant has to clear. In contrast, in the preterm infant weighing less than 1500 g, or in any infant with respiratory symptoms signifying aspiration and pneumonia, mortality is the rule unless systemic treatment is begun.

Mucocutaneous infection (thrush or a monilial diaper rash) is the most likely infection after birth, seen in 4% to 6% of newborns and occurring as early as 4 to 5 days after birth but peaking at 3 to 4 months. Thrush manifests as white, curdlike, pseudomembranous plaques on the oropharynx or posterior pharynx, whereas the diaper dermatitis produces an erythematous, scaly lesion with satellite papules or pustules in the intertriginous areas. The latter may be repetitively reinfected by a gastrointestinal tract reservoir. Therapy in those areas is local. Oral nystatin may be given to treat the thrush. Gentian violet works as efficaciously, but its propensity to stain makes it less popular. For the skin lesions, topical nystatin alone works well, although occasionally it should be combined with oral nystatin to reduce the gastrointestinal tract reservoir and to prevent spillage onto the groin. Once the rash starts spreading beyond the usual area in the diaper, systemic therapy must begin.

Invasive candidiasis is a leading cause of morbidity and mortality in infants of less than 1000 g. Incidence in neonatal centers ranges from 2% to 28%.[53] Systemic disease in these infants, unlike in adults, results in multiple foci of infection. Onset is delayed, usually occurring at several weeks of life, and the duration of candidemia, even with treatment, averages 7 days. Most infants have several positive blood culture results, and 10% experience candidemia for longer than 14 days.[49,54] Infants have a multitude of signs and symptoms including, in order of frequency, respiratory deterioration, apnea and bradycardia, hyperglycemia, a necrotizing enterocolitis–like picture without pneumatosis, skin involvement, temperature instability, and hypotension.[55] Meningitis, once reported in half of infants with systemic candidiasis, now occurs in only 5% to 9%,[49,56] probably due to more aggressive diagnosis and treatment. Roughly half of infants with meningitis will have negative blood culture results and half will have normal CSF parameters.[52,56] Endophthalmitis, once seen in half of infants, again is now relatively uncommon, occurring in fewer than 1%.[57,58] Prognosis is excellent if the infection is treated. However, fungal sepsis in extremely low-birth-weight infants may be associated with increased frequency of threshold retinopathy of prematurity.[59,60] Endocarditis, which may be the source of infected thromboemboli, is associated with the presence of central venous catheters. The prognosis for osteoarthritis or osteomyelitis is also good with treatment. Cutaneous manifestations may include a generalized erythema or subcutaneous abscesses. Infants may be neutropenic or have an extreme leukocytosis. Continued thrombocytopenia is often an indication of ongoing disease. Pneumonitis presents with respiratory deterioration and a bronchopulmonary dysplasia–like picture on chest radiograph. Other infants may develop abdominal distension, guaiac-positive stools, and feeding intolerance but no pneumatosis intestinalis. A few will have hepatic abscesses, diarrhea, or perforation. Mortality is extremely high in those with candidal peritonitis. Urinary tract involvement is found in over half of infants with systemic candidiasis and ranges from a bladder infection to renal abscesses or renal papillary necrosis to a mycetoma or fungal ball in the renal pelvis, possibly resulting in a flank mass. Disease of the urinary tract may be entirely silent or present with hypertension or acute renal failure with oliguria or anuria. Mortality is usually in the range of 20% to 50%, but death or disability ensues in as many as 73% of extremely low-birth-weight infants.[49] Compared with age-matched controls, there is a higher incidence of periventricular leukomalacia, chronic lung disease, severe retinopathy of prematurity, and adverse neurologic outcome at 2 years corrected age.[61]

Candidal species grow readily in cultures of blood or urine or specimens from other normally sterile sites, and yeast or hyphae can be seen on urinalysis. Given the propensity for dissemination, the patient should undergo ultrasonography of the kidneys, echocardiography, and a retinal examination. Fungal stains of skin scrapings can be helpful. A complete blood count and C-reactive protein level may give indirect evidence of infection. A lumbar puncture, together with culture, gram staining and cytologic analysis, is imperative. Overall, it is important to have a high index of suspicion.

Immediate consideration should also be given to the removal of possibly contaminated medical devices, particularly central intravascular catheters. Amphotericin B has been the standard for antifungal therapy for years, but many other agents have been introduced, and few data are available to indicate the advantages of one drug over another, let alone safety, efficacy, dosages, or duration of treatment. CSF penetration of amphotericin B, while better than in adults, is highly variable. This has led a few to suggest the use of 5-fluorocytosine or fluconazole, both of which have good penetration of the CSF, in combination with amphotericin B. Others have successfully treated meningitis with amphotericin B alone. There are three lipid formulations approved by the U.S. Food and Drug Administration for use in adults: amphotericin B lipid complex (ABLC), amphotericin B colloidal dispersion (ABCD), and liposomal amphotericin B (AmBisome). Because higher dosages may be used without toxicity, these preparations may be appropriate for the infant with renal disease or severe nephrotoxicity.[62-64] A few studies have shown fluconazole to be efficacious in the treatment of invasive disease in neonates, equivalent to treatment with amphotericin B.[65,66] Unfortunately, half of *Candida glabrata* and *Candida krusei* isolates are resistant to fluconazole. Fluconazole monotherapy is only recommended in neonates after identification of the fungal organism and determination of its susceptibility. Caspofungin is fungicidal against all candidal species. However, there are only case reports of its use in neonates, and it cannot be recommended at this time.

Prevention is clearly the best treatment for neonatal systemic candidiasis, yet this is also the area of greatest controversy.

Treatment of maternal candidal infections may limit vertical transmission to the neonate. Prevention of horizontal transmission is more difficult. Hand washing does not reduce the recovery of *C. albicans* from medical workers' hands.[67] Removal of artificial fingernails may help. Careful attention to central lines is of benefit, as is attention to limiting exposure to drugs that increase the risk of disease. No consensus has been reached on the use of fluconazole prophylaxis. Some studies have shown a decrease in the incidence of colonization, invasive disease, or mortality.[68-72] Finally, concern remains regarding the risk of isolates developing resistance. A recent metaanalysis of three trials involving over 1600 infants found a decrease in the risk of invasive fungal infection in very low-birth-weight infants with oral-topical antifungal prophylaxis but warned about the major methodologic weaknesses in trials to date.[73] Also, one recent trial comparing fluconazole and nystatin oral prophylaxis had to be halted early due to a significant increase in deaths not related to fungal infections among the nystatin-treated infants.[74] Reports do exist of increased resistance among infants with *C. parapsilosis* infection, a rising form of candidiasis.[75,76]

CONGENITAL CYTOMEGALOVIRUS INFECTION

Cytomegalovirus (CMV) infection is the most frequent congenital infection in humans. The virus is endemic and worldwide and has no seasonal pattern of infection. Typically, after a primary infection, virus is shed for weeks to even years before becoming latent. Periodic episodes of viral shedding occur. The virus consists of three major components: an inner icosahedral or 20-sided capsid containing double-stranded DNA that is similar to that of herpes simplex virus; an amorphous layer consisting of viral proteins and RNA; and an outer envelope. The virus does not code for thymidine kinase, which renders acyclovir ineffective.

Infection with CMV largely depends on socioeconomic status, which reflects crowding. It also increases with parity and number of sexual partners. Finally, seropositivity is much higher among African American and Asian women. Seropositivity occurs in 0.5% to 2.0% of infants in the United States and Western Europe and rises to 50% to 85% among young women, but it is much more prevalent in developing countries and among lower socioeconomic groups, where seropositivity may be as high as 90%. At childbearing age, 2% of women of middle to upper socioeconomic status seroconvert yearly, compared with 6% of those of lower socioeconomic groups.[77] Transplacental transmission of CMV from mother to infant is typical in congenital infection. A primary maternal infection results in transplacental infection in 30% to 40% of infants, with 10% to 15% of them developing symptomatic infection. The later in the pregnancy the seroconversion occurs, the more likely it will result in neonatal infection: 75% of infants are infected in the third trimester. However, the later in the pregnancy the infection occurs, the less likely the infection will be significant in the infant. Recurrent infections in the mother may also occur as a result either of reactivation or reinfection with a different strain.[78] In either instance, transplacental infection still occurs in 1% of infants, but fewer than 1% of the infections are symptomatic. Polymerase chain reaction (PCR) methodology can detect CMV excretion in breast milk in 70% to 90% of women, particularly when the whey portion is tested, and perinatal transmission occurs to 40% to 60% of infants.[79] Excretion occurs among these infected infants from 3 weeks to 3 months after birth. Also, transmission appears to occur readily among young children, and day care is responsible for transmission rates of over 50%, which most likely reflects contamination from saliva on toys and hands. Seroconversion may be as high as 15% to 45% among parents of children attending day care and 11% among women working in day care centers, so that subsequent pregnancies account for nearly one fourth of symptomatic congenital infections in the United States. In contrast, studies of seroconversion among health care workers do not show any risk of nosocomial transmission greater than the risk of acquiring the infection in the community. Yet nosocomial transmission to the infant may occur in the nursery, most likely via contaminated hands or fomites. Finally, infants may be infected as a result of blood transfusion or exchange transfusion. These cases may be largely prevented by using seronegative donors, leukocyte filtration, or frozen, deglycerolized packed red blood cells.

Nearly 90% of congenital infections are asymptomatic and the infants are neither growth restricted nor premature, although 10% to 15% of them are still at risk of later developmental abnormalities, which appear within the first years of life. Among asymptomatic infants, 7.2% will ultimately have hearing loss.[80] Half of these neonates will have bilateral, progressive disease. This progressive loss, however, may be missed by routine nursery screening. A much lower risk (2%) is that of chorioretinitis, which is also usually delayed in onset. A similar number of children may also develop neurologic abnormalities, including microcephaly, neuromuscular motor defects, and mental retardation, or defects in tooth enamel. Cytomegalic inclusion disease is seen in only 5% to 10% of infected newborns and usually occurs as a result of primary infection in the mother around the time of conception (Table 14-1).[81] Mortality, which may reach 20% to 30%, results from liver failure, bleeding, disseminated intravascular coagulation (DIC), and secondary bacterial infection. Some deaths may occur after the neonatal period as a result of the complications of severe neurologic handicap. One half of symptomatic infants have intrauterine growth restriction and one third are prematurely born. Microcephaly may also be seen in half of the infants, along with intracranial calcifications. Hepatomegaly, and even more frequently splenomegaly, are among the most common findings in newborns. Two thirds of the infants develop jaundice, which often persists and becomes increasingly due to a rise in the direct component, and most infants have some rise in liver enzyme levels. Petechiae and even purpura are found in over half. Thrombocytopenia, due to suppression of the megakaryocytes in the bone marrow, may be severe (one third have platelet counts of <10,000). There may also be a Coombs-negative hemolytic anemia. Diffuse interstitial pneumonitis is rare (<1%) and is more commonly seen in perinatally acquired disease. A peculiar defect of the enamel of the primary teeth may be seen in infants. This yellow, soft enamel wears away early, leaving the teeth susceptible to rampant caries. Male infants may also have inguinal hernias. Both the defect in dental enamel and the hernias appear to be teratogenic in nature. A few infants have manifested necrotizing enterocolitis. Sensorineural hearing loss is found in over one third of the infants and, as in asymptomatic infants, may be unilateral or bilateral, profound, and progressive. Chorioretinitis, optic atrophy, and strabismus may be found

Table 14-1.	Sequelae in Children with Congenital Cytomegalovirus Infection According to Type of Maternal Infection		
	Type of Maternal Infection		
Sequela	Primary % (No.)	Recurrent % (No.)	P value
Sensorineural hearing loss	15 (18/120)	5.4 (3/56)	0.05
Bilateral hearing loss	8.3 (10/120)	0 (0/56)	0.02
Speech threshold >60 dB*	7.5 (9/120)	0 (0/56)	0.03
IQ <70	13.2 (9/68)	0 (0/32)	0.03
Chorioretinitis[†]	6.3 (7/112)	1.9 (1/54)	0.20
Other neurologic sequelae[‡]	6.4 (8/125)	1.6 (1/64)	0.13
Microcephaly	4.8 (6/125)	1.6 (1/64)	0.25
Seizures	4.8 (6/125)	0 (0/64)	0.08
Paresis or paralysis	0.8 (1/125)	0 (0/64)	0.66
Death[§]	2.4 (3/125)	0 (0/64)	0.29
Any sequela	24.8 (31/125)	7.8 (5/64)	0.003

From Fowler K, Stagno S, Pass RF, et al: The outcome of congenital cytomegalovirus infection in relation to maternal antibody status, *N Engl J Med* 326:663, 1992.
*For the ear with better hearing.
[†]Three of the seven children with chorioretinitis (43%) in the primary infection group had visual impairment.
[‡]Four of the eight children (50%) had more than one abnormality.
[§]After the newborn period.

in 22%, and the retinitis is more likely to present at the macula than in adults.[82] The outcome is grim, with 90% of infants developing at least one neurologic abnormality. Although microcephaly is a strong predictor of intellectual impairment, intracranial calcifications on computerized tomographic images indicate a risk as high as 90% and are often accompanied by progressive, severe, bilateral hearing loss, optic atrophy, and neuromuscular abnormalities. Ultrasonography may accurately demonstrate calcifications, but magnetic resonance imaging may provide additional findings, such as polymicrogyri, hippocampal dysplasia, and cerebellar hypoplasia.[83]

A perinatal infection may develop in an infant after passage through the birth canal or from breast milk. In the term infant this is usually asymptomatic with little effect on developmental outcome, although such infants may develop a diffuse interstitial pneumonitis. Few require hospitalization and mortality is low. Among preterm infants there is more risk. Transfusion of packed red blood cells may result in a sepsis-like picture with pneumonia, hepatosplenomegaly, thrombocytopenia, and neutropenia, and the mortality may reach 50%. More recently there has been considerable concern regarding breast feeding of preterm infants by seropositive mothers,[79] but most studies

have indicated little long-term developmental effect in infected infants.

Viral isolation in tissue culture, usually from urine or saliva, remains the most sensitive and specific test for diagnosis in the infant. To differentiate congenital infection in the neonate from perinatal infection, virus must be isolated in the first 2 weeks after birth. With hyperimmune sera or monoclonal antibodies, detection may occur within 24 hours. Because immunoglobulin (Ig) G is transplacentally transferred, its detection is not helpful without paired sera, and the measurement of serum IgM is associated with many false negatives. However, PCR amplification for detection of viral DNA has been found to be extremely sensitive for diagnosis in a large range of tissues and secretions, particularly blood and saliva.[84] A new technique is the use of nested PCR to detect viral DNA in dried blood spots that are obtained for metabolic tests after birth.[85] These blood spots may be used in screening or can be tested later to determine whether symptoms such as hearing loss are a result of congenital infection. Once the blood is dried it is no longer infectious. The samples can be shipped easily and stored for years.

Maternal and prenatal diagnosis is more complicated. The mother is usually asymptomatic, so infection is not suspected clinically. Screening thus becomes more important. The detection of IgG does not define whether the mother has a primary infection or a recurrent one. The same is true of isolation of the virus. IgM responses are variable and may be detected for 16 weeks or longer after infection. An IgG avidity assay, based on the determination that antibody is of low avidity in the first months of infection, is particularly effective as a negative predictor up to 21 weeks of pregnancy, but is less so later. However, the most important factor is whether or not the fetus is infected and whether or not that infection is symptomatic. Cordocentesis for fetal blood testing will miss many infected fetuses. IgM appears only after 20 weeks' gestation and is only detected in half of cases. Viral DNA can be detected but the test has a low sensitivity. The standard assay has now become quantitative PCR on amniotic fluid.[86] Ultrasonographic abnormalities may be associated with, but are not diagnostic of, infection and many are transient. These include microcephaly, intracranial calcifications or cysts, intrauterine growth restriction, oligohydramnios or polyhydramnios, pericardial or pleural effusions, hepatic lesions, and hyperechoic abdominal masses.

Because disease is often present for a prolonged period in the fetus and already has deleterious effects, treatment becomes problematic. Clearly the best treatment is prevention of fetal infection. Vaccines are being explored but are not currently available. Recently, hyperimmune globulin was given to 31 women with primary infections in pregnancy and the infant of only one (3%) had disease at birth, developing handicaps by 2 years of age.[87] In contrast, the rate of disease was 50% among the infants of 14 women who did not receive the hyperimmune globulin. Placental thickness, which increases in primary infection, declined after treatment as well.[88] Passive protection after birth is unlikely to be of benefit. In a randomized, controlled trial of intravenous ganciclovir in 100 infants with central nervous system (CNS) disease, the therapy prevented worsening of hearing loss at 6 months and 1 year of age.[89] Fewer developmental delays at 6 and 12 months of age, as measured by Denver developmental tests, were also seen among infants receiving intravenous ganciclovir therapy than among control infants.[90] Treatment of congenital CMV in infants with CNS disease should be considered but needs to

be initiated in the first month of life, and the infants need to be closely monitored for toxicity, particularly neutropenia.

HERPES SIMPLEX

Neonatal herpes simplex virus (HSV) disease has really only been recognized in the last 70 years. This double-stranded DNA virus consists of a dense viral DNA core surrounded by an icosahedral protein capsid, which is further surrounded by an amorphous layer of proteins and an envelope. The herpesviruses are known for their ability to enter a latent state after the primary infection from which an active recurrence may arise, despite the presence of humoral and cellular immunity. There are two antigenic types: HSV-1 is usually found above the waist, whereas HSV-2 is found below the waist and is the most common source of genital and neonatal herpes. Infections with either type are usually asymptomatic. HSV-1 may cause gingivostomatitis in young children and a sore throat or a mononucleosis-like infection in an adult. As with other herpesviruses, seroprevalence is related to socioeconomic status. More than three quarters of lower socioeconomic populations have antibody to HSV-1 in their first decade, as opposed to only one third of those of upper middle socioeconomic groups. HSV-2 is responsible for 80% of genital infections and is usually transmitted by sexual intercourse; thus it most often appears after the second decade and is found in 20% to 25% of individuals. African Americans have a higher rate of infection than whites. Higher rates are also seen in women, who have an 80% risk of infection after a single contact with an infected male. From 1988 to 1994 in the United States, the prevalence of HSV-2 infection was 21%, which represented a significant increase over prior years. In the most recent surveys, from 1999 to 2004, the seroprevalence of HSV-2 dropped to 17%.[91] Of note, HSV-1 is now responsible for a larger proportion of both genital and neonatal disease. HSV-1 genital infections are less likely to recur than HSV-2 genital infections and are usually less severe. Both HSV-1 and HSV-2 are found worldwide, and the only reservoir is in humans. Infection occurs year round and is not seasonal. Host defenses begin in 7 to 10 days, with humoral immunity appearing 2 to 6 weeks later, although this does not prevent recurrences.

Transmission to the neonate most commonly occurs from exposure of the infant to contaminated maternal secretions in the birth canal at delivery. Maternal infection is classified as primary if it is the initial infection with either HSV-1 or HSV-2 and there are no preexisting antibodies to either type. A recurrent infection occurs in an individual with latent infection, whereas an initial nonprimary infection occurs in an individual with preexisting antibodies to the other HSV type. All three types of infection are likely to be asymptomatic. Many infections believed to be new infections in pregnant women are actually reactivations of previously acquired asymptomatic infections. Infection does not appear to be associated with an increase in spontaneous abortion or premature rupture of membranes. Cervical shedding of virus has been demonstrated in 0.56% of women with symptomatic infections and in 0.66% of women with asymptomatic infections. Frequent cervical cultures have failed to detect which mothers will be shedding virus at the time of delivery. It is important to note that over 75% of infected neonates are born to women who have no history or symptoms of HSV infection, nor do their sexual partners. Acquisition of HSV-1 or HSV-2 occurs in 2% of susceptible pregnant women and is evenly distributed throughout the pregnancy.[92] There is up to a 60% risk of neonatal infection when the mother is shedding virus at the time of delivery secondary to a primary infection.[92] The risk falls to 30% if the mother is shedding virus at delivery due to an initial nonprimary infection and to 2% if the mother is shedding virus due to reactivation of infection acquired either before pregnancy or during an earlier trimester. This is primarily due to the larger quantity and duration of viral shedding from the cervix during a primary infection. However, some protection is afforded by preexisting neutralizing transplacental antibodies, so that the infants at highest risk are the ones who are infected at birth or after birth and who are born before transplacental transfer of antibodies. Type-specific maternal antibody testing may be useful in determining the risk of infection of the neonate.[93] The use of invasive monitoring provides a site for viral entry into the fetus, and this site is often the location of initial lesions. An additional risk factor is rupture of membranes longer than 6 hours before delivery in a mother with active cervical lesions. For this reason, many experts recommended that infants of such mothers be delivered via cesarian section—before rupture of membranes, if possible, but at least before 6 hours after rupture.[93] Cesarian section reduces the risk of fetal infection from 7.7% to 1.2%,[94] but does not eliminate the risk entirely. In the United States it is estimated that infection occurs in 1 in 1500 deliveries, resulting in 2200 infected newborns per year.

Intrauterine infection is rare and may result from either ascending infection from the birth canal or transplacental infection. It may also occur in either primary or recurrent maternal infection. These infants are severely affected and have a combination of skin vesicles and scarring, hydranencephaly or microcephaly, and keratoconjunctivitis. Antiviral therapy is futile.

The third route of transmission is postnatal acquisition. Virus may be obtained by breast feeding from an infected breast or being kissed by a family member who has orolabial herpes, usually HSV-1. Nosocomial infection in the nursery is also possible. Prospective hospital studies have demonstrated that as many as one third of employees have a history of nongenital herpes and that twice that many have asymptomatic shedding. It remains controversial whether individuals with labial lesions should be removed from the nursery. Currently they are asked to use face masks and to perform careful hand washing. Individuals with herpetic whitlow (finger lesions) should not be providing direct patient care.

In stark contrast to the case of congenital infection of the newborn with CMV, another herpesvirus, asymptomatic infections with either HSV-1 or HSV-2 are rare. Neonatal disease has been classified, for purposes of describing outcome, into localized skin, eye, and mouth (SEM) disease; encephalitis with or without skin, eye, or mouth involvement (CNS); and disseminated disease, with or without CNS involvement. The National Institute of Allergy and Infectious Diseases Collaborative Antiviral Study Group reported that 34% of neonates had SEM disease at presentation, 34% had CNS disease, and 32% had disseminated disease.[95] Common presenting signs and symptoms include lethargy, temperature instability, conjunctivitis, pneumonia, hepatitis, and DIC. Skin lesions are the most suggestive of HSV infections, but fewer than 30% of infants ever develop such lesions.

Likewise, seizures, focal or generalized, and encephalitis are very indicative.

Symptoms of SEM disease usually appear at 7 to 10 days of life. The most easily recognized skin lesion is the vesicle, which may progress to clusters of vesicles or join with other vesicles to form bullae. Although limited to the skin at first, the lesions tend to progress to more serious disease; this was particularly true before the advent of acyclovir therapy. They are most commonly found on the head of the infant, especially if there was a scalp monitor, but may also be found on the trunk or extremities. Lesions in the mouth presumably are caused by swallowed contaminated amniotic fluid and maternal secretions. Keratoconjunctivitis, chorioretinitis, and cataracts may also develop. Even with antiviral therapy, infants tend to have recurrent skin lesions over several years and some may develop cataracts. Long-term neurologic impairment has also been seen in these infants, probably due to unrecognized CNS disease. This group may experience quadriplegia, microcephaly, and blindness between 6 and 12 months of age.[95] Before the acyclovir era, 30% of these infants progressed to more invasive disease and had neurologic sequelae. With acyclovir therapy, all infants with HSV-1 infection and 95% of those with HSV-2 SEM disease had normal neurologic examination findings at 12 months of age.[96,97]

Isolated CNS disease in the newborn probably represents retrograde axonal transport of the virus in infants who have acquired transplacental neutralizing antibody, which possibly has not allowed hematogenous spread of the virus.[95] In these infants the infection becomes apparent at a slightly older age, after the first week of life—often in the second or third week, but even as late as 6 weeks of life. Nonspecific signs may include temperature instability, lethargy, irritability, and poor feeding. HSV encephalitis should always be considered in the presence of focal or generalized seizures, especially if they are refractory to treatment; a bulging fontanelle; tremors; pyramidal tract signs; and focal neurologic deficits. Skin lesions or vesicles frequently are not found at presentation. The CSF may be normal initially or show only subtle abnormalities. Many infants will have a bloody tap due to CNS hemorrhage. Most commonly the CSF glucose concentration is low and there is a mononuclear pleocytosis. The protein content may show little elevation at

first but rises significantly over time. Computed tomography may show localized or multifocal areas of hemorrhage, edema, and infarct. An electroencephalogram may also help in determining the extent of disease. Brain stem disease results in the death of half of untreated infants.[96] The prognosis of survivors is poor and includes severe psychomotor retardation, blindness, microcephaly, chorioretinitis, and spasticity. Even with antiviral therapy, only 17.5% of infants infected with HSV-2 and 75% of infants infected with HSV-1 have a normal outcome at one year of age.[97]

Most infants with disseminated HSV disease are born to mothers with primary infection and lack transplacental antibody. The resulting viremia in the infant spreads the disease to all organs, usually in the first week of life but also in the first 24 hours. Adrenal hemorrhage and shock with fulminant hepatitis may be prominent. There may be a sepsis-like picture with metabolic acidosis, respiratory distress, DIC, direct hyperbilirubinemia, thrombocytopenia, neutropenia, elevated hepatic enzyme levels, and seizures. A vesicular rash is usually not present at onset, and one third of infants never develop vesicles. Meningoencephalitis develops in the majority of infants. Others may develop an interstitial or hemorrhagic pneumonia or necrotizing enterocolitis with pneumatosis intestinalis. These infants have the highest mortality—more than 80% if untreated, often secondary to DIC or pneumonia—but survivors may have a better neurologic outcome. Although HSV-1 and HSV-2 infection are clinically indistinguishable in disseminated disease, a normal neurologic outcome is more common after antiviral therapy in infants infected with HSV-2 (41%) than in infants infected with HSV-1 (23%).[97]

It is extremely important to have a high index of suspicion for HSV. Enteroviral sepsis is the major differential. Viral isolation by culture remains the standard. Swab specimens for viral isolation should be taken from all skin lesions, the nasopharynx, urine, stool, and conjunctivae. Isolation of the virus from the skin or nasopharynx in the first 24 hours of life may represent transient contamination from birth, so swab specimens should be taken at 24 hours of life in infants born vaginally to mothers with genital lesions or known shedding. Viral typing is important for prediction of survival and neurologic outcome. Analysis as well as viral culture of the CSF is required. The sensitivity and specificity of PCR for viral antigen in the CSF is high. Skin lesions should also be examined by either immunofluorescence or PCR testing. The evaluation should include an ophthalmologic examination, brain imaging, electroencephalography, and audiologic testing. A complete blood count, measurement of hepatic enzyme levels, blood gas analysis, and coagulation studies should also be performed for these infants.

Intravenous acyclovir is the treatment of choice for newborns. Infants should be isolated to prevent nosocomial spread. Oral therapy is not acceptable. Acyclovir is a competitive inhibitor of HSV DNA polymerase and terminates DNA chain elongation. It is activated by HSV thymidine kinase. All infants with HSV disease should be treated with 60 mg/kg/day acyclovir in three divided doses. Infants with SEM disease may be treated for 14 days, but all infants with either CNS or disseminated disease require 21 days of therapy.[98] PCR assessment of the CSF at the end of treatment of encephalitis or meningitis can be used to determine the need for continued therapy in infants whose PCR results remain positive.[99] Adequate hydration is important to prevent nephrotoxicity. Ocular antiviral therapy should be used in the presence of ophthalmic infection, but topical treatment is not necessary for skin lesions because intravenous acyclovir adequately penetrates these lesions. There is no indication that hyperimmune globulin is of benefit. Acyclovir resistance is rare in the non–human immunodeficiency virus–infected newborn.

As discussed, prognosis depends on both the viral antigen type and the location of the infection (SEM disease only, localized CNS infection, or disseminated disease). Further improvements in outcome will require earlier recognition and treatment of infection, but this has not occurred since acyclovir has become available.[96] Poor prognostic signs at the initiation of therapy include prematurity, coma, DIC, and pneumonitis.[96] There is also an association between the frequency of recurrence of skin lesions and the development of late sequelae. A 6-month trial of oral acyclovir suppression did eliminate the recurrence of skin lesions in 81% of treated infants, whereas only 54% of untreated infants escaped recurrence,[97,100] but whether this will improve the long-term outcome is not known. Serial evaluations should include ophthalmologic

and audiologic assessments in addition to neurodevelopmental testing.

Recurrent skin lesions can also be a source of infection. Exclusion from day care is not necessary, however, if the lesions are covered to prevent direct contact with others.

Reducing transmission of HSV to neonates is the ideal, but most women shed virus asymptomatically. Delivery by cesarian section may be beneficial in the presence of maternal genital lesions or symptoms but is not indicated in the absence of lesions, because the risk of transmission to the exposed infant in recurrent infection is less than 3%. A primary maternal infection during pregnancy should be treated. Valacyclovir is now commonly being administered to pregnant women with a history of recurrent genital HSV, beginning at 36 weeks' gestation. Metaanalysis indicates that treatment reduces the risk of HSV recurrences and viral shedding at delivery and the need for cesarean section.[101] It is not known if this therapy also reduces the incidence of neonatal herpetic disease, and its use may give the clinician a false sense of security.[102] The long-term risk to the fetus, particularly the fetal kidney, is not known, although the acyclovir and valacyclovir pregnancy registry has not shown any increase in the rate of birth defects or change in their pattern in infants born to treated women, compared with those born to the general population of pregnant women. The rise of resistant virus in these treated women is also of concern.

HUMAN IMMUNODEFICIENCY VIRUS INFECTION

In the early 1980s, acquired immunodeficiency syndrome (AIDS) was first described in infants and children. Children younger than 13 years infected with human immunodeficiency virus (HIV) account for fewer than 1% of the total number of infected people in the United States. More than 90% of these cases resulted from vertical transmission from infected mothers. Since 1992, the CDC reports a 90% decrease in new infection in children younger than 13 years of age. Only 166 new cases in this age group were reported in 2005.[103] As will be discussed, this nadir was achieved by improved prenatal screening, management of pregnant mothers, and postpartum prophylaxis.

HIV is an RNA retrovirus of the genus *Lentivirus*. The virus primarily targets CD4$^+$ lymphocytes, where it incorporates itself as a provirus into the host cells' genome and is replicated as part of normal host cell DNA replication. Infection is therefore lifelong. Even with the use of potent combination antiretroviral therapy and reduction in HIV RNA serum levels below detectability, latent virus has been demonstrated in peripheral blood monocytes. In active infection, virus can be isolated from a variety of cells, organs, and bodily fluids; however, epidemiologic studies have only demonstrated infectivity from blood, breast milk, cervical secretions, and semen.

Neonatal infection is generally clinically silent. Infants may have nonspecific physical examination findings of hepatosplenomegaly or lymphadenopathy. Oral candidiasis in a neonate does not arouse suspicion for pathologic T-cell dysfunction. Refractory, recurrent oral candidiasis, encephalopathy, developmental delay, poor growth, chronic diarrhea, and parotitis are relatively common findings in infected infants during the first year of life; again, none of these symptoms is particularly specific for HIV infection. Before the improvement in identification of infected mothers, use of highly active antiretroviral therapy (HAART), and initiation of appropriate postnatal prophylaxis for viral and opportunistic infections, pneumonia caused by *Pneumocystis jiroveci* (formerly *Pneumocystis carinii*) accounted for the majority of AIDS-defining illness in the first year of life, with a peak incidence between ages 3 and 6 months.[104] Many infants, however, do not have AIDS-defining opportunistic infection, but rather may experience recurrent serious bacterial infections, including pneumonia, septic arthritis, bacteremia, or meningitis. Although a single occurrence of these infections does not raise suspicion about immunodeficiency, their recurrence should alert the clinician to evaluate the infant's immune system. In general, the likelihood of serious bacterial infection or opportunistic infection correlates inversely with infants' CD4$^+$ counts; without HAART, these counts begin to decline around 3 months of age.[105]

Diagnosis of HIV infection in infants can be made in several ways. Serologic testing is not diagnostic in a neonate, because a positive result on an enzyme immunoassay may simply reflect maternal serologic status due to passive transplacental transfer of IgG antibody. Antibody tests may yield false-negative results if the mother was infected late in pregnancy and had not yet undergone seroconversion. In infants born to HIV-infected mothers, blood should be sent for either HIV DNA PCR testing or HIV RNA PCR assay during the first 48 hours of life. If results are positive, a second sample should be sent for PCR assay to confirm the diagnosis. Once infection has been established, HIV RNA PCR testing is used to monitor the efficacy of therapy, because this test reports back a quantitative result or viral load in copies per milliliter. There are several ways to rule out infection. A negative result on two PCR samples obtained after 1 month and 4 months of life rules out infection. Two negative antibody test results separated by 1 month obtained after 6 months of life or a single negative antibody test result after 12 to 18 months of life excludes infection.[106]

As noted earlier, interruption of vertical transmission has greatly reduced the number of infected children in the United States. Currently, the CDC recommends universal screening of all pregnant women in the first trimester with repeat testing in the third trimester for women felt to be at high risk of infection. In 1994, the Pediatric AIDS Clinical Trials Group Protocol 076 trial demonstrated a 67% reduction in perinatal HIV transmission with use of a zidovudine regimen for mother and infants.[107]

Numerous subsequent studies have looked at a variety of simple and complex regimens testing different antiretroviral agents, timing, and duration, and have examined their efficacy and side effects in pregnant women and their offspring. The routine use of HAART starting in 1996 has enabled physicians to greatly suppress viral burden in infected patients. Several studies have demonstrated the benefit of viral suppression in mothers in preventing vertical transmission to their infants.[108] The CDC currently recommends that pregnant women receive HAART, containing zidovudine if possible, if they require it for their own health or if they have HIV RNA levels of more than 1000 copies/mL.[109] There is no absolute viral threshold that reduces the risk of transmission to zero, and therefore the CDC urges consideration of this regimen for pregnant women even if they have HIV RNA levels of less than 1000 copies/mL. Several studies have shown that elective cesarean delivery in HIV-infected women who have not received HAART and who have not begun labor or had rupture of membranes reduces the rate of vertical transmission by 50%.[110,111] The role of cesarean section in women receiving HAART who have RNA viral loads of less than 1000 copies/mL is controversial, and therefore cesarean section is not recommended for those women. Breast feeding has been a major vehicle of vertical transmission. Studies estimate that between 15% and 40% of vertical transmission worldwide occurs through breast milk. Since 1985, the CDC has recommended that women with HIV avoid breast feeding if they have access to safe, affordable formula[112]; the World Health Organization made a similar recommendation in 2000.[109]

Any infant born to an infected mother should receive antiretroviral therapy as soon as possible after delivery. Antiretroviral therapy administered beyond 48 hours of life is not likely to impact the rate of vertical transmission. The therapeutic regimen should be determined with the help of a pediatric infectious disease specialist and should take into account the mother's viral load and CD4+ count, mode of delivery, and antiretroviral exposure. Exposed infants generally receive antiviral therapy for 4 to 6 weeks unless infection is confirmed. For all exposed infants chemoprophylaxis against *P. jiroveci,* most commonly trimethoprim-sulfamethoxazole, should be initiated at 4 to 6 weeks of life. Prophylaxis should be continued until HIV infection is excluded. The likelihood of vertical transmission can be reduced to less than 1% with the aggressive use of HAART to reduce maternal viral loads below the limits of detection and the use of neonatal antiretroviral prophylaxis. In the most recent guidelines for testing of pregnant mothers and neonates, the CDC recommends that women in labor whose HIV status is unknown be offered rapid antibody testing. If the results are positive, the woman should be offered antiretroviral therapy and cesarean section without waiting for confirmatory test results.[113] This aggressive approach reflects clinical consensus that the risk of exposing an uninfected mother or child to antiretroviral therapy and/or surgery is outweighed by the ability to prevent vertical transmission of this incurable infection. Infants with documented HIV infection should be evaluated and treated by an experienced pediatric infectious disease physician who can monitor response to therapy as well as medication toxicities. Current guidelines suggest that all children younger than 1 year of age receive HAART regardless of viral load or immune status. *Pneumocystis* prophylaxis should be continued until the infant is 12 months of age and has CD4+ counts appropriate for age. The need for chemoprophylaxis against infection with other opportunistic agents, including *Mycobacterium avium-intracellulare* complex, *Toxoplasma gondii,* and various herpesviruses, will be determined by the patients' CD4+ counts and clinical conditions. A discussion of specific HAART regimens is beyond the scope of this chapter. HAART has dramatically increased the life expectancy of infants and children with HIV infection. In the absence of a cure, HIV-infected children may require lifelong therapy with drugs that have been associated with premature coronary artery disease, insulin resistance, and bone fragility. The personal and societal costs of prolonged HAART therapy emphasize the importance of HIV prevention.

GONOCOCCAL INFECTION

Neisseria gonorrhoeae is frequently asymptomatic in women and may therefore be unknowingly transmitted to neonates. Endocervical screening samples should be sent for mothers in the first trimester of pregnancy, and for women at high risk, a second culture should be performed late in the third trimester. Gonococcal infection, whether or not overt clinical symptoms are present, may cause vaginitis, cervicitis, salpingitis, and pelvic inflammatory disease. These conditions may result in neonatal morbidity and mortality directly by infection of the neonate or indirectly by precipitation of preterm labor with its consequent complications.

The most common manifestation of neonatal infection is ophthalmia neonatorum, a severe bacterial ocular infection. Before the routine use of silver nitrate, tetracycline, or erythromycin topical eye preparations, an infant born to a mother with *N. gonorrhoeae* endocervical infection had approximately a 30% chance of developing ocular disease. A premature infant or an infant born a prolonged period after membrane rupture has an even greater risk of developing infection. Signs of infection typically manifest by 48 to 96 hours of life but may occur within hours. Classically, the infant has bilateral lid edema, chemosis, and purulent drainage. Without treatment the infection can result in permanent corneal damage and panophthalmitis with vision loss.

Rarely, disseminated infection with *N. gonorrhoeae* occurs in neonates secondary to bacteremia. The majority of systemically infected infants in the United States are born to mothers who were inadequately screened and who have asymptomatic infection. The most common presentation of disseminated neonatal *N. gonorrhoeae* infection is pyogenic polyarthritis. The infant may have a pseudoparalysis of the affected limb. Even in disseminated disease, meningitis has rarely been reported. Interestingly, the hallmark skin manifestations of disseminated *N. gonorrhoeae* infection seen in adults are not common in bacteremic infants. Localized cellulitis at breaks in the skin, such as pH probe sites, does occur. In the United States, most systemically infected infants do not have ocular disease because of the universal use of topical prophylaxis. The diagnosis of infection at any site is best made by Gram staining and culture of purulent material on appropriate media.

Prevention of neonatal infection is accomplished through appropriate maternal screening, treatment of infected pregnant mothers, and universal ophthalmic prophylaxis. Pregnant women found to have *N. gonorrhoeae* infection should be treated according to current CDC guidelines. Universal ophthalmic prophylaxis effectively prevents ocular disease in over 95% of infants born to infected mothers; however, as noted, the topical therapy does not prevent systemic illness. Infants born to mothers with known *N. gonorrhoeae* infection should receive standard ocular prophylaxis and a single dose of 125 mg of intravenous or intramuscular ceftriaxone. In preterm or low-birth-weight infants, the dose should be 25 mg to 50 mg/kg with a maximum dose of 125 mg.

For any infant with suspected infection, cultures should be performed on blood and CSF as well as samples from any exudate—ocular, skin abscess, or articular. Most infants should be hospitalized to ensure evaluation and therapy. Gonococcal ophthalmia neonatorum should be treated with a single dose of intravenous or intramuscular ceftriaxone at 25 to 50 mg/kg up to a maximum dose of 125 mg. In addition, infants should receive frequent eye irrigation with saline until the discharge has resolved. Topical therapy alone is insufficient to treat established infection and is unnecessary with systemic therapy. In infants with bacteremia or septic arthritis, ceftriaxone or cefotaxime therapy should be administered for 7 days. If cultures of CSF give positive results, the duration of therapy should be 10 to 14 days.[114]

Any infant with documented gonococcal disease should also be evaluated for other common sexually transmitted diseases: syphilis, *Chlamydia trachomatis* infection, HIV infection, and hepatitis B.

CHLAMYDIA TRACHOMATIS INFECTION

Chlamydia trachomatis is an obligate intracellular bacterium. *C. trachomatis* infection is the most common reportable sexually transmitted disease in the United States. The high prevalence of maternal infection coupled with the lack of efficacy of the topical agents recommended as universal ocular prophylaxis for neonates makes *C. trachomatis* the most common cause of ophthalmia neonatorum. A few of the 18 reported serovars are responsible for the majority of genital infections in women and, consequently, in neonates. Transmission is primarily from infected genital secretions but has been reported in infants born via cesarean section to mothers with intact membranes. Infants born to mothers with untreated infection have a 50% likelihood of acquiring infection, with the nasopharynx being the most frequently colonized site. Once infected, infants have between a 25% and 50% chance of developing conjunctivitis and between a 5% and 20% chance of developing pneumonia.

Conjunctivitis typically appears within a few days to weeks after birth, but the timing of infection cannot reliably distinguish *C. trachomatis* infection from gonococcal disease. The symptoms tend to be similar to, although milder than, those seen in gonococcal disease: lid edema, erythema, and purulent exudate. Treatment results in resolution of symptoms within 1 to 2 weeks without permanent sequelae. No treatment or inadequate therapy can result in symptoms for up to a year with the potential for conjunctival scarring or micropannus formation. Diagnosis is confirmed by culture of cells from conjunctival specimens. The test depends on the collection of epithelial cells, because *C. trachomatis* is an intracellular pathogen. Consultation with the hospital microbiologist or infectious disease expert to determine the most appropriate collection methods and culture media is recommended. Staining will reveal intracytoplasmic inclusion in more than 90% of neonatal ocular specimens with confirmation of *C. trachomatis* infection by species-specific monoclonal antibody staining.

Pneumonia caused by *C. trachomatis* typically presents from the late neonatal period through the first 4 months of life with a mild to moderate respiratory illness characterized by persistent staccato cough, tachypnea, and nasal congestion without fever. Physical examination often demonstrates tachypnea and rales but no wheeze. Half of infants with *C. trachomatis* pneumonia have evidence of conjunctivitis. Classically, chest radiography demonstrates bilateral interstitial infiltrates with hyperinflation. Diagnosis of *C. trachomatis* pneumonia is largely clinical. Although in many affected infants cultures of nasopharyngeal specimens will be positive for the organism, the absence of a positive culture finding in samples from this site does not eliminate the possibility of *C. trachomatis* as the responsible pathogen. Elevation of *C. trachomatis*–specific IgM to a titer of 1:32 or higher is diagnostic, but this assay is not always readily or rapidly available. Interestingly, IgM levels do not typically increase in infected infants with isolated ocular disease.

Infants with chlamydial conjunctivitis should be treated with oral erythromycin base or ethylsuccinate, 50 mg/kg/day divided into four doses for 14 days. Azithromycin and clarithromycin are likely to be effective; however, not enough data exist about the proper dosing and duration of therapy to allow them to be recommended for neonatal ocular disease at this time. Pneumonia may be treated with erythromycin in the same manner as ocular disease or may be treated with azithromycin 20 mg/kg/day for 5 days. Outside of the period immediately after birth, sulfonamides may be used if the infant cannot tolerate erythromycin therapy. Up to 20% of treated infants will require a second course of antibiotics. In infants younger than 6 weeks of age, erythromycin therapy has been associated with hypertrophic pyloric stenosis. The American Academy of Pediatrics continues to recommend that neonates with chlamydial disease be treated with erythromycin pending further studies of other potentially effective agents and further delineation of the association between erythromycin and pyloric stenosis.[115] If neonates are treated with erythromycin, the physician should inform the parents of this association and its warning signs.

Disease prevention targets screening of all pregnant women, with treatment of those infected and documentation of cure. Despite the high likelihood of neonatal infection for infants born to untreated or inadequately treated mothers, the routine use of systemic erythromycin therapy for exposed infants is not recommended given the association with the drug and hypertrophic pyloric stenosis. *C. trachomatis* disease, as discussed, is generally not associated with significant morbidity or mortality. Infants should be observed for clinical signs of infection and treated if such signs are present.

SYPHILIS

After World War II, the number of cases of acquired and, consequently, of congenital syphilis declined steadily until the late 1980s and early 1990s, when an epidemic occurred. This epidemic coincided with an increase in the incidence of HIV infection, crack cocaine use, and the poverty rate. By 1998, aggressive public health measures led to a decline in congenital syphilis cases to the current record low level of fewer than 500 cases per year (Fig. 14-2).[116]

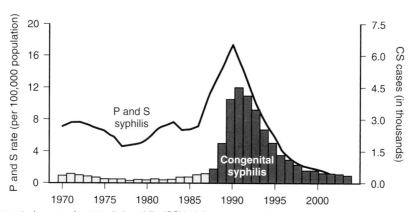

Figure 14-2. Reported cases of congenital syphilis (CS) in infants younger than 1 year of age and rates of primary (P) and secondary (S) syphilis among women in the United States, 1970 to 2004.

The causative organism, *Treponema pallidum*, can cross the placenta at any time during pregnancy and during any stage of maternal disease. Among newly infected women, 40% of pregnancies result in stillbirth, spontaneous abortion, or perinatal death. Women with untreated primary or secondary syphilis have a 60% to 90% chance of transmitting infection to the fetus. Women with early latent and late latent infection have a 40% and 8% chance of transmission, respectively.

By definition, congenital syphilis is a hematogenously spread infection and therefore lacks a primary stage. More than half of infected newborns are asymptomatic at birth. Historically, infection that is detected before a child is 2 years old is referred to as early disease, and infection discovered after 2 years of age is classified as late disease. Early-onset disease typically manifests before an infant is 3 months old.

When symptomatic, infected infants manifest multiorgan involvement consistent with their hematogenously disseminated infection. Neurologic symptoms are usually absent even when the CSF is markedly abnormal. The CSF shows signs of elevated protein or pleocytosis in 50% of symptomatic infants and in up to 10% of asymptomatic infants. Some infants may have pseudoparalysis of an extremity secondary to bony involvement. Long bone radiographs show abnormalities in 95% of symptomatic infants and 20% of asymptomatic infants.[117] The chronic, erosive rhinorrhea of syphilis, "snuffles," is no longer commonly seen. If present, the nasal discharge is highly infectious. Highly symptomatic infants may present with respiratory distress and pulmonary infiltrates referred to as *pneumonia alba*. Nearly all symptomatic infants have hepatomegaly with elevations in serum alkaline phosphatase level. Generalized lymphadenopathy is also common. Many symptomatic infants develop an erythematous, maculopapular rash that becomes coppery and frequently involves their palms and soles. Infants, unlike children and adults with skin involvement, may develop vesicles or bullous lesions, known as *pemphigus syphiliticus*, that tend to rupture and contain numerous infectious organisms. Leukocytosis, anemia, or thrombocytopenia is present in the majority of symptomatic infants.

Late-onset disease presents in children older than 2 years of age. Bony malformations secondary to chronic osteomyelitis include frontal bossing, saber shins, and saddle nose deformity. Dental abnormalities include abnormal molars and notched, small central incisors classically described as *Hutchinson teeth*. Interstitial keratitis presents as unilateral or bilateral photophobia with lacrimation that occurs after the fifth year of life. The symptoms are followed within weeks to months by vascular opacification of the cornea and consequent blindness. Eighth nerve involvement can present at any age with vertigo, progressive hearing loss, and ultimately permanent deafness. The high proportion of asymptomatic infected neonates and the devastating consequences of late-onset disease underscore the importance of screening all women in early pregnancy. All 50 states require serologic testing of women at the beginning of prenatal care.

The definitive diagnosis of syphilis is made by darkfield microscopic identification of spirochetes in exudate or tissue or direct fluorescent antibody testing of such material. These tests can be performed on the placenta or umbilical cord. Unfortunately, neither procedure is particularly sensitive or practical. Serologic screening is generally performed using nontreponemal tests: the rapid plasma reagin (RPR) test and the Venereal Disease Research Laboratory (VDRL) test. These tests detect IgG and IgM to lipoidal antigen from *T. pallidum*. These tests, however, are not specific enough to make a definitive diagnosis. False-positive results can be seen in pregnancy, intravenous drug use, a variety of connective tissue diseases, and viral infection. Nontreponemal antibodies generally appear within 8 weeks of infection and are seen in 100% of patients with secondary or latent syphilis. False-negative results can occur if specimens are drawn too early after infection or if antibody concentrations are extremely high and cause a prozone effect. Titer testing can use serial dilution to provide useful quantitative data about a patient's response to therapy. The same nontreponemal test should be used to follow a patient's titer. The titers typically show a fourfold decrease within 6 months of successful therapy for primary or secondary infection and antibodies are undetectable after a year. Unfortunately, most untreated patients, including those with congenital infection, will become seronegative by nontreponemal testing within 2 years. Only the VDRL test has been approved for detecting spinal fluid infection.

Treponemal tests—the fluorescent treponemal antibody absorption test (FTA-ABS) and the microhemagglutination assay–*Treponema pallidum* (MHA-TP)—are more specific for *T. pallidum* and should be performed to confirm a diagnosis of syphilis in patients with positive results on nontreponemal tests. These tests are qualitative, and results remain positive for life. They are therefore not used to ascertain the treatment status or clinical response of a patient.

An infant born to a mother with a history of syphilis or serologic evidence of syphilis should undergo the same test of nontreponemal antibodies as the mother so that titers can be compared. If the mother's titer has increased fourfold, if the infant's titer is four times higher than the mother's titer, or if the infant has signs or symptoms of infection, further evaluation is warranted. Cord blood is not reliable for serologic diagnosis. Further evaluation should also be initiated if documentation of maternal therapy is unavailable, if insufficient serologic follow-up is available to assess adequacy of therapy, if syphilis during pregnancy was treated with a nonpenicillin regimen,[118] or if syphilis during pregnancy was treated less than 1 month before delivery. In any infant with signs and symptoms of infection, nontreponemal titers four times higher than those of the mother, or positive results on body fluid testing by darkfield microscopy or fluorescent examination, CSF should be sent for VDRL testing, cell count, and measurement of protein concentration. In addition, asymptomatic infants born to inadequately treated mothers should have their CSF examined even if their nontreponemal titers are the same as or less than four times higher than the mother's titer.

Any infant with evidence of infection, positive results on placental or umbilical cord testing by darkfield microscopy or fluorescent technique, a fourfold higher nontreponemal titer than the mother, or positive VDRL results for CSF should be treated with parenteral penicillin G for 10 days. If infection cannot be excluded, the evaluation cannot be completely performed, or follow-up is not ensured, the infant should be treated for 10 days. A negative CSF VDRL result does not exclude congenital neurosyphilis; pleocytosis and elevated protein level should be considered signs of infection. In the case of an asymptomatic infant born to an inadequately treated mother, if physical examination findings, results of laboratory

evaluation including CSF testing, and radiographic findings are normal and appropriate follow-up is expected, some experts would treat with a single intramuscular dose of benzathine penicillin.

The American Academy of Pediatrics recommends that exposed infants undergo nontreponemal serologic follow-up testing at 2 to 4 months, 6 months, and 12 months after treatment or until the titers decline fourfold or are nonreactive. The titers should be nonreactive by 6 months in infants who have been adequately treated or who were uninfected but had transplacentally acquired maternal antibody. Persistently positive titers or increasing titers warrant complete evaluation and 10 days of intravenous penicillin G therapy. Neonates with positive results on VDRL tests of CSF or uninterpretable CSF results should have repeat examinations of their CSF every 6 months until negative.[119]

CASE 1

An infant is born vaginally at 39 weeks to a mother with known gonococcal and chlamydial cervicitis. The mother's HIV status, hepatitis B status, and VDRL status are unknown. The baby receives 0.5% erythromycin ocular ointment and intramuscular vitamin K.

Which of the following is(are) true?

a. The infant has a 30% chance of developing ophthalmia neonatorum from *N. gonorrhoeae* and a 25% chance of developing it from *C. trachomatis*.
b. The infant should receive a 25 to 50 mg/kg dose of intramuscular ceftriaxone.
c. The infant should receive oral erythromycin therapy for 2 weeks.
d. The infant should be given hepatitis B vaccine and hepatitis B immunoglobulin (HBIG) within 12 hours of birth.
The correct answer is *b*.

Standard ocular prophylaxis with 0.5% erythromycin, 1% tetracycline, or 1% silver nitrate is more than 95% effective in preventing gonococcal ophthalmia neonatorum. In the absence of prophylaxis, the neonate would have approximately a 30% likelihood of developing gonococcal disease. This prophylaxis, however, is ineffective in preventing chlamydial disease. Approximately 50% of infants born to mothers with *Chlamydia* infection will have nasopharyngeal infection; half of these infected children will go on to develop ophthalmia neonatorum. Infants born to a mother known to be infected with *N. gonorrhoeae* should receive standard ocular prophylaxis as well as a single dose of intramuscular ceftriaxone at 25 to 50 mg/kg to a maximum dose of 125 mg. This therapy effectively prevents gonococcal ophthalmia neonatorum and disseminated gonococcal disease. *Chlamydia* does not cause disseminated infection. Although 10% of infants born to mothers with chlamydial infection will develop pneumonia, *Chlamydia* does not disseminate or cause acute, vision-threatening ophthalmic disease. The association between neonatal erythromycin exposure and hypertrophic pyloric stenosis combined with the relatively indolent consequences of chlamydial infection preclude the prescription of erythromycin as a prophylactic. In cases of documented chlamydial infection, the benefits of erythromycin outweigh the risks.

Although hepatitis B is readily transmitted vertically, the vaccine is fairly effective in preventing disease. The infant should receive the vaccine within 12 hours of birth while the mother is tested for hepatitis B surface antigen. If she is found to be positive for the antigen, the infant then should receive HBIG. In addition, the mother should be tested for syphilis and HIV infection.

CASE 2

A 3-week-old male infant is brought to the emergency department with vesicular lesions on his thigh and abdomen. The vesicles appear to contain cloudy fluid and are surrounded by an erythematous base. The infant is afebrile and otherwise well appearing.

Which of the following is(are) true?

a. The vesicles should be unroofed to obtain specimens for viral and bacterial culture.
b. The absence of a maternal history of genital HSV infection makes this cause unlikely.
c. Mothers with active, recurrent genital herpes pose the highest risk of vertical transmission.
d. Exudate from the lesions is inadequate to test for HSV.
The correct answers are *a* and *d*.

The differential diagnosis for vesicular lesions includes bacterial impetigo and HSV or varicella-zoster virus infection. If these lesions are prominent in the diaper area, *C. albicans* is also a possibility. Some 60% to 80% of infants with neonatal HSV infection are born to mothers without a clinical history of HSV disease. Although mothers with active, recurrent HSV infection give birth to the majority of infected infants, the risk of transmission to the infant is greatest in a mother with a first-episode primary infection. The latter situation implies a mother without any protective antibodies to HSV. Both culture and antigen testing for HSV rely on the recovery of cells. The base of the vesicle should be scraped for diagnosis.

Gram staining of a sample from a lesion gives a negative result. A direct fluorescent antibody test is positive for HSV-2. Which of the following is(are) true?

a. The infant should undergo lumbar puncture.
b. The infant should be admitted to the hospital for at least 2 weeks of intravenous acyclovir therapy.
c. This patient will likely show an elevation of transaminase levels.
d. If a lumbar puncture is performed and the results are negative, the infant can be managed with oral therapy.
The correct answers are *a*, *b*, and *d*.

Neonatal HSV infection is classically divided into three clinical presentations. The most severe and earliest to present is disseminated disease. This usually manifests in the first week of life with systemic illness and multiorgan involvement, and carries a high mortality. The majority of these patients have significant hepatitis. The next most serious presentation is that of meningoencephalitis. This presentation typically occurs around 3 weeks of age and has clinical manifestations that can be as subtle as fever without a focus or as obvious as severe alterations in mental status and seizures. The gold standard for making this diagnosis has become PCR testing of the CSF. HSV infection is clearly in the differential diagnosis of any neonate with an "aseptic" meningitis. The patient in this case description has the most indolent type of neonatal HSV—SEM disease. The patient should undergo a lumbar puncture, because a positive PCR result on the CSF would have prognostic implications and would extend the duration of therapy. Even if they have a well appearance, if they are not treated systemically, infants with this presentation develop disseminated disease 70% of the time. Acyclovir should be administered intravenously for 2 weeks because of its exceedingly poor oral bioavailability. The dosing and efficacy of newer, more bioavailable antiviral agents for treatment of these infants have not been adequately studied.

CASE 3

The mother of a 42-day-old, 32-week gestation preterm infant asks you about the appropriate timing of immunizations and the need for prophylaxis for respiratory syncytial virus (RSV) infection. The infant currently weighs 2700 g and after going home will continue to receive supplemental oxygen via nasal cannula for chronic lung disease.

Which of the following is(are) true?

a. The infant should receive the same immunizations as any 6-week-old infant.

b. The infant should receive a single 0.25-mL dose of influenza vaccine in January and a second 0.25-mL dose a month later.
c. Whether treatment with monoclonal RSV antibody (palivizumab) is needed in infants such as this 32-week gestation premature infant is controversial.
d. The immunizations should be given when the infant reaches a corrected age of 6 weeks.
   The correct answer is *a.*

Inactivated polio, conjugate pneumococcal, *Haemophilus influenza* B, and DTaP (diphtheria, tetanus, and acellular pertussis) vaccines are all safe and immunogenic in this population. The infant should be immunized as any other infant. If the infant has not already received the first dose hepatitis B vaccine, it would be appropriately given at this point. If an infant weighing less than 2000 g received the first dose of hepatitis B at birth because of maternal risk factors, that dose would not be counted toward the three doses necessary to complete the series. The first counted dose can be given anytime after 4 weeks of age.

Inactivated influenza vaccine should not be administered before 6 months of life. The first time it is to be administered to a child younger than 3 years, the doses would be split up as described in the case description.

Although controversy exists about the need for palivizumab in a healthy infant born after 32 weeks' gestation, consensus exists that infants younger than 2 years of age with chronic lung disease of prematurity who require therapy within 6 months of the start of RSV season should receive antibody prophylaxis for at least the first season.

REFERENCES

The reference list for this chapter can be found online at www.expertconsult.com.

The Heart

Christina M. Phelps, Philip T. Thrush,
and Clifford L. Cua

15

Congenital heart disease is the most common cause of infant death in the United States.[1] In most children, serious heart disease presents during the first month of life. Thus, care for newborns demands an awareness of the prevalence of cardiac defects and the ability to screen appropriately to differentiate infants with cardiac disease from other critically ill newborns. In 2000, the prevalence of congenital heart disease found by a population study in Quebec was 11.89 per 1000 among children and 5.78 per 1000 in the general population. By contrast, the prevalence of severe congenital heart disease was 1.45 per 1000 children and accounted for 12% of all congenital cardiac lesions in children.[2] Advances in fetal and neonatal ultrasonographic screening allow identification of an increasing number of children with congenital heart disease and, more importantly, appropriate counseling for their parents. As many as 60% of newborns admitted to large pediatric cardiac intensive care units have an established diagnosis at the time of birth. Although some studies indicate an important benefit of fetal diagnosis in terms of morbidity and mortality, the unintended result is that in some centers postnatal acute presentations of congenital heart disease are becoming more rare, and this may be detrimental by assuaging fears of congenital heart disease in symptomatic newborns and thus causing delay in care and potentially increased morbidity and mortality. In a large study of neonates in the United Kingdom, up to 25% of children with congenital heart disease were not diagnosed until after discharge from the newborn nursery, and misdiagnosis was found to occur in up to 7 per 100,000 live births in the United States.[3,4]

Careful evaluation of the history, physical examination findings, laboratory data (including the response of upper and lower body blood gas concentrations and arterial oxygen saturation in an enriched oxygen environment), radiographic findings, and results of electrocardiography, echocardiography, and occasionally additional imaging such as cardiac computerized axial tomography (CAT), magnetic resonance imaging (MRI), or invasive cardiac catheterization allows the physician to delineate the specific congenital cardiac defect. When a neonate suspected of having congenital heart disease is being examined, it is important to frame physical and laboratory findings within the context of the transition from fetal to neonatal circulation. This chapter considers the physiology and pathophysiology of the fetal and neonatal cardiovascular systems in newborns with and without heart disease.

PHYSIOLOGY AND PATHOPHYSIOLOGY

FETAL AND PERSOENS NEONATAL CIRCULATIONS

Newborns undergo dramatic changes in the pulmonary and systemic circulations following birth. In the fetus, oxygen-rich blood from the placenta reaches the right atrium via the umbilical vein and shunts preferentially across the foramen ovale to the left ventricle, providing increased oxygen content to the myocardium and brain (Fig. 15-1). A smaller portion of the highly oxygenated blood passes from the right atrium to the right ventricle and bypasses the lungs via the ductus arteriosus to flow to the lower body. Because of this parallel circulation, individual organs may receive blood from both ventricles, and thus the output of the fetal heart is expressed as *combined ventricular output* (CVO). Advances in fetal ultrasonographic techniques have enabled a more accurate determination of human fetal blood flow than was previously available using fetal lamb studies. In the normal human fetus, CVO has been documented by echocardiographic studies to be 450 mL/kg/min.[5]

Approximately 45% (200 mL/kg/min) of this blood perfuses the placenta for oxygen uptake and returns via the umbilical veins. Approximately one half of umbilical venous return enters the inferior vena cava directly through the ductus venosus, thereby bypassing the hepatic microcirculation; the remainder passes primarily through the left lobe of the liver and enters the inferior vena cava via the left hepatic vein. Although venous returns from the lower body, ductus venosus, and hepatic veins all pass into the thoracic inferior vena cava, these streams do not mix completely. There is preferential streaming via the inferior vena cava into various cardiac chambers, with blood from the ductus venosus and left hepatic veins passing preferentially across

the foramen ovale into the left atrium. Oxygenated blood crossing the foramen ovale comprises 76% of the left ventricular output and 33% of combined cardiac output supplying the cerebral and myocardial circulations.[6] Thus, the streaming of blood from the inferior vena cava to the left heart increases the efficiency of oxygen delivery to the most actively metabolizing area of the fetus, the brain. Venous drainage from the right hepatic veins and the abdominal inferior vena cava tends to stream preferentially to the right atrium and right ventricle. Similarly, desaturated superior vena caval return from the cerebral circulation is preferentially directed to the right ventricle through the tricuspid valve. The right ventricle ejects much of this relatively undersaturated blood via the ductus arteriosus back to the placenta. The remainder of the right ventricular output passes into the pulmonary vascular bed. The proportion of CVO to the lungs increases throughout gestation by 60% from 20 to 38 weeks, with pulmonary blood flow accounting for 11% of the CVO.[6,7] Thus, although the circulations are not completely separated, each ventricle primarily performs its postnatal function—the left ventricle delivers blood for oxygen utilization, the right for oxygen uptake.

The left and right ventricles do not eject similar volumes in the fetus. The right ventricle has been shown to be dominant in fetal lamb studies, ejecting almost twice the blood volume ejected by the left ventricle. In human fetuses, the stroke volume of the right ventricle is approximately 28% greater than that of the left ventricle.[5] Left ventricular output is distributed mainly in the upper body, including the brain (approximately 20% of CVO) and the myocardium (3%); the remainder (about 10%) crosses the aortic isthmus to the lower body.

In the fetus, the ductus arteriosus is part of a specialized system of oxygen-sensitive organs and tissues in the body. Blood flow across the ductus arteriosus is 78% of the right ventricular cardiac output and 46% of the CVO.[6] In comparison with the aorta and the pulmonary arteries, it is thicker walled, with a medial layer composed of longitudinal and spiral layers of smooth muscle fibers within concentric layers of elastic tissue and an intimal layer of smooth muscle and endothelial cells.[8-10] Continued patency of the ductus arteriosus throughout gestation is controlled by the relatively low fetal oxygen tension and the inhibition of procontractile

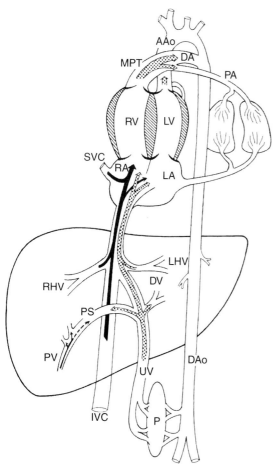

Figure 15-1. Diagrammatic representation of normal fetal circulation. *AAo,* Ascending aorta; *DA,* ductus arteriosus; *DAo,* descending aorta; *DV,* ductus venosus; *IVC,* inferior vena cava; *LA,* left atrium; *LHV,* left hepatic vein; *LV,* left ventricle; *MPT,* main pulmonary trunk; *P,* placenta; *PA,* pulmonary artery; *PS,* portal system; *PV,* portal vein; *RA,* right atrium; *RHV,* right hepatic vein; *RV,* right ventricle; *SVC,* superior vena cava; *UV,* umbilical vein.

mechanisms by vasodilators.[11,12] The vasodilators primarily responsible for ductal patency include prostaglandin and prostacyclin, which interact directly with ductal prostanoid receptors, and to a lesser extent carbon monoxide and nitric oxide.[13,14]

Fetal Echocardiography

The increased availability and use of fetal echocardiography has significant clinical implications postnatally. All echocardiographic techniques (see the later section on echocardiography of the newborn) can be used to produce a fetal echocardiogram. A fetal study is usually performed between 18 and 22 weeks' gestation for optimal imaging. Studies can be carried out earlier in gestation but may need to be repeated to clarify the diagnosis or follow disease progression. A fetal study can be prompted by either maternal or fetal indications (Box 15-1).[15]

Not only can fetal echocardiography be used to diagnose cardiac anatomic defects, but analysis of fetal blood flow patterns in the ductus venosus, umbilical artery, and umbilical vein can provide information on the overall cardiovascular well-being of the fetus.[16] Fetal echocardiography may also have prognostic implications in infants

with congenital diaphragmatic hernia and twin-twin transfusion syndrome (TITS).[17-20] From a cardiac standpoint, fetal echocardiography can accurately diagnose most forms of congenital heart defects and track their evolution in utero (Fig. 15-2). This may improve postnatal morbidity and mortality, especially in newborns with ductal-dependent cardiac defects.[21,22] The level of parental psychological stress, however, appears to be related to the severity of the cardiac defect and not to a prenatal versus postnatal diagnosis.[23] Another recent use of fetal echocardiography is in conjunction with interventional techniques.[24] Interventions have been reported in fetuses with hypoplastic left heart syndrome and restrictive atrial septa,[25] severe aortic stenosis,[26,27] and pulmonary stenosis or atresia.[28] Fetal echocardiography is essential for assisting in these procedures.

Fetal Heart Failure

The parallel nature of the fetal circulation makes it uniquely equipped to tolerate most structural abnormalities of the heart that are life threatening after birth. Even in cases of significant obstruction and falling unilateral ventricular output, the unaffected side of the heart is able to increase its output and fetal blood flow is redistributed so that the unaffected ventricle can produce most, if not all, of the cardiac output.[29] As a result, cardiac shunts, pulmonary overcirculation, and anatomic causes of systemic hypoperfusion generally do not become noteworthy until the infant is born. There are a limited

Box 15-1.	Indications for Fetal Echocardiography
Maternal indications	**Fetal indications**
Family history of congenital heart disease	Abnormal obstetrical ultrasound screen
Metabolic disorders	Extracardiac abnormality
Exposure to teratogens	Chromosomal abnormality
Exposure to prostaglandin synthase inhibitors	Arrhythmia
	Hydrops
Rubella infection	Increased first-trimester nuchal translucency
Autoimmune disease (systemic lupus erythematosus, Sjögren syndrome, etc.)	
	Multiple gestation and suspicion of twin-twin transfusion syndrome
Familial inherited disorders (Marfan syndrome, Noonan syndrome, etc.)	
In vitro fertilization	

From Rychik J, Ayres N, Cuneo B, et al: American Society of Echocardiography guidelines and standards for performance of the fetal echocardiogram, J Am Soc Echocardiogr 17:803, 2004.

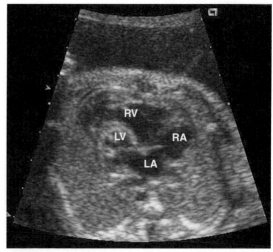

Figure 15-2. Fetal echocardiogram of an infant with a hypoplastic left heart. *LA,* Left atrium; *LV,* left ventricle; *RA,* right atrium; *RV,* right ventricle.

number of cardiovascular causes of fetal distress that may result in the development of hydrops, including arrhythmias, myocardial disease, severe atrioventricular (AV) or semilunar valve insufficiency, and premature constriction of the ductus arteriosus with a restrictive atrial septum. All of these conditions share a final common pathway of elevated ventricular end-diastolic pressure, increased atrial and central venous pressure, and movement of fluid from the capillary bed into fetal tissue.[29]

Sustained tachyarrhythmias (over 200 beats per minute) or bradycardia associated with congenital heart disease are not well tolerated. Tachyarrhythmias may be controlled by administering antiarrhythmic medications to the mother, including digoxin, β-blockers, sotalol, flecainide, and amiodarone. Digoxin is a first-line therapy for short ventriculoatrial supraventricular tachycardia and atrial flutter in the absence of hydrops and is associated with an 80% to 85% success rate in the treatment of fetal supraventricular tachycardia and a 60% to 65% success rate for atrial flutter.[30] Sotalol is another first-line therapy with a 72% conversion rate.[31] Arrhythmia control is likely to be successful if treatment is initiated before the development of hydrops. Successful treatment of supraventricular tachyarrhythmias in the presence of hydrops is more complex and typically requires the use of at least two medications and a longer therapeutic course. Incessant fetal supraventricular tachycardia warrants an attempt at conversion with intraumbilical administration of antiarrhythmic medications. Even with successful treatment, there is an 8% to 30% reported risk of fetal or neonatal mortality.[32-35]

Fetal bradycardia may be associated with significant intrauterine mortality. AV block is caused by maternal autoantibodies in approximately 45% to 48% of cases and can present as early as 18 weeks' gestation.[36,37] There have been reports of successful treatment of early low-grade heart block, with improvement in outcomes, by administration of fluorinated steroids to the mother.[37,38] β-Sympathomimetic agents, intravenous immunoglobulins, and direct fetal pacing are also being used as therapies for autoimmune-mediated fetal AV heart block. Another 45% to 48% of fetal AV block is associated with structural heart disease (most commonly left atrial isomerism and congenitally corrected transposition of the great arteries). Unfortunately, even with aggressive intervention, survival of infants with AV block associated with structural heart disease is particularly dismal, with a 75% to 90% incidence of fetal or neonatal demise.[36]

Structural heart disease is the most common cause of fetal heart failure and may lead to significant mortality without intervention. Some fetuses with severe semilunar valve stenosis are candidates for an attempt at intrauterine valvuloplasty to stabilize the patient's condition and ideally improve long-term surgical options.[26,27] Early delivery with immediate intervention is often the best management strategy for fetuses who show symptoms associated with specific structural heart defects such as ductus arteriosus restriction, Ebstein anomaly of the tricuspid valve, or tricuspid valve dysplasia with significant tricuspid insufficiency.[36]

Circulatory Changes After Birth

By the end of the third trimester, the fetal pulmonary circulation begins to demonstrate vasoreactivity and responsiveness to maternal hyperoxygenation.[39] The onset of breathing produces a dramatic increase in pulmonary blood flow (from 11% of the CVO to a full cardiac output) and a decrease in pulmonary vascular resistance. With the onset of ventilation, air replaces intraalveolar fluid and local oxygen concentration increases markedly, both of which may directly dilate the pulmonary vascular smooth muscle or cause the release of vasodilating substances. Bradykinin, a potent pulmonary vasodilator, is released when the lungs are exposed to oxygen; bradykinin, in turn, stimulates endothelial cell production of nitric oxide, a potent vasodilator. Prostacyclin (prostaglandin I_2), a pulmonary vasodilator derived from the metabolism of arachidonic acid, is released when the lung is mechanically ventilated (not necessarily oxygenated) or exposed to other vasoactive substances such as bradykinin or angiotensin II. Inhibiting prostaglandin production by administering a cyclooxygenase inhibitor (such as indomethacin) attenuates the normal ventilation-induced decline in pulmonary vascular resistance, which further supports the role of these vasoactive substances in the establishment of a normal pulmonary circulation after birth. The increase in pulmonary blood flow greatly alters the venous return to the left atrium and consequently the left ventricular preload. Left ventricular cardiac output increases from an estimated 179 mL/min/kg to approximately 240 mL/min/kg within the first 2 hours after birth due to increased stroke volume.[40] As the ductus arteriosus closes and the left-to-right shunt diminishes, left ventricular output falls to approximately 190 mL/min/kg.[40]

The initial dramatic decrease in pulmonary vascular resistance is secondary to relaxation of the resistance vessels. There is then a slow, progressive decline over the next 2 to 6 weeks of life as these pulmonary arterioles remodel from their fetal pattern, in which a large amount of smooth muscle is present in the medial layer, to the adult pattern, with very little muscle in the media. The development of the "physiologic anemia" that normally occurs during this time decreases the viscosity of the blood perfusing the lungs, which decreases shear stress and also contributes to the overall decrease in pulmonary vascular resistance.

Closure of the Foramen Ovale

Functional closure of the foramen ovale occurs after the placenta is removed from the circulation. With clamping of the umbilical cord, blood flow through the inferior vena cava to both atria decreases dramatically. Initiation of breathing increases blood flow through the pulmonary bed to the left atrium. These changes result in a left atrial pressure that now exceeds the right atrial pressure, which causes the valvelike flap of the foramen ovale to close. Although functional closure of the foramen ovale occurs in most infants, anatomic closure is not always complete. As a result any action that raises right atrial pressure to the point that it equals or exceeds left atrial pressure can result in a right-to-left shunt across the foramen ovale. Likewise, in conditions that have large left-to-right shunts, such as a large patent ductus arteriosus (PDA) or ventricular septal defect (VSD), the left atrium may become dilated, which results in stretching of the atrial septum and incompetence of the foramen ovale and a left-to-right shunt. In many adults, despite the events leading to functional foramen closure, a probe-patent foramen may persist.

Closure of the Ductus Arteriosus

Closure of the ductus arteriosus is a more complex phenomenon. The media of the ductus arteriosus contains smooth muscle in a spiral configuration that is maintained in a relaxed state, primarily by the action of prostaglandins. Constriction and closure after birth reflect removal of the stimuli that maintain relaxation and the addition of factors that produce active constriction. Circulating prostaglandin E_2 (PGE_2) concentrations in the fetus are high because of the very low pulmonary blood flow. With clamping of the placenta, the source of prostaglandin E_2 is removed. With inspiration, there is a dramatic increase in pulmonary blood flow and an abrupt increase in oxygen tension that inhibits ductal smooth muscle voltage-dependent potassium channels and results in an influx of calcium and ductal constriction.[12] In addition, the remaining prostaglandin E_2 (is almost completely metabolized as it passes through the pulmonary circulation, which results in a rapid decrease in serum levels of prostaglandin E_2 and allows active constriction of the ductus arteriosus to be unopposed. The ductus arteriosus constricts rapidly; in mature infants, functional closure generally occurs within 10 to 15 hours after birth. Permanent closure by intimal cushion formation, intimal proliferation, fibrosis, and thrombosis may take several weeks.[41]

MYOCARDIAL PERFORMANCE AND CARDIAC OUTPUT

Fetal myocardium differs from neonatal and adult myocardium in several important ways. The primary fuel for fetal myocardium is almost exclusively glucose in contrast to the adult heart, which can use fatty acids as a significant energy source. In addition, especially early in gestation, the fetal heart grows by hyperplasia of the myocardial cells in contrast with the newborn heart, in which the myocardium grows by hypertrophy. Fetal myocardium also functions distinctly by developing less active tension for a given stretch than does adult myocardium and therefore has less ability to contract. Thus, ventricular output can be increased only modestly by volume loading and only at relatively low atrial pressures; unlike in the adult, output increases only slightly at levels more than 2 to 4 mm Hg above baseline. Inotropic stimulation of the fetal myocardium also increases cardiac output relatively little. This inability to respond to changes in preload and in the inotropic state is related in part to immaturity of muscle structure. Early in gestation, there are relatively fewer contractile elements, an immature sarcoplasmic reticulum with lower affinity for calcium binding and a some what chaotic overall arrangement of fibers with considerable interstitial tissue. Toward term, more contractile elements are present, and these are more mature and are arranged in a more orderly fashion. Another factor limiting fetal myocardial performance is incomplete sympathetic innervation, which limits response to inotropic stimulation. The fetus is best able to increase ventricular output by increasing its heart rate. There is a linear relationship between ventricular output and heart rate up to about 250 beats per minute; thereafter, ventricular output reaches a plateau and even starts to decline. As heart rate goes below the normal range, ventricular output decreases dramatically because of the limited ability to increase stroke volume. As a result the fetal myocardium is operating under a high-volume load and responds poorly to any increase in ventricular afterload. Although adrenergic support can be supplied either by circulating catecholamines or through neural pathways, the overall quantitative response may be less than in the adult. The control of cardiac rate and the distribution of cardiac output are the major mechanisms for maintenance of circulatory function.

As discussed previously, the left ventricular cardiac output increases dramatically within the first 2 hours after birth and remains elevated for several weeks before decreasing to approximately 190 mL/min/kg.[40] Because of the high resting values in the period immediately after birth, ventricular output can be increased only modestly by volume loading or inotropic stimulation with dopamine and dobutamine. The neonatal myocardium remains sensitive to the administration of the calcium ion and responds positively to the lusitropic effects of milrinone. After the initial newborn period, resting values decrease progressively, and ventricular output can be increased much more effectively.

Normal Physiologic Data in the Newborn

The normal physiologic values in the heart and great vessels are shown in Figure 15-3. Pulmonary arterial pressures in the newborn are variable but generally decrease to half of systemic pressure within 8 to 12 hours and to one third of systemic pressure within a day or so. Over the next 4 weeks, there is a further slow, progressive decline to adult levels.

The oxygen saturation on the right side of the heart is approximately 60% to 70%;

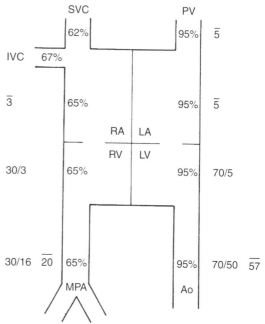

Figure 15-3. Representative blood oxygen saturation (%) and pressure (mm Hg) in various cardiac chambers and vessels in the normal newborn infant. *Ao,* Aorta; *IVC,* inferior vena cava; *LA,* left atrium; *LV,* left ventricle; *MPA,* main pulmonary artery; *PV,* pulmonary vein; *RA,* right atrium; *RV,* right ventricle; *SVC,* superior vena cava.

that on the left side of the heart is 92% to 95%. The oxygen saturations may be used to determine the direction of shunting within the heart or great vessels. For example, an increased saturation in the right atrium suggests a left-to-right shunt at the atrial level; a decreased saturation in the left atrium in a neonate with otherwise healthy lungs indicates a right-to-left shunt at the atrial level.

Physical Factors That Control Blood Flow

Flow (*Q*) through a vascular bed is governed by the resistance to flow (*R*) and the pressure decrease across the bed (*ΔP*) (Ohm's law).

$$Q = \frac{\Delta P}{R}$$

Furthermore, by application of Poiseuille's law, resistance to flow is directly related to the viscosity of the blood and inversely related to the cross-sectional area of the bed (radius).

An appreciation of the general relationship of pressure, resistance, and flow is important in understanding the pathophysiology and natural history of various congenital heart defects.

Blood flows where resistance is least.

Vascular resistance is calculated from the formula

$$Q = \frac{\Delta P}{R}$$

For the systemic circulation, the ΔP (pressure decrease) is systemic arterial pressure (SAP) minus systemic venous pressure (SVP); for the pulmonary circulation, the ΔP is pulmonary arterial pressure (PAP) minus pulmonary venous pressure (PVP).

$$\text{Pulmonary vascular resistance (PVR)} = \frac{\text{PAP} - \text{PVP}}{\text{Pulmonary flow}}$$

$$\text{Systemic vascular resistance (SVR)} = \frac{\text{SAP} - \text{SVP}}{\text{Systemic flow}}$$

If the pressure decrease is measured in millimeters of mercury and the flow is measured in liters per minute per square meter, then the calculated vascular resistance is considered in *resistance units*. One resistance (or Wood) unit is equal to 80 dyne • sec/cm^5. The maximum normal PVR is 2.5 to 3 units, and the maximum normal SVR is 15 to 20 units.

Peripheral vascular resistance is not the only type of resistance that will affect flow. For example, a narrowed valve provides more resistance to blood flow than does a wide open valve; a small VSD provides more resistance to blood flow than does a large VSD; and a thick, noncompliant ventricular chamber provides more resistance to blood flow than does a thinner, more compliant ventricular chamber.

If two similar cardiac chambers or arteries (one left-sided or systemic and the other right-sided or pulmonary) communicate with each other and the opening between them is so large that there is little or no resistance to blood flow, the defect is considered *nonrestrictive*. The pressures on each side of the opening are fully transmitted and approximately equal. If the opening is small (*restrictive*), there is resistance to blood flow, and the pressures are not fully transmitted. In the presence of a nonrestrictive defect, the resistances to outflow (downstream resistance) from each of the two communicating chambers determine the direction of blood flow. For example, with a large VSD in which ventricular pressures are equal, pulmonary vascular resistance is usually lower than systemic vascular resistance, and pulmonary blood flow is greater than systemic blood flow; that is, a left-to-right

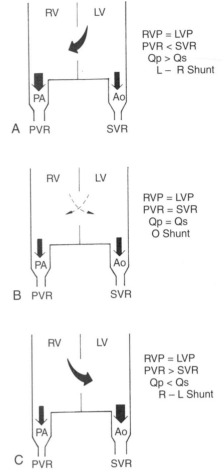

Figure 15-4. Diagrammatic representation of intracardiac shunting patterns as related to outflow resistances of the two sides of the heart. *Ao,* Aorta; *L,* left; *LV,* left ventricle; *LVP,* left ventricular pressure; *PA,* pulmonary artery; *PVR,* pulmonary vascular resistance; *Qp,* pulmonary blood flow; *Qs,* systemic blood flow; *R,* right; *RV,* right ventricle; *RVP,* right ventricular pressure; *SVR,* systemic vascular resistance.

shunt is present (Fig. 15-4, *A*). Because the flows and shunting pattern depend on the relationship of the downstream pulmonary and systemic vascular resistances, these are called *dependent shunts*. When the two resistances are equal, no shunt occurs (see Fig. 15-4, *B*). When resistance to outflow of the right ventricle exceeds that of the left ventricle (see Fig. 15-4, *C*)—as might occur with the development of pulmonary vascular disease or, more commonly, when there is an associated pulmonic stenosis (tetralogy of Fallot)—right-to-left shunting is present. When there is a communication between the two sides of the heart at different anatomic levels (e.g., arteriovenous malformation, left ventricular–right atrial communication), the pressure difference between the two chambers or vessels, rather than down-stream resistance, dictates the magnitude of the shunt; these are called *obligatory shunts*. For example, in a left ventricular–right atrial shunt, blood shunts continuously through the defect because the left ventricular pressure is always higher than right atrial pressure, regardless of the distal pulmonary and systemic vascular resistances.

It is customary to relate the cardiac outputs and pressures in each side of the heart. Thus, if there is three times as much flow into the pulmonary artery as into the aorta, there is a 3 to 1 pulmonary-to-systemic flow ratio. If the pressure in the pulmonary artery is 60 mm Hg and that in the aorta is 90 mm Hg, pulmonary hypertension is at two thirds of the systemic level.

PHYSICAL EXAMINATION

It is imperative to perform a complete physical examination of all neonates and to monitor for ongoing changes suggestive of pathologic conditions. Some studies have begun to advocate using pulse oximetry to screen all newborns. In 2009 the American Academy of Pediatrics and the American Heart Association issued a scientific statement regarding the usefulness of pulse oximetry in clinical practice. The statement authors concluded that additional studies were needed before the use of pulse oximetry in all newborns could be recommended as a standard of care.[42] In an infant who is not transitioning in a normal fashion, however, pulse oximetry may be used in concert with physical examination findings to suggest the need for supplementary testing.

The neonate with congenital heart disease must be differentiated from infants with other acute illnesses. Likewise, an infant with known heart disease remains susceptible to other disease processes, including bacterial sepsis, anemia, and pulmonary disease. Acutely ill infants may have several simultaneous working diagnoses while caregivers are stabilizing their physiologic condition. In these instances, some additional factors may suggest cardiac abnormalities. Dysmorphic or syndromic features in any neonate should prompt the clinician to pay particular attention to the cardiovascular system as the infant transitions to postnatal life.

CYANOSIS

Central cyanosis indicates a reduced arterial blood oxygen saturation and is generally visible when reduced hemoglobin in the blood exceeds 5 g/dL (saturation equal to or below 85% in patients with a normal hemoglobin level). If the lungs are functioning normally, the level of systemic arterial blood oxygen saturation depends entirely on the effective pulmonary blood flow—that is, the amount of blood oxygenated by the lungs that subsequently passes into the systemic arterial circulation. Neonates frequently experience acrocyanosis that is unrelated to heart disease. The best method of assessing for central cyanosis in an infant is to look at the tongue. Other diagnostic procedures are needed to determine the cause of the cyanosis. Comparing arterial blood oxygen saturation or Po_2 above and below the ductus arteriosus may be beneficial. In addition, the "hyperoxia" test, or ventilation with a high inspired oxygen concentration, is frequently considered a valuable diagnostic tool. An increase of more than 50 mm Hg (and often much higher) in systemic arterial Po_2 is seen in infants with primary pulmonary problems (especially because high levels of oxygen tend to dilate the pulmonary arterioles and decrease the pulmonary arterial pressures). A Pao_2 of less than 100 mm Hg in an enriched oxygen environment indicates congenital heart disease until proven otherwise and should prompt an echocardiographic examination and the initiation of prostaglandin E_2 therapy. Frequently the practicalities adhere less to the textbook: a significant increase in systemic arterial blood oxygen tension or saturation can occur in cyanotic heart disease as long as effective pulmonary blood flow is reasonable. Therefore, a Pao_2 of 100 to 250 mm Hg may be suggestive of congenital heart disease and warrants additional investigation. A Pao_2 above 250 mm Hg makes life-threatening cyanotic heart disease less likely. If a hyperoxia test is performed, direct oxygen measurements should be made simultaneously in the upper and lower body to exaggerate any potential difference and thus help to delineate the presence of a right-to-left ductal shunt. The measurement of upper and lower body saturation during crying can also help to exaggerate potential differences due to ductal shunting.

RESPIRATORY DISTRESS

Most infants with mild arterial oxygen desaturation are tachypneic because of chemoreceptor stimulation but show little or no respiratory distress. Congenital heart disease that presents with respiratory distress is very difficult to diagnose in infants: their symptoms are usually more insidious and less dramatic than cyanosis, the differential diagnosis is broader, and the yield of heart disease is much less, which lowers one's index of suspicion. When a physician sees a newborn lying in a crib, blue and comfortable, the diagnosis is almost always cardiac disease; when the infant is acyanotic, tachypneic, and showing retractions, it is usually not. Infants with respiratory distress usually have modest degrees of systemic blood oxygen desaturation, depending on the type of circulatory derangement and the severity of pulmonary edema. The respiratory distress is related to decreased lung compliance in these patients, and interstitial fluid is usually present. Thus, even with a normal separation of circulations, some degree of hypoxemia is present.

CARDIAC EXAMINATION

Palpation

The cardiac impulse should be palpated. Obvious cardiac malposition in the right chest should be documented and warrants additional evaluation. The right ventricular impulse is dominant in a newborn.

Auscultation

Heart sounds in most newborns with significant congenital heart disease are abnormal. The rapid heart rates of most neonates can make this determination difficult even for the experienced practitioner. Multiple studies have assessed the skill of pediatric cardiologists and general pediatricians in detecting heart disease in inpatient neonatal settings and have found sensitivity rates of 80% to 83% for congenital heart disease.[43-45] A single second sound after the first 12 hours may indicate pulmonary atresia or transposition of the great arteries. The presence of a pulmonary systolic ejection click may be normal in the first hours, but after that any systolic ejection click is abnormal, indicating an abnormal pulmonary or aortic valve, an enlarged pulmonary artery or aorta, or truncus arteriosus. If the infant has pulmonary disease without congenital heart disease and has a narrowly split or single second sound, then a high pulmonary vascular resistance is expected. Although systolic murmurs are more easily distinguished than the first and second heart sounds, they are common during the neonatal period and have historically been reported in up to 60% of healthy newborns.[46] Several recent studies have demonstrated a higher incidence of congenital heart disease in infants with murmurs in the neonatal period. In a study of 7204 consecutively examined newborn infants, fewer than 1% of the neonates were found to have cardiac murmurs. All neonates with cardiac murmurs were referred for echocardiography, and an underlying cardiac malformation was diagnosed in 54% of them.[47] A retrospective review of 20,323 live births over a 3-year period in a hospital in Israel found 170 newborns with an isolated finding of a heart murmur who were referred for echocardiography. Of those infants, 147 (86%) were found to have structural heart defects, including isolated VSD (37%), PDA (23%), and combined VSD and PDA (7%); abnormalities creating left-to-right shunts comprised 66% of the diagnoses.[48] Thus, although any murmur noted in the neonatal period should prompt the practitioner to be suspicious of congenital heart disease, certain murmurs are nearly diagnostic. An S_4 gallop is always abnormal.

ABDOMINAL EXAMINATION

Hepatomegaly is a nonspecific finding that may be indicative of increased central venous pressures. It can be associated with cardiac lesions that volume-load the right side of the heart (such as a systemic arteriovenous malformation, anomalous pulmonary venous return, or right-sided valve insufficiency as seen with Ebstein anomaly and absent pulmonary valve syndrome). Hepatomegaly may also be associated with low-output states such as myocarditis, cardiomyopathy, and tachyarrhythmias.

PERIPHERAL EXAMINATION

It is imperative to palpate femoral and radial pulses in all newborns. Bounding pulses are typically associated with a widened pulse pressure and may be found in congenital abnormalities with increased diastolic pulmonary blood flow. Diminished femoral pulses or brachial-femoral delay may be associated with coarctation of the aorta, hypoplastic left heart syndrome, or an interrupted aortic arch. Inability to palpate pulses in all extremities should prompt the examiner to palpate the right carotid or temporal artery. If these pulses remain intact, the diagnosis would include an aberrant subclavian artery in addition to aortic arch obstruction. If all pulses are severely diminished, the obstruction to blood flow is at the aortic valve or within the left ventricle. Diminished femoral pulses should prompt the clinician to initiate therapy with prostaglandin infusion while awaiting confirmatory imaging or transfer to another center.

IMAGING OF THE NEONATE

Accurately diagnosing the anatomy and physiology of the cardiac defect is a cornerstone of pediatric cardiology. To accomplish these goals, multiple imaging modalities are available. Currently, the most frequently used techniques for imaging the newborn are echocardiography, CAT scans, MRI, and cardiac catheterization. The decision to perform one or more of these studies will depend on the history, clinical examination findings, and clinical course of the patient. With the use of these imaging techniques, a complete assessment of the cardiac defect can be obtained to aid in achieving an optimal outcome.

ECHOCARDIOGRAPHY

Echocardiography remains the main imaging technique in pediatric cardiology.[6] An echocardiogram is likely the first and possibly the only cardiac image that will be obtained to rule in or rule out a cardiac abnormality (Box 15-2). Most clinical and surgical decisions can be made purely from the echocardiographic examination. Advantages of echocardiography include its portability, noninvasive nature, provision of real-time information, and overall ease of use. Disadvantages of echocardiography include limitations in image quality in some clinical circumstances and only fair ability to accurately diagnose certain complicated extracardiac vascular anomalies.

Echocardiography is the application of ultrasound to obtain an image via reflected sound waves. Higher-frequency probes, usually 5 MHz or higher, are used in the newborn since minimal penetration of the sound wave into the patient is needed and the shorter wavelengths allow clearer resolution of the images. Scatter of the ultrasonic wave, which inhibits image quality, usually occurs between interfaces of material that have different densities. Bone and air, when adjacent to soft tissue or fluid, produce significant artifacts, whereas soft tissue next to fluid produces minimal artifacts. For this reason, clinical conditions such as pneumothorax or bronchopulmonary dysplasia may reduce image quality.

A complete and standardized approach is needed for the initial echocardiographic evaluation of the neonate. In the usual examination the probe is placed just to the left of the sternum to obtain parasternal long (Fig. 15-5) and short axial images (Fig. 15-6), at the apex of the heart to obtain an apical four-chamber view (Fig. 15-7), under the xiphoid process to obtain subcostal coronal (Fig. 15-8) and sagittal images (Fig. 15-9), and in the suprasternal notch to obtain suprasternal long (Fig. 15-10) and short axial views (Fig. 15-11). More views may be obtained depending on the complexity of the anatomy. If the heart is displaced as in the case of dextrocardia or congenital diaphragmatic hernia, adjustments of probe position are required. Numerous sweeps with application of M-mode, two-dimensional analysis, Doppler, and color Doppler allow for an inclusive examination that will give anatomic, physiologic, and functional data. For a complete review the reader is referred to recent textbooks on echocardiography in pediatric heart disease.[49,50]

Box 15-2.	**Indications for Initial Echocardiographic Examination of the Neonate**

Syndromes
Trisomy 13
Trisomy 18
Trisomy 21
CHARGE association
VACTERL association
DiGeorge syndrome
Noonan syndrome
Turner syndrome
William syndrome

Nonsyndromes
Congenital diaphragmatic hernia
Omphalocele
Midline abnormality workup
Tracheoesophageal fistula

Other
Unexplained hypoxemia
Abnormal findings on cardiac examination
Perinatal asphyxia
Persistently positive blood culture results
Genetic abnormalities not otherwise specified

CHARGE, Coloboma of the eye, heart disease, atresia choanae mental retardation, genital anomalies, ear anomalies; VACTERL, vertebral anomalies, anal atresia, cardiac anomalies, tracheoesophageal fistula, renal anomalies, limb anomalies.

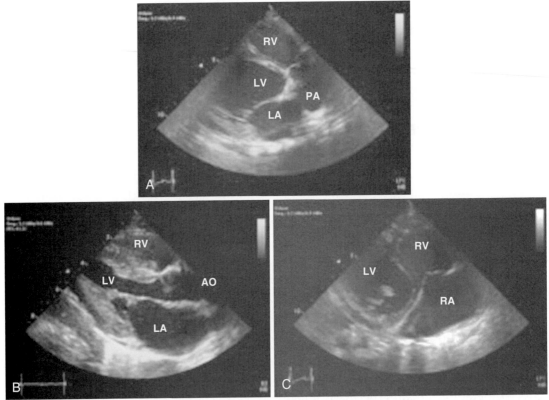

Figure 15-5. Echocardiogram in the parasternal long axis view sweeping anterior **(A)** to posterior **(C)** through the heart. *Ao,* Aorta; *LA,* left atrium; *LV,* left ventricle; *PA,* pulmonary artery; *RA,* right atrium; *RV,* right ventricle.

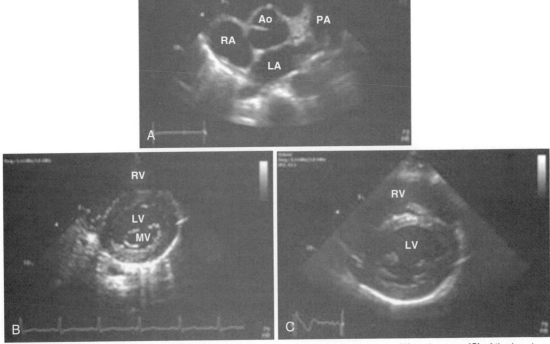

Figure 15-6. Echocardiogram in the parasternal short axis view sweeping from the base **(A)** to the apex **(C)** of the heart. *Ao,* Aorta; *LA,* left atrium; *LV,* left ventricle; *MV,* mitral valve; *PA,* pulmonary artery; *RA,* right atrium; *RV,* right ventricle.

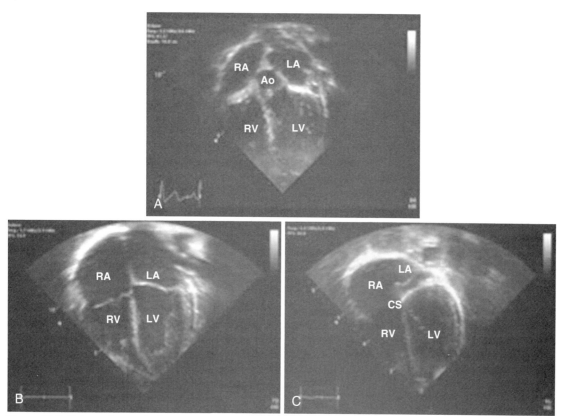

Figure 15-7. Echocardiogram in the apical four-chamber view sweeping anterior **(A)** to posterior **(C)**. *Ao,* Aorta; *CS,* coronary sinus; *LA,* left atrium; *LV,* left ventricle; *RA,* right atrium; *RV,* right ventricle.

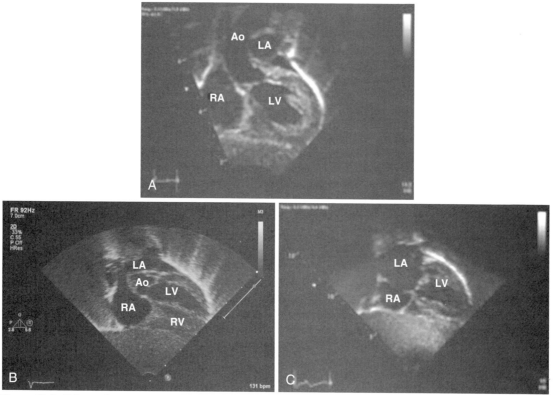

Figure 15-8. Echocardiogram in the subcostal coronal view sweeping anterior **(A)** to posterior **(C)**. *Ao,* Aorta; *LA,* left atrium; *LV,* left ventricle; *RA,* right atrium; *RV,* right ventricle.

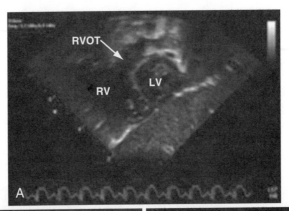

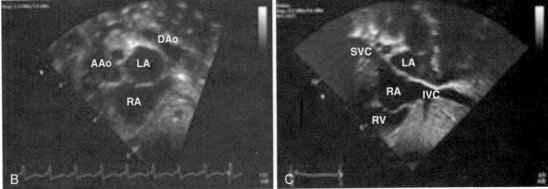

Figure 15-9. Echocardiogram in the subcostal sagittal view sweeping apex **(A)** to base **(C)**. *AAo,* Ascending aorta; *DAo,* descending aorta; *IVC,* inferior vena cava; *LA,* left atrium; *LV,* left ventricle; *RA,* right atrium; *RV,* right ventricle; *RVOT,* right ventricular outflow tract; *SVC,* superior vena cava.

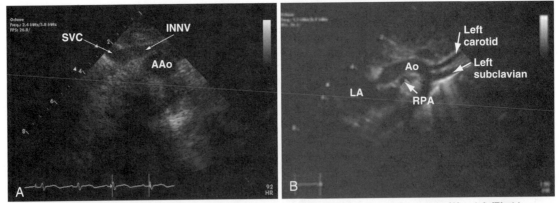

Figure 15-10. Echocardiogram in the suprasternal long axis view sweeping from the patient's right **(A)** to left **(B)** side assuming a left aortic arch. *AAo,* Ascending aorta; *Ao,* aorta; *INNV,* innominate vein; *LA,* left atrium; *RPA,* right pulmonary artery; *SVC,* superior vena cava.

M-Mode Echocardiography

M-mode echocardiography was one of the earliest techniques for evaluating cardiac structures. A single line of interrogation is obtained and plotted over time (Fig. 15-12). Two-dimensional echocardiography has largely replaced this modality, but M-mode is still used, mainly to calculate shortening fraction and measure wall thickness and

chamber size. The image is usually obtained in the parasternal short-axis view at the level of the papillary muscle (see Fig. 15-6). Shortening fraction is defined as follows: [(left ventricular end-diastolic dimension – left ventricular end-systolic dimension)/ left ventricular end-diastolic dimension]. The normal value is above 28%. M-mode echocardiography has long been used to

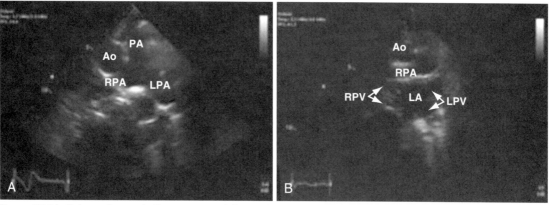

Figure 15-11. Echocardiogram in the suprasternal short axis view sweeping superior **(A)** to inferior **(B)**. *Ao,* Aorta; *LA,* left atrium; *LPA,* left pulmonary artery; *LPV,* left pulmonary vein; *PA,* pulmonary artery; *RPA,* right pulmonary artery; *RPV,* right pulmonary vein.

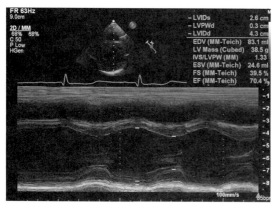

Figure 15-12. M-mode analysis through the left ventricle with a normal shortening fraction of 39%.

estimate cardiac function, but it has limitations, including the fact that only a single plane is used to estimate global function and thus regional wall abnormalities may be missed. In addition, it is fairly preload dependent and does not measure intrinsic myocardial contractility per se. Using shortening fraction to define ventricular function also assumes normal electrical conduction and a circular shape of the left ventricle. Conduction abnormalities or flattening of the interventricular septum that may occur with increased right ventricular volumes due to shunts or elevated right ventricular pressures due to persistent pulmonary hypertension of the newborn (PPHN) may invalidate these measurements. Normative data are available for wall thickness and chamber sizes and are usually referenced to a z score. The z score is simply a normalized value expressed as the number of standard deviations from the mean, and if a z score is within ±2, it is considered normal.

Two-Dimensional Echocardiography

As stated earlier, two-dimensional echocardiography incorporating numerous views is the most common way that a cardiac anatomic diagnosis is made. Systolic function can also be qualitatively and quantitatively assessed. Tracing the left ventricular chamber in end systole and end diastole can give an estimate of ventricular volume, and thus an ejection fraction can be calculated similarly to shortening fraction. In general, an ejection fraction above 50% is considered normal. Not only does two-dimensional echocardiography support anatomic diagnosis and functional analysis, but secondary changes to chamber sizes may give physiologic clues. For example, a PDA may be large by dimensions, but if left-sided structures are not enlarged, there may be minimal left-to-right shunting, possibly because of PPHN or insufficient passage of time for these changes to be noted.

Three-Dimensional Echocardiography

The ability to perform real-time three-dimensional imaging is a relatively new advancement in technology. The benefit of this technology is that it can improve visualization of spatial relationships between structures instead of requiring mental construction of an image from two-dimensional views (Fig. 15-13). Although three-dimensional imaging continues to improve, its practical uses for imaging the newborn are minimal at this time.

Doppler Echocardiography

Use of the Doppler principle allows one to determine the direction and velocity of moving objects being interrogated. Currently, measurement of blood flow velocity and direction is the main use for Doppler analysis, although measurement of myocardial velocity, termed *tissue Doppler imaging,* has recently been introduced as another way to quantify systolic and diastolic function. Color, pulsed wave, and continuous wave Doppler are the three main techniques used for analysis.

Color Doppler simply transforms the image of the interrogated area into colored pixels. By convention, shades of red signify an object moving toward the transducer and shades of blue indicate an object moving away from the transducer. Color Doppler does not necessarily give quantitative information, but it is extremely helpful for identifying minor defects such as a small muscular VSD or PDA that might not easily be seen by standard two-dimensional echocardiography (Fig. 15-14). Color analysis also aides in the qualification of regurgitant jets based on the

width of the regurgitant jet. Stenotic areas are also easily seen with color analysis because the solid red or blue usually becomes multicolor due to the abrupt increase in velocities that occurs in those areas (Fig. 15-15).

Pulse and continuous wave Doppler are simply two technical ways to measure the velocity of the object of interest. Pulse Doppler enables one to interrogate a specific area and define the velocity at that point. The drawback is that high-velocity objects cannot be measured accurately because they will exceed the pulse Doppler capabilities. Continuous wave Doppler can measure high-velocity objects because the system is continuously measuring signals, but it cannot pinpoint the area where the change of velocity occurs. This is important, because the area where the change in velocity occurs is usually the site where a stenosis is located. By convention, objects moving away from the transducer have velocities designated below a baseline and objects with flow toward the transducer have velocities designated above the baseline. It must also be mentioned that the line of interrogation should be as close as possible to parallel to the object of interest or else velocities, and thus also gradients, will be underestimated.

Tissue Doppler imaging (TDI) is a newer technique that measures the velocity of the myocardium via Doppler. The area interrogated is usually the free wall at the level of the AV valves. Three waves are usually obtained via TDI: an e′ wave corresponding to early ventricular relaxation, an a′ wave corresponding to atrial contraction, and an s′ wave corresponding to ventricular systolic function (Fig. 15-16). The e′ and a′

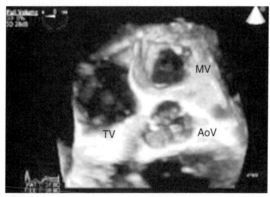

Figure 15-13. Three-dimensional echocardiographic image of the cardiac valves. *Av,* Aortic valve; *MV,* mitral valve; *TV,* tricuspid valve.

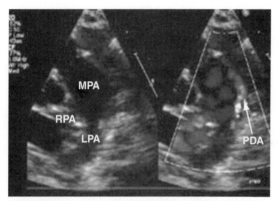

Figure 15-14. Black and white rendition of an image of a small patent ductus arteriosus (PDA) obtained using color Doppler echocardiography. *LPA,* Left pulmonary artery; *MPA,* main pulmonary artery; *RPA,* right pulmonary artery.

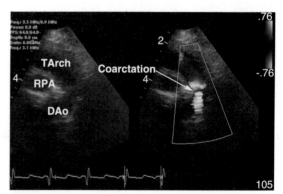

Figure 15-15. Doppler echocardiogram showing a coarctation of the aorta as revealed by color flow aliasing at the coarctation site. *DAo,* Descending aorta; *RPA,* right pulmonary artery; *TArch,* transverse aortic arch.

waves quantify diastolic function, and the s' wave quantifies systolic function.[51] This technique is less preload dependent and therefore may be more useful than other previously described methods. TDI has already been used in patients with broncho-pulmonary dysplasia and congenital dia-phragmatic hernia to assist in quantifying right ventricular function, and use of this technique will likely continue to grow as more data become available.[52-54]

Estimation of pressure gradients between two separate areas is obtained by measuring the blood velocity across the site and using the Bernoulli equation:

$$\Delta P = \tfrac{1}{2}\,\rho\,(v_2 - v_1) + \rho\,f(dv/dt)\,ds + R(\mu)$$

where ΔP is the pressure difference across the stenotic area, ϱ is the density of blood, v_1 and v_2 are the velocities proximal and distal to the stenosis, R is the viscous resistance, and μ is the viscosity of the fluid. The three com-ponents of the formula account for kinetic energy, loss of energy through acceleration

and deceleration of blood, and viscous forces. This formula can be simplified to

$$\Delta P = 4v^2$$

assuming minimal proximal velocity, a dis-crete stenosis, and minimal viscosity. By using all three Doppler techniques and the Bernoulli equation, the physiology can be thus determined (Fig. 15-17). For example, a left-to-right shunt is seen via color Doppler through a PDA with a peak velocity of 3.5 m/sec by continuous wave Doppler. The pressure difference between the aorta and main pul-monary artery is 3.5 m/sec × 3.5 m/sec × 4 = 49 mm Hg. Furthermore, the right ven-tricular systolic pressure can be calculated as aortic systolic pressure minus 49 mm Hg. Similarly, if the tricuspid jet is 2.5 m/sec, the pressure difference between the right atrium and right ventricle is 25 mm Hg. Assuming that a normal right atrial pressure is 5 mm Hg, the right ventricular systolic pressure is approximately 30 mm Hg. Numerous calculations are thus performed to quan-tify the physiology present. This equation will underestimate the gradient if there is a long-segment stenosis or if polycythemia is present because of the simplification. Con-versely, if there is a significant proximal ste-nosis in series, such as a stenotic aortic valve and a coarctation, the proximal velocity must be taken into account or else the distal gradient will be overestimated. In general, a velocity of 1 m/sec or less can be ignored.

Strain and Strain Rate

Strain (ε) is defined as the deformation of an object relative to its original length and is expressed as a percentage. Strain rate is the local rate of deformation or strain (ε) per unit of time and is expressed as inverse seconds.

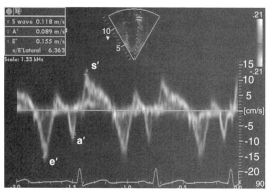

Figure 15-16. Tissue Doppler analysis of the left ventricular free wall at the level of the mitral valve annulus.

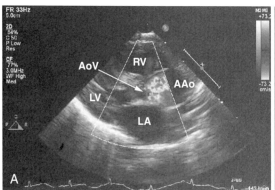
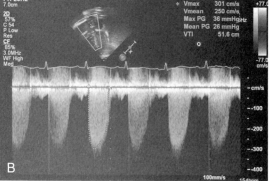

Figure 15-17. Color flow aliasing at the level of a stenotic aortic valve **(A)** with a peak velocity of 3 m/sec by continuous wave Doppler echocardiography estimating a 36 mm Hg gradient **(B)**. *AAo,* Ascending aorta; *AoV,* aortic valve; *LA,* left atrium; *LV,* left ventricle; *RV,* right ventricle.

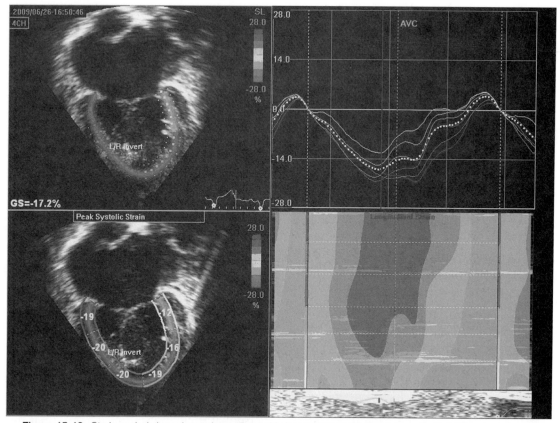

Figure 15-18. Strain analysis based on echocardiographic imaging in a patient with hypoplastic left heart syndrome.

These values can be obtained via TDI or via speckle tracking technology using echocardiography. These parameters are probably the least preload-dependent values obtained via echocardiography and thus are theoretically the best values to quantify contractility and relaxation. This technique does not use geometrical assumptions and therefore is ideal for quantifying function in patients with complex congenital anatomy (Fig. 15-18). Minimal data currently exist in pediatrics, especially for the premature neonate, but like TDI, this technique will probably continue to gain acceptance over time.[55-57]

Transesophageal Echocardiography

Transesophageal echocardiography is simply the application of all the echocardiographic techniques described earlier via a probe inserted down the esophagus. It is rarely indicated for newborns because most, if not all, of the desired images can be obtained using transthoracic echocardiography. Furthermore, neonates would likely need to be intubated for this procedure to secure an airway. If the procedure is needed, probes are currently available for neonates weighing as little as 2.5 kg. Transesophageal echocardiography is most often performed in neonates in conjunction with cardiac catheterization or surgical intervention to give real-time information and aid in the intervention being performed (Fig. 15-19).[58,59]

COMPUTERIZED AXIAL TOMOGRAPHY AND MAGNETIC RESONANCE IMAGING

CAT or MRI scans may add additional information that the echocardiogram cannot provide. As noted earlier, complex extracardiac abnormalities involving pulmonary arteries, pulmonary veins, and the aortic arch may not be well delineated by echocardiography. Mixed total anomalous pulmonary veins and tetralogy of Fallot with multiple aortopulmonary collaterals are just two examples of cardiac defects for which CAT and MRI are superior to echocardiography for defining extracardiac abnormalities (Figs. 15-20 and 21). In addition to anatomic information, both modalities have the ability to provide hemodynamic data, with MRI being superior to CAT in that respect.

In general, MRI is preferable to CAT because of the lack of radiation exposure.

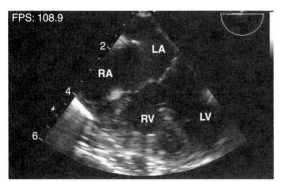

Figure 15-19. Transesophageal echocardiogram in a patient with an atrioventricular septal defect. Note the common atrioventricular valve and the large central defect. *LA,* Left atrium; *LV,* left ventricle; *RA,* right atrium; *RV,* right ventricle.

Since many children with complex cardiac anatomy may undergo multiple imaging and catheterization procedures over a lifetime, minimization of radiation exposure is warranted. CAT customarily requires contrast, which is a relative contraindication in patients with renal insufficiency (Table 15-1). Some concerns have also been raised regarding MRI and use of gadolinium contrast in patients with renal insufficiency associated with nephrogenic systemic fibrosis.[60] Because of this concern, gadolinium is probably best not used in those patients until more data are available. CAT produces images more quickly than MRI; thus in a patient in unstable condition, CAT may be preferable to MRI. CAT scanning is also not as affected by artificial materials such as stents, coils, and so on, compared with MRI. As technology advances, more devices have become MRI compatible. It is essential that whenever an patient may undergo MRI, screening for device compatibility be performed (www.mrisafe.com). Cardiac MRI may not be readily available at some institutions, so the decision regarding type of imaging may be driven by practical considerations.

CARDIAC CATHETERIZATION

Like CAT and MRI studies, catheterization procedures provide excellent images of extracardiac structures. Nonetheless, most anatomic, physiologic, and functional data can be obtained via the imaging modalities previously described. It would be extremely rare to perform a catheterization procedure purely for imaging purposes. Catheterization is reserved for neonates in whom pulmonary vascular resistance measurements are needed or when an intervention is required,

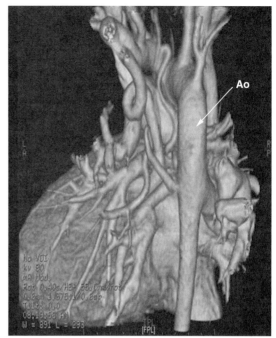

Figure 15-20. Three-dimensional computerized axial tomographic scan reconstruction for a patient with tetralogy of Fallot, pulmonary atresia, and multiple aortopulmonary collaterals. This left posterior oblique view shows multiple collateral vessels arising from the aorta and supplying blood to the small pulmonary arteries. *Ao,* Aorta.

such as balloon atrial septostomy or valvuloplasty.[61] Disadvantages of catheterization include its invasive nature and the radiation and contrast exposure involved (see Table 15-1).

In summary, multiple imaging techniques are available for evaluation of the neonate with suspected heart disease. Echocardiography will likely remain the main modality for the reasons stated earlier, but other techniques may give additive information depending on the clinical situation. Imaging technology will undoubtedly improve over time, but the goal will always remain the same: complete and accurate assessment of anatomy, physiology, and function of the cardiac defect.

DIAGNOSTIC GROUPS OF CONGENITAL HEART DISEASE

The spectrum of neonatal congenital and acquired heart disease is conventionally divided into broad categories based on presentation, unifying pathologic features, and anticipated course. Practically, there can be significant variation in the duration of neonatal transition, which impacts the observed physiology of a given lesion. Ideally, lesions

Table 15-1.	Advantages and Disadvantages of Imaging Techniques			
	Echocardiography	CAT	MRI	Cardiac Catheterization
Portable	Yes	No	No	No
Noninvasive	Yes	Yes	Yes	No
Intracardiac structures	+++	++	+++	+
Hemodynamic assessment	++	+	++	+++
Extracardiac structures	++	+++	+++	+++
Contrast exposure	No	Yes	No	Yes
Radiation exposure	No	Yes	No	Yes
Interventional capability	No	No	No	Yes

CAT, Computerized axial tomography; MRI, magnetic resonance imaging. + to +++, The greater the number of plus signs, the greater the advantage of the test.

can be classified by their primary presenting features: (1) cyanosis caused by obstruction to pulmonary blood flow or poor mixing, (2) hypoperfusion and shock caused by obstruction to systemic blood flow, or (3) mild or no cyanosis with tachypnea and increased pulmonary blood flow. This section discusses these types of presentation, the most common lesions in each, the diagnostic tests necessary to distinguish among the lesions, subsequent therapy, and the differential diagnosis of noncardiac disease.

MILD OR NO CYANOSIS WITH RESPIRATORY DISTRESS AND INCREASED PULMONARY BLOOD FLOW

Infants with a primary presentation of tachypnea secondary to cardiac disease can be categorized into two major subgroups: (1) those with pure left-to-right shunts, in whom the shunt solely consists of pulmonary venous return being directed back to the pulmonary arterial circulation, so that any arterial desaturation is secondary to alveolar fluid or an intrapulmonary shunt; and (2) those with bidirectional shunts (complete mixing lesions), in whom systemic venous blood is also directed back to the systemic arterial circulation, which directly causes some arterial desaturation. Both groups may have elevated pulmonary venous pressures or pulmonary blood flow that causes interstitial edema, at which point respiratory distress becomes apparent.

Some of the most common defects in congenital heart disease, including simple left-to-right shunt lesions (atrial and ventricular septal defects, PDA, endocardial cushion defect, arteriovenous malformations, and aortopulmonary window) as well as more complex complete mixing lesions such as anomalous pulmonary venous connection

and truncus arteriosus, present with respiratory distress in infancy. Often these neonates are asymptomatic immediately after birth. As the pulmonary vascular resistance falls, infants may begin to manifest signs of increased pulmonary blood flow, including tachypnea, tachycardia, diaphoresis, hepatomegaly, and eventually failure to thrive. An exception to this situation is the preterm infant, in whom there may be hemodynamically significant left-to-right shunting within a few days following delivery that contributes to earlier onset of symptoms. When the lung, particularly the pulmonary vascular bed, is underdeveloped or damaged, such as with diaphragmatic hernia, omphalocele, or chronic lung disease, a small shunt seems much larger because of the reduced size of the pulmonary vascular bed in these infants.

The differential diagnosis of infants with respiratory distress includes parenchymal lung disease, an aspiration syndrome, diaphragmatic hernia, pneumonia, and PPHN. The premature infant with resolving respiratory distress syndrome (RDS) who requires increasing respiratory support may have either an increasing ductal shunt or the onset of interstitial lung disease. Thus, several days of careful evaluation may be required before the presence of heart disease is fully appreciated.

Ventricular Septal Defect

An isolated VSD accounts for between 30% and 40% of all congenital heart disease. The majority of isolated VSDs are very small and restrictive. In these infants, the resistance to flow between the left and right ventricles allows the pulmonary vessels to mature normally into adult-type vessels. With a rapid decrease in pulmonary vascular resistance, there is a corresponding decrease in right ventricular pressure, and a left ventricular–right ventricular pressure gradient will arise. Therefore a left-to-right shunt can develop quickly, resulting in a loud (grade 3 to 4/6) systolic murmur that is often present in the newborn period. Despite the low pulmonary vascular resistance, the resistance to flow at the VSD prevents large-volume left-to-right shunting, which averts symptoms of congestive heart failure. Infants with this defect rarely demonstrate pulmonary overcirculation. As a result, most of these defects follow their natural history and close spontaneously, and the remainder rarely require surgical intervention because the defect and resulting additional pulmonary blood flow do not contribute to the development of additional abnormalities.

In a large, nonrestrictive VSD (see Fig. 15-4), the pressure in the right ventricle and pulmonary artery is at systemic levels. If the thick-walled pulmonary vessels matured normally, the vascular resistance would decrease rapidly, and there would be a large left-to-right shunt with left ventricular failure and pulmonary edema. Such a series of events is unusual. In fact, when a large VSD is present, a heart murmur is not usually heard, even in the newborn period. The left-to-right shunt does not develop rapidly, because the pulmonary resistance vessels remain heavily muscular for a longer period than normal and the decrease in pulmonary vascular resistance is delayed. The variation in pulmonary vascular resistance from one child to the next is considerable. In some infants the resistance decreases considerably; in others, hardly at all. When there is a large defect, the shunt is usually maximal by 2 to 3 weeks of age, so that congestive heart failure, when it occurs, is usually present by 4 weeks of age.

Patent Ductus Arteriosus

Persistent patency of the ductus arteriosus beyond the first few days of life accounts for 10% to 15% of all congenital heart defects. Premature infants comprise the majority of patients with persistant patency of the ductus arteriosus. The proportion increases with lower gestational age and weight, with upto 70% of infants born less than 28 weeks of age demonstrating ductal patency.[62] Patency of the ductus arteriosus may result from adverse events such as hypoxia or acidosis in the newborn. Persistent patency of the ductus arteriosus occurs more frequently in premature infants than in full-term infants. The exact mechanisms are not clear. The ductus arteriosus in premature animals is certainly less responsive to the constricting effects of oxygen. The relaxing effects of prostaglandin E_2 and prostacyclin are greater in the immature ductus arteriosus, and the metabolism of prostaglandin E_2 is not efficient. As a result, even the small circulating concentrations of prostaglandin E_2 that may be present in the immature infant can cause the ductus arteriosus to remain in a partially relaxed state. The principles discussed for VSD also apply to PDA. However, because there is length to the ductus arteriosus as well as caliber, resistance to flow is greater. A nonrestrictive PDA is less common, so that systemic-level pulmonary hypertension is also less common.

In a full-term infant with a PDA, the outcome depends on the size of the channel. With the gradual decrease in postnatal pulmonary vascular resistance, a left-to-right shunt develops from aorta to pulmonary artery, which produces excessive pulmonary blood flow, increased pulmonary venous return, and left atrial and ventricular dilatation. A small PDA produces only the typical continuous machinery murmur and full pulses. A moderate to large PDA may produce signs of congestive heart failure as well as a typical continuous murmur and wide pulse pressure (bounding pulse), often in the second month of life. In the healthy term infant, only rarely does heart failure occur in the newborn period.

Patent Ductus Arteriosus in Preterm Infants

As noted earlier, preterm infants, and particularly very low-birth-weight infants, have a significantly increased incidence of persistent PDA compared with their term peers. The PDA of the preterm infant warrants specific discussion, because it may seriously complicate the management of RDS. Although the left ventricle is capable of maintaining near-normal systemic blood flow even with a large left-to-right shunt in the premature infant, the increased intravascular blood volume and the associated increase in interstitial fluid aggravate the respiratory distress already present. If left ventricular oxygen demand exceeds supply, the left ventricle may begin to fail, which raises pulmonary venous pressure and further increases interstitial fluid production. In addition, pulmonary arterial pressures may be elevated because of the nonrestrictive PDA itself or because of pulmonary venous hypertension, which may further decrease lung compliance and exacerbate the pulmonary dysfunction. Thus, a PDA in the presence of RDS may seriously affect pulmonary function by a variety of mechanisms.

The diagnosis of a PDA may be difficult in that tachycardia and an intermittent systolic murmur may be the only auscultatory findings. A wide pulse pressure is often present, as is increased precordial activity. Ventilator therapy and continuous positive airway pressure may mask not only the clinical findings but also the radiographic findings of a PDA. When the chest radiograph shows a large heart and pulmonary venous congestion in the presence of signs of a PDA and a large liver, there is no problem in diagnosis. However, for many reasons, the heart may not be very large, and severe RDS may obscure radiographic findings of cardiomegaly and pulmonary edema. In the premature infant with pulmonary disease, impaired oxygen exchange in the lung may maintain an elevated pulmonary vascular resistance, which masks the presence of PDA. Improvement in the pulmonary disease permits the pulmonary resistance to fall, and signs of a left-to-right ductal shunt to ensue. Thus, a PDA must be suspected in all infants with severe RDS when the illness is protracted, blood gas concentrations suddenly deteriorate and require manipulation of ventilation, or apneic episodes are intensified. Fluid balance must be closely monitored, because excess fluid administration may exacerbate the physiology of a PDA and induce congestive heart failure. Infants must undergo auscultation for murmurs several times each day during the illness and should be briefly removed from the ventilator to permit proper auscultation. Echocardiography and Doppler imaging are diagnostic. Color flow Doppler mapping can detect even a small, hemodynamically insignificant PDA. In the past, a large left atrium-to-aortic ratio, bulging of the atrial septum from left to right indicating increased left atrial pressure, a dilated left ventricle, and the need for severe fluid restriction and diuresis together with failure of aggressive ventilatory management were considered sufficient to suggest that the ductus was hemodynamically significant. Recent studies have determined that conventional echocardiographic markers do not predict outcome or neurodevelopment at 2 years.[45,63-65] As a result, several studies have used biomarkers, including troponin T, brain natriuretic peptide (BNP), and N-terminal pro-BNP, to distinguish a hemodynamically significant PDA.[66-69] The question remains whether infants undergoing treatment for a hemodynamically significant PDA as identified by these markers have improved outcomes compared with peers whose PDAs are identified as significant by conventional methods.

Part of the challenge in identifying infants with a significant PDA is that the management approach to these infants remains controversial. Constriction of the ductus arteriosus in premature infants has been achieved by pharmacologic manipulation using inhibitors of prostaglandin synthesis or by surgical ligation. Permanent closure of the ductus arteriosus requires both effective muscular constriction to block luminal blood flow and anatomic remodeling to prevent later reopening. In the last few years, multiple investigators have looked for ways to determine the appropriate treatment strategy for premature infants with a PDA. To ascertain which patients require treatment, investigators must clearly show a morbidity or mortality risk associated with a PDA in this patient group. Several observational studies have linked a ductus arteriosus in premature infants with increased risk of chronic lung disease, necrotizing enterocolitis, intraventricular hemorrhage, diminished regional cerebral oxygen saturation[63,72] and overall poor neurodevelopmental outcome and mortality.[62,70-71] Both indomethacin and ibuprofen have been studied extensively over the last decade and they have been determined to be equally effective in closing a PDA.[59,68] However, confounding the decision to close the duct are additional data from several studies linking treatment with indomethacin to necrotizing enterocolitis, platelet dysfunction, and renal failure and ibuprofen to pulmonary hypertension and hemorrhage.[71,73-76] Although these risks may be acceptable to physicians facing the significant morbidities associated with intraventricular hemorrhage or necrotizing enterocolitis, a Cochrane review demonstrated that administration of indomethacin at less than 24 hours of life regardless of PDA status is associated with a reduction in the risk of severe intraventricular hemorrhage but has no impact on mortality or severe developmental disability at 18 to 36 months.[77] As a result, several recent studies have challenged the idea that premature neonates should receive prophylactic treatment.

Aortopulmonary Window

An aortopulmonary widow is a relatively uncommon communication between the ascending aorta and the pulmonary trunk differing from a truncus due to the presence of two semilunar valves. The defect, although variable in size, is very proximal and, unlike a PDA, does not have length; thus flow is determined simply by the difference in systemic and pulmonary resistances. As a result, a large left-to-right shunt may develop early in life. Classic cardiac examination findings include a systolic murmur with middiastolic rumble secondary to increased blood flow across the mitral valve. The electrocardiograph (ECG) typically demonstrates left or biventricular hypertrophy. The classic chest radiographic findings include cardiac enlargement with prominence of pulmonary artery and pulmonary vasculature. Due to the magnitude of the shunting that can occur, these patients are often referred for surgical repair at the time of diagnosis to avoid the development of pulmonary vascular disease.

Combined Shunt Defects

Although an isolated VSD, PDA, or atrial septal defect rarely causes symptoms of heart failure in the full-term newborn, combinations of these are more likely to do so. For example, in a term infant with the clinical features of VSD, if cardiac failure and respiratory distress develop in the first week or two of life, an additional shunt or another cardiac or vascular abnormality might be present. In infants beyond the first few days of life, it is important to remember that the closing ductus arteriosus may unmask another lesion such as a coarctation or arch interruption that causes an infant in stable condition to abruptly become symptomatic.

Complete Atrioventricular Septal Defect (Endocardial Cushion Defect)

Endocardial cushion defects are composed of atrial and ventricular septal defects as well as a common atrioventricular valve orifice. In isolation these lesions are rarely associated with cardiac failure in the newborn. Patients with signs of early failure may have a more complex lesion with associated left-sided heart obstruction, valvular insufficiency, or, less commonly, left ventricular-to-right atrial shunting that causes an obligatory shunt (not dependent on pulmonary vascular resistance).

Truncus Arteriosus

Truncus arteriosus is characterized by a single arterial trunk that arises from the heart and gives rise to the aorta, the pulmonary arteries, and the coronary arteries. It occurs in 1% of cases of congenital heart disease and may be fatal by a mean age of 2.5 months if untreated.[78,79] The pathophysiology is variable, but generally, as pulmonary vascular resistance falls in the first days of life, torrential pulmonary blood flow ensues, and the patient rapidly develops significant pulmonary overcirculation and symptoms of heart failure, including tachypnea, failure to thrive, feeding difficulties, and sweating. Due to the excessive pulmonary blood flow, infants with truncus arteriosus are only minimally cyanotic and frequently develop oxygen saturation levels above 90%. If there is proximal pulmonary artery stenosis, the described clinical presentation may be delayed. In the newborn period, classic physical examination findings include a hyperdynamic precordium, a left precordial bulge, a loud single S_2 with an early systolic ejection click, and a systolic ejection murmur along the left sternal border. If the truncal valve is insufficient, an early diastolic decrescendo murmur may be noted at left midsternal border accompanied by signs of heart failure immediately after birth. As pulmonary blood flow increases, the patient develops a wide pulse pressure and bounding pulses due to continuous diastolic flow into the pulmonary arteries and an apical rumble from increased flow across the mitral valve. The ECG frequently demonstrates right, left, or biventricular hypertrophy and should be used to rule out the unusual scenario of myocardial ischemia. Medical management can be extremely challenging if there is no obstruction to pulmonary blood flow and is focused on alleviating symptoms with diuresis, inotropic support to augment cardiac output, and ventilatory support until the patient can undergo definitive surgical repair. Mortality in the first year of life may be higher than 80% without repair.[41] Thus early identification of neonates with truncus arteriosus can be critical to their long-term survival.

Total Anomalous Pulmonary Venous Return

In total anomalous pulmonary venous return (TAPVR), also known as *total anomalous pulmonary venous connection*, both systemic and pulmonary venous flows return to the right atrium, where they mix. There is an obligate right-to-left shunt across the atrial septum that is the only preload to the left side of the heart and provides the systemic cardiac output. Oxygen saturations in all cardiac chambers are identical and are determined by the relative amount of pulmonary blood flow. TAPVR types are classified according to the manner in which blood from the confluence returns to the heart: supracardiac (~50% of cases), cardiac (~25%), infradiaphragmatic (~15%), and mixed (~10%). The location of the defect and the degree of obstruction dictates the presentation of an infant with TAPVR.

The majority of infants with unobstructed venous return have a dramatic increase in pulmonary blood flow as vascular resistances fall over the weeks after birth. As a result, it is not uncommon for pulmonary blood flow to be three or more times that of the preserved systemic circulation. As a result oxygen saturation percentages are typically in the upper 80s and low 90s, and there is no clinically apparent cyanosis. Instead, these infants manifest tachypnea, poor feeding, repeated "respiratory infections," failure to thrive, and clinical signs of heart failure. On physical examination, there is a prominent right ventricular impulse, a widely split S_2 with an accentuated pulmonary component, and an S_3 gallop. There may be a systolic murmur along the left upper sternal border reflective of increased pulmonary blood flow across the pulmonic valve and relative pulmonary stenosis. The ECG characteristically demonstrates a tall, peaked P wave in lead II, right axis deviation, and right ventricular hypertrophy. The chest radiograph shows signs of increased pulmonary blood flow with enlarged right atrium and ventricle, prominent pulmonary artery, and in the case of supracardiac veins draining into the left innominate vein, the "snowman sign" created by the large supracardiac shadow.

In contrast, obstructed TAVPR (Fig. 15-21), which is more common in the infradiaphragmatic type, typically manifests after the first 12 hours of life with rapid progression of increased work of breathing, feeding failure, and cardiorespiratory collapse. The differential diagnosis at the time of presentation often includes PPHN, RDS, pneumonia, pulmonary lymphangiectasia, meconium aspiration, and hypoplastic left heart syndrome. Cardiovascular findings are minimal. The right ventricular impulse is not increased and S_2 is normally split. There may be a soft blowing murmur in the pulmonic area, but the remainder of the cardiac examination yields normal finding. Hepatomegaly is almost always present. The ECG demonstrates right ventricular hypertrophy

with qR in V_3R but may be without tall spiked P waves. The chest radiograph demonstrates pulmonary venous obstruction with diffuse densities in a reticular pattern fanning out from the hilum and obscuring the cardiac borders. The heart is not enlarged. Infants with this defect must be symptomatically supported until a cardiac surgeon is available. Most undergo surgical repair within a few hours of diagnosis. All children with very severe respiratory distress who are candidates for extracorporeal support should undergo echocardiography before initiation of support. The presentations of severe meconium lung disease and severe obstruction in TAPVR are similar and easily confused. This form of TAPVR remains one of the few cardiac surgical emergencies in the newborn.

The most severe form of anomalous venous return is complete atresia of the common pulmonary vein with no definitive egress of blood from the lungs. These infants become profoundly cyanotic immediately after birth and have markedly diminished pulmonary blood flow. There are no significant cardiac examination findings, and the chest radiograph demonstrates

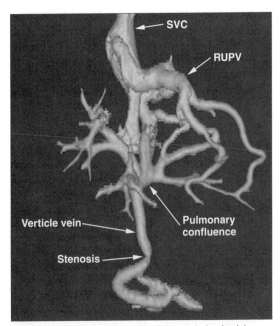

Figure 15-21. Three-dimensional computerized axial tomographic scan reconstruction (posterior view) for a patient with mixed total anomalous pulmonary venous return. The right upper pulmonary vein (RUPV) drains into the superior vena cava (SVC), with the other veins draining into a confluence, then down via a vertical vein into the hepatic veins. Note the narrowing in the vertical vein where a stenosis is present.

severe venous obstruction. Most infants with atretic pulmonary veins die within a few days of life.

Additional Defects

Interference with inflow to the left ventricle, as in congenital mitral stenosis or cor triatriatum, may lead to severe pulmonary venous congestion and respiratory distress but may not compromise systemic perfusion to any major degree. Congenital mitral stenosis may be related to parachute mitral valve or double-orifice mitral valve with chordae that are shortened and deformed and valve leaflets that are thickened and dysplastic. Infants are typically small with growth failure and have wheezing and dyspnea. The cardiac examination demonstrates a rumbling diastolic murmur with an opening snap. Chest radiograph demonstrates left atrial enlargement and pulmonary venous congestion. Infants with cor triatriatum have a similar presentation and in many instances have been diagnosed as having chronic lung disease and have undergone treatment for many months before a congenital cardiac malformation is suspected.

CYANOTIC HEART DISEASE

Central cyanosis indicates reduced arterial blood oxygen saturation and is generally visible when the level of reduced hemoglobin in the blood exceeds 5 g/dL. The typical picture of the infant with cyanotic heart disease is the development of cyanosis in the first few hours of life, which may be noted initially only with crying or feeding, and the absence of respiratory distress. As the ductus arteriosus begins to close, the cyanosis may become progressively more obvious.

There are two major subgroups of lesions that feature cyanosis as the primary finding: (1) lesions with obstruction to pulmonary blood flow, and (2) lesions with normal or increased pulmonary blood flow but with separation of the pulmonary venous return from the systemic arterial circulation. In both subgroups, effective pulmonary blood flow is low. The differential diagnosis of these infants includes mild pulmonary disease, PPHN, abnormalities of the central nervous system, and methemoglobinemia. The initial evaluation usually directs the physician to strongly suspect cardiac disease. The history of the cyanotic infant with heart disease is generally benign, and the pregnancy and delivery uneventful. In contrast, the infant with PPHN often has a history of perinatal distress or meconium aspiration. An exception in the cardiac group is tricuspid insufficiency resulting from myocardial ischemia, in which a history of perinatal asphyxia is common. Additional testing may be beneficial in differentiating pulmonary and cardiac abnormalities. Simultaneous upper and lower extremity pulse oximetry measurements can be diagnostic. If the oxygen saturation in the upper body is lower than that in the lower body, the infant most likely has dextro-transposition with pulmonary hypertension or coarctation of the aorta. In contrast, infants with PPHN have elevated pulmonary vascular resistance, and the ductus arteriosus, if patent, shows right-to-left ductal shunting with subsequent lowering of the blood oxygen saturation or Po_2 in the descending aorta. Chest radiographs taken in the first few days of life usually show normal heart size. Most cyanotic lesions are associated with either a diminutive pulmonary artery (e.g., pulmonary atresia) or one that is transposed to the right; thus the normal pulmonary artery contour at the upper left region of the cardiac silhouette is absent. In addition, the aortic arch should be visualized, because the aorta may descend to the right of the spine in right-sided obstructive lesions (especially if associated with DiGeorge syndrome). Finally, an attempt should be made to evaluate the pulmonary vascularity. Although assessment of pulmonary vascularity radiographically depends on the quality of the image and lung expansion, if there are diminished markings on a good-quality radiograph with normally inflated lungs in the absence of PPHN, there is almost always heart disease.

If the patient is not at a facility where echocardiography can be performed, immediate transfer is mandatory. Stabilization before the transport is of utmost importance: metabolic requirements must be reduced to a minimum to provide adequate substrate delivery, and if oxygen delivery is borderline (measured blood oxygen saturation is ≤80%, Po_2 is ≤30 to 35 mm Hg, or metabolic acidosis is present), prostaglandin E_1 infusion started at 0.05 µg/kg/min and increased to 0.15 µg/kg/min should be initiated. Prostaglandin E_1 effectively dilates the ductus arteriosus to provide adequate pulmonary or systemic blood flow, and the infant's condition can then be stabilized and carefully evaluated if a duct-dependent lesion is present. It is appropriate to administer prostaglandin E_1 to *any infant in whom the diagnosis of cyanotic congenital heart disease is strongly suspected, even before a complete evaluation is performed.* Prostaglandin E_1 has well-defined side effects, such as apnea, jitteriness or even frank seizures, hypotension with peripheral vasodilatation, and a possible increased risk of infection that should be expected by the treating physician. Fluid administration may be necessary after initiation of prostaglandin E_1 treatment to maintain the arterial blood pressure if there is significant systemic vasodilatation, and intubation may be necessary if significant apnea occurs.

Abnormalities of the Tricuspid Valve

Tricuspid atresia is a complete mixing lesion. Because of the atretic valve there is no outlet from the right atrium except across the patent foramen ovale to the left atrium. Blood flow reaches the right ventricle via a VSD that is typically unrestrictive in the neonate. Tricuspid atresia may be associated with normally related or transposed great arteries, and saturations and blood flow depend on the relationship of the great arteries, the size of the VSD, and the presence or absence of semilunar valve stenosis. If pulmonary blood flow is unobstructed, patients may have tachypnea and early heart failure with minimal to no cyanosis. The physical examination is significant for an increased left ventricular impulse (in contrast to other cyanotic heart diseases with increased right ventricular impulses). Depending upon the anatomy, the second heart sound may be single (with atresia of one of the great arteries), normal (in normally related great arteries), or diminished (in transposed great arteries). A murmur may or may not be present depending upon restriction of blood flow through the ventricular septal defect (holosystolic murmur) and the semilunar valves (systolic ejection murmur) and a holosystolic murmur at the left lower sternal border. The ECG may demonstrate left axis deviation and right atrial enlargement. Echocardiography should be performed and, in addition to confirming the diagnosis, will concentrate on assessing the stability of the circulation in the absence of a PDA.

Ebstein anomaly of the tricuspid valve is characterized by the downward displacement of the valve leaflets into the right ventricular cavity. The severity of disease is often dependent on the degree of displacement and the ability of the remaining portion of the right ventricle to generate sufficient force to eject blood into the pulmonary vessels. Newborns may have massive cardiomegaly, marked cyanosis, holosystolic murmurs, a gallop rhythm, hydrops, and pulmonary artery hypoplasia. The ECG will demonstrate right atrial hypertrophy, and there may be associated Wolff-Parkinson-White syndrome (short PR interval and a delta wave). The chest radiograph frequently demonstrates significant cardiomegaly, or "wall-to-wall heart." Infants with severe disease will require prostaglandin to maintain pulmonary blood flow until pulmonary vascular resistance has fallen and the adequacey of the right ventricle and pulmonary valve can be assessed. Many cardiologists adopt a "watch and wait" strategy with these infants in an effort to avoid early surgical intervention and the associated mortality.

Abnormalities of the Right Ventricular Outflow Tract

Tetralogy of Fallot is the signature lesion associated with cyanosis due to decreased pulmonary blood flow. The symptoms and presentation depend on the degree of subpulmonary or pulmonary valve obstruction. Infants with mild obstruction may manifest primarily symptoms of heart failure from the large VSD. Other infants may have severe cyanosis on closure of the ductus arteriosus. "Tet spells" may be associated with vigorous crying—infants are initially hyperpneic and restless with increasing cyanosis. The murmur becomes softer and may disappear entirely during a spell due to the lack of pulmonary blood flow. If untreated, the infant may have a syncopal episode. Treatment for an acute spell involves knee-to-chest positioning, oxygen supplementation, sedation and/or analgesia, administration of β-blockers, and surgical repair to provide a consistent form of pulmonary blood flow.

In cases of absent pulmonary valve syndrome, the hemodynamic pattern is similar to that in tetralogy of Fallot, but there is often severe respiratory distress. The massively dilated pulmonary arteries that are present in this syndrome compress the airways and cause respiratory embarrassment.

Pulmonary atresia with a VSD is a more severe form of tetralogy of Fallot that presents with severe cyanosis shortly after birth. The infant with pulmonary atresia and VSD lacks the prominent pulmonary murmur present in tetralogy of Fallot. The S_1 may be associated with an ejection click secondary to a dilated aortic root. If the patient has additional pulmonary blood flow in the form of collateral vessels from the descending aorta (which may be identified by continuous murmurs auscultated over the patient's back) the infant may have a stable form of pulmonary blood flow. All other infants require treatment with prostaglandin E_2. The ultimate surgical treatment depends on the presence or absence of the native pulmonary arteries and their size.

Neonates with pulmonary atresia with an intact ventricular septum have severe cyanosis that progresses as the ductus arteriosus closes. The S_2 is single and loud. Often there are no other murmurs (or a continuous murmur from the ductus). This defect is dependent on the ductus for pulmonary blood flow. Due to the high-pressure right ventricle, there may be associated coronary artery abnormalities that affect whether surgical palliation via a single ventricle route or orthotopic heart transplantation is recommended.

Transposition of the Great Arteries

Infants with transposition of the great arteries (TGA) show severe cyanosis immediately after birth. Left untreated, these infants rapidly progress from cyanosis to tissue hypoxemia, acidosis, and, if the disorder is unrecognized, death. Unlike infants with other cyanotic congenital heart lesions, these infants have a normal volume of blood passing through the pulmonary bed. However, because the heart is arranged in parallel, infants with TGA have very low effective pulmonary blood flow (deoxygenated blood from the systemic circulation that reaches the pulmonary bed) and effective systemic blood flow (oxygenated blood that perfuses the systemic bed). The degree of mixing between the separate circulations depends on the number and size of the anatomic connections. Blood may shunt at the atrial, ventricular (if a VSD is present), or ductal level. The typical infant with TGA and an intact ventricular septum becomes progressively more hypoxemic as the ductus arteriosus closes secondary to inadequate mixing at the foramen ovale. Frequently these infants are given prostaglandin E_1 until the atrial communication can be enlarged. Although it is unusual to have sufficient mixing at the ductal level, the increased pulmonary blood flow provided by the PDA dilates the left atrium, which allows a larger anatomic left-to-right shunt across the stretched foramen ovale and increased systemic oxygen delivery. Often this is sufficient to avoid acidosis and tissue oxygen debt. Frequently, however, patients with TGA will undergo balloon atrial septostomy either in the cardiac catheterization laboratory or at the bedside. Clinically, the infant with TGA is likely to be male and appear cyanotic but healthy, with a weight appropriate for gestational age. Auscultatory findings may be unremarkable except for a single loud S_2. A nonspecific systolic murmur may be present. Reverse differential cyanosis is rare but is indicative of TGA with a PDA and an associated aortic arch abnormality or pulmonary hypertension. ECG findings may vary considerably, with findings of the initial study often normal for age. In the neonate with TGA and an intact ventricular septum, the chest radiograph may demonstrate a narrowed superior mediastinum with an egg-shaped cardiac silhouette ("egg on a string"), mild cardiomegaly, and increased pulmonary vascular markings. Surgical repair (arterial switch operation) is often undertaken in the first week of life, and most patients are expected to survive to adulthood and lead a normal life.

In summary, an infant with cyanosis and little respiratory distress usually has cardiac disease and requires prompt evaluation and stabilization. When the initial evaluation cannot exclude cardiac disease, it is important to proceed with a complete cardiovascular evaluation. With the dramatic improvements in neonatal surgery and the advent of prostaglandin E_1 therapy, infants with cyanotic heart disease are now expected to survive to lead a more normal life.

SYSTEMIC HYPOPERFUSION

The third common type of presentation of critical heart disease in the newborn is shock due to hypoperfusion. Hypoperfusion is secondary to inadequate ejection of blood into the systemic arterial system, resulting in hypotension and progressive metabolic acidosis. This typically occurs as the ductus arteriosus constricts in a patient with a ductal-dependent systemic circulation but may also be found in infants with lesions in which the function of the left ventricle is seriously impaired without underlying obstruction. The course may be rapidly progressive over the first few hours of life or insidious in onset over the first few weeks. Cardiac lesions in this category include functional abnormalities of the left ventricle such as endocardial fibroelastosis, dilated cardiomyopathy, hypertrophic cardiomyopathy, left ventricular noncompaction, left ventricular outflow tract obstruction, aortic valve stenosis, interruption of the aortic arch, coarctation of the aorta, Shone complex, and hypoplastic left heart syndrome. Systemic hypoperfusion may also be caused by arrhythmias that severely decrease cardiac output in the neonate. Hypoperfusion syndromes often have associated findings, including lethargy, a mottled appearance with pallor and poor pulses, and a degree of systemic arterial desaturation caused by mixing of systemic and pulmonary venous return, and most are associated with respiratory distress secondary to elevated pulmonary venous pressures.

The differential diagnosis of primary noncardiac hypoperfusion is broad and includes sepsis, adrenal insufficiency, anemia, hypovolemia, inborn errors of metabolism, and neurologic instability. In practice, all of these typically have a component of poor cardiac function that improves as the underlying disease is correctly diagnosed and treated. While one works toward a unifying diagnosis for a hypoperfused state, it is important to consider conditions that are most life-threatening if missed. The most frequent misdiagnosis in an infant with heart disease and hypoperfusion is sepsis. Because overwhelming infection is associated with high mortality, it is reasonable to perform a workup for sepsis and even begin specific therapy in any infant with signs of low output, but it is important to consider cardiac disease as well. The most important decision immediately following the diagnosis of left-sided heart disease is to determine whether the left ventricle can sustain systemic cardiac output. If there is any question, the infant should receive prostaglandin therapy to ensure continued patency of the ductus arteriosus until a more thorough assessment can be made.

The history can help distinguish between cardiac and noncardiac disease and differentiate among the specific cardiac lesions. In general, the timing of presentation depends on the role of the ductus and the timing of its closure. There is sometimes a history of perinatal problems. A history of recent viral infection in the mother may be elicited in infants with myocarditis. Fetal hydrops occurs in intrauterine supraventricular tachycardia, cardiomyopathy, premature closure of the foramen ovale, and, on rare occasions, aortic stenosis or hypoplastic left heart syndrome. Maternal diabetes suggests diabetic cardiomyopathy, and a familial history might suggest other forms of cardiomyopathy.

The physical examination uniformly shows a pale, tachypneic, and lethargic infant. It is critical to differentiate sinus tachycardia in a severely stressed infant from an underlying conduction disturbance resulting in poor function. Some arrhythmias may be easily distinguished on telemetry, although a full 12-lead ECG should be obtained to confirm the diagnosis and guide treatment. Peripheral pulses are decreased in low-output states, but a differential pulse or blood pressure between the upper and lower extremities can be diagnostic. In patients with obstruction along the aortic arch or descending aorta (i.e., interrupted aortic arch or coarctation of the aorta), the lower limb pressures will be low in the absence of a nonrestrictive ductus arteriosus. It is important to realize that the left subclavian artery frequently arises at the origin of the coarctation and thus should not be used to represent ascending aortic pressures in coarctation (Fig. 15-22, *A*). Similarly, the right subclavian artery may arise aberrantly from the descending aorta in 0.5% to 2% of the population,[78] which makes assessment of the ascending aorta difficult. However, a difference in intensity between the carotid or temporal artery pulse and the extremity pulses can be a clue to this diagnosis. The precordial impulse is often nonspecific, usually showing a right ventricular heave. The S_2 is single in hypoplastic left heart syndrome, but because of the tachycardia in low-output states, it is often difficult to appreciate a split sound in any of the lesions. Murmurs rarely help the diagnosis in this group: in the presence of severe heart failure, most lesions are not associated with murmurs or have nonspecific ones. Coarctation of the aorta in which a VSD or subaortic stenosis is present is an exception, but critical aortic stenosis may be associated with little or no murmur when the left ventricular output is low. Rales are heard in most low-output states as a result of elevated pulmonary venous pressures.

Arterial blood gas values often indicate a metabolic acidosis at the time of diagnosis. Differential pulse oximetry measurements between the right hand and foot may be helpful. In coarctation or interruption of the aorta, the saturation in the foot will be lower

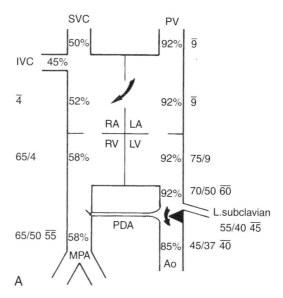

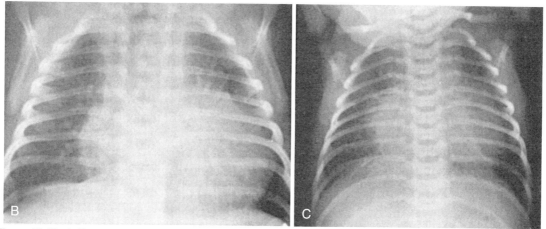

Figure 15-22. A, Representative blood oxygen saturation (%) and pressure (mm Hg) in an infant with coarctation of the aorta. (See Fig. 15-3 for abbreviations.) **B,** Chest radiograph of an infant with coarctation of the aorta. **C,** Chest radiograph of an infant with hypoplastic left heart syndrome. Chest radiographs usually cannot differentiate between left-sided obstructive lesions.

if the ductus is patent because there will be right-to-left shunting from the pulmonary artery to the descending aorta. Conversely, if the saturation is higher in the descending aorta, transposition with PPHN or transposition with interrupted arch should be considered. The chest radiographic study often shows cardiomegaly and interstitial edema in both cardiac and noncardiac lesions once there is severe heart failure and thus is not useful for diagnosis. The ECG is helpful in identifying several lesions. For example, left-sided forces are absent in hypoplastic left heart syndrome; the regular rapid heart rate of supraventricular tachycardia is diagnostic (Fig. 15-23); there are signs of an anterolateral ischemia or infarction in

an anomalous left coronary artery; endocardial fibroelastosis is characterized by prominent Q and R waves in the precordial leads; there usually is marked right ventricular hypertrophy in coarctation of the aorta or critical aortic stenosis; ST-T wave abnormalities are present in myocarditis. The echocardiogram is diagnostic in the obstructive lesions; however, occasionally an isolated aortic coarctation can be masked after the administration of prostaglandin E_1, because the presence of a large PDA decreases the flow through the area. Also, in some patients, ductal tissue wraps around the aorta (so-called "ductal sling"), causing the obstruction when it contracts and the ductus closes. This area can be dilated by

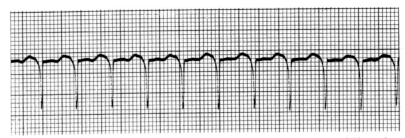

Figure 15-23. Supraventricular tachycardia. Lead II standard electrocardiogram at a speed of 50 mm/sec. Heart rate is 300 beats per minute. No P waves are seen.

administration of prostaglandin E_1, which makes diagnosis problematic in its presence. The echocardiogram is also useful in assessing ventricular performance and the response to therapeutic interventions.

Therapy must be prompt. Once deterioration begins, it is usually rapidly progressive. Initial measures must be directed at the metabolic derangements: partial correction of the metabolic acidosis; maintenance of adequate substrate, hemoglobin, and blood volume; and prompt inotropic support with rapidly acting agents such as dopamine or epinephrine. Prostaglandin E_1 administration is of utmost importance when obstructive lesions are considered; maintaining ductal patency ensures that the lower body will be perfused with blood ejected from the right ventricle through the pulmonary artery. The entire body can be perfused by this route in critical aortic stenosis and hypoplastic left heart syndrome. In left ventricular obstructive lesions, the infant can be maintained on prostaglandin E_1 before surgery. If the diagnosis is in doubt, antibiotics should be instituted after a sepsis workup, and corticosteroids should be considered if adrenal insufficiency is a possibility.

ARRHYTHMIAS IN THE NEONATE

Neonatal arrhythmias are not infrequent, but the clinical significance can vary greatly depending on the diagnosis, which can be difficult to make, especially the differentiation of sinus tachycardia from tachyarrhythmias. Neonatal arrhythmias occur in 1% to 5% of newborns during the first 10 days of life.[80] Neonatal arrhythmias can be classified using various schemes, including bradycardia versus tachycardia and benign versus nonbenign. No single scheme encompasses all aspects of arrhythmias, and often one must use an expanded classification system. The following sections address the various arrhythmias encountered in the neonate.

EXTRASYSTOLES

Premature atrial contractions (PACs) and premature ventricular contractions (PVCs) are common findings in the fetal and newborn period, with PACs being the most common arrhythmia seen in neonates. PACs can be normally conducted, aberrantly conducted, or blocked (Fig. 15-24). Distinguishing between PACs and PVCs can prove difficult for various reasons. The P wave can be superimposed on the preceding T wave, QRS prolongation can be subtle in the newborn, and aberrantly conducted PACs are common. Blocked PACs may mimic sinus bradycardia when atrial bigeminy is present and the P waves are superimposed on the antecedent T wave. These extrasystoles rarely produce symptoms and become less frequent with time. In patients with central venous lines, it is important to ensure that the catheter is not producing right atrial mechanical irritation resulting in PACs. If this is the case, withdrawal of the catheter from the right atrium should result in termination of the arrhythmia.

SINUS BRADYCARDIA, SINUS PAUSES, AND JUNCTIONAL ESCAPE BEATS

Sinus bradycardia, sinus pauses, and junctional escape beats are very common findings in neonates, reported in 19% to 90% of infants.[81] However, the true incidence of these findings is likely unknown, because almost all patients are asymptomatic and only hospitalized infants are typically monitored. These findings are usually transient and rarely symptomatic. In previous studies, sinus bradycardia has been documented by 24-hour Holter monitoring in healthy neonates with rates as low as 42 beats per minute while asleep.[81] However, others have recommended defining sinus bradycardia on Holter monitoring in neonates as 60 beats per minute while asleep and 80 beats per minute while awake.[82,83] These findings are typically secondary to increased

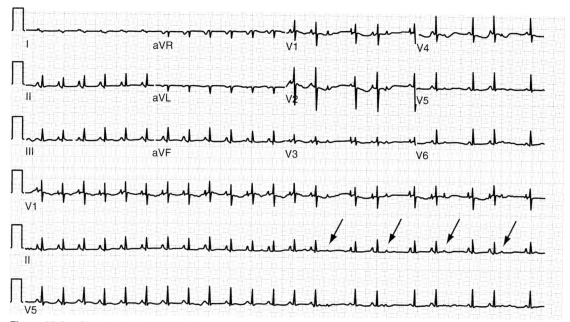

Figure 15-24. Sinus rhythm with blocked premature atrial contractions in an asymptomatic 1-day-old infant. Sinus rhythm precedes atrial trigeminy. Solid arrows indicate blocked premature atrial contractions.

autonomic tone and require no therapy or intervention. However, sinus bradycardia can be a manifestation of a more significant underlying medical condition, such as hypothyroidism, hypoglycemia, hyperkalemia, hypercalcemia, increased intracerebral pressure, or hypoxia.[84] Sinus bradycardia can be seen with airway obstruction, endotracheal intubation, and certain medications, especially sedatives. Finally, infants with long QT syndrome have been shown to have significantly slower sinus rates, and thus any neonate with sinus bradycardia should be evaluated for long QT syndrome.[85]

Treatment for sinus bradycardia is usually directed toward the underlying cause. However, in symptomatic infants, temporary chronotropic and inotropic support may be warranted and can be achieved pharmacologically using various drugs, including isoproterenol, epinephrine, and atropine. Temporary pacing is rarely necessary, and efforts should remain focused on addressing the underlying cause.

SINUS NODE DYSFUNCTION

Sinus node dysfunction can be secondary to direct injury to the sinus node or intrinsic sinus node disease. Sinus node dysfunction often manifests as slow resting heart rate, decreased heart rate variability, decreased peak heart rate, and prolonged sinus pauses. True congenital sinus node dysfunction,

either with or without structural heart disease, is rare and is most likely secondary to sodium channelopathies.[86] More often the disorder is seen following cardiac catheterization procedures, such as balloon atrial septostomy, or cardiac surgery. These procedures can result in direct injury to the sinus node. Although surgery often results in permanent dysfunction, cardiac catheterization procedure–associated sinus node dysfunction is frequently transient. Sinus node dysfunction can be acquired, as seen in cardiomyopathy, various inflammatory diseases (e.g., myocarditis), and genetic syndromes affecting the conduction system, such as sodium channelopathies.

Patients with sinus node dysfunction should be evaluated by 24-hour Holter monitoring to assess degree of bradycardia, frequency and duration of sinus pauses, average heart rate, and associated atrial tachycardias. Escape beats can arise from any cardiac focus, including atrial, junctional, or ventricular, during times of sinus pauses. Depending on the findings, these patients may benefit from pacemaker implantation. Associated atrial tachycardias should also be appropriately treated with antiarrhythmic medications.

ATRIOVENTRICULAR BLOCK

First-Degree Atrioventricular Block

First-degree AV block, also called *first-degree heart block,* is defined as a PR interval longer than the upper limit of normal for a patient's age. The PR interval upper limit of normal is 160 msec in the first 24 hours of life and 140 msec at 1 month of age, although it is variable during the first month of life and continues to vary throughout childhood.[87] The PR interval can be prolonged because of delay in conduction from the sinus node through the atrium, from the atrium to depolarization of the bundle of His, or from depolarization from the bundle of His to initiation of ventricular depolarization. First-degree AV block is typically due to delayed conduction at the level of the AV node. First-degree AV block may be associated with congenital heart disease or may be secondary to an inflammatory process, such as viral myocarditis. Various autoimmune inflammatory disorders, muscular dystrophies, trauma, and pharmacologic therapies (including tricyclic antidepressants, clonidine, and digoxin) can cause a prolonged PR, but these causes are rare in neonates. First-degree AV is often considered a normal variant and does not produce symptoms. No therapy is typically indicated.

Second-Degree Atrioventricular Block (Type I and Type II)

Second-degree AV block is present when there is intermittent failure to conduct atrial impulses to the ventricular conduction system. Second-degree AV block can be further subclassified into Mobitz type I (Wenckebach) and Mobitz type II block. Mobitz type I block is defined by progressive lengthening of the PR interval with eventual loss of conduction to the ventricle of 1 beat. The PR interval of the subsequent conducted atrial impulse is always shorter than the PR interval of the last conducted ventricular beat. Mobitz type II block is defined by abrupt failure to conduct one or more atrial impulses to ventricles without preceding PR prolongation. This block typically occurs below the AV node and can progress acutely to complete heart block.[88] The pattern of type II second-degree AV block can be regular and is described as 2:1, 3:1, and so on. High-grade second-degree AV block is considered 3:1 or higher. This differs from complete heart block by the presence of R-R interval variation or R-R intervals that are multiples of the atrial cycle length.

Type I second-degree AV block is often considered a normal variant and can be seen during periods of sleep in older children. Causes of type I second-degree heart block are similar to those of first-degree heart block. High-grade second-degree heart block has a variety of causes, only a handful of which are seen in the neonatal period, including viral myocarditis, tuberous sclerosis, cardiac surgery, cerebral edema, and certain medications such as antiarrhythmics and digoxin.[89] High-degree second-degree AV block may also be associated with congenital heart disease, typically AV septal defects, levo-TGA, and left atrial isomerism in patients with heterotaxy syndrome. Recent publications have also reported high-grade AV block caused by mutations in the cardiac transcription factors *TBX5* and *NKX2.5*.[90,91]

Therapy is not necessary for Mobitz type I or asymptomatic Mobitz type II second-degree heart block. The mainstay of therapy for patients with symptomatic high-grade heart block is pacemaker implantation, which is discussed in the following section on complete AV block.

Third-Degree or Complete Atrioventricular Block

Third-degree or complete AV block is characterized by a complete lack of conduction of atrial impulses to the ventricles (Fig. 15-25). The P-P intervals are typically constant on electrocardiogram, although they can display some variability due to respirations and vagal tone. The R-R intervals are fixed as well. In contrast to surgical complete heart block, congenital complete heart block can display some variability in the escape rhythm depending on the physiologic conditions.

Complete AV block occurs in approximately 1 of every 20,000 pregnancies.[92] Causes of complete AV block are similar to those for high-grade second-degree AV block. However, in 91% of affected neonates, complete AV block is secondary to neonatal lupus erythematosus.[93] This is caused by transplacental passage of maternal anti-Ro/SSA and/or anti-La/SSB antibodies—autoantibodies often seen in mothers with systemic lupus erythematosus and Sjögren syndrome. Although the mechanism is not completely understood, the condition is thought to be the result of an immune-mediated inflammatory cascade leading to fetal myocardial fibrosis and thus complete heart block. It is important to recognize that the mother may be completely asymptomatic, and the birth of an affected neonate may be the initial sign of maternal systemic

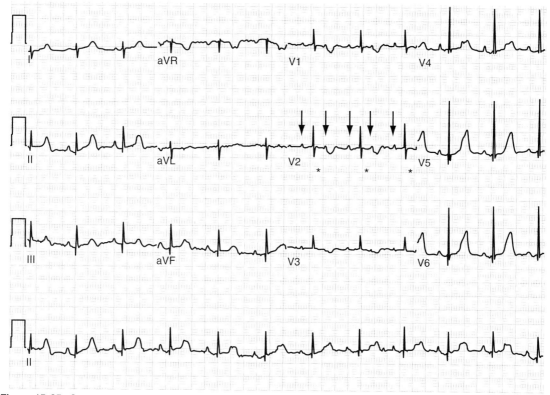

Figure 15-25. Congenital complete atrioventricular block in an asymptomatic 3-week-old infant. Solid black arrows indicate underlying atrial rate of 167 beats per minute. Asterisks denote narrow-complex junctional escape rhythm with a rate of 83 beats per minute.

lupus erythematosus. After the birth of an affected child, the risk of complete AV block in subsequent children is up to 25%.

Although complete heart block is the most concerning ECG finding in neonatal lupus erythematosus, these neonates and infants can display first- and second-degree AV block as well. Fetuses can manifest heart block as early as 16 to 18 weeks' gestation, and first-degree heart block can rapidly progress to complete heart block. The fetus with complete AV block can develop hydrops fetalis, and fetal mortality rate ranges from 15% to 30%.[37] The mortality during the first year of life due to dilated cardiomyopathy is 12% to 41%.[38] Thus, efforts have focused on early identification via fetal echocardiography to identify those infants with early, low-grade heart block. Fluorinated steroids, such as betamethasone and dexamethasone, are not metabolized by the placenta and have been shown to prevent progression of first-degree AV block to complete heart block in fetuses of mothers with anti-Ro/SSA and/or anti-La/SSB antibodies.[37,38]

Although congenital complete heart block is universally irreversible once present,

postoperative AV block may be transient or persistent. Older studies recommended waiting 10 to 14 days for return of AV conduction, but more recent reports suggest that AV conduction is unlikely to return after 7 to 8 days. Current guidelines recommend delaying pacemaker implantation for 7 days from surgery to evaluate for return of AV conduction.[94]

After delivery, all neonates with complete heart block or known exposure to maternal autoantibodies deserve ECG evaluation. All patients with high-grade second-degree AV block or complete AV block ultimately will require permanent pacemaker implantation. Based on current guidelines from the American College of Cardiology, the American Heart Association, and the North American Society for Pacing and Electrophysiology, current class I indications for permanent pacing in neonates with congenital complete AV block include (1) congenital third-degree AV block with a wide QRS escape rhythm, complex ventricular ectopy, or ventricular dysfunction; (2) congenital third-degree AV block with a ventricular rate of less than 50 to 55 beats per minute; and (3) congenital third-degree AV block with congenital heart disease and a ventricular rate of less than 70 beats per minute. Class IIb indications for these neonates include congenital third-degree AV block in an asymptomatic neonate with an acceptable rate, narrow QRS complex, and normal function.[94]

PROLONGED QT

A prolonged QT interval is generally considered to be an interval longer than 460 msec. However, it is important to correct the QT interval for heart rate. This is termed the *corrected QT interval* (QTc). It can be determined by several formulas but is generally calculated using the Bazett formula

$$QTc = QT \text{ interval} / \sqrt{R - R \text{ interval}}$$

where R-R interval is the R-R interval preceding the measured QT interval. Prolonged QTc (≤470 msec) can occur after stressful delivery but usually resolves within 48 to 72 hours.[89] Otherwise QTc prolongation is typically either secondary to a genetic long QT syndrome or caused by medication administration. The QTc can also be prolonged in the presence of hypocalcemia, hypokalemia, and hypomagnesemia. There are several forms of long QT syndrome, including Jervell and Lange-Nielsen syndrome, Romano-Ward syndrome, and long QT syndrome types 1 to 8. These have been mapped to multiple loci and can affect multiple genes. All are inherited in an autosomal dominant pattern except for Jervell and Lange-Nielsen syndrome, which is autosomal recessive. A prolonged QTc places the neonate at risk for bradycardia, torsade de pointes, ventricular tachycardia, and sudden death.

Treatment is aimed at preventing arrhythmias associated with long QT syndromes. All electrolyte levels should be corrected as necessary and any QTc-prolonging medications discontinued if possible. A current list of QTc-prolonging medications can be found at www.qtdrugs.org. Asynchronous cardioversion and magnesium are useful for treatment of torsade de pointes, although cardioversion may not prevent reinitiation of the arrhythmia. The mainstays of therapy for patients with long QT syndromes are β-blockers. Implantation of a cardiac defibrillator is also warranted in patients at high risk and in those who develop torsade de pointes despite receiving β-blocker therapy.

NARROW QRS COMPLEX TACHYCARDIA

Sinus Tachycardia

Sinus tachycardia is a normal variant in neonates and children. In neonates, sinus tachycardia can be difficult to differentiate from arrhythmias because of the ability of the neonatal conduction system to conduct normally at rates upwards of 230 beats per minute. Therefore, it is imperative to differentiate sinus tachycardia from an arrhythmia before any therapy is initiated. Sinus tachycardia is a sign of any condition that requires increased cardiac output. In the newborn, such conditions may include pain, fever, infection, anemia, opiate withdrawal, hyperthyroidism, dehydration, and administration of certain drugs. Treatment should be directed toward the underlying cause.

Supraventricular Tachycardias

Supraventricular tachycardia (SVT) is a general term that encompasses multiple distinct electrophysiologic tachyarrhythmias, two of which are AV reentrant tachycardia (AVRT) and AV nodal reentrant tachycardia (AVNRT). The latter is uncommon in the neonatal period.

Atrioventricular Reentrant Tachycardia

AVRT is the most common cause of tachycardia in the newborn period and accounts for 50% of all pediatric cases of SVT. AVRT is the most common abnormal SVT encountered in the neonatal intensive care unit. AVRT is characterized by a sudden onset and termination, typically normal QRS complexes, and fixed cycle length (R-R interval). The P wave is usually identified following the QRS complex but can be buried in the T wave. It usually has a retrograde morphology (negative in leads II and aVF) (Fig. 15-26). When a bundle branch block is present or when the accessory pathway is used as the antegrade limb of the reentrant circuit, the QRS can be prolonged. This is referred to as *supraventricular tachycardia with aberrancy* and can be extremely difficult to distinguish from ventricular tachycardia. There is typically a 1:1 AV relationship. AVRT is usually seen in a structurally normal heart but can be associated with Ebstein anomaly of the tricuspid valve, congenitally corrected TGA, and hypertrophic cardiomyopathy.

The reentrant circuit requires two limbs—one is the AV node and the other typically is a bypass tract with the ability to conduct either antegrade or retrograde. The bundle

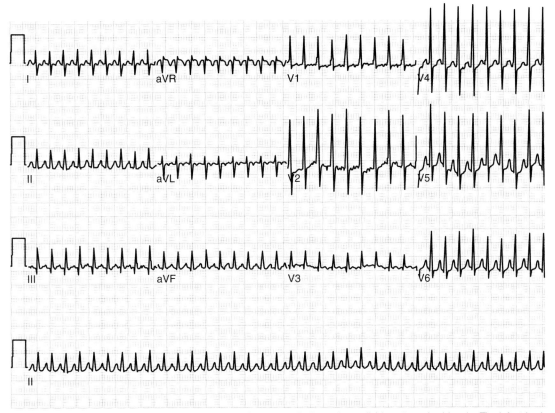

Figure 15-26. Atrioventricular reentrant tachycardia (supraventricular tachycardia) in a 4-week-old male. The infant had manifestations of decreased cardiac output over the preceding 24 hours and showed mild left ventricular dysfunction by echocardiogram. Note that the retrograde P waves are difficult to discern and are buried in the T waves.

of Kent in Wolff-Parkinson-White syndrome (WPW) is one such accessory pathway. "Concealed" pathways are accessory pathways that have the ability to conduct only in a retrograde manner. These accessory pathways electrically link the atrial and ventricular tissue and can occur anywhere along the central fibrous body of the heart. AVRT is frequently triggered by a PAC or PVC. The accessory pathway is typically a source of retrograde conduction, with the AV node serving as the antegrade limb. This is termed *orthodromic reciprocating tachycardia.*

AVRT is typically well tolerated for short periods of time in the neonate. Neonates may be relatively asymptomatic until prolonged tachycardia results in decreased ventricular function. Symptoms can include palpable tachycardia, irritability, tachypnea, poor oral intake, diaphoresis with feeds, and respiratory distress. When decreased ventricular function is present, it usually resolves with adequate treatment of the arrhythmia.

AVRT can be terminated by a multitude of mechanisms. In a patient with AVRT who is in hemodynamically stable condition, vagal maneuvers can be attempted. These can include applying ice to the face for 20 to 30 seconds to elicit the dive reflex, gagging the patient, or inserting a rectal thermometer. Application of pressure over the eyeball or the carotid sinus should be avoided because the former can result in retinal detachment and the latter can result in unilateral occlusion of cerebral blood flow. All of these maneuvers increase vagal tone, which results in decreased AV node conduction. In the event that these maneuvers are unsuccessful, an intravenous bolus of adenosine can be used to block AV node conduction. The initial dose of adenosine is 100 μg/kg and subsequent doses are 200 μg/kg and 400 μg/kg. It is important to immediately follow the rapid intravenous bolus with an adequate saline flush to ensure that the medication reaches the central circulation quickly given the short half-life of adenosine. This can be accomplished by inserting both syringes directly into the same hub or by using a three-way stopcock. A common

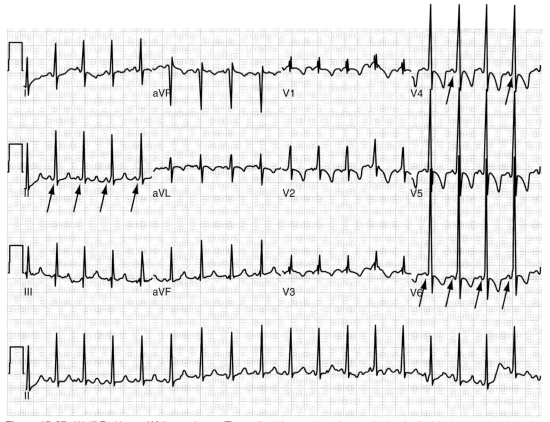

Figure 15-27. Wolff-Parkinson-White syndrome. The patient demonstrated preexcitation (*solid black arrows*) at baseline after conversion to sinus rhythm following administration of adenosine.

cause of failure of adenosine to break SVT is inadequate administration. It is equally important to record the rhythm throughout the administration of adenosine. This allows assessment of the underlying atrial rhythm as well as identification of the mechanism of reinitiation of arrhythmia if it were to recur. If the initial dose of adenosine successfully converts AVRT to sinus rhythm but the arrhythmia recurs, additional doses of adenosine at escalating levels are unlikely to result in sustained sinus rhythm, and additional antiarrhythmic medication is required. Tachycardia can also be terminated by overdrive atrial pacing. This can be accomplished by placing a transesophageal pacing probe and pacing atrially at a rate 10% higher than the SVT rate for approximately 20 seconds. In patients in hemodynamically unstable condition, synchronized cardioversion should be immediately performed to terminate the arrhythmia.

Multiple treatments are available for AVRT. Current first-line therapies for AVRT include digoxin and β-blockers such as propranolol. Digoxin should be avoided

in neonates with WPW because it can potentiate conduction down the accessory pathway by decreasing its refractoriness and lead to ventricular arrhythmias.[95-97] In cases in which digoxin and/or propranolol therapy is unsuccessful, flecainide, amiodarone, and sotalol have been used with success.[98] As the antiarrhythmic properties increase, so do the side effects, and additional monitoring is required. Calcium channel blockers should be avoided in neonates because hemodynamic collapse after administration has been reported. Only in extreme cases is intracardiac electrophysiologic study and accessory pathway ablation necessary. The prognosis for neonates with AVRT is excellent, and most do not require further treatment past 6 to 12 months of age.

Following conversion of SVT to normal sinus rhythm, a baseline electrocardiogram should be obtained to assess for evidence of ventricular preexcitation, which is manifested on the electrocardiogram as a delta wave as in WPW (Fig. 15-27). This is important for initial medical management decisions as outlined previously. The prevalence of WPW is 0.4 to 1 per 1000 in infants and children, and 60% of cases present before 2 months of age.[99] Although patients who manifest WPW during the neonatal period and infancy have a 60% to 90% chance of resolution during the first year of life, one third will experience recurrence of symptoms during the first decade of life, typically around 4 to 6 years of age.[80] Patients demonstrating WPW should undergo screening echocardiography to assess for associated congenital heart disease.

Persistent Junctional Reciprocating Tachycardia

Persistent junctional reciprocating tachycardia (PJRT) is a relatively rare form of reentrant tachycardia. This is an incessant orthodromic tachycardia with anterograde conduction over the AV node and retrograde conduction via an accessory pathway with slow and decremental conduction.[100,101] This arrhythmia can present in utero, in the neonatal period, during childhood, or during adulthood in slower forms of PJRT. Over a long period of time, the incessant tachycardia can lead to tachycardia-induced cardiomyopathy, although this is reversible with rate control. Infants with cardiomyopathy may come to attention due to symptoms of heart failure. During episodes of PJRT, the P wave is characteristically inverted in the inferior leads but may be normal during the brief periods of sinus rhythm. These periods of sinus rhythm are typically no longer than a few beats. Because of the risk of tachycardia-induced cardiomyopathy, aggressive therapy should be initiated for PJRT. β-Blockers have been used with some success but may be inadequate. Success rates of 80% have been reported for the use of amiodarone and verapamil to achieve arrhythmia suppression.[102] PJRT may also resolve spontaneously, although not as frequently as does AVRT. Vaksmann et al observed resolution in 22% of their cohort and in 25% of patients younger than 1 year of age. Unfortunately, the range for resolution of tachycardia was 2 months to 16 years with a median of 5.4 years.[102]

Ectopic Atrial Tachycardia and Chaotic Atrial Tachycardia

Ectopic atrial tachycardia (EAT) is a primary atrial tachycardia resulting from localized automatic foci located in the atria. EAT accounts for 5% to 20% of cases of SVT in pediatric patients and can be present in paroxysmal and permanent forms.[98,103] In this type of tachycardia, there is no reentrant circuit. EAT is usually chronic and incessant. The tachycardia tends to "warm up" and "cool down" rather than showing the abrupt onset and resolution of reentrant tachycardias. EAT typically manifests with heart rates at or just above the upper limit of normal for age. However, the resting heart rate is often more elevated than expected, and the response to exercise is exaggerated.[89] EAT can be distinguished from sinus tachycardia by abnormal P-wave morphology on electrocardiogram. The permanent form can frequently lead to congestive heart failure; otherwise the symptoms can be very subtle, and the clinician must have a high degree of suspicion. Class Ic antiarrhythmics (propafenone and flecainide) and class III antiarrhythmics (sotalol, amiodarone) have been shown to provide effective rhythm control in multiple studies.[104-106] When medication fails, catheter ablation of the automatic focus is a therapeutic option. The chance of spontaneous resolution of EAT is 75% to 95% during the first year of life according to earlier reports.[104,107] A more recent study looked specifically at those patients diagnosed with EAT before 3 years of age (range: 1 day to 2 years; median: 7 days) and found that 78% of patients in this group experienced spontaneous resolution.[108]

Chaotic atrial tachycardia is defined as an atrial tachycardia with at least three P-wave morphologies. The tachycardia rates vary significantly with irregular P-P intervals. Chaotic atrial tachycardia is not typically related to congenital heart disease. However, it has been frequently associated with respiratory illness, especially bronchiolitis caused by respiratory syncytial virus.[77,109] As with EAT, prolonged arrhythmia can result in decreased cardiac function. Treatment options are similar to those for EAT.

Atrial Flutter

Atrial flutter is uncommon in the neonatal period and accounts for approximately 3% of neonatal arrhythmias.[110,111] It is caused by a macro-reentry circuit within the atrial muscle. Atrial flutter is characterized by regular, rapid atrial tachycardia with sawtooth flutter waves (Fig. 15-28). These are typically best appreciated in the inferior leads and tend to have atrial rates of 300 to 600 bpm. AV block is typically present with a 2:1 block, and thus the R-R interval is an integer of the atrial rate. However, the conduction can vary. In the neonatal presentation, atrial flutter is typically not associated with congenital heart disease, but it was seen in conjunction with an atrial septal defect in one study.[112] As with other tachyarrhythmias, neonates in atrial flutter for prolonged periods can show depressed ventricular function. Spontaneous conversion to normal sinus rhythm is common in infants with atrial flutter, occurring in almost 25% of patients. For those who fail to convert to sinus rhythm, direct-current (DC) cardioversion and transesophageal pacing are effective in reestablishing sinus rhythm. Previously, digoxin was the antiarrhythmic medication of choice, but its efficacy has been debated because of the widely variable time between initiation of digoxin therapy and conversion to sinus rhythm.[112-114] Given the likelihood of spontaneous conversion, it is reasonable to monitor an asymptomatic infant for a period of several hours, but cardioversion should be the treatment of choice in symptomatic

neonates. Because atrial flutter is a self-limited process with a low risk of recurrence once sinus rhythm has been established, no further antiarrhythmic medication may be necessary following initial cardioversion.

Junctional Ectopic Tachycardia

Junctional ectopic tachycardia (JET) is an uncommon narrow-complex automatic tachycardia originating in or near the AV node that is typically seen in the early postoperative period in infants and children with congenital heart disease. However, a congenital form of JET can also been encountered in patients who have had no prior surgery. JET is characterized by a narrow-complex tachycardia with rates typically 180 to 240 beats per minute with AV dissociation and a slower atrial rate.[89] Appropriately timed atrial beats conduct normally through the AV node, and this can be an important clue to the diagnosis. Transesophageal atrial electrocardiography may be necessary to confirm the diagnosis. In patients with

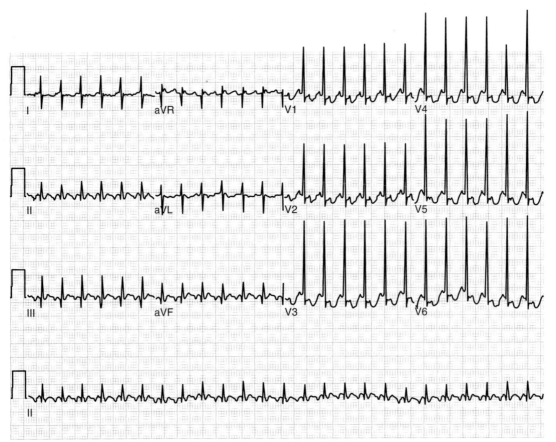

Figure 15-28. Atrial flutter with 2:1 atrioventricular conduction in a 1-day-old infant. Note the sawtooth flutter wave pattern, most evident in the rhythm strip, at a rate of approximately 380 beats per minute and a ventricular rate of approximately 190 beats per minute.

postoperative JET, the atrial electrocardiogram can often be obtained from temporary atrial pacing wires. Congenital JET can present at any age, but when it presents in infancy it can be associated with up to 35% mortality according to one study.[115] Others, however, have reported lower mortality rates of 0% to 4%.[116,117] The cause of congenital JET is poorly understood, but postoperative JET is thought to be secondary to surgical trauma. The hemodynamic significance of JET warrants aggressive therapy. JET is refractory to overdrive pacing, DC cardioversion, and adenosine administration. Class III antiarrhythmics, particularly amiodarone, have been relatively successful in controlling the rhythm. Additional management should focus on withdrawal of inotropic agents when possible and modest cooling. A recent study demonstrated that therapeutic hypothermia resulted in a significant decrease in JET rate and subsequent restoration of AV synchrony, either by reestablishing sinus rhythm or by allowing successful atrial pacing above the JET rate.[118] In patients with persistent JET or failure of amiodarone therapy, it is reasonable to pursue either radiofrequency ablation or cryoablation of the automatic focus. Both modalities have similar success rates (82% to 85%) and recurrence rates (13% to 14%).[117] These procedures may lead to inadvertent high-grade second-degree or complete heart block that necessitates pacemaker implantation.

WIDE QRS COMPLEX TACHYCARDIA

Accelerated Idiopathic Ventricular Rhythm

Accelerated idiopathic ventricular rhythm is a benign arrhythmia occasionally seen in the neonatal period. It is characterized by wide-complex tachycardia with rates no higher than 20% of the preceding sinus rate. Most of these rhythms are less than 200 beats per minute. The QRS is prolonged above the upper limit of normal for age and generally has a left bundle branch morphology. Fusion beats are commonly seen at the onset and termination of the accelerated ventricular rhythm because the rate is similar to the sinus rate. There is no association with congenital heart disease, and the arrhythmia results in no hemodynamic compromise. No further evaluation or therapy is necessary.

Ventricular Tachycardia

Ventricular tachycardia (VT) is defined as three or more consecutive ventricular beats that occur at a rate more than 20% above that of the preceding sinus rhythm (Fig. 15-29). VT is a wide-QRS complex tachycardia, but it is important to distinguish VT from aberrantly conducted SVT, whether caused by rate or antegrade conduction down an accessory pathway such as in WPW. VT can be distinguished by the presence of fusion beats, AV dissociation, and morphology similar to that of PVCs. Unfortunately, neonates and infants tend to have 1:1 retrograde conduction. This means that AV dissociation may not be seen in VT in this population. VT can be monomorphic (a single morphology) or polymorphic (more than one morphology), such as torsade de pointes. It can also be nonsustained, lasting between 3 and 30 beats, or sustained, lasting longer than 30 beats. VT can progress to ventricular fibrillation if left untreated.

The presence of VT requires a thorough evaluation for possible causes. These can include myocarditis, cardiomyopathy, tumors (including hamartoma and rhabdomyoma), myocardial infarction (secondary to anomalous origin of the left coronary artery from the pulmonary artery, maternal cocaine use, or thromboembolism), electrolyte abnormalities, metabolic abnormalities, drug intoxication, and long QT syndrome, to name a few. Initial evaluation should consist of electrocardiography, echocardiography, and possibly cardiac MRI to aid in the diagnosis of cardiac tumors not seen by echocardiography.

The morphology of VT can also be a clue to the underlying diagnosis. Polymorphic VT tends to occur in myocarditis and myocardial infarctions. Incessant VT, defined as VT occurring for more than 10% of a 24-hour period, is often associated with myocarditis and hamartoma.[119]

In patients with sustained VT and hemodynamic compromise, synchronized DC cardioversion is the treatment of choice. In patients who remain in hemodynamically stable condition, initial management may consist of intravenous administration of either procainamide or lidocaine, but pharmacologic therapy is typically initiated after conversion to sinus rhythm. In patients with asymptomatic, nonsustained VT, no underlying cause, and a structurally normal heart, spontaneous resolution is expected, and therefore therapy may not be indicated once conversion to sinus rhythm is achieved.[120] For sustained VT, incessant VT, or rapidly conducting nonsustained VT,

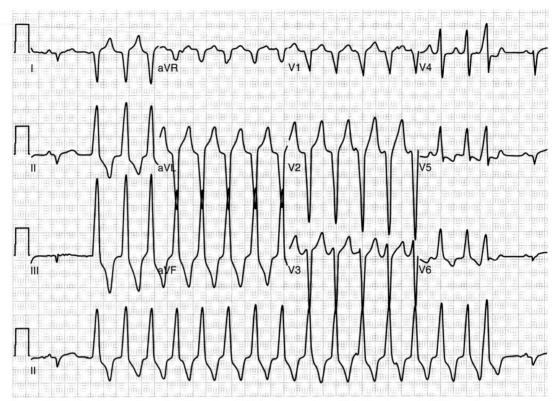

Figure 15-29. Ventricular tachycardia with a rate of 140 beats per minute. Note the change in QRS morphology compared with the sinus beats.

class I, II, and III antiarrhythmic drugs have been used with varying success. Implantation of a cardioverter-defibrillator is typically not indicated in the neonatal period.

SUMMARY OF NEONATAL ARRHYTHMIAS

Arrhythmias are a common problem in the neonatal period. Although AVRT is the most common arrhythmia encountered, most other forms of SVT and VT are rare. The electrocardiogram remains crucial for accurate diagnosis and proper therapeutic intervention. Echocardiographic evaluation is warranted in all neonates with arrhythmias, but most arrhythmias are not associated with congenital heart disease. Finally, although some neonatal arrhythmias, such as PJRT and incessant VT, can be recalcitrant to treat, most are responsive to antiarrhythmic medications and are "outgrown" during the first year of life.

PRACTICAL HINTS

All of the following hints should be used in conjunction with additional data to make a diagnosis of cardiac disease. The adequacy of systemic perfusion, arterial oxygen tension, and results of the cardiac examination should be used in conjunction with heart size, respiratory pattern, and other findings to point toward a diagnosis.

1. Heart sounds are usually abnormal in newborns with a serious congenital heart disease. A single S_2 after the first 12 hours often indicates heart disease, although with rapid heart rates this can be difficult to verify. A well-split S_2 is always abnormal and suggests TAPVR. The presence of a pulmonary systolic ejection click may be normal in the first hours, but after that any systolic ejection click is abnormal, indicating an abnormal pulmonary or aortic valve, an enlarged pulmonary artery or aorta, or truncus arteriosus. If the infant has pulmonary disease without congenital heart disease and has a narrowly split or single S_2, then a high pulmonary vascular resistance is expected.

2. Visible central cyanosis in the early newborn period usually indicates a very low arterial oxygen tension. Even when the clinical judgment is that of only questionable cyanosis, the arterial Po_2 may be very low.

3. Peripheral cyanosis (acrocyanosis) is normal and must be differentiated from central cyanosis. A suspicion of hypoxemia must be verified by arterial blood gas determinations.

4. Measurement of systemic arterial blood gas concentrations while the infant breathes room air and while supplemental oxygen is administered may be helpful in differentiating pulmonary from cardiac cyanosis. A Pao_2 of less than 100 mm Hg in an enriched oxygen environment indicates congenital heart disease until proven otherwise and is an indication for echocardiography and the initiation of prostaglandin E_2 therapy. A Pao_2 of 100 to 250 mm Hg is suggestive of congenital heart disease and warrants additional investigation. A Pao_2 above 250 mm Hg makes life-threatening cyanotic heart disease less likely. In questionable cases, hypoxemia without significant hypercapnia (CO_2 retention) tends to suggest primary cardiac disease. However, pulmonary venous congestion may result in considerable CO_2 retention.

5. Blood gas concentrations determined from heel-stick specimens do not provide accurate measures of the arterial Po_2. However, the error is always on the low side, so that in cyanotic congenital heart disease, a reasonably high Po_2 on a heel-stick sample is reassuring.

6. Transcutaneous Po_2 or oximetric measurements are inaccurate at low levels and in the presence of hypoperfusion. They are valuable for monitoring trends or comparing upper and lower body oxygenation.

7. Oximetric measurements may be beneficial in determining the type of congenital heart disease. Measurements should be taken simultaneously in the right upper and either lower extremity. Cyanosis-desaturation that is equal in the upper and lower extremities can indicate right-sided heart obstruction or TAPVR. Cyanosis-desaturation that is worse in the lower extremity indicates left-sided heart obstruction or suprasystemic pulmonary artery pressures in the face of a PDA. Cyanosis-desaturation that is worse in the upper extremity is diagnostic for dextro-TGA with elevated pulmonary vascular resistance or coarctation until proven otherwise.

8. Femoral or pedal pulses must be carefully and repeatedly palpated in all newborn infants. The pulse may be palpable even with significant coarctation of the aorta while the ductus arteriosus is open, disappearing when the ductus arteriosus closes. Observation of diminished or absent femoral pulses by any examiner requires additional investigation.

9. A high index of suspicion is required to diagnose congenital heart disease early. Careful history taking, physical examination, and laboratory studies—including chest radiographs, ECG, and blood gas or oximetric studies in an enriched oxygen environment—often help to establish the diagnosis. However, two-dimensional echocardiography permits accurate and definitive diagnosis, accomplished without delay.

10. Life-threatening congenital heart disease is sooner or later associated with respiratory distress or frank cyanosis, or both.

11. The presence of a large liver usually indicates systemic venous congestion but does not necessarily point to congestive heart failure. Many conditions in the neonatal period can produce an enlarged liver.

12. On occasion, in the presence of RDS and a PDA, congestive heart failure may be diagnosed without cardiomegaly.

CASE 1

On the day of discharge, the physical examination findings for a full-term baby are significant for a harsh murmur at the lower left sternal border. The examination before this was unremarkable. The child is acyanotic, and the murmur is typical of a VSD with left-to-right shunt.

Is a VSD possible? Why?

A VSD is possible. The left ventricular pressure is not transmitted to the right side through the small restrictive VSD. Therefore, nothing impedes the normal decrease in pulmonary vascular resistance. As the pulmonary vascular resistance decreases, the right ventricular pressure decreases as it would normally. Therefore, there is a large pressure gradient between the ventricles, and an early left-to-right shunt is possible.

Is the defect likely to be small or large?

The shunt rarely becomes large because of the high resistance to flow through the small defect. The major key to suspecting that the defect is small is the early onset of the loud, typical murmur. Also, large defects should not produce a murmur because the pressure equalizes between the right and left ventricle when a large VSD is present.

Is eventual congestive heart failure likely?

Heart failure is not likely when the left-to-right shunt is small.

If the defect was larger, what symptoms would the infant manifest and how would it best initially be managed?

In the setting of a moderate to large defect that permits significant left-to-right shunting, infants manifest several symptoms. Due to the increased pulmonary blood flow, these patients are tachypneic, although they rarely display respiratory distress at rest, and their oxygen saturation is usually 99% to 100% unless they have significant pulmonary flow to produce interstitial edema. They may have minimal to mild retractions. The liver may be felt below the right costal margin. During feedings, these infants may become more tachypneic or diaphoretic, or develop respiratory distress. Because of increased energy demands, they may also demonstrate poor weight gain.

CASE 2

A 40-year-old mother has just delivered a term infant boy. She had little prenatal care and no prenatal testing or ultrasonography. The infant does well and goes to the newborn nursery. On examination, the infant is found to have multiple features consistent with trisomy 21. The cardiac examination is unremarkable, but because occasional PACs are noted on a monitor, an ECG is obtained. This ECG shows normal sinus rhythm with occasional PACs and a leftward/northwest axis.

Given the findings described, does this infant have congenital heart disease?

Yes. The finding of a leftward or northwest axis on ECG is very suspicious for an AV septal (endocardial cushion) defect. The PACs are insignificant and are a common finding in the neonatal period.

Assuming the infant has a complete atrioventricular septal defect (AVSD), does the lack of a murmur surprise you?

No. In this clinical situation, the pulmonary pressures have not fallen, and thus there may be minimal shunting at the level of the VSD component. In patients with trisomy 21, this fall in pulmonary pressures can be delayed or may not occur. Murmurs are not typically heard due to shunting through the atrial septal defect, but in the setting of a large left-to-right shunt at the atrial level, there may be a diastolic rumble associated with relative tricuspid stenosis at the lower left sternal border or a systolic ejection murmur associated with

relative pulmonary stenosis at the left upper sternal border caused by increased flow across either valve. The degree of atrial-level shunting is determined by the ventricular compliance, so in a patient on the first day of life, there is likely minimal shunting because the right ventricle is still relatively stiff and noncompliant.

Echocardiography confirms a balanced complete AVSD with moderate-sized atrial and ventricular septal defect components. As this infant grows, how will the infant's heart disease manifest?

Manifestations will depend on the right-sided pressures. If the pulmonary pressures remain elevated, the infant will be unlikely to develop overcirculation and will remain relatively balanced. The infant may be mildly cyanotic at baseline due to bidirectional shunting at the ventricular level or may become more cyanotic with transient increases in the right-sided pressure, such as during crying. If pulmonary pressures and right-sided pressures fall, the patient is likely to develop VSD-type physiology with increased pulmonary circulation. In this situation, the patient would manifest symptoms similar to those discussed in Case 1 and may require anticongestive therapy.

CASE 3

A 36-week gestation infant is born to a 20-year-old primigravid mother. The mother received minimal prenatal care. The mother's labor was prolonged with rupture of membranes 18 hours before delivery. There is meconium in the fluid, and the infant undergoes suctioning for meconium aspiration following vaginal delivery. He is intubated due to respiratory distress and taken to the neonatal intensive care unit for further management, where oxygen saturation measured on his right hand is 75%. An oxygen saturation probe on his left foot reads 90%.

What is the difference between differential cyanosis and reverse differential cyanosis?

Differential cyanosis is present when the preductal oxygen saturation is higher than the postductal oxygen saturation. Reverse differential cyanosis is present when the preductal oxygen saturation is lower than the postductal oxygen saturation. A PDA is necessary for either form.

What form of differential cyanosis does this patient have and what clinical situations result in this finding?

The patient has reverse differential cyanosis. This type of cyanosis can be seen in TGA with either a significant coarctation or interrupted aortic arch. Obtaining oxygen saturation measurements from the left upper extremity can be helpful in determining the site of either coarctation or interruption. Reverse differential cyanosis can also occur in TGA with supersystemic pulmonary pressures that result in right-to-left shunting across the PDA.

How can these three distinct entities best be identified?

In the neonatal period, echocardiography should be sufficient to determine the presence of coarctation or interruption. Pulmonary pressures can accurately be estimated and flow across the PDA can be determined by color in color flow Doppler echocardiography.

What clinical scenarios can result in differential cyanosis (not reverse)?

Normally related great arteries with a hypoplastic aortic arch, severe coarctation, or interruption can result in differential cyanosis. Also PPHN with normally related great arteries can result in differential cyanosis.

What should be the initial management of this patient with reverse differential cyanosis?

A common theme in all cases of reverse differential cyanosis is the presence of TGA. Initial management should include initiation of prostaglandin E_1 infusion to maintain ductal patency. Additional management may include balloon atrial septostomy to insure adequate mixing before surgical repair or supplemental oxygen or inhaled nitric oxide to help with management of PPHN if appropriate.

CASE 4

A 38-week gestation girl was born to a 30-year-old mother via cesarean section. Pregnancy was uncomplicated. A grade 3/6 systolic ejection murmur heard best at the mid-left sternal border and right sternal border was noted on examination while the infant was in the nursery. Because the infant was feeding well, she was discharged home at 2 days of age on Friday with instructions for follow-up with the pediatrician on Monday. She did well through the weekend, feeding every 3 hours, but on Monday morning she became more irritable, pale, and tachypneic. She was taken immediately to her pediatrician who noted poor pulses, tachycardia, respiratory distress, hepatomegaly, a hyperdynamic right ventricular impulse, and a similar ejection murmur. The infant was subsequently transferred to the emergency department of a tertiary care pediatric hospital.

Can a diagnosis be suggested?

The location of the murmur in the nursery raises suspicion of aortic stenosis. The progression of symptoms is indicative of critical aortic stenosis with duct-dependent systemic blood supply.

What are the effects of aortic valve stenosis in utero on the left ventricle?

Aortic valve stenosis results in increased left ventricular pressure and left ventricular hypertrophy. Increased left ventricular hypertrophy results in decreased left ventricular compliance, which may lead to decreased flow through the left side of the heart if severe enough. If flow through the left side of the heart is too restricted, it can affect the development of "downstream" structures, including left ventricular chamber size, aortic valve annulus size, and the size of the ascending aorta.

Explain the cardiac collapse when this patient was taken to the pediatrician.

The findings this infant exhibited are characteristic of a patient whose left ventricle is unable to handle the entire cardiac output. In this situation, the infant is dependent upon the PDA for systemic circulation. The symptoms of circulatory collapse can occur abruptly as the ductus closes. Inadequate systemic circulation results in poor peripheral pulses. The respiratory symptoms are secondary to pulmonary venous congestion. Tachycardia is a manifestation of the infant's attempt to increase cardiac output (cardiac output = stroke volume × heart rate).

In a patient such as this with severe aortic stenosis, what would one expect to see on the ECG?

Patients with aortic valve stenosis typically demonstrate voltage changes that meet the criteria for left ventricular hypertrophy, although approximately one third of patients with severe aortic stenosis may have a normal ECG. However, the findings of left ventricular hypertrophy, ST depression, and T-wave inversion are fairly specific for severe aortic stenosis.

What initial steps should be taken to stabilize this patient's condition?

This patient is clearly duct dependent, and prostaglandin E_1 infusion should be initiated immediately to restore systemic circulation. Metabolic acid-base derangements must be managed, and the hemoglobin level should be optimized. Echocardiography is essential to accurately establish the diagnosis and identify any associated lesions. This is also important to determine whether the patient may need a two-ventricle repair.

REFERENCES

The reference list for this chapter can be found online at www.expertconsult.com.

The Kidney

16

David N. Kenagy and Beth A. Vogt

Advances in neonatology, perinatology, and molecular genetics have defined new disease processes and raised new questions in the field of nephrology. For example, the advent of prenatal ultrasonography has created questions about the prenatal management of urinary tract anomalies. The use of invasive vascular catheters has led to a new set of complications, including renal artery and aortic thrombosis associated with umbilical artery catheterization. The administration of loop diuretics and steroids to infants with bronchopulmonary dysplasia has led to neonatal nephrocalcinosis. Simultaneously, genetic similarities among children whose conditions were formerly considered phenotypically distinct are redefining congenital anomalies of the kidneys and urinary tract.

This chapter reviews the anatomic and functional development of the kidney, outlines the recommended approach to evaluation of the neonate with suspected renal disease, and comments on the more common nephrologic and urologic problems seen in preterm and term neonates.

ANATOMIC DEVELOPMENT

The definitive mammalian kidney, the metanephros, starts developing at 5 weeks' gestation and begins to produce urine by 10 to 12 weeks' gestation. Development of the metanephros occurs through a series of interactions between the metanephric blastema and the ureteric bud. The ureteric bud progressively branches and grows, eventually forming the ureter, renal pelvis, and intrarenal collecting system.

At the same time, mesenchymal cells of the metanephric blastema are induced by the advancing ureteric bud to differentiate into epithelial cells that eventually become the glomeruli and renal tubules. Foci of metanephric blastema cells interact with the surrounding extracellular matrix and condense adjacent to the branching ureteric bud to form comma-shaped bodies, which then elongate to form S-shaped tubular structures (Fig. 16-1).

The lower portion of the S-shaped structure becomes associated with a tuft of capillaries and forms the glomerulus; the upper portion forms the tubular elements of the nephron.

The complex process of kidney development appears to be under the control of growth factors, a series of key regulatory genes, and renal innervation.[1-3] A number of genes that control DNA transcription are crucial in the control of cellular events in renal development.[2] For example, mutation of the transcription factor gene *PAX 2*, which is normally expressed in developing renal tissue, is associated with a syndrome characterized by vesicoureteral reflux, hypoplastic kidneys, reduced calyces, and optic nerve colobomas.[4] Mutations in another transcriptional factor gene, *WT-1*, results in renal agenesis, which suggests that this gene product may be crucial for outgrowth of the ureteric bud.[5]

FUNCTIONAL DEVELOPMENT

During intrauterine life, the kidneys play a minor role in regulating fetal salt and water balance, because this function is maintained primarily by the placenta. The primary function of the kidneys prenatally is to produce large amounts of hypotonic or isotonic urine to provide adequate amniotic fluid. After birth, a progressive maturation in renal function begins that appears to parallel the neonate's metabolic needs for growth and development. In general, maturation of most renal functions is complete by 2 years of age (Table 16-1).

RENAL BLOOD FLOW

Both absolute renal blood flow and the percentage of cardiac output directed to the kidneys increases steadily with advancing gestational age (see Table 16-1). Renal blood flow in the human fetus and term infant are estimated to be as low as 4% and 6% of the cardiac output, respectively. The relatively low renal blood flow of the neonate is related to high renal vascular resistance caused by increased levels of renin, angiotensin, aldosterone, endothelin, and catecholamines.

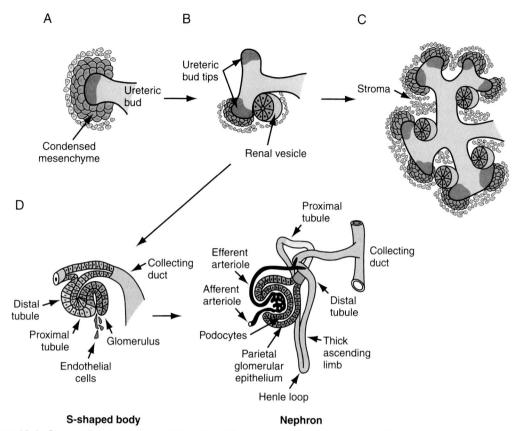

S-shaped body   **Nephron**

Figure 16-1. Stages of nephrogenesis. **A,** Induction of the metanephric mesenchyme by the ureteric bud promotes aggregation of condensed mesenchyme around the tip of the ureteric bud. **B,** Polarized renal vesicles as the mesenchyme transitions to epithelium. **C,** Fusion of renal vesicles occurs with the collecting ducts. **D,** A cleft forms in the renal vesicle, giving rise to the comma-shaped body with formation of a second proximal cleft, the S-Shaped body forms. Invasion of the proximal cleft by angioblasts leads to formation of the glomerulus. *(Redrawn from Dressler GR: The cellular basis of kidney development,* Annu Rev Cell Dev Biol *22:509–529, 2006.)*

Postnatally, there is a sharp increase in renal blood flow, which reaches 8% to 10% of cardiac output at 1 week of life and achieves adult values of 20% to 25% of cardiac output at 2 years of age. This dramatic increase in renal blood flow is related to decreasing renal vascular resistance and increasing cardiac output and perfusion pressure.

In addition to the increase in overall renal blood flow, there is a marked change in distribution of blood flow within the neonatal kidney in the postnatal period. Because of a preferential decrease in vascular resistance in the outer cortex, there is a pronounced increase in superficial renal cortical blood flow.

GLOMERULAR FILTRATION RATE

Glomerular filtration rate (GFR) in the fetal kidney increases with gestational age. By 32 to 34 weeks, a GFR of 14 mL/min/1.73 m^2

is achieved, and the rate further increases to 21 mL/min/1.73 m^2 at term (see Table 16-1). The GFR continues to increase postnatally, achieving adult values of 118 mL/min/1.73 m^2 by age 2 years. In preterm infants born before 34 weeks' gestation, the GFR remains stable until the conceptual age (gestational age plus postnatal age) exceeds 34 weeks, at which time the GFR begins to increase. Although adult values for GFR are attained by 2 years of life in term infants, achievement of adult GFR is delayed in preterm infants, especially in very low-birth-weight infants and infants with nephrocalcinosis.[6]

Several factors are responsible for the postnatal increase in GFR. The increase in GFR during the initial weeks of postnatal life is primarily due to an increase in glomerular perfusion pressure.[7] Subsequent increases in GFR during the first 2 years of life are primarily due to increases in renal

Table 16-1.	Normal Values for Renal Function				
Age	Glomerular Filtration Rate (mL/min/1.73 m^2)	Renal Blood Flow (mL/min/1.73 m^2)	Maximal Urine Osmolality (mOsm/kg)	Serum Creatinine (mg/dL)	Fractional Excretion of Sodium (%)
Newborn					
32-34 wk gestation	14 ± 3	40 ± 6	480	1.3	2-5
Full Term	21 ± 4	88 ± 4	800	1.1	<1
1-2 wk	50 ± 10	220 ± 40	900	0.4	<1
6 mo–1 yr	77 ± 14	352 ± 73	1200	0.2	<1
1-3 yr	96 ± 22	540 ± 118	1400	0.4	<1
Adult	118 ± 18	620 ± 92	1400	0.8-1.5	<1

Adapted from Avner ED, Ellis D, Ichikawa I, et al: Normal neonates and maturational development of homeostatic mechanism. In Ichikawa I, editor: *Pediatric textbook of fluids and electrolytes,* Baltimore, 1990, Williams & Wilkins.

Table 16-2.	Change in Body Water with Maturation		
	% Body Weight		
Age	Extracellular Fluid	Intracellular Fluid	Total Body Fluid
Gestational			
14 wk	65	27	92
28 wk	55	25	80
40 wk	45	30	75
Postnatal			
14 wk	25	40	65

Adapted from Sulyok E: Postnatal adaptation. In Holliday MA, Barratt TM, Avner ED, editors: *Pediatric nephrology,* Baltimore, 1994, Williams & Wilkins.

blood flow and maturation of superficial cortical nephrons, which lead to an increase in glomerular filtration surface area.

During the first week of postnatal life, an infant's GFR passes through three distinct phases to maintain fluid and electrolyte homeostasis. The initial 24 hours of life (prediuretic phase) is characterized by a transitory increase in GFR at 2 to 4 hours of life followed by a return to low baseline GFR and minimal urine output regardless of salt and water intake. This phase may extend up to 36 hours of life in the preterm infant, with delay in onset of the transitory increase in GFR. During the second and third days of life (diuretic phase), the GFR increases rapidly, and the infant experiences diuresis and natriuresis regardless of salt and water intake. By the fourth to fifth day of life (postdiuretic phase), the GFR decreases slightly, then continues to increase slowly with maturation, with salt and water excretion varying according to intake.

Importantly, the duration and timing of these phases differ among infants, so that individualization of fluid and electrolyte

therapy is required. If insensible fluid losses are overestimated during the prediuretic phase, excess fluid intake may result in dilutional hyponatremia. On the other hand, a deficiency in fluid intake during this phase may lead to volume contraction and hypernatremia. During the diuretic phase, hypernatremia may develop as a result of excessive urinary fluid losses.

FLUID COMPARTMENTS

The change in distribution of intracellular fluid (ICF) and extracellular fluid (ECF) in the fetus and newborn infant is summarized in Table 16-2. In the healthy term infant, ECF volume decreases and ICF volume increases in the first few days of life.[8] In the preterm infant, total body water decreases, primarily as a result of ECF losses in the first week of life, a process that is delayed in infants with respiratory distress syndrome. The change in ICF during the first week of life is variable and may be dependent on total energy intake and corresponding change in body weight during this period. For example, in preterm infants with more than a 10%

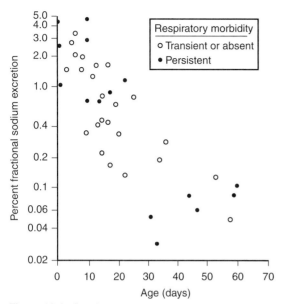

Figure 16-2. Fractional excretion of sodium in neonates born at 28 to 33 weeks of gestation during the first 2 months of life. *(From Ross B, Cowett RM, Oh W: Renal functions of low birth weight infants during the first two months of life,* Pediatr Res *11:1162, 1997.)*

loss in body weight during the first week of life, there is a decrease in ECF without an increase in ICF.

Capillary filtration between the intravascular and interstitial fluid compartments is higher in the neonatal period than it is later in life, which leads to a relatively large interstitial fluid compartment. This phenomenon may be due to a number of factors, including increased hydrostatic pressure, decreased intravascular osmotic pressure, and increased levels of atrial natriuretic factor, vasopressin, and cortisol.[9] The relatively large interstitial fluid compartment enables the neonate to better tolerate hemorrhage because the large volumes of interstitial fluid can shift into the intravascular space, but it may also lead to reduced ability to excrete a free water load.

SODIUM HANDLING

Renal sodium losses are inversely proportional to gestational age, and the fractional excretion of sodium (FE_{Na}) may be as high as 5% to 6% in infants born at 28 weeks' gestation (Fig. 16-2). As a result, preterm infants younger than 35 weeks' gestation may display negative sodium balance and hyponatremia during the initial 2 to 3 weeks of life due to high renal sodium losses and inefficient intestinal sodium absorption.[10] Up to 4 to 5 mEq/kg/day of sodium may be necessary in preterm infants to offset high renal sodium losses during the first few weeks of life.

Healthy term neonates have basal sodium handling similar to that of adults, as demonstrated by an FE_{Na} of less than 1.0%, although a transient increase in FE_{Na} occurs during the second and third days of life (diuretic phase). Urinary sodium losses may be increased in certain conditions, including renal dysplasia, hypoxia, respiratory distress, hyperbilirubinemia, acute tubular necrosis (ATN), polycythemia, increased fluid and salt intake, and the use of theophylline or diuretics.[7] Pharmacologic agents such as dopamine, labetalol, propranolol, captopril, and enalaprilat that influence adrenergic neural pathways in the kidney and the renin-angiotensin axis may also increase urinary sodium losses in the neonate.

The mechanisms responsible for increased urinary sodium losses in the preterm infant are multifactorial. Glomerulotubular imbalance, which occurs when GFR exceeds the reabsorptive capacity of the renal tubules, occurs because of the preponderance of glomeruli compared with tubular structures, renal tubular immaturity, large extracellular volume, and reduced oxygen availability.[11] Decreased renal nerve activity may also contribute; studies in fetal and newborn sheep demonstrate an inverse relationship between renal nerve stimulation and urine sodium excretion.[11] Finally, fetal and postnatal kidneys exhibit diminished responsiveness to aldosterone compared with adult kidneys, which results in the attenuation of sodium reabsorption.[12]

URINARY CONCENTRATION AND DILUTION

As noted in Table 16-1, renal concentrating capacity is low at birth and progressively increases following delivery from 800 mOsm/kg H_2O in the first 2 weeks of life to adult values of 1400 mOsm/kg H_2O between 1 and 3 years of age.[13] This improvement in ability to excrete a concentrated urine is due to increased urea generation, improved end-organ responsiveness to vasopressin, and anatomic maturation of the renal medulla and its vasculature.

The ability of the neonatal kidney to excrete a water load is somewhat limited in comparison with that of the adult kidney. For example, term and premature newborns can dilute their urine to an osmolality of

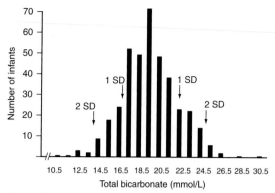

Figure 16-3. Frequency distribution of serum total bicarbonate level in low-birth-weight neonates during the first month of life. *(From Schwartz GJ, Haycock GB, Chir B, et al: Late metabolic acidosis: a reassessment of the definition,* J Pediatr *95:102, 1979.)*

50 mOsm/kg and 70 mOsm/kg, respectively, whereas adults can dilute their urine to 30 mOsm.[13] This inability to maximally dilute the urine is due to reduced GFR as well as to decreased activity of transporters in the early distal tubule (diluting segment), which are most prominent in the preterm infant.[14]

ACID-BASE BALANCE

The range of normal serum bicarbonate levels is lower than that of adults, and infants maintain a mild metabolic acidosis (Fig. 16-3). This limitation in acid-base homeostasis seen in neonates, particularly preterm infants, is related to immaturity of both proximal and distal tubular function.

The proximal tubular bicarbonate threshold, defined as the steady-state serum bicarbonate level above which significant amounts of bicarbonate appear in the urine, is much lower in neonates than in adults, which leads to incomplete bicarbonate reabsorption. The cause of the low proximal tubular bicarbonate threshold is unknown. Studies in the fetal lamb have demonstrated that renal tubular reabsorption of bicarbonate is inversely proportional to ECF volume.[15] Therefore, expanded ECF compartment characteristic of the preterm and term infant may be related to the low renal bicarbonate threshold and low plasma bicarbonate concentration. Limited distal tubular excretion of titratable acid and incomplete development of tubular ammonia production also contribute to the relative metabolic acidosis of the newborn.

Newborn infants may display two forms of acidosis. In the first 24 hours of life, an early type of combined respiratory and metabolic acidosis may develop as a result of stress during birth and disturbances in cardiopulmonary adaptation. Late metabolic acidosis, on the other hand, may develop during the first week of life and is most pronounced in the second and third weeks of life. This type of acidosis is due to an imbalance between net acid input, primarily from dietary protein intake and bone mineralization, and renal capacity for net acid excretion. Late metabolic acidosis may result in poor weight gain or skeletal growth. Late metabolic acidosis usually resolves spontaneously by the end of the first month of life as a result of the rapid postnatal increase in the renal capacity for net acid excretion.

An important consequence of chronic metabolic acidosis in the newborn is enhanced urinary calcium losses, negative calcium balance, and bone demineralization, which may contribute to the phenomenon of osteopenia of prematurity. The mechanism for this process is multifactorial. Acidosis causes release of calcium from bones directly and via parathyroid hormone secretion. Acidosis also inhibits intestinal calcium absorption and impairs 1α-hydroxylation of 25-hydroxyvitamin D. Finally, acidosis increases urinary flow rate and urinary calcium excretion.[16] Therefore, persistent metabolic acidosis should be corrected with sodium bicarbonate, with a goal of achieving a serum bicarbonate level of 17 to 18 mEq/L.

CALCIUM AND PHOSPHORUS BALANCE

Within 24 to 48 hours after birth, the serum calcium concentration decreases, a phenomenon that is most pronounced in preterm infants.[17] Although the exact mechanism of neonatal hypocalcemia is unknown, it appears to be due to suppressed parathyroid hormone secretion and elevated plasma phosphate concentration. In most neonates, the ionized calcium level remains above a physiologically acceptable concentration and the infant experiences no clinical symptoms. Symptomatic hypocalcemia may occur, however, in neonates stressed by illness or in the presence of aggressive fluid administration, diuresis, and sodium supplementation, all of which increase urinary calcium losses.

The normal serum phosphorus level in the newborn ranges from 4.5 to 9.5 mg/dL, whereas adult values are 3.0 to 4.5 mg/dL. The higher serum phosphorus level in the newborn is due to enhanced dietary phosphorus intake, particularly in infants fed cow's milk formulas; lower GFR; and higher tubular reabsorption of phosphorus. Tubular reabsorption of phosphorus is lower, however, in preterm infants and increases progressively during gestation as a result of maturation of renal tubular function. The phosphorus losses seen in premature infants cause relative phosphorus deficiency, which may result in inadequate bone mineralization. For premature infants, therefore, greater attention must be given to nutritional supplies of phosphorus and calcium in enteral and parenteral formulations.

EVALUATION

The evaluation of an infant with suspected renal disease must be comprehensive and begins with a careful history taking and thorough physical examination. Selected laboratory studies may be useful in determining the cause and severity of renal dysfunction. Limited radiologic evaluation may be useful in clarifying renal anatomy and detecting complications of vascular catheters.

HISTORY

Results of prenatal ultrasonography should be carefully reviewed with particular attention to kidney size, echogenicity, malformations, amniotic fluid volume, and bladder size and shape.[18] The presence of unilateral or bilateral small or enlarged kidneys, renal cysts, hydronephrosis, bladder enlargement, or oligohydramnios may suggest significant renal or urologic abnormalities.

The causes of congenital renal disease are multifactorial but may include exposure to teratogens.[19] The antenatal history should be reviewed, with particular attention given to medications, toxins, or unusual exposures during the pregnancy. Congenital renal anomalies have been described in infants with antenatal exposure to angiotensin-converting enzyme inhibitors,[20,21] angiotensin receptor blockers,[21] nonsteroidal antiinflammatory drugs,[19,22] gentamicin, corticosteroids,[23] calcineurin inhibitors,[19] and cocaine.[24]

Review of the family medical history should include information on any prior fetal or neonatal deaths. Although there is no hereditary cause for most congenital renal anomalies, there is a clear genetic basis for certain diseases such as polycystic kidney disease and nephronophthisis.

PHYSICAL EXAMINATION

Evaluation of blood pressure and volume status is critical in the newborn with suspected renal disease. Hypertension may be present in infants with autosomal recessive polycystic kidney disease, acute renal failure, or renovascular or aortic thrombosis. Hypotension, on the other hand, in addition to cardiovascular disorders, may suggest volume depletion, hemorrhage, or sepsis, all of which may lead to acute renal failure. Edema may be seen in acute renal failure, in hydrops fetalis, or with massive urinary protein losses associated with congenital nephrotic syndrome. Ascites may be seen in acute renal failure with volume overload, congenital nephrotic syndrome, or urinary tract obstruction with rupture.

Special attention should be paid to the abdominal examination. In the neonate, the lower pole of both kidneys should be easily palpable because of the neonate's reduced abdominal muscle tone. An abdominal mass present in a newborn should be assumed to involve the urinary tract until proven otherwise, because the majority of neonatal abdominal masses are genitourinary in origin.[25] The most common renal cause of an abdominal mass is hydronephrosis, followed by multicystic dysplastic kidney. Less common causes of an abdominal mass are polycystic kidney disease, renal vein thrombosis, ectopic or fused kidneys, renal hematoma or abscess, and renal tumors. The newborn bladder should be able to be percussed just above the symphysis pubis and, if it is enlarged, lower urinary tract obstruction should be suspected. A palpable prostate in a male newborn is always abnormal and suggests posterior urethral valves. The abdomen should be examined for absence or laxity of the abdominal muscles, which may suggest Eagle-Barrett (prune-belly) syndrome.

A number of anomalies should alert the physician to the possibility of underlying renal defects, including abnormal ears, aniridia, microcephaly, meningomyelocele, pectus excavatum, hemihypertrophy, persistent urachus, bladder or cloacal exstrophy, abnormality of the external genitalia, cryptorchidism, imperforate anus, and limb deformities. A single umbilical artery should raise suspicion of renal disease. In one study, 7% of otherwise normal infants with a single umbilical artery were found to have significant persistent renal anomalies.[26] The utility of screening all infants with a single umbilical artery, however, remains controversial.

A constellation of physical findings called the *Potter sequence* may be seen in infants with bilateral renal agenesis. Lack of fetal renal function results in severe oligohydramnios, which causes fetal deformation by uterine wall compression. The characteristic facial features include wide-set eyes, depressed nasal bridge, beaked nose, receding chin, and posteriorly rotated, low-set ears. Other associated anomalies include a small, compressed chest wall and arthrogryposis. The condition is uniformly fatal. "Potter-like" features may be noted in infants with in utero urinary tract obstruction or chronic amniotic fluid leakage. In this group of infants, pulmonary and renal function are generally not as severely impaired and the prognosis is less grim. In infants with significant renal defects, pneumothorax or pneumomediastinum are common clinical associations related to varying degrees of pulmonary hypoplasia.

URINALYSIS

Twenty-five percent of male infants and 7% of female infants void at the time of delivery. Although 98% of full-term infants void in the first 30 hours of life,[29] a delay in urination for up to 48 hours should not be a cause for immediate concern in the absence of a palpable bladder, abdominal mass, or other signs or symptoms of renal disease. Failure to void for longer than 48 hours should prompt further investigation, including kidney and bladder ultrasonography to rule out urinary tract anomalies.

Evaluation of the urine is a vital part of the examination of any neonate suspected of having a urinary tract abnormality. Collection of an adequate, uncontaminated specimen is difficult in the neonate. A specimen collected by cleaning the perineum and applying a sterile adhesive plastic bag enables analysis of urinary protein or electrolytes. Tests for heme and cultures may give erroneous results. For cultures, bladder catheterization produces a reliable specimen but may be technically difficult in preterm infants. Suprapubic bladder aspiration has been considered the collection method of choice in infants without intraabdominal abnormalities or bleeding disorders, although anecdotal evidence suggests that few clinicians opt for that approach.

Analysis of the urine should include inspection, measurement of specific gravity, urinary dipstick testing, and microscopic analysis. The urine of newborns is usually clear and nearly colorless. Cloudiness may be caused by either urinary tract infection or the presence of crystals. A yellow-brown to deep olive-green color may indicate increasing amounts of conjugated bilirubin. Porphyrins, certain drugs such as phenytoin, bacteria, and urate crystals may stain the diaper pink and be confused with bleeding. Brown urine suggests bleeding from the upper urinary tract, hemoglobinuria, or myoglobinuria.

Urinary specific gravity may be measured using a clinical refractometer or a urinary dipstick. The specific gravity of neonatal urine is usually very low (<1.004) but may be factitiously elevated by high-molecular-weight solutes such as contrast agents, glucose or other reducing substances, or large amounts of protein. Gouyon and Houchan showed that dipstick estimation of urinary specific gravity was an unreliable test of urinary concentrating ability in the neonate and suggested that urinary osmolarity is a more reliable measure of the kidney's concentrating and diluting ability.[30]

Urine dipstick evaluation can detect the presence of heme-containing compounds (red blood cells, myoglobin, and hemoglobin), protein, and glucose. White blood cell products such as leukocyte esterase and nitrite may also be detected by urine dipstick and should raise suspicion of urinary tract infection, which should prompt the clinician to order a urine culture. Microscopic urinalysis should be performed if the urinary dipstick result is abnormal and is useful in detecting the presence of red blood cells, casts, white blood cells, bacteria, and crystals.

LABORATORY EVALUATION

Clinical evaluation of neonatal renal function begins with measurement of serum creatinine level. As discussed previously, normal values for serum creatinine vary with gestational age and postnatal age (see Table 16-1). The serum creatinine level is relatively high at birth, with normal values up to 1.1 mg/dL in term babies and 1.3 mg/dL in preterm infants, but decreases to a mean value of 0.4 mg/dL within the first 2 weeks of life.[13] In general, each doubling of the serum creatinine level represents a 50% reduction in GFR; for example, an increase in creatinine concentration from 0.4 mg/dL to 0.8 mg/dL reflects a 50% reduction in GFR. The Schwartz formula, which estimates GFR using serum creatinine level and body length, has been applied to normal preterm and term infants. Recently, the methodology for measuring serum creatinine has changed from the Jaffe method to one involving the plasma disappearance of iohexol. This has led to a revision of the Schwartz formula for children aged 1 to 16 years.[31] The new formula, which has not yet been studied in term or preterm infants, is as follows:

$$\text{Estimated GFR} = \frac{0.413 \times \text{Height}}{(\text{Cr})}$$

where GFR is expressed in milliliters per minute per 1.73 m^2; height is expressed in centimeters; and creatinine (Cr) concentration is expressed in milligrams per deciliter.

RADIOLOGIC EVALUATION

Renal ultrasonography is the initial procedure of choice in infants with suspected renal disease.[25] Renal ultrasonography offers a noninvasive anatomic evaluation of the urinary tract without the use of contrast agents or radiation exposure. Renal ultrasonography can demonstrate kidney size and morphology, presence of nephrocalcinosis or nephrolithiasis, complications of infection (renal abscess, perinephric abscess), obstruction (hydronephrosis, hydroureter), and bladder morphology.

Voiding cystourethrography is the procedure of choice to evaluate the urethra and bladder and to ascertain the presence or absence of vesicoureteral reflux. This study involves urinary catheterization and instillation of radiopaque dye into the infant's bladder. A voiding cystourethrogram should be considered in all infants with urinary tract obstruction, renal dysplasia or anomaly, or documented urinary tract infection.

Other radiologic tests may occasionally be used for diagnostic purposes in the neonate. A technetium 99m (^{99}mTc) MAG-3 (mercaptoacetyltriglycine) or ^{99}mTc DTPA (diethylene triamine pentaacetic acid) diuretic renal scan may be helpful in confirming urinary tract obstruction in an infant with hydronephrosis or hydroureter on ultrasonography. A renal scan using ^{99}mTc DMSA (dimercaptosuccinic acid) or ^{99}mTc glucoheptonate may help to identify renal scarring related to prior pyelonephritis or umbilical artery catheter–related embolic phenomenon. Computerized tomography may be helpful in evaluating suspected renal abscess, mass, or nephrolithiasis.

SPECIFIC PROBLEMS

HEMATURIA AND PROTEINURIA

At 16 hours of age, a 4300-g 41-week infant born to a mother with gestational diabetes develops macroscopic hematuria. Physical examination reveals a listless, pale infant with a large left flank mass. Urinalysis demonstrates hematuria (4+) with more than 250 red blood cells/mm.[32] Laboratory findings include a hematocrit of 36%, a platelet count of 75,000/mm^3, and a serum creatinine concentration of 1.0 mg/dL. Renal ultrasonography shows an enlarged left kidney with impaired venous flow by Doppler study, consistent with renal vein thrombosis.

The infant is treated conservatively with hydration and careful observation of fluid balance and renal function. Within 48 hours, the macroscopic hematuria resolves and renal function remains stable. Serial ultrasound examinations reveal gradual resolution of the thrombosis over the next 7 days, with improvement in renal venous blood flow. At 6 months of age, the infant's serum creatinine concentration is 0.4 mg/dL and renal ultrasound findings are normal.

Hematuria may be suspected by urinary dipstick testing (microscopic) or visual examination (macroscopic or gross). Confirmation of hematuria requires microscopic examination showing at least 5 red blood cells per high-power field. A positive urinary dipstick result with negative findings on microscopic examination for red blood cells suggests myoglobinuria or hemoglobinuria. Myoglobinuria may be seen in infants with inherited metabolic myopathies, infectious myositis, and rhabdomyolysis related to prolonged seizure activity, corticosteroid use, or direct muscle trauma. Hemoglobinuria may be present in erythroblastosis fetalis and other forms of hemolytic disease.

The most frequent cause of hematuria in the neonate is ATN following birth asphyxia, exposure to nephrotoxic drugs, or sepsis. Another important cause of hematuria is renal vein thrombosis, which must be considered in infants of diabetic mothers and in infants with cyanotic congenital heart disease, polycythemia, or marked dehydration. Other causes of hematuria are urinary tract infection, blood dyscrasias, bladder hemangioma, renal tumor, nephrolithiasis, congenital urinary tract malformations, and cortical necrosis. Glomerulonephritis, which represents a common cause of hematuria in childhood and adolescence, is extremely uncommon in the neonatal population.

Proteinuria is defined as a urinary dipstick reading of 1+ (30 mg/dL) or higher with a specific gravity of 1.015 or less, or a reading of 2+ (100 mg/dL) or higher with a specific gravity of more than 1.015. False-positive dipstick readings for protein may result from very concentrated urine, alkaline urine, infection, and detergents. Average quantitative protein excretion declines with increasing gestational age, from 182 mg/m^2 per 24 hours in premature infants to 145 mg/m^2 per 24 hours in full-term infants to 108 mg/m^2 per 24 hours in infants 2 to 12 months of age.[33]

Common causes of neonatal proteinuria include ATN, fever, dehydration, cardiac failure, high-dose penicillin therapy, and contrast agent administration. Persistent massive proteinuria and edema in a neonate should prompt consideration of congenital nephrotic syndrome, an autosomal recessive disorder characterized by proteinuria, failure to thrive, large placenta, and chronic renal dysfunction.

ACUTE KIDNEY INJURY

A 2300-g female infant is delivered after a 36-week uncomplicated pregnancy. Fetal decelerations were noted before delivery, and a tight nuchal cord is present. Apgar scores are 1 at 1 minute and 4 at 5 minutes. The infant is resuscitated using intubation, compressions, and epinephrine. Arterial blood gas analysis shows a pH of 7.10, P_{CO_2} of 54 mm Hg, and P_{O_2} of 93 mm Hg. Initial laboratory work reveals normal electrolyte levels and a serum creatinine concentration of 0.9 mg/dL.

Over the next 3 days, the infant becomes oliguric, and laboratory results are as follows: Na, 127 mmol/L; K, 6.5 mmol/L; Cl, 106 mmol/L; HCO_3, 15 mmol/L; blood urea nitrogen, 18 mg/dL; and creatinine, 2.0 mg/dL. Urinalysis shows hematuria (2+) and proteinuria (1+). Renal ultrasonography shows hyperechoic parenchyma without evidence of renal dysplasia or obstruction. Peritoneal dialysis is initiated for supportive treatment of presumed ATN. After 10 days, dialysis is discontinued as the infant's renal function recovers. The infant is discharged home at 21 days of age with a serum creatinine concentration of 1.0 mg/dL. Follow-up laboratory work 6 weeks later shows the serum creatinine level to be 0.5 mg/dL.

Acute kidney injury (AKI) is characterized by a sudden impairment in renal function that leads to an inability of the kidneys to excrete nitrogenous wastes. Both the clinical care of infants and studies of AKI are complicated by the difficulty of defining the condition. A consensus definition of AKI based on biomarkers is a serum creatinine level of more than 1.5 mg/dL.[34] Creatinine, however, is a metabolic product of muscle. Normal levels reflect maternal levels initially and fall as the infant's production and excretion find their own steady state. Clinically, oliguric AKI is characterized by a urine flow rate of less than 0.5 to 1 mL/kg/hr, whereas in nonoliguric AKI, urine flow rate is maintained at a higher level. This measure of renal function is unreliable when diuretics have been administered. A prospective study of 229 infants found the incidence of AKI to be 18% among very low-birth-weight infants.[35] The causes of neonatal AKI are multiple and can be divided into prerenal, renal, and postrenal categories (Box 16-1).

| Box 16-1. | Causes of Acute Renal Failure in the Neonate |

Prerenal
Dehydration
Hemorrhage
Sepsis
Necrotizing enterocolitis
Congestive heart failure
Drugs: angiotensin-converting enzyme inhibitors, nonsteroidal antiinflammatory agents, amphotericin, tolazoline

Intrinsic
Acute tubular necrosis
Renal dysplasia
Polycystic kidney disease
Renal vein thrombosis
Uric acid nephropathy
Transient acute renal insufficiency of the newborn

Postrenal
Posterior urethral valves
Bilateral ureteropelvic junction obstruction
Bilateral ureterovesical junction obstruction
Neurogenic bladder
Obstructive nephrolithiasis

EDITORIAL COMMENT: Acute kidney injury (AKI) is a common clinical problem in neonatal intensive care units and is usually associated with a contributing condition such as hypovolemia, hypotension, or hypoxia, often due to sepsis, asphyxia, and heart failure. Attention has been focused on biomarkers for AKI that might enable early recognition and prompt interventions to limit renal injury. The level of neutrophil gelatinase–associated lipocalin (NGAL), and specifically urinary NGAL (UNGAL), predicts renal failure sooner than serum creatinine level, and the immunoassay can be done as quickly as creatinine determination.[36]

Neonatologists tend to focus on the lung, brain, and gastrointestinal tract, giving little attention to the kidney. This needs to change. In the first prospective epidemiologic study addressing AKI in preterm infants with a birth weight of less than 1500 g, 18% of 229 infants manifested AKI when a creatinine-based definition was used.[37] However, because the investigators did not measure serum creatinine concentration in every infant every day, this number may be an underestimate. Furthermore, AKI is a serious condition, and there is an independent association between AKI and mortality when analyzed both by gestational age and by birth weight. Most infants who developed AKI were extremely premature and developed AKI within the first week of life. Sicker babies whose condition was depressed at birth

and who required mechanical ventilation and blood pressure support in addition to umbilical artery catheterization were most likely to manifest AKI. The next steps are to identify early and reliable markers of AKI, intervene appropriately, and improve outcomes. These infants all need long-term follow-up to monitor their renal function and watch for the onset of hypertension.

Prerenal Acute Kidney Injury
Prerenal (functional) AKI is the most common type of AKI in the neonate and accounts for up to 85% of neonatal AKI.[37] Prerenal AKI is characterized by inadequate renal perfusion, which, if promptly treated, is followed by improvement in renal function and urine output. If glomerulotubular injury occurs as a consequence of inadequate renal perfusion, the constellation of clinical and laboratory findings constitute AKI. The most common causes of prerenal AKI are hypotension (dehydration, hemorrhage, septic shock, necrotizing enterocolitis) and renal hypoperfusion (patent ductus arteriosus, congestive heart failure, asphyxia) as well as medications that reduce renal blood flow, such as nonsteroidal antiinflammatory drugs (indomethacin) and angiotensin-converting enzyme inhibitors (enalaprilat).

Intrinsic Acute Kidney Injury
ATN is one of the most common manifestations of intrinsic AKI in neonates. Causes of ATN include perinatal asphyxia, sepsis, cardiac surgery, prolonged prerenal state, and administration of nephrotoxic drugs (indomethacin and aminoglycoside antibiotics). The pathophysiology of ATN is complex and appears to involve renal tubular cellular injury, alterations in adhesion molecules, and changes in renal hemodynamics. Cellular injury results from decreased adenosine triphosphate (ATP), increased intracellular calcium influx, and the destructive action of phospholipases, free radicals, and proteases. Alterations in cellular adhesion molecules lead to sloughing of injured tubular epithelial cells and subsequent luminal obstruction. Increased endothelin as well as decreased prostaglandins and nitric oxide activity result in markedly decreased renal blood flow.

Other less common causes of intrinsic renal failure in the newborn include renal dysplasia, autosomal recessive polycystic kidney disease, and renal vein thrombosis. Uric acid nephropathy may represent an underrecognized cause of AKI in the neonatal population and may occur when uric acid crystals precipitate in the lumen of the nephron following hypoxia, hemolysis, rhabdomyolysis, or cardiac surgery. Finally, neonatal transient renal failure is a poorly understood, rapidly reversible syndrome characterized by oliguric AKI and hyperechogenic renal medullary pyramids on ultrasonography.[38] This syndrome has been reported in otherwise healthy full-term infants with sluggish feeding and is thought to be related to deposition of uric acid crystals and/or Tamm-Horsfall protein in the renal tubular collecting system.

Postrenal Acute Kidney Injury

Postrenal (obstructive) AKI is caused by bilateral obstruction of the urinary tract and can be reversed by relief of the obstruction. Obstructive AKI in the neonate may be related to a variety of congenital urinary tract conditions, including posterior urethral valves, bilateral ureteropelvic or ureterovesical junction obstruction, obstructive nephrolithiasis, or neurogenic bladder. Extrinsic compression of the ureters or bladder by a congenital tumor such as a sacrococcygeal teratoma and intrinsic obstruction by renal calculi or fungus balls are rare causes of obstructive AKI.

Evaluation of the Neonate with Acute Kidney Injury

For neonates with AKI a careful history should be taken that focuses on prenatal ultrasonographic abnormalities, perinatal asphyxia, systemic illness, administration of potentially nephrotoxic drugs, and family history of renal disease. Physical examination should focus on the abdomen, genitalia, and a search for other congenital anomalies or signs of Potter sequence. Levels of electrolytes (including acid-base status), blood urea nitrogen, creatinine, calcium, phosphorus, and uric acid should be monitored at least daily and more frequently if significant metabolic abnormalities are present. Urine should be sent for urinalysis, urine culture, and urine sodium and creatinine determination. Calculation of FE_{Na} may be helpful in differentiating prerenal AKI from intrinsic AKI. This calculation is a sensitive measure of tubular injury.

$$FE_{Na} = \frac{[Na_{urine}] \times [Cr_{plasma}]}{[Na_{plasma}] \times [Cr_{urine}]} \times 100\%$$

Neonates with an FE_{Na} of more than 2.5% to 3.0% generally have intrinsic AKI, whereas those with an FE_{Na} of less than 1.0% have prerenal AKI. Prematurity, however, is associated with immaturity of Na^+,K^+-ATPase, which results in a higher FE_{Na} under normal circumstances. As mentioned earlier, the ability of creatinine concentration to assess glomerular filtration is limited. New biomarkers that are not affected by muscle mass are emerging but have not yet been validated in this population. Of these, neutrophil gelatinase-associated lipocalin (NGAL), kidney injury molecule 1, and cystatin C have been studied in AKI following cardiac surgery.[39]

Renal ultrasonography is helpful in the identification of congenital renal disease and urinary tract obstruction. Voiding cystourethrography should be performed in neonates with suspected posterior urethral valves, vesicoureteral reflux, or bladder abnormality.

Medical Management

If the neonate is oliguric, a urinary catheter should be placed to rule out lower urinary tract obstruction. If there is no improvement in urine output after bladder drainage is established, a fluid challenge of 10 to 20 mL/kg should be administered over 1 to 2 hours to rule out prerenal AKI. A lack of improvement in urine output and serum creatinine concentration after adequate drainage of the urinary tract and volume resuscitation suggests intrinsic AKI, and fluids should be restricted to insensible losses (500 mL/m²) plus urine output and other losses. Daily weights and careful intake and output measurements are optimal to follow volume status.

The goal of medical management of established intrinsic AKI is to provide supportive care until there is spontaneous improvement in the infant's renal function. Nephrotoxic drugs should be discontinued to reduce the risk of additional renal injury. Medications should be adjusted by dose and interval according to the degree of renal dysfunction. Potassium and phosphorus should be restricted in neonates with hyperkalemia or hyperphosphatemia. Metabolic acidosis may require treatment with intravenous or oral sodium bicarbonate. Loop and thiazide diuretics may prove helpful in augmenting urinary flow rate. The role of low-dose dopamine in neonatal AKI management remains unproven.

Renal Replacement Therapy

Renal replacement therapy (RRT) refers to all technologies that substitute for the work of native kidneys. RRT should be considered if maximal medical management fails to maintain acceptable fluid and electrolyte status. The two purposes of RRT are ultrafiltration (removal of water) and dialysis (removal of solutes). Indications for initiation of RRT include hyperkalemia, hyponatremia, acidosis, hypocalcemia, hyperphosphatemia, symptomatic volume overload, uremic symptoms, and inability to provide adequate nutrition (Box 16-2).

Peritoneal dialysis is the most commonly employed renal replacement modality in the neonatal population, because it is less technically difficult and does not require vascular access or anticoagulation. In this procedure, hyperosmolar dialysate is repeatedly infused into and drained out of the peritoneal cavity via a catheter, accomplishing both ultrafiltration and dialysis (Fig. 16-4). Cycle length, dwell volume, and the osmolar concentration of the dialysate can be varied to accomplish the goals of therapy. Relative contraindications to peritoneal dialysis include recent abdominal surgery, necrotizing enterocolitis, pleuroperitoneal leak, and ventriculoperitoneal shunt.

Continuous renal replacement therapy (CRRT) is becoming a more practical option for RRT in children who are in hemodynamically unstable condition.[40] In this procedure, the neonate's blood is continuously circulated through an extracorporeal circuit containing a highly permeable hemofilter. An ultrafiltrate of plasma is removed, and a smaller volume of fluid is returned to the patient. This smaller volume is a physiologic replacement fluid. The two CRRT modalities are continuous venovenous hemofiltration (CVVH) and continuous venovenous hemodialysis (CVVHD). CVVH removes solute by convection, whereas CVVHD removes solute primarily by diffusion. The chief advantage of CRRT is that it allows continuous control of fluid removal, which makes this modality especially useful in the neonate with hemodynamic instability. The main disadvantages are the need to achieve and maintain central vascular access and the need for continuous anticoagulation. Limiting factors are the size of catheter that the child can tolerate and the ability to obtain flow through the catheter without occlusion by thrombi.

Acute hemodialysis is a less commonly employed, but technically feasible, mode of RRT in the neonatal population. Hemodialysis involves intermittent 3- to 4-hour treatments in which fluids and solutes are rapidly removed from the infant using an extracorporeal dialyzer with rapid countercurrent dialysate flow. The chief advantage of hemodialysis is the ability to rapidly remove solutes or fluid, a characteristic that makes this modality the therapy of choice in neonatal hyperammonemia, although CRRT has also been used successfully in the management of inborn errors of metabolism. Critically

Box 16-2.	**Indications for Dialysis**

Hyperkalemia
Hyponatremia
Acidosis
Hypocalcemia
Hyperphosphatemia
Volume overload
Uremic symptoms
Inability to provide adequate nutrition

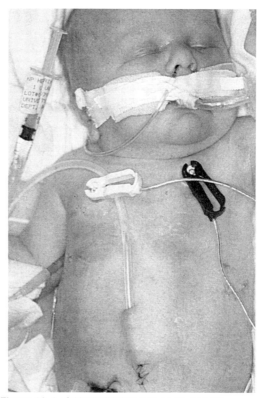

Figure 16-4. Critically ill infant with acute renal failure undergoing treatment with peritoneal dialysis. *(Courtesy Julie H. Corder, PNP, Rainbow Babies and Children's Hospital, Cleveland.)*

ill neonates may experience hemodynamic instability and osmolar shifts with the rapid solute and fluid movement associated with intermittent hemodialysis.

Prognosis

The prognosis for neonates with AKI is variable. In general, infants with prerenal AKI who receive prompt treatment for renal hypoperfusion have an excellent prognosis. The outcome for infants with postrenal AKI related to congenital urinary tract obstruction depends on the degree of associated renal dysplasia. Infants with intrinsic AKI have the poorest prognosis.

Survival differs, depending on the cause of AKI. Blowey et al reported that neonates with renal structural anomalies had a 17% mortality rate, whereas those with ATN had a 55% mortality rate.[41] After adjustment for potential confounders, very low-birth-weight infants with AKI have a higher chance of death, with an adjusted hazard ratio of 2.4 (95% confidence interval: 0.95 to 6.04).[35]

Kidney survival may be improving. In Blowey et al's 1993 study of 23 infants who received peritoneal dialysis in the first month of life, at 1 year 30% were receiving dialysis, 9% had chronic kidney disease, and 26% had made a full renal recovery; 35% died in the neonatal period.[41] In 2003, decreased GFR was reported in 45% of extremely low-birth-weight infants who sustained neonatal AKI.[42] In 2009, Mortazavi et al reported that 76% of Iranian infants who had developed AKI were discharged with normal kidney function and 3% with diminished kidney function.[43] In this population renal disease was due to intrinsic AKI in 52%, prerenal AKI in 42%, and postrenal AKI in 5%. Perinatal asphyxia was present in 30% of the neonates, sepsis in 29%, respiratory distress syndrome in 25%, dehydration in 24%, and heart failure in 21%. Eight-five percent of patients had more than one contributing condition.[43] Risk factors for the development of long-term impairment of GFR include multisystem failure, hypotension, need for pressors, hemodynamic instability, need for mechanical ventilation, and need for dialysis. Therefore, high-risk neonates who appear to have recovered from acute renal failure should be followed carefully over time, because they may be at risk for late development of chronic kidney disease.

HYPERTENSION

A 4500-g term male infant develops respiratory distress and clinical features consistent with pulmonary hypertension of the newborn. Blood pressure is 70/40 mm Hg. Mechanical ventilation is initiated and an umbilical artery catheter is placed to the level of T8. On day 7 of life, the blood pressure is noted to be 116/78 mm Hg.

Serum electrolyte levels are normal and creatinine concentration is 0.7 mg/dL. Ultrasonography reveals an irregularly shaped thrombus measuring 1.5 cm in length in the abdominal aorta, partially occluding the right renal artery. The infant is initially given sodium nitroprusside and furosemide to control blood pressure and is later converted to oral captopril. At 6 months of age, the child's creatinine level is 0.4 mg/dL and a renal ultrasound examination reveals that the right kidney is slightly smaller than the left kidney. By 12 months of age, the infant is successfully weaned off all antihypertensive therapy.

Many factors influence blood pressure in neonates, including gestational age, weight, postconceptual age, anxiety, pain, and level of wakefulness. For example, in term infants, systolic blood pressure is approximately 6 mm Hg higher in awake infants than in asleep infants and may increase by 25% with abdominal palpation, crying, or pain.[44] The gold standard for blood pressure measurement is intraarterial analysis of the waveform. Upper extremity pressures may be overestimated by this technique in older children, but in neonates, the umbilical and peripheral arterial values correlate well.[45] Automated oscillometric methods are easy to use, but accuracy varies among devices. There is a greater likelihood of an elevated pressure when measured by oscillometric devices than when obtained by direct methods.[45] Nwankwo et al suggested a protocol (Box 16-3) for standardizing pressure measurement using oscillometric devices that has been embraced by other experts in pediatric hypertension.[46]

Hypertension occurs in only 0.2% to 3% of neonates.[45] Zubrow et al collected data that show normal neonatal blood pressures according to birth weight, gestational age, and postconceptual age.[47] Normal blood pressures on day 1 of life for newborn infants as a function of birth weight are presented in Figure 16-5.[47]

Wait at least 1.5 hours after a meal or medical intervention.

Place infant in prone or supine position.

Use appropriately sized blood pressure cuff.

Place cuff on right upper arm.

Leave infant undisturbed for 15 minutes after cuff placement.

Ensure that infant is asleep or in quiet awake state.

Take three successive blood pressure readings at 2-minute intervals.

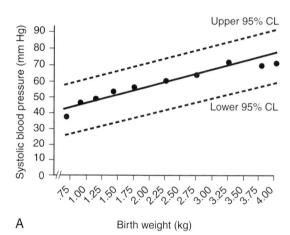

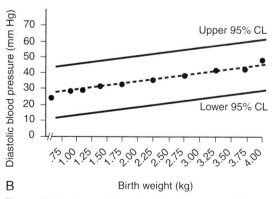

Figure 16-5. Linear relationship between mean systolic **(A)** and diastolic **(B)** blood pressure and birth weight on day 1 of life. *CL,* Confidence limit. *(From Zubrow AB, Hulman S: Determinants of blood pressure in infants admitted to neonatal intensive care units: a prospective multicenter study. Philadelphia Neonatal Blood Pressure Study Group, J Perinatol 15:470, 1995.)*

After birth, the blood pressure in premature infants increases quickly, so that the normal value in a 10-week-old baby born at 28 weeks is not comparable to that of a newborn baby born at 38 weeks.[47] Dionne et al published a table of values (Table 16-3) that is better suited to evaluating blood pressure according to postconceptual age.[45] Hypertension in children is defined as blood pressure elevation above the 95th percentile for peers of similar age, size, and gender. Dionne et al recommend that drug treatment begin when pressures consistently exceed the 99th percentile. For older infants found to be hypertensive following discharge from the neonatal intensive care unit, data generated by the Second Task Force on Hypertension, shown in Figure 16-6, are useful.[48]

Causes of Neonatal Hypertension

Causes of hypertension in the neonate are listed in Box 16-4. Renovascular hypertension is a frequent cause of neonatal hypertension and accounts for up to 90% of cases for which a discrete cause is identified. The most common cause of renovascular hypertension is renal artery thromboembolism related to umbilical artery catheterization, although congenital renal artery stenosis and renal vein thrombosis may also occur. Hypertension may also be seen in infants with hypervolemia related to oliguric acute renal failure. A small proportion of neonatal hypertension is related to structural renal disease, including autosomal recessive polycystic kidney disease and obstructive uropathy. Conditions associated with hypertension include bronchopulmonary dysplasia, patent ductus arteriosus, intraventricular hemorrhage, indwelling umbilical artery catheter, antenatal steroid therapy, maternal hypertension, coarctation of the aorta, medications, endocrine disorders, abdominal wall closure, and extracorporeal membrane oxygenation.[45,49]

Clinical Presentation

The clinical presentation of hypertension in the neonate is variable. Although some babies may be asymptomatic, nonspecific symptoms such as poor feeding, irritability, and lethargy are common. Significant cardiopulmonary symptoms may be present, including tachypnea, cyanosis, impaired perfusion, vasomotor instability, congestive heart failure, cardiomegaly, or hepatosplenomegaly. Neurologic symptoms such as lethargy, coma, tremors, hypertonicity, hypotonicity,

Table 16-3.	Blood Pressure Values in Infants from 26 to 44 Weeks' Postconceptual Age		
Postconceptual Age	**50th Percentile**	**95th Percentile**	**99th Percentile**
44 wk			
SBP	88	105	110
MAP	63	80	85
42 wk			
SBP	85	98	102
MAP	62	76	81
40 wk			
SBP	80	95	100
MAP	60	75	80
38 wk			
SBP	77	92	97
MAP	59	74	79
36 wk			
SBP	72	87	92
MAP	57	72	71
34 wk			
SBP	70	85	90
MAP	50	65	70
32 wk			
SBP	68	83	88
MAP	48	62	69
30 wk			
SBP	65	80	85
MAP	48	65	68
28 wk			
SBP	60	75	80
MAP	45	58	63
26 wk			
SBP	55	72	77
MAP	38	57	63

From Dionne JM, Abitbol CL, Flynn JT: Hypertension in infancy: diagnosis, management and outcome, *Pediatr Nephrol* 27(1):17, 2012.
MAP, Mean arterial pressure; *SBP,* systolic blood pressure.

opisthotonos, asymmetric reflexes, hemiparesis, seizures, and apnea may also occur. Hypertensive retinopathy is uncommon in neonates with hypertension and resolves with control of blood pressure. Renal effects of hypertension may include acute renal failure and sodium wasting related to pressure natriuresis.

Evaluation of the Neonate with Hypertension

Evaluation of the hypertensive newborn begins with a careful history taking and physical examination. Initial laboratory studies should include urinalysis, serum electrolyte levels, blood urea nitrogen level, serum creatinine concentration, and serum calcium level. Ultrasonography of the kidneys with Doppler flow study of the aorta and renal arteries should be performed to rule out a renal artery or aortic thrombus or urinary tract structural anomalies. A finding of unequal kidney size (>1.5 cm difference) should raise suspicion of renal artery disease. Echocardiography should be performed to diagnose aortic coarctation and evaluate left ventricular mass and function. Thyroid function studies and urinary studies for catecholamines, 17-hydroxysteroids, and 17-ketosteroids should be reserved for the rare instances in which results of the aforementioned studies are normal.

Management of the Neonate with Hypertension

Neonates with signs and symptoms of a hypertensive emergency such as cardiopulmonary failure, acute neurologic dysfunction, or renal insufficiency require immediate treatment with intravenous medication. The goal of therapy is a prompt decrease in blood pressure to minimize injury to the brain, heart, and kidneys. Blood pressures should

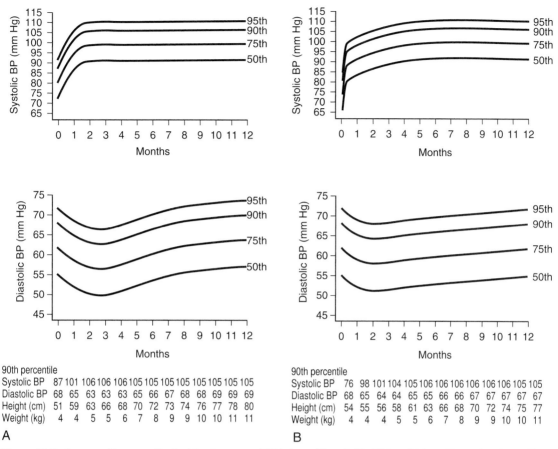

Figure 16-6. Age-specific percentiles for blood pressure (BP) in boys **(A)** and girls **(B)** from birth to 12 months of age. *(From Report of the Second Task Force on Blood Pressure Control in Children—1987. National Heart, Lung, and Blood Institute, Bethesda, Md, Pediatrics 79:1, 1987.)*

Box 16-4. Causes of Neonatal Hypertension

Renovascular disease
- Renal artery thrombosis
- Renal artery stenosis

Congenital renal malformations
- Polycystic kidney disease
- Hydronephrosis

Renal parenchymal disease
- Acute tubular necrosis

Coarctation of the aorta

Other
- Endocrine disorders
- Bronchopulmonary dysplasia
- Drug exposure: cocaine, methadone, corticosteroids, aminophylline
- Abdominal wall closure
- Extracorporeal membrane oxygenation

not be lowered below the 95th percentile until 24 to 48 hours after initiation of therapy to avoid cerebral and optic disc ischemia.

Antihypertensive medications used in the neonate are listed in Table 16-4. Sodium nitroprusside is commonly administered as an intravenous infusion to treat hypertensive emergencies. Alternative intravenous infusions include nicardipine, esmolol, and labetalol. Enalaprilat, an intravenous angiotensin-converting enzyme inhibitor, is effective in reducing blood pressure but must be used with extreme caution because it may cause prolonged hypotension and acute renal failure.[50]

Oral antihypertensive agents are useful in infants with less severe, asymptomatic hypertension or in those whose acute blood pressure elevation has been controlled with intravenous agents and who are ready to transition to long-term therapy. Captopril has a long history of use in neonates.[51] The risk of renal injury or failure has contributed

Table 16-4.	Antihypertensive Medications				
Drug	**Dose**	**Route**	**Dosing Interval**	**Action**	**Comment**
Sodium nitroprusside	0.5-10 µg/kg/min	IV	Continuous infusion	Vasodilator	Thiocyanate toxicity can occur with prolonged use or in renal failure.
Nicardipine	1-4 µg/kg/min	IV	Continuous infusion	Calcium channel blocker	May cause reflex tachycardia.
Esmolol	100-300 µg/kg/min	IV	Continuous infusion	β-Blocker	Very short acting; use constant infusion only.
Labetalol	0.25-3 mg/kg/hr	IV	Continuous infusion	α-, β-Blocker	Heart failure and BPD are relative contraindications.
	0.20-1.0 mg/kg/dose	IV	Bolus q6h		
Diazoxide	2-5 mg/kg/dose	IV	q12h	Vasodilator	Rapid IV bolus.
Hydralazine	0.15-0.6 mg/kg/dose	IV	bolus q4h	Vasodilator	Tachycardia is a frequent side effect.
Enalaprilat	5-30 µg/kg/dose	IV	q8-24h	ACE inhibitor	May cause prolonged hypotension and acute renal failure.
Amlodipine	0.1-0.3 mg/kg/dose	PO	q12h	Calcium channel blocker	Longer acting than isradipine.
Captopril	0.1-0.5 mg/kg/dose (max 2 mg/kg/day)	PO	q8-12h	ACE inhibitor	Drug of choice for most neonatal hypertension; monitor serum creatinine and potassium.
Isradipine	0.05-0.15 mg/kg/dose (max 0.8 mg/kg/day)	PO	q6h	Calcium channel blocker	Suspension may be compounded.
Propranolol	0.5-1.0 mg/kg/dose	PO	q8h	β-blocker	May cause bradycardia; avoid in infants with BPD.
Furosemide	1-2 mg/kg/dose	PO/IV	q8-24h	Loop diuretic	Monitor electrolytes.
Chlorothiazide	5-15 mg/kg/dose 1-4 mg/kg/dose	PO	q12h	Distal tubule diuretic	Monitor electrolytes.

ACE, Angiotensin-converting enzyme; *BPD*, bronchopulmonary dysplasia; *IV*, intravenous; *PO*, oral.

to a greater interest in the use of calcium channel blockers.[45] Hydralazine, a direct vasodilator, is also effective in controlling neonatal hypertension. Diuretics such as furosemide or hydrochlorothiazide may be effective adjunctive agents in infants with volume overload.

The long-term prognosis for children with neonatal hypertension is excellent, particularly for those with hypertension related to an umbilical artery catheter. Of 17 children described by Friedman and Hustead with hypertension diagnosed either in the nursery or by 18 weeks of age after discharge, no children were receiving antihypertensive medication at 24 months of age.[52] Children with hypertension related to other causes, including polycystic kidney disease, coarctation of the aorta, renal artery stenosis, or renal vein thrombosis may have persistent hypertension throughout childhood.

RENAL ARTERY THROMBOSIS

In the neonatal population, renal artery thrombosis is most commonly associated with an indwelling umbilical artery catheter. The incidence of thrombus formation in the aorta in the presence of umbilical artery catheters ranges from 26% when evaluated by ultrasonography to 95% when determined by aortography.[53,54] Risk factors for complications from umbilical artery catheters include maternal diabetes, sepsis, dehydration, birth trauma, perinatal asphyxia, patent ductus arteriosus, and cocaine exposure. Although 30% to 40% of infants with arterial thrombosis may be asymptomatic, hypertension occurs in approximately 25% of patients and may be associated with hematuria, oliguria, renal failure, congestive heart failure, or lower extremity ischemia.

Ultrasonography of the kidneys with Doppler flow study of the aorta and renal arteries is the diagnostic study of choice when renal artery thromboembolism is suspected. In patients with suspected renal artery thromboembolism in whom renal ultrasound and Doppler findings are normal, confirmation with renal radionuclide imaging using either MAG-3 or DTPA may be required. Aortography may be necessary even in the presence of normal ultrasound findings in a sick child with lower extremity vascular insufficiency, congestive heart failure, or acute renal failure.

The primary treatment for hypertension associated with arterial thromboembolism is removal of the umbilical artery catheter and institution of antihypertensive therapy. Heparinization and fibrinolytic therapy are reserved for patients at high risk of complete occlusion or those with oliguric acute renal failure, congestive heart failure, or severe lower extremity ischemia. In these situations, successful use of systemic or intrathrombic urokinase or streptokinase has been reported.[55] Aortic thrombectomy may be necessary in patients in whom anticoagulants and fibrinolytic agents are ineffective, but spontaneous recanalization of an aortic clot with development of collateral circulation around permanently occluded renal arteries has been described.[56]

Although children with renovascular hypertension secondary to renal artery thromboembolism from umbilical artery catheters do not typically require antihypertensive medications beyond 24 months of age, several long-term issues exist. In a report of 12 children studied at a mean follow-up of almost 6 years, Adelman noted that 5 of 11 patients displayed unilateral renal atrophy on ultrasonography or intravenous pyelography despite having normal creatinine clearances.[32] Furthermore, follow-up radionuclide scans continued to show abnormal findings in all patients studied, even in patients without renal atrophy on ultrasonography. The long-term significance of these findings in terms of the likelihood of chronic hypertension or renal insufficiency with prolonged follow-up is unknown.

NEPHROCALCINOSIS

A 5-month-old infant with bronchopulmonary dysplasia who had been born prematurely at 25 weeks was incidentally noted to have medullary nephrocalcinosis on an abdominal ultrasound study. She had required long-term loop diuretic and corticosteroid administration to treat her lung disease. Urinalysis revealed hematuria (1+) with 10 to 15 red blood cells per high-power field. Urine culture yielded no growth. Spot urine calcium-to-creatinine ratio was elevated at 1.65. Loop diuretics were discontinued and chlorothiazide initiated to reduce urinary calcium excretion. Corticosteroids were tapered and discontinued over the next 2 months. Urine calcium-to-creatinine ratio decreased to 0.8 and serial ultrasound examinations showed gradual resolution of nephrocalcinosis. When the infant was 8 months of age, chlorothiazide was discontinued, and at 1 year of age a follow-up renal ultrasound study yielded normal findings.

Renal medullary calcifications in the premature infant were first described in 1982 by Hufnagle et al.[57] Since then, nephrocalcinosis has become a well-known complication in the neonatal population, occurring in 27% to 65% of hospitalized premature infants.[58] Infants with nephrocalcinosis may present with microscopic or gross hematuria, granular material in the diaper, acute renal failure related to ureteral obstruction, or urinary tract infection. Nephrocalcinosis may also be discovered incidentally on abdominal ultrasound examination.

The majority of infants with nephrocalcinosis have had exposure to loop diuretics for management of bronchopulmonary dysplasia. Furosemide and other loop diuretics enhance urinary calcium excretion, which predisposes to deposition of calcium oxalate crystals in the renal interstitium. However, nephrocalcinosis has also been reported in infants with no prior exposure to loop diuretics. Other factors that may contribute to the development of neonatal nephrocalcinosis include fluid restriction; treatment with corticosteroids or xanthine derivatives, which have a hypercalciuric effect; decreased urinary concentration of stone inhibitors such as citrate and magnesium; hyperuricosuria; increased oxalate excretion related to parenteral hyperalimentation; and familial history of nephrolithiasis.[59,60] In infants with nephrocalcinosis or nephrolithiasis, use of agents that increase urinary calcium excretion, such as loop diuretics and corticosteroids, should be minimized or eliminated if possible. A high urinary flow rate should be maintained to reduce the probability of urinary crystallization. Oral calcium supplements should be discontinued, and metabolic acidosis, if present, should be treated with bicarbonate, because chronic acidosis enhances urinary calcium excretion. Thiazide diuretics such as chlorothiazide may be effective in reducing urinary calcium excretion,[57] although serum calcium levels should be monitored closely to avoid hypercalcemia.

The long-term consequences of neonatal nephrocalcinosis are not clearly defined. In approximately 50% of affected infants, nephrocalcinosis spontaneously resolves within 5 to 6 months of discontinuation of diuretics without identifiable adverse consequences.[61] However, infants with nephrocalcinosis may have diminished renal growth and impairment of renal function, although the degree to which nephrocalcinosis causes these sequelae remains uncertain.

> **EDITORIAL COMMENT:** Kist-van Holthe et al[62] looked at the long-term effects of nephrocalcinosis in a prospective study in which they followed a number of preterm infants (<32 weeks' gestation) with and without nephrocalcinosis. They found that even 7½ years later children who had had neonatal nephrocalcinosis showed increased rates of (mild) chronic renal insufficiency. In addition, the investigators found that prematurity itself was associated with small kidneys, high blood pressure, and (distal) tubular dysfunction. Thus it becomes imperative to provide long-term follow-up of blood pressure and renal function in preterm infants, especially those with nephrocalcinosis.

CONGENITAL RENAL DISEASE

> A 2100-g male infant was delivered at 32 weeks after oligohydramnios had been noted in the third trimester. Apgar score was 8 at 1 minute and 9 at 5 minutes. Physical examination yielded normal findings, including absence of abdominal masses. The infant fed poorly and showed decreased activity. Laboratory evaluation revealed a rising serum creatinine level, which reached 4.5 mg/dL on day 6 of life. Renal ultrasonography demonstrated absence of the right kidney and a small, hyperechoic left kidney with several small cortical cysts. Results of voiding cystourethrography were normal.
>
> The infant's diagnosis was chronic kidney disease due to right renal agenesis and left renal dysplasia. A peritoneal dialysis catheter was placed and dialysis initiated. The infant's parents were trained by the nephrology team to perform home dialysis, supply supplemental nasogastric feedings, and administer multiple medications for management of chronic kidney disease. The infant continued on home peritoneal dialysis until 2 years of age, when he received a donor kidney from his mother.

Molecular genetic research reveals that shared genetic defects are associated with phenotypes that were previously considered to be distinctly different conditions. This finding has led to wider use of the term *congenital anomalies of the kidney and urinary tract* (CAKUT) for a spectrum of renal malformations. *CAKUT* refers to conditions as diverse as hypoplasia, hydronephrosis, ureterocele, vesicoureteral reflux, and posterior urethral valves. CAKUT occurs in 1 in 500 live births.[63]

Renal Agenesis

Unilateral renal agenesis occurs in 1 in 500 to 1 in 3200 individuals, whereas bilateral renal agenesis occurs in 1 in 4000 to 1 in 10,000 live births.[64] Renal agenesis occurs when the ureteric bud fails to induce proper differentiation of the metanephric blastema, an event that may be related to both a genetic defect and environmental factors.[63]

Renal agenesis may be seen in infants with VACTERL association (*v*ertebral defects, imperforate *a*nus, *c*ardiac defects, *t*racheoesophageal fistula, *r*adial and renal anomalies, *l*imb anomalies), caudal regression syndrome, branchio-oto-renal syndrome, and multiple chromosomal defects,[64] but it may also be seen in otherwise healthy infants. Because contralateral urinary tract abnormalities, including vesicoureteral reflux, ureteropelvic junction obstruction, renal dysplasia, and ureterocele, occur in up to 90% of individuals with unilateral renal agenesis,[65] a thorough evaluation of the urinary tract including voiding cystourethrography is warranted in all patients.

Renal Dysplasia

Renal dysplasia is characterized by abnormal fetal renal development that leads to replacement of the renal parenchyma by cartilage and disorganized epithelial structures. The pathogenesis of renal dysplasia may involve mutations in developmental genes, altered interaction of the ureteric bud with extracellular matrix, abnormalities of renal growth factors, and urinary tract obstruction.[66]

Renal dysplasia is frequently present in infants with obstructive uropathy and a variety of congenital disorders, including Eagle-Barrett syndrome (prune-belly syndrome); VACTERL association; branchio-oto-renal syndrome; CHARGE syndrome (*c*oloboma of iris, choroid, or retina, *h*eart defects, *a*tresia of the choanae, *r*estricted growth and development, *g*enital anomalies or hypogonadism, *e*ar anomalies or deafness); trisomy 13, 18, and 21; and Jeune syndrome. The function of dysplastic kidneys is variable, and infants with bilateral dysplasia may exhibit signs of renal insufficiency as early as the first few days of life. Concentrating and acidification defects may also be present, whereas hematuria, proteinuria, and hypertension are unusual findings. Progressive renal insufficiency generally develops in children with bilateral renal dysplasia during childhood and adolescence.

Multicystic Dysplastic Kidney

Multicystic dysplastic kidney (MCDK) represents the most severe form of renal dysplasia, in which the kidney consists of a grapelike cluster of cysts devoid of normal renal architecture and function. MCDK is the most common unilateral abdominal mass in the neonatal period, although with the advent of prenatal ultrasonography, the majority of cases are identified prenatally. The incidence of MCDK is estimated at 1 in 4000 live births.[67] MCDK usually occurs as a sporadic event, although it may be seen in conjunction with VACTERL association, branchio-oto-renal syndrome, Williams syndrome, Beckwith-Wiedemann syndrome, trisomy 18, or 49,XXXXX syndrome. The pathophysiology is incompletely understood but may involve failure of the ureteric bud to integrate properly into the metanephros during development. Because contralateral urinary tract abnormalities (reflux, obstruction, dysplasia) are present in up to 50% of patients with unilateral MCDK, a careful evaluation of the urinary tract including voiding cystourethrography is warranted in all patients.

The majority of infants with unilateral MCDKs have an excellent prognosis, because the MCDK generally involutes spontaneously over time, whereas the contralateral kidney grows larger than expected as a result of compensatory hypertrophy.[67] In view of the small but real risk of hypertension and malignancy, children must be followed carefully with serial ultrasound studies and blood pressure monitoring. Some clinicians offer the option of surgical removal of a unilateral MCDK if the MCDK fails to involute, increases in size, or causes any symptoms.

Polycystic Kidney Disease

Both autosomal dominant polycystic kidney disease (ADPKD) and autosomal recessive polycystic kidney disease (ARPKD) may present in the neonatal period. ADPKD has an incidence of 1 in 200 to 1 in 1000 and is the most common inherited renal disease.[68] Mutations in the *PKD1* and *PDK2* genes may trigger ADPKD by altering a multimeric protein complex that plays an important regulatory role in kidney development. The clinical presentation of ADPKD in the neonatal period may vary from a severe form with significant renal failure to asymptomatic renal cysts detected by ultrasonography.

ARPKD is a much less common disorder, with an incidence of 1 in 20,000.[69] The majority of cases present in infancy. Prenatal ultrasonography may show oligohydramnios and bilaterally large, hyperechoic kidneys. Characteristic clinical findings in the neonate include palpable abdominal masses, severe hypertension, pulmonary hypoplasia, congenital hepatic fibrosis, and renal insufficiency. Primary management concerns include control of hypertension, management of renal insufficiency, and provision of ventilatory support.

HYDRONEPHROSIS

> At 20 weeks' gestation, screening ultrasonography reveals moderate bilateral hydronephrosis in a male fetus. Serial ultrasound studies show persistence of the hydronephrosis, development of hydroureters, and a large bladder with a thickened wall. The infant is delivered at 35 weeks' gestation. A bladder catheter is placed immediately to secure adequate bladder drainage. Renal ultrasonography shows moderate bilateral hydronephrosis and hydroureter, a trabeculated bladder, and a dilated proximal urethra. Voiding cystourethrography confirms the diagnosis of posterior urethral valves as well as the presence of bilateral grade III vesicoureteral reflux.
>
> The infant undergoes primary valve ablation to relieve the urinary tract obstruction. Antibiotic prophylaxis is administered to prevent urinary tract infection. Serum creatinine concentration is 1.4 mg/dL at hospital discharge and 0.9 mg/dL at 6 months of age, which suggests chronic kidney disease.

The advent of prenatal ultrasonography has led to detection of hydronephrosis in 0.45% to 4% of all pregnancies.[70,71] Hydronephrosis is defined as dilatation of the upper urinary tract. Prenatal hydronephrosis may be associated with a wide spectrum of conditions ranging in severity from urethral atresia with expected fetal demise to transient physiologic dilatation of the collecting system with expected complete spontaneous resolution.[72] The Society for Fetal Urology uses a grading scale ranging from grade 0 (absent) to grade 4 (most severe) for fetuses of more than 20 weeks' gestation. Measurement of the anterior-posterior diameter of the renal pelvis offers an alternative means to judge the severity of neonatal hydronephrosis.[73,74] There is no firm consensus on which system is more clinically relevant.

Unilateral hydronephrosis with a normal contralateral kidney does not compromise fetal or neonatal survival. Bilateral hydronephrosis, however, carries greater risk. Unilateral hydronephrosis accompanied by contralateral renal dysplasia may have a less favorable outcome. The finding of oligohydramnios may be an early indicator of such a pathologic condition.

Neonates with hydronephrosis identified on prenatal ultrasonography should undergo postnatal ultrasonography within the first week of life. Because the degree of hydronephrosis may be underestimated (as a result of the newborn's low GFR), a second ultrasound study is necessary within several weeks. In infants with only low-grade hydronephrosis on prenatal ultrasonography, postnatal ultrasonography may be postponed until 2 weeks of age if the infant is otherwise well. Further evaluation, including voiding cystourethrography and radionuclide renal scanning, should be coordinated by a pediatric nephrologist or urologist.[71] In 48% of cases of antenatal hydronephrosis, no cause is identified.[70]

Ureteropelvic Junction Obstruction

Ureteropelvic junction obstruction is a common cause of congenital hydronephrosis and may be the result of incomplete recanalization of the proximal ureter, abnormal development of ureteral musculature, abnormal peristalsis, ureteral valves, or polyps. Ureteropelvic junction obstruction is more common in male infants and may be associated with other congenital anomalies, syndromes, or genitourinary malformations. Diagnosis is confirmed by an obstructive pattern on a diuretic-enhanced radionuclide scan. Many clinicians advocate antibiotic prophylaxis to prevent urinary tract infection, although this practice remains somewhat controversial in cases of ureteropelvic junction obstruction without

reflux. Definitive treatment involves surgical repair.

Ureterovesical Junction Obstruction

Ureterovesical junction obstruction is the second most common cause of congenital hydronephrosis and is characterized by hydronephrosis with associated ureteral dilatation. This disorder may be related to underdevelopment of the distal ureter or the presence of a ureterocele. Diagnosis is confirmed by radionuclide scan and voiding cystourethrogram. Ureterovesical junction obstruction is usually not associated with other congenital malformations. Many clinicians advocate antibiotic prophylaxis to prevent urinary tract infection, although this practice remains somewhat controversial in cases of ureterovesical junction obstruction without associated reflux. Definitive treatment involves surgical repair.

Posterior Urethral Valves

Posterior urethral valves are the most common cause of infravesicular urinary tract obstruction, with an incidence of 1 in 5000 to 1 in 8000 males. Prenatal ultrasonography may show hydronephrosis, dilated ureters, thickened trabeculated bladder, dilated proximal urethra, and oligohydramnios. Antenatal presentation may include a palpable, distended bladder; poor urinary stream; and signs and symptoms of renal and pulmonary insufficiency. Voiding cystourethrography is diagnostic for posterior urethral valves and may reveal associated vesicoureteral reflux in 30% of patients.

Treatment is centered on securing adequate drainage of the urinary tract, initially by placement of a urinary catheter and later by primary ablation of the valves, vesicostomy, or upper tract diversion. The long-term outcome for infants with posterior urethral valves depends on the degree of associated renal dysplasia. As many as 30% of boys with posterior urethral valves whose symptoms manifest in infancy are at risk for progressive renal insufficiency in childhood or adolescence.

Eagle-Barrett Syndrome

Eagle-Barrett syndrome, formerly known as *prune-belly syndrome*, is characterized by deficiency of abdominal wall musculature, a dilated nonobstructed urinary tract, and bilateral cryptorchidism. The estimated incidence is 1 in 35,000 to 1 in 50,000 live births, with more than 95% of cases occurring in males. Two current theories of pathogenesis include in utero urinary tract obstruction and a specific mesodermal injury between the fourth and tenth weeks of gestation.

The most common urinary tract abnormalities in infants with Eagle-Barrett syndrome are renal dysplasia or agenesis, vesicoureteral reflux, and a large-capacity, poorly contractile bladder. Cardiac, pulmonary, gastrointestinal, and orthopedic anomalies occur in a large percentage of patients with Eagle-Barrett syndrome. Treatment in the neonatal period involves optimization of urinary tract drainage, management of renal insufficiency, and antibiotic prophylaxis if vesicoureteral reflux is present. Management later in childhood may include surgical repair of reflux, orchiopexy, reconstruction of the abdominal wall, and renal transplantation.

Vesicoureteral Reflux

Vesicoureteral reflux, defined as retrograde propulsion of urine into the upper urinary tract during bladder contraction, is another potential cause of hydronephrosis in the neonate.[75] The underlying pathophysiology of vesicoureteral reflux is believed to be ectopic insertion of the ureter into the bladder wall resulting in a shorter intravesicular ureter, which acts as an incompetent valve during urination. Vesicoureteral reflux appears to have a genetic component, because the incidence of reflux is at least 30% in first-degree relatives. Of infants and children evaluated for their first urinary tract infection, at least one third have vesicoureteral reflux on voiding cystourethrography.

Primary vesicoureteral reflux tends to resolve over time as the intravesical segment of the ureter elongates during growth, with the greatest rate of spontaneous resolution in patients with the lowest grades of reflux. Conservative management involves administration of daily oral antibiotic prophylaxis to prevent urinary tract infection. Surgical repair is considered in children with breakthrough urinary tract infections or high-grade reflux. Newer minimally invasive methods to correct reflux, including endoscopic injection of a dextranomer and hyaluronic acid gel (Deflux), have recently been introduced. Long-term complications of vesicoureteral reflux include hypertension, renal scarring, and chronic kidney disease.

REFERENCES

The reference list for this chapter can be found online at www.expertconsult.com.

Hematologic Problems

17

John Letterio, Sanjay P. Ahuja, and Agne Petrosiute

RED BLOOD CELLS

The great questions of the day are not decided by speeches and majority votes but by blood and iron.

Otto von Bismarck, September 30, 1862

FETAL ERYTHROPOIESIS AND CHANGES IN ERYTHROPOIESIS AFTER BIRTH

Rapid growth during fetal development demands a brisk pace for red blood cell production, and this capacity must expand with the increase in blood volume, which is proportionate to the weight of the fetus. Blood volumes average 80 mL/kg of fetal body weight at term, but the ratio is larger in the preterm fetus (~90 mL/kg). The rapid pace of erythropoiesis is reflected by a rise in hematocrit throughout gestation (from a mean of 40% at 28 weeks of gestation to 50% at term) and by high reticulocyte counts and the presence of circulating nucleated red blood cells at birth.

Hematopoiesis during mammalian embryonic development proceeds from the yolk sac blood island to the aorta-gonad-mesonephros region, the fetal liver, and subsequently the fetal bone marrow, and is tightly regulated by the stromal cells in each of these unique areas that make up the hematopoietic niche[1,2] (Fig. 17-1). Moreover, there are likely distinct myeloid-erythroid progenitors in the early yolk sac niche that may exist transiently and contribute to the unique regulation of the β-globin locus in the mammalian embryo.[3] The control of red blood cell production and progression of fetal erythropoiesis from yolk sac to liver (in utero) to bone marrow at birth is also in part orchestrated by Kruppel-like factors (KLFs) that control cell differentiation and embryonic development. KLF1 (erythroid Kruppel-like factor) is essential during both embryonic and adult erythropoiesis. KLF2 is a positive regulator of the mouse and human embryonic β-globin genes. KLF1 and KLF2 have highly homologous zinc finger DNA-binding domains and have overlapping roles in embryonic erythropoiesis.[4] The ontogeny of fetal erythropoiesis has been reviewed elsewhere.[5]

Fetal erythropoiesis also occurs during chronic bone marrow failure and recovery from marrow suppression. Fetal erythrocytes have hemoglobin F, with more G-γ than A-γ chains, i antigen, large mean corpuscular volume, characteristic enzyme levels, low carbonic anhydrase, low hemoglobin A_2, and short life span. Many of these fetal characteristics are present in the red blood cells of patients with temporary or chronic hematopoietic stress. Chronic fetal erythropoiesis is seen in patients with constitutional aplastic anemia, such as Fanconi anemia or Diamond-Blackfan anemia. Thus fetal erythropoiesis occurs during hematopoietic stress, whether chronic or transient, if there is some marrow activity and may be due to expansion of fetal clones.[6]

Several endogenous proteins contribute to the changes in regulation of erythropoiesis after birth, with erythropoietin being the most recognized. Fetal erythropoiesis is regulated by endogenous (fetal) erythropoietin produced in the liver, but in infancy the main site of production converts to the kidneys. Although the rate of erythropoiesis in the fetus is quite high, serum erythropoietin levels are low, and the erythropoietin response to hypoxia in the fetus and neonate is reduced compared with that in adults. After delivery erythropoietin levels vary among species, which is probably related to the oxygen transport capacity of the hemoglobin mass. In all mammals, hemoglobin level declines following birth and erythropoiesis nearly ceases, which

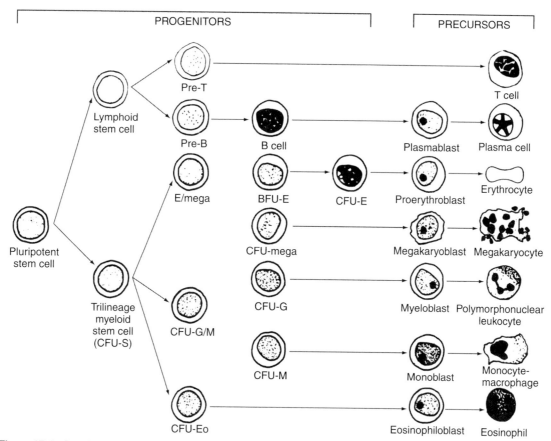

Figure 17-1. Overview of the cellular stages of hematopoiesis. The most primitive pluripotent stem cell is shown at the far left. As hematopoietic progenitor cells differentiate, they become committed to a single lineage. This diagram does not emphasize the large increase in the number of cells (amplification) that occurs in the progenitor and precursor compartments. *BFU*, Burst-forming unit; *CFU*, colony-forming unit; *E*, erythrocyte; *Eo*, eosinophil; *G*, granulocyte; *M*, macrophage; *mega*, megakaryocyte; *S*, stem cell. (From Lipton JW, Nathan DG: The anatomy and physiology of hematopoiesis. In Nathan DG, Oski FA, editors: *Hematology of infancy and childhood*, ed 3, Philadelphia, 1987, Saunders.)

gives rise to "early anemia." Except in humans, erythropoietin levels increase proportionally with the fall in hemoglobin, but there is a discrepancy between the curves for serum immunoreactive erythropoietin and for erythropoiesis-stimulating factors. The latter include other stimulatory factors in addition to erythropoietin. These other factors work in concert with erythropoietin to control erythropoiesis and probably contribute to enhanced erythropoiesis during periods of rapid growth, which is unlikely to be attributable to the same molecular controls that enhance erythropoiesis during periods of stress or hypoxia. For example, it is known that erythropoietin acts in concert with general growth-promoting factors, particularly growth hormone (GH) and the insulin-like growth factors (IGF-I and IGF-II). The erythropoietin and GH/IGF systems are both activated by hypoxia and share similar receptors and pathways.

Recent studies indicate that human fetal and infant growth is stimulated by GH, IGF-I, and IGF-II. Erythropoietin, GH, and IGFs are expressed early in fetal life. IGF-I levels are low in the fetus and increase slowly following birth except in preterm infants, in whom the levels decline. The physiology of erythropoietin during mammalian development has been reviewed elsewhere.[7]

The low level of erythroid production noted earlier persists for over a month following birth, during which time the hematocrit gradually declines. Late in the second or third month of life, the hematocrit approaches 30%. This is commensurate with a rise in serum erythropoietin levels, which prompts a resumption of erythropoiesis and leads to a rise in red blood cell mass. This rise in red blood cell mass keeps pace with rapid overall growth and blood volume, and the hematocrit rises relatively little as a consequence.

Erythropoietin and Neuroprotection in the Neonate

One other aspect of the erythropoietin system that is important to the fetus and newborn deserves mention here. Erythropoietin is a pleiotropic neuroprotective cytokine, and recent studies have shed light on the biological basis of its efficacy in the damaged developing brain. Coordinated expression of erythropoietin ligand and receptor expression occur during central nervous system development to promote neural cell survival. Studies of fetal hypoxia-ischemia in rat models have demonstrated that prenatal third-trimester global hypoxia-ischemia disrupts the developmentally regulated expression of neural cell erythropoietin signaling and predisposes neural cells to death. Furthermore, exposure of the neonate to exogenous sources of recombinant erythropoietin can restore the mismatch of erythropoietin ligand and receptor levels and enhance neural cell survival. The data generated by these studies suggest the potential utility of neonatal recombinant erythropoietin when administered in the days immediately after a global prenatal hypoxic-ischemic insult as a means to rescue neural cells and present a novel clinically relevant paradigm in which the benefits of erythropoietin in the context of a stress are linked to the induction of signaling pathways in both erythroid and non-erythroid lineages.[8,9]

PLACENTAL TRANSFUSION AND DISTRIBUTION OF BLOOD AT BIRTH

The effect of early and late umbilical cord clamping on neonatal hematocrit has been well studied.[10] Delayed cord clamping has been shown to be associated with a higher hematocrit in very low-birth-weight infants, which suggests effective placental transfusion.[11] Several analyses have confirmed that delaying cord clamping (by at least 30 seconds) increases average blood volume across the full range of gestational ages studied.[12] On average, the infant will gain roughly 14 mL/kg of blood during this first 30 seconds, which leads to a blood volume of 89 mL/kg. This process has been termed *placental transfusion*. It occurs due to the continued circulation of blood through the umbilical arteries and veins, and leads to a net shift of blood from the placenta to the newborn infant. At birth, the partition of blood volume between the infant and the fetal placental vasculature is nearly 2:1 (75 mL/kg body weight in the infant and 40 mL/kg in the placenta). If the umbilical cord is not clamped quickly, a major shift in blood can lead to significant effects on blood volume, hematocrit, and hemoglobin concentration during the first days of life. Infants exposed to a significant delay in umbilical cord clamping may experience excessive placental transfusion, with attendant decreases in plasma volume, increased hematocrit, and elevated blood viscosity. Regardless of the extent of placental transfusion, postnatal adjustments of blood volume and hematocrit begin within 15 minutes after birth and continue for several hours. A controlled trial has suggested that delayed cord clamping in very preterm infants may reduce the incidence of intraventricular hemorrhage and late-onset sepsis.[13]

> **EDITORIAL COMMENT:** Delayed cord clamping has continued to show benefits and little, if any, risk in preterm infants.[14,15] The benefits of delayed cord clamping in preterm infants include increased blood volume,[15,16] improved circulatory and respiratory function, reduced need for blood transfusion, improved cerebral oxygenation, and reduced intraventricular hemorrhage and sepsis.[13] The cord blood of extremely preterm infants is a rich source of hematopoietic progenitor cells such as hematopoietic stem cells, endothelial cell precursors, mesenchymal progenitors, and stem cells of multipotent-pluripotent lineage; hence the merit of delayed cord clamping has been magnified. Tolosa et al referred to this aspect of delayed cord clamping as "realizing mankind's first stem cell transfer" and proposed that "it should be encouraged in normal births."[17] The extra endowment of progenitor cells resulting from delayed cord clamping has the potential to both increase red blood cell production and boost host immune defenses through production of leukocytes.
>
> There has been a shift in thinking to explore milking of the umbilical cord as an alternative to delayed cord clamping, which may provide the same benefits without the need to delay resuscitation.

PROPERTIES OF FETAL HEMOGLOBIN AND THE SWITCH TO ADULT HEMOGLOBIN

The different types of human hemoglobin consist of various combinations of the embryonic, fetal, and adult hemoglobin subunits that are present at distinct times during development. This orderly transition from one form of hemoglobin to another represents a major paradigm of developmental biology but remains poorly understood. Studies have pointed to a competition between subunits for more favorable partners with stronger subunit interactions, so that the protein products of gene expression can themselves play a role in the developmental process due to their intrinsic properties.[18] Fetal hemoglobin, or Hb F (two α-globin chains and two γ-globin chains, [$\alpha_2\gamma_2$]), is the main hemoglobin synthesized up to birth, at which point it makes up more than 80% of the hemoglobin in circulating red blood cells. However, Hb F subsequently declines, and adult hemoglobin, Hb A ($\alpha_2\beta_2$), becomes predominant.

The main reason for this shift is the transition from synthesis of mainly γ chains during fetal development to mainly β chains during late gestation, with a concomitant gradual shift from Hb F to Hb A beginning at 34 weeks' gestation. Several studies have indicated that expression of the Hb F subunit γ-globin might also be regulated posttranscriptionally. One recently identified mechanism for posttranscription regulation of gene expression is through the production of micro-RNAs. These micro-RNAs are approximately 22 nucleotides in length and can specifically target messenger RNAs (mRNAs) for selected genes, thus acting as disease modifiers as well as molecules that control gene expression during development and in response to environmental stimuli. A study comparing micro-RNA expression in reticulocytes from cord blood and adult blood revealed several micro-RNAs that were preferentially expressed in adults, among them micro-RNA-96, which appears to directly suppress γ-globin expression and thus contributes to control of Hb F production and its suppression during the switch to postnatal erythropoiesis.[19]

Although new hemoglobin produced during postnatal life is essentially all Hb A, there are exceptions to this rule. Perhaps the most well known is the persistence of Hb F in patients with sickle cell disease and the contribution of Hb F to amelioration of disease severity in these individuals (see later discussion). Hb F expression can be increased during periods of stress erythropoiesis, and in the infant recovering from anemia of prematurity, there is a transient phase in the recovery of erythropoiesis during which Hb F is the predominant hemoglobin synthesized.

Functional Differences of Specific Hemoglobins

The major physiologic function of hemoglobin is to bind oxygen in the lungs and deliver it to the tissues. This function is regulated and/or made efficient by endogenous heterotropic effectors.

Hb A is the major oxygen-binding tetrameric protein found in the blood. It is one of the best-recognized proteins in the human body because of its uniquely bright red color, and its color changes in diseases such as anemia, hypoxia, and cyanide and carbon monoxide poisoning. Hemoglobin has drawn the attention of physicians and physiologists since ancient times. Modern quantitative analysis of the structure and function of hemoglobin started in the late 1800s and early 1900s. Important observations of the hemoglobin allostery have been attributed to Christian Bohr (who reported in 1903 that its oxygen-binding process was sigmoidal or cooperative) and to Bohr, Hasselbalch, and Krogh, who reported in 1904 that the position of the oxygen-binding curve of the blood was sensitive to changes in P_{CO_2} (and H+ or pH), known as the *Bohr effect*. These observations regarding the allosteric behaviors of hemoglobin are reviewed elsewhere.[20]

It is widely recognized that the most important functional difference between Hb F and Hb A is their different oxygen-binding properties. The higher oxygen affinity of Hb F is an advantage to the fetus because of the site of oxygen uptake, the placenta, where the umbilical venous P_{O_2} is just 35 to 40 mm Hg, and represents the highest P_{O_2} in all the fetal circulation. Because the oxygen dissociation curve is "shifted" to the left (because of higher affinity), there is a capacity to maintain a higher O_2 content, but this capacity is no longer needed after birth because the lungs provide an environment with a significantly higher oxygen tension (typically above 75 mm Hg) in the pulmonary capillaries. More importantly, the persistence of Hb F is a disadvantage to the newborn because the release of oxygen in the capillary bed depends on a much lower P_{O_2} for efficient oxygen delivery and maintenance of tissue metabolism, which is in contrast to the dynamics of O_2 release by Hb A. This difference has been shown in clinical investigations to influence morbidity in newborns with cardiopulmonary disease. Studies evaluating the impact of exchange transfusion in extremely premature infants demonstrated a link between improved survival and substantial replacement of Hb F by Hb A, despite the absence of a significant change in hematocrit. This effect is often achieved as a consequence of frequent phlebotomies and multiple small transfusions of packed red blood cells in very low-birth-weight infants.

Hemoglobinopathies

Globin gene mutations are a rare but important cause of cyanosis. Crowley et al identified a missense mutation in the fetal G γ-globin gene (*HBG2*) in a father and daughter with transient neonatal cyanosis and anemia. This newly recognized mutation modifies the ligand-binding pocket of fetal hemoglobin. The mechanisms described include a diminutive effect of the relatively large side chain of methionine on both the affinity of oxygen for binding to the mutant hemoglobin subunit and the rate at which it does so. In addition, the mutant methionine is converted to aspartic acid posttranslationally, probably through oxidative mechanisms. The presence of this polar amino acid in the heme pocket is predicted to enhance hemoglobin denaturation, causing anemia.[21]

Methemoglobinemia

Methemoglobinemia arises from the production of nonfunctional hemoglobin containing oxidized Fe^{3+}, which results in reduced oxygen supply to the tissues and manifests as cyanosis in the patient. It can develop by three distinct mechanisms: genetic mutation resulting in the presence of abnormal hemoglobin, a deficiency of the methemoglobin reductase enzyme, and toxin-induced oxidation of hemoglobin. The normal hemoglobin fold forms a pocket to bind heme and stabilize the complex of heme with molecular oxygen. This process prevents spontaneous oxidation of the Fe^{2+} ion chelated by the heme pyrroles and the globin histidines. In the abnormal M forms of hemoglobin (Hb M) amino acid substitution in or near the heme pocket creates a propensity to form methemoglobin instead of oxyhemoglobin in the presence of molecular oxygen. Under normal conditions, hemoglobin is continually oxidized, but significant accumulation of methemoglobin is prevented by the action of a group of methemoglobin reductase enzymes. In the autosomal recessive form of methemoglobinemia, there is a deficiency of one of these reductase enzymes, which allows accumulation of oxidized Fe^{3+} in methemoglobin. Oxidizing drugs and other toxic chemicals may greatly enhance the normal spontaneous rate of methemoglobin production. If levels of methemoglobin exceed 70% of total hemoglobin, vascular collapse occurs resulting in coma and death. Under these conditions, if the source of toxicity can be eliminated, methemoglobin levels will return to normal. Disorders of oxidized hemoglobin are relatively easily diagnosed and in most cases, except when congenitally defective Hb M is present, can be treated successfully.[22]

ANEMIA

Neonatal anemia is a condition with a diverse etiologic spectrum. To reach an accurate diagnosis, the pediatrician must have some knowledge of the more common causes of low hemoglobin concentrations and hematocrit in the neonate. Proper history taking, physical examination, and interpretation of diagnostic test results can narrow the focus and aid in establishing an accurate diagnosis and in directing the appropriate therapeutic interventions.[23]

HEMORRHAGIC ANEMIAS

Hemorrhagic anemia in a newborn is often heralded by some features of the history or clinical findings that allow time to anticipate and prepare for treatment of the infant. The fetus may lose blood through a variety of routes. Hemorrhage commonly occurs through the placenta into the mother's circulation and may be detected most readily through a Kleihauer-Betke test performed on the mother's blood. For monozygotic twins, there is an additional risk that one fetus may hemorrhage through the placental vascular anastomosis into the other twin (see the section on twin-to-twin transfusion syndrome later in this chapter). The fetus may also bleed through the placenta into the birth canal. In many cases of placental abruption, the vaginal blood contains a mixture of fetal and maternal blood. The fetus may lose a large volume of blood into the fetal placental circulation at the time of birth (see also Chapter 2). All of the latter circumstances have the same effect as hemorrhage. Some of these mechanisms, such as placental abruption and trapping of blood in the placenta by cord compression, also produce asphyxia, and the coexistence of asphyxia with hypovolemia complicates both the assessment and the management of the infant. Even though most newborn babies with asphyxia are not hypovolemic, there is a subset of infants who have lost blood volume around the time of delivery and most also experienced asphyxia.

Before delivery, internal hemorrhage may occur, with the most common type being intraventricular hemorrhage. The true incidence of intracranial hemorrhage is not certain, but in cases of alloimmune thrombocytopenia in which there is severe thrombocytopenia, intracranial hemorrhage may be seen in as many as 20% of cases. Administration of intravenous gammaglobulin (IVIG) and/or corticosteroids to the mother during a subsequent pregnancy with an affected fetus is widely practiced to increase the fetal platelet count and thus avoid intracranial hemorrhage (see later discussion).[24] Internal hemorrhage can also result from trauma around the time of delivery. Important common types of hemorrhage secondary to birth-related trauma are subgaleal hematomas, hepatic subcapsular and mediastinal hematomas, intracerebral and cerebellar hemorrhage, and hematomas in fractured limbs. Adrenal hemorrhage is more common in neonates than in children or adults. The incidence of detected cases ranges from 1.7 to 2.1 per 1000 births. Because adrenal bleeding may remain asymptomatic, the real incidence is probably higher. In published series, the most common clinical feature in infants with adrenal hemorrhage was jaundice, which was observed in 67.6% of cases in at least one series. Thus, it has been suggested that in cases of hyperbilirubinemia of unknown cause, adrenal hemorrhage must be kept in mind.[25]

For hemorrhages that are associated with birth trauma, the occurrence is highest in difficult term deliveries, particularly in infants who are large for gestational age and require multiple applications of vacuum to assist delivery. Splenic rupture is uncommon but may lead to catastrophic intraabdominal hemorrhage in infants with hemophilia and in babies in whom intrauterine splenomegaly develops as a result of erythroblastosis or other causes. Extensive trauma to the perineum in babies born through breech deliveries can lead to hypovolemia and anemia, and these symptoms are typically exaggerated in the preterm infant.

In the newborn the clinical presentation and symptoms associated with fetal hemorrhage are directly related to the interval between hemorrhage and delivery, as well as to the extent of hemorrhage. When the bleed occurs only shortly before birth, there is little time for hemodilution; thus these babies will not be anemic initially and will show few if any signs that would indicate hypovolemia or anemia. The hematocrit will fall during the first hour after delivery, but a rise in reticulocyte count will not typically be seen until the anemia has been present for several days.

When approaching the treatment of hemorrhagic anemia presenting in the newborn period, one needs first to consider any attendant cardiorespiratory effects of blood loss that are present. Because of the capacity for rapid transport of fluid across the placenta and a limitless reservoir for volume replacement, a hemorrhage that occurs sufficiently far in advance of delivery will likely manifest only the consequences of decreased oxygen-carrying capacity from the anemia. This capacity for rapid replacement of volume loss via the placenta is an important safety net for the fetus, who might not otherwise tolerate intermittent hypoxemia during the contractions associated with labor. For any infant known to have chronic in utero anemia, volume expansion must be approached carefully. The infant in this situation is often anemic but has normal intravascular volume. Consequently, additional volume may lead to heart failure secondary to volume overload. For symptomatic infants with chronic anemia, partial exchange transfusion with packed red blood cells can be performed to achieve a desired hematocrit and avoid volume fluctuation and severe volume shifts. The amount to be exchanged depends on both the baby's blood, the severity of the anemia, and the hematocrit of the packed red blood cells, but an exchange of between 30 and 50 mL/kg body weight may be required.

When hemorrhage occurs acutely during delivery, the hematocrit will not fully reflect the degree of blood loss because there has been little hemodilution. In this situation, one will need to aggressively manage shock, paying close attention to the hemodynamic and cardiorespiratory parameters. Measures of metabolic acidosis, capillary filling time, and both arterial and/or central venous pressures are important to monitor, because they will guide the approach and extent of fluid resuscitation. Almost invariably, newborn babies with hypovolemic shock will have experienced some degree of asphyxia, the manifestations of which will influence the assessment of shock. Thus, one must consider this to be an important variable, and it needs rapid attention, so that the treatment of shock must not delay correction of asphyxia. Acute situations may include placenta previa, vasa previa, abruption, or blood loss from the cut umbilical cord. In such cases, immediate volume replacement with blood is preferable because this rapidly enhances oxygen delivery to tissues, which is not the case when crystalloid solutions are used. Anticipation of the need for resuscitation is a key factor, so recognition of maternal vaginal bleeding should be a signal to anticipate for the need for transfusion. Most labor and delivery units have type O Rh-negative uncrossed red blood cells available.[26] The classic approach to shock in the newborn is to transfuse 10 mL/kg of blood over 5 to 10 minutes and to repeat infusions until there are signs of adequate circulation.

Twin-to-Twin Transfusion Syndrome

Twin-to-twin transfusion syndrome (TTTS) is a complication that may occur in monochorionic twins which may originate in either imbalance or abnormality of the single placenta serving two twins. It is a serious complication in 10% to 20% of monozygous twin gestations with an overall incidence (i.e., including those in which it is not a serious complication) of 4% to 35% in the United States.[27] The diagnosis is well established in overt clinical forms through the association of polyuric polyhydramnios and oliguric oligohydramnios. TTTS is a progressive disease in which sudden deterioration in clinical status can occur, leading to the death of a twin. Up to 30% of survivors have abnormal neurologic development as a result of the combination of profound antenatal insult and complications of severe prematurity. Newer treatment options have improved the outcomes.[27]

TTTS results from an unbalanced blood supply through placental anastomoses in monochorionic twins. These anastomoses may be arterial to arterial, but arterial to venous are believed to be responsible for a majority of the cases presenting clinically. TTTS induces growth restriction, renal tubular dysgenesis, and oliguria in the donor and visceromegaly and polyuria in the recipient. Studies have shown a potentially important role of the renin-angiotensin system with upregulation in the donor twin, whereas in recipients, renin expression was virtually absent, possibly because it was downregulated by hypervolemia.[28] In the donor, congestion and hemorrhagic infarction were accompanied by severe glomerular and arterial lesions resembling those observed in polycythemia- or hypertension-induced microangiopathy. Thus, fetal hypertension in the recipient twin in TTTS might be partly mediated by the transfer through the placental vascular shunts of circulating renin produced by the donor.

The degree of transfusion from one twin to the other and the time course of the transfusion may be highly variable. It may begin as early as the second trimester and therefore be long-standing at the time of delivery. In the most severe cases in which the transfusion is of long duration, the donor is substantially anemic and exhibits significantly increased erythropoiesis that can even be present in the dermis ("blueberry muffin baby"); the donor also becomes progressively small for gestational age and develops oligohydramnios. Simultaneously, the recipient twin continues to grow normally and becomes polycythemic; in extreme cases, this progresses to polyhydramnios and potentially to hydrops fetalis. If the growth-restricted twin dies in utero, the risk exists for embolization through vascular anastomoses to the surviving twin as a consequence of intravascular coagulation in the dying twin. Embolization in the surviving twin will have major consequences, often affecting vital organs including the brain, gastrointestinal tract, and kidneys. Postpartum management of liveborn twins affected by this syndrome will be quite complicated, even when the pediatrician is prepared well in advance of delivery. The polycythemic twin will need reduction of the hematocrit, whereas the treatment of the anemic donor is more straightforward. If either of the newborn twins demonstrates evidence of cardiomyopathy, the infant would be intolerant of blood volume shifts and may be particularly sensitive to blood volume expansion, in which instance a partial exchange transfusion is again the preferred approach.

The best treatment in cases of TTTS presenting before 26 weeks of gestation is fetoscopic laser ablation of the intertwin anastomoses on the chorionic plate.[29-31]

EDITORIAL COMMENT: In twin-to-twin transfusion syndrome (TTTS) the likelihood of perinatal survival of at least one twin was not found to vary with severity as classified by Quintero stage (stage I, 92%; stage II, 93%; stage III, 88%; stage IV, 92%).[32] However, dual twin survival did vary by stage (stage I, 79%; stage II, 76%; stage III, 59%; stage IV, 68%; $P < .01$), primarily because stage III TTTS was associated with decreased donor twin survival. Sequential selective laser photocoagulation of communicating vessels in pregnancies with TTTS was associated with higher dual survival and donor twin survival rates compared with a nonsequential technique. Overall survival of one or both twins was 91% and dual twin survival was 72%.

NONHEMORRHAGIC ANEMIAS

Hyperbilirubinemia is far more common and more severe in neonates with hemolytic anemia than in older children. The bilirubin level may increase rapidly in the first hours after birth, so identification of the underlying cause is extremely important. To diagnose the cause of hemolysis, it is essential to obtain good information about any family history of anemia or neonatal jaundice, and without exception, *both* the baby and a blood smear should be examined. Clues to the appropriate diagnostic tests are often present in these smears, suggested by morphologic abnormalities of the red blood cells. It is standard to perform a direct antiglobulin test (DAT, or direct Coombs test), because the majority of hemolytic episodes are a consequence of maternal antibodies that cross the placenta in late gestation and then react with paternal antigen expressed on the infant's erythrocytes. These maternal immunoglobulin G (IgG) alloantibodies against paternal antigen are responsible for most cases of hemolytic disease of the newborn. If the DAT result is negative but hyperbilirubinemia persists and the hematocrit is declining, a more thorough evaluation is required. This typically does not include a bone marrow examination, which is reserved for cases in which anemia is not associated with hemolysis and in which there is evidence suggesting a primary disorder of erythropoiesis.

Hemolytic Anemias

Maternal Antibodies

Fetal-neonatal alloimmune disease is the most common cause of severe hemolytic anemia in an otherwise healthy newborn. Of these disorders, Rh disease remains the most common cause of severe anemia. Anemia varies from mild to severe, the DAT result is strongly positive, and the reticulocyte count is almost uniformly elevated. Antenatal assessment is an important aspect of good management and should include maternal screening and frequent surveillance of fetal well-being. In sensitized pregnancies, vigilance in pursuing these evaluations is essential if one is to define the appropriate time for intervention with premature delivery or intrauterine transfusions.

Hyperbilirubinemia

Hyperbilirubinemia is a problem in the majority of cases of Rh disease, and in patients with the most severe degree of hemolysis, the elevated bilirubin level cannot be managed by phototherapy alone and ultimately requires exchange transfusion. For patients with Rh sensitization and intrapartum asphyxia, correction of anemia is essential to minimize cardiorespiratory distress and is thus an important part of resuscitation in this group of patients. The most extreme cases of Rh sensitization are associated with hydrops fetalis in utero. Antenatal therapies have been implemented to prevent this severe manifestation of alloimmunization, including intrauterine transfusions. Treated infants are born with only mild to moderate anemia, with all of their red blood cells derived from the intrauterine transfusions. In these infants, the DAT finding may often be negative, but the result of the indirect antiglobulin test is strongly positive. Quite frequently, the consequence of intrauterine transfusion is that the newborn will have no reticulocytosis despite moderate anemia, and with the majority of the infant's red blood cells derived from intrauterine transfusions with Rh-negative blood, there is no hemolysis. It is imperative that these infants be watched closely over the first several months, because a late episode of hemolysis and anemia may arise when the donor erythrocytes eventually decline in number. As erythropoiesis begins to accelerate, these infants produce their own Rh-positive blood cells, which are susceptible to attack by residual maternal antibodies. In such infants, the DAT result may remain strongly positive for months and they will require supplemental folic acid to keep pace with the demands of increased erythropoiesis.

EDITORIAL COMMENT: It is truly remarkable that after the discovery of the blood groups in the 1940s, the virtual elimination of erythroblastosis with anti-D globulin took a mere 30 years, and this is one of the more notable accomplishments in modern medicine. Anti-D, a polyclonal immunoglobulin G, is purified from the plasma of D-alloimmunized individuals. It is routinely and effectively used to prevent hemolytic disease of the fetus and newborn caused by the antibody response to the D antigen on fetal red blood cells. This therapy has effectively reduced the number of cases of Rh isoimmunization from 13% to less than 1% and the mortality rate from one in four to fewer than 5%. The residual cases are few and far between and have been attributed mainly to failed maternal prophylaxis caused by improper timing or dosage of immunoglobulin anti-D therapy and by immunization during pregnancy resulting from an early occult fetomaternal hemorrhage (at <28 weeks' gestation). With erythroblastosis, the late-onset anemia may be either hemolytic or hyporegenerative.

Alloimmune Disease

Alloimmune disease may also occur as a consequence of other blood group incompatibilities (anti-c, anti-e, and anti-C in the Rh system and anti-Kell). In alloimmune anemia of the newborn, the level of hemolysis caused by the presence of antibodies to antigens of the Kell blood group system is less than that caused by antibodies to the D antigen of the Rh blood group system, and the numbers of reticulocytes and normoblasts in the baby's circulation are inappropriately low for the degree of anemia. These findings suggest that sensitization to Kell antigens results in suppression of fetal erythropoiesis as well as hemolysis. Vaughan et al compared the ex vivo growth of Kell-positive and Kell-negative hematopoietic progenitor cells from cord blood in the presence of human monoclonal anti-Kell and anti-D antibodies and serum from women with anti-Kell antibodies.[33] The growth of Kell-positive erythroid progenitor cells (erythroid burst-forming units and colony-forming units) from cord blood was markedly inhibited by monoclonal IgG and IgM anti-Kell antibodies in a dose-dependent fashion (range of concentrations: 0.2% to 20%), but monoclonal anti-D antibodies had no effect. The growth of these types of cells from Kell-negative cord blood was not affected by either type of antibody. Neither monoclonal anti-Kell antibodies nor monoclonal anti-D antibodies inhibited the growth of granulocyte or megakaryocyte progenitor cells from cord blood. Serum from 22 women with anti-Kell antibodies inhibited the growth of Kell-positive erythroid burst-forming units and colony-forming units but not of Kell-negative erythroid burst-forming units and colony-forming units (*P* <.001 for the difference between groups). The maternal anti-Kell antibodies had no inhibitory effects on granulocyte-macrophage or megakaryocyte progenitor cells from cord blood. These data indicate that anti-Kell antibodies specifically inhibit the growth of Kell-positive erythroid burst-forming units and colony-forming units, a finding that supports the hypothesis that these antibodies cause fetal anemia by suppressing erythropoiesis at the progenitor cell level.

A third form of alloimmune disease is caused by ABO incompatibility. This is perhaps one of the most frequent causes of hyperbilirubinemia in the newborn but is rarely responsible for a significant hemolytic anemia. The peripheral blood smear of patients with ABO incompatibility shows microspherocytes, and in most cases, the mother is type O, whereas the baby is either type A or type B. The elevation in serum bilirubin concentration typically resolves within 1 to 2 weeks, and it is rare for this form of alloimmune hemolytic disease to result in a drop in hemoglobin level or hematocrit sufficient to require transfusion in the absence of other complicating factors such as infection. Clinical disease rarely occurs in group A mothers with group B babies or in group B mothers with group A babies.

Congenital Infections

Congenital infections may be associated with hemolytic anemias and have most often been observed in the setting of TORCH infections (*t*oxoplasmosis, *r*ubella, *c*ytomegalovirus infections, *h*erpes simplex) as well as syphilis.[34,35] The association of hemolytic anemia with cytomegalovirus infection is well described, and cytomegalovirus infection has been documented as a cause of autoimmune hemolytic anemia in the setting of vertically acquired neonatal infection with human immunodeficiency virus (HIV).[36] Parvovirus B19 has an affinity for erythroid progenitors and produces severe erythroid hypoplasia, with severe infection during fetal development resulting in hydrops fetalis or congenital anemia. Diagnosis is based on examination of bone marrow and virologic studies. Much is known of the pathophysiology of the virus, and studies are in progress to develop a vaccine to prevent this widespread infection. Bacterial infections can precipitate a hemolytic episode, particularly in individuals with glucose-6-phosphate dehydrogenase deficiency, and thus this diagnosis should be considered in the setting of sepsis and severe hemolysis in the neonate.[37]

Enzymopathies

Specific erythrocyte glycolytic enzyme defects can be the cause of hemolytic syndromes in the neonate. Two of the most commonly observed enzymopathies are described in the following sections.

Glucose-6-Phosphate Dehydrogenase Deficiency

Glucose-6-phosphate dehydrogenase (G6PD) deficiency is the most common human enzyme defect and is present in more than 400 million people worldwide.[38] As with sickle cell disease, the global distribution of G6PD is remarkably similar to that of malaria, which lends support to the hypothesis that these red blood cell disorders confer protection against malaria. G6PD deficiency is an X-linked genetic defect caused by mutations in the G6PD gene, which lead to functional variants with many biochemical and clinical phenotypes. Significant deficiency occurs almost exclusively in males. About 140 mutations have been described; most are single-base changes leading to amino acid substitutions. The most common G6PD mutation in North America is the G6PD-A variant, present in approximately 10% of African Americans. Term infants are rarely symptomatic. The most frequent clinical manifestations of G6PD deficiency are neonatal jaundice and acute hemolytic anemia, which are usually triggered by an exogenous agent. Jaundice in the neonate with G6PD deficiency may occur without any known oxidant exposure. In contrast to G6PD-A, G6PD-Canton, a variant common in South China, is commonly associated with significant neonatal jaundice. Some G6PD variants cause chronic hemolysis, which leads to congenital nonspherocytic hemolytic anemia. The most effective management of G6PD deficiency is to prevent hemolysis by avoiding oxidative stress.

Glucose-6-phosphate dehydrogenase is the rate-limiting enzyme in the hexose monophosphate shunt pathway. This pathway is principally important for the production of reduced glutathione, and this antioxidant has a vital role in protecting the red blood cell membrane from oxidant damage. G6PD deficiency is common worldwide, with certain molecular variants associated with neonatal hemolysis and hyperbilirubinemia. A case recently reported in the literature described a novel missense mutation in a white neonate with chronic nonspherocytic hemolytic anemia caused by a class I G6PD deficiency.[39] The missense mutation in exon eight of the G6PD gene (c.827C>T p.Pro276Leu) was associated with severe elevation in serum bilirubin level, which peaked on day 5 at 24 mg/dL with a conjugated bilirubin level of 17 mg/dL. Jaundice resolved within 4 weeks. A detailed work-up failed to reveal other specific factors contributing to cholestasis. Severe hemolytic disease of the newborn may cause cholestasis, even in the absence of associated primary hepatobiliary disease.

The diagnosis of G6PD-deficient hemolytic anemia should be suspected in male infants with evidence of acute hemolytic anemia and a negative result on Coombs test/DAT. Because the reticulocyte has higher levels of G6PD, screening tests for G6PD activity performed on the heels of a hemolytic episode are less reliable and should be repeated 2 to 3 months after an acute hemolytic episode in conjunction with family studies.

Pyruvate Kinase Deficiency

Pyruvate kinase deficiency is a rare cause of neonatal hemolytic jaundice, with a prevalence estimated at 1 case per 20,000 live births in the United States, but with a higher prevalence in the Amish communities in Pennsylvania and Ohio. One report described four neonates with pyruvate kinase deficiency born in a small community of individuals practicing polygamy.[40] All four had early, severe hemolytic jaundice. Pyruvate kinase deficiency should be considered in neonates with early hemolytic, Coombs test–negative, nonspherocytic jaundice, particularly in communities with considerable consanguinity. Such cases should be recognized early and managed aggressively to prevent kernicterus. (See also Chapter 13.)

DEFECTS OF THE RED BLOOD CELL MEMBRANE

Inherited abnormalities of one of the proteins of the red blood cell membrane may be associated with neonatal hemolysis and jaundice. Hereditary spherocytosis is an autosomal dominant condition and the most common of this class of disorders. Most cases of spherocytosis result from decreased production of spectrin. Hereditary spherocytosis, including the very mild or subclinical forms, is the most common cause of nonimmune hemolytic anemia among people of Northern European ancestry, with a prevalence of approximately 1 in 2000. However, very mild forms of the disease may be much more common. Hereditary spherocytosis is inherited in a dominant fashion in 75% of cases; the remaining are truly recessive cases and de novo mutations.[41] A negative family history does not rule out the diagnosis, because new mutations are quite common. Diagnosis may be aided by the evaluation of a peripheral blood smear in infants suspected of one of these disorders of the red blood cell membrane.

OTHER CONGENITAL ANEMIAS

Congenital Dyserythropoietic Anemias

Congenital dyserythropoietic anemias (CDAs) are rare hereditary disorders characterized by ineffective erythropoiesis and by distinct morphologic abnormalities of erythroblasts in the bone marrow. Although historically these disorders have been largely diagnosed through identification of characteristic morphologic aberrations, the recent discovery of underlying etiologic genetic abnormalities has established the usefulness of molecular diagnostic approaches that might serve as rapid tools for the identification of these conditions. The first CDA partly accounted for genetically has been CDA I, for which the responsible gene *CDAN1*, encoding codanin-1, was discovered in 2002. Genetic defects linked to CDA II (*SEC23B*) and a previously unrecognized CDA (*KLF1*) have been identified. *SEC23B* encodes SEC23B, which is a component of the coated vesicles transiting from the endoplasmic reticulum to the *cis* compartment of the Golgi apparatus. *KLF1* encodes the erythroid transcription factor KLF1 (Kruppel-like factor 1), and the recently identified mutation leads to major ultrastructural abnormalities, the persistence of embryonic and fetal hemoglobins, and the absence of some red blood cell membrane proteins. The current understanding of the various CDAs, including genotype-phenotype relationships, has recently been reviewed elsewhere.[42]

Deficiencies of Red Blood Cell Production

Among the anemias that present in the newborn period, those resulting from inadequate production are rare but, when present, may point to one of the rare congenital disorders affecting red blood cell production. These congenital defects of erythropoiesis exhibit a very low prevalence ranging from 4 to 7 per million live births and include Blackfan-Diamond anemia and Fanconi anemia, which are described in the following sections.

Blackfan-Diamond Syndrome

Blackfan-Diamond syndrome (also called *congenital hypoplastic anemia*) is the most common congenital disorder of red blood cell production in the neonate.[43] Infants with Blackfan-Diamond syndrome are often small for gestational age and may have other anomalies (including renal abnormalities) that must be considered when pursuing this diagnosis. Blackfan-Diamond anemia may result in severe fetal anemia requiring transfusion. Although autosomal dominant inheritance of Blackfan-Diamond syndrome is considered uncommon, it has been described[44]; the onset of anemia characteristically occurs within the first year of life, with 10% of cases presenting at birth. Affected infants exhibit variable degrees of anemia, with normal circulating white blood cell and platelet counts. Hydrops fetalis has been reported in rare cases. Among women with this disorder, a percentage are at risk for having an infant with substantial anemia in both the fetal and perinatal periods. Because the penetrance of the disorder is variable, pregnant women with a history of Blackfan-Diamond anemia should be considered at risk. Recommendations for the prenatal management of Blackfan-Diamond syndrome include prepregnancy counseling for parents with Blackfan-Diamond syndrome, detailed and serial fetal ultrasound and echocardiographic studies, cordocentesis if there are signs of anemia, consideration of in utero transfusion, and planned early delivery if the fetus is affected.[44]

Fanconi Anemia

Fanconi anemia is a rare chromosomal instability disorder associated with a variety of developmental abnormalities, bone marrow failure, and predisposition to leukemia and other cancers.[45] The Fanconi anemia gene family is a recently identified addition to the group of genes coding for the complex network of proteins that respond to and repair certain types of DNA damage in the human genome, but little is known about the regulation of this novel group of genes at the DNA level.[46] A homozygous missense mutation in the *RAD51C* gene has been described in a consanguineous family with multiple severe congenital abnormalities characteristic of Fanconi anemia.[47] *RAD51C* is a member of the RAD51-like gene family involved in homologous recombination-mediated DNA repair. The mutation results in loss of *RAD51* focus formation in response to DNA damage and in increased cellular sensitivity to the DNA interstrand cross-linking agent mitomycin C and the topoisomerase-I inhibitor camptothecin. Fanconi anemia generally affects children and results in bone marrow failure requiring blood or marrow transplantation for survival. A unique feature of the condition is the long waiting period, often many years, between genetic diagnosis and treatment, which presents a significant challenge to the family and requires a strong, supportive multidisciplinary approach to care.[48]

ANEMIA SECONDARY TO HEMOGLOBINOPATHIES

Hemoglobinopathies arise from mutations in the globin genes, with the most common hemoglobinopathies resulting from mutations in the β-globin gene. These are typically clinically silent at birth due to the persistence of Hb F but manifest as the expression switches from γ- to β- chain production.

Thalassemias

Mutations in the β-globin gene that lead to a decrease in production are referred to as *β-thalassemias*. The β-thalassemias resulting from large structural deletions of the β-globin gene cluster are a rare familial cause of microcytic anemia and hyperbilirubinemia.[49] Although blood cell counts are normal at birth, this disorder can be detected by demonstrating the absence of Hb A on electrophoresis. In most states, umbilical cord blood is routinely screened to identify infants with thalassemia and other hemoglobin disorders (including sickle cell disease; see later discussion) before they become symptomatic.

α-Thalassemia is one of the most common human genetic disorders and is found extremely frequently in populations in Southeast Asia and southern China, and the expanding populations of Southeast Asian immigrants in the United States, Canada, the United Kingdom, and Europe mean that this disorder is no longer rare in these countries.[50,51] Couples in which both partners carry α^0-thalassemia traits have a 25% risk of producing a fetus affected by homozygous α-thalassemia or hemoglobin Bart's (Hb Bart's) disease, with severe fetal anemia in utero, hydrops fetalis, and stillbirth or early neonatal death, as well as various maternal morbidities.

The α-thalassemias present a different, greater challenge than β-thalassemia to the neonatologist and pediatrician. The α-thalassemias are characterized by the decrease or complete suppression of α-globin polypeptide chains, with reduced or absent synthesis of one to all four α-globin genes. In the fetus, a complete deficiency of chain synthesis results in an absence of Hb F and

the production of Hb Bart's. Hb Bart's is composed of tetrads of the γ-globin chain (γ_4) and exhibits a profoundly abnormal oxygen dissociation curve reflecting the reduced capacity to off-load oxygen at the tissue capillary bed. The gene cluster, which codes for and controls the production of these polypeptides, maps near the telomere of the short arm of chromosome 16 within a G+C-rich and early-replicating DNA region. The genes expressed during the embryonic stage (ζ) or fetal and adult stage (α-2 and α-1) can be modified by point mutations that affect either the processing-translation of mRNA or make the polypeptide chains extremely unstable. Much more frequent are the deletions of variable size (from approximately 3 kilobases to more than 100 kilobases) that remove one or both α genes in *cis* or even the whole gene cluster. Deletions of a single gene are the result of unequal pairing during meiosis, followed by reciprocal recombination. These unequal crossovers, which produce also α-gene triplications and quadruplications, are made possible by the high degree of homology of the two α genes and of their flanking sequences.

The interaction of the different α-thalassemia determinants results in three phenotypes: α-thalassemic trait, clinically silent and presenting with only limited alterations of hematologic parameters; Hb H disease, characterized by the development of a hemolytic anemia of variable degree; and Hb Bart's hydrops fetalis syndrome (lethal), a consequence of compromised oxygen delivery to tissues. The diagnosis of α-thalassemia caused by deletions is based on electrophoretic analysis of genomic DNA digested with restriction enzymes and hybridized with specific molecular probes. Recently, polymerase chain reaction (PCR)–based strategies have replaced Southern blot analysis. Hemoglobin H disease, a mutation of three α-globin genes, is more severe than previously recognized. Anemia, hypersplenism, hemosiderosis, growth failure, and osteoporosis are commonly noted as the patient ages. Infants with one or two functional α-globin genes have microcytosis at birth (mean corpuscular volume is <95) and an elevated percentage of Hb Bart's on electrophoresis. α-Thalassemia major is usually fatal in utero. Surviving newborns who did not undergo intrauterine transfusion often have congenital anomalies and neurocognitive injury. Serious maternal complications often accompany pregnancy. Doppler ultrasonography with intrauterine transfusion ameliorates these complications. The high incidence in selected populations mandates population screening and prenatal diagnosis of couples at risk. Universal newborn screening has been adopted in several regions with DNA confirmatory testing using the methods noted earlier.[52,53]

Sickle Cell Anemia

Sickle cell disease (SCD) is caused by a single point mutation in the β-globin gene that causes the hydrophilic amino acid glutamic acid to be replaced with the hydrophobic amino acid valine at the sixth position. SCD is an autosomal recessive genetic blood disorder with incomplete dominance, characterized by red blood cells that assume an abnormal, rigid, sickle shape.[54] Sickling decreases the cells' flexibility and carries a risk of various complications. The introduction of newborn screening in the United States has had a significant impact on morbidity and mortality from SCD. Historically, the failure to achieve early identification of SCD resulted in a high rate of mortality because of the susceptibility of these patients to overwhelming infection, particularly with encapsulated organisms. Penicillin prophylaxis and the introduction of the pneumococcal vaccine have had an additional impact on the risk of sepsis and mortality in this population.[55] Inheritance of the sickle gene with a thalassemia variant, such as β-thalassemia, can alter the presentation, in part by increasing the relative concentration of Hb S.

ANEMIA OF PREMATURITY

Anemia of prematurity is thought to be principally a direct consequence of delivery before placental iron transport and fetal erythropoiesis are complete and is exaggerated by various factors, including blood losses associated with phlebotomy to obtain samples for laboratory testing, low plasma levels of erythropoietin due to both diminished production and accelerated catabolism, rapid body growth and the need for commensurate increases in red blood cell volume and mass, and disorders causing red blood cell losses due to bleeding and/or hemolysis. Blood losses resulting from the phlebotomy required for frequent laboratory studies can be a frequent cause of anemia of prematurity, despite advances in blood conservation with microsampling methods. The sick preterm infant receiving ventilatory assistance can often have more than 5 mL of blood per day withdrawn for laboratory studies. At this rate, an 800-g infant would lose his or her entire blood volume for laboratory studies in approximately 13 days. Large infants are less affected because of their greater blood volumes.

Rapid somatic growth of the preterm and very low-birth-weight infant also contributes substantially to anemia of prematurity. Very low-birth-weight infants will typically more than double their body weight and blood volume by the time they are ready for discharge from the nursery. In addition to the factors mentioned earlier, possibly the most significant contributing factor to this process is the prolonged cessation of erythropoietin production. As noted previously, reactivation of erythropoietin production in the infant kidney appears to be determined more by a biologic clock than by a response to stress. Indeed, there is no erythropoietin response to even severe anemia until the infant reaches a corrected gestational age of about 34 to 36 weeks. After this time, the erythropoietin system will respond when the hematocrit declines into the range of 25% to 30%. The reticulocyte count will typically rise within 1 week after the increase in erythropoietin production. Because transfusion during this critical period suppresses the release of endogenous erythropoietin, it can delay the recovery from anemia of prematurity, particularly in the seriously ill preterm requiring multiple transfusions, in whom recovery may not be observed until an even later corrected gestational age. Ultimately, it is the tissue oxygen tension that stimulates erythropoietin release, and recipients of multiple transfusions in whom Hb F has largely been replaced by Hb A will be less likely to achieve a low enough tissue oxygenation to stimulate timely or early erythropoietin release.

The treatment for anemia of prematurity has evolved substantially. Because placental iron transport is incomplete in the preterm infant, these babies require supplemental iron to mount an effective erythroid response. Iron stores are largely acquired during the last month of intrauterine life, thus term infants are born with large iron stores. The combination of a lack of these iron stores and a rapid rate of growth (and concomitant increase in blood volume) during the first 6 months of life place the preterm infant at significant risk of anemia of prematurity. Most infants with a birth weight of less than 1000 g are given multiple red blood cell transfusions within the first few weeks of life. Red blood cell transfusions have typically been the mainstay of therapy for anemia of prematurity; recombinant human erythropoietin (rHuEPO) is largely unused because of the view that it fails to substantially diminish red blood cell transfusion needs despite exerting substantial erythropoietic effects on neonatal marrow.[56]

Multiple randomized, controlled trials have shown that treatment of extremely preterm infants with rHuEPO during the period when their endogenous erythropoietin system is inactive stimulates erythropoiesis, maintains a higher hematocrit, and reduces the need for transfusions. Reticulocytosis appears about 1 week after the start of treatment. The main population thought to benefit are those infants born before 30 weeks of gestation, with the smallest, least mature in this group exhibiting the greatest benefit.

Treatment is usually started after the infant has tolerated the introduction of enteral feedings. Large multicenter trials have demonstrated that administration of rHuEPO plus iron supplementation cannot prevent early transfusions, particularly in very low-birth-weight newborns and in infants with severe neonatal diseases. However, this approach may be effective in preventing late transfusions. Doses of 100 U/kg body weight given 5 days per week or 250 U/kg given three times per week are equally effective, and there is no evidence that larger doses are more effective. Current treatment of anemia of prematurity should focus on efforts to minimize factors that reduce erythrocyte mass (phlebotomies, noninvasive procedures) and promote factors that increase it (placental transfusion, adequate nutritional support).[57]

EDITORIAL COMMENT: Extremely low-birth-weight preterm infants often develop anemia of prematurity from frequent and excessive blood draws, a process referred to by Ed Bell as "gradual exsanguination."[58] The hypoproliferative anemia is marked by inadequate production of erythropoietin. Recombinant human erythropoietin (rHuEPO) has been available since 1990, but trials looking at reduction of red blood cell transfusions with rHuEPO achieved limited success. There has been a focus recently on autologous transfusion, blood-sparing technologies, and limitation in the number of donors. Treatment of anemia of prematurity includes red blood cell transfusions, which are given to preterm infants based on indications and

guidelines (hematocrit and hemoglobin levels, ventilation and oxygen needs, apneas and bradycardias, poor weight gain) that are relatively nonspecific.

The need for transfusions can be reduced by limiting phlebotomy losses, providing good nutrition, and using standard guidelines for transfusion based on hemoglobin level or hematocrit. What those guidelines should be is not clear. Analysis of data for the Premature Infants in Need of Transfusion (PINT) trial, which compared management according to restrictive and liberal transfusion guidelines in infants weighing less than 1000 g and used a composite primary outcome of death before home discharge or survival with either severe retinopathy, bronchopulmonary dysplasia, or brain injury on cranial ultrasonography, revealed no statistically significant differences between groups in any secondary outcome.[59] The investigators concluded that in extremely low-birth-weight infants, maintaining a higher hemoglobin level results in more infants receiving transfusions but gives little evidence of benefit. Data on the impact of transfusion practices on long-term outcome are very limited and inconclusive. Until further evidence surfaces, the tendency will probably be to adopt more liberal indications for transfusion. Many centers continue to use the Shannon criteria[60] which call for transfusion in infants if any of the following conditions are met: (1) a requirement for more than 35% inspired oxygen on continuous positive airway pressure (CPAP) or positive pressure ventilation with a mean airway pressure of more than 6 cm H_2O; (2) a requirement for less than 35% inspired oxygen on CPAP or positive pressure ventilation with a mean airway pressure of less than 6 cm H_2O, significant apnea and bradycardia, tachycardia (>180 beats per minute) or a respiratory rate of more than 80 breaths per minute, weight gain of less than 10 g/day over 4 days, or sepsis; or (3) a hematocrit of less than 20%. Valieva et al modified these criteria to be more restrictive because of concerns about complications in the transfused group.[61] Their criteria include the following:

Hematocrit of less than 35% in the first week of life *and* in unstable condition*

Hematocrit of less than 28% in the first week of life *or* in unstable condition*

Hematocrit of less than 20% if older than 1 week of age *and* in stable condition

---

Instability is defined as an increased risk for poor oxygen delivery (e.g., prolonged oxygen desaturation episodes or hypotension requiring treatment).

POLYCYTHEMIA

Several conditions are associated with polycythemia in utero. These include chronic hypoxia due to maternal toxemia and placental insufficiency, placental insufficiency with postmaturity syndrome, pregnancy at high altitudes, pregnancy in a diabetic woman, and trisomy 21. In most instances, newborns who have clinically significant polycythemia have a preexisting high hematocrit in utero due to one of the causes listed previously, which is then exaggerated by excessive placental transfusion at delivery. Conversely, early cord clamping and reduced placental transfusion can lead to a normal hematocrit in an infant who developed polycythemia in utero.

The complications of polycythemia are a consequence of the rise in blood viscosity that occurs as the hematocrit rises, which compromises circulation to a variety of tissues and organs. The clinical manifestations are distinct in each organ system. Skin manifestations include plethora and delayed capillary filling. Renal symptoms include proteinuria and hematuria, and in extreme conditions, renal disease can be indistinguishable from renal vein thrombosis. If the severity of polycythemia is poorly appreciated and early feeding is instituted, infants can develop necrotizing enterocolitis (NEC). The central nervous system manifestations of polycythemia may be mild, including poor feeding, irritability, and an abnormal cry; more concerning cases are those manifesting apnea, seizures, and cerebral infarction.[62]

The diagnosis of polycythemia is not based solely on hematocrit, because there is no precise hematocrit at which symptoms appear in all infants. This is partly due to the fact that other factors affect viscosity in addition to hematocrit. Although symptoms are common when the venous hematocrit exceeds 66%, serious signs of organ dysfunction develop in some infants with lower hematocrits. It is essential that polycythemia be confirmed by measuring the venous blood hematocrit, because capillary values correlate poorly with the central venous hematocrit (capillary hematocrits are generally higher). The treatment for the neonate with polycythemia is partial exchange transfusion in which blood is replaced with a plasma substitute. Isotonic saline, plasma, and a mixture of saline and albumin have all been used with equal efficacy. The goal for the hematocrit is 50%. To achieve this through exchange, the following formula is typically used: $V = [(HCT_1 - HCT_D) \times$ body weight (kg) $\times$ 90 mL]/HCT_1, where V = the exchange volume, HCT_1 is the baby's hematocrit, and HCT_D is the desired hematocrit. The hematocrit must be monitored carefully after this procedure, because it will ultimately rise and if the HCT_D is not reached with the initial volume exchange, it may rise again to a dangerous level.

The greatest dilemma is that posed by the asymptomatic newborn with polycythemia. Although one might advocate observation, the reality that the first manifestations are neurologic argues for early intervention and extremely close observation. Supporting early prophylactic exchange is the observation that the incidence of neurologic handicaps is increased in children who had untreated neonatal polycythemia.[63] However, the benefit of this approach for preventing neurologic complications remains controversial.[64]

ERYTHROCYTE TRANSFUSION IN THE FETUS AND NEWBORN

Packed red blood cell transfusions are often administered to patients in the neonatal intensive care unit (NICU). Infants who have significant cardiopulmonary disease are transfused when they become anemic, because it is thought that a higher oxygen-carrying capacity improves their tolerance of cardiorespiratory distress.[65] Current blood transfusion guidelines are useful in establishing parameters for transfusion, but it is essential that physicians also modify the application of these guidelines based on their own perceptions and assessments in identifying patients in need of a packed red blood cell transfusion. In an evaluation of the influence of caregiver perception and assessment on transfusion practices, neonates who underwent transfusion based on caregivers' perceptions rather than adherence to strict guidelines were more likely to be receiving noninvasive ventilatory support and were more symptomatic. Neonates who improved after transfusion had a lower pretransfusion hematocrit and were more symptomatic compared with the group that did not show clinical improvement. In this study, tachycardia was the most sensitive predictor of benefit from packed red blood cell transfusion.[66]

Extremely low-birth-weight infants are the most heavily transfused, yet the indications for transfusion do continue to represent an area of controversy. A very important concept to which one should always adhere is that there is no single critical hematocrit that always requires transfusion. In reality, there will be a range of critical hematocrits at which transfusion may be required even for an individual patient, and these different thresholds are values that are influenced by the severity of illness. Several studies have suggested an association between red blood cell transfusion and NEC in premature neonates.[67,68] Withholding feeds during transfusion has never been clearly demonstrated to be beneficial but may have a protective effect against the development of NEC. In a retrospective case-control study of premature low-birth-weight infants (<32 weeks' gestation and <2500 g) who developed NEC over a 6-year period (25 infants with NEC and 25 controls who never developed NEC), more infants in the NEC group received transfusions in the 48 to 72 hours preceding diagnosis (56% versus 20% within 48 hours [P = .019] and 64% versus 24% within 72 hours [P = .01]).[68] The total number of transfusions and age of red blood cells were not different in the two groups. The same investigators implemented a policy of withholding feeds during transfusion, and this practice was associated with a decrease in the incidence of NEC from 5.3% to 1.3% (P = .047). These data support the recognized association of NEC with the administration of red blood cell transfusions in the 48 to 72 hours preceding presentation of NEC and provide a rationale for exercising caution in feeding around the time of packed red blood cell transfusions in the neonate.

The risk-to-benefit ratio of blood transfusions for preterm infants will continue to be defined by ongoing experience. Although use of a more restrictive transfusion threshold for hemoglobin level or hematocrit, or both, may decrease the number of blood transfusions in preterm infants, the impact of such an approach on long-term outcomes must be defined.[69,70]

WHITE BLOOD CELLS

But so long as you stimulate the phagocytes, what does it matter which particular sort of serum you use for the purpose?

George Bernard Shaw,
The Doctor's Dilemma

Mature white blood cells are derived from pluripotent hematopoietic stem cells. In early development, hematopoietic stem cells emerge separately from the yolk sac, chorioallantoic placenta, and aorta-gonad-mesonephros region.[71] Following the initial

erythropoietic stage, myeloid progenitor cells can be found in the yolk sac during the third to fourth week of gestation.[72] From the yolk sac, these progenitor cells sequentially migrate to the liver, thymus, and spleen and eventually take up permanent residence in the bone marrow at the eleventh to twelfth week of gestation. Hematopoietic stem cells with self-renewal capacity give rise to pluripotent progenitors that progress to common lymphoid or common myeloid progenitors.[73,74] Common lymphoid progenitors differentiate into natural killer (NK) cells, B lymphocytes, T lymphocytes, and immature lymphoid dendritic cells. Common myeloid progenitors differentiate into granulocytes (neutrophils, eosinophils, and basophils), monocytes, and immature myeloid dendritic cells. Monocytes give rise to tissue macrophages.[73]

The systems mediating innate immunity have qualitative and quantitative deficiencies that affect the newborn's response to infections. For example, neonatal neutrophils ingest and kill bacteria as efficiently as their adult counterparts, but adhesion and subsequent migration of these cells to sites of infection are impaired. The migratory defect of neonatal neutrophils is exacerbated by limited production of the chemoattractant C5a and low generation of C3b, which is necessary for opsonization and phagocytosis. Neutrophil storage pools are rapidly exhausted in the face of serious infection, and the capacity to replenish those stores is limited in the neonate. Acquired immunity in the newborn is affected by qualitative and quantitative deficiencies in lymphoid lineage as well. Cell-mediated killing by NK and cytotoxic T cells is diminished, which leaves the newborn vulnerable to certain viral and intracellular pathogens.[73] The newborn infant produces primarily IgM, and little IgG and IgA, in response to antigenic challenge. Neonatal T and B cells are predominately of a naive phenotype. Since the lymphocyte maturation process is directed largely by cytokines and the capacity of neonatal cells to produce key cytokines such as interleukin-4 and IFN-T interferon-gamma is limited, the acquisition of adult-type functional capabilities is delayed in vivo.

Despite encountering a pathogen-rich environment at the time of birth, most newborn infants, do not become ill. The relative immunodeficiency of the neonate has been viewed by some as an adaptive mechanism to optimize survival by balancing the conflicting immunologic requirements of life in utero with those of the external environment.

NEUTROPHIL DISEASES

NEUTROPENIA

The neutrophil counts in an infant vary by birth weight and postpartum age. For term and near-term infants, values published by Manroe et al are considered appropriate. An absolute neutrophil count (ANC) of 1800 to 5500/µL is seen at birth, and ANC increases by threefold to fivefold over the next 12 to 18 hours of life.[75] By 24 hours of life, the ANC begins to fall, decreasing steadily to 1800 to 7200/µL at 5 days, from then it falls to and remains at 1800 to 5400/µL through 28 days of age. Studies by Mouzinho et al show that normal preterm very low-birth-weight neonates have leukocyte reference ranges that differ significantly from those of older neonates (neutrophil counts have lower minimum values in the former group).[76] Publications recommend using the Mouzinho et al chart for infants of less than 1500 g birth weight and the Manroe et al chart for larger infants (see also Appendix C).[75-78] Studies suggest that neonates with neutrophil counts above 1000/µL are not likely to be at high risk of acquiring a nosocomial infection. Counts below 500/µL (particularly when they remain below 500/µL for many days) are associated with an increased risk for developing a nosocomial infection. Persistent counts between 500 and 1000/µL may pose some intermediate risk.[77,78]

Causes of Neonatal Neutropenia

Box 17-1 lists the most common causes of neutropenia in newborns. In general, neutropenia can be caused by either decreased neutrophil production or increased destruction.

Neutropenia Secondary to Increased Neutrophil Destruction

Alloimmune Neonatal Neutropenia

In alloimmune neonatal neutropenia (ANN) the mother becomes immunized to a father's neutrophil antigen that is expressed on the fetal neutrophils. Subsequently, IgG antibodies directed against fetal neutrophil antigen crosses the placenta and destroys the fetal granulocytes. The severity of neutropenia is influenced by the titer and subclass of the maternal IgG neutrophil antibodies, the phagocytic activity of the infant's

---

Box 17-1. **Causes of Neutropenia in the Neonate**

Increased neutrophil destruction or utilization

Immune
- Alloimmune/isoimmune neutropenia
- Autoimmune neutropenia in the mother

Nonimmune
- Maternal preeclampsia
- Infection: bacterial, viral
- Periventricular hemorrhage
- Asphyxia
- Metabolic disorders

Reduced neutrophil production

Infants of hypertensive mothers
Donors of twin-to-twin transfusion
Nutritional factors
Kostmann disease (severe congenital agranulocytosis)
Pure white cell aplasia
Barth syndrome
Reticular dysgenesis
Hyperimmunoglobulin M syndrome
Shwachman-Diamond syndrome
Dyskeratosis congenita

Mixed causes

Drugs
TORCH infections (*toxoplasmosis*, *rubella*, *cytomegalovirus*, *herpes simplex*)

Excessive neutrophil margination

Pseudoneutropenia
Endotoxin-induced margination

---

reticuloendothelial system, and the capacity of the infant's marrow to compensate for the shortened survival of antibody-coated neutrophils.[79,80] Antineutrophil antibodies have been found in as many as 20% of surveyed pregnant and postpartum women, but studies have documented ANN in 0.2% to 2% of consecutively sampled newborns.[79-82] A wide variety of antigenic targets have been identified, including human neutrophil alloantigen (HNA) groups HNA-1, HNA-2, and HNA-3 as well as NC1, SH, SAR, LAN, LEA, and CN1.[79-83] The role of human leukocyte antigen (HLA) is controversial.[84] Despite all the available data, in nearly half of cases the antigens cannot be recognized.[81,82] Symptomatic infants can manifest delayed separation of the umbilical cord, skin infections, otitis media, or pneumonia within the first 2 weeks of life. Although most infections are mild, overwhelming sepsis is known to occur and is associated with a mortality rate as high as 5% in infants with ANN. When neutropenia is prolonged (>7 days), severe (ANC of <500/μL), or associated with serious infections, ANN can be treated with subcutaneous recombinant human granulocyte colony-stimulating factor (rG-CSF). The use of growth factor in this setting is discussed later in the chapter. Fortunately, in the majority of cases the disorder is self-limiting and resolves over a period of weeks to a few months as levels of the transplacentally acquired maternal antibody diminish.[79-82]

Autoimmune Neutropenia of Infancy

Autoimmune neutropenia of infancy (AIN) is a disorder caused by increased peripheral destruction of neutrophils as a result of antibodies in the infant's blood that are directed against the infant's own neutrophils. It is analogous to immune thrombocytopenic purpura or autoimmune hemolytic anemia. Primary AIN, which is not associated with other diseases such as systemic lupus erythematosus, is often observed in infants and has an incidence of 1 in 100,000.[80] A large number of children with primary AIN show the presence of antibodies specific to HNA-1a or HNA-1b. Less frequently, the antineutrophil autoantibodies recognize adhesion glycoproteins of the CD11/CD18 (HNA-4a, HNA-4b) complex, the CD35 molecule (CR1), and FcγRIIb.[85,86] The origin of these autoantibodies is not known. The mechanism proposed include molecular mimicry of microbial antigens, modification of endogenous antigens as a result of drug exposure, increased or otherwise abnormal expression of HLA antigens, or loss of suppressor activity against self-reactive lymphocyte clones. There have been reported associations with parvovirus B19 infection and exposure to β-lactam antibiotics.[87,88] AIN is usually diagnosed during the first few months of life (3 to 8 months).[85]

Diagnosis of AIN in premature twins has been reported, which suggests that sensitization can occur even in utero.[89] Although there is significant neutropenia at presentation (500 to 1000/μL), the clinical course is usually benign with mild infections.[85,86,90] Severe infectious complications (pneumonia, sepsis, meningitis) are seen in about 12% of these patients.[80,86] AIN resolves spontaneously by the age of 2 or 3 years in 95% of cases.[85,86,90] Therefore most cases require no specific therapy. The usefulness of antibiotic prophylaxis must be assessed on a case-by-case basis. Administration of

rG-CSF is currently the first-line therapy to achieve remission of the neutropenia. Treatment with IVIG is effective in less than 50% of cases and the benefit lasting less than 2 weeks. Steroids have limited effect in immune-mediated neutropenia.[86]

Neonatal Autoimmune Neutropenia

Neonatal autoimmune neutropenia is seen when mothers with autoimmune disease transfer their neutrophil autoantibodies passively to the fetus. Most often, the mother and the infant are neutropenic. The infant's neutropenia is transient and asymptomatic. The recovery process takes a few weeks to a few months and depends on the time it takes to clear IgG antibodies.[81,82]

Neutropenia in Neonates with Sepsis

Neonates have immature granulopoiesis. This frequently results in neutropenia after sepsis, which is likely secondary to exhaustion of the storage and proliferative pools of the bone marrow. Neutropenic septic neonates have a higher mortality rate than nonneutropenic septic neonates.[91,92] Whether growth factor or granulocyte infusions should be used in such a setting remains controversial (see later discussion). Neutropenia commonly occurs in neonates who have NEC as well. In this instance, neutropenia results from increased use and/or destruction in tissues, margination due to endotoxinemia, and increased mobilization of neutrophils into the peritoneum.

Neutropenia Secondary to Decreased Neutrophil Production

Severe Congenital Neutropenia

Severe congenital neutropenia is a genetically heterogeneous bone marrow failure syndrome characterized by maturation arrest of myelopoiesis at the promyelocyte-myelocyte stage. Estimated frequency is approximately 1 to 2 cases per million with equal male-female distribution. Severe congenital neutropenia follows an autosomal dominant or autosomal recessive pattern of inheritance. About 60% of cases are attributable to mutations in the gene for neutrophil elastase (*ELA2*).[93] Less commonly, mutations in *HAX1*, *G6PC3*, and other genes cause this disorder. From early infancy, patients who have severe congenital neutropenia experience bacterial infections. Omphalitis, beginning directly after birth, may be the first symptom; however, otitis media, pneumonitis and infections of the upper respiratory tract, and abscesses of the skin or liver are also common and can lead to the diagnosis of severe congenital neutropenia. Patients with the disorder have severe chronic neutropenia with ANCs continuously below 200/µL; in many cases, peripheral blood neutrophils are completely absent. Peripheral monocytosis or eosinophilia may be present. The bone marrow usually shows a maturation arrest of neutrophil precursors at an early stage (promyelocyte-myelocyte level) with few cells of the neutrophilic series beyond the promyelocyte stage. The use of rG-CSF remains first-line treatment for most patients with severe congenital neutropenia. Transplantation of hematopoietic cells from an HLA-identical sibling is beneficial for patients who are refractory to rG-CSF therapy. Patients who have severe congenital neutropenia are at risk of leukemic transformation, and those who develop myelodysplasia or leukemia should proceed urgently to hematopoietic stem cell transplantation.[78,93]

Shwachman-Diamond Syndrome

Shwachman-Diamond syndrome is an autosomal recessive marrow failure syndrome associated with exocrine pancreatic insufficiency and predisposition to leukemia. Approximately 90% of patients meeting clinical criteria for the diagnosis of Shwachman-Diamond syndrome harbor mutations in the SBDS gene (Shwachman-Bodian-Diamond syndrome) that maps to the 7q11 centromeric region of chromosome 7.[94,95] The initial symptoms typically are diarrhea and failure to thrive beginning in early infancy, and it is truly rare for the disease to present in the neonatal period. Growth failure and metaphyseal chondrodysplasia associated with dwarfism are seen in some patients. The most common hematologic abnormality, affecting 88% to 100% of patients with Shwachman-Diamond syndrome, is neutropenia. Patients with Shwachman-Diamond syndrome are susceptible to recurrent bacterial, viral, and fungal infections; in particular, otitis media, sinusitis, mouth sores, bronchopneumonia, septicemia, osteomyelitis, and skin infections.[94] The illness may progress to bone marrow hypoplasia or dysplasia, leading to moderate thrombocytopenia and anemia. For treatment, rG-CSF has been used. The only definitive therapy for marrow failure, myelodysplasia, or leukemia is hematopoietic cell transplantation.[94,95]

Neutropenia in Neonates with Hypertensive Mothers

Infants born to mothers who have pregnancy-induced hypertension (PIH) or HELLP syndrome (*h*emolysis, *e*levated *l*iver enzymes, and *l*ow *p*latelet count) are observed to have neutropenia in 40% to 50% of cases, with the most severe neutropenia in the very low-birth-weight infants.[78] This type of neutropenia is the result of placental production of an inhibitor of myelopoiesis. It can be severe, with blood neutrophil counts below 500/µL. With no specific treatment, this variety of neutropenia generally resolves in about 72 hours and almost always resolves by the fifth day after birth. Whether a risk of sepsis is associated with neutropenia in infants born to mothers with preeclampsia remains a topic of discussions.[96,97]

Neutropenia in Donor Twins

Neutropenia occurs in the donor twin (the twin who becomes anemic) in twin-to-twin transfusion. It is usually transient. Since the myelopoiesis shifts toward erythropoiesis, neutrophil production decreases, which results in neutropenia. No left shift is present.

Neutropenia in Neonates with Rh Hemolytic Disease

The neutropenia in neonates with Rh hemolytic disease is likely caused by a shift of myelopoiesis toward erythropoiesis, which diminishes neutrophil production. It is usually transient.

Neutropenia Secondary to Mixed Causes

Drugs

Drugs can cause neutropenia through suppressive effects on progenitors, changes in marrow extracellular matrix, development of autoantibodies, and other mechanisms.[78] Ganciclovir has been strongly associated with neutropenia, and cessation of therapy may be necessary.[98] Other drugs used in the NICU that have been implicated in causes of neutropenia include β-lactam antibiotics, thiazide diuretics, and ranitidine.[88]

Infection

Intrauterine cytomegalovirus and rubella virus infections can be associated with neutropenia or pancytopenia. Neutropenia in this instance is likely secondary to splenomegaly; however, there might be an element of decreased production as well.[78,99]

Pseudoneutropenia

Artifactual neutropenia has been described that is caused by ethylenediaminetetraacetic acid (EDTA)–induced neutrophil agglutination in vitro. The condition can be diagnosed by the presence of neutrophil clumps on peripheral smears.

EVALUATION OF THE NEONATE WITH NEUTROPENIA

Neutropenia in the NICU requires little diagnostic evaluation if the cause is clear (e.g., NEC, sepsis, maternal PIH). However, if neutropenia persists more than 3 to 5 days, particularly if the count is less than 500/μL, additional evaluation is needed. Helpful findings on physical examination include characteristic dysmorphic features such as skeletal dysplasia, radial or thumb hypoplasia (congenital bone marrow failure syndromes), hepatosplenomegaly (TORCH syndrome, storage disorders), and skin or hair pigmentary abnormalities (Chédiak-Higashi syndrome). A complete blood count, including microscopic examination of the peripheral blood smear to determine neutrophil morphology, can be useful in identifying congenital neutropenia syndromes. The immature-to-total (I/T) neutrophil ratio can be helpful in differentiating defects in production from destruction of neutrophils. The I/T ratio can be calculated as follows:

$$(Bands + Metamyelocytes + Myelocytes) / (Segmented\ neutrophils + Bands + Metamyelocytes + Myelocytes)$$

A normal or low I/T ratio in the presence of severe neutropenia suggests that the neutropenia is due to decreased production. A very high I/T ratio suggests increased neutrophil production, which implies increased peripheral destruction or tissue recruitment of neutrophils.[78] It is also useful to obtain a complete blood count for the infant's mother. If maternal blood neutrophil concentration is normal, maternal neutrophil antigen typing and antineutrophil antibody screening should be pursued at a reference laboratory highly skilled in detection of neonatal alloimmune neutropenia. A bone marrow study is useful in patients with severe and prolonged neutropenia who were not born to mothers with PIH and in whom alloimmune and maternal autoimmune neutropenia have been excluded.[77]

Management of Neonatal Neutropenia

In ill neutropenic neonates, sepsis should always be suspected and antibiotic therapy initiated promptly. If the neutropenia is severe and prolonged, reverse isolation procedures might be useful. Accepted treatment options for symptomatic neonatal neutropenia are discussed below.

Treatment

Recombinant Granulocyte and Granulocyte-Macrophage Colony-Stimulating Factors

The availability of recombinant myeloid growth factors has provided new strategies in the management of neonatal neutropenia. rG-CSF is structurally identical to the natural human G-CSF and increases the number of circulating neutrophils by stimulating the release of neutrophils from the bone marrow, inducing myeloid proliferation, and reducing neutrophil apoptosis.

Both rG-CSF and recombinant granulocyte-macrophage colony-stimulating factor (rGM-CSF) have been administered as treatment for neonates with neutropenia with varying degrees of success. Calhoun et al have outlined consistent approaches to procedures and practices in neonatal hematology,[100] including one for the use of rG-CSF.

The decision regarding whether to administer rG-CSF to any given neutropenic patient in the NICU must be individualized with consideration of the risks and benefits. The U.S. Food and Drug Administration (FDA) has approved the use of rG-CSF as long-term treatment to reduce the incidence and duration of sequelae of neutropenia (e.g., fever, infections, oropharyngeal ulcers) in symptomatic patients with congenital neutropenia, cyclic neutropenia, or idiopathic neutropenia. The varieties of severe chronic neutropenia for which rG-CSF administration has been best studied are Kostmann syndrome, Shwachman-Diamond syndrome, Barth syndrome, and cyclic hematopoiesis. At this time, it is not clear whether chronic idiopathic neutropenia or neonatal alloimmune neutropenia fit under the FDA indication of severe chronic neutropenia, because although these disorders can be very severe, they are self-limited, and the duration rarely exceeds 6 months. Moreover, administration of rG-CSF to patients with these latter neutropenic disorders has not been tested in randomized placebo-controlled trials.[100] However, these patients generally derive considerable benefit from rG-CSF treatment.[101] In addition to increasing circulating neutrophil numbers by stimulating the release of neutrophils from the bone marrow, rG-CSF downregulates antigen expression, which makes the neutrophils less vulnerable to circulating antibodies. The majority of neonates with either idiopathic or alloimmune forms of neutropenia will respond to doses of 5 to 10 µg/kg given subcutaneously at intervals ranging from every day to less than once per week, as needed, to bring the blood neutrophil concentration to levels above 500 to 1000/µL.[100] It is recommended that rG-CSF be used with caution in patients who have immune-mediated neutropenias caused by antibodies against HNA-2a (NB1), since it has been shown to increase the expression of HNA-2a in healthy adult volunteers. In one case of a neonate who had ANN caused by anti–HNA-2a antibodies, the response was delayed and was achieved only with an unusually high dose.[102] rG-CSF has also been used successfully in patients with neutropenia caused by maternal PIH.[103]

Several studies evaluated the role of rG-CSF therapy in septic neutropenic neonates.[104-108] These were followed by two metaanalyses that examined the efficacy and safety of treatment with hemopoietic colony-stimulating factors (rG-CSF or rGM-CSF) in newborn infants with suspected or proven systemic infection. In a metaanalysis by Bernstein et al,[109] rG-CSF recipients were found to have a lower mortality than did controls. However, when the nonrandomized studies were excluded, the analysis did not remain statistically adequate. More importantly, neutropenia was not defined consistently in the studies reviewed, and therefore the significant reduction in mortality noted when rG-CSF was given to neonates with neutropenia requires further confirmation. A metaanalysis by Carr et al examined the effect of adjuvant G-CSF or GM-CSF treatment on 14- and 28-day overall mortality in neonates with suspected or documented sepsis.[110] A combination of five studies ($n = 194$) in the 28-day mortality analysis showed a reduction in all-cause mortality in treated infants (relative risk: 0.51; 95% confidence interval [CI]: 0.27 to 0.98). When results from three studies ($n = 97$) that were limited to neutropenic infants with systemic infection were analyzed, 14- and 28-day overall mortality was found to be reduced by rG-CSF therapy (relative risk: 0.34; 95% CI: 0.12 to 0.92). Current evidence suggests the need for a multicenter randomized clinical trial demonstrating the clinical efficacy of rG-CSF before this therapy can be universally recommended in the NICU.[111]

EDITORIAL COMMENT: Neonates have a high risk of sepsis if they are either neutropenic or have low concentrations of immunoglobulin. Carr et al reported that early postnatal prophylaxis with granulocyte-macrophage colony-stimulating factor corrects neutropenia but does not reduce sepsis or improve survival and short-term outcomes in extremely preterm neonates.[112] A metaanalysis that included this trial as well as previously reported prophylactic trials showed no survival benefit.[110]

Although administration of granulocyte colony-stimulating factor and granulocyte-macrophage colony-stimulating factor can raise white blood cell counts, this does not translate into fewer infections. Nor is there conclusive evidence that in the face of proven sepsis these cytokines effectively stimulate release of neutrophils and improve outcome. The role of neutrophil transfusions and intravenous immunoglobulin for neutropenic septic babies is still being evaluated.

Intravenous Immunoglobulin

IVIG has been used with success in both ANN and AIN, with a response rate of about 50%.[80-82] However, because of the lack of a titratable dose-response effect and the possibility that IVIG may itself induce neutropenia, this treatment has been used less often than rG-CSF in patients who have immune neutropenia.[80-82]

Granulocyte Transfusions

Current evidence does not show a clear beneficial role for granulocyte transfusion in neonates. Calhoun et al recommend using granulocyte infusions for patients who have early-onset sepsis and shock,[100] are undergoing mechanical ventilation and receiving infusions of pressors, have a blood neutrophil concentration well below 1000/µL with a left shift, and have already received IVIG. A systemic review by Mohan et al found no significant difference in "all-cause mortality during hospital stay" in infants with sepsis and neutropenia who received granulocyte transfusions and those who received placebo or no granulocyte transfusion.[113] Adequately powered multicenter trials of granulocyte transfusion are needed to clarify its role in the treatment of neonates with sepsis and neutropenia.

NEUTROPHILIA

Neutrophilia (defined as >7000 white blood cells/µL in term infants and >13,000 white blood cells/µL in premature infants) typically is a nonspecific response to a stressor.[114] The most common cause of neonatal neutrophilia is infection (Box 17-2). Birth asphyxia and other causes of acute or chronic hypoxia can induce the marrow to prematurely release immature myeloid and erythroid cells into the circulation. Nucleated erythrocytes are registered by electronic cell counters as leukocytes, so it is important to correct for the presence of nucleated red blood cells when interpreting the white blood cell count. Neonatal granulocytosis caused by intrinsic disorders of the marrow is rare. Neonatal leukemia and the transient myeloproliferative disorder seen in infants with trisomy 21 are usually associated with large numbers of circulating immature myeloid cells and with hepatosplenomegaly. The diagnosis is established by bone marrow examination, which should include cytogenetic analysis of unstimulated bone marrow.

NEUTROPHIL FUNCTIONAL DEFECTS

Neutrophil functional defects are uncommon disorders that rarely present in the newborn. Because neonates have inherent functional defects in their polymorphonuclear neutrophils and monocytes, and also have a higher rate of infections than older infants and children, the clinical manifestations characteristic of dysfunctional phagocytosis may be obscured by the already higher infection rates in neonates. Therefore, it is necessary to have a relatively low threshold for specific evaluation of these conditions. Diagnostic evaluation may be difficult because of the limited volume of

blood that can be taken from the neonate for diagnostic studies.[114] For all of these reasons, it is difficult to identify the rare infant in whom infection is due to an inherited defect in neutrophil function.

EOSINOPHILIA

Eosinophilia (most frequently defined as >700 eosinophils/µL[115]) is common in hospitalized neonates of all gestational ages, but there are significant differences in patterns of incidence and severity based on gestational age, with increased incidence and greater severity of eosinophilia in the more immature infants.[116,117] Eosinophilia in neonates has been attributed to a variety of causes (Box 17-3).

When evaluating the infant with eosinophilia, it is helpful to consider the potential differences in etiology for those who are ill versus those who are well.[118] In the latter group, infection should be strongly considered, especially if the complete blood count was obtained because of clinical suspicion of infection. An evaluation for sepsis is appropriate if risk factors or predictors are present, such

---

Box 17-2. **Conditions Associated with Neutrophilia in the Neonate**

Infection
Birth asphyxia
Other causes of acute or chronic hypoxia (pneumothorax, meconium aspiration)
Hemolytic disease
Seizures
Leukemoid reaction
Neonatal leukemia and transient myeloproliferative disorder
Congenital anomalies (tetralogy of Fallot)
Leukocyte adhesion deficiency

Box 17-3. **Conditions Associated with Eosinophilia in the Neonate**

Hematologic disorders
- Hypereosinophilic syndrome
- Eosinophilic leukemoid reaction
- Eosinophilic leukemia
- Thrombocytopenia–absent radius syndrome
- Congenital neutropenia with eosinophilia
Infection
- Bacterial
- Viral
- Fungal
Necrotizing enterocolitis
Immune deficiency disorders
- Congenital immune deficiency syndromes
- Hyperimmunoglobulin E
Familial eosinophilia
Establishment of an anabolic state
Drug reactions
- L-Tryptophan
- Ceftriaxone
Congenital immunodeficiency syndromes
- Hyperimmunoglobulin E
- Omenn syndrome
Cow's milk allergy
Miscellaneous
- Congenital heart disease
- Chronic lung disease

as neutropenia, thrombocytopenia, coagulation dysfunction, hypotension, or respiratory distress. An evaluation for NEC is appropriate if signs consistent with gastrointestinal dysfunction are present. If the neonate with eosinophilia is well, close monitoring for 48 hours is suggested. If the eosinophilia persists, then a search for a specific cause of the eosinophilia should be undertaken.[118]

CHRONIC GRANULOMATOUS DISEASE

Chronic granulomatous disease (CDG) is the most common inherited disorder of leukocyte function. CDG has an X-linked or autosomal recessive inheritance pattern involving defects in genes encoding phox proteins, which are the subunits of phagocyte reduced nicotinamide adenine dinucleotide phosphate oxidase (NADPH oxidase). This results in failure to produce superoxide anion and downstream antimicrobial oxidant metabolites and to activate antimicrobial proteases. Affected patients are susceptible to severe, life-threatening bacterial and fungal infections (such as pneumonia caused by *Aspergillus* or liver abscess caused by *Staphylococcus aureus*) and excessive inflammation characterized by granulomatous enteritis and genitourinary obstruction. Early diagnosis of CGD and rapid treatment of infections are critical. The diagnosis of CGD requires demonstration of defective NADPH oxidase activity in neutrophils. The most common diagnostic assays are the nitroblue tetrazolium dye reduction test (a measure of superoxide anion release) and flow cytometry evaluating dihydrorhodamine 123 (DHR) fluorescence (a measure of intracellular hydrogen peroxide). Infection prophylaxis and interferon-γ administrations have significantly improved the natural history of CGD. Currently, the only cure is allogeneic hematopoietic cell transplantation, although controversy remains as to which patients with CGD should receive a transplant.[119]

LEUKOCYTE ADHESION DEFICIENCY

Leukocyte adhesion deficiency (LAD) exists in two forms. LAD-1 (Mac-1 deficiency) is due to deficiency or dysfunction of leukocyte integrins, and LAD-2 is due to congenital deficiency of selectin function. It is a rare disorder that can present in the neonatal period with severe infections, delayed separation of the umbilical stump, and leukocytosis. Diagnosis is made by flow cytometry (absence of CD11b/CD18 on blood

phagocytic cells in LAD-1 and absence of sialylated CD15 leukocyte antigens in LAD-2).[114,120]

CHÉDIAK-HIGASHI SYNDROME

Chédiak-Higashi syndrome is a rare autosomal recessive disorder caused by mutations in the *LYST* (or *CHS1*) gene. The Chédiak-Higashi syndrome gene affects the synthesis and/or maintenance of storage-secretory granules in various types of cells. Lysosomes of leukocytes and fibroblasts, dense bodies of platelets, azurophilic granules of neutrophils, and melanosomes of melanocytes are generally larger in size and irregular in morphology. Che'diak–Higashi syndrome manifests as recurrent pyogenic infections, oculocutaneous albinism, and giant intracellular granules in blood leukocytes.[114,120]

NEONATAL IMMUNE DEFICIENCIES OF LYMPHOCYTE LINEAGE (T CELL, B CELL, NATURAL KILLER CELL)

It is important for neonatologists and pediatricians to be able to differentiate between immune immaturity and a true primary immunodeficiency that may present during the neonatal period. Failure to identify primary immune deficiency properly can result in delayed diagnosis and treatment, which in turn can affect the outcome of the disease. Examples of specific T-cell and B-cell disorders that are recognizable during early infancy are presented in Table 17-1. Selected deficiencies are discussed in the following sections.

HUMORAL IMMUNE DEFICIENCIES

Antibody deficiencies are often unrecognized during the neonatal period because of the protective effect of passively acquired maternal antibodies. In premature neonates, deficiency secondary to immaturity, as opposed to primary antibody deficiency, makes the diagnosis even more difficult. As the levels of maternal antibodies decline, humoral deficiency in the neonate becomes apparent and can be diagnosed as early as 6 months of age (earlier in the preterm infant).

X-Linked Agammaglobulinemia

X-linked agammaglobulinemia is a defect in B-cell development caused by mutations in a cytoplasmic tyrosine kinase called *Btk* that plays a pivotal role in B-cell development. Patients have a profound hypogammaglobulinemia and markedly reduced numbers or absence of B cells (no CD19- or

Table 17-1.	Most Common Immune Deficiencies Encountered in Neonates	
Type	**Disorder**	**Clinical Features**
Humoral immune deficiencies	X-linked agammaglobulinemia	Upper respiratory infections
	Hyperimmunoglobulin M syndrome	
	Transient hypogammaglobulinemia of infancy	
Predominantly cellular immune deficiencies	Neonatal human immunodeficiency virus infection	
Combined immune deficiencies	Severe combined immunodeficiency	
	Omenn syndrome	
Combined immune deficiency associated with other syndromes	Wiskott-Aldrich syndrome	Eczema, thrombocytopenia, recurrent infections
	DiGeorge syndrome	Characteristic facial features, hypocalcemia, microdeletion of chromosome 22
	Ataxia-telangiectasia	Recurrent infections

CD20-bearing cells).[121] Onset of recurrent bacterial infections is seen in the first 24 months of life. Overwhelming enteroviral sepsis and paralytic ileus following administration of live polio vaccine have been observed in neonates with X-linked agammaglobulinemia. Treatment is with immunoglobulin replacement.[121]

Hyperimmunoglobulin M Syndromes
Hyperimmunoglobulin M syndromes are a heterogeneous group of genetic disorders causing primary immunodeficiency in which defective immunoglobulin class switch recombination leads to deficiency of IgG, IgA, and IgE with preserved or elevated levels of IgM. The most common form of hyperimmunoglobulin M syndrome, accounting for at least 70% of cases of class switch recombination defects, is caused by mutations in the gene encoding the CD40 ligand (*CD40LG*). Clinical problems occur early in life with a median age at diagnosis of younger than 12 months. Two thirds of infants have neutropenia with associated perirectal abscesses and oral ulcers. Patients have increased susceptibility to *Pneumocystis* and other opportunistic organisms (e.g., chronic cryptosporidial infection leading to persistent diarrhea and failure to thrive). The mainstay of treatment for these forms of hyperimmunoglobulin M syndrome is immunoglobulin replacement therapy.[122]

Transient Hypogammaglobulinemia of Infancy
Transient hypogammaglobulinemia of infancy is a common and heterogeneous immune deficiency with indistinct pathophysiology presenting with a delay in maturation of immunoglobulin production in an infant as maternal antibodies disappear. This diagnosis encompasses cases in which serum concentrations of one or more of the three major immunoglobulin classes is more than 2 standard deviations below normal for age in at least two specimens obtained during infancy and the disorder lacks features consistent with other forms of primary immunodeficiency. In transient hypogammaglobulinemia of infancy, there is an extended period of hypogammaglobulinemia, which usually resolves by 30 to 40 months of life. Infants usually remain asymptomatic or develop recurrent sinopulmonary infections, but severe or life-threatening infections are rare.[123]

PREDOMINANTLY CELLULAR IMMUNE DEFICIENCIES
Neonatal HIV infection is discussed in Chapter 14.

COMBINED IMMUNE DEFICIENCIES
T-cell and combined immune deficiencies commonly manifest initially during the neonatal period (secondary to a lack of maternally acquired immunity and a vital T-cell role in immune response). Patients experience severe infections including opportunistic infections (*Pneumocystis jiroveci* [*Pneumocystis carinii*] pneumonia, infection with *Mycobacterium* species, fungal infections), viral infections, and graft-versus-host disease (caused by either maternally derived T cells or transfusions with nonirradiated blood products). Some combined immunodeficiencies present as a part of a syndrome that also includes altered function of other

organ systems (Wiskott-Aldrich syndrome, DiGeorge syndrome, etc.).

Severe Combined Immunodeficiency

Severe combined immunodeficiency (SCID) designates a genetically heterogeneous group of syndromes that have in common a profound disturbance of both T and B cells. At least 15 different molecular defects have now been identified, all of which lead to early death in the absence of therapy.[124,125] The affected genes encode cell surface receptors and other activation signaling molecules (IL2RG, JAK3, IL7R, CD45, CD3 components, FOXN1), T-cell and B-cell antigen receptor gene recombinases (RAG1, RAG2, Artemis, DNA ligase 4), and purine pathway enzymes (adenosine deaminase, purine nucleoside phosphorylase).[125] Typical symptoms of SCID are noted from birth and include recurrent severe infections, chronic diarrhea, and failure to thrive. However, infants may appear normal at birth and have no family history of immunodeficiency. Therefore, infants with severe T-cell deficiencies may not be identified until life-threatening infections occur. Physical examination may reveal thrush and absence of lymphoid tissue. Hypogammaglobulinemia is often present, and T cells are often absent. B-cell and NK cell pattern varies, which results in various SCID phenotypes.[120]

Hematopoietic stem cell transplantation and enzyme replacement (in the case of adenosine deaminase deficiency) have made this previously fatal set of diseases treatable.[125]

If the diagnosis is made early in the first months of life before the onset of serious infections, the long-term prognosis for infants with SCID may be markedly improved (better survival, less morbidity, and lower treatment costs than when SCID is recognized only after the onset of serious infections). Administration of attenuated vaccines that are recommended in early infancy and that can cause serious infection in infants with T-cell lymphopenia should be avoided.

Molecular identification of SCID gene mutations now enables early diagnosis in affected families. Infants with SCID identified because of a family history can undergo prenatal mutation diagnosis and be treated early in life.[125]

Universal newborn screening for SCID has become an important public health goal. As a potential screening tool, a test of T-cell receptor gene excision circles (TRECs) was chosen by some researchers. This test is performed on DNA from the dried blood spots collected for screening newborns. It can identify any infant with profound T-cell lymphopenia and not just infants with SCID. In a study by Routes et al,[126] TREC assay by real-time quantitative PCR was performed on newborn screening cards for newborn infants. Seventeen of 64,397 infants older than 37 weeks' gestation screened using the TREC assay (approximately 0.026%) had TREC values below the cutoff limit (<25 TRECs/µL blood). Eleven infants subsequently underwent a confirmatory flow cytometry screening test, which confirmed the presence of T-cell lymphopenia in 8 infants. The ongoing trials of SCID screening will need to answer questions on optimal screening protocols and the costs of treatment and screening that would provide appropriate information for policy makers deciding among competing health care priorities.[127]

Omenn Syndrome

Omenn syndrome is an autosomal recessive combined immunodeficiency characterized by infiltration of the skin and gastrointestinal tract by activated oligoclonal T lymphocytes. In contrast with other forms of SCID, the total number of circulating T lymphocytes in Omenn syndrome is normal and they show activated phenotype. However, their proliferative response to in vitro stimulation by mitogens and antigens is markedly decreased. In contrast, B cells are usually undetectable both in peripheral blood and in lymphoid tissues, and hypogammaglobulinemia results. A remarkable hypereosinophilia and increased IgE serum levels are observed. T-cell repertoire in Omenn syndrome is highly restricted as well.[128] The most common causes of Omenn syndrome are hypomorphic mutations of the recombination-activating genes. Mutations of the Artemis (*DCLRE1*), *IL7RA*, *RMRP*, *IL2RG*, and *CHD7* genes may also result in the Omenn syndrome phenotype.[129] Patients with Omenn syndrome develop early-onset, generalized, exudative erythrodermia associated with lymphadenopathy, and hepatosplenomegaly. The loss of protein through the skin (and often also due to chronic diarrhea) results in hypoproteinemia and generalized edema. In addition, alopecia is a frequent finding. Many of the clinical features of Omenn syndrome are reminiscent of acute graft-versus-host disease. Because of their unique susceptibility to severe infections, patients with Omenn syndrome inevitably die early in life unless treated with hematopoietic stem cell transplantation.[128]

COMBINED IMMUNE DEFICIENCIES ASSOCIATED WITH OTHER SYNDROMES

Wiskott-Aldrich Syndrome
Wiskott-Aldrich syndrome is discussed later in the section on thrombocytopenia caused by reduced platelet production.

DiGeorge Syndrome
DiGeorge syndrome is caused by a hemizygous deletion of chromosome band 22q11.2. It is extremely common, with nearly 1 in 3000 children affected.[130] Patients display characteristic facies (hypertelorism, short philtrum, low-set ears), cardiac defects, parathyroid hormone deficiency, and immune deficiency. Approximately 20% of patients have no evidence of diminished T-cell numbers, and fewer than 1% have true thymic aplasia requiring transplantation.[130] Based on clinical and immunologic profiles, partial and complete DiGeorge syndrome have been distinguished. In the complete form of DiGeorge syndrome, the thymus is absent. Therefore, T cells are absent or markedly decreased in number, and B cells (although present) make little antibody. Complete DiGeorge syndrome is usually fatal unless treated with thymus transplantation.[130] In partial DiGeorge syndrome, T-cell numbers correlate with the amount of thymus tissue present. T-cell proliferative responses, as well as immunoglobulin levels, are usually normal. However, IgA deficiency, impaired responses to vaccines, and frank hypogammaglobulinemia have been described. Clinical studies show that most patients do not demonstrate a susceptibility to opportunistic infections.[130]

Ataxia-Telangiectasia
Ataxia-telangiectasia is an autosomal recessive disorder that is characterized by early-onset progressive cerebellar ataxia, oculocutaneous telangiectasia, immunodeficiency, and lymphoid tumors.[120,131] Various other abnormalities are also associated with this disorder, including the absence or rudimentary appearance of a thymus, progressive apraxia of eye movements, insulin-resistant diabetes, and clinical and cellular radiosensitivity (higher incidence of malignancies). The gene that is mutated in ataxia-telangiectasia (*ATM*) has been localized to chromosome band 11q22-23.[131]

Immunodeficiency is seen in approximately 70% of patients with ataxia-telangiectasia. T- and B-cell numbers are normal. T cells bearing the γ-δ form of the T-cell receptor constitute up to 50% of T cells (normal: 1% to 5%), and T-cell function is impaired. A varying degree of humoral deficiency (IgA, IgG) is common. Patients usually have bronchopulmonary infections at presentation.[131]

NEONATAL THROMBOCYTOPENIA
Neonatal thrombocytopenia is the most common hematologic problem in the neonate. A normal platelet count in healthy newborn infants irrespective of gestational age is considered to be 150×10^9/L and above.[132-136] Some 1% to 5% of newborns show thrombocytopenia at birth, and 0.1% to 0.5% have severe thrombocytopenia ($<50 \times 10^9$ platelets/L). In contrast, 22% to 35% of all infants admitted to the NICU develop thrombocytopenia, the rate of which increases as gestation age decreases.[134] Christensen et al observed that 73% of extremely low-birth-weight neonates had one or more platelet counts below 150×10^9/L, and 38% of them had a severely low count.[137]

Causes of thrombocytopenia can be classified into those leading to increased platelet destruction (including consumption), those resulting in decreased platelet production, and those involving both.[138] Box 17-4 lists the most common causes of thrombocytopenia in neonates.

Classification can also be based on whether the thrombocytopenia was caused by maternal factors or not.[138] Cause can be predicted by the timing of the onset of thrombocytopenia and its natural history.[132-134] For instance, thrombocytopenia presenting during fetal life is most commonly caused by an alloimmune reaction, congenital infection, or aneuploidy, whereas thrombocytopenia presenting within 72 hours of birth (early-onset neonatal thrombocytopenia) mostly affects preterm neonates born after pregnancies characterized by impaired placental function and/or fetal hypoxia. Neonatal alloimmune or autoimmune thrombocytopenia is common as well. Finally, thrombocytopenia presenting in infants in the NICU after the first 72 hours of life (late-onset

Box 17-4.	Causes of Thrombocytopenia in the Neonate

Increased platelet destruction or consumption
Alloimmune neonatal thrombocytopenia
Autoimmune neonatal thrombocytopenia
Sepsis
Birth trauma
Acidosis/hypoxia
Disseminated intravascular coagulation
Thrombosis
Kasabach-Merritt syndrome
Malignancies (leukemia, etc.)
Cyanotic heart disease

Decreased platelet production
Thrombocytopenia–absent radius syndrome
Congenital amegakaryocytic thrombocytopenia
Amegakaryocytic thrombocytopenia and
    radioulnar synostosis
X-linked macrothrombocytopenia due to
    GATA1 mutation
Fanconi anemia
Wiskott-Aldrich syndrome
Bernard-Soulier syndrome
MYH9-related thrombocytopenias
Chromosomal abnormalities
Preeclampsia

Mixed causes
Maternal medications
Intrauterine growth restriction
TORCH infections (*t*oxoplasmosis, *r*ubella,
    *c*ytomegalovirus, *h*erpes simplex)
Rh disease

neonatal thrombocytopenia) almost always results from late-onset sepsis or NEC.[132-134] When the cause is being sought, the gestational age of the infant is important as well. In one study of extremely low-birth-weight infants, more than 60% of cases of thrombocytopenia were due to infection, disseminated intravascular coagulation, or NEC, and 10% were not explained.[137]

Despite our growing knowledge of neonatal thrombocytopenia, the cause cannot be identified in a significant number of patients.

THROMBOCYTOPENIA DUE TO INCREASED PLATELET DESTRUCTION

Neonatal Alloimmune Thrombocytopenia

Neonatal alloimmune thrombocytopenia (NAIT) is the platelet equivalent of Rh disease. Human platelet antigens (HPAs) are uniquely expressed on platelets, and 16 HPAs have been identified, although fetomaternal incompatibility between only 3 (HPA-1a, HPA-5b, and HPA-15b) cause 95% of cases in white populations. Fetomaternal incompatibility for HPA-1a is the most common and is responsible for 75% of cases in whites.[139] In NAIT the mother is HPA-1a negative and the father is HPA-1a positive, as is the fetus. When the mother is exposed to fetal platelets, anti–HPA-1a antibodies are generated. These antibodies traverse the placenta via the neonatal Fc receptor, as does all maternal IgG, and cause fetal thrombocytopenia.[140] Because of its frequency and severity, NAIT is the most important cause of severe fetal-neonatal thrombocytopenia.

HPA-1a incompatibility occurs in 1 in 350 pregnancies, although thrombocytopenia develops in only 1 in 1000 to 1 in 1500 pregnancies. The ability of an HPA-1a–negative woman to form anti–HPA-1a is class II restricted and is controlled by the HLA-DRB3*0101 allele, so that HLA-DRB3*0101-positive women are 140 times more likely to make anti–HPA-1a than HLA-DRB3*0101-negative women.[141] NAIT is usually suspected in neonates with bleeding or severe, unexplained, and/or isolated postnatal thrombocytopenia. Three criteria distinguish cases of NAIT from other causes of unexplained thrombocytopenia[142]:

1. Severe thrombocytopenia (platelet count of $<50 \times 10^9$/L)
2. Intracranial hemorrhage (ICH) associated with one or more of the following:
   - Apgar score at 1 min of more than 5
   - Birth weight of more than 2200 g
   - Documented antenatal or postnatal bleeding
3. No additional nonhemorrhagic neonatal medical problems

Thrombocytopenia is often extremely severe (platelet count of $<20 \times 10^9$/L) and begins early in gestation. It may result in major bleeding, particularly ICH. Although the incidence of ICH is difficult to ascertain precisely, large series report ICH in 10% to 20% of pregnancies in which NAIT is present.[134] It is reported that 80% of ICH events associated with NAIT occur in utero, with 14% occurring before 20 weeks and a further 28% occurring before 30 weeks.[143] Overall, two thirds of infants with NAIT-associated ICH develop neurodevelopmental problems, approximately half of which are severe (e.g., severe cerebral palsy and/or sensory impairment).[139] The course of NAIT in otherwise well neonates is variable, with thrombocytopenia resolving in most cases within 1 week without long-term sequelae.

Considerable advances have been made in the clinical and laboratory diagnosis of NAIT, and its postnatal and antenatal management. Detailed laboratory investigations are required to confirmation the diagnosis and should be performed by an experienced reference laboratory.

Current consensus is that screening should be performed for HPA-1, HPA-3, and HPA-5 in all cases of potential NAIT and for HPA-4 as well if the patient is of Asian descent. HPA-9 and HPA-15 are the next most commonly involved in antigen incompatibilities. For testing to confirm NAIT, analysis must reveal both a platelet antigen incompatibility between the parents and a maternal antibody directed against that antigen.

Because of the morbidity and mortality associated with NAIT, this disorder requires expert management with close collaboration between fetal medicine specialists, hematologists, and neonatologists.

The mainstay of postnatal management of affected neonates is prompt random-donor platelet transfusion.[144] If promptly available, matched (antigen-negative) platelets are preferred. The latter are platelets from donors negative for HPA-1a or HPA-5b (which are compatible in >90% of NAIT cases, can be given in larger increments, and have a longer half-life). Concentrated maternal platelets can also be used; however, their processing takes at least 12 to 48 hours.

Platelet transfusion is recommended in well term neonates if the count is less than 30×10^9/L unless an ICH is diagnosed, in which case a threshold of 100×10^9/L is used. A higher count, for example 50×10^9/L, may be selected in cases of prematurity, birth asphyxia, or another condition predisposing to ICH.[140]

IVIG can also be infused (effective in at least 75% of cases).[145] The IVIG dose is 1 g/kg/day for 1 to 3 days depending on response. Some centers administer steroids with IVIG.[140] However, with these therapies, platelet count increase is slow (requiring about 48 to 72 hours), and therefore platelet transfusion may still be needed. Head ultrasonography is mandatory for a thrombocytopenic neonate. If NAIT is complicated by even asymptomatic ICH, the target platelet count is higher—more than 100×10^9/L—and management of the next affected pregnancy will be more intensive and start earlier. NAIT often resolves within 2 to 4 weeks.[140,145]

Another important aspect of NAIT care is antenatal management of subsequent pregnancies. If the previously affected sibling had an ICH, the next affected fetus will have early, severe thrombocytopenia and in utero ICH unless effective treatment is provided.[140] Radder et al performed a literature search for ICH cases in untreated NAIT pregnancies.[146] The recurrence rate of ICH in the subsequent offspring of women with a history of NAIT with ICH was 72% (CI: 46% to 98%) when fetal deaths were not included and 79% (CI: 61% to 97%) when they were included. The risk of ICH after a previous occurrence of NAIT without ICH was estimated to be 7% (CI: 0.5% to 13%). The lack of laboratory parameters predictive of severe disease remains one of the major barriers to optimizing antenatal management of NAIT and is an important area for future research.[145] Antenatal treatment intensity depends on the occurrence of ICH and severity of thrombocytopenia in the previous sibling. Maternally administered therapy (maternal IVIG, steroids) should be the first-line approach in all cases. This recommendation is based on data describing the effectiveness and safety of maternal treatment in contrast to the toxicity of serial administration of fetal bovine serum to deliver weekly fetal platelet transfusions. Different centers currently have different strategies based on their own experience and results of published studies.[141,145]

Neonatal Autoimmune Thrombocytopenia

Neonatal autoimmune thrombocytopenia is mediated by the transplacental passage of maternal antiplatelet antibodies. Unlike in NAIT, in this case the antibody responsible binds both maternal and fetal platelets and causes thrombocytopenia in the mother and the neonate.[138] In most instances, the underlying maternal disease is idiopathic thrombocytopenic purpura, but other disorders (e.g., systemic lupus erythematosus) can also produce this syndrome. Maternal platelet autoantibodies occur in 1 to 2 in 1000 pregnancies; however, they are much less likely to cause a clinical problem than NAIT. Thrombocytopenia occurs in only 10% of neonates whose mothers have autoantibodies, and the incidence of ICH is 1% or less. Maternal disease severity and/or platelet count during pregnancy and the occurrence of severe thrombocytopenia in a previous neonate are the most useful indicators of the likelihood that significant fetal and neonatal thrombocytopenia will complicate the current pregnancy.[135,147,148] The platelet count should be determined at birth for all neonates of mothers with autoimmune disease. In neonates with normal platelet counts (>150 × 10⁹/L), no further action is necessary. In those with thrombocytopenia, a platelet count should be repeated after 2 to 3 days, because platelet counts are often at a nadir at this time before rising spontaneously by day 7 in most cases.[134] In a small number of cases thrombocytopenia may persist for several weeks. In this situation, when the thrombocytopenia is severe (platelet count of <30 × 10⁹/L), treatment with IVIG (2 g/kg over 2 to 5 days) may be useful.

Disseminated Intravascular Coagulation

Disseminated intravascular coagulation (DIC) complicates several disease processes (bacterial or viral sepsis, respiratory distress syndrome, meconium aspiration, asphyxia). Thrombocytopenia is a consistent and very early finding in neonates with DIC.[135] Prolonged prothrombin times and partial thromboplastin times, increased levels of fibrin degradation products, increased D-dimer levels, and depletion of fibrinogen are other abnormal laboratory findings usually seen in neonates with DIC. Successful treatment of neonatal DIC depends on the diagnosis and treatment of the underlying disorder. Treatment of the hemostatic abnormalities in neonates with DIC is not clearly established and depends on the clinical manifestations.[135] Exchange transfusions complement administration of platelets and fresh frozen plasma.

Kasabach-Merritt Syndrome

Kasabach-Merritt syndrome typically presents in the neonatal period with profound thrombocytopenia together with microangiopathic anemia, DIC, and an enlarging vascular lesion. Hemangiomas are usually cutaneous, but in 20% there is visceral involvement (e.g., in the liver). Thrombocytopenia in Kasabach-Merritt syndrome is mainly due to the trapping of platelets on the endothelium of the hemangioma.

Usually it is severe, but it is exacerbated in some cases by the development of DIC. Review of the blood film often, although not always, reveals red blood cell fragmentation, which can help in the diagnosis of difficult cases. When treatment is required, administration of steroids followed by interferon and/or vincristine is effective in over 50% of cases, although the mortality is 20% to 30%.[149]

Necrotizing Enterocolitis

NEC frequently causes thrombocytopenia in neonates. In fact, probably 80% to 90% of patients with NEC develop thrombocytopenia (platelet count of <150 × 10⁹/L) as part of the presentation, and many have platelets counts in the range of 30 to 60 × 10⁹/L. Platelet destruction seems to be the primary mechanism.[135]

Thrombosis

Thrombosis can cause thrombocytopenia in a neonate when platelet uptake in the thrombus is more rapid than platelet production. If thrombocytopenia is severe it can be treated by platelet transfusions until the underlying cause of the platelet destruction is removed.[132,135]

THROMBOCYTOPENIA DUE TO DECREASED PLATELET PRODUCTION

Bernard-Soulier Syndrome

Bernard-Soulier syndrome is an autosomal recessive disorder caused by qualitative or quantitative defects in the glycoprotein Ib-IX-V complex. Bernard-Soulier syndrome may present in the neonatal period, although bleeding is not usually severe in neonates. A diagnosis of Bernard-Soulier syndrome is suggested when there is mild to moderate thrombocytopenia together with giant platelets. Treatment by platelet transfusion is effective but should be reserved for cases of life-threatening hemorrhage.[150]

Wiskott-Aldrich Syndrome

Wiskott-Aldrich syndrome, caused by mutations in the Wiskott-Aldrich syndrome gene, is a complex and diverse disorder with X-linked inheritance.[115] Affected boys exhibit microthrombocytopenia with hemorrhagic diathesis in early childhood and variable degrees of eczema, combined immunodeficiency, and increased risk of autoimmunity and lymphoid malignancies. The numbers of T and B lymphocytes decline over the years, and in vitro proliferation of T lymphocytes to specific antigens is reduced. IgA and IgE serum levels are often increased, which reflects immune dysregulation. Unless hematologic and immune reconstitution by hematopoietic stem cell transplantation or gene therapy is achieved, patients with classic Wiskott-Aldrich syndrome tend to develop autoimmune disorders and lymphoma or other malignancies that lead to an early death.[115]

Fanconi Anemia

Fanconi anemia is an autosomal recessive disease characterized by aplastic anemia and congenital abnormalities (absent radii, absent or malformed thumbs, microcephaly, hypogonadism, hypertelorism, gastrointestinal malformations, renal-ureteral malformations, café au lait spots). Hypersensitivity to DNA cross-linking agents like diepoxybutane is often used as a diagnostic test. At birth, the blood count is usually normal, and macrocytosis is often the first detected abnormality. This is typically followed by thrombocytopenia and anemia that progresses to pancytopenia. The majority of patients develop progressive bone marrow failure or acute myelogenous leukemia, of which are diagnosed with peak frequencies at the age of 7 and 10 to 15 years, respectively.[151] Of subjects registered between 1982 and 1992 in the International Fanconi Anemia Registry, several showed hematologic abnormalities during the neonatal period.

Thrombocytopenia–Absent Radius Syndrome

Thrombocytopenia–absent radius (TAR) syndrome is characterized by bilateral absence of the radii with the presence of both thumbs and thrombocytopenia. Thrombocytopenia may be congenital or may develop within the first few weeks to months of life. Patients usually show severe symptomatic thrombocytopenia in the first week of life with increased mortality due to ICH when the platelet count is less than 20×10^9/L. With increasing age, the recurrence of thrombocytopenic episodes decreases, and platelet count can improve to near-normal levels. Leukocytosis and eosinophilia may precede thrombocytopenia. Typically, patients have bilateral aplasia of the radii, but abnormalities involving the lower extremities have also been described. Unlike in Fanconi anemia, thumbs are present bilaterally. Cardiac and facial anomalies, as well as hypoplasia of the cerebellar vermis and corpus callosum, may be present. Symptomatic allergy to cow's milk is present in 47% of individuals with TAR syndrome. Treatment is based on provision of platelet support when needed.[152,153]

Congenital Amegakaryocytic Thrombocytopenia

Congenital amegakaryocytic thrombocytopenia (CAMT) is an autosomal recessive disorder caused by mutations in the thrombopoietin receptor c-Mpl. It presents at birth with severe thrombocytopenia (platelet count of $<50 \times 10^9$/L) with platelets that are of normal size and granularity. Importantly, phenotypic findings in CAMT are usually limited to those related to thrombocytopenia, including cutaneous and intracranial hemorrhages before or after birth. Several patients have been described with clinical features of CAMT who also exhibited growth or developmental delay, strabismus, or central nervous system abnormalities, including cerebellar malformations and cortical dysplasia.[153-155] Reduction or absence of megakaryocytes is seen in the bone marrow with evolution of hypocellular or aplastic bone marrows later in the course. Measurement of plasma thrombopoietin levels is a useful diagnostic assay in the evaluation of congenital thrombocytopenia; however, this assay is not widely available.[154] In children in whom the diagnosis is suspected based on clinical findings, CAMT can be confirmed by identification of homozygous or compound heterozygous mutations in the thrombopoietin receptor c-Mpl. Supportive care for patients with CAMT consists primarily of platelet transfusions. Currently, the only definitive treatment available for the long-term management of patients with CAMT is hematopoietic stem cell transplantation.[153-155]

Amegakaryocytic Thrombocytopenia and Radioulnar Synostosis

Amegakaryocytic thrombocytopenia and radioulnar synostosis is an autosomal dominant disorder associated with *HOXA11* mutation with features that include congenital amegakaryocytic thrombocytopenia, aplastic anemia, proximal radioulnar synostosis, clinodactyly, syndactyly, hip dysplasia, and sensorineural hearing loss.[156] Symptomatic thrombocytopenia with bruising and bleeding is present from birth, necessitating ultimate correction by stem cell transplantation.[157]

MYH9-Related Inherited Thrombocytopenia

MYH9-related inherited thrombocytopenia (MYH9-related disease) is one of the most frequent forms of inherited thrombocytopenia. It is transmitted in an autosomal dominant fashion and derives from mutations of *MYH9*, the gene for the heavy chain of nonmuscle myosin IIA. Patients have congenital macrothrombocytopenia with mild bleeding tendency and may develop kidney dysfunction, deafness, and cataracts later in life. The term *MYH9-related disease* encompasses four autosomal dominant thrombocytopenias that were previously described as distinct disorders: namely, May-Hegglin anomaly, Sebastian syndrome, Fechtner syndrome, and Epstein syndrome. Thrombocytopenia is usually mild and derives from complex defects of megakaryocyte maturation and platelet formation. Usually the presence of giant platelets in peripheral blood raises the suspicion of MYH9-related disease, and a simple immunofluorescence test showing the distribution of nonmuscle myosin heavy chain IIA within neutrophils on blood films confirms the diagnosis. Characteristic Döhle-like bodies are identified in the cytoplasm of neutrophil granulocytes in 42% to 84% of patients.[158]

X-Linked Macrothrombocytopenia

X-linked macrothrombocytopenia caused by mutation in *GATA1* is a recently described isolated X-linked macrothrombocytopenia without anemia (but with some dyserythropoietic features). In this disorder, immature platelets are released into the circulation that have hyperplastic endoplasmic reticulum and a disturbed glycoprotein Ib-V-IX complex with weakened function. The disorder may present with severe thrombocytopenia and profound bleeding at birth.[159,160]

Chromosomal Abnormalities

Infants with chromosomal abnormalities (trisomies of chromosomes 13, 18, or 21; Turner syndrome) can have neonatal thrombocytopenia in addition to the characteristic physical features of these disorders. Although historically trisomy 21 has been associated mostly with other hematologic disorders, such as polycythemia, transient myeloproliferative disorder, and acute leukemia, isolated neonatal thrombocytopenia is a frequent finding. The thrombocytopenia is usually mild to moderate and transient, with resolution at 2 to 3 weeks of life.

Therefore, an extensive evaluation of mild to moderate thrombocytopenia in neonates with Down syndrome is not suggested.

Pregnancy-Induced Hypertension

PIH is a common cause of thrombocytopenia in neonates, but the pathogenesis of the condition is unclear. Possibly, it is the kinetic result of decreased platelet production. Of all infants born to women with PIH, preterm babies are at highest risk of developing thrombocytopenia. The thrombocytopenia presents at birth or in the first few days of life, reaches a nadir on days 2 to 4, and resolves by day 7 to 10.[135]

THROMBOCYTOPENIA DUE TO MIXED CAUSES

Infection

Intrauterine cytomegalovirus infection and rubella can be associated with neutropenia or pancytopenia. Thrombocytopenia is most likely secondary to splenomegaly; however, an element of decreased production might be associated as well.[99]

Intrauterine Growth Restriction

Thrombocytopenia is particularly common in preterm infants who are small for gestational age, but it is relatively uncommon in term infants who are small for gestational age. The cause of the thrombocytopenia is not known. The pathogenesis may involve accelerated platelet removal from the blood or decreased platelet production related to a failure to compensate by increasing production of thrombopoietin.[135]

EVALUATION OF THE NEONATE WITH THROMBOCYTOPENIA

The first step in evaluating a neonate with thrombocytopenia is to classify the thrombocytopenia into one of the categories discussed previously. This involves consideration of the infant's age (early versus late thrombocytopenia), the severity of the thrombocytopenia, the presence of dysmorphic features, the clinical condition (sick versus not sick), and the medications used. In determining the cause of thrombocytopenia in an affected neonate, it is important first to consider conditions that could be life threatening (e.g., infections, DIC, NEC, thrombosis) or that have significant implications for further pregnancies (e.g., alloimmune or autoimmune thrombocytopenia, genetic disorders). If any of these entities is suspected, appropriate diagnostic testing should be conducted promptly (e.g., bacterial or viral cultures, assays for antiplatelet antibodies, chromosome analysis). Once these conditions have been ruled out, other causes of thrombocytopenia (generally more benign) should be considered. Several tests have been used for indirect evaluation of the mechanisms causing thrombocytopenia. Two of them (mean platelet volume and time between transfusions) are easily available to the clinician caring for a thrombocytopenic neonate. A high mean platelet volume usually suggests increased platelet production, presumably as a compensation for accelerated platelet destruction. In cases in which the cause is clearly defined, no further evaluation is necessary unless the thrombocytopenia is especially severe or more prolonged than is expected given the cause identified. A bone marrow evaluation may be warranted in a patient with prolonged and severe thrombocytopenia of unclear cause despite extensive evaluation.[135]

PLATELET TRANSFUSION GUIDELINES

Until data from controlled trials become available, decisions about platelet transfusion in neonates will be based on consensus guidelines.[100] Patients qualifying for a platelet transfusion should receive 10 to 15 mL/kg of cytomegalovirus-negative standard platelet suspension, prepared from a fresh unit of whole blood or by platelet pheresis. This amount should be sufficient to increase the platelet count of a thrombocytopenic infant by approximately 100×10^9/L. No volume-reducing processing is routinely recommended because of the risk of platelet loss, clumping, and dysfunction due to the additional handling.[100]

The decision to administer a prophylactic platelet transfusion should be made on the basis of many factors, including the platelet count, the mechanism responsible for the thrombocytopenia, the medications administered, and the condition of the patient. Usually such decisions are institution-driven, "best-guess" estimates. For patients in the first week of life at greatest risk of hemorrhage (e.g., extremely preterm neonates in unstable condition), administration of prophylactic platelet transfusions at trigger thresholds of up to 50×10^9/L is generally considered to represent acceptable and safe clinical practice. Platelet transfusions in neonates with platelet counts of more than 50×10^9/L should be reserved for patients with active major bleeding, such as new or extending intraventricular hemorrhage or pulmonary, gastrointestinal, or renal hemorrhage.[134,161]

Infants who are being treated with medications known to induce platelet dysfunction (e.g., indomethacin, aspirin, or nitric oxide) should probably be maintained at higher platelet counts than neonates who are not receiving such medications. The same applies to neonates receiving anticoagulants (heparin or low-molecular-weight heparin) or thrombolytic agents (e.g., tissue plasminogen activator), whose risk of bleeding is significantly higher in the presence of thrombocytopenia.[100] As discussed earlier, special consideration should be given to the transfusion of HPA-1b–negative platelets, or platelets obtained from the mother, to neonates with alloimmune thrombocytopenia.

COAGULATION SYSTEM IN THE NEONATE

The human hemostatic system starts developing in utero and continues to develop well into childhood. This system can be thought of as having discrete fluid phase (circulating proteins), cellular (platelets), and vascular (vessel wall) compartments. Although this approach is useful in classifying specific disorders, the component parts of the hemostatic system are functionally and biochemically interrelated. The functional levels of many of the procoagulants, coagulation inhibitors, and fibrinolytic components in the neonate differ from the those in the adult. The component functions reach adult levels by 6 months of age. The pioneering work of Dr. Maureen Andrew in the 1980s elucidated the unique aspects of the neonatal and fetal coagulation system (Fig. 17-2). The term *developmental hemostasis* was used for the first time to describe her work. Even though neonates have different functional levels of all the coagulation components compared with adults, they rarely have problems with bleeding or thrombosis. The differences in prothrombotic and antithrombotic components are uniquely balanced in the neonate, which creates a normal physiologic state. Table 17-2 presents the reference ranges for coagulation test values for healthy full-term neonates and healthy preterm babies.

A number of bleeding and clotting disorders can present in the neonatal period. The following sections briefly review the

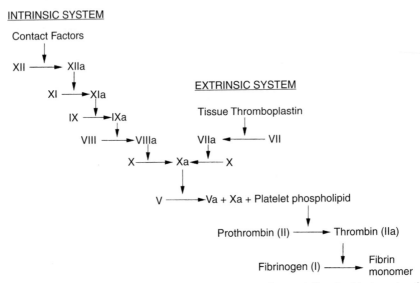

Figure 17-2. Overview of the coagulant proteins of the intrinsic system (*upper left*) and extrinsic system (*upper right*), which both feed into the common pathway (*bottom*).

Table 17-2.	Normal Values for Coagulation Tests in Healthy Full-Term and Premature Infants		
Coagulation Test	**Full-Term Infant**	**Premature Infant**	**Older Child**
Platelets (per µL)	150,000-400,000	150,000-400,000	150,000-400,000
Prothrombin time (sec)	10.1-15.9	10.6-16.2	10.6-11.4
Partial thromboplastin time (sec)	31.3-54.5	27.5-79.4	24-36
Thrombin clotting time (sec)	19-28.3	19.2-30.4	19.8-31.2
Fibrinogen (mg/dL)	167-399	150-373	170-405
Fibrin degradation products (µg/mL)	<10	<10	<10
Factor VIII (U/mL)	0.50-1.78	0.50-2.13	0.59-1.42
Factor IX (U/mL)	0.15-0.91	0.19-0.65	0.47-1.04
von Willebrand factor (U/ml)	0.50-2.87	0.78-2.10	0.60-1.20

presentation, work-up, and initial management of common inherited bleeding and clotting disorders.

INITIAL LABORATORY EVALUATION OF THE NEONATE WITH BLEEDING

About 15% to 30% of patients with inherited bleeding disorders have bleeding symptoms in the neonatal period.[162] Evaluation of a bleeding neonate always begins with taking a detailed maternal and family history. It is important to obtain details about the mother's state of health during pregnancy and labor, including infections, maternal autoimmune disease, and platelet count. Other details about the labor and delivery itself, such as prolonged time between rupture of membranes and delivery, fetal distress, and chorioamnionitis are also important.

Next, history taking for the infant should focus on confirming administration of vitamin K. A detailed family history focusing on the types and severity of any bleeding symptoms, as well as the sex of the affected members, gives valuable information on the type and inheritance pattern of a possible bleeding disorder. However, a third of new cases of severe hemophilia represent new mutations, and therefore no family history of such disorders is present.

Examination of the neonate should quickly differentiate between a well-appearing baby and a sick one. A sick infant may have medical conditions contributing to hemorrhage. Findings of birth trauma, evidence of bruises and petechiae, and presence of flank masses suggestive of renal vein thrombosis should be sought.

Hepatosplenomegaly in a sick neonate may suggest disseminated intrauterine infection. The most common cause of bleeding in healthy infants is thrombocytopenia secondary to transplacental passage of a maternal antiplatelet antibody, sepsis, vitamin K deficiency, or congenital coagulation factor deficiencies. In an otherwise well infant, bleeding from a circumcision site, oozing from the umbilicus, bleeding into the scalp, large cephalhematomas, or ICH may point to coagulation factor deficiencies such as hemophilia or von Willebrand disease, or disorders of platelet numbers such as NAIT. NAIT is the most common cause of severe thrombocytopenia in a well infant, occurring in approximately 1 in 1000 to 2000 births. A detailed description of the causes and investigation of thrombocytopenic bleeding can be found elsewhere in this chapter.

Blood volume in a neonate is low, and hence a small blood loss, even for investigative blood draws, can have major consequences. Judicious use of laboratory tests for screening for underlying bleeding disorders requires partnership with an experienced hematologist specializing in coagulation disorders. If the history and physical examination are not suggestive of a specific disorder, a panel of screening tests should be ordered. These include a complete blood count with review of the peripheral smear, including platelet number and morphology; prothrombin time (PT); activated partial thromboplastin time (APTT); and thrombin time (TT). The results must be compared with the expected normal ranges based on the gestational age of the infant as mentioned previously. References ranges for PT and APTT in healthy term newborns and preterm infants are given in Table 17-2. The PT and APTT measure the overall function of proteins in the coagulation cascade. The PT measures the activities of factors I (fibrinogen), II (prothrombin), V, VII, and X. PT is generally prolonged when the functional activities of one of these factors goes below 30%. The most common cause of isolated prolongation of PT is factor VII deficiency. The APTT measures the functional activities of the factors in the intrinsic arm of the coagulation cascade: namely, VIII, IX, XI, XII, prekallikrein, and high-molecular-weight kininogen. It also measures the functional activities of factors I (fibrinogen), II (prothrombin), and V. Deficiency of any of these factors results in the prolongation of the APTT. The sensitivity and reproducibility of the APTT, unlike those of the PT, depend strongly on the specific reagents used. With most reagents, the APTT is not prolonged unless the factor VIII level is less than 35% (0.35 U/mL). Deficiencies of factor XII, prekallikrein, and high-molecular-weight kininogen result in prolongation of APTT but no clinical bleeding symptoms. Isolated prolongation of the APTT in the neonate is likely due to deficiency of factor VIII, IX, or XI, if contamination with heparin is ruled out. For a child with mild bleeding, if hemophilia is suspected, factor VIII and IX assays must be performed regardless of the APTT value. The APTT is somewhat less sensitive to vitamin K deficiency than the PT. The TT measures the thrombin-induced conversion of fibrinogen to fibrin and hence is useful for investigating the clotting function of fibrinogen in a variety of fibrinogen disorders.

A number of pitfalls exist in performing and interpreting tests such as the PT and APTT. Extreme caution must be taken when sending blood for coagulation testing. The blood sample must be from free-flowing blood without any air bubbles present. Particular attention should be paid to ensuring the 1:10 ratio of the anticoagulant sodium citrate to plasma by filling the tube up to the appropriate mark. Specialized microcollection tubes (1 mL) must be available in the neonatal unit to avoid wastage. Drawing blood from an indwelling catheter is strongly discouraged because it often results in contamination of the sample with heparin and other fluids, which leads to spurious prolongation of clotting times. In neonates with polycythemia (hematocrit of >55%), the amount of citrate should be reduced to maintain the 1:10 ratio of citrate to plasma. This is particularly important in neonates with cyanotic congenital heart disease, who have very high hematocrit values. If the sample is suspected of being contaminated with heparin, measuring TT and reptilase time helps to differentiate between prolongation of APTT due to heparin and prolongation due to other causes. A 1:1 mixing study of the sample with prolonged APTT can also be performed by adding normal plasma to the specimen. If the prolonged APTT corrects, the cause is not heparin contamination.

Other coagulation tests include closure time measured by platelet function analyzer, platelet aggregation test, urea clot solubility, and other coagulation factor assays.

These tests are not useful as screening tests in the neonate and should not be performed unless there is a strong suspicion of a specific disorder. These tests are described in the discussions of the individual bleeding disorders to which they are relevant.

Bleeding in a neonate with thrombocytopenia is discussed in a different section of this chapter.

BLEEDING IN NEONATES WITH NORMAL PLATELET COUNTS

The disorders considered in the differential diagnosis of bleeding in a neonate with a normal platelet count can be broadly classified based on whether the infant appears well or sick. These various disorders are discussed in the following sections. The clinical and laboratory features of these disorders are summarized in Table 17-3.

HEMORRHAGIC DISEASE OF THE NEWBORN (VITAMIN K DEFICIENCY)

Hemorrhagic disease of the newborn (HDN) is defined as hemorrhage from multiple sites on days 1 to 5 in an otherwise healthy infant. It was first described by Townsend[163] in 1894. Vitamin K acts on the precursors of factors II, VII, IX, and X (vitamin K–dependent factors) to generate active procoagulants. Its biochemical function involves creating calcium-binding sites in these proteins by carboxylating specific glutamic acid residues. Levels of the vitamin K–dependent factors are physiologically low in newborns.[164] It is a common practice to routinely administer parenteral vitamin K after birth. Therefore, HDN is a rare condition.

The clinical manifestations of HDN can be of three different types based on the timing and type of bleeding complications. Classic HDN is defined as bleeding on days 2 to 7 of life in breast-fed, healthy, full-term infants.

The bleeding manifestation is usually in the form of oozing from the umbilicus, bleeding from circumcision and puncture sites, ICH, and gastrointestinal hemorrhage. Causes include poor placental transfer of vitamin K, marginal vitamin K content in breast milk (<20 μg/L), inadequate milk intake, and a sterile gut. Vitamin K deficiency bleeding (VKDB) rarely occurs in formula-fed infants because commercially available formulas are supplemented with vitamin K. In the absence of vitamin K prophylaxis, the incidence of VKDB ranges from 0.25% to 1.7%. The incidence depends on the population studied, the supplemental formula used, and the prevalence of breast feeding in the community. Early HDN develops in the first 24 hours of life and is linked to maternal use of specific medications that interfere with vitamin K stores or function, such as some anticonvulsants. Bleeding can be in the form of ICH, gastrointestinal bleeding, or cephalhematomas. Late HDN occurs between weeks 2 and 8 of life and is linked to disorders that compromise ongoing vitamin K supply, such as cystic fibrosis, α_1-antitrypsin deficiency, biliary atresia, and celiac disease. Infants with these disorders are at risk of development of late vitamin K deficiency weeks to months after receiving parenteral vitamin K at birth.

Results of screening laboratory tests reveal a normal platelet count and an abnormal PT and APTT. The PT is often markedly prolonged compared with the APTT. Levels of fibrinogen and fibrin degradation products as well as TT are normal. Other tests that can aid in the diagnosis are specific factor assays, measurement of the levels of decarboxylated forms of vitamin K–dependent factors, assay of protein induced by vitamin K antagonists, and direct measurement of vitamin K levels.

Table 17-3.	Conditions Associated with Bleeding and Normal Platelet Count			
Diagnosis	**Appearance**	**PT**	**APTT**	**Other Useful Tests**
Hemorrhagic disease of the newborn	Well	↑	↑	Fibrinogen; fibrin degradation products
Hepatic disease	Sick	↑	↑	Albumin; fibrinogen; fibrin degradation products; liver function tests
von Willebrand disease*	Well	Normal	Normal or ↑	Bleeding time (see text)
Hemophilia	Well	Normal	↑	Mixing tests; factor VIII and IX assays
Factor XIII deficiency	Well	Normal	Normal	Urea clot solubility
Disorders of platelet function*	Well	Normal	Normal	Bleeding time, platelet aggregometry

*Some patients with these disorders show mild to moderate thrombocytopenia (see text for details).
APTT, Activated partial thromboplastin time; *PT*, prothrombin time.

All newborns suspected of having HDN should be treated with vitamin K immediately pending the results of laboratory tests. For hemorrhages that are not life threatening, parenteral vitamin K can be used to rapidly correct the bleeding diathesis. Vitamin K works within a few hours because it generates active procoagulants from the precursors with no requirement for new protein synthesis. Infants with VKDB should be given vitamin K either subcutaneously or intravenously, depending on the situation. Vitamin K should not be given intramuscularly to infants with VKDB because large hematomas may form at the site of the injection. Intravenous vitamin K should be administered slowly and a test dose should be given, because it may induce an anaphylactoid reaction. For infants with major or life-threatening hemorrhage, fresh frozen plasma should be administered to stop bleeding and increase levels of vitamin K–dependent proteins. Prothrombin complex concentrates, if available, can also be used to treat life-threatening hemorrhages.

A number of special considerations apply to the high-risk newborn. Vitamin K production by bacteria in the gut is reduced by illnesses which require that enteral feedings be delayed or interrupted. Treatment with broad-spectrum antibiotics also decreases vitamin K synthesis. For these reasons, it is highly recommended that vitamin K be administered weekly to infants who are not breast fed and to those who are being treated with parenteral antibiotics.

LIVER DISEASE

Coagulopathy associated with liver disease in newborns is a result of failure of the hepatic synthetic function. There is generalized impairment of hepatic synthesis of proteins, including the coagulation proteins. In a newborn, the problem may be exacerbated, because of the already existing physiologic immaturity of the coagulation system. Common causes of liver dysfunction in newborns are total parenteral nutrition, hypoxia, shock, fetal hydrops, and viral hepatitis. Rarely, genetic diseases such as α_1-antitrypsin deficiency, galactosemia, and tyrosinemia are responsible for the liver impairment.

Laboratory abnormalities induced by acute liver disease include prolongation of the PT and low plasma concentrations of several coagulation proteins, including fibrinogen. Fibrinogen is present at adult levels in newborns and may be a useful marker. The diagnosis is also supported by a low serum albumin level and by abnormal results on liver function studies. Secondary effects of liver disease on platelet number and function also occur in newborns. Secondary vitamin K deficiency may occur as a result of impaired absorption from the small intestine, particularly in infants with intrahepatic and extrahepatic biliary atresia. Supplemental vitamin K should be administered to these infants. Severe bleeding is best treated by infusion of fresh frozen plasma. Cryoprecipitate is indicated for patients with severely reduced fibrinogen levels. Patients with clinical bleeding may benefit temporarily from replacement of coagulation proteins using fresh frozen plasma, cryoprecipitate, or exchange transfusion. Without recovery of hepatic function, however, replacement therapy is futile. Hence, the overall goal should be to identify and reverse the underlying condition.

HEREDITARY COAGULATION FACTOR DEFICIENCIES

A number of hereditary coagulation factor deficiencies can present in the neonatal period. Deficiencies of factors VIII and IX are common and have an X-linked inheritance pattern, whereas deficiencies of factors II, V, VII, XI, and XII, prekallikrein, and high-molecular-weight kininogen are autosomally inherited disorders and are rare, with consanguinity present in many affected families. Rarely, combined deficiencies of factors II, VII, and IX and/or factors V and VIII present in the neonatal period.[165] Only the common inherited coagulation factor deficiencies such as the hemophilias and von Willebrand disease are described here. A detailed discussion of the rarer forms of coagulation factor deficiencies can be found elsewhere.[120]

The Hemophilias

Hemophilia A and hemophilia B are X-linked bleeding disorders caused by congenital deficiencies of proteins in the intrinsic coagulation cascade. Hemophilia A (or classic hemophilia) is due to a deficiency of factor VIII and accounts for 85% of cases. Hemophilia B (Christmas disease) results from absent or decreased factor IX activity and is responsible for the remaining 15% of cases. Hemophilia A and hemophilia B are clinically indistinguishable. The percentage of factor VIII or IX coagulant activity is used to classify the hemophilias as severe (<1%), moderate (1% to 5%), or mild (5% to 15%). Severe factor VIII deficiency is the most common inherited bleeding disorder manifesting in the neonatal period. Although a positive family history is helpful in making the diagnosis, new mutations account for about one third of all cases of factor VIII deficiency. The bleeding symptoms in infants with hemophilia range from mild to catastrophic. Large cohort studies have shown that approximately 10% of children with hemophilia have clinical symptoms in the neonatal period. Approximately 50% of patients with severe hemophilia bleed excessively following circumcision. Other cases present with severe visceral or intracranial hemorrhage after difficult vaginal deliveries. These infants may be acutely ill from hypovolemia or local hemorrhage into vital organs.

The only abnormality in laboratory test results is prolongation of the APTT (to >100 seconds in severe cases). The PT and the platelet count are normal. Specific assays for factors VIII and IX quickly confirm the diagnosis, but these are not available in all laboratories. When hemophilia is suspected in a male infant with a prolonged APTT and factor assays are not immediately available, other studies are helpful. The PTT should be repeated using a 50:50 mix of patient and normal plasma. In hemophilia, the PTT corrects to normal. Even small clinical laboratories often have a stock of factor VIII–deficient plasma. If the PTT corrects with normal plasma, the mixing study is repeated with this factor VIII–deficient plasma. If the PTT corrects to normal, hemophilia A is excluded and hemophilia B is the likely diagnosis. If the PTT does not correct to normal, factor VIII deficiency is the presumptive diagnosis.

Recombinant concentrates of factor VIII or factor IX (produced in vitro using recombinant DNA technology) have been the mainstay for treating bleeding in patients with hemophilia. In the early 1980s, use of lyophilized concentrates was associated with a high incidence of transfusion-transmitted HIV infection. Routine heating of factor concentrates in the manufacturing process has apparently eliminated this problem. The dose of factor VIII or IX used to treat hemorrhagic complications depends on the severity of the bleeding. Life-threatening hemorrhages in infants with hemophilia A should be treated with an initial dose of factor VIII concentrate of 50 U/kg followed either by a continuous infusion of 8 to 10 U/hr or by boluses of 50 U/kg every 8 hours. Infants with hemophilia B who have severe bleeding are given a bolus of 100 to 120 U/kg of factor IX concentrate followed either by a continuous infusion starting at 5 U/kg/hr or by bolus doses given every 12 hours. Lower dosages are recommended for less severe bleeding.[166] The presence of inhibitors is rare in neonates. The duration of replacement therapy is based on the location and extent of the bleeding and on the clinical response of the patient. Less severe hemorrhages (such as those that typically follow circumcision) often resolve after application of pressure to the wound or may require a single bolus dose of 10 to 25 U/kg of factor VIII concentrate or 15 to 30 U/kg of factor IX concentrate. Replacement therapy is not indicated for infants with hemophilia who are not bleeding unless they require surgery. Cryoprecipitate contains factor VIII but not factor IX and can therefore be used to treat bleeding complications in hemophilia A. One unit of cryoprecipitate per 5 kg of body weight increases the factor VIII level by about 40%. The Medical and Scientific Advisory Committee of the National Hemophilia Foundation recommends against the use of cryoprecipitate because it is not a virally inactivated product. Recommended dosages of factor concentrates and cryoprecipitate are presented in Table 17-4.

von Willebrand Disease

Although von Willebrand Disease (VWD) is probably the most common inherited bleeding disorder, it is rarely diagnosed in the nursery. von Willebrand factor is the product of an autosomal gene, and the common form of VWD is transmitted as a dominant condition. von Willebrand factor plays a central role in hemostasis by promoting platelet adherence to the vascular endothelium, a reaction mediated through a specific receptor on the platelet called *glycoprotein Ib*. von Willebrand factor is stored in platelet granules and is also released from the endothelial cell lining of the injured vessel. von Willebrand factor circulates as high-, intermediate-, and low-molecular-weight complexes called *multimers*. In addition to playing a role in platelet adherence, von Willebrand factor associates with and stabilizes factor VIII. This, in turn, delivers factor VIII to sites of vascular injury. Although there is extraordinary clinical heterogeneity in the common, autosomal dominant

Table 17-4.	Products Used in the Treatment of Neonatal Coagulopathies		
Product	**Contents**	**Usual Dose**	**Indications**
Fresh frozen plasma	All factors	10-20 mL/kg	Disseminated intravascular coagulation (DIC), protein C deficiency, liver disease
Cryoprecipitate	Factor VIII, factor XIII, von Willebrand factor, fibrinogen	1 bag (~250 mg fibrinogen, 80-120 U factor VIII)	Factor XIII deficiency, DIC, liver disease, factor VIII deficiency, von Willebrand disease
Factor VIII concentrates	Factor VIII	25-50 U/kg	Factor VIII deficiency
Factor IX concentrates	Factor IX	50-120 U/kg	Factor IX deficiency
Vitamin K		1-2 mg	Vitamin K deficiency
Platelet concentrates	Platelets	1-2 U/5 kg	Thrombocytopenic bleeding

type of VWD, hemorrhage typically occurs in the skin and mucosal surfaces. Screening tests usually reveal a normal PT and platelet count, although some patients have mild thrombocytopenia. The APTT is either normal or mildly prolonged depending on the amount of factor VIII activity. Plasma concentrations of von Willebrand factor are increased in neonates. Therefore, laboratory testing of affected adults in the family is a good initial step in evaluating infants suspected of having VWD. The results may be used to determine the best test (or tests) for the infant. However, even this approach has pitfalls, particularly because pregnancy markedly alters VWF levels, which renders evaluation of the mother unreliable. Some plasma-derived factor VIII concentrates are manufactured so that they also contain von Willebrand factor. These products are an excellent treatment for bleeding complications in neonates with VWD. Cryoprecipitate is another effective therapy for treating hemorrhage in infants with a family history of VWD. Circumcision should not be performed if a parent has VWD. In the absence of significant bleeding, laboratory work-up of infants with a family history of VWD should be deferred until after 6 months of age.

The autosomal recessive form of VWD (type III VWD) is a much rarer and more severe condition. Affected infants have a severe bleeding disorder caused by a combination of profoundly abnormal platelet function and low factor VIII levels, and they require regular treatment with an appropriate von Willebrand factor–containing concentrate.

DISORDERS OF PLATELET FUNCTION

Inherited disorders of platelet function are rare. In general, they present with petechiae, purpura, and bleeding from puncture sites, a circumcision site, and umbilical cord separation. Because these disorders are uncommon and are often inherited as autosomal recessive conditions, a history of consanguinity is especially important. The PT and APTT values are normal. In some disorders (e.g., gray platelet syndrome, Bernard-Soulier syndrome), there is mild thrombocytopenia and the platelets are morphologically abnormal. Careful examination of the blood smear is therefore mandatory whenever an inherited disorder of platelet function is suspected. In certain diseases (e.g., Glanzmann thrombasthenia), both the platelet count and platelet appearance are normal. A hallmark of inherited disorders of platelet function is marked prolongation of the bleeding time. Studies of platelet aggregation in response to various stimuli, antibody staining for antigens expressed on the surface of the platelets, electron microscopy, and molecular analysis are all useful in selected cases. Transfusions of platelet concentrates are given for severe bleeding.

THROMBOSIS

Despite prolongation of the PT and APTT well beyond the normal adult range, many experts in neonatal hematology believe that neonates are better viewed as being in a "hypercoagulable" state. Indeed, thrombotic complications are more common in the neonatal period than at any other time during the first two decades of life and are receiving increased attention as more high-risk patients survive invasive medical interventions. Why newborns experience a relatively high incidence of thrombosis is unknown; however, increased blood viscosity resulting from a high hematocrit at birth may play an important role. Polycythemia may partially account for why infants of diabetic mothers are at high risk of thrombosis. In addition, the levels of protein C, a vitamin K–dependent serine protease, are low at birth. Preterm infants with respiratory distress syndrome have very low levels of antithrombin, increasing their risk of thromboembolic complications.

Although thrombosis is a serious complication in high-risk infants, this problem has received relatively limited attention until recently. Investigators at McMaster University estimated that the incidence of clinically apparent thrombotic episodes was 2.4 per 1000 admissions to the NICU based on a multicenter survey of 97 cases.[167] Ninety percent of cases in their series were associated with the use of indwelling catheters. Twenty-one infants had renal vein thrombosis, 39 had right atrial thrombosis or other major venous thromboses, and 33 had arterial thrombosis. Because severe thrombosis is relatively uncommon in neonates, almost no data from controlled trials are available addressing the efficacy of thrombolytic or anticoagulant therapies.

THROMBOSIS ASSOCIATED WITH INDWELLING CATHETERS

Thromboembolic complications are clearly an important risk associated with the use of venous and arterial catheters. Autopsy studies reveal that 20% to 65% of infants who die with an umbilical venous catheter have an associated thrombus. Use of appropriate technique and proper placement of umbilical venous catheters are crucial to prevention of a thrombus and its possible complications, such as portal vein thrombosis with portal hypertension, splenomegaly, gastric and esophageal varices, and hepatic necrosis. The incidence of asymptomatic clot formation in the aorta is also high. A number of studies have shown that continuous infusion of heparin at a rate of 0.5 to 3.5 U/kg/hr improves catheter patency, reduces the rate of thrombus formation, and decreases the incidence of hypertension.[168] It is uncertain whether higher dosages of heparin provide any additional benefit, and the evidence linking heparin use to intraventricular hemorrhage is weak.[169] Damping of the arterial pressure wave tracing is a frequent early sign of catheter thrombosis. Blanching or cyanosis of a "downstream" anatomic area suggests obstruction. The involved segment may include only the tip of a toe, or it may encompass an entire extremity or even half of the body.

Ultrasonography is a useful, noninvasive initial test and may be followed by arteriography in severe cases.[170] Contrast-enhanced angiography is considered the gold standard for diagnosis of arterial thrombosis. The sensitivity and specificity of Doppler ultrasonography for diagnosis of venous and arterial thrombosis is unknown.

Management of severe thrombosis should be individualized. Systemic heparinization, treatment with fibrinolytic agents, and thrombectomy have all been used.[167,170] In infants without evidence of major vessel obstruction, catheter removal is often followed by resolution of symptoms.

RENAL VEIN THROMBOSIS

Renal vein thrombosis in infants occurs most commonly (80% of cases) in the first month and usually in the first week of life. There is no sex predilection and the left and right sides are equally affected. About 24% of infants have bilateral renal vein thrombosis. The clinical triad of flank mass, hematuria, and mild thrombocytopenia (average platelet counts of 100×10^9/L) is the classical presentation of renal vein thrombosis in the neonatal period. Proteinuria and impaired kidney function are also seen. If the inferior vena cava is involved, cold, cyanotic, and edematous lower limbs can be noted. Doppler ultrasonography is the test of choice for diagnosis. Treatment depends on the extent and severity of involvement. Supportive care alone is sufficient for unilateral renal vein thrombosis with no uremia or extension into the inferior vena cava. However, heparin therapy is usually indicated in infants with unilateral renal vein thrombosis with inferior vena cava extension or bilateral renal vein thrombosis, because the risk of pulmonary embolism and renal failure increases. In cases of bilateral renal vein thrombosis with evidence of renal failure, thrombolytic therapy must be considered. More than 85% of children survive with adequate renal function. Long-term morbidity data are lacking, however.

PROTEIN C DEFICIENCY

Severe protein C deficiency is a recessive disorder associated with catastrophic thrombosis and necrosis of dependent tissues, consumption of coagulation factors, and DIC.[171] A history of consanguinity or thrombotic disease in multiple adult relatives may be elicited. Infants with severe protein C deficiency are severely ill with purpura fulminans—diffuse tissue infarction with secondary hemorrhage, particularly in the skin. The PT and PTT are prolonged, the platelet count and fibrinogen level are reduced, and the level of fibrin degradation products is elevated. An important diagnostic clue that helps distinguish protein C deficiency from DIC is its propensity to be associated with prominent areas of segmental tissue infarction. Although the diagnosis is strongly supported by the demonstration of profoundly reduced levels of protein C, Manco-Johnson et al observed transient reductions in some infants that later improved.[172] Their data emphasize the importance of parental blood studies and serial testing to confirm the diagnosis. Treatment may initially include exchange transfusions, infusions of fresh frozen plasma at 10 to 20 mL/kg every 6 to 12 hours to raise the protein C level and replenish consumed coagulation factors, and heparinization.[173] A protein C concentrate (Ceprotin) has been approved by the FDA for use in the treatment of congenital protein C deficiency. The dose of Ceprotin for acute thrombotic episodes and short-term prophylaxis is 100 to 120 IU/kg in neonates with subsequent doses of 60 to 80 IU/kg every 6 hours and maintenance doses of 45 to 60 IU/kg every 6 to 12 hours.[174] Warfarin is preferred for long-term management, with a target international normalized ratio of 2.5 to 4.5.[173]

FACTOR V LEIDEN

A missense mutation in the factor V gene was first associated with resistance to the action of activated protein C in adults with venous thrombosis. This allele encodes a molecule called *factor V Leiden* that is relatively insensitive to inactivation by protein C and is most prevalent in northern European populations. Individuals who are heterozygous for the factor V Leiden mutation show a five- to ten-fold increase in the incidence of venous thrombosis as young adults, and homozygotes are at very high risk. Pediatric patients with thrombosis have been shown to have a higher than expected incidence of factor V Leiden mutation.[175]

EVALUATION OF INFANTS WITH THROMBOSIS

In general, thrombosis appears to be both underdiagnosed and undertreated in neonates. Symptoms and signs are highly variable and depend on the location and severity of the thrombotic process. Not only do a high percentage of infants with thrombosis have indwelling catheters, but thrombosis often occurs in the context of systemic infection. A constellation of hematuria, abdominal mass, and thrombocytopenia is observed in many infants with renal vein thrombosis. Although the PT, APTT, and platelet count all should be measured, the values of these indicators are frequently unremarkable in infants with thrombosis. The mother should be screened for the presence of antiphospholipid antibodies (lupus anticoagulant), because these may be associated with neonatal thrombosis. In addition, studies should be performed to exclude hereditary conditions, including factor V Leiden mutation, prothrombin gene mutation, and deficiencies of antithrombin III, protein C, and protein S. With the exception of DNA analysis for factor V Leiden mutation and prothrombin gene mutation, all of these tests may be unreliable in the setting of acute thrombosis. For this reason, it is suggested that parents be screened initially with follow-up testing of the infant as indicated. Although contrast angiography is the most definitive modality for demonstrating thrombi, Doppler ultrasonography is preferred by most clinicians because it can be performed at the bedside.[176] Prospective studies have not been reported comparing the sensitivity of contrast angiography and Doppler ultrasonography in infants with thrombosis. It is imperative to use imaging studies to evaluate clinically significant thrombotic events, because this aids in therapeutic decision making and provides a baseline for clinical follow-up. Infants should not be exposed to the risks of systemic anticoagulant therapy unless thrombosis is well documented.

ANTICOAGULANT AND FIBRINOLYTIC THERAPY

The paucity of data from controlled studies and the clinical heterogeneity seen in newborns with thrombosis preclude definitive recommendations regarding which infants are likely to benefit from anticoagulant and fibrinolytic treatment and which agents, doses, and schedule should be used. The following discussion describes the guidelines and therapeutic agents for such therapy. The Children's Thrombophilia Network (800-NO-CLOTS) offers telephone advice on management of infants and children with thrombosis. Although this service is very helpful, its optimal use is in combination with on-site pediatric hematology consultation. To exclude ICH and hemorrhagic infarction, it is essential that central nervous system imaging be performed before systemic anticoagulant or thrombolytic therapy is administered in the NICU.

Heparin is the mainstay of anticoagulant therapy for infants with acute thrombosis. McDonald and Hathaway studied the use of continuous heparin infusions in 15 infants with significant thrombosis.[177] They achieved plasma heparin levels in the therapeutic range at dosages of 16 to 27 U/kg/hr and found that infants who had large thrombi showed the most rapid clearance. Because of the very wide range of normal APTT values, the authors followed micro whole blood clotting times to monitor heparin effects. The recommendation is that heparin therapy begin with a loading dose of 50 U/kg followed by a continuous infusion at 20 U/kg/hr. Heparin treatment should be continued for at least 7 days in infants with significant thrombosis.

The advantages of low-molecular-weight heparin (LMWH) products include a longer plasma half-life than standard heparin, which permits subcutaneous dosing, and less variability in anticoagulant effects in different patients. Given the difficulties in administering and monitoring heparin therapy in neonates, LMWH drugs appear to offer considerable theoretic advantages over standard heparin in managing thrombosis in the NICU. There are important differences in the biochemical mechanisms of action of standard heparin and LMWH (enoxaparin sodium [Lovenox]). In particular, although heparin markedly accelerates the rate of thrombin inactivation through its ability to form a stable ternary complex that includes antithrombin III and thrombin, the major anticoagulant effect of LMWH occurs through antithrombin III–mediated destruction of activated factor X. The APTT is therefore not a useful test for measuring the anticoagulant effects of LMWH, which can be monitored by following anti-factor Xa levels. Studies have begun to elucidate optimal dosing for neonates. In a series that included 7 infants and 18 older children, Massicotte et al found that infants required higher doses of enoxaparin per kilogram to achieve therapeutic anti–factor Xa levels than older children.[178] In a much larger study examining 147 courses of enoxaparin in pediatric patients, the same group reported clinical resolution of thromboembolic events in 84% of patients.[179]

Warfarin is a competitive inhibitor of vitamin K and therefore depresses the levels of active procoagulant factors II, VII, IX, and X and of the anticoagulant proteins C and S. Warfarin is not an appropriate treatment for acute thrombosis, but warfarin administration may be instituted later and used as long-term therapy in some infants with ongoing hypercoagulable disorders. There is little published experience in the use of warfarin in neonates, and dosing is problematic given the rapid growth and dietary changes that occur during the first few months of life.

The fibrinolytic agents urokinase and tissue plasminogen activator (TPA) are used in the acute management of certain types of vascular occlusion in adults.[180] TPA is the most commonly used thrombolytic agent in neonates. The administration of TPA to 23 neonates with venous thrombosis, most of whom were treated for renal vein, atrial, or vena cava thrombosis, resulted in complete clot lysis in 56%, partial lysis in 35%, and no lysis in 9%. Major hemorrhagic complications occurred in three infants (13%), two of whom had ICH. Both infants experiencing ICH were thrombocytopenic.[181-183] An absolute contraindication to the use of TPA in neonates is the presence of ICH or active bleeding from any site. A platelet count above 100,000/µL and fibrinogen level above 100 mg/dL is highly recommended during TPA therapy. Laboratory responses include a decrease in the fibrinogen level and an increase in the D-dimer level. A hematologist with experience in the management of neonatal thrombosis should be consulted when fibrinolytic treatment is considered.

CASE 1

You are called to evaluate a 2-day-old full-term male infant who was noted to have continued oozing from the circumcision site. The nurse provides results for a complete blood count and coagulation studies, which reveal a normal platelet count of 220 x 10⁹/L, a PT of 12.9 seconds (normal for age), and an APTT of 72 seconds (prolonged).

What is your initial approach?

The first goal is to determine whether the baby is a well-appearing or sick-appearing infant. In a sick-appearing infant, DIC or sepsis can cause bleeding. Usually the platelet count is abnormally low in such cases. If the baby appears ill, a sepsis work-up should be performed and parenteral antibiotic therapy should be initiated. The platelet count, as mentioned earlier, is normal in this case. Investigation of bleeding in a well-appearing infant always includes obtaining a detailed family and maternal history. Maternal infection, prolonged period between rupture of the placental membranes and delivery, and maternal idiopathic thrombocytopenic purpura all predispose to bleeding in the neonate. A detailed family history should focus on the type and severity of bleeding in family members with particular emphasis on the sex of the family members affected. This information gives important clues to the inheritance pattern of the bleeding disorders under investigation. If only male members on the maternal side are affected, the diagnosis is most likely one of the hemophilias. If both sexes are affected in the family, one should think of VWD, keeping in mind the autosomal inheritance pattern. Finally, administration of vitamin K should be confirmed in any neonate with bleeding symptoms. Although physical examination may not contribute much to the diagnosis of a bleeding disorder, it is required for completeness.

The baby appears well except for bleeding from the circumcision site. The remainder of the physical examination is unremarkable. Family history is negative for any bleeding symptoms in any of the family members.

What should be done next?

About 15% to 30% of patients with an inherited bleeding disorder come to medical attention in the neonatal period. Moreover, 30% of cases of newly diagnosed hemophilia are caused by a new mutation in patients with no family history of bleeding. In a case such as this, an isolated prolongation of the APTT is suggestive of hemophilia. Ideally, factor VIII and IX assays will be performed to quickly confirm the diagnosis. However, factor assays are not available in all centers and at all times. The APTT test should be repeated using a 50:50 mix of patient and normal plasma. In hemophilia, the APTT corrects to normal. Even small clinical laboratories often have a stock of factor VIII–deficient plasma. If the APTT corrects when the specimen is mixed with normal plasma, the mixing study is repeated with the factor VIII–deficient plasma. If the APTT corrects to normal, hemophilia A is excluded and hemophilia B is the likely diagnosis. If the APTT does not correct to normal, factor VIII deficiency is the presumptive diagnosis.

The baby's APTT corrected to normal when a 50:50 mix of patient and normal plasma was tested. The APTT did not correct to normal when factor VIII–deficient plasma was used, which confirms a diagnosis of factor VIII deficiency, or hemophilia A.

What should be done now?

The baby's diagnosis is severe hemophilia A with a factor VIII level of less than 1%. Infusion of recombinant factor VIII concentrate at a dose of 50 U/kg will raise the plasma factor VIII level by 100% and stop the bleeding from the circumcision site. The baby may need additional smaller doses of the recombinant factor over the next day or two if the oozing from the circumcision site continues.

The mother should be checked to determine if she is a carrier of hemophilia by measuring factor levels and possibly performing genetic mutation analysis. If the mother is a carrier of hemophilia A, there is a 25% chance that a male child in subsequent pregnancies will be affected. If the mother is not a carrier, the baby is deemed to have a new mutation that caused hemophilia.

CASE 2

You are called to evaluate a 12-hour-old infant who was noted to have a petechial rash soon after delivery. A complete blood count is obtained, which reveals a platelet count of 8×10^9/L.

What is your initial approach?

The baby should be examined. The first goal is to determine whether there is clinical evidence of severe pathology (i.e., does the baby look sick?). Thrombocytopenic bleeding may be the first sign of sepsis or NEC. Maternal fever, rupture of the placental membranes a prolonged time before delivery, and premature birth all predispose to invasive infection. If the baby appears ill, a sepsis workup should be performed and parenteral antibiotic therapy should be initiated. Physical examination may disclose other abnormalities that suggest the correct diagnosis. Babies with thrombocytopenia caused by congenital viral infections often show microcephaly and hepatosplenomegaly. Radial and ulnar aplasia or hypoplasia suggests a primary defect in platelet production (e.g., Fanconi anemia or TAR syndrome).

The baby weighs 3450 g and vaginal delivery was uncomplicated. She appears well except for scattered petechiae and bruising from heel-stick and venipuncture sites. The remaining results of the complete blood count are unremarkable (white blood cell count: 10,000/μL with a normal differential; hemoglobin level: 17.2 g/dL).

What should be done next?

Factitious thrombocytopenia should always be considered, but it is unlikely in this case because of the presence of clinical signs. The blood smear should be examined for normal-appearing red and white blood cells and for giant platelets, which, if present, suggest an increased rate of peripheral platelet destruction with the marrow attempting to compensate by releasing young platelets into the circulation. The mother's platelet count should be checked and she should be questioned regarding medication use and any history of idiopathic thrombocytopenia purpura, lupus, or other collagen-vascular disorder. Maternal thrombocytopenia is an important clue that suggests transplacental transmission of maternal antiplatelet IgG autoantibodies. This is a common cause of neonatal thrombocytopenia in babies who appear well.

The baby's blood smear reveals giant platelets and marked thrombocytopenia, but findings are otherwise normal. The mother's platelet count is normal and there is no history suggesting maternal autoimmune disease.

What is the most likely diagnosis and what should be done?

The most likely diagnosis is neonatal alloimmune thrombocytopenia (NAIT). Detailed laboratory investigations are required for confirmation of the diagnosis and should be performed by an experienced reference laboratory. Current consensus is that both parents should be screened for HPA-1, HPA-3, and HPA-5 in all cases of potential NAIT and for HPA-4 as well if the patient is of Asian descent. HPA-9 and HPA-15 are the next most commonly involved in antigen incompatibilities. For testing to confirm NAIT, results must reveal both a platelet antigen incompatibility between the parents and maternal antibody directed against that antigen.

The baby's platelet count should be measured at least daily for the first few days of life, and she should be observed for signs of active hemorrhage.

While discussing the probable diagnosis with the parents, you are called urgently to the nursery because the baby has developed worsening petechiae and gross hematuria. Her vital sign values are stable.

What should be done next?

The baby now has evidence of significant active hemorrhage and should receive a random-donor platelet transfusion promptly. If readily available, matched (antigen-negative) platelets are preferred. The latter are platelets from donors negative for HPA-1. They can be given in larger increments and have a longer half-life. Concentrated washed irradiated maternal platelets can be used as well; however, their processing takes at least 12 to 48 hours.

The baby's platelet count increases and she stops bleeding after she is transfused with HPA-1–negative platelets. The mother is HPA-1 negative. The parents are interested in having other children and are concerned about the risk of recurrence.

What do you tell them?

The risk of severe neonatal hemorrhage in subsequent pregnancies is high. The mother should be followed as a "high-risk" patient. If the previously affected sibling had an ICH, the next affected fetus will have early, severe thrombocytopenia and in utero ICH unless effective treatment is instituted. Recent data indicate that the administration of IVIG to the mother before delivery decreases the incidence of neonatal thrombocytopenia.

CASE 3

You are asked to evaluate a newborn who appears pale shortly after birth and reportedly has a low blood capillary venous hematocrit.

What is your initial approach?

An important first step is to obtain an accurate history of both the prenatal course and the delivery. This should be accompanied by a thorough examination of the newborn that looks for signs of bleeding as well as for organomegaly (increased size of the liver and spleen, in particular).

You learn that this baby boy was born at 39 weeks' gestation and weighs 3700 g. All routine prenatal screening yielded negative results, and the prenatal course was uneventful. The mother is a 28-year-old white female, now gravida 3 para 3, who failed to report for the majority of her routine visits to her obstetrician leading up to this delivery. Her other two children were also term deliveries, and there was no report of problems in the newborn period. You are told that the mother is group O, Rh- negative, that her antibody screen results are negative, and that she did not receive anti-Rh globulin. The delivery was reportedly without complications, and the baby had Apgar scores of 8 and 9 with normal vital sign values at birth. A venous specimen obtained by heel stick at 25 minutes of age showed a hematocrit of 37%, and the test was repeated because of the increase in pallor. Examination shows no petechiae, bruising, or evidence of bleeding, and no splenomegaly or hepatomegaly.

What should be done next?

A thorough review of the available laboratory results is necessary to determine the appropriate tests and the next steps needed to confirm the diagnosis.

A hematocrit of venous blood obtained at 45 minutes was 30%.

What do you consider in your differential diagnosis and what should be done?

A decline in the hematocrit in the newborn period should raise a concern for hemolytic disease. An important consideration is Rh disease, given the maternal blood type and the mother's failure to follow up with her obstetrician during the latter part of gestation. ABO incompatibility and isoimmune disease should also be considered. The quickest way to determine whether these might be a real concern is to perform a DAT (Coombs test), the results of which will invariably be strongly positive in Rh disease. The absence of organomegaly in this instance argues against this possibility; however, it cannot be ruled out on the basis of examination alone, and accurate diagnosis will depend on the results of blood typing on both mother and infant.

You request the tests mentioned. The results of the direct antiglobulin test are negative, the baby's blood type is group O, Rh(D)-positive. The reticulocyte count is 138,000/μL, (4%), and the platelet count is 300 x 10⁹/L, with a normal white blood cell count and differential.

What is the diagnosis? What should be done?

For the reasons discussed earlier (negative result on DAT, absence of splenomegaly, lack of elevated reticulocyte count), this is not a case of Rh disease. It is also clearly not ABO incompatibility, because mother and infant are both blood group O. The negative DAT result also rules out other isoimmune disorders. One could consider G6PD deficiency because this is a male infant, but G6PD deficiency is most common in the African American population, which makes it less likely in this instance. A hint in this case is the low reticulocyte count. This provides a clue that the anemia has an onset and cause that are more acute in nature and could indeed be caused by blood loss, despite the lack of any physical evidence on examination of the baby.

What do you tell the physician requesting the consultation?

The most likely cause, and greatest concern, is that transplacental blood loss occurred. This would place the mother at significant risk of being sensitized to the Rh(D) antigen. This risk is further heightened because she did not receive hyperimmune anti-Rh globulin during pregnancy, but in the setting of a significant bleed even the standard dose may fail to provide sufficient protection from sensitization of the mother to the Rh(D) antigen. In this case, because the mother and infant share the blood group antigen O, the mother's risk of becoming sensitized to D antigen is even greater.[184,185] You should instruct the obstetrician to order a Kleihauer-Betke test on the mother's blood immediately to look for fetal cells. If increased numbers of fetal cells are present, a larger dose of hyperimmune globulin must be given to the mother. One can establish an estimated blood loss based on the baby's blood volume and hematocrit at birth.

REFERENCES

The reference list for this chapter can be found online at www.expertconsult.com.

Brain Disorders of the Fetus and Neonate

18

Mark S. Scher

A physician's knowledge of prenatal brain development in the context of maternal-placental health and disease greatly enhances the neurologic assessment of the newborn.[1] Although acute neurologic signs after birth should be investigated aggressively for peripartum or neonatal causes, pathologic processes may also occur during prenatal life that subsequently modify neonatal brain functions. Any discussion of the neurologic evaluation of the newborn, therefore, must take into account historical and physical examination findings that integrate intrauterine and extrauterine periods, during which inherited and acquired components may synergistically alter fetal brain development in ways specific to gestational maturity. The evaluation of the neonate must consider familial, maternal, fetal, placental, and environmental factors to better determine the developmental niche of the fetus or neonate when stress or disease favorably or unfavorably alters structure and function because of time-sensitive strengths or vulnerabilities.

This chapter begins with a discussion of prenatal brain development, followed by three sections that each highlight a different perspective on accurate neurologic diagnosis: consideration of fetal neurologic consultations in the context of prenatal organ development and disease risk, serial and systematic bedside examinations, and laboratory investigations of the newborn, with emphasis on classic components of neurologic assessment. Finally, selected neurologic conditions are described that underscore the importance of integrating historical and examination findings in the evaluation of brain disorders of the fetus and neonate.

STAGES OF PRENATAL BRAIN DEVELOPMENT

Maturation of the brain is defined through descriptions of sequential and overlapping developmental processes, beginning with conception and involving continual interactions of the gene environment. Beginning during gestation and following trimester-specific stages of development of the embryo and fetus, anatomic, biochemical, and physiologic processes occur: neural induction followed by neuronogenesis, programmed cell death and neuroblast migration, formation of axons and dendrites, continuous energy generation to provide membrane excitability, synaptogenesis, neurotransmitter biosynthesis, and myelination of axons. These prenatal time periods are fundamental for brain development. However, postnatal processes of programmed cell death, continued synaptogenesis, and neurotransmitter maturation highlight important brain maturational events needed for continued preservation of appropriate structure and function.[2] Regional differences in the rate of maturation of the nervous system also must be recognized. Different brain structures do not express equivalent function at specific times during the development of the fetus, premature infant, and full-term neonate. Table 18-1 summarizes the major prenatal developmental sequences in brain maturation that occur in the cerebrum and cerebellum and lists representative disorders at each stage. Both volume and gyral-sulcal complexity increase during prenatal development, with prominent changes in the last 3 months of gestation (Fig. 18-1)[3] reflecting major molecular and histologic maturational changes during the formation of maturing cortical-subcortical cellular connections.

Table 18-1.	Major Stages of Central Nervous System Development			
Stage	**Peak Time of Occurrence**	**Major Morphologic Events in Cerebrum**	**Major Morphologic Events in Cerebellum**	**Main Corresponding Disorders***
Uterine implantation	1 wk			
Separation of three layers	2 wk	Formation of neural plate		Enterogenous cysts and fistulae
Dorsal induction Neurulation	3-4 wk	Formation of neural tube, neural crest, and derivatives Closure of anterior (day 24) and posterior (day 29) neuropores	Paired alar plates	Anencephaly, encephalocele, craniorachischisis, spina bifida, meningocele
Caudal neural tube formation	4-7 wk	Canalization and regressive differentiation of cord	Rhombic lips (day 35), cerebellar plates	Diastematomyelia, Dandy-Walker syndrome, cerebellar hypoplasia
Ventral induction	5-6 wk	Forebrain and face (cranial neural crest) Cleavage of prosencephalon into cerebral vesicles (day 33) Optic placodes (day 26), olfactory placodes Diencephalon	Fusion of cerebellar plates	Holoprosencephaly, median cleft face syndrome
Neuronal and glial proliferation	8-16 wk	Cellular proliferation in ventricular and subventricular zone (interkinetic migration) Early differentiation of neuroblasts and glioblasts	Migration of Purkinje cells (9-10 wk) Migration of external granular layer (10-11 wk)	Microcephaly, megalencephaly
Migration	12-20 wk	Radial migration and accessory pathways (e.g., corpus gangliothalamicum) Formation of corpus callosum	Elaboration of the dendritic tree of Purkinje cells (16-25 wk)	Lissencephaly-pachygyria (types I and II), Zellweger syndrome, glial heterotopia, microgyria (some forms), agenesis of corpus callosum
Organization†	24 wk to postnatal	Late migration (to 5 mo) Alignment, orientation, and layering of cortical neurons Synaptogenesis Glial proliferation-differentiation well into postnatal life	Monolayer of Purkinje cells (16-28 wk) Migration of granules to form internal granular layer (to postnatal life)	Minor cortical dysplasias, dendritic and synaptic abnormalities, microgyria (some forms)
Myelination	24 wk to 2 yr postnatally			Dysmyelination, clastic insults

Adapted from Aicardi J, Bax M, Gillberg C, et al: *Diseases of the nervous system in childhood,* ed 2, New York, 1998, MacKeith Press.
*Disorders do not necessarily correspond to abnormal development. They may also result from secondary destruction or disorganization.
†Programmed cellular death takes place throughout the second half of pregnancy and the first year of extrauterine life.

FETAL NEUROLOGIC CONSULTATIONS

The pediatric neurologist can fulfill a useful role as a subspecialty consultant for the fetus with a suspected brain disorder, given that neurologic disease may occur before the intrapartum period, either from a primary brain disease or secondarily from systemic diseases. Brain disorders detected in the neonatal period may also reflect fetal brain damage that occurred before dysfunction is first documented. Alternatively, medical conditions during the antepartum or intrapartum periods can predispose the fetus or neonate to express brain dysfunction at a later period, with either de novo or compounded brain injury. The pediatric neurologist must therefore consider maternal, placental, and fetal diseases on which a neonatal encephalopathy may be superimposed (Box 18-1). This section describes how the neurologist uses an integrative approach to

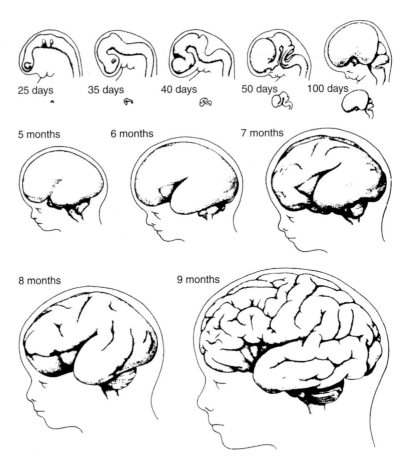

25 days 35 days 40 days 50 days 100 days

5 months 6 months 7 months

8 months 9 months

Figure 18-1. Gyral development in the human brain from 25 days to 9 months. Note the prominent increase in volume and gyral complexity in the last 3 months of gestation. *(From Cowan WM: The development of the brain,* Sci Am *241:113, 1997.)*

fetal neurology, emphasizing perspectives from other subspecialties such as maternal-fetal medicine, pathology, and neonatology, as well as additional pediatric subspecialties. Evaluation of future strategies for either fetal or neonatal brain resuscitation will need to consider the developmental context in which a suspected brain injury occurred during the antepartum, intrapartum, or neonatal period.[4]

TOOLS FOR FETAL NEUROLOGIC DIAGNOSIS

Diagnostic techniques for evaluation of the fetus have improved over the past several decades, providing morphologic, biochemical, and physiologic diagnoses. Many medical conditions can be better documented during the prenatal period.

Indications for the use of these tests are enumerated in both obstetric and pediatric guidelines (Box 18-2).[5,6] Most of the following investigative tools are invasive and have specific indications.

1. Amniocentesis is usually performed at 16 weeks' gestational age or earlier if necessary. Fluid can be used for karyotyping as

well as a variety of biochemical investigations. The most commonly performed tests are α-fetoprotein level and screening studies for specific chromosomopathies or neural tube defects.[7-9] (See Chapter 2.)

2. Chorionic villous sampling can be undertaken at 8 weeks' gestation or beyond, with specimens used for chromosomal studies by direct examination or culture as well as for biochemical analysis.

3. Fetal blood sampling guided by ultrasonography can be performed from 18 weeks' gestation onward to clarify ambiguous amniocentesis or chorionic villous sampling results and diagnose fetal infections, isoimmunization, or other hematologic problems.

4. Ultrasound examination using transvaginal probes can detect structural abnormalities as early as the embryonic period, but abdominal probes are routinely used at 15 to 20 weeks' gestation and the examination can be repeated as required. Evaluation of fetal maturity and the assessment of intrauterine growth are powerful measures for the antenatal diagnosis of many neurologic

Box 18-1.	**Main Causes of Fetal Encephalopathies of Circulatory Origin**

Lesions related to maternal pathologic conditions

Systemic diseases
- Maternal anemia
- Toxemia with chronic hypertension
- Renal diseases
- Repeated seizures during second trimester of pregnancy
- Severe hypoxia

Maternal trauma
- Direct trauma to abdomen
- Maternal accidents

Gas intoxication
- Carbon monoxide intoxication
- Butane intoxication

Lesions related to fetal conditions

Twin gestation (especially with one macerated twin)

Prenatal arterial occlusions

Blood dyscrasias
- Hemolytic disease with or without fetal-maternal blood group incompatibility
- Thrombocytopenia (genetic, isoimmune, or of infective origin)

Nonimmune hydrops fetalis

Lesions related to placental or cord abnormalities

Fetomaternal hemorrhage

Chronic placental insufficiency with fetal distress

Placental abruption

Cord knotting

Adapted from Larroche JC: Fetal encephalopathies of circulatory origin, Biol Neonate 50:61, 1986.

Box 18-2.	**Indications for the Use of Prenatal Diagnostic Tests**

General risk factors*

Maternal age 35 years or older at time of expected delivery[†]

Specific risk factors

Previous child with malformation or chromosomal abnormality

History of stillbirth or neonatal death

Structural abnormality in mother or father (e.g., neural tube defect)

Balanced chromosomal translocation in one parent

Family history of inherited disease in first-degree relatives

Maternal diabetes mellitus, phenylketonuria, exposure to teratogens, or some infectious diseases

Risk factors specific to certain ethnic groups

Tay-Sachs disease (screening in Ashkenazi Jews of Eastern European origin)

Sickle cell disease (screening in African and African American blacks)

Thalassemia (screening in some Mediterranean and some Asian populations)

Modified from D'Alton ME, DeCherney AH: Prenatal diagnosis, N Engl J Med 328:114, 1993, with permission.
*Mostly for chromosomal anomalies.
†Risk of Down syndrome increases significantly after 35 years. Other chromosomal abnormalities are also increasingly common after this age with double or triple the overall risk.

and nonneurologic fetal conditions. Table 18-2 lists selected brain malformations that can be diagnosed antenatally by ultrasonography. Newer techniques using three- and four-dimensional ultrasonography can show cerebral and noncerebral anatomic structures in greater detail.[10] Although abnormal fetal ultrasonographic findings might be discovered fortuitously, previous pregnancy complications or current medical difficulties during early pregnancy usually prompt the proactive performance of one or more studies. In routine practice, the sensitivity of ultrasonography is not uniformly satisfactory, but reliability has improved (Fig. 18-2).[11] The addition of

Doppler-visualized placental and umbilical blood flow adds valuable information regarding fetal stress secondary to uteroplacental insufficiency.[12,13]

5. Fetal neuroimaging provides additional anatomic information for the clinician regarding normal and abnormal structure. Magnetic resonance imaging (MRI) technology provides greater detail regarding gray and white matter structures, and can now detect anatomic correlates of pathophysiologic mechanisms related to asphyxia and/or inflammation that affect water diffusion and lead to edema (e.g., diffusion-weighted imaging).[14-17]

6. Biochemical, cytogenetic, and molecular biological techniques can assess for specific enzymes or other biochemical products that bear a relationship to specific genetic conditions. Techniques of DNA

Table 18-2.	Major Malformations That Can Be Diagnosed Antenatally by Ultrasonography	
Diagnosis	**Earliest Gestational Age at Which Diagnosis Is Possible* (wk)**	**Percentage Diagnosed by 20-24 wk[†]**
Anencephaly	12-16	100
Encephalocele	12-20	75-100
Meningomyelocele	14-32	60-95
Hydrocephalus	20-36	25
Microcephaly[‡]	18-36	25
Callosal agenesis	20	Probably high
Lissencephaly	20	Occasional reports

Adapted from Aicardi J, Bax M, Gillberg C, et al: *Diseases of the nervous system in childhood*, ed 2, New York, 1998, MacKeith Press, with permission.
*Associated malformations are often the most obvious and can lead to discovery of central nervous system abnormalities.
[†]Frequency estimates using best technique available in 1990.
[‡]This group includes cases of lissencephaly, true genetic microcephaly, and microcephaly caused by early destructive lesions.

analysis make possible prenatal diagnosis of specific inherited biochemical abnormalities, detection of mutant genes, and linkage studies with fragment-length polymorphisms or other DNA markers for a specific familial condition.[18]

7. Techniques are available to assess for physiologic fetal well-being versus distress. In utero surveillance of physiologic functions of the fetus can also be achieved using fetal ultrasonography. Specific fetal activities that can be monitored include gross body movements, eye movements, sucking movements, heart rate patterns, and respiratory patterns, and quantitative determination of amniotic fluid volume is possible.[19] Components can be combined to calculate a fetal biophysical score, which may reflect fetal physiologic well-being. Early or midgestation assessments are controversial; during the last trimester, studies of fetal behaviors may help document altered functional brain maturation by defining dysfunctional fetal organization of different behaviors.[20]

8. Intrauterine fetal therapies involve direct intervention on the fetus by a variety of techniques to treat specific conditions.[5,21] For instance, fetal exchange transfusion is used to treat the anemia and secondary consequences of hematologic disorders. Withdrawal of fluid from body cavities (e.g., pleural, peritoneal), catheterization of the bladder, and, in rare situations, fetal surgery for hydrocephalus can be considered.

THE CONSULTATION PROCESS

Advances in neuroscience at the bench and bedside throughout the last several decades have refocused attention on the fetal origins of neonatal brain diseases. Discussions of the causes for fetal and neonatal brain injury have been reviewed. Stevenson et al highlight maternal, placental, and fetal factors that may contribute to encephalopathy and subsequent functional impairments in the newborn.[22] A consensus report by a multidisciplinary task force reviewed medical literature regarding neonatal encephalopathy and cerebral palsy, emphasizing antepartum and intrapartum factors that need to be considered in determining the pathogenesis and pathophysiology of neonatal brain disorders.[23] Pediatric neurologists who provide either fetal or neonatal consultations need to consider antepartum and intrapartum factors when offering recommendations for brain resuscitation to either the perinatologist or neonatologist, as novel therapeutic opportunities are made available.

Initiation of Fetal Neurologic Consultations

A physician's formulation of a medical differential diagnosis always begins with fact finding and incorporates relevant historic information into the diagnostic fabric of the patient's medical presentation.[24] Although the investigation begins with the history of the present illness, consideration of medical and family histories may augment the physician's understanding of the present abnormal medical condition. These general guidelines can be applied to fetal neurologic consultations. The information obtained regarding the preconception and pregnancy health of the mother, fetal well-being, and placental function must always include details of acquired environmental stresses and adverse family medical histories to allow the physician to unravel the diagnostic puzzle.

The pediatric neurologist will be called upon to offer opinions on fetal neurologic issues as part of the interdisciplinary fetal consultation team. Such input may be requested at any time during the mother's pregnancy. This multispecialty team

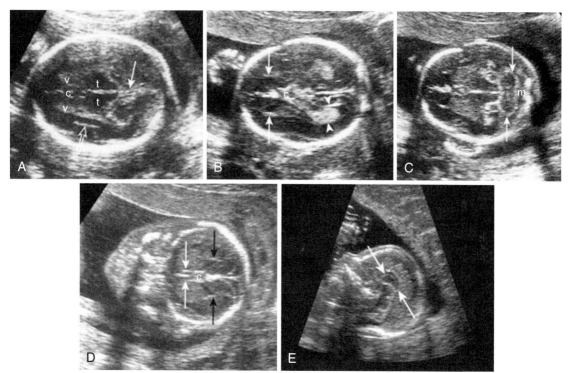

Figure 18-2. Standard planes for viewing cerebral structures. **A,** Thalamic view at 20 menstrual weeks showing thalamus-hypothalamus complex *(t)*, ambient cistern *(solid arrow)*, insula *(open arrow)*, tips of the anterior frontal horns of the lateral ventricles *(v)*, and cavum septi pellucidi *(c)*. **B,** Ventricular view at 18 weeks. The ventricle measurement is indicated *(arrowheads)*. The tips of the anterior frontal horns *(arrows)* and cavum septi pellucidi *(c)* are visible. **C,** Cerebellar view at 18 menstrual weeks. The cerebellar hemispheres *(arrows)* and cisterna magna *(m)* are indicated. **D,** Coronal view at 19 weeks through the coronal suture showing anterior frontal horns *(black arrows)* and large nerve trunks; the fornices *(white arrows)* are clearly visible below the cavum septi pellucidi *(c)*. **E,** Midsagittal view through the metopic suture at 19 weeks showing the normal corpus callosum *(arrows)* containing the cavum septi pellucidi in its arc below the corpus callosum. *(From Rumack CM, Wilson SR, Charboneau JW, et al, editors:* Diagnostic ultrasound, *ed 4, St Louis, 2011, Mosby, Figure 34-2.)*

(sometimes referred to as the *fetal board*) generally holds regular meetings, coordinated by maternal-fetal specialists, to discuss case histories of maternal-fetal pairs. The pediatric neurologist can provide an important perspective to this multidisciplinary group regarding neurologic diagnoses, while also considering input from the perinatologist, neonatologist, and other subspecialists. The pediatric neurologist can clarify findings that may suggest normal variation of the brain rather than a disease entity and provide experienced views regarding long-term prognosis.

The neurologist provides a balanced perspective on a neurologic diagnosis that is based on the structural and functional expressions of a brain disease or anomaly. Although structural brain anomalies, such as myelomeningocele, can be detected by ultrasonography, anticipation of postnatal bulbar dysfunction cannot always be predicted from prenatal imaging in the absence of polyhydramnios. Cranial nerve deficits evident on postnatal examinations will drastically alter the neurologist's prognostic assessment.

Fetal neurologic consultations can also be initiated because of the presence of systemic maternal or fetal disease entities. Hypertensive disorders or autoimmune disorders in the mother during pregnancy, for example, predispose some fetal patients to thrombophilia, and thrombo-occlusive disease occurs in the brains of some children.[25-27] Careful serial documentation of brain structures and cerebrovascular integrity around the circle of Willis by fetal ultrasonography needs to be performed to detect possible blood flow compromise with parenchymal brain injury. Systemic fetal diagnoses such as hydrops fetalis, for example, raise suspicion of cerebrovascular compromise of the fetal brain because of reductions in end-diastolic placental flow documented by ultrasonographic Doppler studies.[28]

Information regarding the structural-functional expression of fetal brain disorders must be communicated by the pediatric neurologist not only to other subspecialists on the fetal board but also to the primary care physician in family practice or pediatrics who will oversee the general health care of the child after birth. Finally, the child neurologist has the opportunity to establish an early relationship (during the prenatal period) with the family of a child with a brain disorder, which will facilitate continuity of care after the birth both in the neonatal unit and the outpatient service.

Timing of Fetal Neurologic Consultations

On occasion, preconceptional consultations will be requested when the medical diagnoses of the parents or other siblings with neurologic disorders may affect the decision making of parents who wish to conceive additional children. More likely, the pediatric neurologist begins the consultation during the second or third trimester, depending on prenatal diagnostic findings supplemented by other information, after referral by the high-risk perinatal service. This consultation may include a review of the results of abdominal imaging, Doppler flow studies showing placental perfusion, nonstress tests to assess state stability in the fetus, and cytogenetic testing interpreted by maternal-fetal specialists and geneticists. Given the greater diagnostic accuracy of genetic screening tests or transvaginal imaging performed during the first trimester, brain disorders may be detected during the embryonic period of development (i.e., sooner than 56 days after conception). At the other extreme, consultations may be initiated only after birth when neurologic problems are first detected or suspected.

The grave prognostic implications of triploidy of chromosomes 13 to 15 or 18, for example, may be pointed out by the geneticist or maternal-fetal specialist, who will ask the neurologist to discuss the low chances for survival and poor quality of life because of associated brain anomalies such as the holoprosencephaly syndromes. Cardiologists and nephrologists may identify anomalies in these organ systems that carry associated risks to the nervous system. The deletion syndrome involving the short arm of chromosome 22 (velocardiofacial syndrome), for instance, is associated with cardiac and other organ system anomalies in addition to those in the central nervous system (CNS) in a percentage of children.[29]

Diagnostic Process of Fetal Neurologic Consultations

Fetal Considerations: CNS-Specific Anomalies

Care of fetal patients with primary CNS anomalies requires input from the neurologic consultant. Estimates are that 50% of all cases presented to a multidisciplinary fetal board involve primary CNS anomalies.[30] An opinion may also be requested from the pediatric neurosurgery service, since surgical intervention after birth may be considered for hydrocephalus or myelodysplasia. Even if the CNS anomaly is the starting point for the multidisciplinary term, a brain anomaly may be a surrogate marker for non-CNS abnormalities or genetic syndromes. For example, the presence of holoprosencephaly may suggest triploidy of chromosomes 13 to 15 or 18, non-CNS organ anomalies (e.g., cardiac lesions), or cholesterol dysmetabolism associated with underdeveloped genitalia (Smith-Lemli-Opitz syndrome).[31]

Structural abnormalities in the brain can be detected by prenatal imaging (See Table 18-2) and represent a spectrum of disorders that involve different parts of the CNS, with implications for involvement of multiple organ systems.[24] Knowledge of prenatal brain development provides perspective regarding timing, pathogenesis, and pathophysiology of congenital or acquired brain lesions. The pediatric neurologist, however, may not always accurately predict postnatal developmental trajectories during fetal consultations. Continuity of care for children with neurologic disorders provides an accurate long-term perspective on functional plasticity at successively older ages.

An example of a more nonspecific, and consequently problematic, prenatal imaging finding is fetal ventriculomegaly. At the initial ultrasonographic study, documentation of enlarged ventricles does not allow immediate insight into whether a progressive process representing hydrocephalus exists or compensatory fetal ventriculomegaly has arisen because of a failure of adequate brain growth with resultant enlargement of the ventricular and cisternal spaces. Hydrocephalus in utero requires serial ultrasonographic evaluations to document progressively decreasing cortical thickness and progressively increasing ventricular size. Only after 24 weeks'

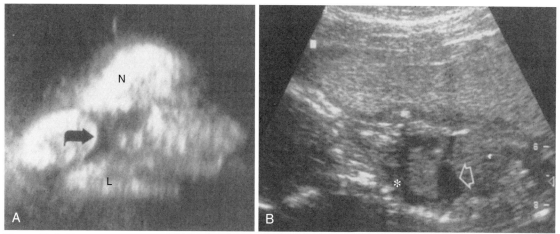

Figure 18-3. Nonneurologic findings on fetal ultrasound images that may suggest brain disease. **A,** Unilateral cleft lip *(arrow)*. *L,* Lip; *N,* nose. **B,** Sagittal view of the fetal trunk. Pleural effusion *(asterisk)* surrounds the fetal lung. Fetal ascites is present *(arrow)*. *(From Sanders RC:* Structural fetal abnormalities, *St Louis, 1996, Mosby.)*

gestation do changes in the occipital-frontal circumference reliably indicate progressive ventriculomegaly suggesting hydrocephalus. Ventriculomegaly is also a nonspecific anatomic finding that can be a marker for associated nervous system anomalies such as myelomeningocele, Dandy-Walker malformation, Chiari malformation, and a variety of genetic syndromes (Fig. 18-3).[32] Fetal MRI may delineate CNS anomalies better than fetal ultrasonography.

Ultrasonographic detection of other major body anomalies as well as cytogenetic and serologic findings from amniocentesis may suggest syndromic, chromosomal, and infectious disorders associated with ventriculomegaly. The perinatal team must develop the best delivery strategy and postnatal treatment of the infant with suspected progressive ventriculomegaly.

A second nonspecific ultrasonographic finding that may suggest a variety of CNS anomalies is the intracranial cystic lesion. Usually detected during the second or third trimester, these lesions can arise from multiple causes ranging from congenital to acquired conditions.[24] When such intracranial lesions have been detected by transabdominal ultrasonography, fetal MRI studies should be performed to more definitively visualize intracranial lesions and surrounding brain structures. One must always distinguish destructive from congenital lesions. A cystic lesion is more likely to be congenital if it occurs during the first half of pregnancy (e.g., encephaloclastic lesions such as schizencephaly or arachnoid cysts)

(Fig. 18-4), whereas acquired lesions from intravascular occlusive events generally occur later during the second half of pregnancy (e.g., encephalomalacia from stroke syndromes associated with maternal preeclampsia or fetal thrombotic vasculopathy of the placenta). Thrombophilia predisposes the fetus to intravascular occlusive events within either the arterial or venous circulation of the brain. Fetal stroke occurs in approximately 1 in 4000 live births and can be associated with multiple maternal, placental, and fetal diseases.[33-37]

Fetal Circulatory and Vascular Disorders
Bothing ischemic and hemorrhagic cerebrovascular lesions can result from circulatory disorders of the mother, fetus, or placenta.

The consequences of intrauterine circulatory and vascular disorders related to systemic diseases of the mother, including maternal anemia, hypertensive disorders of pregnancy, and uncontrolled maternal seizures leading to severe hypoxia, may present only after birth in the immediately neonatal period. Direct trauma to the mother's abdomen, indirect consequences of maternal accidents, and gas intoxication by carbon monoxide or butane poisoning are other examples of maternal pathologic conditions that promote fetal vascular brain injury. Vascular lesions related to fetal conditions include vascular disruptions associated with multiple gestation, particularly when one macerated twin is present (Fig. 18-5); prenatal arterial occlusions caused by altered angiogenesis; blood dyscrasias due to hemolytic disease or thrombocytopenia; and

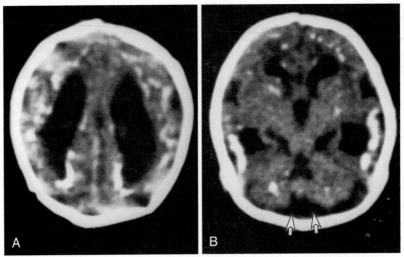

Figure 18-4. Congenital cytomegalovirus infection in a 5-day-old newborn evident on two computed tomographic scans. **A,** Periventricular and diffuse cerebral calcifications and ventriculomegaly. **B,** Cerebellar hypoplasia and large cisterna magna *(arrows). (From Volpe J: Neurology of the newborn, ed 3, Philadelphia, 1995, Saunders, p 680.)*

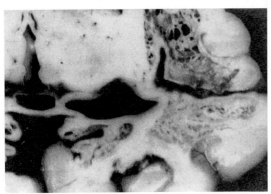

Figure 18-5. Multicystic encephalomalacia in the brain of a monozygotic twin whose stillborn co-twin was macerated. Note honeycomb appearance of subcortical white matter on postmortem examination. *(From Aicardi J, Bax M, Gillberg C, et al: Diseases of the nervous system in childhood, ed 2, New York, 1998, MacKeith Press, p 15.)*

hydrops fetalis with hematologic, infectious, or other congenital causes. Finally, placental or cord anomalies, including fetal-maternal hemorrhage, chronic placental insufficiency with fetal distress, placental abruption, true cord knots, and long or short cords may contribute to vascular compromise in the fetus in either the antepartum or intrapartum period (see Box 18-1).

Circulatory disturbances affect the fetal brain differently depending on the stage of brain development. Brain injuries before the seventieth day in utero result in abnormal migratory patterns of neuronal groups within the white matter or neocortex without major cavitation, whereas later injuries result in

destructive (encephaloclastic) lesions caused by ischemia or hemorrhage. For example, schizencephaly may be the result of faulty vascular supply to the developing neocortex before the seventieth day of gestation, which leads to a "true porencephaly" with an ependymal lined cleft or tract between the intraventricular and subarachnoid spaces.

In general, the migration of neocortical cells, angiogenesis of the blood vessels, and gliogenesis of supportive cellular elements occur in an overlapping manner. Therefore, it may be difficult to predict precisely the specific brain injury because of the unknown timing of the insult or insults that precede or follow critical stages of brain maturation. Circulatory disturbances generally damage the periventricular white matter of the preterm infant. Ischemic or hemorrhagic injuries in the preterm brain tend to occur between 26 and 34 weeks' gestation, whether they occur prenatally in the fetal brain or postnatally in the preterm infant's brain. On the other hand, cortical, subcortical, and basal ganglia regions are more susceptible to injury after 34 weeks' gestation in either the near-term or term infant, because of the more advanced maturation of brain vasculature. These vascular lesions may also be produced before or after birth, depending on the timing of the insult after 36 weeks' gestation. This topic is discussed in greater detail in the section on asphyxia.

Clinical manifestations of fetal circulatory and vascular disorders may be difficult to detect, either before or after birth. The presence of unexpected alterations in fetal movements, as perceived by the mother or with abdominal ultrasonography, may be a helpful sign, but such alternations are observed largely through serendipity. Fetal growth restriction, hydrops fetalis, and hydramnios are examples of other, more obvious suspicious features. Multiple gestation pregnancies and maternal trauma can also be associated with circulatory abnormalities in the fetal brain. However, vascular lesions may result even in the absence of documented maternal, fetal, or placental disorders.

After birth, specific clinical and laboratory findings may suggest in utero brain injury related to circulatory disturbances. Marked neonatal anemia, microcephaly at birth, marked rigidity or spasticity, or isolated seizures in the absence of post–hypoxic-ischemic brain disorder raise suspicions of antepartum disorders. Early neuroimaging (computed tomography [CT] or MRI) within 48 hours after birth should distinguish an acute from a chronic brain lesion. Specific types of CT or MRI images (e.g., inversion-recovery sequences or diffusion-weighted views) may distinguish acute stages of cellular edema with transmembrane diffusion of intercellular and intracellular fluid contents[38,39] (whatever the cause, but presumably after a recently occurring pathogenetic process such as asphyxia, infection, trauma) from gliotic scarring, irregular ventricular borders, ventriculomegaly, or brain maldevelopment, which imply a remote brain injury.

Inherited Metabolic and Neurodegenerative Diseases of Fetal Onset

Although it may be difficult to definitively identify children with metabolic or neurodegenerative disorders during fetal life, certain clues can raise concerns before or after birth.[40] Specific disease entities may present in the neonatal period with hypotonia, decreased levels of arousal, or intractable neonatal seizures inappropriate to events around birth. Decreased arousal or coma after formula feedings may suggest a biochemical disorder involving carbohydrate, protein, or fat metabolism. A constellation of minor brain or somatic anomalies may heighten the physician's clinical suspicions. Limb contractures, an underdeveloped thorax, or decreased muscle mass, for instance, may suggest congenital neuromuscular diseases. Careful ophthalmologic evaluation of

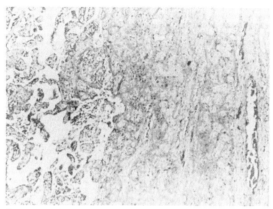

Figure 18-6. Microscopic sample of intervillous region at 20x HxE stain. Chronic placental infarction superimposed on a more recent retroplacental hemorrhage.

the anterior chamber of the eye may document an anterior chamber (i.e., embryotoxon) anomaly associated with peroxisomal diseases, or colobomata of the iris or retina, which represent a nonspecific arrest in ocular development caused by either metabolic and genetic or developmental disorders. Association with nonimmune hydrops or intrauterine growth restriction may also be a clue to the diagnosis. Careful inspection of placental specimens may document destructive lesions, vascular lesions, congenital anomalies, or storage material that reflects the timing or cause of disease states (Fig. 18-6).

Fetal Considerations: Non-CNS Anomalies

The fetus with brain disorders may initially show abnormalities of other organs. Important diagnostic clues for the fetal or neurologic consultant are provided by a variety of systemic fetal conditions, as suggested by Table 18-3. Regardless of which organ system is the starting point for a multidisciplinary medical discussion, associations with the nervous system must be considered, because non-CNS anomalies may be surrogate markers for CNS disease. Seventy-eight percent of fetal neurologic consultations provided to 166 maternal-fetal pairs involved systemic disease conditions, with or without CNS anomalies.[30] For example, children with the midgut anomaly omphalocele can have associated neural tube defects.[41]

Generalized systemic medical conditions also predispose the fetal brain to harmful effects. For example, multiple gestation pregnancies may result in twin-to-twin transfusion syndrome, which is seen in 5% to 15%

Table 18-3.	Nonneurologic Findings Associated with Neurologic Diagnoses
Nonneurologic Finding	**Neurologic Diagnosis**
Cardiac rhabdomyoma	Tuberous sclerosis
Hypoplastic left heart syndrome	Brain malformations (e.g., microgyria, agenesis of corpus callosum)
Multicystic dysplastic kidney	Brain malformations with specific genetic syndromes vs. destructive brain lesions
Diaphragmatic hernia	Brain malformations (e.g., cerebellar hypoplasia)
Polyhydramnios	Brain malformations with genetic syndromes or destructive brain lesions
Hydrops fetalis	Congenital syndromes (e.g., Turner syndrome) or destructive brain lesions, usually of vascular or infectious origin (e.g., asphyxia, parvovirus infection, metabolic disorders)
Cleft lip and palate	Midline brain malformations (e.g., holoprosencephaly)
Arthrogryposis	Neuromuscular disease or destructive brain lesions (e.g., congenital muscular dystrophies)
Multiple gestation pregnancy	Destructive brain lesions of white or gray matter (e.g., periventricular leukomalacia)
Omphalocele/gastroschisis	Neural tube defects

of all twin pregnancies,[42,43] with the most severe form occurring in 1% of monochorionic gestations. Twin-to-twin transfusion syndrome has hematologic consequences that lead to overperfusion or underperfusion of the siblings. Polycythemia and hydrops fetalis are two possible complications, and these conditions predispose the unborn child to cerebrovascular injury from hypoperfusion caused by either hyperviscosity or ischemia, possibly with accompanying thrombophilia. Significant growth discrepancy with growth restriction in the donor twin may result. End-diastolic volume, as determined by Doppler flow ultrasonography, may become compromised, with loss of placental flow to one or both twins. If one twin dies in utero, the surviving fetus will have a significantly increased risk of cerebrovascular injuries and may later exhibit cerebral palsy. Associated placental abnormalities also have been described in children who experienced brain injury manifesting as motor deficits.[44,45]

Another systemic presentation of fetal disease with adverse consequences to the brain is hydrops fetalis. The diagnosis of hydrops fetalis requires documentation of fluid accumulation in serous cavities and edema of the soft tissues of the fetus, which can be documented by transabdominal ultrasonography (Fig. 18-3) (see also Chapter 2). Most clinical series include isolated fetal ascites in the definition of hydrops fetalis, with an incidence of approximately 1 in 2500. The causes of most cases of hydrops fetalis remain nonspecific, involving maternal, fetal, or placental disorders. Associated conditions include congenital heart disease, triploidy, Turner syndrome, cystic hygroma, twin pregnancies, hematologic disorders, diaphragmatic hernia, gastrointestinal problems, maternal diabetes, placental-cord diseases, congenital infections, and inborn errors of metabolism.

Hydrops fetalis is an important pathologic condition that may predispose the child to fetal or neonatal encephalopathies. Cerebral injury and genetic or metabolic diseases of the brain may present in general as hydrops fetalis on fetal ultrasonography. Fetal brain vasculopathies may manifest as stroke syndromes or intracranial hemorrhage in patients with hydrops fetalis. Neonatal encephalopathies expressed after birth in neonates with hydrops fetalis may also reflect remote fetal brain injury, usually from hypoperfusion or thrombo-occlusive disease that occurred during the third trimester due to hydrops fetalis.

Infectious Diseases

Both the embryo (<8 weeks' gestation) and fetus (>8 weeks' gestation) are vulnerable to a number of infectious agents. Infections during the first and early second trimesters result in congenital malformations more commonly than in destructive lesions. Later infections during the third trimester generally result in destructive changes in the brain. The inflammatory response provoked by infectious agents leads to glial scarring of the brain, usually after 26 to 28 weeks' gestation.

The brain may appear markedly atrophic, with calcification of neurotic areas, as documented by CT scans of the head after birth (see also Chapter 14). Major destructive lesions may also be noted on fetal sonograms or neonatal neuroimaging scans (see Fig. 18-4). The most common infections that can affect fetal brain integrity and development are those caused by cytomegalovirus, rubella virus, herpes simplex virus, *Toxoplasma gondii, Treponema pallidum,* and human immunodeficiency virus (HIV).

Clinical manifestations in the neonate of fetal infectious disease may include organomegaly, intrauterine growth restriction, jaundice, microcephaly, intracranial calcification, osseous lesions, encephalitis, and chorioretinitis, particularly with cytomegalovirus infection.[46,47] Specifically for rubella, any combination of brain, eye, heart, or ear involvement is possible, and some infants may show irritability, lethargy, and hypotonia at birth, whereas others experience only hearing loss, depending on when the fetus was infected. Infants with herpes simplex infections may be acutely ill during the period immediately after delivery or may become symptomatic over the first several weeks of life.[48,49] Intractable seizures and coma may also highlight their neonatal clinical course. Congenital toxoplasmosis can take a severe neonatal form that includes hepatosplenomegaly, fever, and purpura. Ventricular dilatation may exist in utero, as documented by fetal ultrasonography, and chorioretinitis is a common feature seen on retinal examination in the newborn period. The clinical presentation of an infant with congenital syphilis also includes hepatosplenomegaly, retinitis, and osteochondritis, but these may appear only after several months of life, along with irritability, vomiting, cranial nerve deficits, and chronic hydrocephalus. HIV infection can be transmitted as early as 15 weeks' gestation; most HIV-infected neonates are asymptomatic with positive serologic results for up to several years.[50] Diagnosis in the neonatal period is generally difficult. However, some infants receive a large viral load in utero and may be born prematurely with microcephaly and calcification of the basal ganglia.

Less common viruses that also affect the brain but have no consistent pattern of fetal injury include influenza virus, measles virus, hepatitis virus, variola virus, and enteroviruses and adenoviruses. Infection with one virus, parvovirus B19, has been associated with nonimmune hydrops fetalis and may indirectly affect fetal brain integrity by causing uteroplacental insufficiency leading to vasculopathies.

Exogenous and Endogenous Toxic Disorders
Although the placenta is usually an effective barrier between maternal and fetal circulations, specific exogenous or endogenous toxins may nonetheless reach the fetus to produce malformations or destructive disturbances, depending on the timing of the toxin exposure. Examples of such exogenous agents are therapeutic agents, industrial pollutants, and recreational substances. Some of the main agents producing neurologic injury are listed in Table 18-4, which also describes the various patterns of damage that may occur. An example of endogenous toxicity is maternal diabetes mellitus. All forms of diabetes may produce problems for the fetus and neonate. Careful control of maternal diabetes can prevent most major congenital malformations of the brain and spinal cord, yet developmental and destructive insults can result during fetal life, during parturition, or after birth, including immaturity of brain development, sacral agenesis, intracranial venous thromboses from hyperviscosity-polycythemia syndrome, and peripheral nerve injury from shoulder dystocia caused by impaction of a hypotonic-macrosomic fetus against the pelvic inlet during delivery. Postnatal polycythemia, hypoglycemia, and hypocalcemia all may result in neonatal seizures or coma, or both.

Immunologic and Blood Disorders in the Fetus
Blood type incompatibility has classically been associated with erythroblastosis fetalis and can be prevented by isoimmunization and the administration of globulins. Blood dyscrasias of either an immune or a nonimmune origin can also contribute to hydrops fetalis; the association of hydrops fetalis with cerebrovascular lesions in the fetus was described earlier. Nonimmune hydrops fetalis may occur after infection with parvovirus B19 or as a result of various inherited metabolic disorders, cardiac diseases, or chromosomal diseases such as Turner syndrome. Fetal-maternal and twin-to-twin transfusion syndromes are also frequently implicated in fetal brain disease, which usually results from ischemic or hemorrhagic injuries caused by venous stasis (i.e., hyperviscosity-polycythemia syndrome) or arterial ischemia (i.e., anemia). Intrauterine thrombocytopenia resulting from isoimmunization against fetal platelets or idiopathic causes may produce fetal brain damage.[51,52] The inflammatory process has been implicated in cerebral palsy.

Intrauterine Growth Restriction
Fetal growth restriction increases the risk of neurologic problems. Intrauterine growth

Table 18-4.	Main Substances That Can Be Transmitted from Mother to Fetus and Produce Neurologic Damage	
Category	**Pattern of Damage**	
THERAPEUTIC AGENTS		
Antiepileptic drugs (phenytoin, barbiturates, carbamazepine, diones, sodium valproate)	Fetal growth restriction, small head, dysmorphism of face and fingers, clefts, congenital heart disease, and other defects	
Benzodiazepines	Poorly defined	
Warfarin and other Coumarin derivatives	Punctate chondrodystrophy, deafness	
Vitamin A	Hydrocephalus, ear, and heart anomalies (uncertain)	
Retinoic acid, isotretinoin	Central nervous system migration disorder	
INDUSTRIAL POLLUTANTS		
Methylmercury	Abnormal neuronal migration, deranged cortical organization	
Polychlorinated biphenyls (PCBs)	Microcephaly, large fontanelles, behavioral disturbances	
Carbon monoxide	Hypoxic-ischemic lesions	
RECREATIONAL SUBSTANCES		
Alcohol	Fetal growth restriction, facial dysmorphism, brain malformations with excess neuronal migration, and other central nervous system defects	
Narcotics (heroin, codeine, methadone) Other street drugs (amphetamines, pyribenzamine, phencyclidine) Cocaine	Virtually all such substances may produce fetal growth restriction, and narcotics may produce withdrawal symptoms in neonates. In addition, cocaine can induce placental abruption and fetal death and may be responsible for skull and brain malformations and vascular damage with infarcts or hemorrhage.	
Toluene and other inhalants	Microcephaly, minor craniofacial anomalies, limb anomalies	
Tobacco	Fetal growth restriction, possible effects on cognitive development	

Adapted from Aicardi J, Bax M, Gillberg C, et al: *Diseases of the nervous system in childhood*, ed 2, New York, 1998, MacKeith Press.

restriction is defined in various ways, usually as somatic growth that is less than the 2nd percentile or at least 2 standard deviations less than the mean for gestational age (see also Chapter 5). Symmetric growth restriction and asymmetric growth restriction imply different time courses for a disease state. A fetus with early gestational disorders from chromosomal or syndromic conditions is more likely to demonstrate balanced growth restriction (i.e., both head and somatic growth compromised). Asymmetric growth restriction occurs during the last trimester in response to acquired deficits, which tend to spare head growth. Infants who are small for gestational age as a compensatory response to stress in utero may escape subsequent neurologic sequelae, whereas other infants with intrauterine growth restriction may experience brain injury. However, a subset of infants with more subtle reductions in somatic dimensions (i.e., lower ponderal index) may have more pervasive disorders or diseases that occur closer to parturition. The fetus with intrauterine growth restriction exhibits malformations or dysmorphic syndromes at a much higher rate than the general population (5% to 15%). Therefore, the possible association of intrauterine growth restriction and brain injury should be considered in the context of other historical and physical examination factors.

Maternal-Placental Considerations

Fetal neurologic consultations can be initiated because of maternal disorders such as diabetes mellitus, pregnancy-induced hypertension, or specific organ diseases. A woman's history of miscarriages in early pregnancy may suggest genetic or acquired risks to the fetus resulting from inherited forms of thrombophilia or recurring infection. Thrombo-occlusive disease (e.g., stroke, heart disease) at younger ages in family members also suggests the possibility of these disease entities in the mother.

Placental anomalies also suggest increased risks to the fetus. An abnormally large or small placenta, anomalies of the umbilical cord, and structural anomalies to the placenta may adversely affect fetal well-being. Velamentous insertion of the cord, for example, puts the child at risk for later exsanguination if umbilical vessels separate during the delivery process. Vascular changes within maternal or fetal placental vascular beds, such as chorioangiosis, maternal floor infarction, and fetal thrombotic vasculopathy, imply hypoperfusion of the fetus.[53,54]

Consultations during the Peripartum and Neonatal Periods

Knowledge of adverse events around the puerperal period is important to the pediatric neurologist who later participates in neurointensive neonatal consultation.[55] The mother's report of the quality and quantity of fetal movements before the onset of labor, as well as specific information from fetal surveillance close to and during labor, need to be considered. Abnormal findings on nonstress tests and biophysical profiles may provide important clues to fetal distress during the period preceding or during parturition. Accurate information regarding the length of labor and delivery and any associated complications must be provided for the neurologist's consideration. Fetal heart rate patterns, scalp and cord pH values, Apgar scores, and the degree of neonatal resuscitative efforts can help characterize an evolving neonatal brain disorder in the context of adverse conditions before and during labor and delivery. Fetal distress, as reflected by fetal heart rate abnormalities, uncommonly indicates intrapartum brain injury and instead usually reflects antepartum causes.[56,57] For the individual neonate, however, severe and abrupt changes in markers of fetal well-being, such as scalp pH or fetal heart rate, denote risks for acute brain injury.

During the period immediately after birth, the neurologist must be cognizant of the infant's extrauterine adaptation following the stresses of labor and delivery. Altered arousal, altered muscle tone, and seizures are the three principal clinical components of an evolving encephalopathy and sometimes occur after a stressful experience during parturition.[24] However, the infant's initial metabolic acidosis, neonatal depression, and hypotonia may not evolve into a persistently altered state of depressed arousal, hypotonia, and seizures.[58] Rapid resolution of metabolic acidosis and improvement in Apgar scores without the need for resuscitation indicate that a neonatal encephalopathy is less likely to develop. Specific examination findings may preferentially reflect fetal brain disorders even in the encephalopathic newborn. Intrauterine growth restriction, joint contractures, and hydrops fetalis are examples of clinical findings that suggest longer-standing fetal diseases, which predispose

the fetus to intrapartum distress and neonatal depression with hypotonia immediately after birth and during delivery room stabilization. The rapid expression of hypertonicity, sometimes with cortical thumbs, in an initially neurologically depressed neonate who rapidly returns to wakefulness after vigorous resuscitation usually suggests chronic fetal neurologic disorder.

By contrast, after an intrapartum asphyxial stress as documented by severe metabolic acidosis at birth (pH of <7.00), a depressed 10-minute Apgar score (<3), sustained hypotonia, and unresponsiveness with seizures throughout the next 3 to 7 days suggest an evolving hypoxic ischemic encephalopathy.[23] These general encephalopathic features consisting of a depressed sensorium and hypotonia (with or without seizures), however, may also be expressed by infants with fetal (i.e., antepartum) brain injury that is superimposed on neonatal brain dysfunction after a stressful labor and delivery.[22-24] It may be impossible in a particular infant to differentiate neonatal encephalopathy from preexisting antepartum brain injury that occurred only hours to a few days before the start of active labor. A presumption of fetal brain injury might be supported by the presence of preexisting maternal disease, chronic placental-cord abnormalities, specific persistent neuroimaging findings, or neuropathologic findings on postmortem examination.[59,60] Intrapartum asphyxial stress certainly can add further brain injury to previous damage in some infants. Newer neuroimaging techniques using diffusion-weighted MRI and magnetic resonance spectroscopy may help establish the timing of injury that occurred closer to events during labor and delivery.[14,61-63]

The pediatric neurologist must unify all pertinent data from the antepartum, peripartum, and neonatal periods to arrive at the most accurate interpretation of the neonatal neurologic examination findings. Comparisons between prenatal brain images (obtained via abdominal ultrasonography or fetal MRI) and postnatal images are essential. Diffusion-weighted MRI images may help identify any acute or subacute cerebral edema. Although fetal MRI provides better resolution of brain structures than abdominal ultrasonography, continued brain development in utero may mislead the neurologist, who consequently offers inaccurate or incomplete anatomic diagnoses after birth. The postnatal evaluation of the infant must be incorporated into the neurologic consultation. Phenotypic features of either genetic or acquired medical conditions may not have been appreciated during fetal life.

Neurointensive care recommendations by the pediatric neurologist will involve recommendations for neuroimaging studies, neurophysiologic testing with electroencephalography or evoked potentials, as well as biochemical studies to investigate metabolic disturbances. Pathologic examination of the placenta and umbilical cord during the first day of life are essential to provide additional information on the etiology and timing of a fetal or neonatal brain disorder. All recommendations will be integrated with those of the neonatal team.

APPROACH TO NEUROLOGIC EXAMINATION OF THE NEWBORN

Although the nervous system of the newborn is structurally and functionally immature, general strategies for performing a neurologic examination should parallel the bedside approach used with the older infant and child.[1,64,65] Neuronal networks in the neonatal brain with limited dendritic and synaptic interconnections, as well as immature myelination patterns, contribute to the expression of immature neurologic function. Clinical neurologic signs therefore reflect subcortical structures to a larger extent and cortical function to a more limited extent. Judicious coordination of careful neurologic clinical examination and neurobehavioral state assessment, with electroencephalographic (EEG) and polygraphic analyses, can provide better assessment of brain function.

To reinforce the discussion in the previous section concerning fetal brain development and the unique susceptibilities of the fetal brain to maldevelopment or injury, the present discussion of the clinical evaluation of the newborn explores how the newborn's clinical repertoire reflects prenatal, peripartum, and postnatal disease processes.

Systematic neonatal examination techniques must be followed in a sequential and repetitive fashion, emphasizing specific levels of the neuraxis (Box 18-3). The preterm infant has a more limited clinical repertoire because of greater immaturity; yet, serial examinations can optimize the validity of normal or suspicious findings. Knowledge of the evolution of signs and symptoms over the early postnatal period can contribute to

---

Box 18-3.	Basic Elements of the Neonatal Neurologic Examination

Level of alertness
Cranial nerves
- Olfaction (I)
- Vision (II)
- Optic fundi (II)
- Pupils (III)
- Extraocular movements (III, IV, VI)
- Facial sensation and masticatory power (V)
- Facial motility (VII)
- Audition (VIII)
- Sucking and swallowing (V, VII, IX, X, XII)
- Sternocleidomastoid function (XI)
- Tongue function (XII)
- Taste (VII, IX)
Motor function
- Tone and posture
- Motility and power
- Tendon reflexes and plantar response
- Primary neonatal reflexes
  Moro reflex
  Palmar grasp
  Tonic neck response
Sensory function

Adapted from Volpe JJ: Neurology of the newborn, ed 3, Philadelphia, 1995, Saunders, p 95.

---

the clinician's diagnostic and prognostic abilities. Abnormalities found on neurologic examination reflect the moment-to-moment functional integrity of the infant and may have little bearing on the location or extent of brain damage that occurred during fetal or neonatal life; this becomes more demonstrable only at older ages.

ESTIMATION OF GESTATIONAL AGE

Estimation of the maturity of an infant is crucial to understanding the neurodevelopmental niche in which the infant is situated when an examination is performed. Responses to the neonatal neurologic examination change with the infant's maturational level. Disease entities also express different characteristics in newborns who are born appropriate for gestational age compared with those who are small for gestational age. Finally, specific types of insults to the brain have varying impact on different parts of the nervous system, depending on the child's gestational maturity.[1]

The most useful historical data for estimating gestational age, especially in preterm infants, is the date of the mother's last menstrual period. Techniques for estimating gestational maturity by clinical examination are based on careful anthropometric measurements such as body weight, length, and head circumference, as well as observations of external characteristics such as body hair, skin texture, skin creases, and areola size. Ponderal index and body mass index reference curves for large neonatal populations identify more pervasive expressions of growth restriction not detected using standard growth curves.[66] Laboratory evaluations also provide estimates of maturity; these include radiographic studies of bone growth, neurophysiologic measures of EEG or nerve conduction velocities,[67] and neuroimaging descriptions of sulcal, gyral, and myelination features.[68]

CHARACTERISTICS OF THE HEAD

Examination of the head focuses on four areas: skin characteristics, head circumference, shape of the head, and rate of head growth.

The skin should be carefully inspected for the presence of (1) dimples or tracts, which can be associated with brain malformations; (2) subcutaneous masses that reflect trauma, tumors, or encephaloceles; and (3) cutaneous lesions, which may be associated with specific congenital vascular abnormalities or neurocutaneous syndromes, such as Sturge-Weber syndrome, linear sebaceous nevus syndrome, or incontinentia pigmenti. Description of skin lesions may help diagnose a medical condition with important manifestations in the brain. For instance, the port wine stain of Sturge-Weber syndrome can be associated with abnormalities in choroidal vessels in the eye and meninges, which may result in glaucoma and cortical lesions. Skin lesions may evolve with maturation. For example, pale macular lesions present in Sturge-Weber syndrome become more deeply stained red or purple with age (Fig. 18-7).[69]

Head circumference should be considered as a surrogate measure of brain and cerebrospinal fluid (CSF) volumes. Generalized or localized scalp edema affects the accuracy of the head circumference measurement. True macrocephaly or microcephaly can be estimated by determining whether the child's head size is larger than the 97th percentile or smaller than the 3rd percentile, respectively.

The shape of the head also requires careful inspection. Skull deformities may result

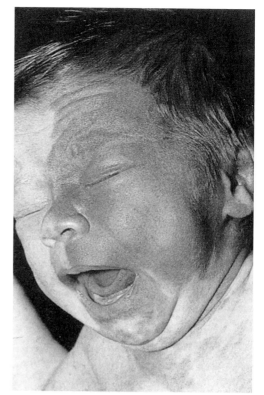

Figure 18-7. Angiomata characteristic of Sturge-Weber syndrome in a newborn.

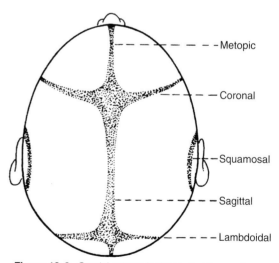

Figure 18-8. Cranial sutures in the skull of the newborn.

from acquired or congenital processes. Molding of the skull may be caused by a difficult vaginal descent and extraction. Scalp edema, cephalohematomas, or subgaleal hematomas may have occurred. Knowledge of all cranial sutures is necessary (Fig. 18-8). Craniosynostosis (premature closure of a cranial suture) may be a congenital cause of a malformed shape. Sagittal synostosis is

Table 18-5.	Major Features of Neonatal Behavioral States in Term Infants			
	Eyes Open	**Respiration Regular**	**Gross Movements**	**Vocalization**
State 1	−	+	−	−
State 2	−	−	±	−
State 3	+	+	−	−
State 4	+	−	+	−
State 5	±	−	+	+

Adapted from Volpe JJ: *Neurology of the newborn,* ed 3, Philadelphia, 1995, Saunders, with permission.
Data from Pryds O, Greisen G, Lou H, et al: Heterogeneity of cerebral vasoreactivity in preterm infants supported by mechanical ventilation, *J Pediatr* 115:638, 1989.
−, Absent; +, present; ±, present or absent.

the most common type, leading to an elongated shape with a high forehead. Different head shapes result from closure of coronal, metopic, or lambdoidal sutures; several sutures may also be fused. Genetic disorders or endocrinologic syndromes such as Treacher Collins syndrome and congenital hypothyroidism can be associated with craniosynostosis.

Finally, the rate of head growth is extremely important to note on serial examinations. Appropriate postnatal growth rates are difficult to define, but certain generalities should be considered. Modest head shrinkage, reflected by overriding sutures, can be seen during the first several days in the near-term or term infant. Increases in head growth by a mean of approximately 0.5 cm in the second week, 0.75 in the third week, and 1 cm per week thereafter, should be expected for a healthy premature infant.[70] The clinician must recognize that a sick preterm infant with systemic disease may require initial time for "catch-up" head growth, which may exceed the expected rate. However, extremes of growth arrest or excessive growth must be considered as part of a pathologic process (e.g., continued nutritional deprivation, genetic influences, or progressive hydrocephalus). The possibility of a pathologic condition should be considered in all infants with changes in head growth that are more than 2 standard deviations above or below the mean for all infants at that corrected age.

Among newborns of extremely low gestational age, microcephaly at 2 years, but not at birth, is associated with motor and cognitive impairment at age 2 years.[71]

Comparison of relative head and face proportions may help elucidate genetic or acquired syndromes or conditions. For example, squaring of the forehead with frontal bossing may support a diagnosis of hydrocephalus, rickets, or skeletal dysplasias. Underdevelopment of the mandibular structures suggests congenital syndromes such as Pierre Robin sequence.

LEVELS OF ALERTNESS

As with a patient at any older age, the formal neurologic examination of the newborn should include an assessment of the level of alertness. Terms such as *state* or *vigilance* have been used in defining criteria for level of alertness, and these criteria usually describe the two initial states of quiet (state 1) and active (state 2) sleep, followed by progressively increased levels of arousal from an awake-sleep transition (state 3) through quiet wakefulness (state 4) and vigorous crying with wakefulness (state 5).[72,73] The infant varies in levels of alertness depending on feeding or environmental stimuli, as well as disease states. Behavioral or polygraphic criteria help define these state transitions (Table 18-5).[74] Recent events in the nursery, such as exposure to painful procedures, bathing, feeding, or medication administration, also affect the infant's state of alertness. Scores on qualitative scales of arousal and attention in the neonate and infant have important prognostic implications.[75]

Abnormalities in levels of alertness are one of the more common neurologic deficits noted in the newborn period. Such abnormalities may be subtle, and their detection requires consideration of environmental influences as well as the maturity of the infant. General categories of increased or decreased levels of arousal include hyperalertness, lethargy, stupor, and coma. The appearance of the infant in a resting state, his or her arousal response, and the quality and quantity of motor responses allow the examiner to estimate whether the infant should be considered normally alert versus hyperalert and irritable versus stuporous versus asleep. Exaggerated, diminished or absent arousal responses and reduced motor responses are noted in the infant who is abnormally hyperalert or lethargic. The distinction between stupor and coma is also based on the quality and quantity of motor responses relative to the infant's gestational maturity. After 28 weeks' gestational age, stimulation consistently results in the infant's waking for several minutes. By 32 weeks' gestational age, no stimulation is needed for arousal. After 36 weeks' gestational age, increased alertness is readily observed, and well-formed sleep-wake cycles are noted by term age.[74] In general, the examiner should assume bilateral cortical dysfunction or subcortical disturbance of the reticular activating system within the gray matter of the diencephalon, midbrain, and upper pons if wakefulness cannot be achieved, even with vigorous stimulation. Diffuse or multifocal disease processes, including those with infectious, vascular, dysgenetic, metabolic, or toxic causes, can result in altered arousal.

CRANIAL NERVES

There are 12 pairs of cranial nerves that are identified by their specific functions within the cortex and brain stem. Cranial nerve functions and abnormalities referable to a particular region of the brain are elaborated in the following sections.

Olfaction (I)

Olfaction is often ignored in the neurologic evaluation of the neonate, but it may be affected by various disease conditions.[76,77] A sensory stimulus such as a cotton pledget soaked with peppermint extract elicits a consistent response in an infant of 30 to 32 weeks' gestational age, with a sucking arousal or withdrawal response; more immature infants normally lack this response. Olfactory discrimination has been demonstrated in the newborn, who prefers odors from the mother, and rapid associative learning occurs within 48 hours. An absence of this response should be considered in infants in whom the olfactory bulbs and tracts may not have developed, as is sometimes noted in disturbances of midline brain development such as holoprosencephaly. This condition could be present in infants of diabetic mothers, who have a higher risk of this type of brain anomaly.

Vision (II)

Specific visual responses are subserved by the second cranial nerves. Blinking to light begins by approximately 25 to 26 weeks of gestation[78]; by 32 weeks, infants sustain prolonged eye closure as long as the light source remains present. By 34 weeks of gestation, infants can track a large red object, and by 37 weeks, they can follow ambient light. Optokinetic nystagmus elicited by a rotating drum or striped cloth may be seen after 36 weeks' gestational age. Anatomic localization for visual fixation and following responses does not require the occipital cortex and may be subserved by subcortical structures such as the superior colliculus of the midbrain and the pulvinar, which link with the retina and optic nerves.

It is far more difficult to study the visual abilities of acuity, color perception, contrast sensitivity, and visual discrimination in the newborn. Estimations of these responses can be obtained by careful observation of functional abilities using age-specific visual fixation devices.[79] By 35 weeks' gestational age, newborns prefer complex patterns with curved contours over straight lines. However, acuity, binocular visual acuity, and appreciation of depth perception vary widely in the newborn, and these rapidly improve only during the first 3 to 4 postnatal months.[80] Therefore, the evaluation of visual function may be hampered by the difficulty of assessing these visual functions at the bedside. Nonetheless, infants with periventricular leukomalacia involving parieto-occipital regions exhibit delayed visual acuity when studied later in infancy.[81]

Funduscopic examination of cranial nerve II is an extremely valuable aspect of the neurologic assessment of the newborn. Alterations in the color, depth of cup, and circumference of the optic discs may reflect significant disease processes. Careful inspection of the anterior chamber, retinal grounds, and external eye structures by a pediatric ophthalmologist is essential. Corneal clouding, glaucoma, cataracts, colobomata, and chorioretinitis are examples of ophthalmologic findings that have clinical importance for both acquired and genetic fetal disorders. Indirect ophthalmologic evaluation by the pediatric ophthalmologist more fully examines the fundus, particularly the posterior pole of the retinal surface. Major abnormalities of the optic fundus during the newborn period include colobomata, optic disc hypoplasia or atrophy (Fig. 18-9), retinal and preretinal hemorrhages, chorioretinitis, retinopathy of prematurity, and retinoblastoma.

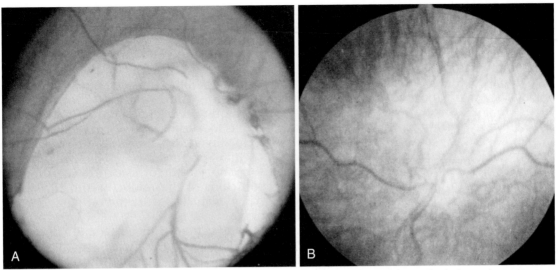

Figure 18-9. A, Coloboma of optic nerve, retina, and choroid. Yellow-white sclera is visible, and retinal vessels can be seen coursing through the coloboma. There is malformation resulting from faulty closure of the fetal fissure within the first month of gestation. **B,** Hypoplasia of the optic disc, which is half the normal size.

Congenital malformations associated with optic disc hypoplasia usually occur early during the first trimester of pregnancy (e.g., septo-optic dysplasia, agenesis of the corpus callosum). As many as 50% of affected infants subsequently exhibit other neurologic disorders. Atrophy suggests an acquired injury or ongoing metabolic or degenerative process. Retinal hemorrhages may suggest increased ocular venous pressure, blood dyscrasias, or asphyxia, but they can also be present in 20% to 40% of all newborns. Chorioretinitis may suggest a congenital infection, and retinopathy of prematurity is characterized by dilatation and tortuosity of vessels resulting from a variety of causes in premature infants.[82] The uncommon presentation of retinoblastoma or an embryotoxon would be helpful in the diagnosis of a neoplasm or a genetic or metabolic disease, respectively. Retinoblastoma in neonates usually presents with a white pupil and strabismus. Embryotoxon signifies an arrest in development within the anterior chamber, which requires documentation with an indirect ophthalmoscope.

Pupils (II and III)
Pupillary function is associated with both the second and third cranial nerves and appears by 30 weeks' gestational age, with consistent responses occurring between 30 and 32 weeks of gestation. Abnormalities in function of the pupillary pathways are reflected by changes in the overall size and symmetry of the pupils; bilateral cortical disease such as asphyxia and medication effects must be considered. Unilateral changes may imply autonomic dysfunction in central or peripheral nerve portions of the pupillary pathways. These can be associated with brachial plexus injuries, with herniation involving unilateral mass lesions (such as from infarction or intracranial hemorrhage), and with the mass effect of supratentorial brain structures along the course of the third cranial nerve in which the parasympathetic fibers are encased.[1]

Extraocular Movements (III, IV, and VI)
Attention must be directed to the infant's eye position, spontaneous eye movements, and movements elicited by oculovestibular maneuvers (i.e., doll's eye reflex) or oculolocaloric testing (i.e., cold or warm water response). Three cranial nerves interconnect within the brain stem to subserve these functions, and the doll's eye reflex can be observed in the infant as early as 25 weeks' gestational age. The eyes normally move conjugately in the direction opposite head movement, depending on the infant's degree of prematurity.[83] Caloric stimulation can be performed after 30 weeks, and spontaneous roving eye movements are expected after 32 weeks.

Abnormalities in extraocular movements include dysconjugate gaze, skew or downward deviation, and opsoclonus. These disorders of ocular motility can be seen in healthy neonates[84] and usually resolve over the first 6 months of life, but they may indicate persistent gaze palsies related to ocular strabismus or intracranial diseases in the brain stem or cortical visual pathways. Intermittent abnormal eye movements may also be associated with seizure abnormalities. Some nonseizure pathologic processes associated with abnormal eye movements are hydrocephalus, mass lesions, and genetic and metabolic diseases.

Facial Sensation and Masticatory Power (V)

The trigeminal nerve has both sensory and motor components. Facial sensation is best assessed by eliciting facial grimaces to noxious stimuli. The three divisions of the trigeminal nerve must be distinguished from the first and second cervical root sensory distributions over the posterior scalp and neck, respectively. Masseter and pterygoid muscle strength also reflect fifth nerve motor function and may be affected if the neonate exhibits suck and swallow abnormalities. Corneal reflexes are also subserved by the autonomic pathway in the fifth cranial nerve, which becomes functional by the twenty-fifth to twenty-sixth week of gestation.

Facial Motility (VII)

Facial nerve function involves the amplitude and symmetry of both spontaneous and sensation-elicited facial movements. Major causes of facial weakness in the neonatal period arise at all levels of the neuraxis (i.e., cerebral, nuclear, peripheral nerve, neuromuscular junction, and muscle). For example, bilateral facial weakness may be secondary to severe hypoxic-ischemic encephalopathy, but bilateral or unilateral facial weakness may also be associated with brain stem hypoplasia or aplasia of the motor nuclear groups in a disorder known as *Möbius syndrome*. Injury to the facial nerve may also occur during labor or delivery as a result of compression of the face against the maternal sacrum or forceps compression. Finally, weakness at either the neuromuscular junction or the muscle may be associated with congenital myasthenia, myopathies, or mitochondrial disorders. Asymmetry of the infant's face while crying may be associated with hypoplasia or absence of a specific muscle, the depressor angularis oris, on the side of the face that does not depress.

Auditory (VIII)

A startle reaction or blink in response to loud sudden noise is present at 28 weeks' gestational age. The lemniscal or auditory pathway that subserves this sensory function is functionally active early in the third trimester of development.[78] Auditory acuity, localization, and discrimination are present in the neonate. Detection of significant hearing deficits may be quite important in the examination of the neonate. Four categories of disorders causing nerve VIII disturbances are familial forms of deafness, bilirubin-induced injury to the auditory pathway, congenital infections, and congenital defects of the head and neck. Premature infants have a distinctly increased incidence of significant hearing loss.[1] The full-term infant may experience hearing loss from asphyxia-related causes that occur any time during the perinatal period; for example, one specific pulmonary problem, *persistent pulmonary hypertension of the newborn*, may result in peripheral injury to nerve VIII. Measurement of the brain stem auditory evoked response may more precisely localize the site of the deficit to the peripheral nerve or auditory pathway.[85]

Sucking and Swallowing (V, VII, IX, X, and XII)

Sucking involves coordinated action of breathing, sucking, and swallowing, with two coordinated phases that are linked in a synchronous action. The swallow response has a voluntary phase followed by an involuntary phase, both of which physiologically improve with maturity. Although rooting occurs as early as 28 weeks of gestation, the synchronous action of swallowing does not appear until 30 to 34 weeks and is not coordinated with breathing until 37 weeks. Gag reflexes subserved by cranial nerves IX and X are essential for the response of the posterior pharyngeal muscles, particularly to close the larynx and prevent aspiration; the gag reflex appears at 28 weeks' gestational age.[86] Disturbances affecting suck and swallow functions may originate throughout the neuraxis, ranging from the cerebral cortex through the brain stem nuclear groups to peripheral nerve, neuromuscular junction, and muscle levels.[1]

Sternocleidomastoid Function (XI)

The function of the sternocleidomastoid muscle, which allows flexion and rotation of the neck and head, is mediated by cranial nerve XI. Disorders in this function are usually related to a contracture or weakness of the muscle, such as from fetal positioning or trauma to the muscle. There are also infants with congenital torticollis that reflects congenital, musculoskeletal, and brain abnormalities referable to the cervicomedullary junction. Malformations during the embryonic or fetal periods can result in specific anomalies. Careful inspection of the posterior occiput of the skull, neck, and scapulae should be integrated into consideration of cranial nerve XI function. Associated anomalies such as a deep posterior occipital shelf, torticollis, or elevated and internally rotated scapulae may be markers for Chiari malformation, Klippel-Feil syndrome, Sprengel deformity, syringobulbia, or basilar impression.

Tongue Function (XII)

Tongue movements are usually best assessed by observing spontaneous tongue movements or the infant's suck on the examiner's fingertip. Abnormalities in tongue function usually involve neurons of the hypoglossal nerve or muscle. Atrophy or fasciculations may suggest a pathologic condition in the brain stem nuclear group subserving tongue movement, ranging from congenital conditions (e.g., progressive spinal muscular atrophy) to destructive processes (e.g., brain stem infarction). The size of the tongue may imply syndromic or metabolic disorders (e.g., macroglossia with hypothyroidism, Beckwith-Wiedemann syndrome, or specific lysosomal storage diseases). The clinician should also consider that the tongue may appear enlarged because the oral cavity is reduced in size due to hypognathism (e.g., Pierre Robin syndrome).

MOTOR EXAMINATION

Major features of the motor examination of the newborn involve descriptions of muscle tone, posture of limbs, motility, muscular power, deep tendon reflexes, and plantar responses. As with all aspects of the neurologic examination, observations of motor function take into account gestational maturity, level of alertness, and findings of serial examinations. Medications, feeding, disease states, and presence of noxious stimuli must also be considered, because they affect the neonate's motor responses.

Tone and Posture

Tone is best assessed by passively manipulating the limbs with the head in the midline. It is important to avoid head turning, which elicits a tonic neck reflex and gives a false sense of asymmetry in tone. Eighty percent of infants spontaneously prefer right-sided head turning. Developmental aspects of tone have been carefully documented by earlier researchers; in general, a caudal to rostral progression in tone development occurs with increasing gestational maturity. Minimal resistance is present at 28 weeks of gestation. By 32 weeks, distinct flexor tone begins in the lower extremities. By 36 weeks, flexor tone is prominent in the lower extremities and palpable in the upper extremities. When an infant's level of maturity is assessed, observations of tone and posture imply measurement or observation of the angle of a limb around a joint, both at rest and with gentle traction.[87,88]

The quantity, quality, and symmetry of motility and muscular power are also important aspects of the motor examination. The initial myoclonic movements of the preterm infant evolve into larger-amplitude, slower movements in the near-term and term infant. Also, as the infant matures, alternating rather than symmetric movements begin to be observed. By term, an awake infant has the ability to momentarily lift the head off the chest and hold it upright for several seconds while being supported in a vertical position.[78]

Deep Tendon Reflexes and Plantar Responses

Deep tendon reflexes are initially elicited in the preterm infant after 32 to 34 weeks' gestational age. Pectoralis, biceps, brachioradialis, knee, and ankle reflexes should be assessed. Symmetric ankle clonus of 5 to 10 beats may be an acceptable finding in a healthy full-term newborn. The plantar response is usually extensor in the newborn; therefore, it is assigned a pathologic significance only if asymmetry is noted.

In general, abnormalities found on motor examination include altered muscle tone with or without weakness, abnormalities in deep tendon reflexes and plantar responses, and abnormal spontaneous movements. A brief description of these abnormalities follows.

One must always consider normal maturational changes in motility, tone, and reflexes before ascribing pathologic significance. Therefore, the presence of low tone or hypotonia—the most common motor abnormality in neonates—must be considered with respect to possible patterns of muscle weakness that usually are present

Table 18-6.	Main Causes of Generalized Hypotonia in the Newborn Infant	
Site of Major Abnormality	**Disorder**
Anterior horn cell	Spinal muscular atrophy
	Other anterior horn cell disease (in association with cerebellar atrophy)
Peripheral nerves or roots	Congenital polyneuropathies (several types)
Muscle	Congenital muscular dystrophy (several types, including Fukuyama type and "occidental" types with and without merosin deficiency)
	Congenital myotonic dystrophy
	Congenital myopathies
	Central core disease
	Centronuclear myopathy
	Nemaline myopathy
	Congenital fiber-type disproportion
	Other structural myopathies
	Glycogen storage diseases types II and III
	Mitochondrial myopathies (deficit in cytochrome *c* oxidase)
	Types of mitochondrial myopathies
	Severe type
	Transient type
Neuromuscular junction	Neonatal myasthenia (infants of myasthenic mothers)
	Congenital myasthenia and myasthenic syndromes (several types)
	Infantile botulism
Central nervous system	Hypoxic-ischemic encephalopathy
	Brain malformations (including trisomy 21)
	Hemorrhagic and other brain damage
	Drug intoxication
Mixed origin (mainly central nervous system)	Zellweger syndrome and related peroxisomal disorders
	Prader-Willi syndrome
	Hypothyroidism
Connective tissue abnormality	Marfan syndrome
	Ehlers-Danlos syndrome

Adapted from Aicardi J, Bax M, Gillberg C, et al: *Diseases of the nervous system in childhood*, ed 2, New York, 1998, MacKeith Press.

with low tone. Levels of the neuraxis that may be involved in hypotonia include focal or bilateral cerebral areas, brain stem, spinal cord, low motor neuron, nerve root, peripheral nerve, neuromuscular junction, and muscle (Table 18-6).[1] Focal injury to the cerebrum results in contralateral hemiparesis. Parasagittal cerebral injury, usually from asphyxia, affects the border zone vascular regions over the cerebral convexities, which results in weakness of the upper extremities more than the lower extremities. Periventricular injury, primarily located in deep white matter structures, largely affects tone and strength in the lower extremities. Spinal cord involvement usually spares the face and other functions of cranial nerves while involving sphincteric as well as motor and sensory functions below the site of the spinal lesion. Other lower motor neuron effects include primarily focal weakness situated in nerve roots or, more commonly, generalized weakness localized to the peripheral nerve, neuromuscular junction, or muscular levels.

Hypertonia is a less common feature of neonatal neurologic disease, but it is one that may have important significance. Three forms of hypertonia can be expressed by neonates as observed in older children and adults.[89] Spastic, rigid, and dystonic forms of hypertonia may reflect acute or chronic processes, depending on the history of the present illness as well as examination findings. Increased tone in the newborn period is commonly noted after acute illnesses such as mild acute postasphyxial dysfunction, meningitis, or subarachnoid hemorrhage. However, remote intrauterine damage from injury or malformation earlier in gestation may be expressed as hypertonia. The chronic phase of bilirubin encephalopathy, prenatal substance exposure (e.g., cocaine and amphetamines), and continuous muscle fiber activity (Isaac syndrome) are other clinical conditions in the newborn that are also associated with hypertonicity. An unusual genetic or familial syndrome known as *hyperexplexia* may also be expressed in an infant as increased muscle tone, usually triggered by tactile stimuli.

Abnormalities in deep tendon reflexes and plantar responses also follow the general rule of localization at the site of neurologic injury above or below the motor neuron level. Preserved reflexes are seen with pathologic processes above the lower motor neuron unit, that is, lesions of the cerebrum down to the anterior horn cell of the spinal cord. Diseases in the lower motor neuron unit, below the anterior horn cell at the peripheral nerve, neuromuscular junction, or muscle levels, result in absent or diminished reflexes. Unlike in children older than 1 year, plantar responses (i.e., Babinski sign) are, in general, extensor and therefore are clinically helpful only if they are asymmetric.

Spontaneous Abnormal Movements

There are a variety of movement disorders that may suggest neurologic abnormalities: tremulousness, myoclonus, dystonia, excessive startle responses, fasciculations, and complex movements all can be expressed by the neonate. Tremulousness is a common feature associated with a brain disorder after asphyxial stress, metabolic disturbances such as hypocalcemia and hypoglycemia, or drug withdrawal. Fasciculations are associated with lower motor neuron disease, particularly that involving anterior horn cells of the spinal cord. Excessive startle reactions are noted with metabolic, genetic, or familial disturbances, and myoclonus can be seen in various diseases affecting multiple levels of the neuroaxis.[90] One striking movement disorder has been observed in preterm infants following severe bronchopulmonary dysplasia at near-term or term corrected age, as well as after bilirubin encephalopathy. Athetotic, choreiform, and dystonic movements have been described that reflect neuronal injury in the basal ganglia or extrapyramidal pathways connected to these midline gray matter structures. These extrapyramidal movements can also be expressed after asphyxial, inflammatory, or traumatic injury to basal ganglia and associated pathways.

EDITORIAL COMMENT: Prechtl et al described general movements that are part of the spontaneous movement repertoire and persist from early fetal life onward until the end of the first half-year of life.[20,73,74,88] General movements involve the whole body in a variable sequence of arm, leg, neck, and trunk movements. They wax and wane in intensity, force, and speed, and they have a gradual beginning and end. If the nervous system is injured, general movements lose their complex and variable character and become monotonous and poor.

So-called "fidgety" movements are small movements of the neck, trunk, and limbs that are of moderate speed with variable acceleration and occur in all directions. Normally, they are the predominant movement pattern in an awake infant at 3 to 5 months. Paucity of such movements may be seen in preterm infants and are a bad prognostic sign.

Two specific abnormal general movement patterns reliably predict later cerebral palsy: (1) a persistent pattern of cramped-synchronized general movements; the movements appear rigid and lack the normal smooth and fluent character, and limb and trunk muscles contract and relax almost simultaneously and (2) the absence of general movements of fidgety character. The assessment of general movements is quick, noninvasive, even nonintrusive, and cost effective compared with other techniques such as MRI, brain ultrasonography, and traditional neurologic examination. A systematic review indicated that the qualitative assessment of general movements, especially during the fidgety movements period, can be used as a prognostic tool to identify infants with neurodevelopmental disabilities.[91,92]

Primitive Fetal and Neonatal Reflexes

There are numerous primitive reflexes whose assessment is a valuable aspect of the neonatal neurologic examination. Five major responses to be elicited include the Moro reflex, palmar and plantar grasp, tonic neck responses, placing reflex, and stepping reflex.[78]

The Moro reflex appears between 28 and 32 weeks' gestational age and is well established by 37 weeks; it is no longer active after 4 months of corrected age. The palmar grasp also appears at 28 weeks' gestational age, becomes well established by 32 weeks, and disappears by 2 months of age. The tonic neck reflex does not appear until 35 weeks' gestational age and is well established at 1 month, but disappears by 5 to 7 months. Placing and stepping reflexes are usually elicited by 37 weeks' gestational age and later become integrated with supporting reflexes after 2 months of age.

Abnormal results on primitive reflex testing usually involve reproducible asymmetry or the incomplete or exaggerated response of a reflex. Asymmetry of any of the reflexes may reflect a cortical, brain stem, plexus, or peripheral nerve disease. The complete repertoire of reflexes should be tested to ascertain whether dysfunction of the upper or lower motor unit exists.

SENSORY EXAMINATION

Although sensory examination is an extremely important part of the newborn neurologic examination, alerting and withdrawal responses are the most practical expressions of both cortical and peripheral sensory abilities. Serial pinpricks over the medial aspect of the extremity should result in a response that can be described in terms of latency, limb movement, facial reaction, localization, and habituation.[1] A lower level of response as well as an exaggerated response should be noted. Some major generalizations provide guidance in evaluating abnormalities in the sensory examination. Most illustrative are the sensory deficits in infants with brachial plexus injuries, which occur in a segmental manner depending on which portion of the plexus has been injured. A spinal cord injury should be considered if an abrupt change in sensory threshold can be appreciated over the thorax, trunk, and legs. Genetic syndromes involving the sensory system rarely present in the newborn period. One example of a genetic disorder that encompasses peripheral sensory and autonomic nervous systems as well as higher cortical structures is Riley-Day syndrome, or familial dysautonomia. Current classification systems place this disease into the category of hereditary sensory neuropathies. These infants characteristically display irritability, lack the ability to express tears, fail to maintain temperature, demonstrate areflexia on tendon reflex testing, and lack fungiform papillae on the posterior part of the tongue.

IMPORTANCE OF SERIAL NEONATAL NEUROLOGIC EXAMINATIONS

Although the neurologic examination is more limited in the newborn infant than in older children and adults, it remains an essential aspect of neurologic diagnosis in the newborn, on which formulations of diagnostic and therapeutic strategies are based. Examination findings documented shortly after birth should be compared with later signs, since neurologic adaptation occurs after a stressful delivery, a resuscitative procedure, or the acute phase of an illness or injury. Also, the neurologic examination permits evaluation of functions that may be subcortical. Constellations of abnormal neurologic findings persisting over time are strong predictors of neurologic deficits at older ages. Specific clinical abnormalities predict the more commonly static motor encephalopathies, collectively referred to as *cerebral palsy*. Various abnormalities of limb, neck, or trunk tone (Fig. 18-10); diminished cry; weak or absent suck and swallow; the need for gavage or tube feeding; and diminished levels of activity or arousal are associated with substantially increased risk of death or disability. Consideration of both clinical and laboratory findings provides the

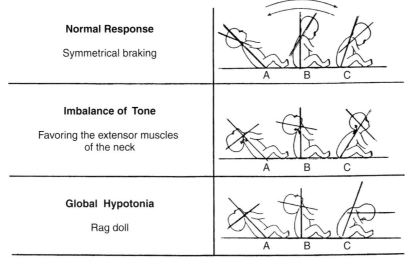

Raise To Sit Maneuver and Return Backward
Figure 18-10. Abnormalities of active tone in the neonate at term.

clinician with compelling bedside evidence of possible neurologic abnormalities. These same clinical findings may also reflect progressive degenerative or metabolic disease that masquerades as asphyxial symptoms and signs.[93]

ADDITIONAL EVALUATIONS OF THE NEWBORN INFANT

After maternal, fetal, and neonatal histories are obtained and a careful bedside examination is performed, neonatal neurologic assessment must then include judicious use of specialized studies that assess the structural and functional integrity of the infant's nervous system. Two diagnostic modalities are tests of structure and tests of function. Several important points should be kept in mind. The early and repetitive use of specialized studies may not only shed light on the severity of the encephalopathic state but also elucidate aspects of cause and timing during fetal life. Structural and functional studies are complementary and are therefore useful when combined with historical and clinical data. Furthermore, serial laboratory studies may provide insight into the persistence or resolution of a pathologic process in the brain as a function of gestational age and the adaptation of brain function to either stress or injury.

CEREBROSPINAL FLUID EXAMINATION

Examination of the CSF is one important aspect of neurologic evaluation of the newborn. The principal components of this specific fluid examination include measurement of intracranial pressure, assessment of the color of the spinal fluid (e.g., bloody or xanthochromic), examination for turbidity (indicative of purulence), performance of red and white blood cell counts and neutrophil differential count, measurement of concentrations of protein and glucose, and testing for microorganisms as well as specific metabolites. Normal values for preterm and full-term neonates have been studied (See also Appendix C), but the following points should be kept in mind. The clinical suspicion of meningitis should always be part of the general concern for clinical sepsis. The CSF might be infected despite the absence of infection in the peripheral blood. Values for blood cells, protein, and glucose in the CSF may be difficult to interpret, and clinical findings may need to be preferentially considered. The documentation of xanthochromia on careful examination of the supernatant after centrifugation, particularly when accompanied by an elevated CSF protein level, strongly suggests the possibility of an intracranial hemorrhage. The presence of nucleated red blood cells in the spinal fluid as well as the peripheral blood may point to an intrauterine pathologic process of longer duration than the peripartum period. (See Appendix C.)

DIAGNOSTIC IMAGING OF THE NEONATAL BRAIN

Important tools have been developed to assist in the structural assessment of the immature brain: cranial ultrasonography, CT, MRI, magnetic resonance spectroscopy, and positron emission tomography. During the neonatal period, the clinical usefulness of positron emission tomography is limited.

Cranial Ultrasonography

Ultrasonography is a rapid, noninvasive, cribside imaging technique that has been the method of choice for detecting and following the evolution of specific brain lesions. Excellent reviews are available for consultation.[1,14,39] Clinicians should be aware of the limits of visibility and accuracy in the images, which are confined primarily to the periventricular regions and ventricular space within the brain. Identification of normal features, including the ventricular outline, choroid plexus, and thalami, should initially be mastered (Fig. 18-11, *A*). Visualization of the germinal matrix, intraventricular hemorrhage (see Fig. 18-11, *B*), periventricular echodensities in the white matter (see Fig. 18-11, *C*), and intraparenchymal echodensities are the principal abnormalities. Normal ultrasound examination results do not rule out the presence of cortical injury or malformation. Brain lesions in intraparenchymal subcortical or meningeal locations are not readily detected. Furthermore, visualization of posterior fossa structures is more limited.

Computed Tomography

CT of the neonatal brain continues to have important applications in neonatal neurologic assessment, despite the greater availability of MRI. Two conditions—acute hemorrhage and intracerebral calcifications—may be better visualized by CT than by MRI during the neonatal period (see Fig. 18-4). It is also somewhat

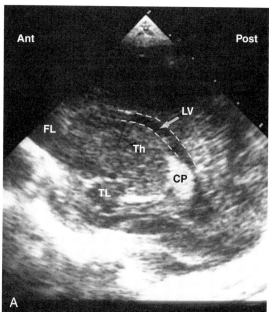

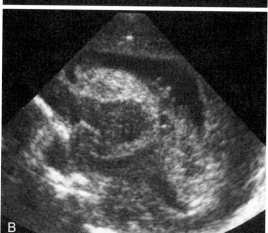

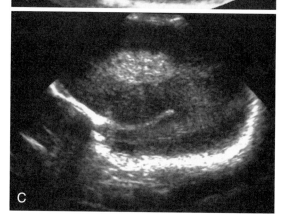

Figure 18-11. A, Normal lateral ventricle. A sagittal view obtained through an open fontanelle clearly shows the frontal lobe *(FL)*, lateral ventricle *(LV)*, thalamus *(Th)*, temporal lobe *(TL)*, and choroid plexus *(CP)*. *Ant,* Anterior; *Post,* posterior. **B,** Grade III intraventricular hemorrhage. Longitudinal view through the left lateral ventricle shows intraventricular hemorrhage and ventriculomegaly. **C,** Periventricular leukomalacia. Longitudinal view through the right hemisphere demonstrates increased echogenicity in the frontal-parietal region. *(**A,** From Mettler FA Jr, editor:* Essentials of radiology, *ed 2, Philadelphia, 2004, Saunders, Figure 9-1;* **B** *and* **C,** *from Martin RJ, Fanaroff AA, Walsh MC, editors:* Fanaroff and Martin's neonatal-perinatal medicine, *ed 9, St Louis, 2011, Mosby, Figures 37-45 and 37-47.)*

Magnetic Resonance Imaging

Even though the indications for MRI are essentially the same as for CT in the newborn, the higher resolution of MRI permits more sensitive assessment of white and gray matter structures; specific radiologic features such as acute hemorrhage and calcifications may not be as readily discernible as with CT. Newer signal-processing techniques in MRI provide better discrimination of regional developmental changes in white and gray matter structures, localization of pathologic processes to specific regions such as the basal ganglia, and detection of early cytotoxic changes with diffusion of water into the extracellular space (Fig. 18-12). Identification of normal age-specific aspects of brain development must first be mastered,[94] particularly the process of myelination. T_1- and T_2-weighted imaging (for increased and decreased white matter signals, respectively), as well as diffusion-weighted imaging, are currently recommended. Morphometric measurements provide quantitative estimates of either developmental or destructive changes. Newer research techniques using structural MRI, functional MRI, and tractography will provide additional insight into the pathogenesis and timing of insults.[95-97]

Magnetic Resonance Spectroscopy

Magnetic resonance spectroscopy is a new method for the measurement of energy metabolism; it can be sensitive in situations in which impaired energy metabolism is suspected (Fig. 18-13). This technique may be particularly useful in detecting more pervasive, less severe lesions that are more

easier to obtain a CT scan than an MRI scan; however, the limited resolution of CT clearly is a factor. Early ischemic injuries and more subtle malformations are generally not as well localized using CT.

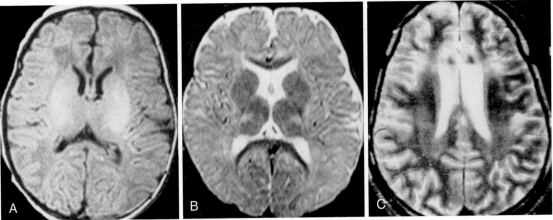

Figure 18-12. Hypoxic-ischemic encephalopathy in a term infant demonstrated by magnetic resonance imaging. **A,** Intense T_2-weighted signal from basal ganglia on axial cuts. **B,** Extensive low T_1-weighted signal from basal ganglia and thalami. **C,** Multifocal cortical-subcortical damage in another infant. *(From Aicardi J, Bax M, Gillberg C, et al: Diseases of the nervous system in childhood, ed 2, New York, 1998, MacKeith Press.)*

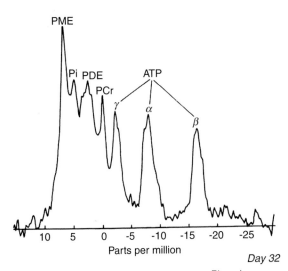

Figure 18-13. Nuclear magnetic resonance Phosphorus p137 spectrum for a normal infant showing individual peaks. *ATP,* Adenosine triphosphate; *PCr,* phosphocreatine; *PDE,* phosphodiesterase; *Pi,* inorganic phosphates; *PME,* phosphomonoesterase. *(From Volpe J: Neurology of the newborn, ed 3, Philadelphia, 1995, Saunders.)*

localized and are not identified by ultrasonography or conventional MRI.[98]

FUNCTIONAL BRAIN ASSESSMENTS

Electroencephalography

EEG is an extremely sensitive technique during the neonatal period for confirming the clinical suspicion of neonatal seizures as well as providing accurate information regarding maturation of regional and hemispheric brain function.[67] Combined EEG-polysomnographic recordings can better assess sleep state transitions and brain organization, which have an important bearing on predicting brain integrity. Serial measurements in EEG-sleep studies document important maturational changes (Fig. 18-14), which can be analyzed visually by a specialist with expertise in interpreting such recordings or digitally by computerized systems that quantitate and correlate data for multiple neuronal systems, such as EEG power, cardiorespiratory regularity, eye movements, and motility.[99] Newer analysis strategies that examine the complexity of physiologic biosignals using nonlinear algorithms such as correlation dimension will offer greater appreciation of the maturation and organization of the brain.[100]

Amplitude-integrated EEG has been "rediscovered" as a bedside screening tool to assist in global hemispheric detection of seizures or brain dysfunction.[101] Studies that compare amplitude-integrated EEG with conventional EEG are needed to properly integrate these tools into the ongoing care of the sick neonate.[102]

Evoked Potentials

Three types of short-latency sensory evoked potentials can be useful for evaluation of the newborn. Brain stem auditory evoked responses can objectively assess the function of the auditory pathways in infants suspected of abnormalities of the cranial nerve VIII or brain stem.[103] Visual evoked responses are useful to screen for major visual pathway disturbances.[104] Somatosensory evoked potentials can preferentially monitor the motor pathways that may be involved in specific disease states.[85]

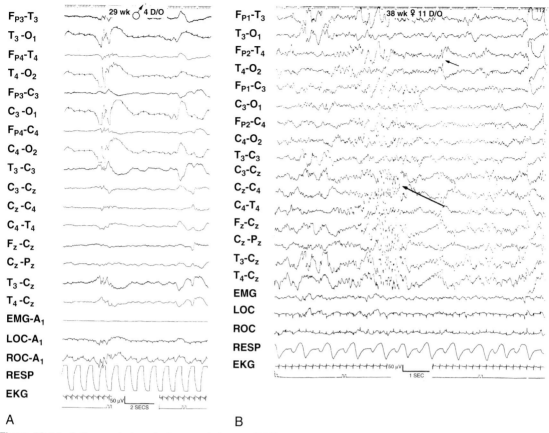

Figure 18-14. A, Segment of an electroencephalogram (EEG) for a healthy 4-day-old preterm infant of 29 weeks' gestational age demonstrating a discontinuous background with discrete regional patterns characteristic of this postconceptual age. **B,** Segment of an EEG for a 38-week gestational age, 11-day-old female infant demonstrating normal patterns, including prominent rhythmic theta and alpha activity at the midline *(long arrow)* and isolated sharp waves in the right temporal region *(small arrow).*

Electromyography and Nerve Conduction Velocity Studies

On rare occasions, electromyelography and nerve conduction velocity studies may be helpful in the newborn nursery.[105] These methods are particularly applicable in infants with suspected myopathic or motor neuron diseases before a muscle or nerve biopsy is considered. For instance, with the simultaneous administration of neostigmine or edrophonium, electromyelography may be used to diagnose congenital and neonatal forms of myasthenia gravis. Assessment of peripheral nerve or nerve root function using nerve conduction velocities can grade the severity of a neurologic lesion at the facial nerve, brachial plexus, or other peripheral nerve location.

PLACENTAL EXAMINATION

Incorporating information from the gross and microscopic examinations of placental and cord specimens can be extremely helpful in assessing the cause and timing of disease states in the newborn.[44,45] The placental weight may not correlate with the weight of the infant; placental weights above the 10th percentile for gestational age or below the 10th percentile for infant weight may suggest placental insufficiency. Body-to-placenta weight ratios are sensitive markers of long-term stress in disease studies.[106,107] Cord length as well as cord abnormalities such as true knots and anomalous development of the cord may also offer insights into fetal and neonatal neurologic diseases. Abnormally short cords imply paucity of fetal movements, whereas excessively long cords can be associated with an increased risk of cord entanglement and resultant occlusion before or during parturition.

Microscopic evaluation of the placenta may reveal acute hemorrhage, villous edema, or the presence of purulent material, which possibly suggests acute or subacute pathologic processes. Alterations in the size or development of the placental cotyledons, more longstanding vascular changes with or without infarction of the placenta, and deeply stained layers of the amnion and chorion with meconium within macrophages may be relevant to fetal or maternal disease processes. These pathologic features have relevance to both the pathogenesis and timing of disorders that ultimately may affect the fetal brain (see Fig. 18-6).

REPRESENTATIVE FETAL AND NEONATAL NEUROLOGIC DISEASES

The discussion in this section of selected disease processes affecting the fetus and neonate reinforces the previous sections pertaining to history taking, neurologic examination, and laboratory assessment. The four disease topics covered illustrate the overlapping nature of the neonatal clinical signs and symptoms that reflect the cause and timing of neurologic disease in the newborn. Hypoxia-ischemia–induced brain dysfunction or injury, cerebrovascular lesions, and neonatal seizures are commonly overlapping clinicopathologic entities in the newborn period (Table 18-7). The final topic is hypotonia, which is another major clinical sign that has an extensive differential diagnosis and may occur in other infants in addition to those who experienced asphyxia.

HYPOXIC-ISCHEMIC ENCEPHALOPATHY

Hypoxic-ischemic encephalopathy (HIE) occurs in 1.5 per 1000 live births and is the single most important fetal or neonatal disease state.[1] Yet in defining HIE, it is difficult to determine the role of events during the intrauterine or peripartum period that result in neurologic dysfunction and to establish the presence or timing of brain injury. Fetal brain disorders that occur before labor and delivery may also cause or contribute to the condition of an infant who manifests post-asphyxial encephalopathy syndrome after birth. The clinician must also recognize that HIE reflects a neurologic condition of dysfunction with or without coincident or subsequent damage. Scoring systems to aid in predicting death or disability are being continually reassessed.[108]

The definition of asphyxia implies two overlapping mechanisms: (1) hypoxia, or reduced supply of oxygen in the blood; and (2) ischemia, or reduced perfusion of blood flow. The conventional method of identifying an asphyxial state is to perform blood gas analysis to document metabolic acidosis; specific values for Pco_2, Po_2, bicarbonate, and base excess must also be considered. A greater degree of acidosis may imply increased production of lactate from incomplete catabolism of glucose (i.e., metabolic acidosis), although hypercarbia from respiratory insufficiency may also explain an acidotic state (i.e., respiratory acidosis), which is associated with less morbidity. Metabolic acidosis eventually depletes high-energy stores of phosphate, which ultimately results in cellular dysfunction because of inadequate energy production. The initial stage of HIE is one of cellular dysfunction. Two successive stages in the pathophysiologic process of HIE occur over several hours, during which time excessive membrane depolarization and release of excitatory amino acid neurotransmitters (e.g., glutamate) lead to calcium influx mediated by *N*-methyl-D-aspartate (NMDA) and α-amino-3-hydroxy-5-methyl-4-isoxazole propionic acid (AMPA) membrane receptors.[109] With an accumulation of cytosolic calcium, intracellular activation of lipases, proteases, and nucleases results in further injury to essential cellular proteins. Free radicals are also generated as a direct or indirect result of increased cytosolic calcium and nitric oxide. This entire cascade ultimately produces membrane injury, cytocellular disruption, and finally cell disintegration. Several therapeutic options are being considered that might abort this cytotoxic cascade, including use of calcium channel blockers,[110] excitatory amino acid antagonists (e.g., magnesium),[111] inhibitors of nitric oxide synthesis, free radical scavengers,[110] and agents that inhibit free radical formation such as allopurinol. Moderate hypothermia produced by either total body cooling or direct brain cooling has proven to be beneficial.[112-114]

EDITORIAL COMMENT: PREDICTORS OF OUTCOME: An Apgar score at 10 minutes provides useful prognostic data before other evaluations are available for infants with hypoxic-ischemic encephalopathy.[115] Death or moderate to severe disability is common, but not uniform, when the Apgar score is less than 3; caution is needed before a specific time interval is adopted to guide duration of resuscitation.

Table 18-7. Clinical Features and Ultimate Outcome in Four Types of Perinatal Brain Damage

Gestational Age	Timing	Risk Situations	Anatomic Findings	Acute Clinical Features	Confirmed by	Late Outcome
HYPOXIC-ISCHEMIC ENCEPHALOPATHY (SEVERE)						
Full term or after term	Intrapartum or immediately postnatal	Acute birth asphyxia (placental abruption, hemorrhage, cord compression, mechanical injury) Prolonged subacute asphyxia (prenatal or intrapartum) Inadequate resuscitation	Brain edema, massive cellular necrosis (cortex, basal ganglia, brain stem), ± hemorrhage (intraventricular, subdural, or intracerebral)	Major CNS depression, repeated seizures (often subtle in comatose child), ± brain stem signs (no spontaneous respiration, no suck) Usually systemic signs of acute hypoxia-ischemia (e.g., acute renal tubular necrosis, paralytic ileus)	EEG findings: critical and severe interictal abnormalities Ultrasound and CT scan findings: edema ± hemorrhage within first week Cerebral necrosis of various degrees and localization, but imaging findings often normal acutely	Severe sequelae in 50% of survivors, with microcephaly, multiple handicaps, ± epilepsy Motor handicap always more severe than cognitive handicap Less severe degree of neuromotor, sensorial, intellectual, or behavioral deficit in others Normal or subnormal outcome possible
HYPOXIC-ISCHEMIC ENCEPHALOPATHY (MODERATE OR MILD)						
Same as above	Same as above	Same circumstances as above but less severe and for shorter duration	Brain edema ± cellular damage ± subarachnoid hemorrhage	In moderate cases, CNS depression ± isolated seizures In mild cases, hyperexcitability and tone abnormalities (no depression, no seizures)	EEG findings: moderate or no abnormalities Ultrasound findings: usually normal Purely clinical diagnosis based on signs within first week of life	Any type of permanent deficit, including cerebral palsy in about 20% of moderate cases Normalization fast and complete in most mild cases and about 50% of moderate cases Minimal brain dysfunction at school age in about 30% of moderate cases
PERIVENTRICULAR LEUKOMALACIA						
Any age	Any time (prenatal or postnatal)	Chronic fetal distress (± intrauterine growth restriction) Low CBF Acute hypotension (may be associated with apneic spell and bradycardia, cardiac arrest, or hemorrhagic shock) Chorioamnionitis	Ischemic necrosis of periventricular white matter (centrum semiovale, corona radiata, occipital and temporal zones) Coagulation necrosis in acute stage ± hemorrhage Cavitation and gliosis later Distribution often asymmetric	CNS depression within first week Poor visual pursuit and poor axial tone at 40 wk corrected age	Ultrasound findings: periventricular leukomalacia including echogenicity Organization within 1 mo: porencephalic cysts ± ventricular enlargement caused by cerebral atrophy	Persisting neurologic findings (including typical spastic diplegia) ± sensorial and intellectual deficit of various degrees

Continued

Table 18-7.   Clinical Features and Ultimate Outcome in Four Types of Perinatal Brain Damage—cont'd

Gestational Age	Timing	Risk Situations	Anatomic Findings	Acute Clinical Features	Confirmed by	Late Outcome
INTRAVENTRICULAR HEMORRHAGE						
Prematurity (<34 wk)	Postnatal (first week of life)	Immaturity + respiratory distress syndrome leading to hypoxia, hypercarbia, unstable CBF Pneumothorax	Hemorrhage in germinal matrix (grade I) Intraventricular hemorrhage without ventriculomegaly (grade II) Intraventricular hemorrhage with ventriculomegaly (grade III) Hemorrhagic venous infarction (grade IV)	Major CNS depression ± seizure, onset at birth or later Nonspecific and unexplained deterioration Often silent	Ultrasound findings: resorption of blood in about 10 days Normalization in grades I and II Organization of periventricular leukomalacia often associated with grade III within 1 mo (see earlier)	Usually excellent in grades I and II Poor or very poor in grade III, especially when associated with extensive periventricular leukomalacia Possible hydrocephalus (10%-30% risk)
CEREBRAL INFARCTION (ARTERIAL TERRITORY)						
Any age (frequently full term)	Mainly prenatal; can occur intrapartum or in first 24 hr	Embolization in twin-to-twin transfusion, placental abnormality Thrombophilia Thrombosis in disseminated intravascular coagulation, sepsis, maternal cocaine use Often no predisposing factors Low risk full term	Infarction of both white matter and cortex in arterial distribution Contraction of affected area, multiple cystic degeneration Middle cerebral artery most common site (2 times more than other arteries) Left hemisphere mainly (3 times more than right)	Repeated focal seizures within first 3 days No major depression Asymmetric findings in case of middle cerebral artery	CT scan within 48 hr of birth: wedge-shaped area of low attenuation with irregular margins; findings may be normal if scan too soon after actual infarction Rescanning a few months later to evaluate actual loss of tissue EEG findings: focal seizures	Improvement of neuromotor function in first year, with mild residual hemiparesis (usually can walk alone) Mild mental deficit or none No speech disorder, usually Epilepsy uncommon

CBF, Cerebral blood flow; *CNS,* central nervous system; *CT,* computed tomography; *EEG,* electroencephalogram.

EDITORIAL COMMENT: Neonatal Hypothermia for Hypoxic-Ischemic Encephalopathy: The neuroprotective effects of hypothermia reflect antagonism of multiple cascades of events that contribute to brain injury. A Cochrane review analyzed eight randomized controlled trials that compared the use of therapeutic hypothermia with standard care in 638 moderately or severely encephalopathic infants without recognizable major congenital anomalies.[116] Therapeutic hypothermia resulted in a statistically significant and clinically important reduction in the combined outcomes of mortality or major neurodevelopmental disability to 18 months of age. Minor adverse effects of hypothermia included a borderline significant increase in the need for inotrope support and a significant increase in thrombocytopenia.

Many important questions regarding the optimal therapeutic use of hypothermia remain to be answered. But independent metaanalyses of the published trials now indicate a consistent, robust beneficial effect of therapeutic hypothermia for moderate to severe neonatal encephalopathy, with a mean number needed to treat of 6 to 8 to reduce disability and 14 to reduce mortality (Fig. 18-15).[117] Despite significant reductions in cerebral palsy and fewer survivors with a mental and psychomotor developmental index of less than 70, almost half of the survivors are still neurologically impaired. Complementary agents will have to be identified to further improve the outcome. Such trials are in progress, as is long-term follow-up for the initial trials.

In summary, for infants with hypoxic-ischemic encephalopathy, moderate hypothermia is associated with a consistent reduction in death and neurologic impairment at 18 months. Hypoxic-ischemic encephalopathy is often unanticipated and unavoidable, and may occur in any obstetric setting. Pediatricians and other providers based in community hospitals play a critical role in the initial assessment, recognition, and stabilization of infants who may be candidates for therapeutic hypothermia.[118]

Neuropathology

Two general forms of brain damage from HIE have been described in experimental animal models. The acute total asphyxial model usually leads to death because of circulatory collapse or the pattern of brain injury; these immature animals are usually stillborn or die shortly after birth. A small number may survive and have evidence of predominantly brain stem and diencephalic damage. Symmetric lesions within the brain stem, basal ganglia, and spinal cord structures are noted on postmortem examination. MRI studies have also documented this pattern of injury in neonates who die or experience severe sequelae after HIE (see Fig. 18-12).[119]

A partial prolonged model of HIE-induced brain damage has also been described. In this model, brain lesions are more diffuse within the cortex, subcortical white matter, and basal ganglia.

Clinical settings in which these two hypothetical forms of asphyxial situations can occur include the antepartum, intrapartum, and neonatal periods. The following sections provide a brief discussion of the common brain lesions associated with asphyxia.

Periventricular Leukomalacia

The most commonly occurring lesion associated with HIE in the preterm infant is

Study or subgroup	Hypothermia		Normothermia		Risk ratio (95% CI)	Weight (%)	Risk ratio (95% CI)
	Events	Total	Events	Total			
TOBY	74	163	86	162		39.0	0.86 (0.68 to 1.07)
NICHD	45	102	64	106		28.3	0.73 (0.56 to 0.95)
Cool Cap	59	116	73	118		32.7	0.82 (0.65 to 1.03)
Total (95% CI)		381		386		100.00	0.81 (0.71 to 0.93)
Total events	178		223				

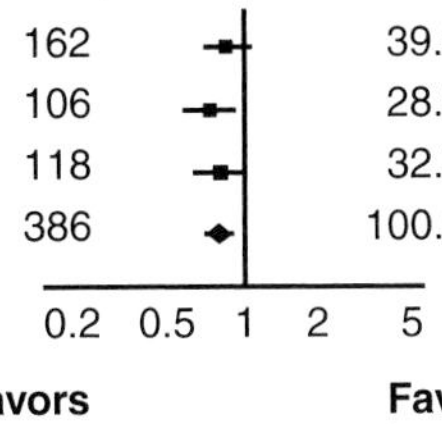

0.2 0.5 1 2 5

Favors hypothermia   Favors normothermia

Figure 18-15. Forest plot of the effect of therapeutic hypothermia compared with standard care (normothermia) on death or disability ("events"). All infants randomly assigned to either study arm were included in the analysis. A Mantel-Haenszel fixed effects model was used to calculate risk ratios and 95% confidence intervals (CIs). Test for heterogeneity: $\chi^2 = 0.82$; degrees of freedom = 2 ($P = .66$); $I^2 = 0\%$. Test for overall effect: $Z = 3.03$ ($P = .002$). Studies shown are the Total Body Hypothermia (TOBY) trial,[167] the National Institute of Child Health and Human Development (NICHD) trial,[114] and the CoolCap trial.[112] *(From Edwards AD, Brocklehurst P, Gunn AJ, et al: Neurological outcomes at 18 months of age after moderate hypothermia for perinatal hypoxic ischaemic encephalopathy: synthesis and meta-analysis of trial data, BMJ 340:C363, 2010.)*

periventricular leukomalacia (PVL). PVL is characterized by symmetric bilateral lesions that result from coagulation necrosis. The lesions are located adjacent to the external angles of the lateral ventricle, with or without cavitation. Extensive lesions produce multicystic encephalomalacia. The occurrence of PVL is directly related to the immaturity of the vascular supply to the central white matter of the preterm brain. Arterial end zones lack adequate collateral blood flow to the deep white matter. PVL is often associated with periventricular-intraventricular hemorrhage.[120] Many pathophysiologic conditions may contribute to this white matter necrosis, but usually it results from either decreases in systemic blood pressure or harmful effects of the inflammatory process. Systemic hypotension immediately results in a decrease in cerebral blood flow, because the immature cerebral vasculature reactivity in the premature brain causes a pressure-passive state of brain hemodynamics.[121] This physiologic immaturity of the preterm infant brain is in contrast to the mature cerebral blood flow response of the term infant, who can better maintain adequate cerebral perfusion over a wider range of systemic blood pressure values. PVL may also result after the elaboration of vasoactive cellular byproducts (e.g., inflammatory mediators) in response to infection or inflammation.[122] Such endotoxic agents contribute to cerebrovascular occlusion and consequent ischemia-induced injury in combination with asphyxia. Release of inflammatory mediators may also occur with infection, even in the absence of circulatory disturbances associated with asphyxia. The final common pathway to injury of immature neurons (pro-oligodendrocytes) can be pathogenetic mechanisms causing asphyxia and/or infection.[123]

Selective Neuronal Necrosis

In near-term and term infants who experience HIE, cortical and basal ganglia injury can occur, including subcortical white matter lesions with selective or extensive gyral involvement. Neuronal necrosis may be localized, multifocal, or diffuse and is generally greater in the left hemisphere than in the right.[1] Cellular necrosis occurs with reactive astrocytic gliosis and resultant laminar injury to the cortical mantle, which results in alterations in gyral thickness (ulegyria) after destruction of layers of gray matter. End zone perfusion between territories

of major intracerebral arteries is also more likely to be compromised in the brain of the term newborn, with injuries resulting in these specific vascular regions within the cortex.

Parasagittal Pattern of Injury

A parasagittal pattern of injury can result after HIE, contributing to a specific pattern of motor deficits in the proximal upper extremities, referable to the motor strip in each cerebral hemisphere. Although uncommon, these lesions have been demonstrated on neuroimaging studies.

Lesions of the Basal Ganglia

Lesions within the basal ganglia are another important type of brain injury that can result after HIE in the near-term or term infant brain. Status marmoratus (a marbleized appearance of injury caused by patterns of increased myelination in the caudate, putamen, and thalamus) has been classically described by neuropathologists. These deep gray matter structures possess a high concentration of excitatory neurotransmitters; consequently, these brain regions are vulnerable to the cytotoxic cascade that results after release of the neurotransmitters into the extracellular space, which leads to further neuronal injury and death.

Focal Cerebral Lesions

Focal lesions in the brain may be caused by arterial infarction, usually within border zone territories between major cerebral arteries. Thrombotic or embolic infarctions may occur, which can convert from ischemic to hemorrhagic lesions.[34,35,38]

Clinical and Neuroimaging Correlates of Hypoxic-Ischemic Encephalopathy

As described earlier, it is difficult for the clinician to distinguish fetal distress that occurs because of events during labor and delivery from brain injury that occurred during the antepartum period.[23] In some neonates, despite classic signs of intrauterine fetal distress, neither neurologic symptoms nor acute brain injury is noted after birth. Infants who are asymptomatic at birth may have already sustained brain injury before parturition. Even though fetal surveillance techniques detect the presence of fetal distress (as documented by electronic fetal monitoring of the heart and fetal scalp pH monitoring) and, after birth, clinical signs of depressed arousal and muscle tone in the neonate indicate an encephalopathy, these expressions of dysfunction may be related to a brain injury that occurred before fetal distress was first noted.[124]

Symptoms and signs of HIE are also different in preterm and term infants. For the near-term or term infant, three general grades of encephalopathy have been described.[125] Stage I HIE syndrome is a mild form in which the infant is hyperalert and tremulous during the first 24 hours, with excessive responsiveness to external stimulation. Muscle tone is generally increased, and tendon reflexes are hyperactive. Stage II, or moderate, HIE syndrome is characterized by stupor or lethargy lasting at least 24 to 48 hours. The infant can be aroused and then shows tremulousness, but muscle tone is generally decreased after birth, although dystonic hypertonia may be seen with tactile stimulation. Weakness is noted in the shoulder and proximal arm muscles. The clinical condition of the infant may worsen or improve within 48 to 72 hours, and seizures may or may not occur. In stage III, or severe, HIE the infant is usually stuporous or comatose, and seizures develop within the first 24 to 48 hours of life. Seizures are difficult to distinguish from nonepileptic seizure-like events, as discussed later in the section on neonatal seizures. In infants who are profoundly hypotonic, unresponsive, and dependent on ventilatory support, cranial nerve abnormalities and other focal motor abnormalities may be present, with a full, bulging fontanelle suggesting increased intracranial pressure. Such infants have the highest likelihood of neurologic sequelae or death.

The preterm infant with HIE, on the other hand, may exhibit fewer clinical signs. The preterm infant with stage III HIE may appear ill based on respiratory distress, sepsis, or other organ system problems, but the neurologic manifestations of HIE are more difficult to ascertain because the infant's immaturity hinders the clinical expression of neurologic function. Stages I and II HIE are much less well defined in preterm infants.

Neurophysiologic and Neuroimaging Correlates of Hypoxic-Ischemic Encephalopathy

EEG can be useful in determining the progression of HIE and the findings may have strong prognostic significance. For moderate to severe HIE, the EEG background abnormalities include suppression of electrical activity (i.e., frequency and amplitude of waveforms) or a burst suppression pattern. The expression of continuous EEG rhythms with age-appropriate patterns that spontaneously change between active and quiet sleep states carries a more favorable prognosis. Immature patterns on the EEG without amplitude-frequency suppression or burst suppression patterns on the EEG may suggest a more chronic in utero HIE process.[67]

Neuroimaging techniques can document the structural injury associated with HIE as well as suggest the timing of the injury. The ultrasonographic appearance of PVL in preterm infants has been extensively studied. Well-defined areas of echodensity along the lateral ventricle appear between 7 and 14 days after a presumed asphyxial insult.[122] These echodensities generally disappear or are replaced by small cysts over subsequent weeks. More sophisticated neuroimaging techniques (e.g., CT and MRI) document more details of neuroanatomy and pathologic features.[39,126] Cortical enhancement, particularly in the depths of the sulci and of lesions within the basal ganglia, indicates brain lesions associated with HIE in the near-term and term infant. Chronic changes include calcifications. Other abnormalities such as focal ischemic lesions in the border zone between major cerebral arteries are more readily documented by either CT or MRI scans. Certain features on neuroimaging may suggest a more remote occurrence of a brain injury caused by an asphyxial insult during the antepartum rather than the peripartum period. Cerebral atrophy or well-formed cystic cavitation at the time of birth seen on ultrasound, CT, or MRI scans signifies the process of liquefaction necrosis, which requires 2 to 6 weeks during intrauterine life to appear. Irregularity of the ventricular borders, white matter multicystic lesions, and the appearance of basal ganglia calcification or overall brain atrophy also suggest more chronic injuries. Therefore, despite the clinical expression of HIE, brain injury may have already resulted from clinically silent events before the onset of fetal distress. This possibility has obvious implications for the choice of therapeutic interventions to treat HIE. The use of glutamate antagonists, for instance, may not be recommended in an infant who has already experienced remote intrauterine asphyxia. Conversely, those infants with well-documented intrapartum or postnatal disorders may experience HIE brain injury, which may respond to therapeutic strategies for brain resuscitation.[127]

Table 18-8.	**Classification of Severity of Periventricular-Intraventricular Hemorrhage**	
Severity	Staging of Papile et al (1978)[129]	Staging of Volpe (1995)[1]
Grade I	Subependymal bleeding only	Subependymal bleeding only, or <10% of ventricular area filled with blood
Grade II	<50% of ventricular area filled with blood; no ventricular dilation	10%-50% of ventricular area filled with blood
Grade III	>50% of ventricular area filled with blood; blood in white matter of centrum semiovale; ventricular dilation	>50% of ventricular area filled with blood; ventricular dilation

EDITORIAL COMMENT: *Cerebral palsy* is an umbrella term encompassing a group of nonprogressive, noncontagious motor conditions that cause physical disability in human development chiefly in the various areas of body movement. Most publications address the high rates and risk of cerebral palsy associated with preterm delivery. Nonetheless, numerically it is term and near-term infants who account for the majority of cases of cerebral palsy despite their significantly lower risk. The risk of cerebral palsy is lowest at 40 weeks, with the higher risks at 37 weeks and at 42 weeks or later.

CEREBROVASCULAR LESIONS OF THE NEONATE

Cerebrovascular lesions occur in both the preterm and full-term brain as a result of varying pathologic processes (e.g., asphyxia), infection, or blood disorders.[34,35,38] Two manifestations of cerebrovascular disease processes may occur: intracranial hemorrhage (ICH) and intracranial occlusive lesions.

The demographics of ICH have changed considerably over the past several decades. Two specific forms of ICH have decreased in occurrence: subdural hemorrhage in term infants and intraventricular hemorrhage in preterm infants. In general, however, brain injuries related to cerebrovascular lesions remain important structural correlates of neurologic sequelae.

Periventricular-Intraventricular Hemorrhage

Periventricular-intraventricular hemorrhage (PIVH) is the most frequent type of intracranial hemorrhage in the neonate and overwhelmingly occurs in preterm infants (60% in infants weighing <1000 g compared with 40% in larger infants).[128] In preterm infants PIVH originates primarily in the subependymal germinal matrix, a highly vascular area that gives rise to neurons and glia during brain maturation.[1] The germinal matrix eventually is resorbed into the head of the caudate. Hemorrhages within the subependymal region may be clinically silent, even if ventricular dilatation occurs. Intraventricular hemorrhage results when venous stasis causes the ependymal lining to rupture, with extravasation of blood that may extend into the ventricular space. The severity of PIVH is graded based on the presence of ventriculomegaly and amount of intraventricular blood (see Fig. 18-11, *B* and Table 18-8).[129] Although PIVH is a hemorrhagic event with leakage of blood due to rupture of the thin endothelial lining of vessels within the germinal matrix, the hemorrhage originates because of venous stasis. More severe venous stasis affects blood drainage more proximally within the terminal vein or the medullary veins of the deep white matter below the developing neocortex. A hemorrhagic infarction may then result and is graded as the most severe form of intraventricular hemorrhage, documented as a parenchymal hemorrhage within a region of ischemia on neuroimaging or postmortem examination. Whereas a symmetric ischemic pattern of injury is noted with PVL, which is in an arterial distribution, the venous infarction associated with PIVH is asymmetric and may be extensive with accompanying ventriculomegaly.

PIVH may subsequently give rise to hydrocephalus as a result of posthemorrhagic adhesive arachnoiditis. Although compensatory ventriculomegaly is expected to occur during the first several weeks after hemorrhage, the time course for the establishment of progressive hydrocephalus is unknown. Both the initial hemorrhagic venous infarction and progressive hydrocephalus contribute to long-term neurologic sequelae.

Periventricular Leukomalacia

PVL is an ischemic mechanism in the preterm brain that was described previously in the section on asphyxia. The tissue destruction that follows an ischemic event caused by either asphyxia or inflammation[130] results in gliosis with or without cavitation, usually limited to the white matter region within the trigone of the white matter, above the occipital horns, along the optic radiations, or more anteriorly along the body and frontal horns of the lateral ventricles. Twenty-five percent of children with PVL also experience PIVH; extensive forms of PVL produce multicystic encephalomalacia. Unlike the asymmetric presentation in PIVH, PVL lesions are largely symmetric (see Fig. 18-11, *C*).

Other Intracranial Hemorrhages in the Neonate

Other hemorrhagic events in the brain occur less commonly. Subdural hemorrhage results from tentorial tears after rupture of the straight sinus, vein of Galen, or small afferent veins. Subdural hemorrhages are mainly of traumatic origin in term infants of higher birth weights. Posterior fossae subdural hemorrhage may also occur as a result of excessive head molding in the vertex presentation or after excessive traction on the skull of the infant in a breech presentation.[1,82]

A third form of hemorrhage occurs within the cerebellar tissue within the posterior fossae, either after asphyxia or as a result of mechanical trauma from occipital osteodiastasis or traumatic cerebellar injury.[131]

EDITORIAL COMMENT: Advances in imaging, including cranial ultrasonography and magnetic resonance imaging, have resulted in increased recognition of cerebellar hemorrhage.[132] The impact of cerebellar hemorrhage is becoming apparent, and 40% of infants with such hemorrhage demonstrate neurologic abnormalities. Hemorrhage seen only on magnetic resonance imaging is associated with a much more favorable outcome than that visible on ultrasonography. Cerebellar injury in term infants is linked with a broad spectrum of neurodevelopmental disabilities, particularly in infants with large cerebellar lesions. Cerebellar injury in preterm infants is associated with impaired growth of the uninjured contralateral cerebral hemisphere with significant impairment evident as early as term-equivalent age.[133,134]

Other intraparenchymal hemorrhage within the cortex can occur in either term or preterm infants, usually in association with subarachnoid hemorrhage.

Thalamic hemorrhage is an uncommon but potentially devastating form of intraparenchymal hemorrhage that is more commonly seen in term infants.

Primary subarachnoid hemorrhage is perhaps the most common form of intracranial hemorrhage and occurs even after seemingly nontraumatic deliveries.[82] The true incidence of subarachnoid hemorrhage remains elusive because many infants remain asymptomatic and the incidence of neurologic sequelae is generally low.

The field of neonatal neurology, and specifically its focus on the premature infant, had its inception in neuropathologic studies. Since then, the development of advanced imaging techniques has guided our developing understanding of the etiology and nature of neonatal brain injury. Brain injury in premature infants is of enormous public health importance because of the large number of such infants who survive with serious neurodevelopmental disability, including major cognitive deficits and motor disability. Cognitive deficits without major motor deficits are the most common neurodevelopmental sequelae in preterm infants, affecting 50% of infants with a birth weight below 1000 g. This type of brain injury is generally thought to consist primarily of PVL, a distinctive form of cerebral white matter injury. Important new work using MRI and neuropathologic techniques to study brain disease in survivors of preterm birth shows that PVL is frequently accompanied by neuronal-axonal disease affecting the cerebral white matter, thalamus, basal ganglia, cerebral cortex, brain stem, and cerebellum. This constellation of PVL and neuronal-axonal disease is sufficiently distinctive to be termed *encephalopathy of prematurity*. Volpe's thesis is that "the encephalopathy of prematurity is a complex amalgam of primary destructive disease and secondary maturational, developmental and trophic disturbances."[135,136]

NEONATAL SEIZURES

Neonatal seizures remain one of the few neurologic emergencies, and this condition may indicate significant dysfunction or damage to the immature nervous system both on a remote and on an acute basis.[4,94,137-141] Advances in neurophysiologic monitoring of the high-risk infant have spurred the development of an integrated classification of both clinical and electrographic criteria for diagnosis of seizures.[142] Synchronized video

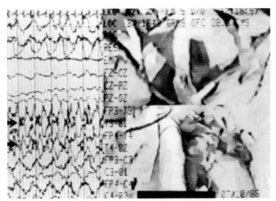

Figure 18-16. Segment of a video electroencephalogram for a 32-week gestational age, 5-day-old female with electroclinical seizures characterized by bitemporal electrographic discharges coincident with tonic posturing to the left.

EEG-polygraphic techniques as well as computer-assisted analyses allow the clinician to better characterize suspicious clinical behaviors that may or may not be associated with coincident surface-generated electrographic seizures (Fig. 18-16). Nonetheless, because of the reliance on detecting suspicious clinical behaviors, recognition of neonatal seizures is still hampered by both overestimation and underestimation of their occurrence. Clinical criteria for suspected seizures may not easily distinguish seizure activity from either normal or pathologic nonepileptic behavior; coincident EEG is needed to best define the diagnosis. Subclinical EEG seizures may also occur that escape detection by clinical observation alone. Conversely, EEG criteria may not adequately recognize ictal patterns that originate from subcortical brain regions, but no universal classification based on clinical criteria can distinguish subcortical seizures from nonepileptic paroxysmal activity, although there is speculation regarding electroclinical disassociation. Certain clinically apparent seizures originate in subcortical structures and only intermittently propagate to the cortical surface where EEG electrodes can readily record electrographic seizures. One pragmatic approach to the diagnosis and management of neonatal seizures is therefore based on the documentation of seizures by surface-recorded EEG studies. A therapeutic end point for the use of antiepileptic medications can be more practically achieved using EEG documentation, because clinical signs may be absent, minimal, or nonepileptic in origin.

Extremely low-birth-weight infants with clinical seizures are at increased risk of an adverse neurodevelopmental outcome, independent of multiple confounding factors.

Seizure Detection: Clinical versus Electroencephalographic Criteria

Neonates are unable to sustain generalized tonic followed by clonic seizures as observed in older patients, although separately occurring generalized tonic and clonic events do appear, even in the same neonate. Most seizures are brief and subtle, and consequently are expressed as clinical behaviors that are unusual to recognize. Five clinical categories of neonatal seizures have been described.[1] Several caveats should be mentioned before these five clinical categories are reviewed.[143] First, the clinician should be suspicious of any abnormal repetitive stereotypic behavior that could represent a possible seizure. Second, certain behaviors such as orbital and buccolingual movements, tonic posturing, and myoclonus can be associated with either normal neonatal sleep behaviors or nonepileptic pathologic behaviors. Third, clinical events may have only an inconsistent relationship to coincident electrographic seizures.

Subtle or Fragmentary Seizures

Subtle or fragmentary seizures constitute the most frequently observed clinical group of seizure-like phenomena and may be characterized by repetitive facial activity, unusual bicycling or pedaling movements, momentary fixation of gaze, or autonomic dysfunction. Specific autonomic signs such as apnea are rarely seen in isolation but usually occur in the context of other seizure phenomena in the same neonate. Even though these clinical expressions appear unimpressive, they may reflect significant brain dysfunction or injury. An inconsistent relationship between specific subtle behaviors and EEG seizures has been documented using synchronized video EEG-polygraphic recordings, which emphasizes the need for further classification.[144] It is generally considered standard practice to require that suspicious clinical behaviors occurring in close temporal proximity to EEG seizure patterns be considered indicative of seizure.

Clonic Seizures

Clonic seizures are characterized by rhythmic movements of muscle groups in a focal or multifocal distribution. Rapid followed by slow movement phases distinguish clonic movements from the symmetric to-and-fro movements of nonepileptic tremulousness or jitteriness.[145,146] Whereas gentle flexion of the extremity can suppress tremors, this is not possible with clonic seizure activity. The clonic event may involve any muscle group of the face, limbs, or torso. Focal clonic seizures may be associated with localized brain injury, but they can also accompany generalized cerebral disturbances.[147,148] Following seizures, newborns may also have a transient period of paresis or paralysis, called *Todd's phenomenon.*

Tonic Seizures
Tonic seizures are characterized by sustained flexion or extension of either axial or appendicular muscle groups, such as decerebration or dystonic posturing (see Fig. 18-16). Focal head or eye turning or tonic flexion or extension of an extremity exemplifies tonic seizures. Although some tonic behaviors are coincident with EEG seizures, there is a high false-positive correlation, with tonic behavior occurring in the absence of concurrent electrical seizure activity.

Myoclonic Seizures
Myoclonic movements are rapid, isolated jerks involving the midline musculature or a single extremity either in a generalized or multifocal fashion. Unlike the movements in clonic seizures, which show fast and slow phases, myoclonic movements lack a two-phase movement. Healthy preterm and term infants may demonstrate abundant myoclonic movements during either sleep or wakefulness.[145,146] However, sick neonates may also exhibit myoclonus, which is either verified as seizure activity by EEG or determined to be a manifestation of nonepileptic abnormal motor activity.[90]

Electroencephalographic Seizure Criteria
EEG remains an invaluable tool for the assessment of both ictal and interictal cerebral activity, as expressed on surface recordings. Although an EEG finding is rarely pathognomonic for a particular disease, important information about the presence and severity of a brain disorder with or without seizures can be gained from careful visual interpretation.[67] Major EEG background rhythm disturbances in the absence of seizures carry major prognostic implications for compromised outcome. Specific interictal EEG abnormalities on serial EEG recordings offer invaluable information to the clinician regarding the presence, severity, and persistence of an encephalopathic state in the neonate.

Interictal EEG Patterns. Background EEG abnormalities have prognostic significance for both preterm and full-term infants.[149,150] Such patterns include burst suppression, electrocerebral inactivity, low voltage invariant, and persistent multifocal sharp wave abnormalities (Fig. 18-17). Other interictal EEG abnormalities, such as disparity in the maturity of EEG and polygraphic activities, also have prognostic importance but require greater skill in visual analysis to identify.[67]

Ictal EEG Patterns. Ictal EEG patterns in the newborn are composed of repetitive waveforms of a certain minimum duration and similar morphology that evolve in response to frequency, amplitude, and electric field. The electroencephalographer can readily identify seizures that are at least 10 seconds in duration.[151] Four categories of ictal patterns have traditionally been described: focal ictal patterns with normal background, focal ictal patterns with abnormal background, focal monorhythmic periodic patterns of various frequencies, and multifocal ictal patterns.

Neonatal encephalopathies should be characterized in functional terms based on both interictal and ictal abnormalities and on severity and persistence over time.[152] The persistence of abnormal patterns in serial studies is more significantly correlated with neurologic sequelae, although EEG patterns rarely denote a particular disease state. Brain lesions documented on neuroimaging or postmortem examination may have had an electrographic signature on EEG studies on an acute, subacute, or chronic basis. Therefore, EEG patterns must be analyzed in the context of history, clinical findings, laboratory information, and neuroimaging.

Clinical Correlates of Neonatal Seizures
Neonatal seizures are not disease specific and may be caused by a number of medical conditions. Establishing a specific reason for seizures in any infant is essential both for treatment and for prediction of neurologic outcome. Neonates with an encephalopathy or brain disorder may or may not have seizures, and they commonly come to attention because of a variety of disturbances.[67]

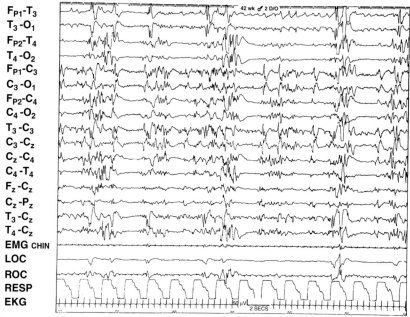

Figure 18-17. Segment of an electroencephalogram for a 42-week gestational age, 2-day-old male infant demonstrating a burst suppression pattern with multifocal sharp waves and attenuation of activity in the right temporal and midline (T_4 and C_z) region.

Asphyxia

Postasphyxial encephalopathy, the principal disorder during which neonatal seizures may occur, can also be accompanied by hypoglycemia, hypocalcemia, cerebrovascular accidents, or intraparenchymal hemorrhage. These latter conditions, individually or in combination, can contribute to seizures.

Most neonates experience asphyxia either before or during parturition. In only 10% of affected neonates does asphyxia result from postnatal causes. Intrauterine factors leading to asphyxia before or during labor and delivery compromise gas exchange or glucose movement across the placenta. These factors may be maternal (e.g., toxemia) or uteroplacental (e.g., placental abruption or cord compression) in origin. However, other maternal conditions such as antepartum trauma or infection not only are associated with acquired brain insults from asphyxia but also may contribute to the formation of congenital malformations during early pregnancy, as detected by fetal ultrasonography or cranial imaging of the infant immediately after birth. Respiratory distress syndrome, pulmonary hypertension of the newborn, and severe right-to-left cardiac shunts associated with congenital heart disease are other major causes of postnatal

asphyxia in a newborn who may also experience seizures. Therefore, the events that lead to asphyxia must be considered in the context of the findings of the maternal, placental, and neonatal examinations, as well as the corroborative laboratory results. Adverse events during labor and delivery may reflect longer-standing maternal, placental, or cord disorders that contribute to postnatal seizures, hypotonia, or coma. HIE, including neonatal seizures, develops in only 45% of infants who experience asphyxia at the time of birth.[122] Similarly, meconium staining of skin, placental tissue, or cord tissue can occur in asymptomatic infants with or without intrauterine insults. Distribution of meconium-laden macrophages throughout the placental amnion generally indicates fetal distress in the antepartum period.[153] Placental weights lower than the 10th or higher than the 90th percentile, altered placental villous morphology, lymphocytic infiltration, and erythroblastic proliferation in the villi indicate longer-term stress to the fetus, whether or not seizures occur during the period immediately after birth in a neonate who is neurologically depressed. In neonates with EEG-confirmed seizures, the odds that antepartum placental lesions would be identified increased by a factor of 12 as postconceptual age increased by

15 weeks.[60] Other findings on neurologic examination, such as hypertonia, joint contractures without profoundly depressed consciousness, seizures within the first hours after delivery, growth restriction, and neuroimaging evidence of encephalomalacia, separately or collectively point to the antepartum period as the time when brain injury occurred.

Hypoglycemia

Low blood glucose levels can result in seizures, either in association with asphyxia or as a separate metabolic consequence of the hypoglycemia. Infants of diabetic or toxemic mothers, those born as one of multiple gestation siblings, and, rarely, those with metabolic diseases may also have hypoglycemia. (See Chapter 12.)

Hypocalcemia

Whereas hypoglycemia may be associated with seizures in neonates with asphyxia, hypocalcemia may be seen in the context of trauma, hemolytic disease, or metabolic disease. Hypomagnesemia may also occur in infants with hypocalcemia. Rarely, a form of hypocalcemia may be caused by congenital hypoparathyroidism or may occur with delayed onset in an infant who received a high-phosphate infant formula. Congenital cardiac lesions have been found in some infants with seizures caused by hypocalcemia or hypomagnesemia.[154] (See Chapter 12.)

Cerebrovascular Lesions

Intracranial hemorrhage as well as ischemic cerebrovascular lesions can occur as a result of asphyxia, trauma, or infection, or in association with developmental or congenital lesions. PIVH in the preterm infant who also has seizures has already been discussed.[155] However, full-term infants with seizures may also have intraventricular hemorrhage, usually arising within the choroid plexus or thalamus. Intracranial hemorrhage at other sites (e.g., subdural space, subarachnoid space, or into the parenchyma) can also be associated with seizures that occur together with or independently of postasphyxial encephalopathy.

Arterial and venous infarctions have been noted in neonates with seizures.[147,148] Cerebral infarctions can occur during the antepartum, intrapartum, or neonatal periods from diverse causes such as persistent pulmonary hypertension, polycythemia, and hypertensive encephalopathy. When isolated seizures occur in neonates with no accompanying encephalopathy, the cause can be timed to the antepartum period.[156]

Infection

CNS infection acquired in utero or postnatally may give rise to neonatal seizures. Congenital infections that are usually associated with a severe encephalitis are also accompanied by seizures and major interictal EEG background disturbances. For instance, neonatal herpes encephalitis is associated with severe ictal and interictal EEG pattern abnormalities consisting of multifocal seizures as well as multifocal periodic discharges.[49] Acquired in utero or postnatal bacterial infections caused by *Escherichia coli* or group B streptococci may result in neonatal seizures. *Listeria monocytogenes* and mycoplasma infections can also produce areas of lymphocytic infiltration and resultant encephalomalacia.

Central Nervous System Malformations

Brain lesions that result from either genetic or acquired defects during early fetal brain development also contribute to neonatal seizures (Fig. 18-18). Such lesions include microgyria, heterotopia, and lissencephaly. Other dysgenic CNS conditions such as holoprosencephaly, schizencephaly, and congenital hydrocephalus may also be associated with neonatal seizures.

Inborn Errors of Metabolism

Inherited biochemical defects are rare causes of neonatal seizures.[141] Peculiar body odors, intractable seizures that occur later in the newborn period, and persistently elevated lactate, pyruvate, ammonia, or amino acid levels in the blood may reflect inherited biochemical disorders rather than transient postasphyxial insults. Neonates with metabolic disease may also have otherwise normal prenatal and delivery histories. The emergence of food intolerance, increasing lethargy, and late onset of seizures may be the only indication of an inborn error of metabolism. Certain conditions are responsive to supplementation or dietary alteration; for example, vitamin B_6 dependency is a rare form of metabolic disturbance that can lead to intractable seizures which are unresponsive to conventional antiepileptic medication.[157] Glucose transporter deficiency syndromes are suspected when CSF levels of glucose are low, and some

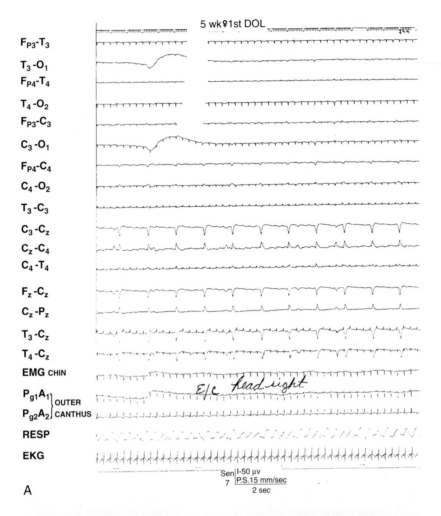

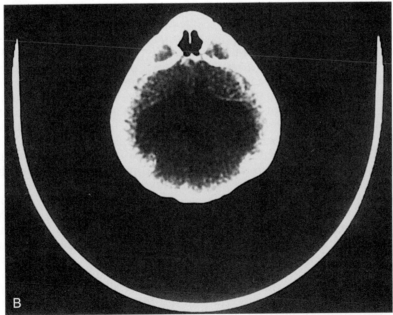

Figure 18-18. A, Segment of an electroencephalogram (EEG) for a 35-week gestational age, 1-day-old female infant with periodic discharges at the midline (C_z). **B,** Computed tomographic scan documenting a lobar holoprosencephaly in the same infant.

patients may respond to the ketogenic diet regimen.[158]

Neonatal Epileptic Syndromes
Few clinical situations involving neonatal seizures represent a chronic epilepsy syndrome. Most seizures in newborns reflect transient disturbances that resolve over days (e.g., asphyxia, metabolic-toxic conditions, infections). Rarely, a newborn has an ongoing epileptic condition that is independent of, but perhaps is triggered by, adverse events during fetal or neonatal life. A rare form of familial neonatal seizures has been described with an autosomal dominant inheritance pattern.[159] The diagnosis requires careful exclusion of acquired causes. In two pedigrees the genetic defect for this condition was assigned to two genetic loci on chromosome 20. Although most newborns with the disorder respond promptly to antiepileptic drug treatment and develop in an age-appropriate manner, some children experience delay at older ages. A defect in potassium-dependent channel kinetics has been described.

Other rare epileptic states include progressive syndromes associated with severe myoclonic seizures and progressive developmental delay. These children have been described as having an early infantile epileptic encephalopathy (Ohtahara syndrome) and usually have severe brain dysgenesis.

Treatment of Neonatal Seizures
Before antiepileptic medications are administered, an acute rapid infusion of glucose or other electrolytes such as calcium or magnesium should be considered. Low magnesium level and altered sodium metabolism are less common causes of neonatal seizures and do not require antiepileptic medications.[141]

Questions persist with respect to when, how, and for how long to administer antiepileptic medications to neonates who experience seizures. Some believe that neonates should undergo treatment only when the clinical signs of seizure are recognized and that brief electrographic seizures need not be treated. Others argue that this practice may be potentially harmful because undetected repetitive or continuous electrographic seizures may adversely affect the metabolism and cellular integrity of the immature brain. Consensus is lacking on the need for treatment when clinical seizure phenomena are minimal or absent.[143]

Major antiepileptic drug classes have been used to treat neonatal seizures. Phenobarbital is the most commonly used antiepileptic medication, with a recommended loading dose of 20 mg/kg and a maintenance dosage of 3 to 5 mg/kg/day. Half-life of the drug is long, 40 to 200 hours.

Phenytoin is the second most commonly used medication for the treatment of seizures. A loading dose of phenytoin is 15 to 20 mg/kg and a maintenance dosage is 4 to 8 mg/kg/day. Maintenance doses may be given intravenously or orally; however, oral absorption can be erratic.[160]

Some clinicians prefer to use benzodiazepines for the acute treatment of seizures, particularly when phenobarbital or phenytoin is no longer effective. Lorazepam is one choice in this class of medication, and the recommended intravenous dose is 0.1 mg/kg.[160] Other benzodiazepines such as diazepam or midazolam, which vary in half-life, have also been used (Table 18-9). Benzodiazepines are not typically used for maintenance therapy because of the potential for tolerance and side effects.

For refractory seizures, new agents are available that have been used with some success as adjuvant therapy. Levetiracetam is the most common of these new agents, but its safety and efficacy data in neonates are limited. The small studies that have been done suggest that it prevents neurodegeneration better than other agents. Dosing begins at 10 mg/kg every 24 hours and can be increased to a maximum of 60 mg/kg/day. Mild sedation is the only side effect that has been observed.[161,162]

Free or unbound drug fractions have been suggested to affect the efficacy and potential toxicity of antiepileptic drugs in pediatric populations, including the neonatal population. Binding of drugs can be altered significantly in neonates with seizures, particularly in sick neonates with metabolic dysfunction. Biochemical alterations may cause toxic side effects by increasing the free fraction of the drug, which readily affects cardiovascular or respiratory function. Regular monitoring of serum drug levels (free and total) along with assessment of seizure control may improve the titration of antiepileptic drugs.[163]

The decision to maintain or discontinue antiepileptic drug treatment is fraught with uncertainty.[141] Practice varies widely, with discontinuation of long-term therapy occurring from 1 week to 12 months after

Table 18-9. Treatment of Neonatal Seizures with Antiepileptic Medications

	Phenobarbital	Phenytoin	Lorazepam	Midazolam	Diazepam	Levetiracetam
Delivery route	IV, IM, PO	IV, PO	IV	IV	IV	IV, PO
Initial loading dose	20 mg/kg IV	15-20 mg/kg IV	0.1 mg/kg	0.15 mg/kg	0.1 mg/kg	
Rate of administration	Give IV dose over 10-15 min	Give IV dose over 30 min Max infusion rate of 0.5 mg/kg/min	Slow push	Slow push over at least 5 min	Give IV dose over 3-5 min	Give IV dose over 15 min
Maintenance dosage	3-5 mg/kg every 24 hr IV, IM or PO	4-8 mg/kg every 24 hr IV or PO	Repeat dose prn based on response	Repeat dose prn based on response	Repeat dose prn based on response	10-60 mg/kg/day divided every 12-24 hr
Timing of first maintenance dose	12-24 hr after loading	12-24 hr after loading				
Therapeutic level	20-40 μg/mL	Total drug concentration: first week 6-15 μg/mL then 10-20 μg/mL				
Serum half-life	Varies from 40 to 200 hr depending on age and duration of drug usage	18-60 hr, decreasing with age	40 hr	4-22 hr	50-95 hr	18 hr in neonates, decreasing to 6 hr by 6 mo of age
Possible adverse effects	Sedation, respiratory depression (at serum concentrations >60 μg/mL)	Bradycardia, arrhythmias, hypotension during infusion	Respiratory depression, myoclonic jerking	Respiratory depression, hypotension, myoclonic jerking	Respiratory depression, hypotension	Sedation, irritability

IM, Intramuscular; *IV,* intravenous; *PO,* by mouth; *prn,* as needed.

the last seizure. Because there is the potential for antiepileptic medications to damage the developing nervous system, prompt discontinuation in the late neonatal period or early infancy is recommended. This is especially true for infants who show no demonstrable brain lesions on cranial imaging, who exhibit appropriate findings on neurologic examination, and who express normal interictal EEG background patterns.[1]

Despite the urgent need to establish the cause of a seizure, several unique aspects of neonatal seizures impede prompt diagnosis and treatment. There are a number of etiologic possibilities for neonatal seizures, and the efficacy of conventional antiepileptic drugs in controlling seizures remains controversial. Neonatal seizures can reflect either acute or remote disease processes or can result from a series of insults that began in the antepartum period and extend to include events during the intrapartum or postnatal periods. This knowledge of the acute or chronic causes of neonatal seizures will alter the clinician's choice of an antiepileptic treatment in the future. Neurorescue protective therapy such as hypothermia can be helpful, as can combinations of drugs that prevent seizures from arising in immature neuronal pathways that are injured, namely, phenobarbital and levetiracetam.

HYPOTONIA

Evaluation of tone in the neonate requires considerable experience and perseverance by the clinician.[164] The earlier section on clinical examination techniques discussed evaluation of the motor system and evaluation of the infant with altered tone, principally hypotonia and, less commonly, hypertonia (Fig. 18-19). Clearly, the approach to the diagnosis of hypotonia requires an understanding of the neuroanatomic locations in the neuraxis that may be responsible for producing low tone in the neonate. Such locations include the cerebrum, spinal cord, peripheral nerve, and neuromuscular junction or muscle (see Table 18-6). The clinical approach to hypotonia in the neonate is summarized in Table 18-10. Most hypotonic neonates have disorders of the cerebrum. In these situations, hypotonia is usually not accompanied by profound weakness, and other signs of brain dysfunction such as lethargy, swallowing difficulties, and abnormal primitive reflexes are present. Hypotonia can be one prominent clinical

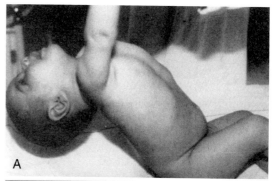
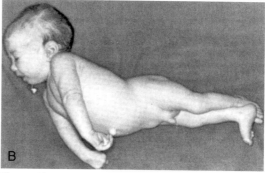

Figure 18-19. A, Three-month-old infant with marked hypotonia resulting from neuromuscular disease. **B,** Decerebrate posturing after severe asphyxia in a term infant.

manifestation of HIE (as discussed previously) or of other acute forms of neonatal disease with metabolic or infectious causes. Other cerebral causes of hypotonia are congenital infections and genetic diseases, including inherited disorders of metabolism involving glucose, amino acids, fatty acids, or peroxisomal pathways.

Peripheral causes of neonatal hypotonia also usually result in greater degrees of weakness, often including respiratory and swallowing difficulties. In cases of hypotonia associated with anterior horn cell disease (i.e., progressive spinal muscular atrophy), infants are alert and their behavior is otherwise normal. In other clinical situations, such as neonatal myotonic dystrophy or Prader-Willi syndrome, there may be a mixture of central and peripheral involvement in motor pathways, causing hypotonia as well as other disorders of cerebral or systemic function.[120,165]

Neonatal myasthenia gravis should be considered in neonates who are the offspring of myasthenic mothers and who have hypotonia located at the neuromuscular junction. These infants exhibit cranial nerve deficits such as facial diparesis, ptosis, and ophthalmoplegia, as well as respiratory depression.[166] Exogenous causes of hypotonia include the

Table 18-10. Approach to Diagnosis of Hypotonia

Anatomic Site	Pathogenesis	Clinical Features							Laboratory Aids			
		Alertness	Cry	Eye Movements	Tongue Fasciculation	Deep Tendon Reflexes	Muscle Bulk	Electromyography	Muscle Biopsy	Muscle Enzyme (CPK)*	Neostigmine
Cerebral	Malformation Hemorrhage Hypoxia-ischemia Metabolic disorder Infection Drugs	Poor	Poor	Occasionally abnormal	No	Normal or increased	Normal	Normal	Normal	Normal	Negative
Spinal cord	Injury	Good	Normal	Normal	No	Decreased or increased	Normal	Normal	Normal	Normal	Negative
Anterior horn cell	Spinal muscular atrophy† (Werdnig-Hoffmann disease)	Good	Normal or weak	Normal	Yes	Absent	Decreased	Neurogenic pattern	Neurogenic group	Normal	Negative
Neuromuscular junction	Neonatal myasthenia gravis	Good	Weak	Abnormal	No	Normal	Normal	± Normal	Normal	Normal	Negative
Muscle	Congenital myopathy Myotonic dystrophy‡ Glycogen storage disease	Good	Good	Normal	No	Decreased or normal	Decreased	Myopathic pattern	Myopathic change	Normal or elevated	Positive

*CPK level is grossly elevated in Duchenne dystrophy, which does not usually manifest as hypotonia in neonates.
†Molecular diagnosis identifies survival motor neuron (SMN) gene deletions or mutations by analysis of blood, amniotic fluid, or tissue.
‡Molecular diagnosis of myotonic dystrophy identifies cytosine–thymine–guanine triplet repeat expansion.
CPK, Creatine phosphokinase.

administration of drugs to the mother, such as inappropriate systemic or local injections of anesthetics that pass to the infant through the placental circulation or are introduced directly into the infant's scalp at the time of administration of paracervical or pudendal blocks. These medications may cause a characteristic syndrome of hypotonia, respiratory depression, and seizures during the first day of life. Administration of magnesium or aminoglycoside may result in transient neuromuscular dysfunction leading to profound weakness and hypotonia.

Connective tissue abnormalities also may be associated with low tone, particularly those involving mesenchymal tissue, such as in Marfan syndrome and Ehlers-Danlos syndrome.

Myopathies associated with either specific muscular dystrophies or congenital myopathies can present with neonatal hypotonia and are generally accompanied by some degree of weakness or decrease in muscle bulk. A mixture of lower and upper motor neuron diseases is noted in certain congenital muscular dystrophies, as well as in mitochondrial myopathies.

QUESTIONS

A full-term newborn whose mother had premature rupture of membranes and a fever to 39° C has a bulging fontanelle, seizures, and irritability. Spinal fluid shows evidence of 100 white blood cells μL and elevation of the CSF protein level to 200 μg/dL. Is this evidence of intracranial hemorrhage, meningitis, or ganglioneuroma?

The infant has an increased risk of infection because of premature rupture of membranes in a mother with probable chorioamnionitis. Careful examination of the placenta reveals lymphocytic infiltration, villous edema, and intravascular thrombin deposition. The CSF findings are typical of meningitis.

A growth-restricted newborn of 37 weeks' gestation shows irritability, hypotonia, hepatosplenomegaly, and chorioretinitis. Congenital infection is suspected. Should the attending neonatologist obtain a cerebral CT scan rather than an MRI scan?

A CT scan better documents calcifications associated with congenital infection, so CT is appropriate. An MRI study would otherwise be preferred for an infant suspected to have brain lesions that require higher resolution to document structural anomalies or injury.

A full-term infant who is clearly awake does not move below the neck except for fine myoclonic movements of the fingers and toes, and shows fasciculations of the tongue. What study should the neonatologist request?

A specific serum-based genetic study to diagnose spinal muscular atrophy should be ordered.

Anterior horn cell disease (i.e., spinal muscular atrophy, historically called *Werdnig-Hoffmann disease*) can be expeditiously diagnosed by genetic analysis using a serum sample to document a deletional defect on chromosome 7. This genetic study has largely replaced the more laborious and indirect diagnostic investigations, including electromyography and muscle biopsy, which lack genetic specificity.

Fasciculation is best evaluated with the tongue at rest.

True or False

A newborn who is in neurologically depressed condition at the time of birth with evidence of fetal acidosis, low Apgar scores, and neonatal seizures has always experienced asphyxia during the intrapartum period.

Asphyxia in the neonate, as documented by clinical and laboratory examination, can have antepartum as well as intrapartum causes. Even though the infant may become symptomatic during a problematic labor and delivery that leads to asphyxia, the intrapartum period may not be the time during which brain damage occurred. Therefore, the statement is false.

True or False

An elongated head shape in a preterm infant who is a corrected age of 44 weeks suggests craniosynostosis, and a neurosurgical referral should be made immediately.

Even though craniosynostosis must be suspected in a child with an abnormal head shape, premature infants commonly experience inhibition of lateral head growth because the head is turned to either side in contact with the mattress. In most of these infants, no premature closure of the sagittal suture can be documented. The Back to Sleep campaign has dramatically decreased the incidence of sudden infant death syndrome; however, its sequela of deformational plagiocephaly has today reached epidemic proportions. Other factors associated with nonsynostotic occipital plagiocephaly are multiple gestations and torticollis. Breast feeding, because of frequent positioning changes, has a protective effect. Plagiocephaly, literally "skull asymmetry," is seen characteristically with unilateral coronal or lambdoidal synostosis. Premature closure of a unilateral coronal suture, anterior plagiocephaly, occurs in 1 in 10,000 live births and is characterized by flattening of the forehead and elevation of the eyebrow on the affected side. Fortunately most clinicians have learned to clinically distinguish deformational plagiocephaly, associated with sleeping in the supine position, from craniosynostosis, so that unnecessary surgical correction is prevented. Therefore, the statement is false.

True or False

A 37-week gestational age female neonate showed spontaneous lateral eye movements, buccolingual and orbital twitching, irregular respirations, and low tone. This constellation of signs occurred intermittently over a 15- to 20-minute period followed by cessation of these movements, resumption of regular cardiorespiratory rates, and increased muscle tone. A concurrent EEG recording would most likely have documented neonatal seizures during the period when the twitching and other signs occurred.

These observations represent appropriate clinical phenomena associated with active (rapid eye movement) sleep followed by quiet (non–rapid eye movement) sleep in a near-term infant. The movements during rapid eye movement sleep may superficially resemble seizures but have no EEG correlate; therefore, the statement is false.

True or False

A cranial ultrasound scan documents bilateral echodensities surrounding the ventricular outline. In addition, the echodensity extends into the left brain substance with high-density signal within the ventricular space. The neuroimaging report concludes that both intraventricular hemorrhage and periventricular leukomalacia occurred in this preterm infant. Is this possible?

These two forms of cerebrovascular lesions can occur in the same preterm infant. The statement is true.

CASE 1

A 2300-g male infant was born at term to a 34-year-old mother who had multiple urinary tract infections during pregnancy. The mother had a fever 24 hours before delivery and foul-smelling amniotic fluid was noted after artificial rupture of membranes. During labor, electronic fetal monitoring showed fetal distress as evidenced by minimal heart rate variability and transient bradycardic episodes to 100 beats per minute on three occasions before delivery. The infant's condition appeared depressed at birth and he had Apgar scores of 1, 3, and 8 at 1, 5, and 10 minutes of life. The cord pH was 7.12 and the base excess was −11. After resuscitation the infant became irritable and hypertonic with back arching on stimulation. The vernix of the infant was noted to be foul smelling.

Did the mother's urinary tract infections contribute to the infant's neonatal encephalopathy?

Although the infant's condition was depressed at birth, the degree of metabolic acidosis and the rapid response to resuscitative effort suggests that other reasons should be considered for the infant's subsequent neurologic abnormalities and irritability and hypertonia. The mother's frequent urinary tract infections, the foul-smelling amniotic fluid on rupture of the membranes, and the malodorous vernix of the infant all point to the probable occurrence of chorioamnionitis.

What diagnostic steps are indicated?

In the context of infection, the infant should be aggressively evaluated for a systemic and/or CNS infection. The cellular blood count showed an elevated white cell count of 20,200/µL but there was no differential shift to the left. Culture was performed on all body fluids, including tracheal aspirate, blood, spinal fluid, and urine, as well as on nasopharyngeal, skin, and throat specimens. Blood glucose, calcium, potassium, and sodium levels were measured, and blood gas analysis, chest radiography and urinalysis were performed.

Results of all the aforementioned studies were normal. The CSF was clear with two white blood cells per µL, both lymphocytes. The CSF glucose level was 90 mg/dL, blood glucose level was 110 mg/dL, and the CSF protein level was 94 mg/dL. The Gram stain of the spinal fluid was also negative for organisms.

Histologic evaluation of the placenta documented severe chorioamnionitis and funisitis.

Despite the negative culture results, should this infant be presumptively treated for infection?

Definitely. This infant should be treated for bacterial meningitis given the clinical picture described. The presence of hypertonia, particularly with dystonic posturing on stimulation, may suggest abnormal function of the CNS, particularly if the fontanelle is full and bulging. Infection may be present even in the absence of positive culture results. The mother's frequent urinary tract infections and clinical evidence of chorioamnionitis supported by histologic examination of the placenta puts the infant at high risk of infection.

Chorioamnionitis seldom causes systemic inflammation in the mother. However, ascending maternal infections frequently lead to a systemic fetal inflammatory reaction manifested by funisitis and elevated levels of proinflammatory cytokines. The fetal inflammatory response is considered to be the counterpart of the systemic inflammatory response syndrome. Furthermore, antenatal exposure to inflammation may masquerade as an asphyxial insult and puts the extremely premature neonate at high risk of worsening pulmonary, neurologic, and other organ development. Bronchopulmonary dysplasia is more common following the fetal inflammatory reaction. Surprisingly, the presence of chorioamnionitis may be associated with a lower rate of neonatal mortality in extremely premature newborns.

CASE 2

A male infant was delivered at 37 weeks' gestation by cesarean section to a 32-year-old gravida 2, para 0 woman. She had a previous pregnancy that spontaneously terminated at 3 months' gestation. The mother has a diagnosis of inflammatory bowel disease, specifically ulcerative colitis. Throughout pregnancy her inflammatory bowel disease was quiescent until shortly before delivery when she had a clinical flare consisting of bloody diarrhea and fever. Although the evaluation for infection yielded negative results, she was given broad-spectrum antibiotics as well as sulfasalazine (Azulfidine) and steroids. Over the subsequent 4 to 5 days her clinical symptoms of inflammatory bowel disease resolved. After the sixth day of treatment she spontaneously went into labor. Fetal heart monitoring showed late decelerations 1 hour before delivery, consisting of bradycardia into the range of 90 to 100 beats per minute. Apgar scores were 7 at 1 minute and 9 at 5 minutes. The infant required deep suctioning and supplemental oxygen for 3 minutes. He was examined and the findings were normal, and he was taken to a well-child nursery. He was observed and showed no problems until 2 days of age, when cyanosis with apnea was noted in association with left arm clonic activity that could not be suppressed by the extremities. An EEG was obtained, which documented focal electrographic seizures coincident with the clonic activity. CT was performed

and revealed a right hemispheric hypodensity in the distribution of the right middle cerebral artery. Seizures continued until two antiepileptic medications were administered. A diffusion-weighted MRI scan was subsequently obtained 1 day after the onset of seizures and documented an abnormal area in the right hemisphere in the distribution of the right middle cerebral artery. An echocardiogram, complete blood count, blood chemistry panel including coagulation studies, CSF analysis, and drug screen all showed normal results.

No subsequent seizures were noted, and the infant was discharged on day 8 of life with normal results on neurologic examination. Subsequent evaluations by the pediatrician and consulting pediatric neurologist indicated that head circumference remained within the normal range, although the infant showed asymmetry of spontaneous movements, which were decreased on the left compared with the right. Reflexes as well as passive muscle tone were also increased on the left. After placement in a sitting position, the infant lacked a lateral prop developmental reflex when leaned to the left. At 9 to 10 months of age he had an asymmetric parachute reflex, with absence on the left. He continued to demonstrate delay in meeting motor milestones. An MRI scan in the second year of life documented a left porencephaly. He is now 7 years of age and requires special education classes as well as preventative treatment for seizures, which recurred at 4 years of age.

When did the brain injury occur?

The specific cerebrovascular injury in this child fits within the diagnostic entity of stroke syndrome. His stroke event was ischemic with no hemorrhagic component. The event more likely than not occurred before delivery. Given the mother's inflammatory bowel disease with an active phase of ulcerative colitis, there is the possibility of an acquired thrombophilia that may have led to occlusion of the right middle cerebral artery due to thrombosis on the fetal surface of the placenta. This possibility is supported by placental findings showing a fetal thrombotic vasculopathy. Despite evidence of transient fetal distress, there was no depression at birth and no evidence of a neonatal encephalopathy at the time of delivery or during the first 2 days of life until the onset of seizures. Seizures can occur following a symptom-free period after delivery in the absence of encephalopathy. After experiencing seizures, the infant required a prompt evaluation for infection, intracranial hemorrhage, and drug withdrawal, given the onset of the seizures in the newborn period without preexisting or concurrent encephalopathic findings. Once results of these evaluations were found to be negative, then the possibility of a focal brain disorder secondary to stroke syndrome, as indicated by neuroimaging and

EEG studies, had to be pursued. Before the availability of neuroimaging, children with stroke syndrome were classically identified during infancy based on congenital hemiparesis, and such children are at high risk of epilepsy as well as cognitive and behavioral deficits at older ages.

Why were results of the initial neurologic examinations normal until 2 days of age?

The infant lacked a brain disorder following a normal delivery and before 2 days of age. The stroke event had occurred in utero if signs or symptoms were present in the first 2 days, then a more recent injury would have reflected acute brain destruction, cerebral edema, and possible associated hemorrhage.

Could the stroke syndrome have occurred during the intrapartum period rather than during the antepartum period?

Although fetal distress was noted, no depression was observed at birth. Seizures then were noted at 2 days of age in the absence of any previous alterations in tone or arousal consistent with a neonatal encephalopathy. The abnormality seen initially on the head CT scan and then on the brain MRI scan suggested that the stroke occurred before the intrapartum period. The lack of convincing signs of neonatal encephalopathy placed the timing of this injury to days before delivery.

Why did the infant appear normal at the time of discharge in the newborn period only to show developmental delay at a later time?

The immaturity of the brain during the early months of life does not allow clinical expression of deficits in children who later demonstrate static motor enceph-

alopathies (i.e., cerebral palsy). Good documentation of clinical abnormalities is important to allow an early intervention strategy to be offered.

Can stroke syndromes be prevented in the fetus and neonate?

Women at increased risk of thrombophilia, including those with known genetic or acquired risk factors for stroke syndromes, may be treated prophylactically with low-dose aspirin or heparin. There are no guarantees that this approach will be successful. There is evidence that women with active inflammatory bowel disease may develop thrombophilia, which can impact the fetus, as occurred in this case.

Could earlier intervention to address developmental difficulties have made a difference?

Early intervention programs provide additional stimulation and prevent contractures from abnormal hypertonicity of the legs. Monitoring of developmental progress may provide an incentive for parents to supplement stimulation at an earlier time and on a more frequent basis. It is unclear whether this early interventional strategy lessens the risk of later learning disabilities and behavioral problems.

REFERENCES

The reference list for this chapter can be found online at www.expertconsult.com.

The Outcome of Neonatal Intensive Care

Maureen Hack

19

Technical advances and improvements in perinatal care have been mainly responsible for the improved survival of high-risk neonates (Fig. 19-1, Table 19-1, and Appendix C). A major concern persists, however, that neonatal intensive care results in an increase in the number of permanently handicapped children.

The initial follow-up studies of preterm infants in the early 1970s described a decrease in unfavorable neurodevelopmental sequelae compared with the era before neonatal intensive care. Despite the continued decrease in mortality rates, the incidence of neurosensory and developmental handicaps initially remained constant in the 1980s; however, morbidity increased in the 1990s following a further decrease in mortality, which was associated with antenatal steroid and surfactant therapies introduced in the early 1990s. These treatments resulted in the survival of high-risk infants who previously would have died. Furthermore postnatal steroid therapy, which was widely used to prevent or treat bronchopulmonary dysplasia, resulted in higher rates of cerebral palsy.[1-3] The absolute number of both healthy and neurologically impaired children in the population thus increased in the 1990s.[3] Additional morbidity resulted from increased infection, necrotizing enterocolitis, and poor physical growth in infants of extremely low birth weight (<1 kg) and short gestation (<26 weeks).[3-5]

Since 2000, the outcomes of children with a birth weight of less than 1 kg have improved; this improvement has resulted from a significant decrease in nosocomial infections and intraventricular hemorrhage, together with a decrease in the use of postnatal steroid therapy.[6]

When outcome results are evaluated, considerable variation is noted in the results cited in different reports. One reason is that selection of patients by birth weight does not guarantee a homogeneous group, and populations studied in one center may differ considerably from those studied in another center. There are several causes for these differences. One of the most important factors is the pattern of referral to the neonatal intensive care unit (NICU). Units that receive admissions from numerous outlying hospitals have a selected population that may contain a disproportionate number of the sickest babies or may include only those infants deemed well enough to transport. In addition, patients treated in an "inborn" unit have the advantage of consistent and, presumably, good obstetric care coupled with the opportunity for immediate postnatal resuscitation and management. Inadequate resuscitation at birth and prolonged hypoxia and acidemia, together with the cold stress associated with transport that may be seen in referred patients, influence not only the outcome in the period immediately after birth but also the type and frequency of developmental sequelae. Other factors that may influence outcome include (1) the socioeconomic profile of the parents, (2) the proportion of infants with intrauterine growth restriction, (3) the incidence of extreme prematurity, (4) a selective admission policy, (5) a selective treatment policy, and (6) changes in therapy during the study period.

The major clinical outcomes that are important to preterm infants and their families are not only survival, but survival accompanied by normal long-term neurodevelopment. These goals are not easily attainable; however, the landscape has improved

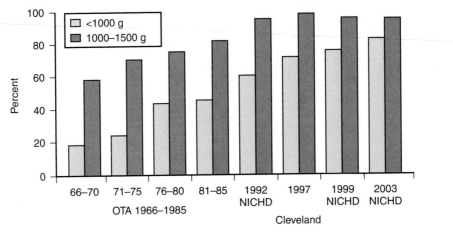

Figure 19-1. Trends in Survival. Improvement in survival of low-birth-weight infants. *(Data for 1966 to 1985 from U.S. Congress, Office of Technology Assessment [OTA]: Neonatal intensive care for low-birthweight infants: cost and effectiveness, Health Technology Case Study 38, Washington, DC, 1987, U.S. Congress; data for 1992, 1999, and 2003 from Stevenson DK, Wright LL, Lemons JA, et al: Very low birth weight outcomes of the National Institute of Child Health and Human Development [NICHD] Neonatal Research Network, January 1993 through December 1994, Am J Obstet Gynecol 179:1632, 1998; and Fanaroff AA, Stoll BJ, Wright LL, et al; NICHD Neonatal Research Network: Trends in neonatal morbidity and mortality for very low birthweight infants, Am J Obstet Gynecol 196[2]:147, e1, 2007; data for 1997 from Rainbow Babies and Children's Hospital, Cleveland.)*

Table 19-1.	Survival and Neurodevelopmental Impairment (NDI) according to Gestational Age		
Gestational Age (wk)	**Survival (%)**	**NDI (%)**	**Survival Without NDI (%)**
22	5	80	1
23	26	65	9
24	56	50	28
25	76	39	46

Adapted from Tyson JE, Parikh NA, Langer J, et al for the National Institute of Child Health and Human Development Neonatal Research Network: Intensive care for extreme prematurity—moving beyond gestational age, *N Engl J Med* 358:1672, 2008.

over the past two decades, and there are now more intact survivors who attend mainstream schools and ultimately live independently. How to preserve brain function and permit normal brain development ex utero remain enormous challenges. The period between 20 and 32 weeks after conception is one of rapid brain growth and development. Illness, hemorrhage, ischemia, metabolic disturbances such as hypoglycemia, hyperbilirubinemia, undernutrition, and infection during this time may compromise neurodevelopment. Indeed, events leading to the premature birth such as chorioamnionitis may have stimulated the release of cytokines that in turn injure the developing brain. Scores of publications continue to demonstrate inferior intellect and function in the most immature babies compared with their term peers.

EDITORIAL COMMENT: Follow-up of graduates from the intensive care unit has shed the orphan role it had for so long and is now a genuine and legitimate component of neonatology. Indeed, neurodevelopmental status on follow-up has become an integral part of the primary outcome measure in most prospective randomized interventional trials involving both term and preterm infants. Absence of harm and normal long-term neurodevelopment are the desired outcome.

Measures of outcomes of neonatal care include the rate of mortality before and after discharge from the neonatal intensive care nursery, rate of rehospitalizations, and incidence of chronic medical conditions such as asthma and growth failure. Neurodevelopmental sequelae include subnormal and borderline cognitive (mental)

Box 19-1.	Measures of Very Low-Birth-Weight Outcome

Survival
- To discharge
- After discharge

Medical morbidity
- Rehospitalization
- Chronic lung disease
- Growth failure

Neurodevelopmental outcome
- Motor dysfunction (cerebral palsy)
- Mental retardation
- Seizures
- Vision problems
- Hearing disorders
- Behavioral problems
- School-age outcomes

Functional outcomes
- Health or illness
- Activity and skills of daily living
- Ambulation
- Need for technologic aids (gastric tube, oxygen)
- Need for special services

Quality of life

Impact on family

Cost of care

Box 19-2.	Factors Affecting Outcomes for the Very Low-Birth-Weight Infant

Birth weight <750 g or <26 weeks' gestation
Periventricular hemorrhage (grade III or IV)
Periventricular leukomalacia or other echodense lesions
Persistent ventricular dilatation
Neonatal seizures
Chronic lung disease
Neonatal meningitis
Subnormal head circumference
Poverty or parental deprivation
Congenital malformations

function and neurosensory deficits such as cerebral palsy, deafness, and blindness. These sequelae have traditionally been used as outcome measures.[7] Other outcomes include functional abilities and the ability to perform the activities of daily living.[8-10] Additional measures involve special health care requirements such as the need for technologic aids, frequent physician visits and medications for chronic conditions, occupational and physical therapy, and special education and counseling.[8] Other measures may include impact on the family, quality of life,[11] and cost of care.

Regional outcome studies provide the most accurate data because they include all infants born in a region rather than hospital-based results. Such studies have rarely been undertaken in the United States, although they have been performed in Canada, the United Kingdom, and Australia.[1] Results may also be reported from multigroup studies or randomized controlled trials of various therapies[12-14] (Box 19-1).

The risk of neurodevelopmental problems increases as birth weight and gestational age decrease. Additional risk factors include the occurrence of neonatal seizures; severe periventricular hemorrhage[13,15]; periventricular leukomalacia[16]; bronchopulmonary dysplasia, defined as an oxygen requirement at 36 weeks' postconceptional age; and severe intrauterine or neonatal growth failure, specifically a subnormal head circumference (≤2 standard deviations [SDs] from the mean) at discharge. Children born to mothers who have a low educational level or live in poverty demonstrate the additional detrimental effects of the environment. Among term-born children, risk factors for later neurologic and developmental sequelae also include perinatal asphyxia, neonatal seizures, an abnormal neurologic finding at discharge, and persistent pulmonary hypertension requiring prolonged ventilator therapy, nitric oxide therapy, or extracorporeal membrane oxygenation.[17] Children born with multiple major malformations also constitute a group that generally has a poor developmental outcome (Box 19-2).

IMPORTANCE OF FOLLOW-UP FOR HIGH-RISK INFANTS

Follow-up clinics should be an integral part of every NICU. Specialized care for problems of growth, sequelae of bronchopulmonary dysplasia, and adaptation is best provided within the setting of a neonatal follow-up program. This care should initially be provided by the neonatal department and then gradually transferred to developmental and educational specialists. The initial continuity of care is important to the family, who will find reassurance in the fact that the same people who were responsible for the life-saving decisions early in the infant's life are continuing to assume responsibility for the child's adaptation into home life. There is also a moral obligation to maintain this contact. Furthermore, even if the neonatologist does not continue the follow-up for an extended period, he or she will benefit greatly by maintaining contact with the nursery graduates and recognizing the sequelae of the early neonatal interventions.

When growth and neurodevelopmental outcomes are assessed, it is important to correct the child's age to account for the preterm birth. This should be done at least until the child is 3 years of age. For extremely immature infants (i.e., those born at 23 to 25 weeks' gestation), such age correction may be necessary until at least 5 years of age.

MINOR TRANSIENT PROBLEMS

The first few months after the neonate's discharge can be considered a period of convalescence for the infant and parents as well. Many infants have minor problems specifically related to being born preterm, but these may seem major problems to their parents. These problems include anemia of prematurity, umbilical and inguinal hernias, relatively large, dolichocephalic, "preemie-shaped" heads, and subtle behavioral differences. Most healthy preterm infants are discharged home at 36 to 37 weeks' gestational age (or when they weigh about 1.9 kg). At this age they still tend to sleep most of the day, waking only for feedings; to feed slowly and not always to demonstrate hunger; to sometimes be jittery; and to have "preemie" vocalizations, which include grunts and a relatively high-pitched cry.

TRANSIENT NEUROLOGIC ABNORMALITY

There is a very high incidence of transient neurologic abnormality during the first year of life, ranging from 40% to 80% among preterm infants. These include abnormalities of muscle tone such as hypotonia or hypertonia. Such abnormalities present as poor head control at 40 weeks' corrected age (the expected term date), poor back support at 4 to 8 months, and sometimes a slight increase in the tone of the upper extremities. Because there is normally some degree of hypertonia during the first 3 months after term, it is difficult to diagnose the early developing spasticity related to cerebral palsy. Children in whom cerebral palsy later develops show hypotonia (poor head control and back support) initially and only later manifest spasticity of the extremities combined with truncal hypotonia. Spasticity during the first 3 to 4 months of life is an indicator of poor prognosis. Mild hypertonia or hypotonia persisting at 8 months usually resolves by the second year of life. Persistence of primitive reflexes beyond 4 months' corrected age might be a sign of early cerebral palsy. Major neurologic handicap presents during the first 6 to 8 months after term in about 10% of newborns in the most high-risk categories; however, 90% of high-risk newborns will be or become neurologically normal after the first year of life.

PERSISTENT NEUROLOGIC SEQUELAE

Major neurologic handicap can usually be defined during the latter part of the first year of life or even earlier if severe. It is usually classified as cerebral palsy (spastic diplegia, spastic quadriplegia, or spastic hemiplegia or paresis); hydrocephalus (with or without accompanying cerebral palsy or sensory deficits); blindness (usually caused by retinopathy of prematurity); or deafness. Blindness currently occurs very rarely because laser treatment or cryotherapy for severe retinopathy of prematurity may prevent the progression of this disease. The developmental and intellectual outcomes differ according to the severity of cerebral palsy. For example, children with spastic quadriplegia usually have severe mental retardation, whereas children with spastic diplegia or hemiplegia may have relatively intact mental functioning. Mental functioning is not always measurable in these children until after 2 to 3 years of age.

EDITORIAL COMMENT: *Cerebral palsy* is an umbrella term encompassing a group of nonprogressive, noncontagious motor conditions that cause physical disability in human development, chiefly in the various areas of body movement. Most health care providers are familiar with the high rates and risk of cerebral palsy in preterm infants. Nonetheless, numerically it is term and near-term infants who account for the majority of cases of cerebral palsy despite their significantly lower risk.

PHYSICAL SEQUELAE AND CHRONIC DISEASE

Chronic diseases of prematurity, mainly chronic lung disease (bronchopulmonary dysplasia), gradually resolve during infancy, although children with bronchopulmonary dysplasia have higher rates of recurrent respiratory infections and asthma during childhood. Scars from various neonatal surgical procedures (tracheotomy, thoracocentesis, Broviac lines, shunt procedures) tend to fade gradually and appear less significant as the child grows. There is, however, a high rate of rehospitalization, especially for those children of extremely low birth weight who have bronchopulmonary dysplasia or neurologic sequelae. Fifty percent of children with chronic lung disease may be hospitalized in the first year after discharge. Many hospitalizations that occur in winter have been due to respiratory syncytial virus infections. These may be minimized with respiratory syncytial virus immunization. Children with neurologic sequelae such as cerebral palsy or hydrocephalus also have a higher rate of rehospitalization for shunt complications, orthopedic correction of spasticity, and eye surgery for strabismus.

PHYSICAL GROWTH

Intrauterine and/or neonatal growth restriction is present in many very low-birth-weight neonates who require intensive care and a prolonged hospitalization. For infants born at a size appropriate for gestational age, poor neonatal growth is related to inadequate nutrition during the neonatal period, to increased caloric requirements associated with breathing in chronic lung disease, to poor feeding in neurologically impaired children, and to the lack of parental care or an optimal environment for growth in the nursery. As these conditions gradually resolve, and when an optimal home environment is provided, catch-up of growth may occur during childhood. However, many of these infants still remain subnormal in weight and height in their third year. Growth attainment after discharge is a very good measure of physical, neurologic, and environmental well-being. To promote optimal catch-up growth, neonatal nutrition needs to be maximized and sufficient calories provided during the recovery phase. This is especially important because catch-up of head circumference in both appropriate for gestational age and small for gestational age infants may occur during the first 6 to 12 months' after term.

The prognosis for catch-up growth is less optimal in infants born small for gestational age after intrauterine growth failure, because their initial period of growth failure occurred relatively early in gestation and extended for a longer time during the critical perinatal period of growth.

Predictors of poor catch-up growth include severe intrauterine growth failure, severe neonatal complications including bronchopulmonary dysplasia following prolonged ventilator and oxygen dependence, necrotizing enterocolitis requiring surgery, and neurologic impairment such as cerebral palsy. Neurologically impaired children may also show failure to thrive after the neonatal discharge. The genetic potential for growth as measured by midparental height also plays a role in the potential for catch-up growth.[18]

Use of increased-calorie formulas providing 22 calories per ounce and increased calcium might enhance growth during the first few months after discharge home; however, there are no reported studies of the longer-term effect of such formulas on growth to the second year of life and thereafter.

Extremely low-birth-weight infants with chronic lung disease (bronchopulmonary dysplasia) who can feed orally may be discharged home with oxygen supplementation when they are in stable condition. These infants need close follow-up with pediatric pulmonary specialists or neonatologists with expertise and interest in pulmonary follow-up care. As the infant is gradually weaned from oxygen, close attention needs to be paid to optimizing growth with the use of increased-calorie formulas and to the gradual weaning of any medications the child might be receiving such as diuretics or antireflux medication. Such children also require respiratory syncytial virus immunization in winter.

Most neurologic or physical problems resolve or become permanent during the first year of life. Furthermore, during the second year of life, the environmental effects of parental education and social class begin to influence the outcome measures. Clinical follow-up is essential for all high-risk infants during this period. After the first year, the new problems that become evident may include subtle motor, visuomotor, and behavioral difficulties. These are best diagnosed and treated in an educational rather than a medical setting.

It is very important to pay attention to the mother's and father's well-being, their support systems, and their ability to care for the infant. Maternal depression is fairly prevalent following the birth of preterm and/or chronically ill infants.

FOLLOW-UP—WHO, WHAT, HOW, AND WHEN

Infants at highest risk should be followed. These include infants who had severe asphyxia complicated by seizures or signs of brain edema, periventricular or other intracranial injury, meningitis, or multisystem congenital malformations; infants who required ventilatory assistance; and those born with very low birth weights (especially those weighing <1 kg) or at 23 to 25 weeks' gestation).[19]

Growth (weight, height, and head circumference), neurologic development, psychomotor development, ophthalmologic status, vision, and hearing should all be examined on a regular basis.

TIMING OF FOLLOW-UP VISITS

The initial follow-up visit should be 7 to 10 days after the neonatal discharge. This is essential to evaluate how the infant is adapting to the home environment. This visit usually occurs around the time of the expected date of delivery. A clinic visit at 4 months' corrected age is important to document problems of inadequate catch-up growth and severe neurologic abnormality that might require intervention or physical therapy.

Eight months' corrected age is a good time to identify the presence of developing cerebral palsy or other neurologic abnormality. It is also an excellent time for the first developmental assessment (preferably using the Bayley Scales of Infant Development). At this age, infants show very little outward stranger anxiety and are most cooperative. Some physicians, however, prefer to perform the first developmental assessment at 12 months of age.

The Bayley score attained at 8 to 12 months' corrected age tends to decrease by the second year (partly as a function of the test and partly because of the increased effect of the environment) and is not of great prognostic significance. However, low scores (<80) are predictive of poor later functioning, as is cerebral palsy. By 18 to 24 months' corrected age, most transient neurologic findings have resolved, and the neurologically abnormal child may show adaptation to neurologic sequelae. Furthermore, most of the potential catch-up growth has been achieved, although catch-up growth may occur into the adolescent years. During the second year of life the mental scale of the Bayley scales provides some assessment of the child's cognitive performance, although these scales have very poor prognostic validity for IQ measurement at school age.[20] Cognitive function is not easily measured before 1 year of age, because the test is based mainly on motor function. Children who

have a Mental Development Index (MDI) score of less than 70 at 18 to 24 months' corrected age and do not have cerebral palsy may have higher IQ scores on testing at school age, although they tend to have poorer school functioning than children who have a normal Mental Development Index score (>70) at 18 to 24 months of age.

Beyond the age of 3 years, other tests may be performed. These tests further validate the child's mental abilities. Language may also be measurable at this age. From 4 years of age, more subtle neurologic, visuomotor, and behavioral difficulties are measurable. These difficulties affect school performance even in children who have normal intelligence.[19,21]

NEUROSENSORY AND DEVELOPMENTAL ASSESSMENT

Neurodevelopmental handicap is usually defined in children who have a neurologic abnormality or a developmental quotient or IQ of less than 80. Some researchers include only a subnormal IQ (<70), whereas others include all children with an IQ less than 1 SD from the norm (IQ of <85). Neurologic abnormality is usually classified by neurologic diagnosis, which can include hypotonia or hypertonia, cerebral palsy (spastic diplegia or quadriplegia), hydrocephalus, blindness, or deafness.

The neurologic examination during infancy is best based on changes in muscle tone that occur during the first year of life. The scale developed by Amiel-Tison measures the progressive increase in active muscle tone (head control, back support, sitting, standing, and walking) together with the concomitant decrease in passive muscle tone that occurs during infancy.[22] Furthermore, it documents visual and auditory responses and some primitive reflexes. This method gives a qualitative assessment of neurologic integrity, which is defined as normal, suspect, or abnormal during the first year after term. The Amiel-Tison method of evaluation extends into early childhood.[22]

Short-term outcome studies of preterm infants who sustained a neonatal grade IV intraventricular hemorrhage (also known as *periventricular hemorrhagic infarction*) have reported a high rate of cerebral palsy ranging from 40% to 85%; however, there has been no consensus regarding cognitive outcome, with normal cognition noted in 20% to 79%.[23] Roze et al prospectively collected a cohort of preterm infants with periventricular hemorrhagic infarction to determine motor,[24] cognitive, and behavioral outcome at school age and to identify cerebral risk factors for adverse outcome. Of 38 infants, 15 (39%) died. Twenty-one of the 23 survivors were included in the follow-up. The investigators concluded that "the majority of surviving preterm children with periventricular hemorrhagic infarction had cerebral palsy with limited functional impairment at school age. Intelligence was within 1 SD of the norm of preterm children without lesions in 60% to 80% of the children. Verbal memory, in particular, was affected. Behavioral and executive function problems occurred slightly more than in preterm infants without lesions. The functional outcome at school age of preterm children with periventricular hemorrhagic infarction is better than previously thought." Papile notes, "Roze et al's study points out one of the major shortcomings of infant neurodevelopmental testing. Because successful completion of many test items relies heavily on motor function, the scores achieved by preterm infants with motor impairment such as cerebral palsy underestimate their true ability and may lead to an unduly pessimistic view regarding their ultimate outcome".[25]

Psychomotor Developmental Tests
The Bayley Scales of Infant Development are the recognized standard for measuring infant development and may be used between early infancy and 42 months of age. Separate motor and mental scales each yield a developmental index with a mean of 100. The scales were revised and restandardized in 1993 and more recently in 2006. In the first year, motor skills are weighted heavily, even in the mental scale, but by the second year, cognitive functions, including speech and behavior, may be more reliably measured. The 2006 edition of the test has three scales that measure cognitive, language, and motor development as well as two scales that measure social-emotional development and adaptive behavior as reported by a parent.

In the preschool years and into adolescence, the following tests are often used both clinically and for research:
- The *Stanford-Binet Intelligence Scale* is used from age 2 years into the elementary school years. It provides a measure of intelligence that is highly correlated with school performance.
- The *Wechsler scales* (Wechsler Preschool and Primary Scale of Intelligence—Third Edition for preschoolers and Wechsler Intelligence Scale for Children—Fourth Edition for ages 6 to 16 years) yield verbal, performance, and full-scale scores with means of 100.
- The *Kaufman Assessment Battery for Children* is used between the ages of 3 and 10 years. Like the Stanford-Binet and Wechsler tests, it has a number of subscales to assess various components of intelligence.
- The *McCarthy Scales of Children's Abilities* provide measures of cognitive, perceptual-performance, and quantitative abilities in children between ages 2½ and 8 years as well as a composite score (comparable to an IQ) and measures of motor and memory functions. However, this test has not been restandardized since 1972, and it is likely that the norms are outdated.
- The *Denver Developmental Screening Test* is used as a clinical screening tool in the first 6 years. It is not highly sensitive and fails to identify a significant number of at-risk children. Because it is not a quantitative assessment, it is rarely used for research to document outcomes in specific high-risk populations.

Visual Testing
An ophthalmologic examination should be performed on all high-risk infants before discharge. Infants younger than 30 to 32 weeks' gestation should have been followed with serial examinations in the nursery for signs of developing retinopathy of prematurity. Those who have residual findings at discharge or who have undergone laser therapy or cryotherapy should be followed by an ophthalmologist until the abnormal findings resolve. All children should undergo a repeat eye examination between 12 and 24 months of age. Infants of extremely low birth weight or gestational age who have had severe retinopathy of prematurity might require correction with glasses during infancy or early childhood.

Hearing
Hearing should be screened before the infant's discharge from the NICU. This may be done by measuring base-of-brain evoked responses or otoacoustic emissions. Hearing should be reexamined between 12 and 24 months of age, because the most common

Table 19-2.	Outcome Variables at 18 to 24 Months' Corrected Age			
		Gestational Age (wk)		
Birth Weight 501-800 g		**23**	**24**	**25**
Total followed (N)	1000	77	323	554
Severe disability	9%-37%	34%	22%-45%	12%-35%
Cerebral palsy	5%-37%		11%-15%	3%-20%
Subnormal cognitive (Mental Development Index of <70)	13%-47%		14%-39%	10%-30%
Blindness	2%-25%		0%-9%	3%-10%
Deafness	0%-7%			

Adapted from Hack M, Fanaroff AA: Outcomes of children of extremely low birthweight and gestational age in the 1990s, *Semin Neonatol* 5:89, 2000.

cause of hearing loss is upper respiratory tract and middle ear infections, which may occur during the first 2 years of life.

EARLY INTERVENTION

Early environmental enrichment with close attention to the family's needs may improve the developmental outcome of all children, including infants with normal birth weight as well as low birth weight and low gestational age, and especially of children in disadvantaged homes.[26] Studies of early intervention have, however, shown a decrease in beneficial effects after discontinuation of the intervention. Initial home visits during early childhood by experienced nurses are also important for surveillance of the child's growth and medical needs, for education concerning preterm behavior and development, and for support of the mother. Such home visits can gradually be phased out as the mother becomes more confident and when the child becomes enrolled in an educational enrichment program, if available.

POINTS TO REMEMBER

1. Correct for gestational age (preterm birth) until at least 3 years of age.
2. Do not emphasize to the parents the many abnormalities observed during the 3-month postdischarge period of convalescence, because most are transient and have little prognostic significance.
3. Be available, be honest, be optimistic. After the initial diagnosis of abnormality is made, most children show improvement, restitution, and growth.
4. The majority of high-risk children do well.
5. In some cases, the diagnosis of cerebral palsy, hydrocephalus, or blindness is made during the first year of life. Early intervention and supportive psychological help that can be facilitated by the follow-up clinic are crucial.
6. Except when a severe neurologic or sensory disorder persists, ultimate development depends on parental education, social class, the child's genetic potential, and the environment. For children of extremely low birth weight and short gestation, neonatal risk factors tend to predominate.[3]
7. The functional capacity attained is more important than the medical diagnosis of abnormality.

EARLY CHILDHOOD OUTCOMES

A summary of some outcome variables for extremely immature and low-birth-weight infants is presented in Table 19-2. The importance of early identification of developmental deficits to plan and establish early appropriate interventions should be emphasized. Developmental outcomes of children are influenced by many risk factors, including social, genetic, and biologic ones.

EDITORIAL COMMENT: Hintz et al compared neurodevelopmental outcomes at 18 to 22 months' corrected age for infants born with extremely low birth weight at an estimated gestational age of less than 25 weeks during two periods: 1999 to 2001 (epoch 1) and 2002 to 2004 (epoch 2).[27] Infant survival in epoch 1 (35.4%) and epoch 2 (32.3%) was similar. Cesarean delivery, surgery for patent ductus arteriosus, and late sepsis were more common in epoch 2, but postnatal steroid use was dramatically reduced (63.5% in epoch 1 versus 32.8% in epoch 2; *P* <.0001). Moderate to severe cerebral palsy was diagnosed in 11% and the Mental Developmental Index was less than 70 in 50% of surviving infants in epoch 1, whereas cerebral palsy in 15% and a Mental Developmental Index of less than 70 in 59% were noted in epoch 2. Hence, adverse outcomes were common in both epochs and were unchanged between the two periods.

SCHOOL-AGE OUTCOMES

At school age, children are required to conform to formal learning in a classroom. Many have difficulty in this regard because of attention and other neuropsychologic deficits, including poor memory, visuomotor, and fine and gross motor function, and difficulty with spatial concepts and executive function.[28] Children who were born preterm are often also shy and withdrawn and have social difficulties as well as behavioral problems, including attention-deficit/hyperactivity disorder and symptoms of depression or anxiety.

EDITORIAL COMMENT: The EPICure study is an ongoing longitudinal evaluation of extremely premature infants born in the United Kingdom and the Republic of Ireland between March and December 1995. The cohort consists of the 308 children who were 20 to 25 weeks' gestational age at birth and survived beyond the first year after birth. Johnson et al assessed the academic attainment and special educational needs in 219 (71%) of these children at 11 years of age and compared them with those of 153 classmates born at term using standardized tests of cognitive ability and academic attainment and teacher reports of school performance and special educational needs.[29] Extremely preterm children had significantly lower scores than classmates on cognitive ability (−20 points; 95% confidence interval [CI]: −23 to −17), reading (−18 points; 95% CI: −22 to −15), and mathematics (−27 points; 95% CI: −31 to −23). Twenty nine (13%) extremely preterm children attended special schools. Among extremely preterm children in mainstream schools, 105 (57%) had special educational needs and 103 (55%) required special educational needs resource provision. Teachers rated 50% of extremely preterm children as having below average attainment compared with 5% of classmates. Overall 40% of the cohort has moderate to severe cognitive impairment (>2 SD from the mean) compared with 1.3% of classmates. Boys were twice as likely as girls to have a serious impairment, but the prevalence was not significantly different for children born at 23, 24, and 25 weeks of gestation. Extremely preterm children who entered compulsory education an academic year early because of preterm birth had similar academic attainment but required more special educational needs support. The investigators concluded that survivors of extremely preterm birth remain at high risk of learning impairments and poor academic attainment in middle childhood. Papile noted, "The high prevalence of intellectual and learning difficulties suggests that a disruption/delay of global brain development rather than a specific lesion may be the underlying cause".[25]

Taylor et al reviewed the topic of mathematics deficiencies in children with very low birth weight or very preterm birth.[30] They noted that children with birth weights of less than 1.5 kg and those with a gestational age of less than 32 weeks have more mathematics disabilities or deficiencies and higher rates of mathematics learning disabilities than normal-birth-weight, term-born children. They commented, "mathematics disabilities or deficiencies are found even in children without global disorders in cognition or neurosensory status even when IQ is controlled, and they are associated with other learning problems and weaknesses in perceptual motor abilities and executive function. Factors related to poorer mathematics outcomes include lower birth weight and gestational age, neonatal complications, and possible abnormalities in brain structure." Little is known about mathematics disabilities or deficiencies. Thus, although the outcomes have improved overall, there is no room for complacency. Understanding the mechanisms of injury may help to provide the solutions, because neuroplasticity is known to permit the neonatal brain to move a given function to a different location as a consequence of normal experience or brain damage.

YOUNG ADULT OUTCOMES

The initial survivors of the early years of neonatal intensive care in the 1970s are now adults. The results, to date, reveal that although these individuals may have a lower IQ on formal testing and fewer attend college than normal-birth-weight, term-born controls, they function fairly well and with few exceptions are satisfied with their health-related quality of life, which when studied is similar to that of controls.[31] Very low-birth-weight young adults also demonstrate less risk-taking behavior than normal-birth-weight controls, including alcohol use, drug abuse, and delinquent activities. Rates of attention-deficit/hyperactivity disorder tend to decrease during young adulthood, although symptoms of depression and withdrawal have been reported in women.[31]

Overwhelming evidence is accumulating that the neurodevelopmental consequences of extremely preterm birth extend far beyond the confines of cerebral palsy (a static lesion) and intellectual delay. Problems in attention, executive function, memory, spatial skills, fine and gross motor function, speech and language, visual integration, and mathematics, together with behavioral disorders, are common. *Executive function* refers to a collection of processes that are responsible for purposeful, goal-directed behavior, such as planning, setting goals, initiating, using problem-solving strategies, and monitoring thoughts and behavior. Executive functioning is important for a child's intellectual development, behavior, emotional control, and social interaction. Luu et al evaluated executive and memory function in 337 adolescents born preterm compared with that in term-born controls at 16 years.[32] After adolescents with neurosensory disabilities and those with an IQ of less than 70 were excluded, adolescents born preterm, compared with term controls, were found to show deficits in executive function on tasks of verbal fluency, inhibition, cognitive flexibility, planning and organization, and working memory as well as verbal and visuospatial memory. The presence of these deficits was associated with severe brain injury as detected by neonatal ultrasonography and lower maternal educational level. This implies that providing a more stimulating and enriched home environment may be of some benefit in averting executive function deficits.

REFERENCES

The reference list for this chapter can be found online at www.expertconsult.com.

Ethical Issues in the Perinatal Period

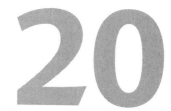

Jonathan M. Fanaroff and
Lawrence J. Nelson

Despite great advances in perinatal medicine, not all newborns born alive can stay alive or survive without experiencing severe—perhaps even devastating—physical and mental problems. This is particularly true for extremely preterm infants (approximately 24 to 27 weeks' gestation), who have a survival rate of approximately 75%.[1] Thus, many extremely low-birth-weight infants can and do survive despite being born much too soon, although they often experience significant long-term problems such as chronic lung disease, short gut syndrome, neurologic and cognitive abnormalities, poor growth, blindness, and chronic illness.[2]

In at least some of these cases, physicians, nurses, or parents raise questions about whether initial or continued aggressive treatment is ethically correct, who should make these decisions, and what criteria they should use. These questions have been publicly asked and answered in a variety of ways since 1973 when Duff and Campbell acknowledged that they, their neonatal intensive care unit (NICU) staff, and the involved parents allowed some infants to die because of their poor chances of survival or of having a reasonable quality of life.[3] No single standard of care exists in this area, and indeed one commentator has noted that this area of bioethics remains "as intractable today as it was 30 years ago, when it began to be publicly discussed."[4] Studies have shown what clinical experience and common sense posit: physicians' practices regarding the use or withholding of resuscitative therapy in the NICU are not consistent.[5]

This chapter explores some answers to these enduring and fundamental questions by presenting and commenting on an actual case. In doing so, it considers the most pressing questions and dominant myths about forgoing treatment of newborns and briefly explains why the myths should be discarded by ethical and humane practitioners of neonatal medicine. These myths deserve attention because they are both widely held and dangerous to the interests of infants, parents, and medicine. Unnecessary legalism, improper disenfranchisement of parents, simplistic reliance on a single popular standard of questionable meaning, and rejection of quality-of-life considerations are still the deepest and most insidious traps into which physicians and nurses caring for newborns fall.

THE CASE

Mark and Karla Miller filed a negligence lawsuit against a hospital, Women's Hospital of Texas, and the company that owns the hospital, Columbia/HCA Healthcare Corporation, following the premature birth of their daughter, Sydney. She was born at 23 weeks' gestation and weighed 615 g. The parents claimed that the hospital had "callously ignored the couple's request not to artificially prolong the child's life at birth" and that resuscitating such an underdeveloped baby amounted to "medical experimentation on humans." They also accused the hospital of being motivated to impose treatment to collect the large revenues that would thereby be generated.

Mrs. Miller had developed chorioamnionitis, and she was hospitalized. "With her own life in potential danger, she and her husband agreed with the doctor to induce labor." They were notified about the "uncertain odds of survival in such a young pregnancy" and the "baby's unlikely prospects for survival so early in pregnancy." After "much agonizing," they decided to have the baby delivered (following induction) but "to let nature take its course." According to the parents' lawyer, they saw it as "God's will" if the newborn had "not developed to the extent that it could survive without artificial means"; they wanted no "special heroics" performed. The parents claimed they had repeatedly requested that doctors not resuscitate the newborn if she had not developed adequately to sustain life on her own.

Although the obstetrician and neonatologist agreed with the parents that comfort care was a very reasonable option, the hospital administrator of the NICU allegedly told the father that the hospital had a policy requiring resuscitation of any infant that weighed more than 500 g, although she was never able to produce a written policy to this effect. She also allegedly informed the father that "his only option would be to take his wife to another hospital, which he could not risk because of her condition." When the father said he would be in the delivery room and would stop physicians from performing resuscitation, this administrator said police would be called to remove him from the premises.

The hospital disputed the parents' version of the facts and claimed it had an ethical and legal obligation to keep the baby alive. It denied that treatment decisions were related to financial considerations, that its administrator had made any threats or statement to the father as he had alleged, and that it had any responsibility for medical decisions that were made by the physicians and family involved. It claimed that the attending physicians had drafted a "birth plan" with the parents' full consent and produced several consent forms signed by the father for medical services.

Furthermore, the father allegedly never questioned the physician's actions to keep the child alive either in the delivery room or later. The hospital also asserted that the physicians honored the parents' decision not to restart the infant's heart if she went into arrest. However, she had a heartbeat when born, although her "lungs and other vital organs" were not working at birth, and received vigorous treatment.

Sydney was born with her eyelids fused shut and is legally blind. She remained hospitalized for nearly a year at a cost of about $1 million. She is severely brain damaged and requires extensive care, because she is almost totally incapacitated. Her mother ended her career as an equities fund broker to care for her daughter full time because the family could not afford the $200,000 annual cost of professional care.

Eleven days after the start of the trial and after 2 days of deliberations, the jury returned a $42.9 million verdict against the hospital and Columbia/HCA by a vote of 10 to 2: $29.4 million for the costs of the child's past and future medical care and $13.5 million in punitive damages. Pretrial interest of $22.4 million on the damages awarded made the total verdict worth $65.3 million. The parents' lawyer stated that the key issue was "who will make the basic medical decisions—families or medical specialists who do not have to live with the consequences." One juror reported that he and other jurors believed the Millers

rather than the hospital and that there was evidence that indicated "arrogance" on the part of the hospital and Columbia/HCA.

Defense witnesses had testified that the care delivered to both the mother and infant met the applicable standard of care and that "the newborn's condition was adequate enough to require them to try to sustain life." These witnesses also stated that denying "proper care could subject the doctors to penalties and sanctions, or even suit alleging negligence."

The case generated considerable attention, and one can read the large punitive damage award as a clear signal by the jury that it supported the parents in this case and disapproved of the actions of the hospital. In the end, however, the Millers did not receive any compensation because the verdict was overturned on appeal, with the Texas Supreme Court creating an "emergent circumstances" exception whereby a physician in Texas may resuscitate an infant in the delivery room without first obtaining parental consent.[4] The sharp difference between the opinion of the jury and the reasoning of the court raise a number of important ethical questions.

This case report is based on four articles published in the Houston Chronicle on January 6, 1998 (Section A, p. 9), January 17, 1998 (Section A, p. 1), January 31, 1998 (Section A, p. 29), and April 18, 1998 (Section A, p. 36). Unless otherwise indicated, all direct quotes are taken from these articles.

DISCUSSION

Is there a legal and ethical obligation to resuscitate all newborns and continue providing treatment until a child is imminently dying?

Some, perhaps many, physicians and nurses believe that no choice exists but to resuscitate every newborn infant in the delivery room, no matter how small, and continue aggressive medical treatment in the NICU until he or she is headed inevitably and imminently toward death. Once the infant has shown itself to be close to death despite aggressive medical management, then and only then can physicians and parents choose to withhold or withdraw life-sustaining treatment.

First, it is incorrect to claim either that all infants are in fact resuscitated at birth or that the standard of care requires that they be resuscitated. In one cross-cultural study of neonatal deaths, 29 of the 183 neonatal deaths (16%) occurred in infants who received comfort care instead of cardiopulmonary resuscitation at delivery.[6] Other articles in the medical literature support the position that resuscitation in the delivery room is not professionally and ethically required in all cases.[5] In addition, the Neonatal Resuscitation Program, created jointly by the American Academy of Pediatrics and the American Heart Association, specifically recognizes that there are situations in which it is ethical not to initiate resuscitation.[7]

Second, it is false to claim on the merits that a strict ethical and legal obligation exists to resuscitate every newborn regardless of his or her condition, prognosis, or parental desires about resuscitation. For example, if prenatal testing and ultrasonography had unambiguously detected anencephaly, the parents had given their informed consent to nontreatment, and this condition was clearly present at birth, no obligation to resuscitate such an infant would exist because of his or her permanent unconsciousness, the nature of the anomaly, and the reasonableness of the parents' determination of what they feel is in the best interests of the child.

In other words, there may be cases in which enough can be known about a child's diagnosis and prognosis before birth that a parental decision to decline aggressive resuscitation is morally justified and within the bounds of parental discretion. Such cases are likely to involve an infant with one of the following diagnoses: confirmed gestational age of less than 23 weeks or a birth weight of less than 400 g, anencephaly, and confirmed lethal genetic disorder or malformation.

On the other hand, an extremely premature infant can be born alive with no prenatal indication of any specific anomaly or disease, and his or her medical condition and prognosis might be so uncertain that the attending physicians cannot honestly assess the particular child's prospects for survival and outcome at birth. In this situation or a similar one, the physicians and nurses could conclude that they were under an ethical obligation to resuscitate the child initially because of uncertainty about his or her true diagnosis and prognosis. If this is the case, however, they would also be obligated promptly to ascertain more accurately the particular child's medical condition and the prospects for a life not characterized by excessive pain, burdensome interventions, or inability to consciously interact with others.

From this point of view, the absence of reasonably accurate medical information at birth needed to ground the value judgment that must inevitably be made about forgoing treatment renders a parental decision against initial resuscitation uninformed, poorly (if at all) justified, and not prima facie morally binding on the health care providers. Even assuming the validity of this rationale, it still remains true that after more clinical information has been gathered and more deliberation has occurred, the physicians, nurses, and hospital should then respect parental decisions to forgo further treatment in appropriate cases.

The father in the Miller case testified that both the obstetrician and the neonatologist were bleak about the future prospects for their child. The Millers were told that the hospital had "never had such a premature infant live and that anything they did to sustain the infant's life would be guesswork." The Neonatal Resuscitation Program explicitly recognizes that parents have the primary role in determining what is in the best interests of their child. Their decision, however, must be based on the best information available, which may not be obtainable until after delivery. In general, infants who will die tend to declare themselves early, although this period has grown increasingly longer, from 2 to 3 days in the early 1990s to 10 days in 2001.[8] Waiting a few days to reflect on forgoing treatment may generate more clinical information and greater predictability about the child's diagnosis and prognosis.

Whatever the merits of this brief moral analysis, it is a myth that the *law* requires all infants to receive aggressive resuscitation and treatment until they are imminently dying. The ultimate source of this myth is the so-called "Baby Doe" law, the Child Abuse Amendments of 1984.[9] These amendments to the Child Abuse Prevention and Treatment Act (CAPTA)[10] and the implementing regulations issued by the Department of Health and Human Services (DHHS)[11] constitute the Baby Doe laws that are currently in effect in the United States. These laws require each state to establish certain procedures for reporting alleged instances of "medical neglect," including the withholding of "medically indicated treatment," to local child protective services and for investigating such reports—*if* the state wishes to receive federal child abuse prevention grants. On their face, the DHHS regulations permit treatment to be forgone only in very limited circumstances.

Many physicians are under the impression that the Baby Doe law directly imposes on them certain duties to care for newborns and that they will suffer federal penalties if they fail to do so. These laws, however, do *not* apply directly to physicians or parents of critically ill newborns; they only require states receiving federal funds to do certain things. The obligation of individual medical professionals to report instances of child abuse or neglect, including medical neglect, arises out of the law of an individual state, not the federal Baby Doe law. The substantive legal standards applicable to a determination of whether a particular decision by a physician and parents to forgo life-sustaining treatment of a newborn as unacceptable are established by state law, not by the Baby Doe law.

State law typically does not contain explicit or detailed standards for determining when treatment is being improperly withheld or withdrawn from a child. California, for example, requires physicians and other licensed providers to report as child neglect parental refusals of "adequate medical care," but not when the parents have made an "informed and appropriate medical decision" after consulting with a physician who has actually examined the child.[12] Because there is no statutory definition of "informed and appropriate medical decision," the practical meaning of the term is left to clinicians, who must decide whether an "inappropriate" medical decision has been made and consequently whether they are going to make a report to child protective services.

The legacy of the Baby Doe law has been mixed. Shortly after its passage, one veteran clinician lamented that the Baby Doe law was "usually taken as a mandate to rescue many infants by the application of available technology, even though families and their health and other advisors often hold that quality of life and other considerations, including staggering costs and low benefits, clearly support a different choice."

He accused an influential portion of the medical profession of helping the federal government to create "a law, which, chiefly on ideological or biological grounds, often mandates treatment that careful reflection by those most intimately involved finds inappropriate."[13]

In addition, at least one court has interpreted CAPTA to mean that resuscitation is required even for a 23-week infant. In *Montalvo v Borkovec*, a negligence suit was brought by the parents of Emanuel Vila against the obstetrician and neonatologist for resuscitating him after he was born at 23 weeks weighing 679 g.[14] The parents claimed that they were not sufficiently informed of the risk of disability to Emanuel and therefore the consent for his birth (via cesarean section) and resuscitation was not informed. The Court of Appeals of Wisconsin, however, sharply disagreed that informed consent was necessary:

> First, requiring the informed consent process here presumes that a right to decide not to resuscitate the newly born child or to withhold life-sustaining medical care actually existed. This premise is faulty.

The court went on to interpret CAPTA to mean that, under these circumstances, the parents "did not have the right to withhold or withdraw immediate postnatal care from him."[14] As a state appellate court decision, it may not have much impact outside of Wisconsin. Nevertheless, if similar reasoning is adopted by the courts, it would effectively remove decision making from the parent-physician dyad.

Not only have legal cases addressed the issue, but legislation was passed in 2002 that has led to some confusion with respect to the treatment of extremely premature or disabled infants. The Born-Alive Infants Protection Act, Public Law No. 107-207, was passed by Congress in 2002. The law states that infants who are born alive, no matter what the circumstances or stage of development, are "persons who are entitled to the protections of the law." The Neonatal Resuscitation Program Steering Committee does not believe that the law should "in any way affect the approach that physicians currently follow with respect to the extremely premature infant."[15] There are concerns, however, that the law may "potentially resurrect dormant governmental oversight of newborn-treatment decisions and thus may have influence over normative neonatal practice."[16]

Parents of extremely sick newborns such as those in the Miller and Montalvo cases often want no "special heroics" (a vague and ambiguous phrase that always needs specific interpretation and explanation) even at birth because they are afraid that once the physicians start to treat, they will refuse to stop until the child is literally a few minutes or hours from death. Ultimately, however, careful attention to the humane and compassionate treatment of disabled and severely ill newborns is the caregiver's primary ethical duty. To the extent that excessive fear of legal liabilities in the past has led physicians to overtreat infants with very poor prognoses and thereby cause them (and others) suffering with no corresponding benefit, or to disenfranchise parents from giving informed consent to the treatment of their infants because "the law" has made the decision for them, we all have been done a profound disservice, most especially the infants who are supposed to be the ones served by the physicians who care for them.

Should physicians or hospitals, rather than parents, make decisions to forgo resuscitation or treatment of an extremely low-birth-weight newborn?

Parents of severely ill newborns are frequently disenfranchised, in whole or in part, from participating in the decisions pertaining to their child's medical treatment. There are a number of reasons for this phenomenon. First, as discussed earlier, physicians are intimidated by what they often misunderstand to be the legal restrictions on forgoing treatment of a newborn. In fairness, they also are probably genuinely puzzled about the ethics of the matter. As a result, though, they have serious trouble identifying the legal and ethical boundaries of medical and parental discretion in deciding to let a newborn die by forgoing life-sustaining treatment.[17] Peremptorily ignoring parental requests to consider forgoing treatment or adopting a policy of never forgoing treatment before a child's death is inevitable and imminent eliminates the need to confront and practically resolve the underlying ethical issue.[18]

Second, at least some physicians simply consider themselves to be best qualified and solely responsible for determining the medical fate of their infant patients. Indeed, in one survey of neonatologists only about one third responded that parental preference would influence their decision on delivery room resuscitation.[5]

Third, many physicians and nurses assume that parents of severely ill newborns are so influenced by anxiety, grief, and guilt that they could not possibly make good decisions about their child's fate. They may even distrust the motives and character of any parent who wants anything other than full, aggressive treatment. Finally, physicians and nurses commonly experience serious difficulty both coping with the inherent

uncertainty of their diagnoses and prognoses and trying to explain this uncertainty to parents.

Whatever its causes, routine disqualification of parents from participating in the medical treatment plans for their newborns is wrong. Parents have rather broad legal and moral authority to give or withhold their consent to treatment of their children, although this authority is certainly *not* unlimited. The President's Commission for the Study of Ethical Problems in Medicine and Biomedical and Behavioral Research rightly notes that there is a presumption, strong but rebuttable, that parents are the appropriate decision makers for their infants. Traditional law concerning the family, buttressed by the emerging constitutional right of privacy, protects a substantial role for parental discretion for parents.[19]

Similarly, the U.S. Supreme Court has affirmed that the "decision to provide or withhold medically indicated treatment is, except in highly unusual circumstances, made by the parents or legal guardian."[20]

Parents have unique natural bonds of love for and loyalty to a child. The child is their flesh and blood and exists in a family they have created. Of course, not all parents treat their children properly, and they can make unacceptably poor decisions about treatment in some cases. Nevertheless, in the absence of strong evidence to the contrary, one must assume that the parents are the proper decision makers. Furthermore, there is no assurance that strangers—be they physicians, nurses, judges, or lawyers—who have no bonds of love or loyalty to a child, will make a better decision about treatment than the parents.[17]

Assuming it is true that the Millers had repeatedly requested that physicians not resuscitate their child if she had not developed adequately to sustain her own life and that the hospital (and presumably the attending physicians and nurses as well) "callously disregarded the couple's request," then the health care providers improperly ignored the parents' presumptive moral and legal authority to make medical decisions for their child. Even if the providers conscientiously disagree with the parents, they have the obligation to express the factual and moral grounds for their disagreement clearly and plainly. More important, they are obliged to disclose whether and under what circumstances they will honor parental decisions to refuse treatment. Even though ultimately overturned, the jury's verdict should serve as a stern warning to physicians, nurses, and hospitals that ignoring parental wishes, particularly in an arrogant and peremptory manner, does not sit well with the public and may carry legal consequences.

One important principle of pediatric ethics is that physicians, nurses, and other clinicians do have independent ethical obligations to the child. Clinicians are not just the tools of the parents' wishes; they are moral agents who bear responsibility for the child as well. The medical team, together with the child's parents, should be deciding how best to care for a severely ill newborn. Clinicians should provide parents with honest and accurate disclosure of both the child's medical diagnosis and prognosis (with any attendant uncertainty) and their own carefully thought out recommendation for a plan of action in light of relevant ethical, medical, and legal considerations. But they may not simply ignore the parents. The jury's verdict in the Miller case shows that members of the public will not automatically defer to the clinicians or hospital and permit them to act arrogantly toward parents who, quite literally, have to live with the consequences of all the medical decisions that are made on behalf of their children.

EDITORIAL COMMENT: Although in the Miller case the parents did not wish resuscitation, often the parents demand resuscitation against the advice of the physician. It is important to appreciate that parents are moving away from a tacit acceptance of physician determination of lethality; they want more say, more information, and more time. In addition, a powerful influence on parents' decisions is being exerted by information on the Internet, which tends to engender an expectation that full resuscitation is a reasonable approach. This does not mean that parents have the only voice. Ceding authority for ethically troubling issues out of respect for parental autonomy can lead to an "ethic of abdication" of professional obligation to the newborn infant (and the parents). We do need to avoid characterizing these types of conflict as clashes in abstract principles—between respect for parental autonomy and physician beneficence—and learn how to harmonize these principles.

J. Hellmann, MBBCh, FRCPC, MHSc

Assuming, then, that decisions to forgo treatment of severely ill newborns ought to be in the hands of the attending clinicians *and* of the child's parents—and *not* the law

except in very rare cases—there remains the question of what standards should be used to make such decisions.

Is the "best interests of the child" the only standard that should be used in making decisions to forgo treatment of newborns and does it have a clear and generally accepted meaning?

The "best interests of the child" constitutes the single most popular principle brought to bear on the controversial subject of forgoing life-sustaining treatment of a child. Many commentators believe that the infant's best interests is the *sole* ethical criterion upon which to base an ethically defensible decision, although these same people disagree on unavoidably related subjects such as which infants should be treated, which conditions count as exceptions to the general duty to preserve life, and whether parents, physicians, and/or ethics committees ought to have a major role in the decision.[21]

Although the standard has remained a cornerstone of pediatric ethics, commentators have long questioned its coherence and adequacy as a substantive ethical principle. Over two decades ago Brody criticized the best interests standard as trying not only to make a very complex matter simple, but also magically to avoid abuse of parental discretion in deciding against treatment (as occurred in the original Baby Doe of Bloomington case).[22] Brody sees decisions to forgo treatment of newborns as inherently complex in light of (1) the near impossibility of having a reliable prognosis, (2) the medical and social differences between newborns and adults, (3) the difficulty predicting which medical interventions will help and which will hurt the child, and (4) the vast differences among families in adapting to the substantial changes that must occur in the life of a family with a severely ill newborn. His analysis of the best interests standard remains insightful and relevant even today and deserves careful consideration.

Among other things, Brody's criticism of the best interests standard rests upon the following factors: (1) an infant's interests are unknowable, (2) the best interests standard can yield results that seem inhumane, and (3) the interests of persons other than the infant deserve consideration at least in certain circumstances.

With respect to the first factor, Brody argues that once we move beyond basic needs such as food and shelter, we cannot really know what is in someone's interests without knowing a good deal about that person's individual plans and desires about life. But a newborn has no such plans or desires. He offers the example of two neonatologists arguing over how aggressively to treat an infant born with a high meningomyelocele and hydrocephalus. One argues that the infant's best interests are served by early surgical intervention, noting the high probability of death or life with worse neurodevelopmental outcome without surgery. She cites the occasional success story of an infant with an equally severe defect who turned out to have only mild cognitive and physical impairment. The other argues that an early death is in the infant's best interests and points to the very high odds of major mental and physical handicap, plus the need for repeated, painful surgeries to treat the condition and its sequelae. Brody correctly points out that what these physicians are really arguing about is what *they* think ought to be done. The phrase "the infant's best interests" is a rhetorical flourish that does no useful work in the discussion.

Second, the best interests standard can yield inhumane or unjust results because it implies that whenever the benefits of treatment outweigh burdens even to a slight degree, that fact alone fixes an obligation to treat—even if the benefits are minuscule or the burdens horrendous. He cites the case of children so severely impaired as to be unable to recognize other people or form any human relationship, who can perceive only primitive sensations such as light and color, but show no sign of suffering. Because such children get some primitive pleasure out of living and suffer little, a best interests analysis would require that any newborn with such a future have its life prolonged, even by invasive or aggressive means. Brody claims that to save a child in order to let it live such a life "may well do nothing of real, substantial benefit for the child."

Finally, Brody agrees with Strong[23] that the refusal to consider any interests other than the infant's own is an arbitrary rather than a principled ethical choice, although this refusal is required by the best interests standard. In the many cases in which treatment will result in clear and substantial benefits to the infant, then its interests override those of others. However, in other cases in which the benefit to the infant is less or more questionable, then the interests of the family ought to be factored into the decision.

In summary, despite its popularity and frequent invocation, the best interests standard as traditionally understood is not necessarily either the best or the most intelligible one to use in making ethical decisions concerning newborns. Physicians, other clinicians, and parents should be considering a complex set of factors when making decisions about newborns and should be careful in concluding just what the "best interests of the infant" may mean in any given case.

Is the present and future quality of an infant's life relevant to a decision to forgo resuscitation or life-sustaining treatment of a premature or seriously ill newborn?

It is a myth that an infant's quality of life is utterly irrelevant to a decision to forgo treatment, although this claim is false only in its extreme form. The appeal to quality of life can be both false and pernicious when it is made in a manner that sanctions nontreatment of children who are only mildly physically or intellectually impaired, or when it is taken to mean that the simple presence of physical disability or mental retardation is a sufficient reason to deny treatment. Denying medically needed treatment to a child *simply* because the child has Down syndrome (trisomy 21) or some form of spina bifida *is* a misuse of quality of life as an ethically proper consideration in forgoing treatment.

The alleged complete irrelevance of quality-of-life considerations is false, however, and moreover potentially inhumane, when it is taken to mean that the life expectancy of a child, his or her level of physical and intellectual functioning, and the relative burdens and benefits of treatment make no difference whatsoever when parents and clinicians decide to intervene medically. The irrelevance of quality of life is typically embedded in the application of a "medical benefit" standard, which holds that medical intervention must occur when it is likely, in the exercise of reasonable medical judgment, to bring about its intended medical result. The use of such a medical benefit standard not only blindly falls into the trap of the technologic imperative (whatever can be done, should be done), but also denies that medicine is an enterprise devoted to benefitting an individual person whose life in the world cannot be reduced to the technical "success" of an operation, a medicine, or a machine. Put differently, people are not meant to be the passive objects of medical technology.

Consider the generally accepted view that newborns with anencephaly should not receive any life-prolonging treatment other than basic supportive care. This view is usually justified on the basis that children lacking a cerebral cortex are irreversibly dying and should not have their agony prolonged. However, on closer analysis, this justification is flawed in several ways. First, although it is true that such infants cannot live indefinitely, it is not true that their deaths are necessarily imminent. Most anencephalic infants die *quickly* precisely because they do not receive any treatment, which is a human choice rather than a fact of nature. Indeed, some babies with anencephaly have lived for several years. Thus, if we choose to, we could keep at least some of these infants alive for quite some time.

Second, because anencephalic infants are permanently unconscious, they experience neither agony nor pain nor anything else during their lives. Deciding not to treat them aggressively does not truly spare them any unpleasantness. More honestly put, it is ethically proper not to resuscitate and treat such newborns aggressively precisely because they have no ability to survive indefinitely and no capability of experiencing even primitive human interaction. In other words, they have an unacceptably poor quality of life.

Paradoxically, the Baby Doe law and its implementing regulations contain an *express* condemnation of quality-of-life considerations and yet also contain two exceptions to the general duty to preserve an infant's life that rest upon quality of life. The first exception approves of forgoing treatment when the infant is "chronically and irreversibly comatose." Because some of these infants could live indefinitely and the exception does not depend upon their imminent demise, the only justification left for not treating them is their poor quality of life: unconscious infants have no potential for human life as we understand it, and thus there is no ethical obligation to prolong their lives.

The second exception encompasses treatment that would be "virtually futile in terms of the survival of the infant and the treatment itself under such circumstances would be inhumane." Thus, treatment can be withheld because the infant's quality of life would be seriously compromised by the pain and burden of intervention and the lack of compensating benefit. At bottom, medical procedures are "inhumane" and contraindicated only because of certain features pertaining directly to the infant's quality of life.

Although quality of life may be relevant, physicians need to be extremely careful about their own personal biases. Empirical studies of children with cerebral palsy using self-reported quality-of-life questionnaires found that they had scores comparable to those of their peers without cerebral palsy.[24] These results are similar to those of other studies which have shown that neonatal "survivors who subsequently develop impairment may live happier lives than doctors imagine."[25]

In summary, virtually all medical interventions have some risk attached: pain, side effects, complications, even death. As noted by the American Medical Association Code of Medical Ethics, determining what is in the best interests of a seriously ill newborn involves a number of difficult considerations, including the following:

- The chance that the therapy will succeed
- The risks involved in treatment and nontreatment
- The degree to which the therapy, if successful, will extend life
- The pain and discomfort associated with the therapy
- The anticipated quality of life of the newborn with and without treatment[26]

Although for many people, a life worth living should hold at least some potential for interaction with others, this potential does not have to be that for normal or near normal intelligence. In addition, physicians must be very careful not to underestimate the quality of someone's life. Quality of life is not an inherently dirty or discriminatory concept, although it does contain potential danger. But this is true of medicine itself: it can do great good, but it can also cause bitter suffering and loss. We should not abandon medicine because its results are not always happy. Nor should we abandon the quest to determine what is best for a newborn just because doing so is challenging.

REFERENCES

The reference list for this chapter can be found online at www.expertconsult.com.

Drugs Used for Emergency and Cardiac Indications in Newborns

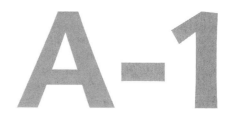

Jacquelyn McClary

Agent	Dosage	Comments
Adenosine (Adenocard)	50 µg/kg rapid IV (over 1-2 sec) followed immediately by NS flush Increase dose every 2 min by 50-µg/kg increments if no response; max dose 250 µg/kg	Facial flushing, irritability, and transient arrhythmias (asystole) may occur. Apnea in a premature infant has been reported. Monitor ECG and blood pressure continuously during administration.
Alprostadil (prostaglandin E1)	Starting dose: 0.05-0.1 µg/kg/min continuous IV infusion Maintenance dose: after response observed titrate down to lowest effective dose, which may be as low as 0.01 µg/kg/min	May cause apnea, fever, hypotension, and flushing.
Amiodarone	Loading dose: 5 mg/kg IV over 30-60 min Maintenance dose: 7-15 µg/kg/min continuous IV infusion	Monitor ECG and blood pressure continuously for bradycardia and hypotension. Administration into central line preferred to minimize risk of extravasation.
Atropine	0.01-0.03 mg/kg IV push or IM Repeat every 10-15 min to max 0.04 mg/kg May be given via endotracheal tube	Low dosages may result in paradoxical bradycardia.
Calcium chloride 10% (27 mg elemental Ca^{2+} per mL)	35-70 mg/kg (0.35-0.7 mL/kg), 10-20 mg/kg elemental calcium IV over 10-30 min	Dilute with NS to a final concentration of 20 mg/mL. Stop infusion if HR <100. Extravasation may lead to tissue necrosis.
Calcium gluconate 10% (9.3 mg Ca^{2+} per mL)	Emergency dose: 100-200 mg/kg (1-2 mL/kg), 10-20 mg/kg elemental calcium IV over 10-30 min Maintenance dose in IV fluids: 200-800 mg/kg/day (20-80 mg/kg/day elemental calcium)	Dilute with NS to a final concentration of 50 mg/mL. Stop infusion if HR <100. Extravasation may lead to tissue necrosis.
Digoxin	Loading dose (digitalization): divided into 3 doses over 24 hr given by slow IV push or PO PMA ≤29 wk: 15 µg/kg IV or 20 µg/kg PO PMA 30-36 wk: 20 µg/kg IV or 25 µg/kg PO PMA 37-48 wk: 30 µg/kg IV or 40 µg/kg PO PMA ≥49 wk: 40 µg/kg IV or 50 µg/kg PO Maintenance dose: PMA ≤29 wk: 4 µg/kg IV or 5 µg/kg PO q24h PMA 30-36 wk: 5 µg/kg IV or 6 µg/kg PO q24h PMA 37-48 wk: 4 µg/kg IV or 5 µg/kg PO q12h PMA ≥49 wk: 5 µg/kg IV or 6 µg/kg PO q12h	Avoid hypokalemia, hypomagnesemia, hypocalcemia, and hypercalcemia. Assess renal function. Monitor HR rate and heart rhythm. Follow serum drug concentrations with a target range of 1-2 ng/mL.
Dobutamine	2-25 µg/kg/min continuous IV infusion	Tachycardia may occur at high dosages. Hypotension risk increases in hypovolemic patients. Tissue ischemia with extravasation; inject phentolamine into affected area as soon as possible.

Continued

Agent	Dosage	Comments
Dopamine	2-20 µg/kg/min continuous IV infusion "Renal dose": 2-5 µg/kg/min Cardiac stimulation: 5-15 µg/kg/min Vasoconstriction: >5 µg/kg/min	Pharmacologic effect is dose dependent. Extravasation may lead to necrosis; inject phentolamine into affected area as soon as possible.
Epinephrine	Emergency dose: 0.01-0.03 mg/kg (0.1-0.3 mL/kg of 1:10,000 concentration) IV push; 0.1 mg/kg ET followed by 1 mL NS Continuous IV infusion: 0.02-1 µg/kg/min	Monitor HR and blood pressure continuously. Infiltration may cause tissue necrosis; inject phentolamine into affected area as soon as possible.
Esmolol (Brevibloc)	Supraventricular tachycardia: 100 µg/kg/min continuous IV infusion; increase by 50-100 µg/kg/min every 5 min; usual max 200 µg/kg/min Postoperative hypertension: 50 µg/kg/min continuous IV infusion; increase by 25-50 µg/kg/min every 5 min; usual max 200 µg/kg/min	Monitor ECG continuously. May cause hypotension at high dosages.
Hydralazine (Apresoline)	0.1-0.5 mg/kg/dose IV or IM q6-8h; increase gradually to max 2 mg/kg/dose q6h 0.25-1 mg/kg/dose PO q6-8h, or twice the IV dose	Administration with a β-blocker may increase antihypertensive effect and decrease the hydralazine dose required.
Ibuprofen lysine (NeoProfen)	First dose: 10 mg/kg IV over 15 min Second and third doses (starting 24 hr after first dose): 5 mg/kg IV over 15 min q24h	Monitor urine output and signs of bleeding.
Indomethacin (Indocin)	3 doses given IV over 30 min q12-24h Age at first dose determines dosing regimen: <48 hr: 0.2/0.1/0.1 mg/kg 2-7 days: 0.2/0.2/0.2 mg/kg >7 days: 0.2/0.25/0.25 mg/kg Prolonged treatment option: 0.2 mg/kg q24h for 5-7 days	Monitor urine output, electrolytes, blood urea nitrogen, creatinine, and platelet count. Monitor for signs of bleeding.
Isoproterenol (Isuprel)	0.05-0.5 µg/kg/min continuous IV infusion; max dose 2 µg/kg/min	May cause arrhythmias and hypoxemia. Correct acidosis prior to starting therapy.
Lidocaine	Bolus dose: 0.5-1.0 mg/kg IV push over 5 min; may repeat every 10 min to a max of 5 mg/kg Continuous IV infusion: 10-50 µg/kg/min	May cause CNS toxicity—monitor for seizures, apnea, respiratory depression. High dosages may cause bradycardia, heart block, hypotension—monitor ECG, HR, and blood pressure continuously. Contraindicated in cardiac failure and heart block.
Milrinone (Primacor)	Loading dose: 50-75 µg/kg/min over 15-60 min Continuous IV infusion: 0.25-0.75 µg/kg/min	Loading dose optional based on status of patient. Correct hypovolemia prior to initiation of therapy. Blood pressure may decrease 5%-9% after loading dose and HR may increase 5%-10%.
Naloxone (Narcan)	0.1 mg/kg IV push repeated every 2-3 min until opioid effect reversed; may need to repeat doses every 20-60 min; may be given IM, SC, or ET, but not recommended due to delayed onset of action	Not recommended as part of the initial resuscitation of newborns with respiratory depression.
Neostigmine (Prostigmin)	0.04-0.08 mg/kg slow IV push (IM and SC administration have delayed onset of action)	Give in addition to atropine 0.02 mg/kg to reverse neuromuscular blockade.
Nicardipine (Cardene)	0.5 µg/kg/min continuous IV infusion; titrate up to 2 µg/kg/min	Monitor blood pressure, HR, and heart rhythm continuously. May take up to 2 days to see final effect of dose.
Procainamide (Pronestyl)	Bolus dose: 7-10 mg/kg IV over 1 hr Continuous IV infusion: 20-80 µg/kg/min	Monitor for hypotension (increased with rapid infusion), bradycardia, arrhythmias. Monitor serum levels, especially in patients with hepatic or renal impairment, or those receiving high dosages. Monitor CBC for neutropenia, thrombocytopenia regularly.

Agent	Dosage	Comments
Propranolol (Inderal)	0.01 mg/kg/dose IV push over 10 min q6h; titrate up to max 0.15 mg/kg/dose q6h 0.25 mg/kg/dose PO q6h; titrate up to max 3.5 mg/kg/dose q6h	Monitor ECG continuously during acute treatment of arrhythmias. Monitor blood glucose for hypoglycemia. Monitor blood pressure.
Sodium nitroprusside (Nipride)	0.25-0.5 μg/kg/min continuous IV infusion; titrate up every 20 min. Usual maintenance dose is <2 μg/kg/min Hypertensive crisis: doses up to 10 μg/kg/min can be used for no longer than 10 min	Monitor HR and intraarterial blood pressure continuously. May produce severe hypotension and cyanide/thiocyanate toxicity; increased risk of toxicity with prolonged treatment, high dosages, and renal or hepatic impairment. Protect drug from light.

CBC, Complete blood count; *CNS,* central nervous system; *ECG,* electrocardiogram; *ET,* endotracheal tube; *HR,* heart rate; *IM,* intramuscular; *IV,* intravenous; *max,* maximum; *NS,* normal saline; *PMA,* postmenstrual age; *PO,* by mouth; *q,* every; *SC,* subcutaneous.

Drug Dosing Table

 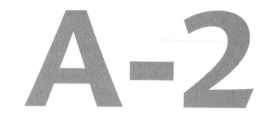

Jacquelyn McClary

Medication (Trade Name)/Route of Administration	Mechanism of Action/Dosing	Important Adverse Events	Special Considerations
Acetaminophen (Tylenol) PO/PR	Inhibits prostaglandin synthesis in central nervous system. Peripherally blocks pain impulse generation. Inhibits hypothalamic thermal regulating center. PO: 10-15 mg/kg q4-6h PR: 15-20 mg/kg q6-8h	Liver toxicity in overdose (acute or chronic)	Rectal administration results in prolonged, variable absorption. Elimination prolonged in patients with liver dysfunction.
Acyclovir (Zovirax) IV	Inhibits DNA synthesis and viral replication by incorporation into viral DNA. IV: 20 mg/kg q8h	Renal dysfunction, neutropenia	Maintain proper hydration, monitor renal function. Consider prolonging dosing interval in infants of <34 wk PMA or with significant renal or hepatic impairment.
Adenosine (Adenocard) IV	Slows AV conduction, thereby interrupting reentry pathway and restoring normal sinus rhythm. IV: 50 µg/kg initially; increase in 50-µg/kg increments and repeat every 2 min to max dose of 250 µg/kg	Momentary complete heart block after administration Bronchoconstriction in patients with reactive airway disease	Administer over 1-2 sec and as close to IV insertion site as possible; follow immediately with NS flush. Contraindicated in patients with second- or third-degree heart block. Methylxanthines diminish effect of adenosine and therefore larger doses may be needed.
Albuterol (Proventil, Ventolin) PO/Neb/MDI	β_2-agonist that relaxes bronchial smooth muscle. Neb: 0.1-0.5 mg/kg q2-6h MDI: 1 actuation q2-6h PO: 0.1-0.3 mg/kg/dose q6-8h	Tachycardia, hypokalemia with continuous administration	Oral administration may be associated with more systemic adverse events.
Alprostadil (prostaglandin E_1) (Prostin VR) IV	Prostaglandin E_1 analog that produces direct vasodilation of vascular and ductus arteriosus smooth muscle. IV: 0.05-0.1 µg/kg/min via continuous infusion; maintenance doses may be as low as 0.01 µg/kg/min	Hypotension, flushing, bradycardia, fever, apnea	Apnea occurs in ~10%-12% of neonates within first hour of infusion.

Amikacin (Amikin) IM/IV	Inhibits bacterial protein synthesis by inhibiting 50S ribosomal subunit.
	
	PMA ≤29 wk:
	  0-7 days old: 18 mg/kg q48h
	  8-28 days old: 15 mg/kg q36h
	  ≥29 days old: 15 mg/kg q24h
	PMA 30-34 wk:
	  0-7 days old: 18 mg/kg q36h
	  ≥8 days old: 15 mg/kg q24h
	PMA ≥35 wk: 15 mg/kg q24h
		Nephrotoxic, ototoxic, additive neuromuscular blockade with neuromuscular blocking agents	Monitor serum concentrations. Therapeutic peak serum concentration is 20 to 30 µg/mL. Therapeutic trough serum concentration is <10 µg/mL. Should not be concurrently administered in same IV line with extended-spectrum penicillins (possible inactivation). Synergistic antibacterial actions with penicillins and other antibiotics.

Medication (Trade Name)/Route of Administration	Mechanism of Action/Dosing	Important Adverse Events	Special Considerations
Amiodarone (Cordarone, Pacerone) IV/PO	Inhibits adrenergic stimulation, prolongs action potential and refractory period in myocardial tissue, decreases AV conduction and sinus node function. IV: 5 mg/kg loading dose followed by maintenance infusion of 7-15 µg/kg/min PO: 5-10 mg/kg q12h after 24-48 hr of IV therapy	Hypotension, bradycardia, AV block, pneumonitis, pulmonary fibrosis, liver injury	Hyperthyroidism or hypothyroidism may occur with long-term use.
Ammonium chloride IV/PO	Increases acidity by increasing concentration of free hydrogen ions, which combine with bicarbonate ion to form CO_2 and water; net result is replacement of bicarbonate ions with chloride ions. IV/PO: 75-150 mg/kg/day divided q6-8h	Metabolic acidosis, hyperchloremia	Use only as alternative supplement after sodium and potassium supplementation have been optimized.
Amphotericin B (Amphocin, Fungizone) Amphotericin B lipid complex (Abelcet) Amphotericin B liposome (AmBisome) IV	Binds to fungal ergosterol, compromising fungal cell wall integrity. Amphotericin B: 1-1.5 mg/kg q24h over 2-6 hr Amphotericin B lipid complex: 5 mg/kg q24h over 2 hr Amphotericin B liposome: 5-7 mg/kg q24h over 2 hr	Hypomagnesemia, hypokalemia nephrotoxicity, fever, chills, thrombocytopenia	Monitor renal function, electrolytes. Adjust dosing interval if serum creatinine increases >0.4 mg/dL from baseline. Less nephrotoxicity with lipid and liposome formulations.

Ampicillin (Omnipen, Polycillin, Principen) IM/IV	Inhibits bacterial cell wall synthesis by binding to specific penicillin-binding proteins. Causes cell wall death resulting in bacteriocidal activity.
	
	PMA ≤29 wk:
	  0-28 days old: 25-50 mg/kg q12h
	  >28 days old: 25-50 mg/kg q8h
	PMA 30-36 wk:
	  0-14 days old: 25-50 mg/kg q12h
	  >14 days old: 25-50 mg/kg q8h
	PMA 37-44 wk:
	  0-7 days old: 25-50 mg/kg q12h
	  >7 days old: 25-50 mg/kg q8h
	PMA ≥45 wk: 25-50 mg/kg q6h
		CNS excitation or seizure activity with very large doses	For GBS bacteremia dosages may be increased to 200 mg/kg/day. For GBS meningitis dosages may be increased to 300-400 mg/kg/day and doses given at more frequent intervals.

Atropine PO/IV/IM/ET	Competitively inhibits actions of acetylcholine in secretory glands, smooth muscle, and CNS. PO: 0.02 mg/kg q4-6h; increase gradually to max 0.09 mg/kg/dose IV/IM: 0.01-0.03 mg/kg over 1 min; may repeat every 10-15 min (max dose 0.04 mg/kg) ET: 0.01-0.03 mg/kg followed by 1 mL NS	Tachycardia, arrhythmias, urinary retention, decreased GI motility	Administer rapidly and undiluted. Small doses may result in paradoxical bradycardia.
Azithromycin (Zithromax) PO/IV	Inhibits bacterial protein synthesis by binding to 50S ribosomal subunit. PO: 10 mg/kg q24h × 5 days IV: 5-10 mg/kg q24h	Diarrhea, rash, blood in stool	Recommended PO dosing is for treatment of pertussis. IV dosing not well studied in pediatric patients.

Continued

Medication (Trade Name)/Route of Administration	Mechanism of Action/Dosing	Important Adverse Events	Special Considerations

Aztreonam (Azactam) IM/IV	Inhibits bacterial cell wall synthesis and causes cell wall destruction by binding to penicillin-binding proteins.
	
	PMA ≤29 wk:
	  0-28 days old: 30 mg/kg q12h
	  >28 days old: 30 mg/kg q8h
	PMA 30-36 wk:
	  0-14 days old: 30 mg/kg q12h
	  >14 days old: 30 mg/kg q8h
	PMA 37-44 wk:
	  0-7 days old: 30 mg/kg q12h
	  >7 days old: 30 mg/kg q8h
	PMA ≥45 wk: 30 mg/kg q6h
		Hypoglycemia, eosinophilia, elevated transaminases	Contains L-arginine—provide adequate glucose to avoid hypoglycemia.

Beractant (Survanta) IT	Modified bovine pulmonary surfactant analog. Replaces deficient or ineffective endogenous lung surfactant. IT: 4 mL/kg divided into 4 aliquots administered as soon as possible after birth; repeat up to 3 doses within 48 hr of life if needed, no more frequently than q6h	Reflux of surfactant up ET, decreased oxygenation, bradycardia	For IT administration only. Suspension should be at room temperature before administering. Do not artificially warm. Swirl suspension; do not shake or filter suspension. Continuously monitor heart rate and oxygen saturation during administration.

Bumetanide (Bumex) PO/IM/IV	Inhibits chloride and sodium reabsorption in ascending loop of Henle and proximal renal tubule, causing increased excretion of water and electrolytes.
	
	PO/IM/IV: 0.005-0.1 mg/kg
	  <34 wk, 0-2 mo old: q24h
	  <34 wk, >2 mo old: q12h
	  ≥34 wk, 0-1 mo old: q24h
	  ≥34 wk, >1 mo old: q12h
		Hypomagnesemia, hyponatremia, hypokalemia, metabolic hypochloremic alkalosis	Higher dosages required with abnormal renal function or congestive heart failure. May displace bilirubin at high dosages or with long duration of therapy.

Caffeine citrate (Cafcit) PO/IV	Stimulates central inspiratory drive and improves skeletal muscle contraction. Loading dose: 20-25 mg/kg Maintenance dose: 5-10 mg/kg q24h	Tachycardia, cardiac dysrhythmias, insomnia, GI disturbances, gastroesophageal reflux	Therapeutic trough serum concentration range is 5-25 μg/mL; toxicity is associated with serum concentrations of >40-50 μg/mL. Monitoring serum concentrations not typically necessary at recommended dosages.
Calfactant (Infasurf) IT	Natural surfactant extracted from calf lung. Replaces deficient or ineffective endogenous lung surfactant. IT: 3 mL/kg divided into 2 aliquots administered as soon as possible after birth; repeat up to 3 doses if needed, no more frequently than q12h	Reflux of surfactant up ET, decreased oxygenation, bradycardia	For IT administration only. Suspension should be at room temperature before administering. Do not artificially warm. Swirl suspension; do not shake or filter suspension. Continuously monitor heart rate and oxygen saturation during administration.
Captopril (Capoten) PO	Competitively inhibits angiotensin-converting enzyme. Initial dose: 0.01-0.05 mg/kg q8-12h; adjust dose based on response Max dose: 0.5 mg/kg q6-24h	Decreased cerebral or renal blood flow, hyperkalemia	Monitor renal function. Onset of action is 15 min and peak effect is 30-90 min after dosing.
Caspofungin (Cancidas) IV	Inhibits synthesis of essential cell wall component in susceptible fungi. IV: 25 mg/m^2 q24h	Thrombophlebitis, hypercalcemia, hypokalemia, increased liver enzymes	Monitor electrolytes and hepatic transaminases.

Medication (Trade Name)/Route of Administration	Mechanism of Action/Dosing	Important Adverse Events	Special Considerations

Cefazolin (Ancef, Kefzol) IM/IV	Inhibits bacterial cell wall synthesis by binding to penicillin-binding proteins.
	
	PMA ≤29 wk:
	  0-28 days old: 25 mg/kg q12h
	  >28 days old: 25 mg/kg q8h
	PMA 30-36 wk:
	  0-14 days old: 25 mg/kg q12h
	  >14 days old: 25 mg/kg q8h
	PMA 37-44 wk:
	  0-7 days old: 25 mg/kg q12h
	  >7 days old: 25 mg/kg q8h
	PMA ≥45 wk: 25 mg/kg q6h
		Phlebitis, eosinophilia	Poor CNS penetration. Often used for perioperative infection prophylaxis.

Cefepime (Maxipime) IM/IV	Inhibits bacterial cell wall synthesis by binding to penicillin-binding proteins.
	
	Mild to moderate infections:
	  ≤28 days old: 30 mg/kg q12h
	  >28 days old: 50 mg/kg q12h
	Meningitis and severe infections:
	  50 mg/kg q12h
		Eosinophilia, elevated hepatic transaminases	Widely distributed in body tissues and fluids, including CNS.

Cefotaxime (Claforan) IM/IV	Inhibits bacterial cell wall synthesis by binding to penicillin-binding proteins.
	
	PMA ≤29 wk:
	  0-28 days old: 50 mg/kg q12h
	  >28 days old: 50 mg/kg q8h
	PMA 30-36 wk:
	  0-14 days old: 50 mg/kg q12h
	  >14 days old: 50 mg/kg q8h
	PMA 37-44 wk:
	  0-7 days old: 50 mg/kg q12h
	  >7 days old: 50 mg/kg q8h
	PMA ≥45 wk: 50 mg/kg q6h
		Leukopenia, granulocytopenia, eosinophilia	Widely distributed in CSF and other tissues.

Cefoxitin (Mefoxin) IM/IV	Inhibits bacterial cell wall synthesis by binding to penicillin-binding proteins.
	
	PMA ≤29 wk:
	  0-28 days old: 25-33 mg/kg q12h
	  >28 days old: 25-33 mg/kg q8h
	PMA 30-36 wk:
	  0-14 days old: 25-33 mg/kg q12h
	  >14 days old: 25-33 mg/kg q8h
	PMA 37-44 wk:
	  0-7 days old: 25-33 mg/kg q12h
	  >7 days old: 25-33 mg/kg q8h
	PMA ≥45 wk: 25-33 mg/kg q6h
		Eosinophilia, elevated hepatic transaminases	Use often limited to skin, intraabdominal, and urinary tract infections.

Ceftazidime (Fortaz) IM/IV	Inhibits bacterial cell wall synthesis by binding to penicillin-binding proteins.
	
	PMA ≤29 wk:
	  0-28 days old: 30 mg/kg q12h
	  >28 days old: 30 mg/kg q8h
	PMA 30-36 wk:
	  0-14 days old: 30 mg/kg q12h
	  >14 days old: 30 mg/kg q8h
	PMA 37-44 wk:
	  0-7 days old: 30 mg/kg q12h
	  >7 days old: 30 mg/kg q8h
	PMA ≥45 wk: 30 mg/kg q8h
		Eosinophilia, elevated hepatic transaminases	Widely distributed in body tissues and fluids. Synergistic with aminoglycosides.

Ceftriaxone (Rocephin) IM/IV	Inhibits bacterial cell wall synthesis by binding to penicillin-binding proteins. Sepsis: 50 mg/kg q24h Meningitis: 100 mg/kg loading dose, then 80 mg/kg q24h	Increased bleeding time, leukopenia, eosinophilia, transient gall bladder precipitations	Displaces bilirubin from albumin binding sites—not recommended for use in neonates with hyperbilirubinemia. Contraindicated with concurrent administration of calcium-containing solutions.

Continued

Medication (Trade Name)/Route of Administration	Mechanism of Action/Dosing	Important Adverse Events	Special Considerations
Chlorothiazide (Diuril) PO/IV	Inhibits Na reabsorption in distal renal tubules causing increased excretion of sodium, chloride, potassium, bicarbonate, magnesium, phosphate, calcium, and water. PO: 10-20 mg/kg q12h IV: 2-10 mg/kg q12h	Hypochloremic metabolic alkalosis, fluid and electrolyte disorders, hyperglycemia	Synergistic effect with loop diuretics (e.g., furosemide) or spironolactone. Monitor serum electrolytes closely.
Cholecalciferol (vitamin D_3, D-Vi-Sol) PO	Vitamin D supplementation is used to stimulate or support skeletal growth. Supplementation: 400 U q24h Vitamin D deficiency: 400-1000 U q24h	Signs of toxicity due to hypercalcemia (vomiting, nephrocalcinosis, arrhythmia)	Monitor 25-hydroxyvitamin D concentrations, particularly in neonates receiving higher dosages. Monitor calcium and phosphorous levels.

Clindamycin (Cleocin) PO/IM/IV	Inhibits bacterial protein synthesis by reversibly binding to 50S ribosome subunit.
	
	PMA ≤29 wk:
	    0-28 days old: 5-7.5 mg/kg q12h
	    >28 days old: 5-7.5 mg/kg q8h
	PMA 30-36 wk:
	    0-14 days old: 5-7.5 mg/kg q12h
	    >14 days old: 5-7.5 mg/kg q8h
	PMA 37-44 wk:
	    0-7 days old: 5-7.5 mg/kg q12h
	    >7 days old: 5-7.5 mg/kg q8h
	PMA ≥45 wk: 5-7.5 mg/kg q6h
		Clostridium difficile-associated diarrhea, pseudomembranous colitis, phlebitis at site of injection	Increase dosing interval in the presence of significant liver dysfunction.

Dexamethasone (Decadron) PO/IV/IM	Decreases inflammation by suppressing proinflammatory mediators. Facilitation of ventilator weaning: 0.01-0.075 mg/kg q12h Airway edema: 0.25-0.5 mg/kg q8h; max dose 1 mg/kg/day	Hypertension, hyperglycemia, GI bleeding or perforation, growth inhibition	For ventilator weaning, 10-day DART trial protocol is commonly used. Typically airway edema treatment limited to 3 doses.
Diazoxide (Proglycem) PO	Inhibits insulin release from pancreas. PO: 2-5 mg/kg q8h	Sodium and fluid retention, pulmonary hypertension, cardiac failure	Alcohol content of oral suspension is 7.25%; GI upset and abdominal distension are common.
Digoxin (Lanoxin) PO/IV	Reversibly binds to Na-K-Ca pump and increases calcium influx within myocardial cells, which results in increase in force of myocardial contraction. See Appendix A-1 for dosing.	Atrial and ventricular arrhythmias	Hypokalemia, hypomagnesemia, hypermagnesemia, and hypercalcemia predispose patients to digoxin toxicity. Follow serum drug concentrations with target range of 1-2 ng/mL.
Dobutamine IV	Reversibly binds to and stimulates β_1-adrenergic receptor, causing increased contractility and heart rate. Continuous IV infusion: 2-25 μg/kg/min	Hypotension in setting of hypovolemia, tachycardia, arrhythmias, phlebitis	Correct hypovolemia before initiation of therapy if possible. Use phentolamine for treatment of extravasation.
Dopamine IV	Stimulates α- and β-adrenergic and dopaminergic receptors, which results in cardiac stimulation, increased renal blood flow, and vasoconstriction. Continuous IV infusion: 2-20 μg/kg/min	Hypertension, tachycardia, phlebitis	Pharmacologic effect is dose dependent. Use phentolamine for treatment of extravasation.
Dornase alfa (Pulmozyme) Neb	Selectively cleaves DNA, which reduces mucous viscosity in pulmonary secretions. Neb: 1.25-2.5 mL q12-24h	Desaturation, airway obstruction	Each single-dose ampule contains 2.5 mg/2.5 mL dornase alfa.

Medication (Trade Name)/Route of Administration	Mechanism of Action/Dosing	Important Adverse Events	Special Considerations
Enalapril (PO) (Vasotec) Enalaprilat (IV)	Exerts blood pressure and cardiac effects through competitive inhibition of angiotensin-converting enzyme. PO: 0.04-0.15 mg/kg q6-24h IV: 0.005-0.01 mg/kg q8-24h	Reflex tachycardia, renal dysfunction, hyperkalemia	Monitor renal function. Begin at low doses q24h and titrate up based on response.

Enoxaparin (Lovenox) SC	Potentiates antithrombin III activity and inactivates anticoagulation factor Xa.
	
	Throm basis treatment:
	  Term: 1.7 mg/kg q12h
	  Preterm: 2 mg/kg q12h
	Prophylaxis: <3 months: 0.75 mg/kg q12h ≥3 months: 0.5 mg/kg q12h
		Intracranial hemorrhage, GI bleeding, hematoma at injection site	Monitor Xa levels 4 hr after a dose; target range is 0.5-1 U/ml for treatment and 0.1-0.4 U/mL for prophylaxis. Therapeutic dosages in preterm neonates are widely variable. Renally cleared; reduced dosages required in renal dysfunction. Call 1-800-NOCLOTS for dosing assistance.

Epinephrine (Adrenalin) IV/ET	Stimulates α- and β-adrenergic receptors, which results in cardiac stimulation and dilation of skeletal muscle vasculature. IV: 0.01-0.03 mg/kg/dose q3-5min Continuous IV infusion: 0.02-1 μg/kg/min ET: 0.1 mg/kg followed by 1 mL NS	Hypertension, tachycardia, arrhythmias, phlebitis, renal vascular ischemia	Correct acidosis before administration if possible. Use phentolamine for treatment of extravasation.
Epoetin alfa (Epogen, Procrit) IV/SC	Synthetic analog of erythropoietin that stimulates erythropoiesis. IV/SC: 400-500 U/kg 3 times per week	Neutropenia	Subcutaneous route preferred. Continue therapy until hematocrit is ≥35% (usually 2-4 wk). Consider administration of iron if iron stores are not adequate.

Erythromycin (Eryped, E.E.S.) PO/IV	Inhibits bacterial protein synthesis by reversibly binding to 50S ribosome subunit.
	
	PO erythromycin ethylsuccinate:
	  Infection: 10-12.5 mg/kg q6h
	  Gastric motility: 10 mg/kg q6h × 48 hr, then 4 mg/kg q6h
	IV erythromycin lactobionate:
	5-10 mg/kg q6h
		Bradycardia and hypotension during IV administration, phlebitis, diarrhea, abdominal pain	Administer PO with feeds to reduce GI side effects and increase absorption.

Esmolol (Brevibloc) IV	Competitively blocks response to β_1-adrenergic stimulation with minimal effect on β_2-adrenergic receptors. Supraventricular tachycardia: 100 μg/kg/min continuous IV infusion; increase by 50-100 μg/kg/min every 5 min to usual max 200 μg/kg/min Postoperative hypertension: 50 μg/kg/min continuous IV infusion; increase by 25-50 μg/kg/min every 5 min to usual max 200 μg/kg/min	Hypotension, tissue necrosis	Use phentolamine for treatment of extravasation.
Famotidine (Pepcid) PO/IV	Competitively inhibits histamine receptors in gastric parietal cells, which results in inhibition of gastric acid secretion. PO: 0.5-1 mg/kg q24h IV: 0.25-0.5 mg/kg q24h	Late-onset bacterial or fungal sepsis	Oral suspension contains sodium benzoate.
Fentanyl (Sublimaze) IV	Binds with opioid μ receptors in CNS to decrease pain. IV push: 1-4 μg/kg q2-4h Continuous IV infusion: 0.5-5 μg/kg/hr	Respiratory depression, chest wall rigidity, urinary retention	Dependence may occur with long-term administration. Effects reversed by naloxone. Approximately 100 times more potent than morphine.

Continued

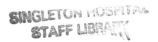

Medication (Trade Name)/Route of Administration	Mechanism of Action/Dosing	Important Adverse Events	Special Considerations
Ferrous sulfate (Fer-In-Sol) PO	Repletes diminished iron stores and is incorporated into hemoglobin. Routine supplementation: 2-4 mg/kg/day divided q12-24h Patients receiving erythropoietin: 6 mg/kg/day divided q12-24h	Constipation, discolored stool	Infants who have received multiple recent blood transfusions are at risk of iron overload—typically no supplementation is required.

Fluconazole (Diflucan) PO/IV	Reversibly binds to fungal cytochrome P-450, inhibiting sterol C-14 α-demethylation and decreasing ergosterol synthesis, which ultimately inhibits cell membrane formation.
	
	Invasive candidiasis
	Loading dose (IV/PO): 12-25 mg/kg
	Maintenance dose (IV/PO):
	  PMA ≤29 wk:
	    0-14 days old: 6-12 mg/kg q48h
	    >14 days old: 6-12 mg/kg q24h
	  PMA >30 wk:
	    0-7 days old: 6-12 mg/kg q48h
	    >7 days old: 6-12 mg/kg q24h
	Thrush
	6 mg/kg PO × 1 dose, then 3 mg/kg PO q24h
		Increased liver enzymes	Limited data for higher dosages—consider using in severe infection or if fungal strain has high minimum inhibitory concentration.
			Extend dosing interval in setting of renal dysfunction.

Flumazenil (Romazicon) IV/IN/PR	Antagonizes effect of benzodiazepines on GABA/benzodiazepine receptors. IV: 5-10 μg/kg over 15 sec; repeat q45sec to max cumulative dose of 50 μg/kg or 1 mg (whichever is smaller) IN: 20 μg/kg per nostril PR: 15-30 μg/kg; repeat q15-20min	Hypotension, seizures	Seizures most common in patients receiving benzodiazepines for long-term sedation.
Fosphenytoin (Cerebyx) IV/IM	Phenytoin prodrug. Increases efflux or decreases influx of sodium ions across cell membranes in motor cortex, which results in neuronal membrane stabilization. Dosing expressed in phenytoin equivalents (PE): Fosphenytoin 1 mg PE = phenytoin 1 mg Loading dose: 15-20 mg PE/kg Maintenance dose: 4-8 mg PE/kg q24h	Hypotension, venous irritation	May administer much more rapidly than phenytoin, up to 1.5 mg/kg/min. Term infants >1 wk of age may need higher dosages at more frequent intervals (8 mg PE/kg q8h). Displaces bilirubin from protein binding sites. Target serum phenytoin levels are 6-20 μg/mL.
Furosemide (Lasix) PO/IV/IM	Inhibits chloride and sodium reabsorption in ascending loop of Henle and proximal renal tubule, which causes increased excretion of water and electrolytes. IV: 1-2 mg/kg/dose q6-48h PO: 1-4 mg/kg/dose q6-48h	Hypochloremic alkalosis, hyponatremia, hypokalemia, hypercalciuria and renal calculi, ototoxicity	Has synergistic effect with proximal and distal tubule inhibitors (e.g., thiazides). Monitor electrolytes closely. Risk of ototoxicity increased in neonates also receiving aminoglycosides.
Ganciclovir (Cytovene-IV)	Competes for incorporation into viral DNA and interferes with viral DNA chain elongation, which results in inhibition of viral replication. Acute infection: 6 mg/kg IV q12h Chronic suppression: 30-40 mg/kg PO q8h	Thrombocytopenia, anemia, neutropenia	Treat acute infections for minimum of 6 wk. Monitor complete blood count results 2-3 times per week for first 3 wk, then weekly if infant's condition is stable. Cut dose in half for neutropenia (<500 cells/mm^3). Discontinue if neutropenia does not resolve.

Medication (Trade Name)/Route of Administration	Mechanism of Action/Dosing	Important Adverse Events	Special Considerations
Gentamicin IV/IM	Inhibits bacterial protein synthesis by inhibiting 30S and 50S ribosomal subunits, which results in defective bacterial cell membrane. PMA <35 wk: 4 mg/kg q24h PMA ≥35 wk: 5 mg/kg q24h	Nephrotoxicity, ototoxicity (increased risk with concurrent use of other nephrotoxic or ototoxic drugs)	Monitor serum trough concentration before third dose if treating for >48 hr. Target trough concentration is <1 µg/mL. Extend dosing interval if trough is >1 µg/mL. Should not be concurrently administered in same IV line with extended-spectrum penicillin.
Glucagon IV/IM/SC	Increases hepatic glycogenolysis and gluconeogenesis, which causes increase in blood glucose. 0.2 mg/kg up to max dose of 1 mg; repeat q20min prn	Tachycardia, GI disturbances, rebound hypoglycemia	Rise in blood glucose lasts about 2 hr.
Heparin IV	Potentiates action of antithrombin III, inactivates thrombin, inhibits conversion of fibrinogen to fibrin. Loading dose: 75 U/kg IV push Maintenance dose: 28 U/kg/hr Continuous IV infusion—adjust based on APTT; target range dependent on indication	Hemorrhage, thrombocytopenia	Effects reversible with protamine. Monitor platelet levels closely. Nontherapeutic doses added to TPN or IV fluids to maintain patency of lines (0.5-1 U/mL).
Hyaluronidase (Amphadase, Vitrase) SC	Modifies permeability of connective tissue and increases distribution and absorption of locally injected substances. SC: 150 U as 5 separate injections around extravasation site	Erythema	Administer as soon as possible after extravasation. Not for use with extravasation of vasoactive agents.
Hydralazine (Apresoline) PO/IV	Produces direct vasodilation of arterioles causing decreased systemic resistance. PO: 0.25-1 mg/kg q6-8h IV: 0.1-0.5 mg/kg q6-8h gradually increased to max of 2 mg/kg q6h	Agranulocytosis, hypotension, tachycardia	If used with β-blocker expect reduction in hydralazine dose required.
Hydrochlorothiazide (Microzide) PO	Inhibits Na reabsorption in distal renal tubules, which causes increased excretion of water and electrolytes. PO: 1-2 mg/kg q12h	Hypochloremic metabolic alkalosis, hypokalemia, hypouricemia, hyperglycemia	Has synergistic effect with loop diuretics (e.g., furosemide). Administer with food to improve absorption.
Hydrocortisone (Solu-Cortef) PO/IV	Corticosteroid that decreases inflammation by suppressing migration and decreasing capillary permeability of proinflammatory mediators. Stress dose: 20-30 mg/m^2/day divided q8-12h Physiologic dose: 7-9 mg/m^2/day divided q8-12h Facilitation of ventilator weaning: 0.2-2 mg/kg q12h	Possible aggravation of fluid retention, pituitary-adrenal axis suppression, hyperglycemia, hypertension, GI perforation (increased risk if given with indomethacin)	For ventilator weaning start at high dosages and wean over 10 days. Taper stress dose and physiologic dose based on patient response and condition.
Ibuprofen lysine (NeoProfen) IV	Inhibits prostaglandin synthesis by decreasing cyclooxygenase activity. Dose 1: 10 mg/kg Doses 2 and 3 starting 24 hr after dose 1: 5 mg/kg q24h	GI perforation, renal impairment, impaired platelet function	Monitor urine output, BUN, and serum creatinine. Verify adequate platelet count before administration. Monitor for signs of bleeding.

Continued

Medication (Trade Name)/Route of Administration	Mechanism of Action/Dosing	Important Adverse Events	Special Considerations
Imipenem/cilastatin (Primaxin) IV/IM	Inhibits bacterial cell wall synthesis by binding to penicillin-binding proteins. IV/IM: 20-25 mg/kg q12h	Seizures in patients with meningitis or renal dysfunction, increased platelet count, eosinophilia, elevated liver enzymes	Cilastatin prevents renal metabolism of imipenem, but has no antibacterial activity. IM route limited to mild to moderate infections. Restricted to treatment of non-CNS infections. Clearance is directly related to renal function.

Indomethacin (Indocin) IV	Inhibits prostaglandin synthesis by decreasing cyclooxygenase activity.
	
	Dose 1: 0.2 mg/kg followed by:
	  Postnatal age <48 hr at time of dose 1: 0.1 mg/kg q12-24h for 2 doses
	  Postnatal age 2-7 days at time of dose 1: 0.2 mg/kg q12-24h for 2 doses
	  Postnatal age >7 days at time of dose 1: 0.25 mg/kg q12-24h for 2 doses
		Oliguria, anuria, GI perforation, impaired platelet function	Monitor urine output, BUN, and serum creatinine—extend dosing interval if severe oliguria occurs.
			Verify adequate platelet count before administration.
			Monitor for signs of bleeding.

Insulin (Humulin R) IV/SC	Regulates metabolism of macronutrients and facilitates glucose transport into muscle, adipose, and other tissues. SC: 0.1-0.2 U/kg q6-12h Continuous IV infusion: 0.01-0.1 U/kg/hr	Hypoglycemia and associated signs and symptoms	Assess blood glucose every 15-30 min after starting infusion and after any changes. To avoid binding of insulin to tubing, fill IV tubing with insulin solution and wait 20 min before starting infusion.
Intravenous immune globulin (IVIG) (Gamunex, Flebogamma, Carimune NF) IV	Concentrated form of immunoglobulin G antibodies for replacement therapy. Standard dose: 500-750 mg/kg Neonatal alloimmune thrombocytopenia: 400-1000 mg/kg	Hypotension, renal dysfunction, phlebitis	Monitor heart rate and blood pressure during infusion. If infusion not well tolerated, decrease in rate may be warranted. In most cases a single dose is sufficient, but doses may be repeated every 24 hr.
Ipratropium (Atrovent) Neb/MDI	Bronchodilator that blocks acetylcholine action in bronchial smooth muscle. MDI: 2-4 puffs q6-8h Neb: 75-175 μg (0.4-0.9 mL) q6-8h		Neonatal lung models suggest better drug delivery with spacer and MDI than with nebulizer.
Iron dextran IV (IN Fed)	Replaces iron and allows for transportation of oxygen via hemoglobin. IV: 0.4-1 mg/kg q24h	Hypotension, respiratory distress, delayed fever or agitation (24-48 hr after administration), phlebitis	Add to TPN solution and infuse continuously if possible. If intermittent infusion necessary, dilute each dose (1-10 mg/mL) and administer over 1 hr. Longer infusion times can be used if intolerance occurs.
Lamivudine (3TC, Epivir) PO	Antiretroviral agent that inhibits reverse transcription via viral DNA chain termination. PO: 2 mg/kg q12h	Lactic acidosis, elevated hepatic enzymes	Used in combination with zidovudine for prevention of mother-to-child HIV transmission. Consider consulting infectious disease specialist for specific antiretroviral regimen recommendations. Monitor liver enzymes regularly if long-term treatment required.

Medication (Trade Name)/Route of Administration	Mechanism of Action/Dosing	Important Adverse Events	Special Considerations
Lansoprazole (Prevacid) PO	Inhibits proton pump and leads to decreased gastric acid secretion. PO: 1 mg/kg q24h	Increased trans-aminases with prolonged therapy	Dosages up to 2 mg/kg/day have been used in refractory cases. Monitor liver function with prolonged therapy.
Levetiracetam (Keppra) IV/PO	Exact mechanism unknown, but activity may include blocking GABA-ergic inhibitory transmission and inhibiting voltage-dependent calcium channels. IV/PO: 10 mg/kg q12-24h titrated up every 1-2 wk to max of 30 mg/kg q12h Administer q24h in neonates and q12h in infants	Sedation, irritabil-ity, GI distur-bances, phlebitis	Second-line therapy for seizures refractory to phenobarbital or other antiepileptics.
Levothyroxine (Synthroid) PO/IV	Replacement therapy for thyroid hor-mone involved in normal metabolism, growth, and synthesis. PO: 10-14 µg/kg q24h IV: 5-8 µg/kg q24h	Tachycardia, fever, GI distur-bances	Adjust PO dose in 12.5-µg increments and always round up. For oral doses crush tablet and suspend in small amount of sterile water, breast milk, or formula and use immediately. Do not use IV formulation for PO administration.

Linezolid (Zyvox) PO/IV	Inhibits initiation of bacterial protein synthesis by binding to 50S ribosome subunit.
	
	Preterm ≤1 wk of age:
	  PO/IV: 10 mg/kg q12h
	Full term or preterm >1 wk of age:
	  PO/IV: 10 mg/kg q8h
		Elevated transam-inases, diarrhea, anemia, thrombo-cytopenia	Limit use to infections caused by gram-positive organisms that are refractory to treatment with vancomycin.

Lorazepam (Ativan) PO/IV/IM	Binds to GABA receptor, enhancing effects of GABA, which is the major inhibitory neurotransmitter. PO/IV/IM: 0.05-0.01 mg/kg repeated based on clinical response	Hypotension, respiratory depression, rhyth-mic myoclonic jerking, phlebitis	Injectable form contains benzyl alcohol, polyethylene glycol, and propylene glycol. Use limited to acute manage-ment of seizures refractory to conventional therapy.

Meropenem (Merrem) IV	Inhibits bacterial cell wall synthe-sis by binding to penicillin-binding proteins.
	GA <32 wk:
	  0-14 days old: 20 mg/kg q12h
	  >14 days old: 20 mg/kg q8h
	GA ≥32 wk:
	  0-7 days old: 20 mg/kg q12h
	  >7 days old: 20 mg/kg q8h
		Thrombocytosis, eosinophilia, phlebitis	Limit use to treatment of severe infections resistant to other antibiotics; use of broad-spectrum antibiotics increases risk of fungal infection and pseudomembranous colitis.

Methadone (Dolophine) IV/PO	Binds to opiate receptors in CNS, altering perception of and response to pain. IV/PO: 0.05-0.2 mg/kg q6-24h	Respiratory depression, abdominal disten-sion, delayed gastric emptying	Start with lower doses at more frequent intervals and titrate up as needed based on NAS scores. Wean doses 10%-20% per week, adjusted based on withdrawal symptoms. Extend dosing interval first until administration is every 12 hr, then wean dose. Long elimination half-life requires slow weaning.
Metoclopramide (Reglan) PO/IV	Dopamine receptor antagonist that promotes gastric emptying and accelerates intestinal transit time. PO/IV: 0.033-0.1 mg/kg q8h	Extrapyramidal symptoms, dys-tonic reactions	Extrapyramidal symptoms more likely at higher dosages or with prolonged use.

Continued

Medication (Trade Name)/Route of Administration	Mechanism of Action/Dosing	Important Adverse Events	Special Considerations
Metronidazole (Flagyl) PO/IV	Breaks helical structure of DNA, which results in inhibition of protein synthesis and cell death. Loading dose: 15 mg/kg Maintenance dose: PMA ≤29 wk: 0-28 days old: 7.5 mg/kg q48h >28 days old: 7.5 mg/kg q24h PMA 30-36 wk: 0-14 days old: 7.5 mg/kg q24h >14 days old: 7.5 mg/kg q12h PMA 37-44 wk: 0-7 days old: 7.5 mg/kg q24h >7 days old: 7.5 mg/kg q12h PMA ≥45 wk: 7.5 mg/kg q8h	GI disturbances, neutropenia, thrombocytopenia	
Micafungin (Mycamine) IV	Inhibits synthesis of essential cell wall components of susceptible fungi, which results in osmotic stress and lysis of the fungal cell. IV: 7-10 mg/kg q24h	Hypokalemia, hypernatremia, thrombocytopenia, elevated liver enzymes	Use higher dose (10 mg/kg) for meningitis and neonates of <27 wk GA and <14 days of age.
Midazolam (Versed) PO/IV/IM/IN/SL	Binds to receptors for GABA, the major inhibitory neurotransmitter, which enhances effects of GABA. IV push/IM: 0.05-0.15 mg/kg q2-4h prn Continuous IV infusion: 0.01-0.06 mg/kg/hr, titrated as needed IN/SL: 0.2 mg/kg PO: 0.25 mg/kg	Hypotension, respiratory depression, myoclonus	Used most often for sedation, but can also be used for refractory seizures. Prolonged or repeated use may have detrimental effects on neurodevelopmental outcomes. Respiratory depression more common when administered with narcotics. Preservative-free injection available.
Milrinone (Primacor) IV	Inhibits phosphodiesterase III, which potentiates delivery of calcium to the myocardium and results in a positive inotropic effect. Also causes relaxation of vascular muscle and vasodilatation. Loading dose: 50-75 μg/kg/min Continuous IV infusion: 0.25-0.75 μg/kg/min	Thrombocytopenia, arrhythmias, tachycardia, hypotension	Loading dose optional based on status of patient. Correct hypovolemia before initiation. Blood pressure may decrease 5%-9% after loading dose and heart rate may increase 5%-10%.
Morphine (Astramorph, Duramorph) PO/IV/IM/SC	Binds to opiate receptors in the CNS, altering perception of and response to pain. *Analgesia* IV/IM/SC: 0.05-0.2 mg/kg q4h prn Continuous IV infusion: 10-20 μg/kg/hr, titrated as needed PO: 0.15-0.3 mg/kg q4h prn (or 3 times IV dose) *NAS* PO: 0.03-0.1 mg/kg q3h, increase as needed to control withdrawal	Hypotension, vasodilation, flushing, pruritus, respiratory depression, GI disturbances	Closely monitor respiratory rate, blood pressure, heart rate, oxygen saturation, and bowel sounds. Metabolized to an active metabolite that is renally excreted. Effects reversed by naloxone. When used for NAS, wean 10%-20% daily as tolerated.

Medication (Trade Name)/Route of Administration	Mechanism of Action/Dosing	Important Adverse Events	Special Considerations
Nafcillin IV/IM	Inhibits bacterial cell wall synthesis by binding to penicillin-binding proteins. Sepsis: 25 mg/kg Meningitis: 50 mg/kg PMA ≤29 wk: 0-28 days old: q12h >28 days old: q8h PMA 30-36 wk: 0-14 days old: q12h >14 days old: q8h PMA 37-44 wk: 0-7 days old: q12h >7 days old: q8h PMA ≥45 wk: q6h	Extravasation, GI disturbances, acute interstitial nephritis	Increase dosing interval in the presence of hepatic dysfunction.
Naloxone (Narcan) IV/IM/SC	Competes and displaces narcotics at narcotic receptor sites. IV/IM: 0.1 mg/kg q2-3min prn		Half-life of naloxone may be shorter than that of opioids; therefore, repeating doses every 1-2 hr may be necessary. May precipitate withdrawal symptoms in neonates receiving long-term opioid therapy.
Neostigmine (Prostigmin) IV/IM/SC	Inhibits hydrolysis of acetylcholine, which facilitates cholinergic activity. IV: 0.04-0.08 mg/kg	Bradycardia, hypotension	Use for reversal of nondepolarizing neuromuscular blockade. Administer with 0.02 mg/kg atropine to minimize bradycardia.
Nevirapine (Viramune) PO	Antiretroviral agent that inhibits reverse transcriptase and disrupts life cycle of the virus. PO: 2 mg/kg × 1 dose as soon as possible after birth	GI disturbances, eosinophilia, neutropenia, hepatoxicity, granulocytopenia	Used in combination with zidovudine for prevention of mother-to-child HIV transmission. Consider consulting infectious disease specialist for specific recommendations on antiretroviral regimen and treatment beyond 1 dose.
Nystatin (Nystop) PO, topical	Binds to sterols in fungal cell membranes and increases permeability, which allows leakage of cellular contents. Topical: q6h PO: Preterm: 0.5 mL (50,000 U) to each side of mouth q6h Term: 1 mL (100,000 U) to each side of mouth q6h	Rash due to inactive ingredients in topical product	Continue treatment for 3 days after symptoms resolve.
Omeprazole (Prilosec) PO	Inhibits proton pump, which results in decreased gastric acid secretion. PO: 0.5-1.5 mg/kg q24h	Mild increase in transaminases with prolonged therapy	Monitor liver function with prolonged therapy.
Oxacillin IV/IM	Inhibits bacterial cell wall synthesis by binding to penicillin-binding proteins. Sepsis: 25 mg/kg Meningitis: 50 mg/kg PMA ≤29 wk: 0-28 days old: q12h >28 days old: q8h PMA 30-36 wk: 0-14 days old: q12h >14 days old: q8h PMA 37-44 wk: 0-7 days old: q12h >7 days old: q8h PMA ≥45 wk: q6h	Thrombocytopenia, leukopenia, eosinophilia, neutropenia, acute interstitial nephritis, extravasation, elevated liver enzymes	Poor CSF penetration. Consider extending dosing interval in the presence of poor renal function.

Continued

Medication (Trade Name)/Route of Administration	Mechanism of Action/Dosing	Important Adverse Events	Special Considerations
Palivizumab (Synagis) IM	Monoclonal antibody that neutralizes and inhibits respiratory syncytial virus (RSV). IM: 15 mg/kg every month during RSV season	Swelling at injection site, fever, upper respiratory tract infection	Immunoprophylaxis against RSV infection in high-risk infants; not effective for treatment of RSV disease.
Pancuronium (Pavulon) IV	Blocks acetylcholine from binding to motor end plate receptors, which inhibits depolarization and causes neuromuscular blockade. IV push: 0.04-0.15 mg/kg q1-2h	Tachycardia, changes in blood pressure	Use with sedatives and analgesics. Provide eye lubrication. Contains benzyl alcohol.
Papaverine IV	Smooth muscle spasmolytic that produces generalized smooth muscle relaxation and vasodilation. Continuous IV infusion: 30 mg per 250 mL arterial catheter solution; infuse at 1 mL/hr	Chronic hepatitis with long-term therapy	Prolongs patency of peripheral arterial catheter. Use with caution in first days of life in infants at risk of developing intracranial hemorrhage.

Penicillin G IV/IM	Inhibits bacterial cell wall synthesis by binding to penicillin-binding proteins.
	
	Meningitis: 75,000-100,000 U/kg
	Bacteremia: 25,000-50,000 U/kg
	PMA ≤29 wk:
	  0-28 days old: q12h
	  >28 days old: q8h
	PMA 30-36 wk:
	  0-14 days old: q12h
	  >14 days old: q8h
	PMA 37-44 wk:
	  0-7 days old: q12h
	  >7 days old: q8h
	PMA ≥45 wk: q6h
	GBS or gonococcal bacteremia:
	  200,000 U/kg/day divided q6-8h
	GBS or gonococcal meningitis:
	  500,000 U/kg/day divided q6-8h
	Congenital syphilis: 50,000 U/kg IV q12h for first 7 days, then q8h or 50,000 U/kg IM q24h
		Extravasation, **cardiorespiratory arrest and death if IM form given IV**	Use only aqueous penicillin for IV administration.
			Use procaine or benzathine penicillin for IM administration.
			Treat congenital syphilis for 10 days.

Phenobarbital (Luminal) PO/IV/IM	Binds to GABA receptor and enhances GABA activity, which results in depressed CNS activity. Loading dose: 20 mg/kg IV; repeat 5-10 mg/kg prn to total 40 mg/kg Maintenance dose: 3-5 mg/kg q24h IV, IM, or PO	Extravasation, respiratory depression, sedation, elevated liver enzymes	Begin maintenance dose 12-24 hr after loading dose. Avoid IM administration for loading dose due to erratic absorption and slower onset of action. Target serum concentration is 15-40 µg/mL; increased sedation at concentrations of >40 µg/mL and increased respiratory depression at concentrations of >60 µg/mL.
Phentolamine SC	Blocks α-adrenergic receptors and reverses vasoconstriction caused by extravasation. SC: 1-5 mL of 0.5 mg/mL solution		Amount injected into extravasation site depends on size of infiltrate. Use for extravasation of vasoconstrictive agents (dopamine, epinephrine, etc.).

Medication (Trade Name)/Route of Administration	Mechanism of Action/Dosing	Important Adverse Events	Special Considerations
Phenytoin (Dilantin) PO/IV	Stabilizes neuronal membranes and decreases seizure activity by altering sodium ion transport across cell membranes in the motor cortex. Loading dose: 15-20 mg/kg IV Maintenance dose: 4-8 mg/kg IV or PO q24h	Bradycardia, arrhythmia, and hypotension during infusion; extravasation; rickets; nystagmus; gingivitis	Infuse slowly at maximum rate of 0.5 mg/kg/min. Do not administer IM. Higher dosages (up to 8 mg/kg q8h) may be needed after 1 wk of age. Target total serum concentration is 6-15 μg/mL in first few weeks of life, then 10-20 μg/mL. Target free serum concentration is 1-2 μg/mL. Administer oral doses at same time daily with regard to meals. Injectable form contains alcohol and propylene glycol.

Piperacillin/tazobactam (Zosyn) IV	Inhibits bacterial cell wall synthesis by binding to penicillin-binding proteins. Tazobactam binds to β-lactamases and prevents degradation of piperacillin.
	
	IV: 50-100 mg/kg
	PMA $\leq$29 wk:
	  0-28 days old: q12h
	  >28 days old: q8h
	PMA 30-36 wk:
	  0-14 days old: q12h
	  >14 days old: q8h
	PMA 37-44 wk:
	  0-7 days old: q12h
	  >7 days old: q8h
	PMA $\geq$45 wk: q8h
		Eosinophilia, hyperbilirubinemia, elevated liver enzymes	Limited CNS penetration; avoid use if meningitis suspected.

Poractant alfa (Curosurf) IT	Natural surfactant extracted from porcine lung. Replaces deficient or ineffective endogenous lung surfactant. Initial dose: 2.5 mL/kg administered as soon as possible after birth Repeat doses: 1.25 mL/kg q12h prn × 2 doses	Reflux of surfactant up ET, decreased oxygenation, bradycardia	For IT administration only. Suspension should be at room temperature before administering. Do not artificially warm. Swirl suspension; do not shake or filter suspension. Continuously monitor heart rate and oxygen saturation during administration.
Propranolol (Inderal) PO/IV	Blocks stimulation of β_1- and β_2-adrenergic receptors, which results in decreased heart rate, myocardial contractility, and blood pressure. IV: 0.01 mg/kg q6h; increase prn to max 0.15 mg/kg q6h PO: 0.25 mg/kg q6h; increase prn to max 3.5 mg/kg q6h	Bradycardia, bronchospasm, hypoglycemia, hypotension	Rebound tachycardia occurs with abrupt discontinuation. Hypotension increased with underlying myocardial dysfunction.
Protamine IV	Combines with heparin to form complex with no anticoagulant activity. Dose based on time since last heparin dose: <30 min: 1 mg per 100 U heparin received 30-60 min: 0.5-0.75 mg per 100 U heparin received 60-120 min: 0.375-0.5 mg per 100 U heparin received >120 min: 0.25-0.375 mg per 100 U heparin received Max dose: 50 mg	Hypotension, bradycardia, bleeding problems	Infusion rate should not exceed 5 mg/min. Increased risk of bleeding and severe adverse reactions with high dose, rapid administration, or repeated doses.

Continued

Medication (Trade Name)/Route of Administration	Mechanism of Action/Dosing	Important Adverse Events	Special Considerations
Ranitidine (Zantac) PO/IV	Competitively inhibits histamine receptors in gastric parietal cells, which results in inhibition of gastric acid secretion. IV, term: 1.5 mg/kg q8h IV, preterm: 0.5 mg/kg q12h Continuous IV infusion: 0.04-0.1 mg/kg/hr PO: 2 mg/kg q8h	Thrombocytopenia, bradycardia, late-onset bacterial or fungal sepsis	Oral solution contains 7.5% alcohol.

Rifampin (Rifadin) PO/IV	Inhibits bacterial RNA synthesis by binding to β subunit of DNA-dependent RNA polymerase, thereby inhibiting RNA transcription.
	
	Treatment
	  IV: 5-10 mg/kg q12h
	  PO: 10-20 mg/kg q24h
	Prophylaxis
	Meningococcus: 5 mg/kg PO q12h × 2 days
	Haemophilus influenzae type B: 10 mg/kg PO q24h × 4 days
		Extravasation, elevated hepatic transaminases, thrombocytopenia	Causes orange-red discoloration of urine, sputum, tears, and other bodily fluids.
			Do not use as monotherapy due to quick development of resistance.

Rocuronium (Zemuron) IV	Binds to cholinergic receptor sites and blocks neural transmission at myoneural junction. IV: 0.3-0.6 mg/kg over 5-10 sec	Increased pulmonary vascular resistance	Must be given with adequate analgesia and sedation. Primarily used before intubation due to rapid onset and short duration of action.
Sildenafil (Revatio) PO/IV	Phosphodiesterase type-5 inhibitor that causes vasodilation in the pulmonary vasculature. IV: 0.25-1 mg/kg q6-12h PO: 0.5-2 mg/kg q6-12h	Worsening oxygenation, hypotension	Start therapy with lower dosages and titrate slowly based on oxygenation and blood pressure. Pharmacokinetics in neonates is not well defined. Data for neonates are limited and use is considered experimental.
Sodium bicarbonate IV	Dissociates to provide bicarbonate ion, which neutralizes hydrogen ion and raises blood and urinary pH. Usual dosage: 1-2 mEq/kg Based on base deficit: HCO_3 needed (mEq) = HCO_3 deficit (mEq/L) × (0.3 × weight in kg) Administer ½ calculated dose then reassess	Tissue necrosis, hypocalcemia, hypokalemia, hypernatremia	Administer 1-2 mEq/kg over at least 30 min. Maximum concentration used in neonates is 0.5 mEq/mL (4.2%). Do not administer with calcium- or phosphate-containing solutions. Not recommended for use in neonatal resuscitation.
Sotalol (Betapace) PO	Blocks stimulation of β_1- and β_2-adrenergic receptors, which results in decreased heart rate and AV node conduction. Prolongs refractory period of atrial muscle, ventricular muscle, and AV accessory pathways. PO: 1 mg/kg q12h; increase every 3 days until stable rhythm maintained to max dose of 4 mg/kg q12h	Arrhythmias (sinoatrial block, AV block, torsade de pointes, ventricular ectopic activity), hypotension, dyspnea	Continuous cardiac monitoring required for at least 3 days at maintenance dose. High dosages increase risk of torsade de pointes.
Spironolactone (Aldactone) PO	Competes for aldosterone receptors in distal renal tubules, increasing sodium, chloride, and water excretion while conserving potassium and hydrogen ions. PO: 1-3 mg/kg q24h	Hyperkalemia, GI upset	Significantly less diuretic effect than thiazide and loop diuretics; use only in combination with other diuretics. May help to decrease potassium losses secondary to use of other diuretics.

Medication (Trade Name)/Route of Administration	Mechanism of Action/Dosing	Important Adverse Events	Special Considerations
Ticarcillin/clavulanate (Timentin) IV	Inhibits bacterial cell wall synthesis by binding to penicillin-binding proteins. Clavulanic acid binds to β-lactamases and prevents degradation of ticarcillin. IV: 75-100 mg/kg PMA ≤29 wk: 0-28 days old: q12h >28 days old: q8h PMA 30-36 wk: 0-14 days old: q12h >14 days old: q8h PMA 37-44 wk: 0-7 days old: q12h >7 days old: q8h PMA ≥45 wk: q6h	Eosinophilia, hyperbilirubinemia, hypernatremia, elevated liver enzymes	Limited CNS penetration; avoid use if meningitis suspected.
Tobramycin IV/IM	Inhibits bacterial protein synthesis by inhibiting 30S and 50S ribosomal subunits, which results in defective bacterial cell membrane. PMA <35 wk: 4 mg/kg q24h PMA ≥35 wk: 5 mg/kg q24h	Nephrotoxicity, ototoxicity (increased risk with concurrent use of other nephrotoxic or ototoxic drugs)	Monitor serum trough concentration before third dose if treating for >48 hr. Target trough concentration is <1 μg/mL. Extend dosing interval if trough is >1 μg/mL. Should not be concurrently administered in same IV line with extended-spectrum penicillin.
Ursodiol (Actigall) PO	Reduces secretion of cholesterol from liver and reabsorption of cholesterol by intestines, which results in decreased cholesterol in bile and bile stones. PO: 10-15 mg/kg q12h	Abdominal pain, constipation, flatulence, nausea and vomiting	Administer with food.
Valganciclovir (Valcyte) PO	Rapidly metabolized to the active component ganciclovir, which competes for incorporation into viral DNA, interferes with viral DNA chain elongation, and thus inhibits viral replication. PO: 16 mg/kg q12h	Thrombocytopenia, neutropenia, anemia	Treat acute infections for minimum of 6 wk. Hold dose for ANC of <500 cells/mm^3 until ANC is >750 cells/mm^3. If ANC falls again to <750 cells/mm^3 reduce dose by 50%. If ANC falls to <500 cells/mm^3 discontinue drug.
Vancomycin (Vancocin) IV	Inhibits bacterial cell wall synthesis and alters bacterial cell membrane permeability. Meningitis: 15 mg/kg Bacteremia: 10 mg/kg PMA ≤29 wk: 0-14 days old: q18h >14 days old: q12h PMA 30-36 wk: 0-14 days old: q12h >14 days old: q8h PMA 37-44 wk: 0-7 days old: q12h >7 days old: q8h PMA ≥45 wk: q6h	Nephrotoxicity and ototoxicity (increased with aminoglycoside therapy), phlebitis, neutropenia	Serum trough concentrations correlate best with both efficacy and toxicity. Target serum trough concentration is 5-15 μg/mL. Concentrations up to 20 μg/mL have been targeted in severe infections.
Vecuronium (Norcuron) IV	Inhibits depolarization by blocking acetylcholine from binding to motor end plate receptors. IV push: 0.03-0.15 mg/kg q1-2h Continuous IV infusion: 0.06-0.1 mg/kg/hr	Bradycardia and hypotension when used with narcotics	Must be given with adequate sedation and analgesia. Provide eye lubrication.

Continued

Medication (Trade Name)/Route of Administration	Mechanism of Action/Dosing	Important Adverse Events	Special Considerations
Vitamin A (Aquasol A) IM	Retinol metabolites exhibit potent effects on gene expression and on lung growth and development. IM: 5000 U 3 times per week × 4 wk	Signs and symptoms of toxicity include lethargy, hepatomegaly, edema, bony tenderness, mucocutaneous lesions	Use in premature infants at highest risk of developing chronic lung disease.

Vitamin K (Mephyton, phytonadione) IM/IV	Promotes formation of clotting factors II, VII, IX, and X in the liver.
	
	Prophylaxis of hemorrhagic disease
	  Term: 0.5-1 mg IM
	  Preterm (<32 wk):
	    <1000 g: 0.3 mg/kg IM
	    ≥1000 g: 0.5 mg IM
	Treatment of hemorrhagic disease:
	  1-10 mg slow IV push
	Treatment of clotting deficiency:
	  1-10 mg IM or IV push
		Pain and swelling at IM injection site	Administer IV doses very slowly, not to exceed 1 mg/min. Severe reactions have been reported very rarely in adults.

Zidovudine (AZT) (Retrovir) IV/PO	Phosphorylated to its active metabolite, which is incorporated into HIV by reverse transcriptase; inhibits HIV viral polymerases and DNA synthesis.
	
	IV: 1.5 mg/kg
	PO: 2 mg/kg
	PMA ≤29 wk:
	  0-28 days old: q12h
	  >28 days old: q8h
	PMA 30-34 wk:
	  0-14 days old: q12h
	  >14 days old: q8h
	PMA ≥35 wk: q6h
		Anemia, neutropenia, thrombocytopenia	Begin within 6-12 hr of birth and continue for at least 6 wk. Consider consulting infectious disease specialist for specific antiretroviral regimen recommendations.

Adapted from Thomson Reuters Clinical Editorial Staff: *NeoFax*, Ann Arbor, Mich, 2011, Thomson Reuters; and Taketomo CK, Hodding JH, Kraus DM: *Pediatric dosage handbook,* ed 17, Hudson, Ohio, 2010-2011, Lexi-Comp.

ANc, Absolute neutrophil count; *APTT,* activated partial thromboplastin time; *AV,* atrioventricular; *BUN,* blood urea nitrogen; *CNS,* central nervous system; *CSF,* cerebrospinal fluid; *DART,* Dexamethasone—A Randomized Trial (multicenter study of low-dose dexamethasone therapy); *ET,* endotracheal tube; *GA,* gestational age; *GABA,* γ-aminobutyric acid; *GBS,* group B streptococcus; *GI,* gastrointestinal; *HIV,* human immunodeficiency virus; *IM,* intramuscular; *IN,* intranasal; *IT,* intratracheal; *IV,* intravenous; *max,* maximum; *MDI,* metered dose inhaler; *NAS,* neonatal abstinence syndrome; *Neb,* nebulizer; *NS,* normal saline; *PMA,* postmenstrual age; *PO,* by mouth; *PR,* per rectum; *prn,* as needed; *q,* every; *SC,* subcutaneous; *SL,* sublingual; *TPN,* total parenteral nutrition.

Drug Compatibility

Jacquelyn McClary and Leta Houston Hickey

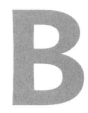

Name	Dosage	Indications	Side Effects	Compatibility	Considerations
Alprostadil (prostaglandin E_1)	Initial dose: 0.05-0.1 μg/kg/min Maintenance dose: 0.01-0.1 μg/kg/min	Maintain patency of ductus arteriosus	Apnea, hypotension, hyperthermia, seizures, diarrhea, flushing, bradycardia	*Solution:* D_5W, NS *Y-site:* TPN, heparin, gentamicin, dopamine, dobutamine, furosemide *Incompatible:* fat emulsion	Give through UAC only if absolutely necessary and if flow is not interrupted by obtaining laboratory specimens. Requires constant, patent IV access.
Dobutamine	2-25 μg/kg/min	Hypoperfusion or hypotension related to myocardial dysfunction	Tachycardia at high dosages, arrhythmia, hypertension, increased myocardial oxygen consumption, tissue ischemia with infiltration	*Solution:* D_5W, NS *Y-site:* TPN, fat emulsion, alprostadil, dopamine, gentamicin, morphine *Incompatible:* ampicillin, sodium bicarbonate	Correct hypovolemia prior to initiation of treatment. Monitor BP and HR continuously. Pink discoloration is not significant.
Dopamine	2-20 μg/kg/min	Hypotension	Tissue sloughing with infiltration, arrhythmias, increased pulmonary artery pressure	*Solution:* D_5W, NS *Y-site:* TPN, fat emulsion, alprostadil, dobutamine, gentamicin, heparin, morphine *Incompatible:* ampicillin, indomethacin, sodium bicarbonate	Use 1-5 mL of phentolamine 0.5 mg/mL for extravasation. Monitor BP and HR continuously. Check urine output and peripheral perfusion frequently. Protect from light. Do not use if solution is darker than slightly yellow.
Epinephrine	0.02-1 μg/kg/min	Asystole, severe bradycardia	Tachycardia, hypertension, arrhythmias, tremors, decreased renal and splanchnic blood flow, ischemia and necrosis of tissue if IV infiltration occurs	*Solution:* D_5W, $D_{10}W$, NS *Y-site:* TPN, heparin, gentamicin, dopamine, dobutamine *Incompatible:* fat emulsion, hyaluronidase, phenobarbital	Never give through UAC or other artery. Discard if brown or pink color observed. Attempt to correct any acidosis before infusion begins. Protect from light.
Milrinone	Loading dose: 50-75 μg/kg over 60 min (optional) Maintenance dose: 0.25-0.75 μg/kg/min	Low cardiac output	Decreased BP after loading dose, increased HR, arrhythmias, thrombocytopenia	*Solution:* D_5W, NS *Y-site:* TPN, ampicillin, dopamine, gentamicin, morphine, sodium bicarbonate *Incompatible:* fat emulsion, furosemide	Correct hypovolemia prior to initiation of therapy. Monitor HR and BP continuously. Monitor fluid and electrolyte changes. Assess renal function regularly. Monitor platelets.

Continued

Name	Dosage	Indications	Side Effects	Compatibility	Considerations
Sodium nitro-prusside (Nipride)	Initial dose: 0.25-0.5 μg/kg/min Maintenance dose: usually <2 μg/kg/min	Hyper-tension, afterload reduction in refractory congestive heart failure	Hypotension, decreased thyroid function, possible cyanide or thiocya-nate toxicity, local tissue necrosis	*Solution:* D$_5$W, NS **only** *Y-site:* TPN, fat emul-sion, heparin, gen-tamicin, morphine, dopamine *Incompatible:* ampicil-lin, hydralazine	Monitor BP and HR continuously. Assess renal and hepatic function daily. Follow cyanide and thiocyanate levels—levels should be <200 ng/mL and <50 μg/mL, respectively. Administer via periph-eral IV or central venous catheter. Protect from light with opaque material. Discard tubing after 24 hr. Slight brownish color is common and not significant.

BP, Blood pressure; *D$_5$W,* 5% dextrose in water; *D$_{10}$W,* 10% dextrose in water; *HR,* heart rate; *IV,* intravenous; *NS,* normal saline; *TPN,* total parenteral nutrition; *UAC,* umbilical artery catheter.

Normal Values

Mary Elaine Patrinos

C

CHEMISTRY VALUES

Table C-1. Blood Chemistry Values in Premature Infants during the First 7 Weeks of Life (Birth Weight 1500–1750 g)

Constituent	Age 1 Week		Age 3 Weeks		Age 5 Weeks		Age 7 Weeks	
	Mean ± SD	Range	Mean ± SD	Range	Mean ± SD	Range	Mean ± SD	Range
Na (mEq/L)	139.6 ± 3.2	133–146	136.3 ± 2.9	129–142	136.8 ± 2.5	133–148	137.2 ± 1.8	133–142
K (mEq/L)	5.6 ± 0.5	4.6–6.7	5.8 ± 0.6	4.5–7.1	5.5 ± 0.6	4.5–6.6	5.7 ± 0.5	4.6–7.1
Cl (mEq/L)	108.2 ± 3.7	100–117	108.3 ± 3.9	102–116	107.0 ± 3.5	100–115	107.0 ± 3.3	101–115
CO_2 (mmol/L)	20.3 ± 2.8	13.8–27.1	18.4 ± 3.5	12.4–26.2	20.4 ± 3.4	12.5–26.1	20.6 ± 3.1	13.7–26.9
Ca (mg/dL)	9.2 ± 1.1	6.1–11.6	9.6 ± 0.5	8.1–11.0	9.4 ± 0.5	8.6–10.5	9.5 ± 0.7	8.6–10.8
P (mg/dL)	7.6 ± 1.1	5.4–10.9	7.5 ± 0.7	6.2–8.7	7.0 ± 0.6	5.6–7.9	6.8 ± 0.8	4.2–8.2
BUN (mg/dL)	9.3 ± 5.2	3.1–25.5	13.3 ± 7.8	2.1–31.4	13.3 ± 7.1	2.0–26.5	13.4 ± 6.7	2.5–30.5
Total protein (g/dL)	5.49 ± 0.42	4.40–6.26	5.38 ± 0.48	4.28–6.70	4.98 ± 0.50	4.14–6.90	4.93 ± 0.61	4.02–5.86
Albumin (g/dL)	3.85 ± 0.30	3.28–4.50	3.92 ± 0.42	3.16–5.26	3.73 ± 0.34	3.20–4.34	3.89 ± 0.53	3.40–4.60
Globulin (g/dL)	1.58 ± 0.33	0.88–2.20	1.44 ± 0.63	0.62–2.90	1.17 ± 0.49	0.48–1.48	1.12 ± 0.33	0.5–2.60
Hb (g/dL)	17.8 ± 2.7	11.4–24.8	14.7 ± 2.1	9.0–19.4	11.5 ± 2.0	7.2–18.6	10.0 ± 1.3	7.5–13.9

Adapted from Thomas J, Reichelderfer T: Premature infants: analysis of serum during the first seven weeks, *Clin Chem* 14:272, 1968.
BUN, Blood urea nitrogen; *Hb,* hemoglobin; *SD,* standard deviation.

Table C-2.	Measured Variables in Cord and Whole Venous Blood in Healthy Term Neonates			
	Cord Blood		**2- to 4-Hour Blood**	
	Mean ± SD	**Range**	**Mean ± SD**	**Range**
pH	7.35 ± 0.05	7.19-7.42	7.36 ± 0.04	7.27-7.45
Pco_2 (mm Hg)	40 ± 6	24.5-56.7	43 ± 7	30-65
Hct (%)	48 ± 5	37-60	57 ± 5	42-67
Hb (g/L)	1.65 ± 0.16	1.29-2.06	1.90 ± 0.22	0.88-2.3
Na^+ (mmol/L)	138 ± 3	129-144	137 ± 3	130-142
K^+ (mmol/L)	5.3 ± 1.3	3.4-9.9	5.2 ± 0.5	4.4-6.4
Cl^- (mmol/L)	107 ± 4	100-121	111 ± 5	105-125
iCa (mmol/L)	1.15 ± 0.35	0.21-1.5	1.13 ± 0.08	0.9-1.3
iMg (mmol/L)	0.28 ± 0.06	0.09-0.39	0.30 ± 0.05	0.23-0.46
Glucose (mmol/L)	4.16 ± 1.05	0.16-6.66	3.50 ± 0.67	5.11-16.10
Glucose (mg/dL)	75 ± 19	2.9-120	63 ± 12	29-92
Lactate (mmol/L)	4.6 ± 1.9	1.1-9.6	3.9 ± 1.5	1.6-9.8
BUN (mmol/L)	2.14 ± 0.61	1.07-3.57	2.53 ± 0.71	1.43-4.28
BUN (mg/dL)	6.0 ± 1.7	3.0-10.0	7.1 ± 2.0	4-12

From Dollberg S, Bauer R, Lubetzky R, et al: A reappraisal of neonatal blood chemistry reference ranges using the Nova M electrodes, *Am J Perinatol* 18:433, 2001.
BUN, Blood urea nitrogen; *Hb,* hemoglobin; *Hct,* hematocrit; *iCa,* ionized calcium; *iMg,* ionized magnesium; *SD,* standard deviation.

Table C-3.	Plasma Ammonia Levels in Preterm Infants of ≤32 Weeks' Gestational Age	
	Ammonia Level*	
Age (days)	**µmol/L**	**µg/dL**
Birth	71 ± 26	121 ± 45[†]
1	69 ± 22	117 ± 37
3	60 ± 19	103 ± 33
7	42 ± 14	72 ± 24
14	42 ± 18	72 ± 30
21	43 ± 16	73 ± 28
28	42 ± 15	72 ± 25
Term infants at birth	45 ± 9	77 ± 16

Modified from Usmanii SS, Cavaliere T, Casatelli J, et al: Plasma ammonia levels in very low birth weight preterm infants, *J Pediatr* 123:798, 1993.
*Values represent mean ± 1 standard deviation unit.
[†]Plasma ammonia level declines significantly from birth to 7 days of age ($P < .01$).

Table C-4.	Liver Function Test Values	
Test	**Age**	**Value**
Albumin (g/L)	0-5 days (<2.5 kg)	20-36
	0-5 days (>2.5 kg)	26-36
	1-30 days	26-43
	31-182 days	28-46
	183-365 days	28-48
Prothrombin time (sec)	1 day (30-36 wk of gestation)	10.6-16.2
	5 days (30-36 wk of gestation)	10.0-15.3
	30 days (30-36 wk of gestation)	10.0-13.6
	90 days (30-36 wk of gestation)	10.0-14.6
	180 days (30-36 wk of gestation)	10.0-15.0
	1 day	11.6-14.4
	5 days	10.9-13.9
	30 days	10.6-13.1
	90 days	10.8-13.1
	180 days	11.5-13.1
Partial thromboplastin time (sec)	1 day (30-36 wk of gestation)	27.5-79.4
	5 days (30-36 wk of gestation)	26.9-74.1
	30 days (30-36 wk of gestation)	26.9-62.5
	90 days (30-36 wk of gestation)	28.3-50.7
	180 days (30-36 wk of gestation)	21.7-53.3
	1 day	37.1-48.7
	5 days	34.0-51.2
	30 days	33.0-47.8
	90 days	30.6-43.6
	180 days	31.8-39.2
Ammonia (μmol/L)	1-90 days	42-144
	3-11 mo	34-133
Aspartate aminotransferase (U/L)	0-5 days	35-140
	1-3 yr	20-60
Alanine aminotransferase (U/L)	0-5 days	6-50
	1-30 days	1-25
	31-365 days	3-35
Alkaline phosphatase (U/L)	0-5 days	110-300
	1-30 days	48-406
	31-365 days	82-383
γ-Glutamyltransferase (U/L)	0-5 days	34-263
	1-182 days	12-132
	183-365 days	1-39

Adapted from Rosenthal P: Assessing liver function and hyperbilirubinemia in the newborn. National Academy of Clinical Biochemistry, *Clin Chem* 43:228, 1997.
For full-term infants unless otherwise noted.

Table C-5.	Plasma-Serum Amino Acid Levels in Premature and Term Newborns (μmol/L)		
Amino Acid	**Premature (First Day)**	**Newborn (Before First Feeding)**	**16 Days to 4 Months**
Taurine	105-255	101-181	
Hydroxyproline	0-80	0	
Aspartic acid	0-20	4-12	17-21
Threonine	155-275	196-238	141-213
Serine	195-345	129-197	104-158
Aspartate + Glutamate	655-1155	623-895	
Proline	155-305	155-305	141-245
Glutamic acid	30-100	27-77	
Glycine	185-735	274-412	178-248
Alanine	325-425	274-384	239-345
Valine	80-180	97-175	123-199
Cystine	55-75	49-75	33-51
Methionine	30-40	21-37	15-21
Isoleucine	20-60	31-47	31-47
Leucine	45-95	55-89	56-98
Tyrosine	20-220	53-85	33-75
Phenylalanine	70-110	64-92	45-65
Ornithine	70-110	66-116	37-61
Lysine	130-250	154-246	117-163
Histidine	30-70	61-93	64-92
Arginine	30-70	37-71	53-71
Tryptophan	15-45	15-45	
Citrulline	8.5-23.7	10.8-21.1	
Ethanolamine	13.4-10.5	32.7-72	
α-Amino-*n*-butyric acid	0-29	8.7-20.4	

From Behrman RE: *Neonatal-perinatal medicine: diseases of the fetus and infant,* ed 2, St Louis, 1977, Mosby, Appendix Table 20. Data from Dickinson JC, Rosenblum H, Hamilton PB: Ion exchange chromatography of the free amino acids in the plasma of the newborn infant, *Pediatrics* 36:2, 1965; and Dickinson JC, Rosenblum H, Hamilton PB: Ion exchange chromotography of the free amino acids in the plasma of infants under 2,500 gm at birth, *Pediatrics* 45:606, 1970.

Table C-6.	Reference Serum Amino Acid Concentrations That Have Been Proposed as Standards for Neonates (µmol/L)	
Amino Acid	**Term Infant Fed Human Milk**	**Cord Blood**
Isoleucine	26-93	21-76
Leucine	53-169	47-120
Lysine	80-231	181-456
Methionine	22-50	8-42
Phenylalanine	22-71	24-87
Threonine	34-168	108-327
Tryptophan	18-101	19-98
Valine	88-222	98-276
Alanine	125-647	186-494
Arginine	42-148	28-162
Aspartic acid	5-51	18 ± 17
Glutamic acid	24-243	92 ± 57
Glycine	77-376	123-312
Histidine	34-119	42-136
Proline	82-319	72-278
Serine	0-326	57-174
Taurine	1-167	41-461
Tyrosine	38-119	34-83
Cystine	35-132	4-37

Modified from Hanning RM, Zlotkin SH: Amino acid and protein needs of the neonate: effects of excess and deficiency, *Semin Perinatol* 13:131, 1989. See also Moro G, Minoli I, Boehm G, et al: Postprandial plasma amino acids in preterm infants: influence of the protein source, *Acta Paediatr* 88:885, 1999.

Table C-7.	Reference Intervals for Urine Amino Acid Excretion in Untimed Samples (mmol per mol creatinine)	
Amino Acid	**0-1 Months (Mean)**	**1-12 Months (Mean)**
Aspartic acid	9-57 (23)	10-69 (26)
Glutamic acid	31-96 (54)	24-102 (50)
α-Aminoadipic acid	7-96 (26)	7-110 (29)
Hydroxyproline	11-556 (100)	5-238 (34)
Phosphoethanol-amine	13-167 (46)	12-216 (51)
Serine	48-509 (156)	34-329 (51)
Asparagine	15-223 (58)	18-197 (59)
Glycine	127-2042 (510)	133-894 (345)
Glutamine	37-600 (148)	63-446 (168)
β-Alanine	2-41 (8)	2-38 (8)
Taurine*	12-1057	10-809
Histidine	23-676 (125)	69-392 (164)
Citrulline	1-18 (5)	2-46 (9)
Threonine	9-337 (56)	12-145 (41)
Alanine	34-358 (109)	27-313 (93)
β-Aminoisobutyric acid	0-520 (14)	5-258 (36)
Carnosine	3-184 (21)	8-160 (36)
Arginine	0-81 (10)	0-40 (5)
Proline	3-257 (29)	2-90 (14)
1-Methylhistidine	0-78 (7)	0-98 (7)
3-Methylhistidine	5-85 (20)	10-95 (31)
Ethanolamine	33-253 (91)	57-221 (112)
Aminobutyric acid	1-43 (5)	1-58 (7)
Tyrosine	5-74 (19)	12-64 (28)
Valine	3-34 (10)	3-43 (11)
Methionine	2-24 (7)	2-18 (6)
Cystathionine	1-26 (6)	1-11 (4)
Cystine	5-109 (24)	2-42 (10)
Isoleucine	2-37 (8)	2-21 (6)
Leucine	4-84 (17)	4-72 (17)
Hydroxylysine	3-49 (11)	2-50 (9)
Phenylalanine	2-49 (9)	7-42 (17)
Tryptophan	1-46 (8)	3-37 (10)
Ornithine	2-37 (8)	2-19 (6)
Lysine	6-464 (54)	4-80 (18)
No. of subjects (male/female)	20 (11/9)	30 (16/14)

Modified from Venta R: Year-long validation study and reference values for urinary amino acids using a reverse-phase HPLC method, *Clin Chem* 47:575, 2001.
*Observed ranges.

HEMATOLOGIC VALUES

Table C-8. Red Blood Cell Parameters of Infants with Very Low Birth Weight during the First 6 Weeks of Life Derived from Arterial or Venous but Not Capillary Blood Samples

Day of Life	No. of Infants	Percentile								
		3	5	10	25	Median	75	90	95	97
Hemoglobin (g/dL)										
3*	559	11.0	11.6	12.5	14.0	15.6	17.1	18.5	19.3	19.8
12-14	203	10.1	10.8	11.1	12.5	14.4	15.7	17.4	18.4	18.9
24-26	192	8.5	8.9	9.7	10.9	12.4	14.2	15.6	16.5	16.8
40-42	150	7.8	7.9	8.4	9.3	10.6	12.4	13.8	14.9	15.4
Hematocrit (%)										
3	561	35	36	39	43	47	52	56	59	60
12-14	205	30	32	34	39	44	48	53	55	56
24-26	196	25	27	29	32	39	44	48	50	52
40-42	152	24	24	26	28	33	38	44	47	48
Red blood cells (10^{12}/L)										
3	364	3.2	3.3	3.5	3.8	4.2	4.6	4.9	5.1	5.3
12-14	196	2.9	3.0	3.2	3.5	4.1	4.6	5.2	5.5	5.6
24-26	188	2.6	2.6	2.8	3.2	3.8	4.4	4.8	5.2	5.3
40-42	148	2.5	2.5	2.6	3.0	3.4	4.1	4.6	4.8	4.9
Corrected reticulocytes (%)										
3	283	0.6	0.7	1.9	4.2	7.1	12.0	20.0	24.1	27.8
12-14	139	0.3	0.3	0.5	0.8	1.7	2.7	5.7	7.3	9.6
24-26	140	0.2	0.3	0.5	0.8	1.5	2.6	4.7	6.4	8.6
40-42	114	0.3	0.4	0.6	1.0	1.8	3.4	5.6	8.3	9.5

From Obladen M, Diepold K, Maier RF; European Multicenter rhEPO Study Group: Venous and arterial hematologic profiles of very low birth weight infants, *Pediatrics* 106:709, 2000.

*On day 3, all infants are included regardless of the use of antenatal steroids and transfusions up to that time. Thereafter, infants who did not receive erythropoietin were studied regardless of the use of antibiotics and steroids.

| Table C-9. | Reference Values for Nucleated Red Blood Cell (NRBC) Count from Umbilical Vein Sampling at Birth in 695 Newborns Divided into Four Groups According to Gestational Age |

| | | Birth Weight (g) | | Gestational Age (wk) | | NRBC* | | |
	No. of Newborns	Mean ± SD	25th-75th Percentiles	Mean ± SD	25th-75th Percentiles	Mean ± SD	Median	25th-75th Percentiles
Group 1	120	954 ± 234	780-1105	26.7 ± 1	26-28	5643 ± 7228	2601	1147-7790
Group 2	128	1413 ± 398	1100-1720	30.4 ± 1	29-31	3328 ± 3577	1901	492-5970
Group 3	215	2189 ± 473	1940-2520	34.7 ± 1	34-36	1099 ± 1275	696	0-1672
Group 4	232	3201 ± 669	2905-3590	38.6 ± 1	38-40	442 ± 807	0	0-638

Adapted from Perrone S, Vezzosi P, Longini M, et al: Nucleated red blood cell count in term and preterm newborns: reference values at birth, *Arch Dis Child Fetal Neonatal Ed* 90:F174, 2005.
*Absolute count (NRBCs/mm^3).
SD, Standard deviation.

Table C-10.	Hematologic Values in the First Weeks of Life Related to Gestational Maturity

MEAN CORPUSCULAR HEMOGLOBIN CONCENTRATION (%)*

	3 days	1 Week	2 Weeks	3 Weeks	4 Weeks	6 Weeks	8 Weeks	10 Weeks
<1500 g, 28-32 wk	32	32	32	33	33	33	33	32
1500-2000 g, 32-36 wk	32	32	32	33	33	33	33	32
2000-2500 g, 36-40 wk	32	32	33	33	33	33	33	33
>2500 g, Term	32	33	33	33	33	33	33	33

HEMOGLOBIN (g/dL)—MEAN (SD)

	3 days	1 Week	2 Weeks	3 Weeks	4 Weeks	6 Weeks	8 Weeks	10 Weeks
<1500 g, 28-32 wk	17.5 (1.5)	15.5 (1.5)	13.5 (1.1)	11.5 (1.0)	10.0 (0.9)	8.5 (0.5)	8.5 (0.5)	9.0 (0.5)
1500-2000 g, 32-36 wk	19.0 (2.0)	16.5 (1.5)	14.5 (1.1)	13.0 (1.1)	12.0 (1.0)	9.5 (0.8)	9.5 (0.5)	9.5 (0.5)
2000-2500 g, 36-40 wk	19.0 (2.0)	16.5 (1.5)	15.0 (1.5)	14.0 (1.1)	12.5 (1.0)	10.5 (0.9)	10.5 (0.9)	11.0 (1.0)
>2500 g, Term	19.0 (2.0)	17.0 (1.5)	15.5 (1.5)	14.0 (1.1)	12.5 (1.0)	11.0 (1.0)	11.5 (1.0)	12.0 (1.0)

HEMATOCRIT (%)—MEAN (SD)

	3 days	1 Week	2 Weeks	3 Weeks	4 Weeks	6 Weeks	8 Weeks	10 Weeks
<1500 g, 28-32 wk	54 (5)	48 (5)	42 (4)	35 (4)	30 (3)	25 (2)	25 (2)	28 (3)
1500-2000 g, 32-36 wk	59 (6)	51 (5)	44 (5)	39 (4)	36 (4)	28 (3)	28 (3)	29 (3)
2000-2500 g, 36-40 wk	59 (6)	51 (5)	45 (5)	43 (4)	37 (4)	31 (3)	31 (3)	33 (3)
>2500 g, Term	59 (6)	51 (5)	46 (5)	43 (4)	37 (4)	33 (3)	34 (3)	36 (3)

RETICULOCYTE COUNT (%)—MEAN (SD)

	3 days	1 Week	2 Weeks	4 Weeks	6 Weeks	8 Weeks	10 Weeks
<1500 g 28-32 wk	8.0 (3.5)	3.0 (1.0)	3.0 (1.0)	6.0 (2.0)	11.0 (3.5)	8.5 (3.5)	7.0 (3.0)
1500-2000 g 32-36 wk	6.0 (2.0)	3.0 (1.0)	2.5 (1.0)	3.0 (1.0)	6.0 (2.0)	5.0 (1.5)	4.5 (1.5)
2000-2500 g 36-40 wk	4.0 (1.0)	3.0 (1.0)	2.5 (1.0)	2.0 (1.0)	3.0 (1.0)	3.0 (1.0)	3.0 (1.0)
>2500 g Term	4.0 (1.5)	3.0 (1.0)	2.0 (1.0)	2.0 (1.0)	2.0 (0.5)	2.0 (0.5)	2.0 (0.5)

*Mean corpuscular volume (MCV) and mean corpuscular hemoglobin (MCH) in cubic micrometers and picograms, respectively, depend on red cell counts that are not generally reliable.
SD, Standard deviation.

Table C-11.	Mean Hematocrit by Age in Hours and Gestational Age		
	Gestational Age (wk)		
Age (hr)	**35-42**	**29-34**	**22-28**
0	51	50	45
1	52	50	44
2	54	50	42
3	53	50	41
4	53	48	39

Data for three groups of neonates are shown (*N* = 23,534), categorized by gestational age.
Modified from Jopling J, Henry E, Wiedmeier SE, et al: Reference ranges for hematocrit and blood hemoglobin concentration during the neonatal period: data from a multihospital health care system, *Pediatrics* 123(2):e333, 2009.

Table C-12.	White Cell and Differential Counts in Premature Infants					
	Birth Weight <1500 g			**Birth Weight 1500-2500 g**		
	Age in Weeks			**Age in Weeks**		
	1	**2**	**4**	**1**	**2**	**4**
Total count ($\times 10^3/mm^3$)						
Mean	16.8	15.4	12.1	13.0	10.0	8.4
Range	6.1-32.8	10.4-21.3	8.7-17.2	6.7-14.7	7.0-14.1	5.8-12.4
Percentage of total polymorphs						
Segmented	54	45	40	55	43	41
Unsegmented	7	6	5	8	8	6
Eosinophils	2	3	3	2	3	3
Basophils	1	1	1	1	1	1
Monocytes	6	10	10	5	9	11
Lymphocytes	30	35	41	9	36	38

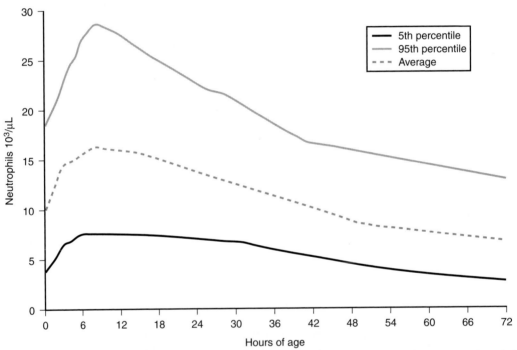

Figure C-1. Neutrophils per microliter of blood during the first 72 hours after birth in term and near-term (>36 weeks' gestation) neonates. A total of 12,149 values were obtained for the analysis. The 5th percentile, the mean, and the 95th percentile values are shown. *(From Schmutz N, Henry E, Jopling J, et al: Expected ranges for blood neutrophil concentrations of neonates: the Manroe and Mouzinho charts revisited,* J Perinatol *28:275, 2008.)*

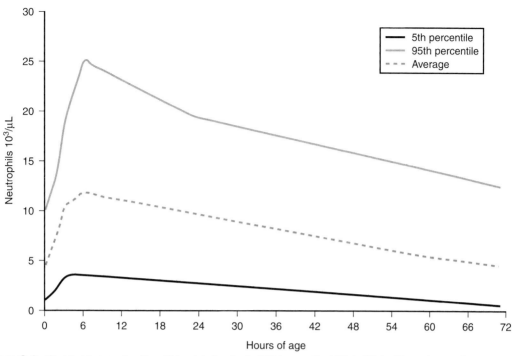

Figure C-2. Neutrophils per microliter of blood during the first 72 hours after birth in 28- to 36-week gestation preterm neonates. A total of 8896 values were obtained for the analysis. The 5th percentile, the mean, and the 95th percentile values are shown. *(From Schmutz N, Henry E, Jopling J, et al: Expected ranges for blood neutrophil concentrations of neonates: the Manroe and Mouzinho charts revisited,* J Perinatol *28:275, 2008.)*

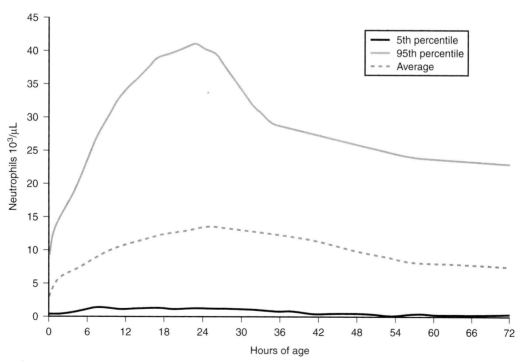

Figure C-3. Neutrophils per microliter of blood during the first 72 hours after birth in preterm neonates of less than 28 weeks' gestation. A total of 852 values were obtained for the analysis. The 5th percentile, the mean, and the 95th percentile values are shown. *(From Schmutz N, Henry E, Jopling J, et al: Expected ranges for blood neutrophil concentrations of neonates: the Manroe and Mouzinho charts revisited,* J Perinatol *28:275, 2008.)*

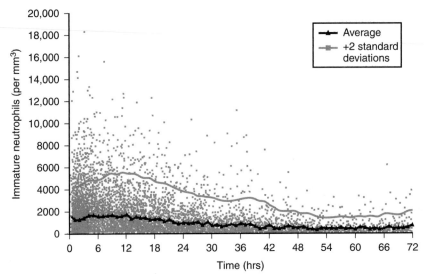

Figure C-4. Immature neutrophils (band neutrophils plus metamyelocytes) per microliter of blood during the first 72 hours after birth in term and near-term (>36 weeks' gestation) neonates. A total of 12,857 values were obtained for the analysis. Values for the average and 2 standard deviations above the mean are shown. *(From Schmutz N, Henry E, Jopling J, et al: Expected ranges for blood neutrophil concentrations of neonates: the Manroe and Mouzinho charts revisited, J Perinatol 28:275, 2008.)*

CEREBROSPINAL FLUID VALUES

Table C-13.   Cerebrospinal Fluid Values in Infants with Birth Weight of 1000 Grams or Less

| | Postnatal Age (Days) | | | | | |
| | 0-7 | | 8-28 | | 29-84 | |
	Mean ± SD	Range	Mean ± SD	Range	Mean ± SD	Range
Birthweight (g)	822 ± 116	630-980	752 ± 112	550-970	750 ± 120	550-907
Gestational age at birth (wk)	26 ± 1.2	24-27	26 ± 1.5	24-28	26 ± 1.0	24-27
Leukocytes/µL	3 ± 3	1-8	4 ± 4	0-14	4 ± 3	0-11
Erythrocytes/µL	335 ± 709	0-1780	1465 ± 4062	0-19050	808 ± 1843	0-6850
Polymorphonuclear cells (%)	11 ± 20	0-50	8 ± 17	0-66	2 ± 9	0-36
Glucose (mg/dL)	70 ± 17	41-89	68 ± 48	33-217	49 ± 22	29-90
Protein (mg/dL)	162 ± 37	115-222	159 ± 77	95-370	137 ± 61	76-260

Modified from Rodriguez AF, Kaplan SL, Mason EO Jr: Cerebrospinal fluid values in the very low birth weight infant, *J Pediatr* 116:971, 1990.
SD, Standard deviation.

Table C-14.	Cerebrospinal Fluid Values in Infants with Birth Weight of 1000 to 1500 Grams					
	Postnatal Age (Days)					
	0-7		**8-28**		**29-84**	
	Mean ± SD	**Range**	**Mean ± SD**	**Range**	**Mean ± SD**	**Range**
Birth weight (g)	1428 ± 107	1180-1500	1245 ± 162	1020-1480	1211 ± 86	1080-1300
Gestational age at birth (wk)	31 ± 1.5	28-33	29 ± 1.2	27-31	29 ± 0.7	27-29
Leukocytes/μL	4 ± 4	1-10	7 ± 11	0-44	8 ± 8	0-23
Erythrocytes/μL	407 ± 853	0-2450	1101 ± 2643	0-9750	661 ± 1198	0-3800
Polymorphonuclear cells (%)	4 ± 10	0-28	10 ± 19	0-60	11 ± 19	0-48
Glucose (mg/dL)	74 ± 19	50-96	59 ± 23	39-109	47 ± 13	31-76
Protein (mg/dL)	136 ± 35	85-176	137 ± 46	54-227	122 ± 47	45-187

Modified from Rodriguez AF, Kaplan SL, Mason EO Jr: Cerebrospinal fluid values in the very low birth weight infant, *J Pediatr* 116:971, 1990.
SD, Standard deviation.

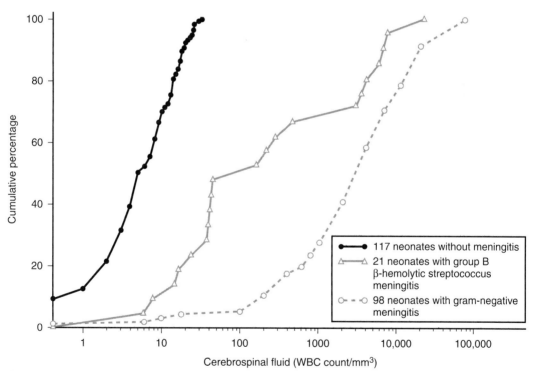

Figure C-5. Comparison of cerebrospinal fluid white blood cell (WBC) counts in neonates with and without meningitis.

Table C-15.   Cerebrospinal Fluid Values in Term Neonates*

Week	Age (days)	No. of Neonates	White Blood Cells (per µL)					Protein (mg/dL)	Glucose (mg/dL)
			Mean ± SD	95% CI	Median	Range	90th Percentile	Mean ± SD	Mean ± SD
1	0-7	17	15.3 ± 30.3	12.5-18.1	6	1-130	18	80.8 ± 30.8	45.9 ± 7.5
2	8-14	33	5.4 ± 4.4	4.6-6.1	6	0-18	10	69 ± 22.6	54.3 ± 17
3	15-21	25	7.7 ± 12.1	6.3-9.1	4	0-62	12.5	59.8 ± 23.4	46.8 ± 8.8
4	22-30	33	4.8 ± 3.4	4.1-5.4	4	0-18	8	54.1 ± 16.2	54.1 ± 16.2
All		108	7.3 ± 13.9	6.6-8	4	0-130	11	64.2 ± 24.2	51.2 ± 12.9

Modified from Rodriguez AF, Kaplan SL, Mason EO Jr: Cerebrospinal fluid values in the very low birth weight infant, *J Pediatr* 116:971, 1990.
*All neonates tested were suspected of having an infection, but no central nervous system infection was found.
CI, Confidence interval; *SD,* standard deviation.

PHYSIOLOGIC PARAMETERS
GROWTH CHARTS

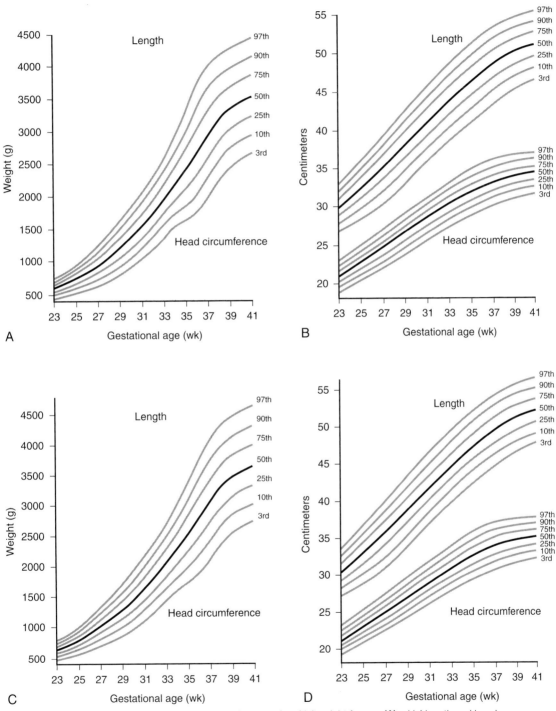

Figure C-6. New gender-specific intrauterine growth curves for girls' weight for age **(A)**, girls' length and head circumference for age **(B)**, boys' weight for age **(C)**, and boys' length and head circumference for age **(D)**. The 3rd and 97th percentile values on all curves for 23 weeks should be interpreted cautiously because of the small sample size; for boys' head circumference at 24 weeks, all percentile curves should be interpreted cautiously, because the distribution of data is skewed left. *(Adapted from Groveman SA: New preterm infant growth curves: influence of gender and race on birth size, master's thesis, Philadelphia, 2008, Drexel University.)*

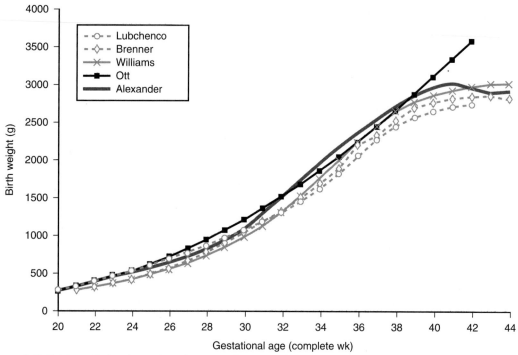

Figure C-7. Fetal growth data from selected sources. *(Data from Lubchenko LO, Hansman C, Dressler M, et al: Intrauterine growth as estimated from liveborn birth-weight data at 24 to 42 weeks of gestation,* Pediatrics *32:793, 1963; Brenner WE, Edelman DA, Hendricks CH: A standard of fetal growth for the United States of America,* Am J Obstet Gynecol *126:555, 1976; Williams RL: Intrauterine growth curves: Intra- and international comparisons with different ethnic groups in california,* Prevent Med *4:163, 1975; Ott W: Intrauterine growth retardation and preterm delivery,* Am J Obstet Gynecol *168:1710, 1993; Alexander GR, Himes JH, Kaufman RB, et al: A United States reference for fetal growth,* Obstet Gynecol *87:163, 1996.)*

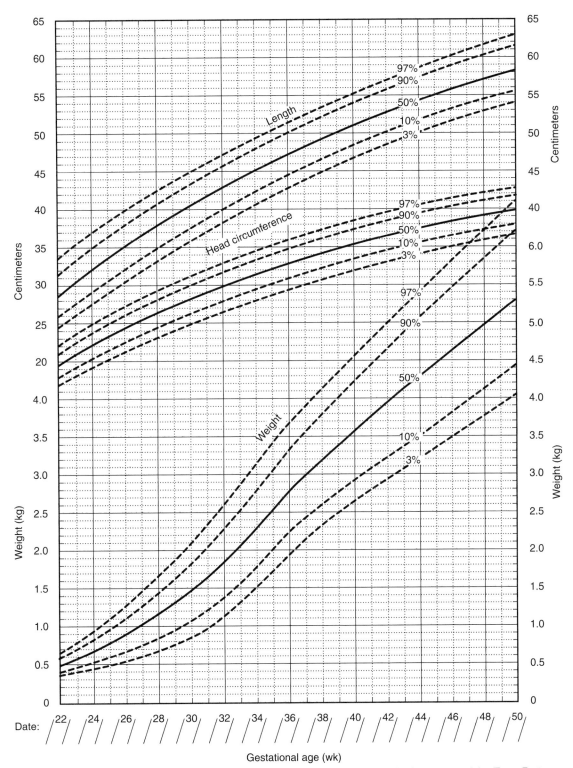

Figure C-8. Fetal-infant growth chart developed through a meta-analysis of published reference materials. *(From Fenton TR: A new growth chart for preterm babies: Babson and Benda's chart updated with recent data and a new format,* BMC Pediatr *3:13, 2003.)*

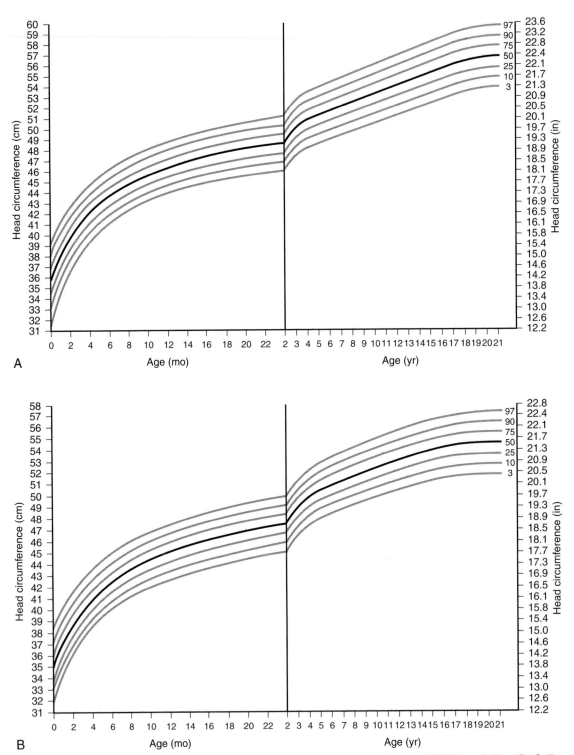

Figure C-9. Proposed occipitofrontal circumference growth curves for males **(A)** and females **(B)**. *(From Rollins JD, Collins JS, Holden KR: United States head circumference growth reference charts: birth to 21 years,* J Pediatr *156[6]:907, 2010.)*

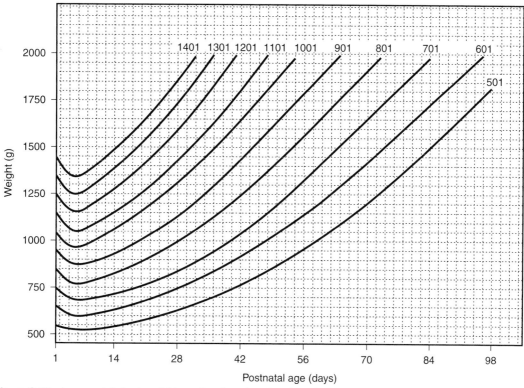

Figure C-10. Average daily body weight as a function of postnatal age in days for infants stratified by 100-g birth-weight intervals. *(From Ehrenkranz RA, Younes N, Lemons JA, et al: Longitudinal growth of hospitalized very low birth weight infants,* Pediatrics *104:280, 1999.)*

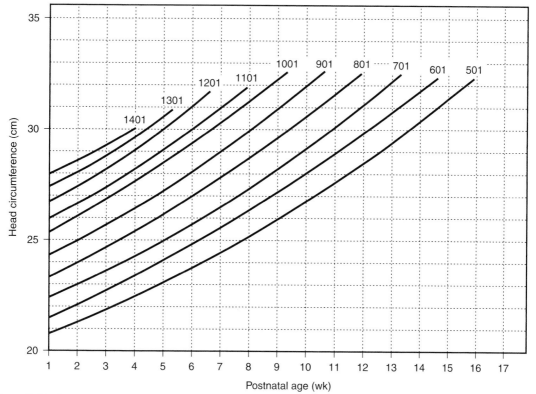

Figure C-11. Average weekly head circumference as a function of postnatal age in weeks for infants stratified by 100-g birth-weight intervals. *(From Ehrenkranz RA, Younes N, Lemons JA, et al: Longitudinal growth of hospitalized very low birth weight infants,* Pediatrics *104:280, 1999.)*

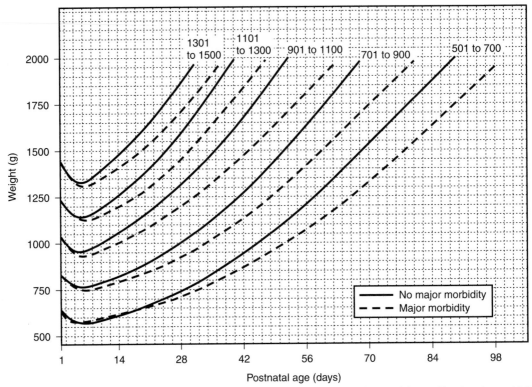

Figure C-12. Growth curves of infants with major morbidities *(dashed lines)* and reference infants without major morbidities *(solid line)* as a function of postnatal age in days. The infants are stratified by 200-g birth-weight intervals. Reference group infants without major morbidities were appropriate size for gestational age and survived to discharge without development of chronic lung disease, severe intraventricular hemorrhage, necrotizing enterocolitis, or late-onset sepsis. *(From Ehrenkranz RA, Younes N, Lemons JA, et al: Longitudinal growth of hospitalized very low birth weight infants,* Pediatrics *104:280, 1999.)*

TIME OF FIRST VOID AND STOOL

Table C-16.	Time of First Void and Stool							

Time of First Void by 920 Full-Term Infants				Time of Passage of First Stool by 920 Full-Term Infants			
Time	**No.**	**%**	**Cumulative %**	**Time**	**No.**	**%**	**Cumulative %**
Delivery room	139	15.1	15.1	Delivery room	210	22.8	22.8
Hours				Hours			
1-24	743	80.8	95.9	1-24	674	73.3	96.1
24-48	35	3.8	99.7	24-48	35	3.8	99.9
>48	3	0.3	100.0	>48	1	0.1	100.0

Time of First Void by 280 Premature Infants				Time of Passage of First Stool by 280 Premature Infants			
Time	**No.**	**%**	**Cumulative %**	**Time**	**No.**	**%**	**Cumulative %**
Delivery room	62	22.1	22.1	Delivery room	30	10.7	10.7
Hours				Hours			
1-24	201	71.8	93.9	1-24	191	68.2	78.9
24-48	17	6.1	100.0	24-48	46	16.4	95.3
>48				>48	13	4.7	100.0

Adapted from Sherry S, Kramer I: The time of passage of the first stool and first urine by the newborn infant, *J Pediatr* 46:158, 1955; Kramer I, Sherry S: The time of passage of the first stool and urine by the premature infant, *J Pediatr* 51:353, 1957; and Clark D: Times of first void and stool in 500 newborns, *Pediatrics* 60:457, 1977.

BLOOD PRESSURE

Table C-17.	Mean Arterial Blood Pressure (MAP) by Birth Weight		
	Mean MAP ± SD		
Birth Weight (g)	**Day 3**	**Day 17**	**Day 31**
501-750	38 ± 8	44 ± 8	46 ± 11
751-1000	43 ± 9	45 ± 7	47 ± 9
1001-1250	43 ± 8	46 ± 9	48 ± 8
1251-1500	45 ± 8	47 ± 8	47 ± 9

From Fanaroff AA, Wright E for the NICHD Neonatal Research Network Bethesda, MD: Profiles of mean arterial blood pressure (MAP) for infants weighing 501-1500 grams, *Pediatr Res* 27:205A, 1990.
SD, Standard deviation.

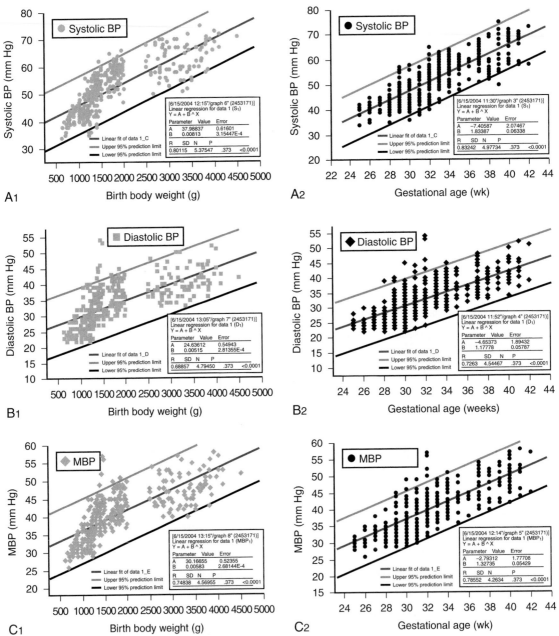

Figure C-13. Linear regression of systolic blood pressure **(top row)**, diastolic blood pressure **(middle row)**, and mean blood pressure **(bottom row)** on birth weight **(left column)** and gestational age **(right column)** on day 1 of life, with 95% confidence limits *(upper and lower solid lines)*. The 95% confidence limits approximate ±2 standard deviations (SDs) from the mean. *BP,* Blood pressure; *MBP,* mean blood pressure. *(From Pejovic B, Peco-Antic A, Marinkoviv-Eri J: Blood pressure in non-critically ill preterm and full-term neonates,* Pediatr Nephrol 22:249, 2007.)

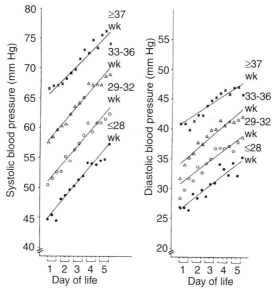

Figure C-14. Systolic blood pressure and diastolic blood pressure in the first 5 days of life, with each day subdivided into 8-hour periods. Infants are stratified by gestational age into four groups: 28 weeks or less (*n* = 33), 29 to 32 weeks (*n* = 73), 33 to 36 weeks (*n* = 100), and 37 weeks or more (*n* = 110). *(From Zubrow AB, Hulman S, Kushner H, et al: Determinants of blood pressure in infants admitted to neonatal intensive care units: a prospective multicenter study. Philadelphia Neonatal Blood Pressure Study Group,* J Perinatol *15:470, 1995.)*

MORBIDITY AND MORTALITY

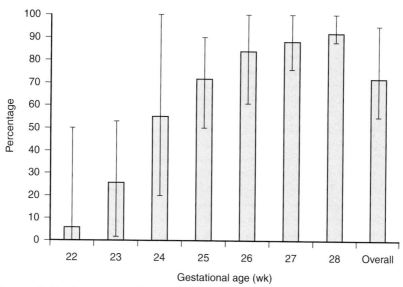

Figure C-15. Mean survival to discharge as a function of gestational age for 9575 low-birth-weight infants born in National Institute of Child Health and Human Development Neonatal Research Network centers between January 1, 2003 and December 31, 2007. The thin lines indicate ranges across centers. *(From Stoll BJ, Hansen NI, Bell EF, et al for the Eunice Kennedy Shriver National Institute of Child Health and Human Development Neonatal Research Network: Neonatal outcomes of extremely preterm infants from the NICHD Neonatal Research Network,* Pediatrics *126:443, 2010.)*

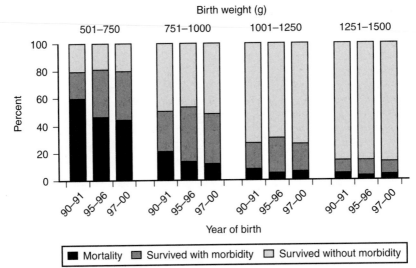

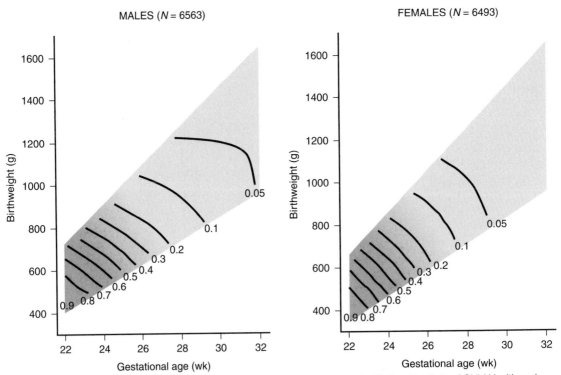

Figure C-16. Comparison of mortality, morbidity, and morbidity-free survival for very low-birth-weight infants cared for in 12 National Institute of Child Health and Human Development Neonatal Research Network centers in 1990 to 1991, 1995 to 1996, and 1997 to 2000. Data are for singleton infants born in the centers and stratified by 250-g birth weight intervals. *(From Fanaroff AA, Stoll BJ, Wright LL, et al for the NICHD Neonatal Research Network: Trends in neonatal morbidity and mortality for very low birthweight infants. Am J Obstet Gynecol 196:147.e1-e8, 2007.)*

Figure C-17. Mortality rates by birth weight, gestational age, and gender from the National Institute of Child Health and Human Development from 1997 to 2002. The upper and lower limits of the shaded areas are the 95th and 5th percentiles, respectively, for birth weight for each gestational age. The curved lines indicate combinations of birth weight and gestational age with the same estimated probability of mortality (10% to 90%). The gradation in shading denotes the change in estimated probability of death: dark shading indicates combinations of lower gestational ages and birth weights associated with greater likelihood of death; light shading indicates combinations of higher gestational ages and birth weights associated with lower likelihood of death. The methods used underestimate mortality at 22 and 23 weeks for infants with a birth weight of up to 600 g. *(From Fanaroff AA, Stoll BJ, Wright LL, et al for the NICHD Neonatal Research Network: Trends in neonatal morbidity and mortality for very low birthweight infants, Am J Obstet Gynecol 196:147.e1-e8, 2007.)*

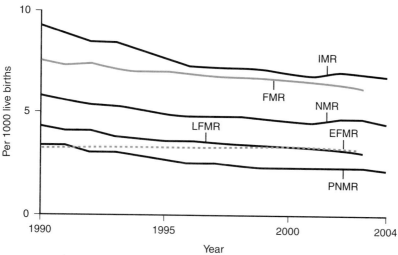

Figure C-18. Fetal, neonatal, and infant mortality rates in the United States from 1990 to 2004 (final data). *EFMR,* Early fetal mortality rate—early fetal deaths (20-27 weeks' gestation) per 1000 live births plus fetal deaths; *FMR,* fetal mortality rate—fetal deaths per 1000 live births plus fetal deaths; *IMR,* infant mortality rate—infant deaths per 1000 live births; *LFMR,* late fetal mortality rate—late fetal deaths (≥28 weeks' gestation) per 1000 live births plus fetal deaths; *NMR,* neonatal mortality rate—neonatal deaths per 1000 live births; *PNMR,* postneonatal mortality rate—postneonatal deaths per 1000 live births. *(From Hamilton BE, Miniño AM, Martin JA, et al: Annual summary of vital statistics: 2005, Pediatrics 119:345, 2007.) For comparison, in 2008: IMR = 6.59 deaths per 1000 live births; NMR = 4.27 per 1000 live births. (From Annual Summary of Vital Statistics 2008.)*

Umbilical Vessel Catheterization

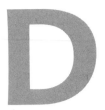

Ricardo J. Rodriguez

Use of central catheters requires careful consideration of the risks involved (Box D-1). The relatively easy access to the umbilical vessels makes these vessels a very good option for central access in emergency situations. A central catheter inserted into the aorta via an umbilical artery may be required in the management of the sick neonate for monitoring of blood pressure, intermittent blood sampling to check acid-base status, and, while in place, infusion of parenteral fluids and medications.

Umbilical artery catheters must be precisely located. A major objective is to avoid the origin of the renal arteries, because a catheter may occlude a renal artery and catheters in the area may produce thrombosis.[1] Both situations can result in renal infarction. Some prefer to position the catheter in the midthoracic aorta (high); others prefer to locate the catheter tip between L3 and L4 (low). Thrombotic complications are reported with both high and low placement.[2] Resolution of the thrombus or development of collateral circulation generally occurs, even when extensive thrombosis (e.g., aorta distal to renal arteries, common iliac) has been documented.[1,3] Occasionally a neonatal death is considered a direct consequence of complications related to umbilical vessel catheterization.[4] Hypertension in the neonate following use of high umbilical artery catheters has been described. However, in a prospective study, the incidence of hypertension was similar with low and high catheters.[5]

Hemorrhage, either resulting from loose connections or careless use of the stopcocks or occurring at the time of removal, is a major complication of arterial catheters. Another major complication is thrombus formation with release of microemboli into the systemic circulation. It is speculated that the catheter tip can traumatize the vessel wall, which may release tissue thromboplastin and activate intravascular coagulation. Alternatively, the presence of the catheter itself may produce clot formation. More rare complications include intimal flap formation and aneurysmatic dilatation of the abdominal artery. Ultrasonographic examination of the abdominal aorta and its branches is indicated when any of these complications is suspected.

Arterial blood samples may be obtained by multiple arterial punctures (of the radial artery) or an indwelling radial artery cannula as the method of choice or in cases in which umbilical artery catheterization is unsuccessful.[6,7]

In general, umbilical vein catheterization is technically easier. However, it should be avoided except when immediate access to a vein is needed because of an unexpected emergency (e.g., the need for delivery room resuscitation), because complications may be serious and difficult to avoid. An

---

Box D-1. Catheter Complications

Hemorrhage
Perforation into
- Peritoneal cavity
- Urachus
- Pericardium

Hepatic laceration
Thrombi and emboli
- Splenic vein thrombus or embolus
- Displacement of thrombus in ductus venosus
- Pulmonary infarction (pulmonary vein thrombus)

Retained broken-off catheter fragment
Calcification of portal vein or umbilical vein

Adapted from Oestreich AE: Umbilical vein catheterization—appropriate and inappropriate placement, Pediatr Radiol 40:1941, 2010.

umbilical vein catheter tip may locate in a branch of the portal vein and lead to areas of liver necrosis without perforation of the vein wall following infusions of hypertonic solutions, such as sodium bicarbonate and hypertonic glucose. Portal vein thrombosis and aseptic abscess formation have also occurred with and without infection. In addition, spontaneous perforation of the colon after exchange transfusion via an umbilical vein catheter has been reported. Radiographic verification of catheter tip location was not performed in any of these cases; most likely, the catheter tip was in the portal vein, and the cause of perforation was local necrosis of the bowel wall following hemorrhagic infarction as a result of retrograde microemboli or obstructive hemodynamic changes. A more rare complication, air embolism in the portal system, has also been observed.

In the first hour or so of life in a normal term infant, or for many hours and occasionally for many days in a sick or preterm infant, an umbilical vein catheter may be passed through the ductus venosus into the inferior vena cava.

Depending on the circumstances and preference of the physician, exchange transfusions can be done using either vessel or both, but not by infusing into the artery.

The umbilical vessel catheter should be removed as soon as possible and a peripheral intravenous line substituted, if necessary. In an undistressed newborn infant requiring parenteral fluids, under no circumstances should an umbilical vessel catheter be used when a peripheral intravenous line could be started via a scalp vein or an extremity vein. In the extremely low-birth-weight group, in whom parenteral nutrition is essential until enteral feeds are established, common practice is to routinely place percutaneous indwelling central catheters and remove umbilical lines as soon as possible.

TECHNIQUE OF CATHETERIZATION

In the small premature infant, the entire catheterization should be done as an operating room procedure with the infant in an incubator or under a radiant warmer to prevent hypothermia. In the delivery room, a radiant heater should be used.

When not precluded by an emergency (e.g., acute asphyxia), the following protocol should be followed. The operator carefully scrubs hands and arms to the elbows and puts on sterile gloves. A 3.5F or 4F (for infants weighing <1500 g) or a 5F catheter with rounded tip, which has a radiopaque line and end hole (Argyle umbilical artery catheter, coridien, mausfield, MASS) is attached to a syringe by a three-way stopcock. The system is filled with heparinized saline solution (1 U heparin per milliliter of normal or half-normal saline). (Box D-2 lists the equipment found on the catheterization tray.) Before the procedure is begun, the length of the catheter to be inserted should be marked according to the location desired (Figs. D-1 and D-2). After the umbilical stump and surrounding abdominal wall are carefully prepared with an antiseptic solution, sterile towels are placed around the stump and a circumcision drape is placed with the hole over the stump. The base of the cord is loosely tied with umbilical tape, with care taken to avoid the skin. The cord stump is then grasped and cut perpendicular to its axis to within approximately 1.5 cm of the abdominal wall with a surgical blade. The exposed vessels are identified—thin-walled oval vein and two smaller thick-walled round arteries with tightly constricted lumens. Occasionally, only one artery is present. The cord is stabilized by grasping the Wharton jelly with one or two Kelly clamps.

The lumen of the vessel to be used is gently dilated with curved Iris dressing forceps or a small obturator (Fig. D-3, *A* and *B*). The catheter is then inserted and gently advanced. Obstruction at the level of the abdominal wall may be relieved by applying gentle traction on the umbilical cord stump accompanied by steady but gentle pressure for about 30 seconds. During umbilical artery catheterization, obstruction may also occur at the level of the bladder. It may be

	Equipment Found on the Umbilical Catheterization Tray at University Hospitals Case Medical Center, Cleveland, Ohio
Box D-2.	

2 Iris dressing forceps, 4-inch curved
1 Iris dressing forceps, 4-inch straight
2 Halsted mosquito forceps, 4-inch curved
2 Halsted mosquito forceps, 4-inch straight
1 Derf needle holder, 4.75 inches
1 Iris scissors, 4.5 inches
1 Operating scissors, 5.5 inches
1 Medicine cup
4 Gauze preparation sponges, 3 × 3 inch
1 Huck towel, folded
1 Steam chemical integrator

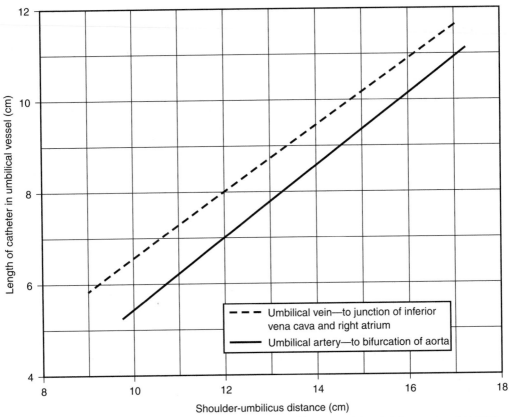

Figure D-1. Determination of the length of catheter to be inserted for appropriate arterial or venous placement. The length of the catheter read from the diagram is to the umbilical ring; the length of the umbilical cord stump present must be added. The shoulder-umbilicus distance is the perpendicular distance between parallel lines at the level of the umbilicus and through the distal ends of the clavicles. *(Adapted from data in Dunn P: Localization of the umbilical catheter by post-mortem measurement,* Arch Dis Child *41:69, 1966.)*

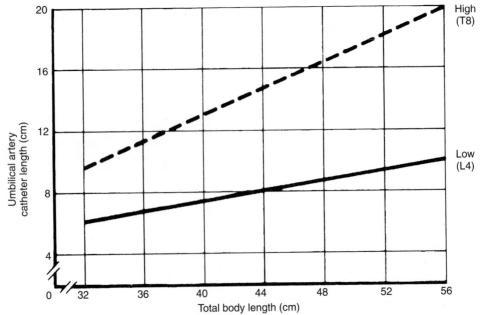

Figure D-2. Catheter position determined from total body length. *(Modified from Rosenfield W, Biagtan J, Schaeffer H, et al: A new graph for insertion of umbilical artery catheters,* J Pediatr *96:735, 1980.)*

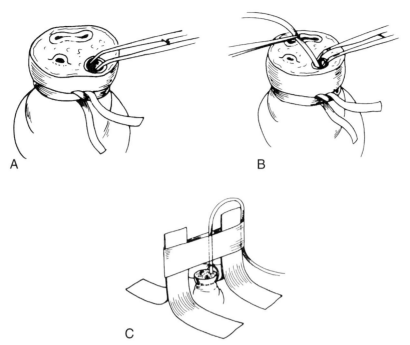

Figure D-3. A, Cross section of the umbilical cord showing tie in place and dilatation of artery with Iris forceps. **B,** Insertion of catheter into umbilical artery. **C,** Bridge technique used to secure catheter after suturing. A purse string suture is used that incorporates all three vessels. A square knot is tied at the base of the catheter, and a second knot is tied 1 cm above the base. The tape bridge further ensures against the line's becoming dislodged.

overcome by application of gentle, steady pressure for 30 seconds. Alternatively, marked resistance may be found where the umbilical artery meets the internal iliac artery (usually at 5 cm). The operator should avoid applying undue pressure to overcome this point of resistance because of the possibility of perforation of the vessel and severe hemorrhage. If continued resistance is met, the other artery should be used. If at any point during or after the line placement persistent blanching or cyanosis of the ipsilateral or contralateral extremity is observed, the catheter should be promptly removed. Cyanosis involving the toes or part of the foot on the side of the catheter may be relieved by warming the contralateral foot; if this is not successful, the catheter should be removed. Both lower extremities and buttocks should be carefully watched for alterations in blood supply when an umbilical artery catheter is in place.

If an umbilical vein catheterization is performed, the next site of obstruction after the abdominal wall is the portal system. (The catheter meets resistance several centimeters before the distance marked on the catheter is reached.) The catheter should be withdrawn several centimeters, gently rotated, and reinserted in an attempt to get the tip through the ductus venosus into the inferior vena cava. Gentle application of caudal traction to the umbilical cord stump sometimes facilitates the introduction of an umbilical venous line. Occasionally it is not possible to get the catheter into the inferior vena cava for anatomic reasons, and vigorous attempts to advance the catheter are to be avoided.

An umbilical vessel catheter should be tied in place with a silk suture around the vessel and catheter and sutured to the umbilical stump or taped to the abdominal wall. Disastrous hemorrhage can occur if the catheter is inadvertently pulled out or the stopcocks are disconnected by the activity of the infant. The position of the catheter must be identified by radiography immediately after insertion. It is important that the umbilical vein catheter tip be at least well into the ductus venosus (Fig. D-4) to protect the portal system from receiving hypertonic solutions.

If the radiograph obtained after umbilical vessel catheterization indicates that the catheter has been inserted too far, it may be gently withdrawn an estimated amount for appropriate placement. If the catheter is not in far enough, it must be completely withdrawn and a new sterile one inserted after the area is appropriately prepared again.

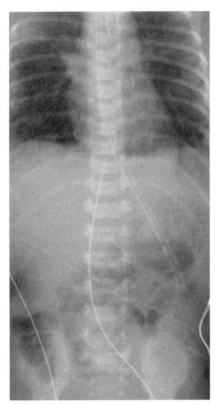

Figure D-4. Anteroposterior radiographic image showing the preferred location of the umbilical vein catheter tip at the most superior portion of the inferior vena cava, where it receives the hepatic veins and the ductus venosus and is about to empty into the right atrium. *(From Oestreich AE: Umbilical vein catheterization—appropriate and inappropriate placement,* Pediatr Radiol *40:1941, 2010.)*

REFERENCES

The reference list for this appendix can be found online at www.expertconsult.com.

Conversion Charts

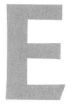

Table E-1. Conversion of Pounds and Ounces to Grams

Pounds	Ounces															
	0	**1**	**2**	**3**	**4**	**5**	**6**	**7**	**8**	**9**	**10**	**11**	**12**	**13**	**14**	**15**
0	—	28	57	85	113	142	170	198	227	255	283	312	340	369	397	425
1	454	482	510	539	567	595	624	652	680	709	737	765	794	822	850	879
2	907	936	964	992	1021	1049	1077	1106	1134	1162	1191	1219	1247	1276	1304	1332
3	1361	1389	1417	1446	1474	1503	1531	1559	1588	1616	1644	1673	1701	1729	1758	1786
4	1814	1843	1871	1899	1928	1956	1984	2013	2041	2070	2098	2126	2155	2183	2211	2240
5	2268	2296	2325	2353	2381	2410	2438	2466	2495	2523	2551	2580	2608	2637	2665	2693
6	2722	2750	2778	2807	2835	2863	2892	2920	2948	2977	3005	3033	3062	3090	3118	3147
7	3175	3203	3232	3260	3289	3317	3345	3374	3402	3430	3459	3487	3515	3544	3572	3600
8	3629	3657	3685	3714	3742	3770	3799	3827	3856	3884	3912	3941	3969	3997	4026	4054
9	4082	4111	4139	4167	4196	4224	4252	4281	4309	4337	4366	4394	4423	4451	4479	4508
10	4536	4564	4593	4621	4649	4678	4706	4734	4763	4791	4819	4848	4876	4904	4933	4961
11	4990	5018	5046	5075	5103	5131	5160	5188	5216	5245	5273	5301	5330	5358	5386	5415
12	5443	5471	5500	5528	5557	5585	5613	5642	5670	5698	5727	5755	5783	5812	5840	5868
13	5897	5925	5953	5982	6010	6038	6067	6095	6123	6152	6180	6209	6237	6265	6294	6322
14	6350	6379	6407	6435	6464	6492	6520	6549	6577	6605	6634	6662	6690	6719	6747	6776
15	6804	6832	6860	6889	6917	6945	6973	7002	7030	7059	7087	7115	7144	7172	7201	7228
16	7257	7286	7313	7342	7371	7399	7427	7456	7484	7512	7541	7569	7597	7626	7654	7682
17	7711	7739	7768	7796	7824	7853	7881	7909	7938	7966	7994	8023	8051	8079	8108	8136
18	8165	8192	8221	8249	8278	8306	8335	8363	8391	8420	8448	8476	8504	8533	8561	8590
19	8618	8646	8675	8703	8731	8760	8788	8816	8845	8873	8902	8930	8958	8987	9015	9043
20	9072	9100	9128	9157	9185	9213	9242	9270	9298	9327	9355	9383	9412	9440	9469	9497
21	9525	9554	9582	9610	9639	9667	9695	9724	9752	9780	9809	9837	9865	9894	9922	9950
22	9979	10,007	10,036	10,064	10,092	10,120	10,149	10,177	10,206	10,234	10,262	10,291	10,319	10,347	10,376	10,404

Table E-2.	Conversion to International System (SI) Units			
Component	**Conventional Unit**	**× Conversion Factor**	**=**	**SI Unit**
CLINICAL HEMATOLOGY				
Erythrocytes	per mm^3	1		10^6/L
Hematocrit	%	0.01		(1) volume of RBCs/volume of whole blood
Hemoglobin	g/dL	10		g/L
Leukocytes	per mm^3	1		10^6/L
Mean corpuscular hemoglobin concentration (MCHC)	g/dL	10		g/L
Mean corpuscular volume (MCV)	μm^3	1		fL
Platelet count	10^3/mm^3	1		10^9/L
Reticulocyte count	%	10		10^{-3}
CLINICAL CHEMISTRY				
Acetone	mg/dL	0.1722		mmol/L
Albumin	g/dL	10		g/L
Aldosterone	ng/dL	27.74		pmol/L
Ammonia (as nitrogen)	μg/dL	0.7139		μmol/L
Bicarbonate	mEq/L	1		mmol/L
Bilirubin	mg/dL	17.1		μmol/L
Calcium	mg/dL	0.2495		mmol/L
Calcium ion	mEq/L	0.50		mmol/L
Carotenes	μg/dL	0.01836		μmol/L
Ceruloplasmin	mg/dL	10.0		mg/L
Chloride	mEq/L	1		mmol/L
Cholesterol	mg/dL	0.02586		mmol/L
Complement, C3 or C4	mg/dL	0.01		g/L
Copper	μg/dL	0.1574		μmol/L
Cortisol	μg/dL	27.59		nmol/L
Creatine	mg/dL	76.25		μmol/L
Creatinine	mg/dL	88.40		μmol/L
Digoxin	ng/mL	1.281		nmol/L
Epinephrine	pg/mL	5.458		pmol/L
Fatty acids	mg/dL	10.0		mg/L
Ferritin	ng/mL	1		μg/L
α-Fetoprotein	ng/mL	1		μg/L
Fibrinogen	mg/dL	0.01		g/L
Folate	ng/mL	2.266		nmol/L
Fructose	mg/dL	0.05551		mmol/L
Galactose	mg/dL	0.05551		mmol/L
Gases				
Po$_2$	mm Hg (= torr)	0.1333		kPa
Pco$_2$	mm Hg (= torr)	0.1333		kPa
Glucagon	pg/mL	1		ng/L
Glucose	mg/dL	0.05551		mmol/L
Glycerol	mg/dL	0.1086		mmol/L
Growth hormone	ng/mL	1		μg/L
Haptoglobin	mg/dL	0.01		g/L
Hemoglobin	g/dL	10		g/L
Insulin	μg/L	172.2		pmol/L
	mU/L	7.175		pmol/L
Iron	μg/dL	0.1791		μmol/L
Iron-binding capacity	μg/dL	0.1791		μmol/L
Lactate	mEq/L	1		mmol/L
Lead	μg/dL	0.04826		μmol/L
Lipoproteins	mg/dL	0.02586		mmol/L
Magnesium	mg/dL	0.4114		mmol/L
	mEq/L	0.50		mmol/L
Osmolality	mOsm/kg H$_2$O	1		mmol/kg H$_2$O
Phenobarbital	mg/dL	43.06		μmol/L

Table E-2. Conversion to International System (SI) Units—cont'd

Component	Conventional Unit	×	Conversion Factor	=	SI Unit
Phenytoin	mg/L		3.964		µmol/L
Phosphate	mg/dL		0.3229		mmol/L
Potassium	mEq/L		1		mmol/L
	mg/dL		0.2558		mmol/L
Protein	g/dL		10.0		g/L
Pyruvate	mg/dL		113.6		µmol/L
Sodium ion	mEq/L		1		mmol/L
Steroids					
17-hydroxycorticosteroids	mg/24 hr		2.759		µmol/day
17-ketosteroids	mg/24 hr		3.467		µmol/day
Testosterone	ng/mL		3.467		nmol/L
Theophylline	mg/L		5.550		µmol/L
THYROID TESTS					
Thyroid-stimulating hormone	µU/mL		1		mU/L
Thyroxine (T_4)	µg/dL		12.87		nmol/L
Thyroxine free	ng/dL		12.87		pmol/L
Triiodothyronine (T_3)	ng/dL		0.01536		nmol/L
Transferrin	mg/dL		0.01		g/L
Triglycerides	mg/dL		0.01129		mmol/L
Urea nitrogen	mg/dL		0.3570		mmol/L
Uric acid (urate)	mg/dL		59.48		µmol/L
Vitamin A (retinol)	µg/dL		0.03491		µmol/L
Vitamin B_{12}	pg/mL		0.7378		pmol/L
Vitamin C (ascorbic acid)	mg/dL		56.78		µmol/L
Vitamin D					
Cholecalciferol	µg/mL		2.599		nmol/L
25 OH-cholecalciferol	ng/mL		2.496		nmol/L
Vitamin (Eα-tocopherol)	mg/dL		23.22		µmol/L
D-Xylose	mg/dL		0.06661		mmol/L
Zinc	µg/dL		0.1530		µmol/L
ENERGY	kcal (kilocalorie)		4.1868		kJ (kilojoule)
BLOOD PRESSURE	mm Hg (= torr)		1.333		mbar

Modified from Young DS: Implementation of SI units for clinical laboratory data. Style specifications and conversion tables, *Ann Intern Med* 106:114, 1987.
RBC, Red blood cell.

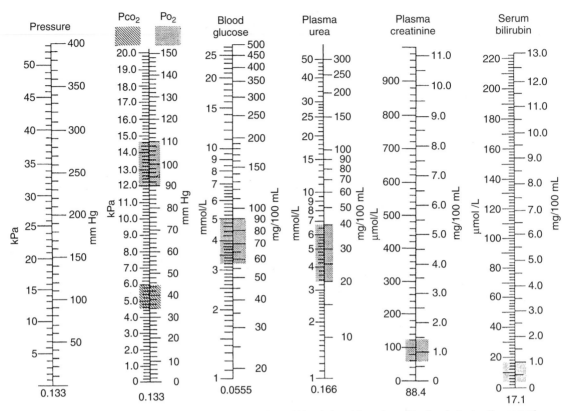

Figure E-1. Conversion chart for pressure, gases, and selected blood chemistry values. Shading indicates the normal range where appropriate. To convert from an old (conventional) unit *(right side of each scale)* to a new (SI) unit *(left side of each scale)*, multiply by the conversion factor at the foot of each column. *(Modified from Halliday HL, McClure G, Reid M:* Handbook of neonatal intensive care, *ed 2, Philadelphia, 1985, Saunders.)*

Selected Radiology
of the Newborn

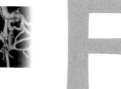

Sheila C. Berlin

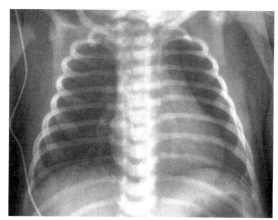

Figure F-1. Newborn chest radiograph showing normal findings.

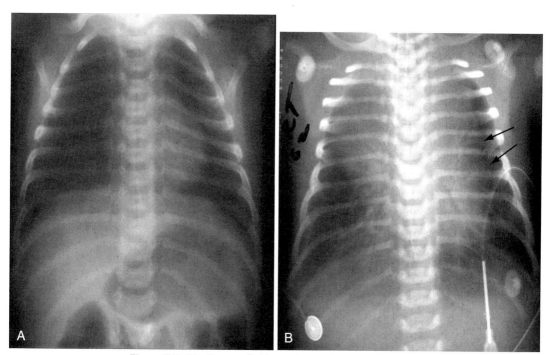

Figure F-2. The thymus. **A,** Absent thymus. **B,** Thymus *(arrows).*

All figures courtesy of Sheila Berlin, MD.

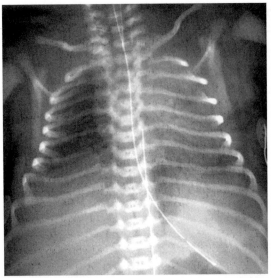

Figure F-3. Pulmonary hypoplasia accompanied by a bell-shaped thorax.

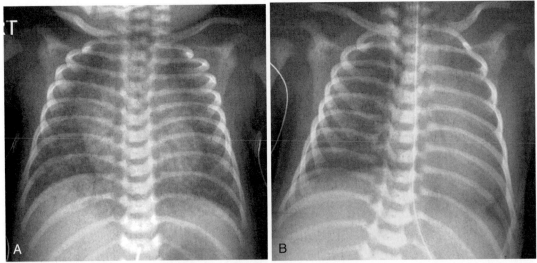

Figure F-4. Transient tachypnea of the newborn. Initial chest radiography demonstrates increased interstitial and alveolar opacity that clears by 48 hours of age. **A,** Radiograph at 4 hours of age. **B,** Radiograph at 48 hours of age.

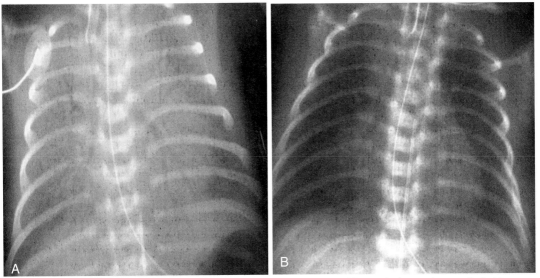

Figure F-5. Respiratory distress syndrome. Chest radiography demonstrates diffuse reticulogranular opacity that improves following surfactant therapy. **A,** Air bronchograms and bilateral symmetric lung consolidation ("white out") before treatment with surfactant. **B,** Improved aeration following surfactant administration.

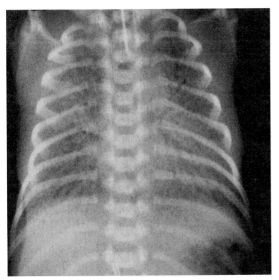

Figure F-6. Pulmonary interstitial emphysema. Note the characteristic tortuous tubular and cystic lucencies.

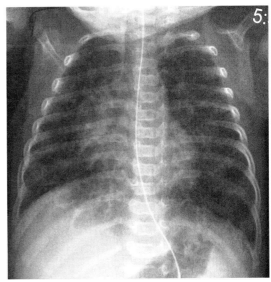

Figure F-7. Chronic lung disease/bronchopulmonary dysplasia. Coarse reticular disease and hyperinflation are present.

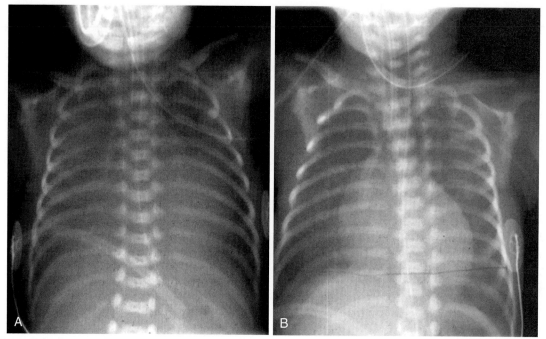

Figure F-8. Congestive heart failure before and after treatment with furosemide (Lasix). Bilateral alveolar infiltrates improve with treatment. **A,** Before furosemide. **B,** After furosemide.

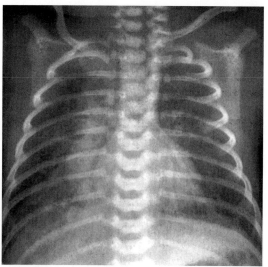

Figure F-9. Neonatal pneumonia. Bilateral interstitial and alveolar infiltrates as well as fluid in the minor fissure are present.

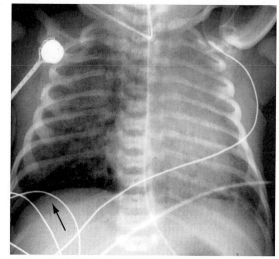

Figure F-10. Meconium aspiration syndrome with pneumothorax. Bilateral asymmetric alveolar infiltrates as well as right pneumothorax *(arrow)* are noted.

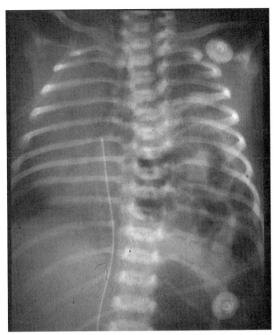

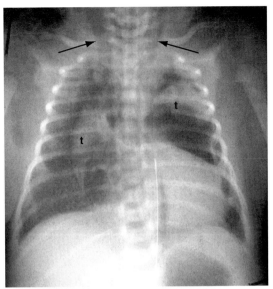

Figure F-12. Pneumomediastinum with air tracking into neck *(arrows)*. Characteristic elevation of both lobes of the thymus *(t)* is noted.

Figure F-11. Congenital diaphragmatic hernia. Note bowel in left chest with mediastinum shifted to right.

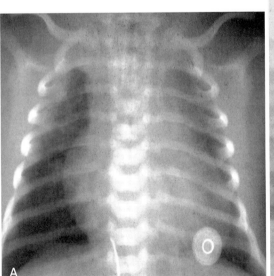

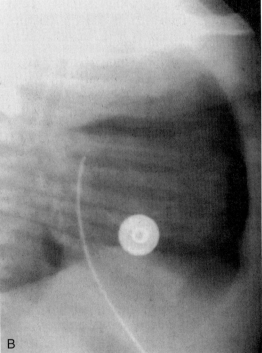

Figure F-13. Pneumothorax. **A,** Hyperlucency of the right lower hemithorax. **B,** Cross-table lateral view demonstrating a pneumothorax with absence of lung markings between the anterior margin of the lung *(arrows)* and chest wall.

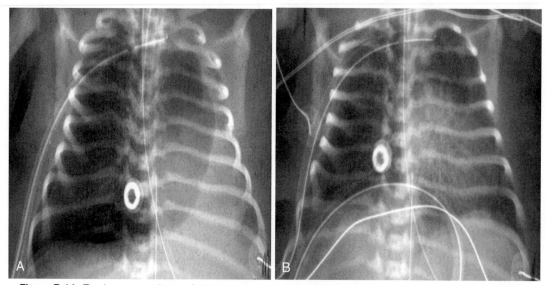

Figure F-14. Tension pneumothorax. **A,** Note mediastinal shift and compressive atelectasis of the left lung. **B,** The mediastinum returns to midline with effective decompression.

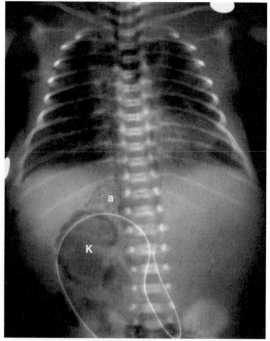

Figure F-15. Pneumoretroperitoneum. Note outline of the right kidney *(K)* and adrenal gland *(a)* by retroperitoneal air.

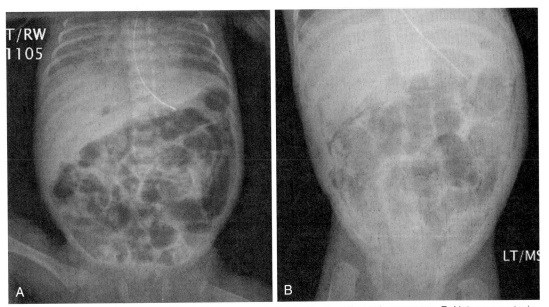

Figure F-16. Necrotizing enterocolitis. **A,** Note pneumatosis intestinalis and portal venous gas. **B,** Note pneumatosis intestinalis and free air under the liver.

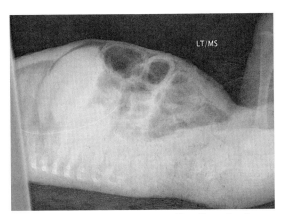

Figure F-17. Necrotizing enterocolitis with perforation. Cross-table lateral view shows free air over the anterior margin of the liver.

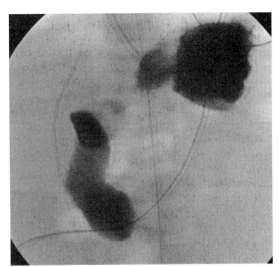

Figure F-18. Malrotation of bowel. Spot film from an upper gastrointestinal series shows a high grade of obstruction and a duodenal-jejunal junction to the right of midline and far below the pylorus.

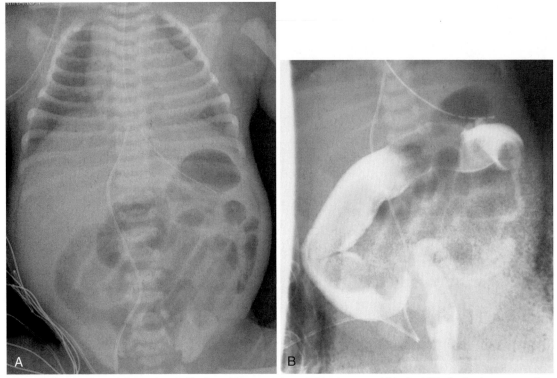

Figure F-19. Distal bowel obstruction. **A,** The bowel loops are elongated and appeared "stacked." **B,** Contrast enema confirms a small left colon.

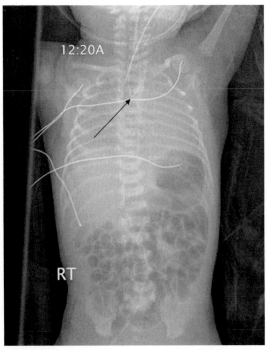

Figure F-20. Esophageal atresia with fistula. Note nasogastric tube coiled at obstruction *(arrow)* and air in the stomach and bowel from a tracheoesophageal fistula.

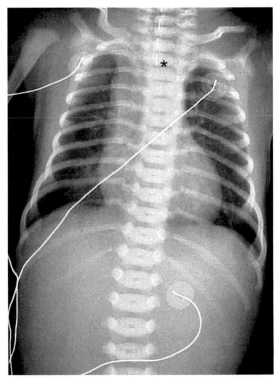

Figure F-21. Esophageal atresia without fistula. Note tip of nasogastric tube at the level of the esophageal pouch *(asterisk)* and gasless abdomen.

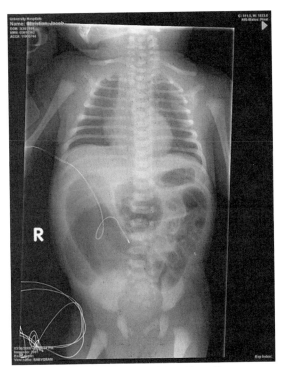

Figure F-22. Imperforate anus. Dilated bowel loops suggest a distal obstruction. No gas overlies the rectum.

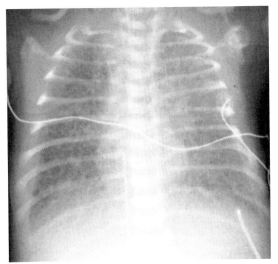

Figure F-24. Total anomalous pulmonary venous return (infracardiac). There is interstitial edema with pleural effusions. Note characteristic normal-sized heart.

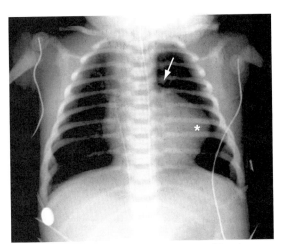

Figure F-23. Tetralogy of Fallot. Boot-shaped heart reflects hypoplasia of the main pulmonary artery segment *(arrow)* and right ventricular hypertrophy *(asterisk)*. Vascular markings are decreased.

Index

Page numbers followed by "b" indicate boxes; "f" figures; "t" tables.